Handbook of Liaison Psychiatry

Liaison psychiatry, the recognition and management of psychiatric problems in the general medical setting, is an essential component of many doctors' work. Depression, anxiety and somatization disorders occur in about 50% of cases presenting to primary care physicians. The *Handbook of Liaison Psychiatry* is a comprehensive reference book for this fast growing subspeciality. A team of experts in the field cover the full range of issues, from establishing a service and outlining the commonest problems encountered in general hospital and primary care, to assessment and treatment guidelines, working with specific units within the hospital setting, disaster planning and legal-ethical considerations. It will be essential reading for doctors and other professionals concerned with the psychological health of patients in acute general hospitals and in primary care.

Geoffrey Lloyd is Visiting Consultant Psychiatrist at the Priory Hospital North London.

Elspeth Guthrie is Honorary Professor of Psychological Medicine and Medical Psychotherapy at the University of Manchester, and Consultant in Psychological Medicine at the Manchester Royal Infirmary.

Handbook of
Liaison Psychiatry

Edited by

Geoffrey Lloyd

and

Elspeth Guthrie

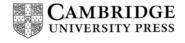

CAMBRIDGE
UNIVERSITY PRESS

CAMBRIDGE UNIVERSITY PRESS
Cambridge, New York, Melbourne, Madrid, Cape Town, Singapore, São Paulo

Cambridge University Press
The Edinburgh Building, Cambridge CB2 2RU, UK

Published in the United States of America by Cambridge University Press, New York

www.cambridge.org
Information on in this title: www.cambridge.org/9780521826372

First published 2007

Printed in the United Kingdom at the University Press, Cambridge

A catalogue record for this publication is available from the British Library

Library of Congress Cataloguing in Publication data

Handbook of liaison psychiatry / edited by Geoffrey Lloyd and Elspeth Guthrie.
    p. ; cm.
  Includes bibliographical references and index.
  ISBN-13: 978-0-521-82637-2 (hardback)
  ISBN-10: 0-521-82637-3 (hardback)
    1.   Consultation-liaison psychiatry—Handbooks, manuals, etc. I. Lloyd, Geoffrey Gower. II. Guthrie,
Elspeth.
    [DNLM: 1. Psychiatry—methods.   2. Referral and Consultation.   WM 64 H2355 2007] III.   Title.

    RC455.2.C65H36 2007
    616.89—dc22

                                                                                2006100689

ISBN-13   978-0-521-82637-2 hardback
ISBN-10   0-521-82637-3 hardback

Contents

List of contributors   *page* ix

Preface   xiii

Part I   Basic skills

1   The development of general hospital psychiatry   3
Richard Mayou

2   Establishing a service   24
Stella Morris

3   Legal and ethical issues in liaison psychiatry   47
Eleanor Feldman

4   Understanding psychological reactions to physical illness   64
Geoffrey Lloyd

5   Detection of psychiatric disorders in the general hospital   83
Damien Longson

6   The role of the nurse in liaison psychiatry   102
Anthony Harrison

Part II   Common psychiatric problems across the general hospital

7   Functional somatic syndromes   125
Lisa Page and Simon Wessely

8   Alcohol problems in the general hospital   149
Jonathan Chick

9   Drug misuse in medical patients   180
Ilana Crome and Hamid Ghodse

10   Sexual problems in medical patients   221
Michael King

11   Suicide and deliberate self-harm   245
Julia Sinclair and Keith Hawton

12   Delirium   270
Paul Gill, Marco Rigatelli and Silvia Ferrari

13   Childhood experiences   290
Mark Berelowitz

Part III   Working with specific units

14   Neurological disorders   305
Alan Carson, Adam Zeman, Lynn Myles and Michael Sharpe

15   Cardiorespiratory disorders   365
Christopher Bass

16   Gastrointestinal disorders   390
Elspeth Guthrie

17   Liver disorders   416
Geoffrey Lloyd

18   Endocrine disorders   432
Antonio Lobo, M. Jesús Pérez-Echeverría and Antonio Campayo

19   Diabetes   454
Khalida Ismail and Robert Peveler

20   HIV and AIDS   474
Russell Foster and Ian Everall

21   Renal disease   506
Janet Butler

22   Musculo-skeletal disorders   527
Chris Dickens and Graham Ash

23   Oncology   547
Geoffrey Lloyd

24   Head and neck cancer   564
      Gerry Humphris

25   Palliative care   592
      Matthew Hotopf and Max Henderson

26   Cosmetic procedures   617
      David Veale

27   Perinatal and gynaecological disorders   632
      Kathryn M. Abel

28   The intensive care unit   673
      Simon Turner, Daniel Conway, Jane Eddleston and Elspeth Guthrie

29   The burns unit   697
      Jonathan I. Bisson

30   Psychocutaneous disorders   714
      Nora Turjanski

31   Genitourinary disorders   733
      David Osborn

32   The emergency department   751
      Andrew Hodgkiss

Part IV   Treatment

33   Psychopharmacological treatment in liaison psychiatry   763
      Ulrik Fredrik Malt and Geoffrey Lloyd

34   The role of psychological treatments   795
      Elspeth Guthrie and Tom Sensky

35   Problem cases   818
      Damien Longson and Sarah Burlinson

Part V   Different treatment settings

36   Developing links with primary care   847
      Richard Morriss, Linda Gask, Christopher Dowrick, Peter Salmon and Sarah Peters

37   Frequent attenders in primary care   871
      Navneet Kapur

38   Major disaster planning   896
       Jonathan I. Bisson, Jim Bolton, Kevin Mackway-Jones and Elspeth Guthrie

       Index   913

List of contributors

EDITORS
Geoffrey Lloyd
Priory Hospital North London
Elspeth Guthrie
University of Manchester

CONTRIBUTORS

Kathryn Abel
University of Manchester

Graham Ash
Ormskirk & District General Hospital

Christopher Bass
John Radcliffe Hospital, Oxford

Mark Berelowitz
Royal Free Hospital, London

Jonathan Bisson
University of Wales Hospital, Cardiff

Jim Bolton
St Helier Hospital, Surrey

Sarah Burlinson
Royal Oldham Hospital

Janet Butler
University of Southampton

Antonio Campayo
University of Zaragoza

Alan Carson
University of Edinburgh

Jonathan Chick
Royal Edinburgh Hospital

Daniel Conway
Manchester Royal Infirmary

Ilana Crome
Keele University Medical School (Harplands Campus), Stoke on Trent

Chris Dickens
University of Manchester

Christopher Dowrick
University of Liverpool

Jane Eddleston
Manchester Royal Infirmary

Ian Everall
University of California, San Diego

Eleanor Feldman
John Radcliffe Hospital, Oxford

Silvia Ferrari
Universita de Modena

Russell Foster
Institute of Psychiatry, King's College
  London

Linda Gask
University of Manchester

Hamid Ghodse
St George's Hospital Medical School,
  University of London

Paul Gill
The Longley Centre, Sheffield

Elspeth Guthrie
University of Manchester

Anthony Harrison
Avon and Wiltshire Partnership Mental
  Health NHS Trust, Bath

Keith Hawton
University of Oxford

Max Henderson
Institute of Psychiatry, King's College
  London

Andrew Hodgkiss
St Thomas' Hospital, London

Matthew Hotopf
Institute of Psychiatry, King's College
  London

Gerry Humphris
University of St Andrews

Khalida Ismail
Institute of Psychiatry, King's College,
  London

Navneet Kapur
University of Manchester

Michael King
Royal Free & University College Medical
  School, London

Geoffrey Lloyd
Priory Hospital North London

Antonio Lobo
University of Zaragoza

Damien Longson
North Manchester General Hospital

Kevin Mackway-Jones
Manchester Royal Infirmary

Ulrich Frederick Malt
University of Oslo

Richard Mayou
University of Oxford

Stella Morris
Hull Royal Infirmary

Richard Morriss
University of Nottingham

Lyn Myles
University of Edinburgh

David Osborn
Royal Free and University College Medical
  School, London

Lisa Page
Institute of Psychiatry, Kings College
  London

M. Jesús Pérez-Echeverría
University of Zaragoza

Sarah Peters
University of Liverpool and Royal Liverpool
  Hospital

Robert Peveler
University of Southampton

Marco Rigatelli
Universita de Modena

Peter Salmon
University of Liverpool

Tom Sensky
West Middlesex University Hospital

Michael Sharpe
University of Edinburgh

Julia Sinclair
University of Oxford

Nora Turjanski
Royal Free Hospital, London

Simon Turner
Stepping Hill Hospital, Stockport

David Veale
Institute of Psychiatry, King's College
  London; Priory Hospital North London

Simon Wessely
Institute of Psychiatry, King's College
  London

Adam Zeman
Peninsula Medical School, Universities of
  Exeter and Plymouth

Preface

The provision of psychiatric services to general hospitals has increased considerably during the last 10 years. New consultant posts have been created, multidisciplinary teams have been established and junior doctors are acquiring experience in an area of psychiatry hitherto denied them. Clinical psychologists have long made significant contributions to this field. They have recently been joined by an expanding number of nurses who have made major improvements particularly to the management of patients with acute behavioural disturbances and of those who have deliberately harmed themselves. But expansion has been uneven, concentrated on university-linked hospitals and dependent on the creative energies of individual clinicians. Many district hospitals in the UK and elsewhere still have a very rudimentary psychiatric service even though the high prevalence of psychiatric disorders in general hospital patients is now widely acknowledged.

This area of clinical practice is known by various terms — liaison psychiatry, consultation-liaison psychiatry, psychological medicine or psychosomatic medicine. Indeed the latter term has been revived by the American Board of Medical Specialties which now recognizes it as a new psychiatric subspeciality with its own training programme and certification examination. Whatever term is used in a particular country the clinical problems are similar, being concerned with the diagnosis and management of patients with combined medical and psychiatric problems and those whose psychiatric disorder presents with physical symptoms. The ultimate goal is to improve the quality of care and the outcome of patients attending general hospitals.

This book aims to provide clinicians from a variety of backgrounds with sufficient information to develop the necessary skills. It covers a wide range of medical specialities and clinical settings. It is concerned predominantly with adult patients although the implications of illness on children are also considered. Within the adult population no age discrimination is made. Our aim has been to cover psychiatric problems throughout the entire spectrum from early adulthood to old age. We have also aimed to transcend national boundaries and hope the book will be relevant to clinicians wherever they practise.

The pattern of medical care is changing steadily. More treatment is being conducted in day-patient or outpatient facilities. Those who are admitted to hospital stay for a shorter duration than was the case only a few years ago. These changes create problems for liaison psychiatrists and the provision of treatment needs to evolve accordingly. More clinical work will be provided in outpatient clinics, in conjunction with specialists from other disciplines. Treatment commenced in a hospital environment will be continued in primary care alongside the patient's primary care doctor. However, whatever the setting, the diagnostic and therapeutic skills required remain the same.

A further challenge for liaison psychiatry arises from uncertainties about the funding and management of clinical services. Where medical and psychiatric services are funded separately it is not clear which budget should fund liaison psychiatry. There is a danger that liaison psychiatry will be neglected unless the case for the service is presented persuasively to comissioners. A model which works in one hospital or community setting may not be appropriate in another. Arrangements need to be made which are flexible and responsive to local requirements. It is important that for each service a managerial and funding policy is established, which is agreed by managers of medical and psychiatric services and by those responsible for commissioning healthcare in general.

Although we intend the book to have an international appeal it undoubtedly has a British emphasis with significant contributions from continental Europe. We believe its contents reflect liaison psychiatry as it is currently practised in many parts of the world. We hope it will help clinicians to develop services further and particularly to establish services where none exist at present.

GEOFFREY LLOYD, London

ELSPETH GUTHRIE, Manchester
June 2006

Part I

Basic skills

The development of general hospital psychiatry

Richard Mayou

General hospital psychiatry is the practice of psychiatry in a particular type of medical setting, whilst liaison psychiatry (the principal focus of this chapter) refers to the clinical expertise and practice relating to psychological and psychiatric problems and treatments in patients presenting to general medical care. Whilst this subject matter has been a part of medicine from the earliest time, its history as a recognized specialist interest is inextricably part of the complicated evolution of psychiatry as a speciality and its at times troubled relationship with the rest of medicine (Shorter 1997). Although now firmly established and expanding, its precise role is uncertain, insecure and misunderstood at least as much within psychiatry as within general medicine. This history cannot be understood as a separate identifiable theme and must be seen as part of the whole social history of medical practice and the rather recent evolution of current patterns of health (Mayou 1989).

This chapter focuses on liaison (or consultation liaison) psychiatry. Although mainly based on historical evidence from the United Kingdom, the central ideas are applicable to the histories of liaison psychiatry in other developed countries. Most other histories of liaison psychiatry have concentrated on North American developments in the last 70 years (Lipowski & Wise 2002; Schwab 1989). Although these have been influential, there is a need for a much more long-term view of the wider relationships between psychiatry and general medicine. The main themes of the chapter can be summarized:

1. Psychological care has always been implicit in the practice of good medicine.
2. In the nineteenth century separate special interests in mental illness (the alienists) and in nervous disorders emerged and gradually became more established. The former was based in large new asylums; the latter

Handbook of Liaison Psychiatry, ed. Geoffrey Lloyd and Elspeth Guthrie. Published by Cambridge University Press. © Cambridge University Press 2007.

was initially provided by physicians interested in treating 'nervous' problems within the general hospital and later by specialists in psychological medicine.

3. During the twentieth century these two approaches became a single new speciality of psychiatry which was increasingly seen as a part of medicine. During the second half of the century a very few psychiatrists (now calling themselves liaison psychiatrists) concentrated on the general hospital consultations, predominantly with inpatients, and on the teaching of colleagues and students.

4. Liaison psychiatry has become a substantial body of expertise largely practised in the general hospital by a small minority of psychiatrists but which relates to a very substantial proportion of medical problems.

5. Since liaison relates to an interface of physical and mental care across the whole range of medical problems, it cannot be precisely defined in terms of particular clinical disorders, settings, or types of care. It is a speciality positioned uncomfortably between psychiatry and medicine and unfortunately not fully accepted by either.

6. Despite an increasingly robust evidence-base on epidemiology, the nature and course of clinical problems and the effectiveness of treatments, psychiatric, psychological and behavioural methods are underused in general medical care by both specialists and non-specialists.

Early history

For most of history both body and mind have been cared for together, apart from a small minority of the most disturbed. The first hospital as we know it in England was St Bartholomew's, established in 1123. In the medieval period mentally ill people were commonly treated in hospitals and religious institutions (Porter 1987; Shorter 1997). Few of these institutions survived the Reformation. In the eighteenth century most of the voluntary hospitals established in many British towns specifically excluded lunatics. Inevitably some patients with physical problems developed certifiable mental illness during their admissions; most were rapidly discharged, although some were transferred to private institutions for the insane and later to asylums. The first general hospital in Britain to admit lunatics to a special ward was Guy's in 1728. There were a small number of others, but none survived beyond the mid nineteenth century. There were similar experiments in other countries.

Some forms of what we would now see as psychiatric disorder have always been accepted in the general hospital, for example functional nervous symptoms, odd behaviour, delirium and complications of physical illness and childbirth. There are many records of admissions for hysteria, hypochondriasis and apparently functional somatic symptoms in surviving eighteenth- and nineteenth-century admission and discharge books. It was also recognized that there were small numbers of disturbed patients who could not be managed in normal settings. Some hospitals had private rooms or special areas for disturbed patients with delirium or puerperal fever. Doctors accepted these problems as part of their responsibility. Alcohol was often mentioned as a cause of physical problems and delirium tremens one of the most frequent explanations for disturbed behaviour. A very small number of general hospitals established special wards for such patients. Records show an even wider range of psychological disorder amongst those attending outpatient clinics (Mayou 1989).

The beginnings of specialization

Asylum psychiatrists (alienists)

The segregation of the mentally ill into large new asylums in the nineteenth century was associated with the development of two groups of specialists – alienists (Porter 1987) and those interested in nervous disorders. This resulted in the development of procedures within the new general hospitals to identify and to transfer disturbed patients to asylums. In a rather small number of general hospitals there were pioneering attempts at the end of the nineteenth century to establish specialist psychiatric care. A few asylum doctors also began to offer early and voluntary treatment of psychiatric illness and less serious disorders. This was very often within outpatient clinics established within general hospitals.

Nervous disorder

Separately, physicians based in general hospitals began to identify and to treat nervous patients and this became a particular interest of some physicians and of the developing speciality of neurology. The role of neurologists is well illustrated in the accounts, especially from North America, of neurasthenia and of the rest cure (Wessely *et al.* 1998). However, the neurologists' initial enthusiasm was not maintained as they became more and more interested in neurological disorders defined by pathology. There was a similar decline in interest amongst general physicians. This left a small number of general hospital physicians who practised what, in Britain, became known as psychological medicine; a new form of psychiatry associated especially with the teaching hospitals in Britain, Europe, North America and elsewhere. Some of these psychiatric specialists in nervous disorder travelled widely in the United States and Europe and became interested in new psychodynamic methods of treatment.

Psychological medicine specialists generally saw themselves as very much apart from alienists working in large and remote asylums. There were, however, signs that there could be a coming together. Some specialist out-patient clinics were established in general hospitals and a few medical schools eventually began to see psychiatry as a subject that might develop on a new and more academic basis, alongside other specialities. Even so, it was many years before nervous patients found it in any way acceptable to be referred to psychiatrists.

These developments occurred against a background of wider change in ideas about mental disorder and its management. A high and conspicuous prevalence of psychological problems during the 1914—18 war had a large influence on care and attitudes. It became obvious that in wartime there were many disabling problems which did not have physical causes but whose psychological under-standing was quite different to the narrow concepts and practice of asylum-based psychiatry. From the beginning of the war, many soldiers began to report symptoms of what came to be known as 'shell shock'. There was considerable clinical innovation, although psychiatrists contributed much less to routine military medicine than did other doctors and psychologists (Shephard 2000). More generally, research by the first cardiologists on another very common syndrome, 'soldier's heart', also contributed to developing understanding of anxiety disorder and neurosis, as recently identified and described by Freud. These new ideas and interests in psychological treatments were especially influential on the wider intellectual culture, as is evident from novels, memoirs and literary criticism of the period. The new ideas about mental disorder were soon also reflected in post-war textbooks and journals and in clinical practice so that in the 1920s and 1930s many physicians emphasized psychological care.

Psychiatry in the general hospital

General hospital specialist psychiatry

In the first half of the twentieth century psychiatric care expanded very slowly within the general hospitals. In Britain, this meant outpatient psychological medicine in the teaching hospitals using methods promoted by the new specialist and academic Maudsley Hospital (founded 1923), and by a small number of pioneering asylums. Influential specialists in psychological medicine, such as Sir Aubrey Lewis, saw psychiatry as a medical speciality which should have a substantial presence in teaching hospitals and in other large general hospitals. These views were not always accepted by mental hospital doctors who saw reformed asylums as a more appropriate therapeutic setting. However, in the 1930s there were some experimental developments in psychiatric inpatient care in general hospitals, usually for the care of the severely mentally ill, but sometimes also offering opportunities to treat less severe nervous disorder and psychological complications of physical illness. In the teaching hospitals such wards or the availability of small numbers of psychiatric beds within medical wards offered the opportunity for limited amounts of teaching.

There were several other major influences on continuing change – psychosomatic medicine, the extensive consequences of the Second World War for medical practice, and North American psychiatric consultation units.

Psychosomatic medicine

Psychosomatic medicine – the idea that psychological factors are important in the aetiology and course of many physical disorders – arose from psychodynamic theory and practice in the early twentieth century. It became influential in the 1930s, especially in the United States and in German-speaking countries. In the latter it has continued to flourish as a distinct medical speciality, separate to both psychiatry and internal medicine. Elsewhere it failed to survive the 1940s and 1950s and the beginnings of a more scientifically and evidence-based approach to medical practice.

Outside German-speaking countries few psychiatrists now see psychosomatic theory as useful. The emphasis on the interaction of physical and psychological processes is beneficial, but simplistic assumptions about possible psychological causes of physical disorder (such as stress and overwork) still hinder professional and public understanding. Psychosomatic medicine has had a lasting legacy within medicine in promoting greater understanding of the psychological aspects of physical symptoms and disorders and, more generally, cultural attitudes as shown in literature and art throughout the twentieth century. Even more important have been wider developments in psychodynamic, cognitive and behavioural understanding and treatment of 'neurotic' disorders.

Psychiatry during and after the Second World War (1939–1945)

The Second World War had at least as great an impact on psychiatry as the First World War. Wartime experience in emergency hospitals of the treatment of neurotic conditions changed the views on the scope and methods of psychiatry. Psychological treatment became generally more acceptable and new physical treatments offered answers to illnesses previously dealt with only by chronic institutional care. Anxiety, depression and other common disorders were more widely recognized and seen as deserving of treatment both by doctors in general and by psychiatrists who, with a wider view of their role, no longer wished to limit themselves to the care of patients admitted compulsorily to asylums.

The changes in patterns of healthcare after the end of the Second World War accompanied rapid scientific advancement and increasing specialization. The asylums began to close. Psychiatry returned to some extent to the general hospital and it became more unified, reconciling the alienists and the specialists in psychological medicine. It seemed for a while that psychiatry was rejoining the rest of medicine. In Britain, there was a coming together of academically minded psychiatrists at both the Maudsley Hospital and also in the undergraduate teaching hospitals with asylum psychiatry, which was developing social and physical methods of treatment and moving increasingly into community outpatient care (Mayou 1989). General hospital psychiatry largely came to mean the provision of specialist psychiatry within the general hospital, remaining clinically and very often managerially separate. Psychological medicine was ready to be renamed liaison psychiatry.

Consultation liaison

The practice of liaison psychiatry evolved in the first half of the twentieth century well before it was given the name. Hindsight allows us to see general hospital and liaison psychiatry services being established around the world, developing in response to local demands and in ways that reflected individual enthusiasms. Most aimed to help with the most conspicuous problems of disturbed and difficult patients. Only tiny proportions of the overall morbidity were recognized (let alone referred and treated) at a time when psychiatric epidemiology was increasingly showing the scale and range of psychiatric issues in all medical settings.

American histories of liaison psychiatry have focused on the influence of a small number of large innovative services in the 1930s, and more recent literature has continued to be dominated by a small number of people working in particularly well-resourced departments. This emphasis is misleading since it ignores the contributions made by many other psychiatrists providing simpler forms of consultation in the United States and around the world. Thus in the 1980s, whilst those working in large centres continued to suggest that 5% of general hospital admissions would benefit from assessment by the consultation liaison psychiatrist, it was apparent that real rates of referral were far lower, well below 1% in the United States (Wallen *et al.* 1987) and lower in other countries.

Consultation and liaison as a specialist interest

The practice of consultation liaison has developed alongside changing methods in psychiatric and psychological treatment as a part of the whole range of psychiatric care.

The United States

In the United States what we now know as consultation-liaison psychiatry is usually dated to pioneering services in the 1930s and particularly to five units established with grants from the Rockefeller Foundation which were intended to stimulate collaboration between psychiatrists and other physicians. They provided consultation and teaching to medical students and staff. The term liaison psychiatry was also introduced for a variety of models involving both psychiatrists and physicians and, in a few instances, based in departments of medicine. Between 1935 and 1960 services were established in many teaching hospitals with a variety of models depending on local enthusiasms and opportunities. However, these developments remained isolated (Wallen *et al.* 1987) and there was no book published or comprehensive review of the subject made until the mid 1960s.

In 1974 the psychiatry education branch of the National Institute of Mental Health (NIMH) decided to support the development and expansion of consultation liaison services throughout the United States (Lipowski & Wise 2002; Schwab 1989). This decision was based on the view that in the future healthcare delivery should be mainly in primary care and that doctors needed appropriate training in psychosocial and psychiatric problems. Many of those involved were influenced by the writings and teaching of George Engel and his colleagues at Rochester in New York State on what they called the biopsychosocial approach (see White 2005). As liaison psychiatry prospered in the 1970s and 1980s, there were widening differences of opinion about methods (Lipowski 1967). The consultation model focused on assessment and treatment of individual patients, whereas the liaison model had a more ambitious role of working with and through medical teams. There was however no agreed conceptual basis and the advocates of consultation and of liaison engaged in bitter controversy, a controversy that reflected extremes of practice rather than the everyday practice of a few specialists in small units. In the end, the increasing financial difficulties resulting from the end of Federal funding favoured consultation programmes, which were easier to fund. Eventually, consultation and liaison combined as a new entity – consultation-liaison psychiatry (CL).

Whilst there has been great innovation and enthusiasm in liaison psychiatry in the United States, as shown by the rest of this chapter and by references throughout this book, most services have remained small. However, there is now a large body of research and clinical evidence to guide practice (see Levenson 2005). Many services have suffered cuts in funding and lack of support from both psychiatry and medicine. The majority of services continue to focus on traditional inpatient consultation (Kornfeld 2002) and very few CL psychiatrists have time for research or teaching. Despite these setbacks there has been significant political progress in achieving recognition as a special interest and in 2003 sub-speciality status was eventually recognized by the American Board of Medical Specialists (ABMS) with support from both the American Psychiatric Association and the American Board of Psychiatry and Neurology. The name of this sub-speciality, debated fruitlessly for many years, is Psychosomatic Medicine. It seems unlikely that this reversion to a controversial historical term will prove satisfactory. Even if less obscure than consultation liaison, it will be no more meaningful or popular with medical colleagues or with patients.

Liaison psychiatry in the UK

After the Second World War consultation became more firmly established, either as informal referrals to individual psychiatrists or by emergency requests to duty doctors. It became essential to involve psychiatrists in any transfer to psychiatric hospital and, at the same time, psychiatrists were increasingly invited to give their opinions on less severe problems. A few hospitals began more organized consultation services, for example at Guy's Hospital. A more elaborate liaison service was established in 1961 at the Middlesex Hospital by Sir Denis Hill and colleagues, modelled on the biopsychosocial approach developed in Rochester by Romano and Engel, in which psychiatrists had liaison attachments to individual medical units (Mayou 1989; White 2005).

New generations of psychiatrists were heavily influenced by North American experience and, inevitably, they took on the terminology of consultation-liaison psychiatry, which in the UK was eventually abbreviated to the no more meaningful 'liaison psychiatry'. As soon as the new name was publicized it was recognized that it was unsatisfactory and that its only advantage was to get away from terms such as psychosomatic which were discredited or seen as having too many alternative meanings.

The literature from the late 1960s until recently assumed that liaison psychiatry should be concerned with acute problems amongst medical inpatients. It recognized that, even in the small number of large centres, referral rates were low, especially as compared with the increasing epidemiological evidence that psychiatric disorder is extremely common amongst hospital inpatients. However, psychological medicine outpatient clinics continued in some teaching centres. Additionally psychiatrists became involved in the assessment of patients who had attempted suicide and who were being seen in increasing numbers in emergency departments. The abolition of suicide as a criminal offence and government recommendations about psychiatric assessment resulted in changes in practice, especially in teaching hospitals.

Developments in the last 20 years have been substantially associated with the work of the Royal College of Psychiatrists' Liaison Group (now Faculty) (Lloyd 2001). Formed in 1983 by a small number of psychiatrists particularly interested in working in the general hospital, it rapidly gathered support and has been responsible for promoting clinical practice, training and research (Guthrie 1998; Mayou & Lloyd 1985). Progress has been steady but slow; there is continuing concern about the lack of acceptance, both within the rest of medicine and within psychiatry, but there have been solid achievements in terms of the number of services, acceptance as a central part of psychiatric training, in collaboration with medical and other groups, and a significant increase in research output. Progress has been aided by increasing contact and collaboration with colleagues in Europe and elsewhere.

Inevitably clinical developments have depended on individual initiatives and local planning and have been largely separate from increasing knowledge of epidemiology, aetiology and treatment effectiveness. Few services have been evaluated. Increasing national and local efforts to define patterns of service and

Table 1.1. Estimate of size of liaison service and workload for a multidisciplinary liaison team for a district general hospital with 600 beds serving a catchment area of 250 000.

Composition of liaison psychiatry service	Number
Consultant liaison psychiatrist	1
Senior house officer	1
Liaison nurses	5
Health psychologist/clinical psychologist	1–2
Secretary	1
Estimated workload of patients seen	Annual rate
Deliberate self-harm	500
A&E episodes	200
Ward referrals	200
Outpatient contacts of patients seen	Annual rate
New	100–150
Follow-up	500
Specialized liaison contracts with one or two specific units	100

Source: Royal College of Physicians and the Royal College of Psychiatrists (2003).

training have largely been based on clinical experience. Table 1.1 reproduces current recommendations for a basic liaison service. The suggested resources are small in relation to the many functions discussed in this book, but do represent realistic and achievable medium-term goals, goals backed by the Royal Colleges of Physicians and Psychiatrists (Royal College of Physicians and the Royal College of Psychiatrists 2003).

International comparisons

This chapter has so far taken the examples of the United States and the UK. Wider international comparisons do not obscure similarities; there may be much greater variation within countries than there is between equivalent types of institution in different countries. Despite large differences in healthcare systems a liaison psychiatrist travelling around the world can expect much of what he sees to be familiar (Mayou & Huyse 1991).

A survey of European centres which had participated in research on inpatient referral patterns described these services in broad clusters according to size and setting (Huyse *et al.* 2000a). There were differences in the size of service and the seniority and experience of staff and whether they were based on a single psychiatric discipline or were multidisciplinary. There was no clear relationship between the size of the hospital and the size of the liaison service. Analysis of inpatient referrals to these hospitals (Huyse *et al.* 2000b) found differences in whether services saw patients with deliberate self-harm and substance abuse. German psychosomatic services saw virtually no such patients, whilst in many other countries such patients made up a quarter to a third of all referred patients. There were few other consistent differences. It was evident that most services saw a high proportion of elderly patients.

Reviews based on informal surveys have reached similar conclusions (Huyse *et al.* 2002; Mayou & Huyse 1991). The most conspicuous international difference is the well-established speciality of psychosomatic medicine in most German-speaking countries. This was founded, and has continued, as a separate speciality outside the formal organization of psychiatry and with close links to internal medicine. Predominantly an inpatient service concerned with complicated interaction of psychiatric and physical disorder, it has been less concerned with consultation. It has had a complicated relationship with psychiatry, which has preserved close links with neurology.

The differences between Europe, Australasia, Japan and other countries largely reflect differences in public funding, patterns of healthcare and the extent of national psychiatric organization. In almost all countries there are similar issues about the role of liaison psychiatry, about the difficulties in achieving adequate funding and recognition, and uncertainty about the future. Despite difficulties and setbacks, the general experience has been that liaison psychiatry is slowly expanding. It is increasingly recognized as a sub-speciality and there are now many enthusiastic national groups which have played influential roles in promoting services for teaching and research.

The wide variation in current practice

The difficulty in describing the current state of liaison psychiatry is the same as that of describing its history; it is not a clearly definable area of interest or practice but a range of expertise across the whole interface of psychiatry and medicine (Table 1.2). It covers problems that are at least as numerous as those that are the subject matter of specialist psychiatry. In addition, it goes well beyond concern with diagnosable psychiatric disorder in that the interaction of psychosocial and physical vulnerability is generally clinically significant. Psychiatric, behavioural and psychological expertise may be highly effective even when there is no disorder in terms of Diagnostic and Statistical Manual (DSM) or International Classification of Disease (ICD) criteria. Although liaison psychiatry is usually seen as a small sub-speciality, its subject matter and political significance is very large.

The difficult task of describing current practice by liaison psychiatrists is made more difficult in that it is also practised by those who see themselves primarily as members of other sub-specialities – child psychiatry, old-age psychiatry, substance abuse, general psychiatry; in fact the whole range of psychiatric specialties. Does this mean that more mainstream psychiatrists who deny the relevance of a special interest of liaison psychiatry are right? Is consultation liaison no more than what all good psychiatrists should take for granted? There is overwhelming clinical evidence that the answers to these

Table 1.2. Types of medical problem.

Psychological complications of medical disorder
Cognitive impairment associated with medical disorder
Functional symptoms
Abnormal behaviour leading to psychiatric complications:
– deliberate self-harm
– substance abuse
– eating disorder
Physical and psychiatric disorder occurring at the same time

questions is no. Psychiatrists who have not trained in the special interest of consultation liaison are poor at recognizing, assessing and treating the problems that are the routine subjects of liaison psychiatrists. There is a separate expertise that requires knowledge and expertise of physical symptoms and disorder. This might mean the need for special interests in liaison within general adult psychiatry and child psychiatry, whereas the practice of old-age psychiatry and learning disability probably requires expertise in the management of physical problems as a basic skill.

Over time it is possible to identify general trends and trends which go beyond the basic model in Table 1.1:

- initial focus on inpatient consultation
- larger services with multidisciplinary staff
- services for different hospital settings (e.g. emergency care) and specialities (e.g. obstetric and cancer liaison)
- services for specific medical problems that call for collaborative planning, training and supervision of the medical team, liaison and consultation by the liaison team
- increased interest in the treatment of functional symptoms
- increased services for outpatients
- links with primary care
- provision of training and supervision for most hospital medical and surgical clinical teams.

There is no single or correct pattern of service delivery. What is important is that within local organization of medical and psychological care the expertise of liaison psychiatry is deployed to greatest effect in the direct care of patients and in the training and support of others involved in care. It is a message that liaison psychiatry has not yet managed to convey. Several overlapping issues are discussed below.

Types of clinical problem

Services vary in the extent to which they aim to provide for the types of problem listed in Table 1.2. Perhaps the greatest change has been the increasing interest in functional symptoms (medically unexplained symptoms) which make up a high proportion of attenders in all medical settings. Such problems have become a large part of many liaison services and especially in those that emphasize outpatient care.

Clinical methods: consultation and liaison

Consultation is frequently with the individual patient, but the focus may also be on others involved (Table 1.3). Particular approaches to consultation that have

Table 1.3. The focus of care.

Patient
Family
Those treating patient — training and supervision
Those treating patient — medication
Establishing and planning services

Table 1.4. Models for consultation.

1. Patient-oriented consultation included not only a diagnostic interview and assessment but also a psychodynamic evaluation of the patient's personality and reaction to illness (Lipowski 1967).
2. Crisis-oriented, therapeutic consultation involved a rapid assessment of the patient's problems and coping style, as well as incisive therapeutic intervention by the consultant (Weisman & Hackett 1960); this model was inspired by Lindemann's crisis theory (Satin & Lindemann 1982).
3. Consultee-oriented consultation focused on the consultee's problem with a given patient (Schiff & Pilot 1959).
4. Situation-oriented consultation was concerned with the interaction between the patient and the clinical team (Greenberg 1960).
5. Expanded psychiatric consultation involved the patient as a central figure in an operational group that included the patient, the clinical staff, other patients, and the patient's family (Meyer & Mendelson 1961).

Source: Lipowski & Wise (2002).

been especially explored and described in the American literature are listed in Table 1.4.

Liaison psychiatry, like most forms of psychiatry, involves many ways of working. It may be focused upon the individual patient, the family, or one of those providing treatment. It can involve relatively limited consultation with patients and those important to them, or a rather different approach which emphasizes liaison with medical teams. In the earlier days, and especially in a small number of well-staffed units, there was argument, indeed controversy, about these methods, which was seen as reflecting fundamental alternatives. This debate was most vigorous and personalized in the United States, but as time has passed, experience and the awareness of the great limitations of staffing have largely overtaken the debate. Consultation is predominant whilst close links and liaison with clinical teams are seen as desirable. There are very few services which are able to provide both consultation and more than a minimum of liaison links with other medical and surgical specialities.

Table 1.5. Types of service.

Consultation by on-call general psychiatrist
Single discipline psychiatric consultation
Multidisciplinary consultation
Multidisciplinary consultation and liaison

Service models

Delivery of a consultation service depends upon a conceptual approach and even more on the available resources. Larger and ambitious services tend to be multidisciplinary and to be able to offer a wider range of services by staff of different levels of seniority and types of skill (Table 1.5).

In terms of organization, consultation and liaison services range from the single-handed and often remote consultant, to multidisciplinary teams. The latter are generally seen as being desirable and tend to be recommended by reviewers and in the plans of national organizations.

Working in varied medical settings

The provision of specialist psychiatry in general hospitals is outside the scope of this chapter.

Table 1.6 lists the commonest ways in which liaison psychiatry is practised in medical settings (Sharpe *et al.* 2000). The items on the list are not alternatives and indeed an ideal service might provide most of these. In practice, services do as much as they can in terms of resources they have and the opportunities within their local healthcare organizations. Much is determined by local circumstance and by the particular interests of medical and surgical colleagues.

Consultation with inpatients remains central to liaison psychiatry. It often involves liaison with particularly interested medical and surgical staff.

Special inpatient units for collaborative management of medical and psychiatric problems are uncommon, apart from the many psychosomatic units in German-speaking countries. Proposals in the United States of various models of medical psychiatric units have made little progress, mainly because it is difficult to solve the problems of funding and who should have clinical responsibility.

Increasingly, consultation-liaison psychiatrists spend their time in outpatient clinics seeing referrals from medical colleagues or from primary care (Bass *et al.* 2002; Dolinar 1993). There are many forms of practice, reflecting various degrees of collaboration with other specialities. These have been poorly described compared with inpatient consultation, even though they relate to the vast majority of patients with psychological and medical problems in medical care.

Table 1.6. Ways of working.

Inpatients
Specialist psychiatric beds in general hospitals
Consultation in medical and surgical units
Liaison with medical and surgical staff
Medical-psychiatric units (USA)
Psychosomatic units (Germany)

Outpatients
The general psychiatry unit in the general hospital
Specialist psychiatry outpatient service
Providing consultation to outpatients
Liaison with specific medical and surgical clinics
An integrated medical-psychiatric clinic

The considerable interest in more collaborative programmes of care for those with chronic conditions, for example stepped care and patient-centred care (see White 2005) offers new opportunities to psychiatrists if they can show a greater political will.

Psychiatric problems are prominent in emergency department care in terms of acutely presenting major psychiatric disorder, deliberate self-harm, and psychiatric complications of medical symptoms and disorders. They are often seen as an important part of liaison psychiatry (Storer 2000), but elsewhere liaison psychiatrists take little part in such emergency care, which is seen as relating more closely to general psychiatry. There is potentially substantial scope for the involvement of liaison psychiatry in the management of psychological issues associated with the wide range of physical and psychiatric presentations, for example in relation to acute functional syndromes, trauma, and bereaved relatives.

A further large area of interest is that of liaison with primary care. It is seen as a major part of the activity of consultation liaison in North America, as is reflected in the regular special section in *General Hospital Psychiatry*. Elsewhere such liaison may be seen as a responsibility of general, rather than liaison, psychiatrists (Bower & Gask 2002). It is a particular problem of the term liaison psychiatry that liaison is part of all psychiatry, indeed of much of medicine. Whatever the model, it is important that patients with complex physical and psychological problems can obtain access to liaison psychiatry teams that have the experience and resources to provide more specialized assessment and treatment.

Services for children (Knapp & Harris 1998a, b) are necessarily separate to those for adults. The overlap in relation to old-age psychiatry is less clear because of varying interest by old-age psychiatrists, and because the high age of many general hospital attenders means that liaison psychiatrists spend much of their time with such patients. There is also overlap in the management of substance abuse in general medical settings. Specialists in this area do have particular clinical skills and access to resources. They see a relatively small number of patients and there is a need for collaboration with liaison psychiatry colleagues.

Sub-specialization within liaison psychiatry

The complexity of liaison psychiatry provision is increased by the development of specific types of liaison with medical, surgical and other specialities (Table 1.7). Some of these see themselves as sub-specialities in their own right, sometimes within liaison psychiatry but sometimes as separate to it, for example, cancer care (Holland 2002), palliative care (Barraclough 2000), and obstetrics liaison. It is unfortunate that psychiatrists with very similar clinical expertise sometimes see themselves as having very little in common and fail to profit from the advantages of being part of a larger, more influential, grouping. Many of these types of service are described elsewhere in this book.

Working with other disciplines

Liaison psychiatry is similar to other aspects of medical care. It is increasingly seen as relating to the role of other disciplines. As elsewhere, this can be as part of a single team or it can result in rivalry whereby competition for the same patient limits effective care.

Psychiatric nurses are usually seen as important in large consultation liaison units, their roles varying from assistants to those with their own individual skills

Table 1.7. Sub-specialities.

Paediatrics
Geriatric medicine
Cancer (psycho-oncology)
Obstetrics
Gynaecology
Palliative care
Medical genetics
Chronic pain
Emergency care (deliberate self-harm)
Neuropsychiatry

and roles. The literature on the particular roles of nurses is limited. In line with general developments within the nursing profession it can be expected that nurses will both seek and find independent roles; this may well be associated with tensions and uncertainty in multidisciplinary working. It remains uncertain as to how the parallel skills of liaison psychiatry, clinical psychologists and behavioural medicine will expand and how they may work together or compete as rivals (see Chapter 6).

Behavioural medicine frequently implies services substantially independent of psychiatry. They are most common in countries with large numbers of qualified clinical psychologists such as the United States and the Netherlands. There is an increasing body of high-quality research relating especially to developing and evaluating assessment and treatment (Keefe *et al.* 2002; Looper & Kirmayer 2002).

Academic issues

Liaison psychiatry developed initially mainly within teaching settings, and its rapid growth in the United States reflected current views on medical education. Since then liaison psychiatrists have seen themselves as having an important contribution to make in teaching students, doctors and other professions.

Research

As with almost all clinical services, the development of liaison psychiatry has so far been based on enthusiasm and experience rather than evidence of epidemiology, aetiology or the effectiveness of treatment. However, research by liaison psychiatrists and by psychologists and others has expanded. It has increasingly applied standard methodologies developed elsewhere to the description of clinical problems, to their epidemiology and aetiology, and to the development and evaluation of treatment. Research output remains modest, reflecting the small number of liaison psychiatrists and the preoccupation of academic departments of psychiatry (and those who fund them) with more obvious psychiatric disorders. The most substantial research has come from other disciplines, especially clinical and health psychologists.

Teaching

Teaching medical students and, more recently, other professional groups has always been a major justification for liaison psychiatry. Indeed in the United States it was the reason for major funding and expansion in the 1970s. As with all aspects of liaison psychiatry, progress over the last 30 years can be viewed as encouraging or disappointingly slow. It is evident that liaison psychiatry has become more prominent in the training of medical students and that it has even had some influence on training in other specialities. On the other hand, surveys and generally reported clinical experience suggest that the amount and quality of teaching about the psychological and behavioural aspects of medical problems is very modest as compared with the clinical significance of the issues.

A review of US medical schools found very variable coverage of what they referred to as psychosomatic medicine topics (Waldstein *et al.* 2001). In general, the amount of teaching was small in terms of number of hours. Student response was mixed. Perceived barriers to teaching included limited resources, student faculty resistance, and a lack of continuity among courses.

The development of liaison psychiatry and behavioural medicine teaching in post-graduate training for psychiatry and for other specialities has also been slow (Lloyd 2001). In a number of countries it has achieved an established position within psychiatric training and also in some other specialities, especially primary care.

Conclusions

Review of the history of what is now termed liaison or consultation-liaison psychiatry shows that the psychological aspects of medicine have until recently been seen as an integral part of good medical care. With progressive specialization and sub-specialization, the separation of medicine from psychiatry is again becoming more apparent and the subject matter of liaison has become a specialist interest at the arbitrary and varying interface of mind and body.

Although the scope and methods are ill-defined, clinical experience and epidemiology have demonstrated the large scale of the clinical problems concerned. It is also evident that successful care depends on specialist expertise which goes well beyond the skills of the more general psychiatric specialities. There are many possible ways of organizing effective psychological input, and liaison psychiatry must be able to respond vigorously in ways that meet local opportunities.

This chapter and this book refer to liaison psychiatry. This term arose in North America and the frequent hybrid version (consultation-liaison psychiatry) reflects historical controversy. Unfortunately these terms have little meaning to anyone who is not familiar with the parochial history. Finding an alternative has not been easy because a number of the possible names have already been used in different ways and have powerful and unacceptable connotations. This understandable failure to find a better name is not an adequate reason for not making a change. 'Liaison psychiatry' is incomprehensible to fellow psychiatrists and to medical colleagues. It severely handicaps the task of publicizing a clinically important activity.

Although the history of liaison psychiatry as a special interest (or sub-speciality) is rather brief and progress has been relatively slow, it is now well established and widely accepted. It is now undeniable that there is a need for special expertise in the management of complex problems involving psychological and physical issues. Whilst it is still seen as marginal and of low priority by many within medicine and within mainstream psychiatry, this book provides substantial evidence as a base for continuing clinical and academic progress. Liaison psychiatry will need determination and political skill if it is to achieve the role that it deserves in new multidisciplinary patterns of delivering health care.

REFERENCES

Barraclough, J. (2000). Liaison psychiatry in palliative care. In *Liaison Psychiatry; Planning Services for Specialist Settings*, ed. R. Peveler, E. Feldman and T. Friedman. London: Gaskell, pp. 163–79.

Bass, C., Bolton, J. and Wilkinson, P. (2002). Referrals to a liaison psychiatry out-patient clinic in a UK general hospital: a report on 900 cases. *Acta Psychiatry Scandinavia*, **105**, 117–25.

Bower, P. and Gask, L. (2002). The changing nature of consultation-liaison in primary care: bridging the gap between research and practice. *General Hospital Psychiatry*, **24**, 63–70.

Dolinar, L. J. (1993). A historical review of outpatient consultation-liaison psychiatry. *General Hospital Psychiatry*, **15**, 363–8.

Greenberg, I. M. (1960). Approaches to psychiatric consultation in a research hospital setting. *Archives of General Psychiatry*, **3**, 691–7.

Guthrie, E. (1998). Development of liaison psychiatry. Real expansion or a bubble that is about to burst? *Psychiatric Bulletin*, **22**, 291–3.

Holland, J. C. (2002). History of psycho-oncology: overcoming attitudinal and conceptual barriers. *Psychosomatic Medicine*, **64**, 206–21.

Huyse, F. J., Herzog, T., Lobo, A., *et al.* (2000a). European Consultation-Liaison Psychiatric Services: the ECLW collaborative study. *Acta Psychiatry Scandinavia*, **101**, 1–7.

Huyse, F. J., Herzog, T., Lobo, A., *et al.* (2000b). European consultation-liaison services and their user populations: the European Consultation-Liaison Workgroup Collaborative Study. *Psychosomatics*, **41**(4) 330–8.

Huyse, F. J., Herzog, T. and Malt, U. F. (2002). International perspectives on consultation-liaison psychiatry. In *American Psychiatry Publishing Textbook of Consultation-Liaison Psychiatry: Psychiatry in the Medically Ill*, 2nd edn, ed. M. G. Wise and J. R. Rundell. Washington, DC: American Psychiatric Publishing.

Keefe, F. J., Buffington, A. L. H., Studts, J. L., *et al.* (2002). Behavioral medicine: 2002 and beyond. *Journal of Consulting and Clinical Psychology*, **70**(3), 852–6.

Knapp, P. K. and Harris, E. S. (1998a). Consultation-liaison in child psychiatry: a review of the past 10 years. Part I: clinical findings. *Journal of the American Academy of Child and Adolescent Psychiatry*, **37**(1), 17–25.

Knapp, P. K. and Harris, E. S. (1998b). Consultation-liaison in child psychiatry: a review of the past 10 years. Part II: research on treatment approaches and outcomes. *Journal of the American Academy of Child and Adolescent Psychology*, **37**(2), 139−46.

Kornfeld, D. S. (2002). Consultation-liaison psychiatry: contributions to medical practice. *American Journal of Psychology*, **159**, 1964−72.

Levenson, J., ed. (2005). *Textbook of Psychosomatic Medicine*. Washington, DC: American Psychiatric Publishing.

Lipowski, Z. J. (1967). Review of consultation psychiatry and *psychosomatic* medicine, 1: general principles. *Psychosomatic Medicine*, **29**, 153−71.

Lipowski, Z. J. and Wise, T. N. (2002). History of consultation-liaison psychiatry. In *Textbook of Consultation-Liaison Psychiatry: Psychiatry in the Medically Ill*, 2nd edn, ed. M. G. Wise and J. R. Rundell. Washington, DC: American Psychiatric Publishing, pp. 3−11.

Lloyd, G. G. (2001). Origins of a section: liaison psychiatry in the College. *Psychiatric Bulletin*, pp. 313−15.

Looper, K. J. and Kirmayer, L. J. (2002). Behavioral medicine approaches to somatoform disorders. *Journal of Consulting and Clinical Psychology*, **70**, 810−27.

Mayou, R. A. (1989). The history of general hospital psychiatry. *British Journal of Psychiatry*, **155**, 764−76.

Mayou, R. A. and Huyse, F. (1991). European workgroup for consultation liaison psychiatry. Consultation liaison psychiatry in Western Europe. *General Hospital Psychiatry*, **13**, 188−208.

Mayou, R. and Lloyd, G. (1985). A survey of liaison psychiatry in the United Kingdom and Eire. *Bulletin of the Royal College of Psychiatrists*, **9**, 214−17.

Meyer, E. and Mendelson, M. (1961). Psychiatric consultations with patients on medical and surgical wards: patterns and processes. *Psychiatry*, **24**, 197−220.

Porter, R. (1987). *A Social History of Madness: Stories of the Insane*. London. George Weidenfeld and Nicolson.

Royal College of Physicians and the Royal College of Psychiatrists (2003). *The Psychological Care of Medical patients: A Practical Guide. A Report by Joint Working Party of the Royal College of Physicians and the Royal College of Psychiatrists*, 2nd edn. London.

Satin, D. G. and Lindemann, E. (1982). The humanist and the era of community mental health. *Proceedings of the American Philosophical Society*, **126**, 229−48.

Schiff, S. K. and Pilot, M. L. (1959). An approach to psychiatric consultation in the general hospital. *Archives of General Psychiatry*, **1**, 349−57.

Schwab, J. J. (1989). Consultation-liaison psychiatry: a historical overview. *Psychosomatics*, **30**(3), 245−54.

Sharpe, M., Protheroe, D. and House, A. (2000). Joint working with physicians and surgeons. In *Liaison Psychiatry; Planning Services for Specialist Settings*, ed. R. Peveler, E. Feldman and T. Friedman. London: Gaskell, pp. 195−206.

Shephard, B. (2000). *A War of Nerves*. London: Jonathan Cape.

Shorter, E. (1997). *A History of Psychiatry*. New York: John Wiley and Sons.

Storer, D. (2000). Liaison psychiatry in the accident and emergency department. In *Liaison Psychiatry; Planning Services for Specialist Settings*, ed. R. Peveler, E. Feldman and T. Friedman. London: Gaskell, pp. 14−26.

Waldstein, S. R., Neumann, S. A., Drossman, D. A., *et al.* (2001). Teaching psychosomatic (biopsychosocial) medicine in United States medical schools: survey findings. *Psychosomatic Medicine*, **63**, 335–43.

Wallen, J., Pincus, H. A., Goldman, H. H., *et al.* (1987). Psychiatric consultations in short-term general hospitals. *Archives of General Psychiatry*, **44**, 163–8.

Weisman, A. D. and Hackett, T. P. (1960). Organization and function of a psychiatric consultation service. *International Record of Medicine*, **173**(306), 311.

Wessely, S., Hotopf, M. and Sharpe, M. (1998). *Chronic Fatigue and its Syndromes*. Oxford: OUP.

White, P., ed. (2005). *Biopsychosocial Medicine: an Integrated Approach to Understanding Illness*. Oxford: Oxford University Press.

2

Establishing a service

Stella Morris

Introduction

Throughout the UK the provision of liaison services is variable both in terms of the existence of specialized teams based in the general hospital and the model of service delivered. The need for liaison psychiatric services has been documented (Benjamin *et al.* 1994; Royal College of Physicians and Royal College of Psychiatrists 1995, 2003; Royal College of Psychiatrists 2005), and the joint report by the Royal Colleges of Physicians and Psychiatrists (2003) proposes that this is best met via specialized multidisciplinary services based in the general hospital. This chapter leads on from previous work (Benjamin *et al.* 1994) in giving a more practical focus and detailing a step-by-step approach of how to establish a service. The chapter will be a useful starting point for trainees in psychiatry hoping to become consultants in liaison psychiatry and to establish a new unit. Likewise it will prove helpful to consultants in general psychiatry (some of whom may wish to move across to liaison psychiatry), health service managers and other clinicians who wish to develop such a service. Although the chapter is written from the perspective of a service for patients aged 16–65, the principles can equally be applied to service developments for children or older adults.

The chapter is divided into several sections. First, the initial negotiations are described, focusing on whom to involve and pertinent issues to discuss. Second, the likely demand on a proposed service is examined and examples of the referral rates to three current UK services illustrate the variability in demand and the importance of allowing for local needs and circumstances. Third, different service models are reviewed and their advantages and disadvantages in relation to different clinical settings are discussed. Fourth, the composition and size of the multidisciplinary team are considered. Fifth, job descriptions together with factors

Handbook of Liaison Psychiatry, ed. Geoffrey Lloyd and Elspeth Guthrie. Published by Cambridge University Press. © Cambridge University Press 2007.

determining how the weekly programmed activities (PAs) may be spent are reviewed. Sixth, possible management arrangements for the proposed service and strategies to obtain funding are discussed, and lastly an example of a business case is given.

Initial negotiations

Prior to any service becoming clinically active a vast amount of preparatory work has to take place. The need for a liaison psychiatry service must be established and this, together with feasibility and benefits of providing such a service, has to be clearly demonstrated in a business case to be submitted to the relevant funding bodies.

Whom to meet

Before the business case is written it will have been necessary to hold many meetings with a wide variety of people to discuss the proposed service. There will be a range of stakeholders and local partners who will need to be influenced and their support harnessed. The project is unlikely to be successful unless there is support from senior clinicians and health service managers within both the acute hospital trust and the usually separate mental health trust. It is essential that a dedicated person is identified to lead the process. If this is a health service manager they will require input from relevant and interested clinical parties, for example from the trainee hoping to become a consultant in liaison psychiatry or another clinician who perceives the need and realizes the importance of such a service.

It is not possible to be prescriptive about whom to include in the initial negotiations since this will vary depending on local circumstances and whether the service is for children and adolescents, people of working age or older adults. Initial negotiations will have to involve senior managers from within the acute hospital and mental health trusts, such as chief executives and medical directors. Senior clinicians from within the acute hospital trust who are interested in such a service or work in areas of high psychiatric morbidity (e.g. neurology, gastroenterology) should be approached. The clinical lead or equivalent in general adult psychiatry should be consulted and it is helpful to meet with the head of clinical psychology. Clinical psychologists are able to provide a unique and important contribution to any liaison service. It is therefore important to gain their support and involvement to prevent tensions and professional rivalries from affecting the successful development of the service. In addition a senior individual within social services should be approached who may consider funding any proposed social work posts. Extensive discussions should also take place at an early stage with potential commissioning and funding bodies to determine their level of support. Currently in the UK the main commissioners and funding bodies for secondary health services are the primary care trusts (PCTs). As there is an increasing shift of resources from secondary to primary care there will also need to be discussions with general practitioners (GPs) and practice-based commissioners to explore links with primary care. Finally, there may be useful allies within local patient/carer groups, and their support and influence should be sought. The acute and mental health trusts should have information about local groups including how to engage with them.

The discussions

Discussions are likely to take place over many months and their content will have common themes. The mental health trust will almost certainly be providing some sort of psychiatric service to the acute hospital, if only in the form of an emergency crisis service to the Accident and Emergency (A&E) department. It is important to find out which services are already in existence in the general hospital for patients with psychiatric/psychological problems and to try to establish their strengths and weaknesses. In this context it is worthwhile enquiring whether there have been any local or regional reviews of existing psychiatric services, which may have highlighted good and bad practice. An example could be a review of services to the A&E department which may have shown the unacceptable length of time that patients must wait for a psychiatrist based in the community to attend, or the number of patients who do not receive a specialist psychosocial assessment following self-harm. If there are deficiencies and inequalities in a service that is being provided then any business case should address these and show how the new development in liaison psychiatry will deal with these problems.

However, if an element of service provision is working well then there is a strong argument not to change it. Duplication of services must also be avoided and this may arise where there is an active clinical health psychology department. Where this is the case there may be an opportunity for some integration, joint working and cross-referral. Clear guidelines regarding referral criteria to each service must be established.

It is crucial to establish from these discussions what is needed or wanted (and these may not be the same) from a proposed liaison psychiatry service. It would therefore make little sense to propose a development in psycho-oncology if an improved psychiatric service to the A&E department is paramount.

The individuals involved in these discussions may know little about liaison psychiatry and what an effective service is able to offer. They will need to be informed and convinced about the high prevalence of psychiatric conditions in the general hospital, the problems with poor detection, the clinical effectiveness of various treatments and the potential of a liaison psychiatry service to reduce healthcare utilization, hospital admissions and lengths of hospital stays (Benjamin *et al.* 1994; Peveler *et al.* 2000; Royal College of Physicians and Royal College of Psychiatrists 1995, 2003; Royal College of Psychiatrists 2005, 2006). The financial restraints within the NHS are evident to managers and clinicians alike. With the advent of the National Service Framework (NSF) for mental health in England (Department of Health 1999), funding for mental health services is linked to the service developments highlighted within that document and has since been refined by further government publications, targets and standards that are regularly published. Little attention was given within the NSF to liaison psychiatry except for self-harm services and the advent of the National Collaborating Centre for Mental Health (NICE) guidelines for the management of self-harm (British Psychological Society and Royal College of Psychiatrists 2004) has brought this further to the fore.

Discussions should also focus on how a liaison service can assist in achieving relevant government recommendations and targets for both the mental health but importantly the acute trust and others stakeholders. These targets will change, but at the time of writing the reduction of waiting lists within the acute trust is a government priority. Consequently, showing how a liaison service may impact on a medical or surgical waiting list would be a useful strategy. Therefore, focusing on how a liaison service will help others achieve their objectives of certain government targets will be a crucial approach. In addition to the references already given, other useful documents to help inform these discussions are listed at the end of the chapter (Department of Health 2000a, b, c, 2001a, b; Royal College of Psychiatrists 1997, 2004a, b). The Department of Health documents are pertinent to readers from the UK, but readers from other countries should refer to relevant publications from their own governments or organizations.

Estimating the demand

Before any business case for a service can be written it is important to have some idea of the likely numbers of referrals to the service so that these can be matched with resources. There are two ways of trying to estimate the referral rates. First, one can attempt to estimate the need using prevalence data from research studies. Such studies have indicated that the prevalence of psychiatric/psychological problems in medical and surgical patients is high (Feldman *et al.* 1987; Royal College of Physicians and Royal College of Psychiatrists 1995, 2003; van Hemert *et al.* 1993). However, prevalence data will not represent the number of patients who will actually be detected by physicians and surgeons, the number that would then be referred or the number of patients that would attend for appointments. Therefore to estimate the number of referrals to a service based on this method is likely to be inaccurate and would not help to plan a realistic service.

The other approach is to look at existing liaison psychiatry services, especially those that serve a similar-sized population and have a similar number of general hospital beds. By knowing the number of referrals per annum it will be possible to estimate the number of referrals on a weekly basis and, depending on the service model employed (see below), to estimate the resources that will be required. Trying to match resources to demands is not an exact science and is always a dynamic process. It is inevitable that as resources increase so too will the number of referrals and similarly as the service becomes more established the number of referrals will rise. It is therefore better when establishing a service to be cautious initially and to aim to restrict referrals.

In addition to this approach, the Royal Colleges' report (Royal College of Physicians and Royal College of Psychiatrists 2003) estimates the likely workload and the likely size and composition of a liaison team to deal with this workload in an established service in a general hospital with 600 beds serving a population of 250 000 (Table 2.1). This estimate of demand is based on previous work by House and Hodgson (Benjamin *et al.* 1994).

Below are three examples of current UK services in liaison psychiatry. The three services are very different and serve to demonstrate the variation in services in

Table 2.1. Estimate of size of liaison service and workload for a multidisciplinary liaison team for a general hospital with 600 beds serving a population of 250 000, together with estimate of size of required liaison team.

Source of referral	Annual rates
Self-harm	500
A&E referrals	200
Ward referrals	200
New outpatient referrals	100–150
Follow-ups	500
Specialized new outpatient contacts	100

Composition of team	Number
Consultant	1
SHO	1
Liaison nurses	5
Health psychologist/clinical psychologist	1–2
Secretary	1

Source: Royal College of Physicians and Royal College of Psychiatrists (2003). Reproduced with permission from Royal College of Psychiatrists.

terms of referral numbers, source of referrals and size and composition of liaison teams. Comparison of these services to the college estimates (Table 2.1) illustrates that whilst the latter are a useful guide, in practice, many factors seem to influence source and rates of referrals and team size and skill mix.

Table 2.2 shows the annual referral rates to the service in Hull. There are three aspects to the service in Hull, the general liaison service, the A&E mental health

Table 2.2. Annual referral rates to the Hull Royal Infirmary service 2005/2006; 800 beds, 600 000 population (some regional specialities serving 1.2 million) and size and composition of team.

Source of referral	Annual rates
Self-harm	725[a]
A&E referrals	80[a]
Ward referrals	91[a]
New outpatient referrals	178
Specialized new outpatient referrals (gynaecology)	46
Chronic fatigue syndrome referrals	171

Composition of team	Number
A&E mental health team	
Band 8 clinical nurse specialist/manager	0.5
Band 6 nurses	2.4
Consultant psychiatrist	0.1
Specialist social worker	1.0
Secretary	0.5
General liaison service	
Consultant psychiatrist	0.6
Senior lecturer	0.6
Specialist registrar	1.0
Senior house officer	1.0
Band 7 nurses (CBT[b])	1.6
Band 7 occupational therapist	0.6
Secretary/administrative support	2.2
Chronic fatigue syndrome service	
Consultant psychiatrist	0.5
Consultant physician	0.2
Band 6 nurse	1.0
Band 6 occupational therapist	0.4
Physiotherapist	0.2
Secretary	1.0

Notes: [a]Number of patients actually assessed; [b]CBT: cognitive behaviour therapist.

team and chronic fatigue syndrome service. All three aspects have slightly different referral criteria. The general liaison service is an outpatient, tertiary referral service covering only one of the two main general hospitals in the city. The hospital covered hosts the A&E department and the regional neurosciences and renal medicine departments. The general liaison service is offered to patients aged 16–65 years and patients aged above and below these 'cut-offs' are directed to the relevant child or older adult services. It has limited medical input to the A&E team. One consultant planned activity (PA) per week is allocated to this work and other medical input is on an ad hoc basis. The senior lecturer has a special interest in neuropsychiatry and provides medical input to the local Huntington's disease team.

The general liaison service offers both assessments and treatments. Approximately 75% of patients who are assessed are taken on for treatment by the multidisciplinary team, since local services to which patients could be referred for further management are very limited. The team does not have adequate resources to deal with the numbers of referrals, hence a long waiting list operates for the initial assessment of non-urgent cases.

The A&E mental health team assesses patients in A&E from age 16 upwards and has no upper age limit. It is an assessment and treatment service (brief and longer term therapies) and operates an extended hours service 9 am–8 pm Monday to Friday. With the advent of the extended hours service the referrals from the A&E department to the Crisis Resolution Service, which provides the out-of-hours service, have reduced by 25%.

The chronic fatigue syndrome service was established two years ago and accepts referrals aged 16–65 years from primary care and both of the general hospitals in the city. It offers assessments and interventions, the latter being on an individual and group basis.

Table 2.3 shows the annual referrals to the liaison service in Middlesbrough. Liaison Psychiatry covers the James Cook University Hospital with 800 beds, which is a large university teaching hospital serving the needs of the local population of 296 000. It is also a cancer centre for 1 million people and a neurology/neurosurgery centre for 1 million people. It houses the regional spinal injuries centre and there are two rehabilitation hospitals and a hospice. The self-harm service uses brief therapy as a tool for therapy during the assessment. Each individual receives a customized package of care on discharge. This service operates seven days per week from 9 am to 5 pm. The liaison work is more of the consultation type due to the paucity of staffing. There are many aspects of the work that remain underdeveloped due to lack of funding.

Tables 2.4, 2.5 and 2.6 describe the service in Leeds. This is a flagship service which has been established for over 20 years. The liaison services in the two main

Table 2.3. Annual referral rates to the Middlesbrough service 2005/2006; 800 beds, 296 000 population (some regional specialities serving approximately 1 million), and size and composition of the team for the Middlesbrough service.

Source of referral	Annual rates
Self-harm	1450[a]
A&E referrals	37[a]
Ward referrals	192
New outpatient referrals	61
Specialized new outpatient contacts (neurology/spinal injuries)	20

Composition of team	Number
Self-harm	
Social workers	1.5
Band 6 nurses	3.0
Vacant post	1.0
Liaison service	
Consultant	1.0
Staff-grade psychiatrist	0.8
Nurse consultant	1.0
Band 7 nurse/manager	1.0
Department secretaries	2.0

Note: [a]This figure includes those patients who were referred but self-discharged prior to assessment. With the implementation of an integrated care pathway for self-harm the majority of patients presenting with self-harm are assessed by the self-harm team with few patients being seen by the out-of-hours service.

hospitals (St James' University Hospital (SJUH) with 1102 beds and Leeds General Infirmary (LGI) with 1218 beds) combined in the year 2000. The service provides both assessment and interventions and has a dedicated inpatient unit based at LGI with eight beds plus a group treatment programme (including groups for pain management, living with chronic illness, depression, etc.). The self-harm assessments at SJUH are provided by senior house officers (SHOs) on a rotational basis as well as one whole-time equivalent (wte) band 7 nurse and one wte social worker. At the LGI these are carried out by SHOs working in the liaison psychiatry department together with one wte social worker, 0.8 wte band 7 nurse and 0.6 wte band 6 nurse. In both of the A&E departments there are also two wte band 6 nurses *in situ* dealing with A&E referrals. They work 2–10 pm Monday to Friday with no cover for sick leave or annual leave. There are three band 7 nurses offering follow-up to the patients seen in A&E across both sites. Resources are not commensurate for the number of referrals, especially the self-harm work. The liaison

Table 2.4. Annual referral rates to the Leeds service 2005/2006; 2320 beds, 750 000 local population, 2.2 million for Leeds Metropolitan District (regional and supraregional services serving a population > 2.2 million).

Source of referral	Annual rates
Leeds General Infirmary (LGI)	
Self-harm	1000[a]
A&E	1044[b]
Ward referrals	456
St James' University Hospital (SJUH)	
Self-harm	1095[a]
A&E	520[b]
Ward referrals	225
New outpatient referrals (LGI and SJUH)	1280
Chronic fatigue syndrome referrals	600

Notes: [a]Actual number of patients assessed by the self-harm team who operate Monday to Friday 9 am–5 pm; [b]Actual number of patients assessed by the A&E team who work Monday to Friday 2 pm–10 pm.

Table 2.5. Leeds General Infirmary Site: size and composition of team.

Composition of team	Number
A&E and self-harm team	
Social worker	1.0
Band 7 nurses	1.8
Band 6 nurses	2.6
Liaison service	
Consultant psychiatrists	2.0
Senior house officers	3.0
Specialist registrars	2.0
Clinical team manager	1.0
Band 8b nurses (0.5 cognitive behavioural therapist)	3.5
Social worker	1.0
Ward staff	
Band 6 nurses	1.6
Band 5 nurses	6.6
Band 2 healthcare workers	2.0
Band 6 occupational therapists	0.5
Band 5 occupational therapists	1.0
Band 6 physiotherapist	0.5

Table 2.6. St James' University Hospital: size and composition of team.

Composition of team	Number
A&E and self-harm team	
Social worker	1.0
Band 7 nurses	3.0
Band 6 nurses	2.0
Liaison service	
Consultants	2.0
Senior house officer	1.0
Specialist registrar	1.0
Band 8b nurse (cognitive behaviour therapist)	0.5
Band 7 nurse	1.0
Social worker	0.5
Band 6 occupational therapist	0.75
Chronic fatigue syndrome service	
Clinical team manager	1.0
Administrator	1.0
Consultant occupational therapist	1.0
Consultant paediatrician	0.1
Nurse specialist (cognitive behavioural therapist)	1.0
Consultant psychiatrist	0.5
Specialist registrar	1.0
Band 6 nurse	1.0
Staff-grade psychiatrist	0.8
Dietitian	0.2
Welfare rights advisor	0.1
Paediatric psychologist	0.2
Band 6 physiotherapist	1.0
Band 3 physiotherapist	1.0
Band 6 occupational therapist	3.0
Band 5 occupational therapist	2.0
Secretary	1.0
Clinic clerk	0.81

service also provides some input to the other four hospitals city-wide (with a total of 694 beds) but there are no designated resources for this work and so it is impossible to provide a particularly comprehensive service.

Therefore in order to try and provide an adequate and feasible service the elements that need to be known are:

• the number of referrals to an existing liaison psychiatry service in a similar setting (population size and number of general hospital beds)

- the type of service (see below, The proposed service) that will be provided as this will influence the numbers of referrals and the size of caseloads carried by team members and hence the size of team required.

Whilst this may be a useful method for estimating demand it is important to recognize that the referral rates will only be approximations of the demand. This is because there is variability within different medical and surgical teams and A&E departments in recognizing patient needs and referring on to the liaison services.

The proposed service

The type of service reflected in the business case will depend on many factors and will become clear through the discussions that take place. Ultimately the type of service that develops will depend on the financial resources available. Whatever type of service is proposed in the business case it is essential that the location of the service is within the acute general hospital even if the service is to offer GP-based clinics. This is because:

- it helps to reduce the stigmatization of referral to a psychiatric service
- it will enable the liaison psychiatry service to be seen as part of the general hospital offering integrated care
- problems often arise acutely and need to be dealt with promptly. With general psychiatric services in the UK usually being community based and geographically separate, there can be considerable delay before psychiatric teams can physically get to the general hospital
- patients who attend the general hospital on a regular basis (for example those receiving regular haemodialysis) often find it easier to be seen for their psychiatric care when they attend for their physical treatment so that they do not have to make separate journeys
- if the service is based in the general hospital it will facilitate the co-ordination of psychological services to the general hospital and is likely to make the referral process less complicated. Ideally all referrals for assessment should be made via a single point of contact.

Some thought should be given to the name of the proposed department. Department of Psychological Medicine suggests a more integrated approach to care than Department of Liaison Psychiatry. It may also be more acceptable to clinical psychology colleagues who will hopefully be working in the department.

Service model

There are many factors to be considered when deciding upon the type of service to be established. The service may offer unrestricted access to all departments in the general hospital, or access may be restricted. The advantages and disadvantages of unrestricted and restricted services are discussed together with ways of limiting access. Other factors to be considered include whether the service will offer assessments only or both assessments and interventions. Finally, the provision of designated beds on the general hospital site is discussed.

Unrestricted versus restricted service model

The business case may outline a bid for a service which accepts referrals from all hospital departments and primary care (making the service a secondary referral service). By making access equitable all potential referrers should be satisfied that a service is being offered to their patients. However, as it is difficult to predict the number of referrals, the biggest danger with this model is being 'swamped' by referrals and not being able to deal with them effectively. This could mean that the department gains a poor reputation in the early stages of its development. Furthermore if team members are put under unreasonable pressure to assess and treat more patients they may become dissatisfied and leave. Recruitment may be difficult in these circumstances making the situation deteriorate further. It is unlikely, particularly in the present financial climate in the UK, that a bid for this type of service provision would be successful and a restricted initial service with a phased approach to development is likely to be the preferred option. This would enable the service to become established and evaluated.

The service may be restricted in a number of ways and these restrictions will be reflected in the referral criteria and/or service level agreement. Referrals can be restricted as follows:

1. Number of referrals accepted — a limit may be put on the number of referrals accepted per annum and this will be reflected in any service level agreement.
2. Referrals only accepted from certain clinical specialties — the service might only take referrals from certain specialities. These may be specialities with known high psychiatric/psychological morbidity, e.g. neurology or oncology, or specialities where the clinicians have been interested in and supportive of the development of such a service. The service may initially only accept referrals from A&E, including self-harm referrals. A variation on this theme is to only accept ward referrals or to only accept outpatient referrals.
3. Secondary or tertiary referral service — the service may be a secondary referral service and accept referrals from primary care as well as the general hospital, or a tertiary service whereby only referrals from clinicians within the hospital are accepted. The disadvantage of the former is high demand as discussed above. Some restriction can be put on the number of referrals if the service accepts tertiary referrals only, and this may particularly apply to a large teaching hospital serving a sizeable population.

Assessment service or assessment and intervention service

Choosing between an assessment-only or assessment and intervention service is an important decision because it will strongly influence the throughput of patients, the caseloads carried by team members and the size of the multidisciplinary team. An assessment service would provide initial assessments only with subsequent referral of patients or discharge. An assessment and intervention service provides assessments and also interventions for appropriate patients. The decision concerning intervention will be influenced by the availability of other services to which patients can be referred. The treatments offered by a liaison psychiatry service are often psychotherapeutic in nature and if there is good access to these services then the liaison multidisciplinary team could be smaller, focusing more on assessments and seeing more new referrals. If the service is to offer both assessments and treatments then a larger team will be required or a smaller number of referrals accepted.

There are strong arguments for the liaison psychiatry service having a multidisciplinary team that is able to offer the appropriate treatments in the departmental base. Patients may be less inclined to attend a separate department of clinical psychology or psychotherapy or the local community mental health team, which is likely to be located away from the general hospital, because of travelling or perceived stigma. Further, a liaison psychiatry service is a specialist service which offers specialist assessments and treatments and generic services may not be able to manage patients as effectively. The management of a patient's care is usually easier for the patient/carer and the professionals involved when all of the treatment can be provided by a single multidisciplinary team which has the necessary skills, rather than the patient being managed by two or more separate teams or departments which may be geographically separate. Finally, job satisfaction for all team members is likely to be greater where the service model offers both assessments and treatments. The main disadvantage of this model is that it is time consuming and the throughput of patients slower. The danger is that it becomes harder for the team to respond to more urgent referrals and a waiting list develops for non-urgent cases.

The types of treatments offered will depend on the focus of the department. For example the treatments offered within a psycho-oncology service will be different from the treatments offered to patients with medically unexplained symptoms. The latter are generally more time consuming and labour intensive and often require a rehabilitation approach. Therefore if the service is going to offer treatments, consideration needs to be given regarding the types of conditions the department will focus on, the treatments that will be offered and the required skill mix of the multidisciplinary team. To some extent this issue is closely linked to referral criteria, which are discussed later.

Inpatient liaison psychiatry beds

The provision of liaison psychiatry beds based in a designated unit or area (e.g. on the neurology ward) on the general hospital site with appropriately trained staff needs to be considered. Such a facility will have considerable cost implications. However, it is a useful provision for managing patients with severe comorbid psychiatric and medical conditions, e.g. a diabetic patient with many complications including renal failure who is on dialysis and has a severe mood disorder and is suicidal, or a patient with severe Parkinson's disease who becomes psychotic. Patients with severe somatoform disorders who may be significantly under-functioning can be assessed and rehabilitation embarked upon in a designated unit. If this facility is not provided then consideration should be given to where patients who require psychiatric admission will be managed. The liaison psychiatrist will therefore need to have access via colleagues in general adult psychiatry to beds on a psychiatric unit, or alternatively to admit under the care of one of the physicians or surgeons to a general hospital bed with the liaison service providing psychiatric input. In reality if there are not designated beds, where a patient is managed will depend on the clinical picture and whether the psychiatric or the medical needs are greatest. The provision of designated liaison psychiatry beds on the general hospital site could become a future service development once an outpatient service has become established.

Referral criteria

The referral criteria will reflect the type of service that is being proposed in the business case and will strongly determine the numbers of patients being referred. Below are examples of referral criteria to different types of services, a comprehensive multidisciplinary liaison psychiatry service offering both assessments and interventions, and a more limited service offering only assessments. Whatever type of service is proposed it is important to have easy referral mechanisms. A single referral point is preferable with postal, faxed and telephone referrals accepted.

Comprehensive service

- Age range 16–65 years (guidelines required about referrals received below and above age limits, e.g. to be referred on to relevant services).
- Inpatients and outpatients from the general hospital accepted. There should be some guidelines about how quickly inpatients will be seen, e.g. the same day or within 24 hours. Psychiatric emergencies will need to be seen as quickly as possible and the team should be organized to respond accordingly.
- Referrals from primary care accepted.

- Provision of a service to the A&E department including self-harm (guidelines required about response times).
- Core outpatient work, offering assessment and treatment, focusing on
  - medically unexplained symptoms,
  - psychological/psychiatric problems associated with physical illness,
  - neuropsychiatric problems.
- Exclusions (these patients may undergo an initial assessment but are excluded from treatment because there will be other services within the mental health trust to whom they can be referred)
  - chronic psychotic disorders,
  - recurrent uni- and bipolar disorders,
  - primary psychosexual problems,
  - primary drugs and alcohol problems,
  - primary eating disorders.

Limited service

- Age range 16–65 years (guidelines as above)
- Inpatients only from the general hospital accepted for assessment (guidelines required as before about response times).
- Provision of a service to the A&E department including self-harm (guidelines required as above).
- Exclusions as above.

The multidisciplinary team

The liaison psychiatry team based within a general hospital is no different from a community psychiatric team covering a sector and should likewise be operating in a multidisciplinary way. As with any multidisciplinary team the emphasis has to be on skill mix rather than professional background

Skill mix

Skills will be required in interviewing and assessment and in providing psychological therapies such as problem solving, interpersonal therapy and cognitive behavioural therapy. Ideally a liaison psychiatry team should be made up of a consultant with specialist training in liaison psychiatry, junior psychiatrists in training, liaison psychiatry nurses, occupational therapists, clinical psychologists, social workers, physiotherapists and administrative/secretarial support. In general the liaison psychiatry nurses need to have specialist knowledge and the more senior the banding (7 or 8) the more independently they are able to practise.

At bands 7 and 8 it is likely that they will be able to manage more complex cases and they may well have gone on to undertake additional training, for example in cognitive behaviour therapy. These types of skills are invaluable within a liaison psychiatry team. In addition to senior nurses an outpatient service will benefit by having junior nurses (band 5 or 6) who can provide ongoing monitoring and support. An increasing role of psychiatric nurses is in the assessment and ongoing management of patients who have self-harmed. With appropriate training and supervision psychiatric nurses can undertake a significant amount of the self-harm work. Psychologists can provide skilled assessments and specialist psychotherapies and neuropsychologists are valuable in the assessment and management of patients with neuropsychiatric disorders. In addition a liaison psychiatry team can be greatly enhanced by having therapists who are able to offer a rehabilitation approach such as an occupational therapist and physiotherapist. These team members are extremely valuable in providing behavioural treatments for patients who are underfunctioning and in the management of patients with somatoform disorders.

The liaison psychiatrist appointed to develop a multidisciplinary liaison psychiatry team should be involved in the recruitment process of other team members. This can prove useful in identifying candidates with the appropriate training and skills.

Size of team

It is very difficult to be definitive about the size of the multidisciplinary team. To some extent the size has to be dynamic and inevitably if there are more resources then there will be more demand placed on the team. In planning the size of a team the principal factors to be considered are:

- estimated number of referrals
- the service model that is to be adopted.

Ultimately the size of the team will be determined by the finances available and often the demand has to be adjusted via the referral criteria or service level agreements in order to meet these resources.

Job description and outline of job plan for a consultant in liaison psychiatry

The joint guidance on the employment of consultant psychiatrists is a helpful document and includes guidance on job descriptions, contracts and the principal duties of a consultant (Department of Health 2005).

Within the job plan there needs to be a dedicated number of programmed activities (PAs) for clinical work (e.g. 7.5 in a 10 PA job), time for teaching (which may be an important component of the job, particularly in the initial stages of any service being developed) and research (if this is desired), for providing educational supervision to trainees and appropriate time for administration and management. The latter should include regular meetings with managers from both trusts but should also allow time to enable the job holder to develop the service. In this context adequate time must be allocated for evaluation and audit of the service, the results of which will be essential for service development. Service development together with evaluation and audit can be very time consuming but it is core business and there must be dedicated time to perform this. Time must also be put aside for continuing professional development (CPD). If the post is half-time and split with general psychiatry the liaison PAs must be protected. Such a job is unlikely to be 'workable' and will not be approved by the regional advisor if there are fewer than five liaison PAs (which will need to include clinical and supporting PAs) in a 10-PA job. Therefore there needs to be careful negotiation so that a sensible and workable job plan is developed.

The clinical PAs can be spent in a variety of different ways and may well change as the service evolves. How they are spent will also depend on the service model that is employed but there will always be clinical PAs spent having face-to-face contact, writing up notes, telephone calls and dictating letters. One clinical PA may be spent usefully each week meeting with the multidisciplinary team to discuss new referrals and patient management. An important aspect of clinical work will be clinical supervision of other team members/trainees, e.g. in the area of self-harm, and appropriate time must be allocated for this. Some liaison psychiatrists spend time participating in ward rounds or multidisciplinary meetings with other specialities. Joint clinics may be established whereby the liaison psychiatrist sits in a clinic with another consultant colleague and patients are seen together. These types of clinic are often good for facilitating the referral, possibly engaging the patient and for allowing an exchange of information. However, their disadvantage is that they are time consuming. Another variant of the joint clinic is where the liaison psychiatrist sees patients in a separate room but at the same time as a particular medical or surgical clinic is occurring. In this way the psychiatrist can be seen as part of that team. This variant of the joint clinic also promotes good communication between specialities. Finally, as acute trust services may be devolved to primary care there might be opportunities to establish some clinics in GP surgeries.

Management and funding issues

There is often debate about which trust, mental health or acute hospital, should manage a liaison psychiatry service. The joint report from the Royal College of Psychiatrists and the Royal College of Physicians (2003) recommends that liaison services should be managed and funded by the acute hospital trust. This is because issues faced by liaison services may be better understood by or are more relevant to the acute trust and the latter is the main beneficiary of the service. Ultimately, the decision may be pragmatic and depend on which trust is the most interested in establishing and developing the service and will most actively support develop-ments and business cases that are submitted. If the liaison psychiatry service is to be managed by the acute trust then there is a danger of professional isolation for all team members and so special arrangements need to be in place to avoid this and to allow professional training to continue. In addition, clinical governance issues need to be reflected appropriately and mechanisms need to be in place to allow cross-referral of patients to and from general psychiatric services and, where necessary, to allow patients to be admitted to psychiatric beds. If the mental health trust takes overall management responsibility, there is a risk that the liaison service will be neglected by the acute trust. In addition it may also be neglected by the mental health trust because much of the work of a liaison service (apart from self-harm) will not be considered core business. Which ever trust manages the liaison service it is good to establish joint management meetings to include managers from both trusts and the consultant liaison psychiatrist. These will ensure that effective links are established between the two trusts, to enable developments to be planned jointly and to maintain the profile of the liaison service with the acute trust. Inevitably there are likely to be wide local variations in management arrangements.

Funding arrangements will likewise be subject to local arrangements. It is absolutely essential to engage with the commissioning and funding bodies, currently the PCTs, at an early stage of any proposed liaison psychiatry development. There is a real need to keep abreast of changes within the NHS and new government targets and initiatives that are introduced, to see how pertinent they are to liaison psychiatry. In reality a liaison psychiatry service is unlikely to be funded unless it can impact on these targets and initiatives. Funding opportunities may arise from within various networks that have been established to offer a collaborative and multiagency approach to commissioning and delivering certain services (e.g. emergency care and diabetes). These networks could be approached if the proposed liaison service will impact on their outcomes. Further opportunities for funding may arise with the proposed move towards practice-based commissioning, which could provide liaison services who can offer specialist services in primary care, e.g. for patients with somatoform disorders and frequent attenders, a unique opportunity to develop. If the acute trust is to submit the business case for the new liaison psychiatry development it will have to compete with all of the other business cases being submitted by that organization. The liaison psychiatry business case may not seem as important or as relevant as a business case for more renal dialysis machines or another consultant anaesthetist. Hence there is a need to make managers in the acute trust aware of the benefits of a liaison psychiatry service and in particular the positive impact a liaison service can have on helping the acute trust to achieve certain targets.

The acute trust managers also need to appreciate that as more developments occur within the acute trust, e.g. an increase of neurologists or gastroenterologists, there will be a potential for the number of referrals to the liaison psychiatry service to increase. Therefore in the business cases for these other services there should be some provision for additional liaison psychiatry funding. By using this mechanism money should accrue for liaison psychiatry, allowing the service to develop and meet the increasing demands.

The further development of an existing liaison service should ideally be driven by the speciality requiring the input. In collaboration with the liaison service the speciality should develop a business case and submit this through the business planning forum of the acute trust. Sometimes the expansion of established units occurs through opportunistic growth when money becomes available. The liaison psychiatrist needs to have good networks in place, particularly within the acute trust, and also the PCTs, to be able to take advantage of these sorts of opportunities.

Business case

The business case will be the culmination of many months' work. It describes the service that needs to be developed, provides arguments to support the development and states the cost implications. Below is an example of a business case, however the format is likely to differ depending on local preferences and it is wise to ask commissioners for their preferred format.

Name of service:

Submitted by:

1. *Aims of proposal*
   To establish a Department of Psychological Medicine/Liaison Psychiatry in *Another General Hospital/Another Acute Trust,* to provide *an assessment service* or to provide an *assessment and treatment service.*

2. *Objectives of the department*
   This will be dependent on the discussions that have taken place but could include a brief description of the clinical service that will be provided, the teaching and supervisory role of the department and how relevant government targets will be met.

3. *Context*
   a. *National*   Under this subheading there should be a description of the psychiatric morbidity in the general hospital, the problems with under-detection and the benefits of providing a service. There may follow a description of other services nationally. Reference should be made to the importance of psychiatric/psychological input in the general hospital as mentioned in any of the National Service Frameworks, government documents and Royal College reports.
   b. *Local*   There should be a description of the gaps and deficiencies in the acute trust regarding psychiatric/psychological input and any inequalities or delays obtaining such input. Reference should be made to any local reviews of services to the general hospital which have indicated the gaps, deficiencies and inequalities.
4. *Proposal*
   a. *Service model*
      (i) Unrestricted versus restricted access (may be phased development over five years and sequential developments should be shown)
      (ii) assessment-only or assessment and intervention service
      (iii) outpatient only or service to have designated inpatient beds in the general hospital.
   b. *The multidisciplinary team*: the size and composition will depend on the service model and estimated number of referrals.
   c. *Location*: must be in the general hospital. The type and amount of accommodation required needs to be specified.
   d. *Brief operational policy*: this should give an outline of the referral criteria, how the service will be accessed, the types of conditions that will be treated and the interventions that will be used, links with other services, the use of the Care Programme Approach (CPA) and managerial arrangements. It is important to emphasize in the proposal that the service will be patient centred and there will be partnership work.
5. *Benefits and outcome*
   This should include a description of the benefits to the patients, carers and the acute trust and how national and local priorities will be addressed.
6. *Evaluation*
   There is a need to collect data systematically to provide continuing evidence of clinical activity and to aid in further service developments. Such data are important for performance management agendas and consultant appraisals. There should be a description of the routine information that will be collected, e.g. number of referrals per annum, number of referrals from different specialities, number of patients actually seen, number of patients taken on

for treatment, number of patients appropriately discharged from the referring clinics, etc. The importance of patient and carer feedback through patient satisfaction surveys should be considered as part of any evaluation. Details of any audit that will be undertaken should be given.

7. *Appendix*

Breakdown of costs to include personnel (clinical and secretarial together with oncosts, e.g., tax and employee and employer national insurance contributions, travel and study leave expenses), consumables and overheads.

Conclusions

Securing funding for new developments within the health service is challenging, particularly for developments such as liaison psychiatry. These are unlikely to be successful unless they can address national and local priorities. Once a service is set up the reputation of the department can be greatly enhanced by the consultant and department keeping a high profile in both the acute trust and also within primary care. A liaison psychiatry service needs to be seen and heard. Presenting cases at the general hospital 'grand rounds', attending wards to see inpatient referrals, maintaining telephone contact with medical and surgical and GP colleagues about patients seen, and being involved in the teaching programmes for junior doctors in medicine and surgery are all ways of maintaining a high profile. It is important to be proactive, flexible and helpful. Although referral criteria are very important there may be times when the referral rules need to be broken and a particular patient assessed in the department. This can be a very good public relations exercise but it is important not to do it too often. It is absolutely essential for the consultant in liaison psychiatry to develop good relationships with consultant colleagues in the general hospital to gain their support.

Finally the newly appointed consultant may well be a 'lone voice in the wilderness' of the general hospital and will need to establish good support networks both professionally and personally. The advice and support of a more senior colleague in liaison psychiatry who may well be based in another town or city is likely to be beneficial. Mentoring arrangements should be established from an early stage.

Acknowledgements

I wish to thank the following: Dr Amanda Gash (Consultant Liaison Psychiatrist, St Lukes Hospital, Middlesbrough) and Dr Peter Trigwell (Consultant Liaison Psychiatrist, Leeds General Infirmary) for providing data about their respective services in *Estimating the demand*, Mrs Angie Mason (Director of Nursing and Service Delivery, Humber Mental Health Teaching NHS Trust) and

Dr Ivana S Markova (Senior Lecturer in Psychiatry and Honorary Consultant Liaison Psychiatrist, Hull Royal Infirmary) for their helpful comments.

REFERENCES

Benjamin, S., House, A. and Jenkins, P. ed. (1994). *Liaison Psychiatry: Defining Needs and Planning Services.* London: Gaskell.

British Psychological Society and Royal College of Psychiatrists (2004). *Self Harm. The Short Term Physical and Psychological Management and Secondary Prevention of Self Harm in Primary and Secondary Care.* Commissioned by the National Collaborating Centre for Mental Health (NICE).

Department of Health (DOH) (1999). *National Service Framework for Mental Health.* London: DOH.

Department of Health (DOH) (2000a). *The NHS Plan.* London: DOH.

Department of Health (DOH) (2000b). *National Cancer Plan.* London: DOH. (This includes 'A policy framework for commissioning cancer services', 1995).

Department of Health (DOH) (2000c). *National Service Framework for Coronary Heart Disease.* London: DOH.

Department of Health (DOH) (2001a). *National Service Framework for Diabetes.* London: DOH.

Department of Health (DOH) (2001b). *National Service Framework for Older Adults.* London: DOH.

Department of Health (DOH) (2005). *Joint Guidance on the Employment of Consultant Psychiatrists.* London: DOH.

Feldman, E., Mayou, R., Hawton, K., *et al.* (1987). Psychiatric disorder in medical inpatients. *Quarterly Journal of Medicine,* **63**, 405–12.

Peveler, R., Feldman, E. and Friedman, T. ed. (2000). *Liaison Psychiatry: Planning Services for Specialist Settings.* London: Gaskell.

Royal College of Physicians and Royal College of Psychiatrists (1995). *The Psychological Care of Medical Patients: Recognition of Need and Service Provision.* CR 35, London: Royal College of Physicians and Royal College of Psychiatrists.

Royal College of Physicians and Royal College of Psychiatrists (2003). *The Psychological Care of Medical Patients: A Practical Guide.* London: Royal College of Physicians and Royal College of Psychiatrists.

Royal College of Psychiatrists (1997). *Report of the Working Party on the Psychological Care of Surgical Patients.* CR 55, London: Royal College of Psychiatrists.

Royal College of Psychiatrists (2004a). *Assessment Following Self Harm in Adults.* CR 122, London: Royal College of Psychiatrists.

Royal College of Psychiatrists (2004b). *Psychiatric Services to Accident and Emergency Departments.* CR 118, London: Royal College of Psychiatrists.

Royal College of Psychiatrists (2005). *Who Cares Wins. Improving the Outcome for Older People Admitted to the General Hospital: Guidelines for the Development of Liaison Mental Health Services for Older People.* London: Royal College of Psychiatrists.

Royal College of Psychiatrists (2006). *Liaison Psychiatry Service Development Report.* London: Royal College of Psychiatrists.

Van Hemert, A. M., Hengeveld, M. W., Bolk, J. H., *et al.* (1993). Psychiatric disorder in relation to medical illness among patients in a general medical outpatient clinic. *Psychological Medicine*, **23**, 167–73.

Useful websites

Royal College of Psychiatrists: www.rcpsych.ac.uk

UK Department of Health: www.doh.gov.uk

National Institute for Health and Clinical Excellence: www.nice.org.uk

3

Legal and ethical issues in liaison psychiatry: treatment refusal and euthanasia

Eleanor Feldman

Introduction

Liaison psychiatrists are frequently asked to advise when patients refuse consent to medical intervention, especially when possible mental disorder, or other emotional or mental disturbance, may play a part in that refusal. The aim of this chapter is to give practising clinicians a framework for understanding legal issues surrounding refusal of treatment in the general hospital context. This will be achieved by a discussion of the legal position in one jurisdiction with which the author has a working knowledge (England and Wales), followed by a series of cases and commentaries that serve to illustrate the kinds of problems that commonly arise. Readers working in jurisdictions other than England and Wales should seek guidance from their hospital's legal advisers as to how the same issues are dealt with in their country.

The legal position in England and Wales

Statute law

The Mental Health Act 1983 (MHA), allows for the legal detention and treatment of persons with mental disorder where admission for that disorder is considered necessary in the interest of their health or safety, or for the protection of others, and where they are unable or unwilling to consent to such admission. The use of the MHA enables patients to be detained in hospital and to be treated, against their will, for their mental disorder, whereas it does not sanction treatment for physical

Handbook of Liaison Psychiatry, ed. Geoffrey Lloyd and Elspeth Guthrie. Published by Cambridge University Press. © Cambridge University Press 2007.

disorders unconnected to the mental disorder, even where the patient is unable or unwilling to give consent. In such cases, practitioners would have to look to other authorities such as Common Law or a declaration by the courts, and the hospital would normally be expected to take legal advice (Mental Health Act Commission Guidance note GN1/2001 2001). For situations that arise commonly and predictably, it is helpful for a hospital to have formulated a policy in conjunction with its legal advisers to help clinicians feel confident in dealing with these matters.

The role of the Mental Health Act (MHA) in the general hospital

Non-psychiatrists in general hospitals are frequently unaware of the limitations of the MHA with respect to issues of non-consent, and may erroneously expect that it normally has a role where there is refusal of treatment for physical health in persons with mental disorder. Nevertheless, it is important to understand where the statute law does apply and if there are special considerations in a general hospital environment.

In legal terms the MHA is an 'enabling' act which means it need not be used in all possible instances where it could conceivably apply, but its use provides certain legal safeguards for patients and for staff responsible for the patients subject to the MHA. Protections for patients include close monitoring and regular inspections by the MHA Commission, and rights to appeals and tribunals. MHA section 139 protects staff such that no civil or criminal proceedings are allowed against persons in pursuance of the Act unless they could be shown to be acting in bad faith or without reasonable care. Civil proceedings require the leave of the High Court and criminal proceedings require the consent of the Director of Public Prosecutions.

Whilst any mental disorder can fall within the remit of the MHA, in practice there are common circumstances where restraint and treatment are applied without recourse to the Act. In these situations, the actions performed (if carried out without the real consent of the patient) can only be defended if within the scope of the Common Law.

In the MHA, mental disorder is defined very broadly: MHA section 1 (2) states: ' "mental disorder" means mental illness, arrested or incomplete development of mind, psychopathic disorder and any other disorder or disability of mind and "mentally disordered" shall be construed accordingly', and hence this may include temporary states of mental disturbance such as delirium and intoxication, as well as more prolonged conditions such as dementia and brain damage. Use of the MHA would be unusual in these conditions in general acute psychiatric practice with the exception of drug-induced psychosis, whereas in general hospital psychiatric practice, the MHA is more likely to be temporarily applied to patients with organic brain disorders in circumstances of risk to self or others. Although MHA section 1(3) states that the Act cannot be applied to persons by 'reason only of promiscuity or other immoral conduct, sexual deviancy or dependence on alcohol or drugs', it should be noted in particular that someone who is intoxicated with alcohol or drugs may legitimately be subject to the MHA, including for the intoxication itself (e.g. amphetamine psychosis), so long as there are current grounds for intervention other than alcohol or drug addiction alone.

The use of the medical holding order

The Mental Health Act, section 5(2), contains a short-term holding order for 72 hours that may be used to detain an existing hospital inpatient. However, it may not be used in an Accident and Emergency (A&E) department, which is regarded as an outpatient setting. Someone who is not already a hospital inpatient may only be detained under MHA sections 2, 3 or 4. Where an A&E department has an associated ward, MHA section 5(2) may be applied to patients who have already been admitted and came in voluntarily.

Unlike patients detained under MHA section 2, 3 or 4, those held under MHA section 5(2) may not be transferred to another hospital and there are no powers to treat. A similar, short-term, holding order is available under MHA section 5(4), but as a registered mental nurse may only use it, it is unlikely to be used in a general hospital.

The MHA section 5(2) power may be used by the registered medical practitioner in charge of a patient's treatment. This person is known as the Responsible Medical Officer (RMO), and is the consultant in charge of the case. There is nothing in the MHA to confine the role of the RMO to a psychiatrist. However, where a person is receiving treatment for a mental disorder it is desirable that the medical practitioner in charge of that part of their treatment be a psychiatrist.

In general hospitals, the initials RMO are frequently applied to the resident medical officer who is usually only of senior house officer grade. It is therefore very important to be clear that, where the term RMO is used in connection with the MHA, it always denotes the consultant with medical responsibility for the case.

The MHA permits the RMO to nominate a deputy, who must be a registered medical practitioner (and not, therefore, a preregistration house officer). Therefore, a consultant physician or surgeon who finds him/herself acting as a patient's RMO may nominate his/her own junior as a deputy for the purposes of the MHA. However, it is not a good practice if junior physicians or surgeons are left to invoke the powers of section 5(2) when they and their seniors are unclear about the precise nature and scope of the powers.

The code of practice on the use of the MHA 1983 (Department of Health and Welsh Office 1999) states that a RMO who is not a psychiatrist should make immediate contact with a psychiatrist when s/he has made use of his/her MHA section 5(2) power (NB not the nominated deputy).

The MHA Commission has issued further guidance on this point for general hospitals as follows:

It is good practice for general hospitals to have a service level agreement in place which allows the care and treatment for the mental disorder to be given under the direction of a consultant psychiatrist from a psychiatric unit. Where such good practice is adhered to, the consultant psychiatrist who takes responsibility for the treatment of the mental disorder that has led to detention should be considered to be RMO for the purposes of the Act.

If a non-psychiatrist does assume responsibility as RMO, he or she should ensure that all relevant staff are aware of the implications of Part IV of the Act, which deals with consent to treatment. Guidance can be found in Chapters 15 and 16 of the Code of Practice. (Mental Health Act Commission Guidance note GN1/2001 2001)

Section 63

Under Part IV of the MHA 1983, section 63 states that 'the consent of a patient shall not be required for any medical treatment given to him for the mental disorder from which he is suffering, not being treatment falling within section 57 or 58 above [these are special treatments requiring consent and/or a second opinion including ECT and psychosurgery]. If the treatment is given under the direction of the responsible medical officer.' The MHA Code of Practice (Department of Health and Welsh Office 1999) further states 'for the purposes of the Act, medical treatment includes nursing and care, habilitation and rehabilitation under medical supervision, i.e. the broad range of activities aimed at alleviating, or preventing a deterioration of, the patient's mental disorder.

In the case of a patient detained under MHA 1983, treatment may be given to him/her under section 63 of that Act for any physical illness or disease that is so integral to the mental disorder as to make such treatment a necessary part of the treatment of that mental disorder. However, in order for such treatment to be lawful, the form of mental disorder which it is proposed be addressed in this way must in the first instance be such as to warrant detention, and the patient should be classified as suffering from that form of mental disorder in his/her detention documentation (*R (on the application of B)* v. *Ashworth Hospital Authority* 2003).

Following the case of *B* v. *Croydon Health Authority* 1994, section 63 may also be extended to cover treatment of the consequences of the mental disorder for which the person has been placed under the MHA section. The consequence in the case of Ms B was self-starvation requiring re-feeding in someone under section 3 for treatment of a borderline personality disorder. This extension could also apply to someone who had self-injured or self-poisoned. Hence, if a patient is already subject to an MHA section allowing treatment for a specified mental disorder, they can also be treated under the MHA for self-harmful acts consequent upon that same disorder. In practice, this extension is of limited assistance, as the vast majority of self-harming persons are not appropriately subject to the MHA, and those who are, unless they are already under an MHA order allowing treatment when they commit the act of self-harm, will usually require their emergency medical intervention before the process of instituting an appropriate MHA order can be completed.

Necessity

The courts have recognized the existence of a Common Law principle of 'necessity', and extend it to cover situations where action is required to assist another person without his or her consent. Although such a situation will often be some form of emergency (or 'urgent necessity'), the power to intervene is not created by that urgency, but derived from the principle of necessity. In practice, there is usually a period when patients who are about to be made subject to the MHA will have to be restrained before the formalities of the Act can be completed. It is also quite common for such patients to require some sedation prior to the completion of formalities. Such actions will be defensible if carried out as a necessity and using the minimal intervention required; this might include the use of drugs. Actions performed out of necessity should not continue for an unreasonable length of time, but progress should be made either to a situation of consent or to the use of powers under the MHA. It is not possible to define precisely what is a reasonable or unreasonable length of time, as this would vary with the particular circumstances of each case.

The use of the place of safety order and the role of the police

MHA section 136 empowers a police constable to detain and take to a place of safety someone found in a public place who appears to be suffering from a mental disorder. It may not be used as an emergency admission section. Its purpose is to enable someone to be assessed in safety for possible admission under the MHA. There are no statutory documents covering the MHA section 136 power, but many NHS trusts and police forces have developed their own forms to record its use.

A person should only be brought to hospital under MHA 1983, section 136 if the hospital has been designated for that purpose. In fact, in many areas it is the police station or a special area in a psychiatric unit that is a designated place of safety. A&E departments are often ill equipped for use as places of safety. They may be unsuited to receive people with severe mental disturbance and their use for that purpose may put others at great risk. In any locality, the places of safety that may be used under MHA section 136 should be agreed between NHS trusts responsible for general non-psychiatric hospitals, those that provide psychiatric services, and the police. In addition, the police should be invited to state in what circumstances they will assist in the removal of dangerous persons, and what they would do to assist hospital staff in circumstances where they have brought a dangerous person to a general hospital for medical assessment and/or care that is not possible elsewhere. Police should use the A&E department for the patient if they believe this is necessary for medical reasons (e.g. the patient has taken a drug overdose).

Managerial arrangements for the MHA

Where a NHS trust does not normally provide inpatient psychiatric services, it may wish to make arrangements for any MHA functions to be performed on its behalf by a NHS trust that does provide inpatient psychiatric services. This will be particularly so for the receipt, scrutiny, and if necessary, rectification of the admission papers, and where the two NHS trusts share the same hospital site. However even where one NHS trust delegates its functions in this way, it will remain responsible for their performance.

Where staff of a non-psychiatric NHS trust may need to perform some MHA functions, it is important that they receive specialist training in that regard and that their performance of those functions is subject to regular specialist review.

Non-psychiatric NHS trusts should consider issuing guidance to their clinical and security staff about the measures that may be taken, and those that are prohibited, in respect of patients who are incapable of consenting to medical treatment. Guidance will need regular review to keep abreast of changes in the law. To ensure its application, trusts should provide appropriate training for staff.

The Common Law

The Common Law is made up of principles identified by judges to meet the needs of particular cases; it can be found published in law reports as judges' statements at the end of cases. This judge-made law is in contrast to statute law passed by Parliament. Once Common Law principles have been stated, their application to future cases should follow. Common Law has the advantage that it can respond to new developments much more quickly than can the processes that create statute law. Clinicians may experience a disadvantage in that the Common Law may change without their knowledge; hence the need for continuing legal advice and review.

In England and Wales a Mental Capacity Act (2005) became law in April 2005, which enshrined in statute law many of the principles set out previously in the Common Law. However the Act is yet to come into force and until it does principles enshrined in Common Law still pertain. Many countries will have different systems in place for determining capacity to refuse medical treatment. This chapter describes both the Common Law principles that preceded the new act, and the new act itself.

Relevant Common Law principles

It is helpful to consider five principles:
1. Assumption of capacity in adults
2. Best interests
3. Duty of care
4. Necessity
5. Bolam/Bolitho test.

Assumption of capacity in adults

Every adult who has reached the age of majority (18 years) has, a priori, the right and capacity to decide whether or not he/she will accept medical treatment, even if a refusal may risk permanent damage to his/her physical or mental health, or even lead to premature death. The reasons for the refusal are irrelevant. Capacity is a legal concept and concerns an individual's ability to understand what is being proposed to them and the consequences of either refusing or accepting the advice given, and weigh it in the balance to arrive at a decision. In law, preregistration house officers are not considered qualified to assess a patient's capacity to accept or refuse treatment, but any registered medical practitioner could be called upon to give evidence on this (British Medical Association and Law Society 1995). Where mental disorder is present or likely, psychiatric opinion is necessary for a detailed assessment of capacity, for example in a patient who may be suicidal.

In 2002, the UK media gave much publicity to a case in point, so that UK professionals have since become much more aware of the force of this aspect of the law. Ms B was a seriously physically disabled patient who wanted life-sustaining artificial ventilation turned off but the intensivists looking after her were not willing to do this, in spite of psychiatric opinion that she had full capacity. Ms B was found also by the court to have full mental capacity. The judge, Dame Butler-Sloss, stated that once it was established that Ms B had the necessary mental capacity to give or refuse consent to life-sustaining medical treatment, the artificial ventilation became an unlawful trespass. Moreover, if there was no disagreement about capacity but the doctors were for any reason unable to carry out the patient's wishes, it was their duty to find other doctors who would do so (*Re B (consent to treatment: capacity)* 2002). Ms B was subsequently transferred to another hospital where artificial ventilation was suspended and she died.

How to assess capacity

A series of cases in the 1990s have established the principles underlying the modern general law on mental capacity. The following cases are particularly helpful:

In *Re C*, a 68-year-old man whom surgeons considered to need amputation of a gangrenous leg to be necessary to prevent imminent death, and who was already under a treatment order of the MHA for chronic schizophrenia, was judged by the court to have the mental capacity to refuse the amputation (*Re C (adult: refusal of medical treatment)* 1994). The fact of his requiring compulsory treatment under the MHA was not evidence in itself that he was mentally incompetent to make decisions about his physical health. The judge, Justice Thorpe, adopted a three-stage test for establishing a patient's capacity to decide:

1. Could the patient comprehend and retain the necessary information?
2. Was he able to believe it?
3. Was he able to weigh the information, balancing risks and needs, so as to arrive at a choice?

In *Re MB*, a 23-year-old pregnant woman was 40 weeks pregnant and the baby was in a breech position, necessitating a Caesarean section delivery (*Re MB (an adult: medical treatment)* 1997). The woman suffered with a needle phobia and initially refused the Caesarean section because of anxiety about intravenous access for the anaesthesia and then, after some changing of her mind and when in the operating theatre itself, she also refused anaesthesia by mask and the surgery. The health authority that day sought a declaration from the courts to proceed and this was granted. MB then instructed her lawyers to appeal that evening, but the following day she agreed to the procedures and a healthy baby was delivered. At the appeal against the declaration, points made by Dame Butler-Sloss with respect to capacity reiterated Lord Donaldson's earlier judgment in *Re T* that the graver the consequences of the decision, the commensurately greater the level of competence required to take the decision, and that temporary factors such as confusion, shock, fatigue, pain, or drugs may completely erode capacity, but that those concerned must be satisfied that such factors are operating to such a degree that the ability to decide is absent (*Re T (adult: refusal of medical treatment)* 1992). Following *Re MB*, another such influence may be panic induced by fear. Again, careful scrutiny of the evidence is necessary because fear of an operation may be a rational decision for refusal to undergo it. Fear may also, however, paralyse the will and thus destroy the capacity to make a decision.

The situation for minors

Those under the age of 18 do not have the same rights at law as adults. It is capacity, rather than chronological age, that determines whether a child or young person can legally give valid consent to medical interventions. In England and Wales, mentally competent 16- and 17-year-olds can give consent in their own right without reference to their parents or legal guardian (Gillick competence), but their refusal can be overridden in law by parents, legal guardians or the High Court.

Best interests

After an appropriate assessment of capacity has been made, if an individual is judged to lack capacity to make the decision in question, doctors have a duty to see that any act or omission taken on that person's behalf with regard to their health must be in that person's best interests. The Law Commission has recommended that in deciding what is in a person's best interests consideration should be given to:

- the past and present wishes of the individual
- the need to maximize as much as possible the person's participation in the decision
- the views of others as to the person's wishes and feelings
- the need to adopt the course of action least restrictive of the individual's freedom (British Medical Association and Law Society 1995).

Best interests extend beyond purely medical considerations to incorporate broader ethical, moral and welfare considerations (*Re S (adult patient's best interests)* 2000).

Duty of care

Common Law imposes a duty of care on all professional staff to all persons within a hospital. By assuming the responsibility of a particular clinical staff appointment, an individual undertakes to provide proper care to those needing it. Staff may be negligent by omission. Actions involving the use of reasonable restraint and driven by professional responsibility in circumstances of necessity are supported by Common Law.

As well as individual staff, hospitals also have duties, for example to provide security staff who are properly trained to assist with aggressive uncooperative patients in an emergency department, and the hospital must ensure that such staff are authorized to act if necessary. Many hospitals experience problems with fulfilling this duty because they fail to train security staff in this role, and commonly such staff may be disinclined to assist in necessary restraint, as they believe that they will be exposed to the risk of litigation for assault and battery. This is a key area for improved staff training and the involvement of the hospital's risk management advisers.

The Bolam test

Where clinical decisions are being made, an individual clinician's competence will be judged against what is considered reasonable and proper by a body of responsible doctors at that time, as ascertained in court from expert testimony, i.e. the Bolam test (*Bolam* v. *Friern Hospital Management Committee* 1957). The Bolam test has been qualified more recently by the House of Lords decision in the case of *Bolitho* v. *City and Hackney HA* (1997), such that the decision of the doctor must be reasonable and responsible (defensible logically), or the judge may still find against.

Official guidance on consent

The Department of Health issued a *Reference Guide to Consent for Examination or Treatment* in March 2001 (see www.dh.gov.uk/assetRoot/04/01/90/79/0401/ 9079.pdf). The General Medical Council has also issued guidance on the ethical considerations with respect to seeking patient's consent (GMC 1999) and set out standards of practice expected of doctors when they consider whether to withhold or withdraw life-prolonging treatments (GMC 2002). These documents are consistent with the advice given above. Moreover, to quote the Department of Health guidance:

Case law on consent has evolved significantly over the last decade. Further legal developments may occur after this guidance has been issued, and health professionals must remember their duty to keep themselves informed of legal developments that may have a bearing on their practice. Legal advice should always be sought if there is any doubt about the legal validity of a proposed intervention. While much of the case law refers specifically to doctors, the same principles will apply to other health professionals involved in examining or treating patients.

The Mental Capacity Act 2005

In April 2005, a new Act to deal with issues related to capacity gained parliamentary approval in England and Wales, and will come into force in April 2007. An incapacity act has already been introduced in Scotland. The Mental Capacity Act 2005 for England and Wales provides a statutory framework to empower and protect vulnerable people who are not able to make their own decisions. It enables people to plan ahead for a time when they may lose capacity. It will enable doctors in England and Wales to have a legal framework to provide treatment to people who lack capacity if such treatment is in the patient's best interests.

The Act is underpinned by a set of five key principles stated at Section 1:

1. A presumption of capacity – every adult has the right to make his or her own decisions and must be assumed to have capacity to do so unless it is proved otherwise.
2. The right for individuals to be supported to make their own decisions – people must be given all appropriate help before anyone concludes that they cannot make their own decisions.
3. Individuals must retain the right to make what might be seen as eccentric or unwise decisions.
4. Best interests – anything done for or on behalf of people without capacity must be in their best interests.
5. Least restrictive intervention – anything done for or on behalf of people without capacity should be the least restrictive of their basic rights and freedoms.

Assessing lack of capacity

The Act sets out a single clear test for assessing whether a person lacks capacity to take a particular decision at a particular time. For the purposes of the Act, a person lacks capacity in relation to a matter if at the material time he/she is unable to make a decision for him/herself in relation to the matter because of an impairment of, or a disturbance in the functioning of, the mind or brain. It does not matter whether the impairment or disturbance is permanent or temporary. The test for capacity is essentially the same as that already outlined above.

The principle of best interests

This is incorporated into the Act in that everything that is done for or on behalf of a person who lacks capacity must be in that person's best interests. The Act allows a person to appoint an attorney to act on their behalf if they should lose capacity in the future. The Act allows people to let an attorney not only make legal and financial decisions for them but also health and welfare decisions.

Advanced decisions

The Act allows for an individual to make advanced decisions in relation to medical treatment within a legal framework. An advanced decision can be made by anyone over the age of 18 years, provided he or she has the capacity to do so. The decision will enable the individual to refuse a specified treatment should he or she be unable to consent to that treatment at the time it is required. Anyone can withdraw an advanced decision at any time, if they have the capacity to do so. A withdrawal does not need to be in writing.

Euthanasia requests

In those countries where physician-assisted suicide is legal, liaison psychiatrists may be involved in assessment to ensure that the person making the request has the requisite capacity to opt for this course of action. In the Netherlands, the Burial Act was amended in November 1993 to allow assisted suicide, and the Royal Dutch Medical Association has procedural guidelines to ensure that the request originates from a longstanding and well-considered wish to die.

Bannink and colleagues describe the helpful inclusion of psychiatric consultation to determine whether appeals for euthanasia were influenced by psychiatric problems (Bannink *et al.* 2000); of 22 cases seen by a psychiatrist, 10 individuals were thought to have a long-lasting and well-considered wish that did not originate from intolerable pain or the undue influence of others, in 6 the psychiatrist established that the wish had not been fully considered, and in another 6, the patients were found not mentally competent either because of cognitive impairment or depression. It appears that the psychiatrist did not influence the outcome in the majority of cases, but in 2 of the patients lacking mental capacity, the physician had been prepared to comply with the requests for euthanasia and so the psychiatric involvement changed the policy; this did not delay the patients' deaths, only the manner of their dying. The authors conclude that standard psychiatric consultation need not be mandatory, but the benefits of the expertise and support of a consultant psychiatrist in improving the quality of decision-making need to be balanced against the disadvantages of using a psychiatrist as the final gatekeeper.

In England and Wales, the High Court in London considered the case of Mrs Dianne Pretty in 2001 and concluded that public opinion was not yet ready to legalize assisted suicide (Dyer 2001). The debate, however, is unlikely to go away.

The law applied to clinical situations

Having covered the principles underlying the relevant law in the jurisdiction of England and Wales, it is helpful to consider their practical application in a number of case vignettes. All the cases have been invented for illustrative purposes. The advice given is not intended to be prescriptive, but to provide an illustration of how principles discussed in the section may be applied in practice. In the law, as in medicine, there is always a place for considered judgment according to the particular circumstances of each case.

Acute organic brain syndrome

A 54-year-old male on the high-dependency unit is recovering from a cardiac arrest that required prolonged resuscitation. As he emerges from several days of coma, he becomes acutely distressed, disorientated and paranoid. He requires heparin for his prosthetic heart valves, and antiarrhythmic drugs, but refuses to have either and is walking about, dressed and demanding to leave. He has already tried to push past you and the nursing staff. You assess that the only way to help him is to restrain and sedate him against his will, keeping him on the high-dependency medical unit.

Comment

This man's refusal is not based on any real understanding of his circumstances and, in delirium, he has no grasp of his risk; it is very clearly in his best interests for him to be detained and sedated so that he can have life-saving treatments. Any reasonable layperson would not dispute this man's need for treatment and would consider hospital staff negligent if they knowingly allowed him to leave and failed to do whatever was necessary to help him.

The MHA could be applied for detention and sedation to treat the delirium (a form of mental disorder), but delirium is not a situation in which the MHA is commonly used. Such patients are more often detained and treated without recourse to the MHA in view of the evident lack of capacity to give meaningful consent or refusal, the transient nature of the disturbance, and the (so far) undisputed need for intervention. However, if strong measures are required, such as the use of psychiatric nursing staff to pin this man to his bed whilst he is forcibly injected with a sedative drug, or if the situation persists over a prolonged period, it may be advisable to use the MHA. The section should be cancelled as soon as the patient has recovered mentally. When the new Mental Capacity Act comes into force, this man's treatment would be covered by this new act.

Treatments other than sedation in this case are not authorized by the MHA, but are justifiably given in a legal sense if the post-registration physician directing the treatment has judged that the patient does not have the capacity to make a meaningful refusal. The same legal decision could also apply to the use of sedation, in which case a psychiatrist need not be involved as, in law, any registered medical practitioner may be considered able to judge a patient's capacity to consent (British Medical Association and Law Society 1995). This does not apply to patients detained under the MHA after the first three months of treatment; only the RMO is then judged to be able to determine a patient's capacity to consent. In relation to the new Mental Capacity Act, all medical treatment could be given provided it was in the patient's best interests.

Patient refusing medical intervention after deliberate self-harm

A 30-year-old male is brought to the A&E department following an overdose of 70 paracetamol tablets taken four hours prior to arrival at hospital. There is no history available and the patient refuses to say anything about himself other than he wants to be left alone to die. He refuses to give blood for a paracetamol level and refuses any medical intervention. Can medical treatment be given without his consent?

Comment

This illustrates a fairly common scenario. The patient presents the medical staff with the dilemma of whether they should assume he has full capacity to refuse medical treatment, in which case they might leave him to suffer the consequences of liver failure, possibly death, or whether they should act out of necessity and as part of their duty of care to treat someone in whom capacity may reasonably be in doubt and where the patient could be mentally ill. A psychiatrist may attend as an emergency to give a further opinion on the issue of capacity but the MHA will not assist with respect to treatment for the poisoning. Doctors in such cases need to consider most carefully whether there is reasonable doubt with respect to such a patient's capacity to make a fully informed and reasoned choice in such a grave matter; if there is, they should proceed with whatever action is needed, as a matter of urgent necessity, and in his best interests to save his life. This is defensible under the Common Law.

To date, commonly occurring cases of this type have tended to be dealt with without application to the courts for assistance and so there are currently no exact precedents either way, but the cases of *Re T* and *Re MB* are particularly instructive (*Re T (adult: refusal of medical treatment)* 1992; *Re MB (an adult: medical treatment)* 1997). However, if time allows, doctors and health authorities should not hesitate to seek a court declaration and courts do have the discretion to grant interim declarations. The practice to be followed for this is set out in *St George's Healthcare NHS Trust* v. *S* (1998). In extreme emergencies, where there is no time to seek the assistance of the court, any doubt that may exist about a patient's capacity to decide that is not resolvable by available further medical opinions must be resolved in favour of society's interest in upholding the concept that all human life is sacred and that it should be preserved if at all possible. It is very unclear with this scenario whether the new Mental Capacity Act could be used. The Act clearly allows for temporary states of incapacity, but it remains to be seen whether it would be invoked in such a situation.

Intoxicated patient refusing to co-operate with assessment following deliberate self-harm

A young adult male is brought to the A&E department by paramedics who found him lying in a doorway with a suicide note and an empty bottle of paracetamol. He is intoxicated with alcohol, belligerent, refuses to talk and is making moves to leave. There is no other information and staff have to make a decision as to whether or not to let him go.

Comment

This case typifies a common clinical problem faced by A&E staff and their covering psychiatrists. If there is sufficient concern to warrant detaining this patient for further assessment of a possible underlying mental disorder, then use of the MHA is certainly justified. The fact that the patient is intoxicated is not an obstacle to the use of the MHA, as the Act is not being used to detain or treat someone because of alcohol abuse or dependence alone (a use of the MHA excluded under section 1(3)), but because of the concern that there may be an underlying mental disorder which is temporarily obscured by intoxication and lack of co-operation.

Anorexia nervosa patient *in extremis* and refusing food

A 19-year-old female weighing only 4 st has been admitted to the acute medical unit. She consents to a saline drip, but not to any parenteral feeding. She is close to death from starvation.

Comment

The MHA is frequently used in relation to patients with anorexia who are close to death to authorize feeding as part of the psychiatric as well as part of their physical treatment. Experts in eating disorders regard refeeding as an essential first step in the psychiatric treatment, as starvation itself produces distorted thinking. There are legal precedents to support this view, notably *Re KB*. The Mental Health Act Commission has issued guidance on this particular topic that discusses the legal issues in more detail (Mental Health Act Commission Guidance Note 3 1999).

Patient with schizophrenia refusing surgery, but accepting other medical care

A 59-year-old male with chronic schizophrenia is a long-stay patient under section 3. He develops a gangrenous foot and the surgeon's advice is to proceed to amputation. The patient refuses surgery on the grounds that he does not want an amputation, but he agrees to antibiotics and all other forms of treatment. The surgeon asks if the operation can be carried out as part of treatment under section 3 and he impresses upon the psychiatrist his conviction that the patient is likely to die without the amputation. The psychiatrist assesses the man as having capacity to refuse the amputation.

Comment

The MHA does not apply to the treatment of the physical disorder in this case as it is not in any way related to the mental disorder; medical opinion here is that amputation of the leg would not improve his schizophrenia (indeed it could make it worse). As the patient is considered to have the capacity to refuse this particular treatment, then his doctors must abide by his wishes.

Best interests in an incapacitated dying man

A 64-year-old man with end-stage chronic bronchitis is disorientated and violent on the acute medical ward, throwing cups about and swearing at staff. Sedation would be dangerous. He has a history of an aggressive personality and has been well known to the chest clinic over many years. He has never complied well with treatment and neglects himself at home. He has been admitted with a further acute exacerbation of his end-stage chronic bronchitis and is repeatedly demanding to go home, but his family want him to stay in hospital, as he cannot manage at home. He does not appreciate that he will die very quickly at home, but is dying anyway, and is not aware of this in spite of being told.

Comment

This man lacks capacity as he is unable to register or retain the information regarding his medical situation, neither appreciating that he is close to death now, nor that he would die even more quickly at home. The difficulty in proceeding with this patient lies mostly in determining his best interests. He is dying anyway and the physician's view is that there is only minor and temporary medical gain likely in his physical condition if he remained in hospital. Although not fully aware of his situation, he is consistent in stating his wish to be at home and cannot be pacified any other way, and so his doctors attempt to seek a way of helping him die more peacefully at home whilst supporting his family in understanding that he is close to death, unlikely to improve, and that overall his best interests now lie in granting him his dying wish.

Acknowledgement

The author is grateful to the Mental Health Act Commission for advice.

REFERENCES

B v. *Croydon Health Authority* 1994 22 BMLR 13

Bannink, M., Van Gool, A. R., van der Heide, A, *et al.* (2000). Psychiatric consultation and quality of decision making in euthanasia. *Lancet*, **356**, 2067–8.

Bolam v. *Friern Hospital Management Committee.* [1957] 2 All ER 118–28 at 122

Bolitho v. *City and Hackney HA* [1997] 4 All ER 771

British Medical Association. (1995). *Advance Statements About Medical Treatment. Code of Practice with Explanatory Notes. Report of the British Medical Association.* London: BMJ Publishing Group.

British Medical Association and Law Society. (1995). *Assessment of Mental Capacity: Guidance for Doctors and Lawyers.* London: British Medical Association.

Department of Health and Welsh Office. (1999). *Code of Practice Mental Health Act 1983.* London: HMSO.

Department of Health. (2001). *Reference Guide to Consent to Examination or Treatment* (www.dh.gov.uk/assetRoot/04/01/90/79/0401/9079.pdf).

Dyer, C. (2001). High Court throws out 'suicide aid' case. *British Medical Journal*, **323**, 953.

General Medical Council. (1999). *Seeking Patient's Consent: the Ethical Considerations.* London: GMC.

General Medical Council. (2002). *Withholding or Withdrawing Life-prolonging Treatments: Good Practice in Decision-making.* London: GMC.

Kennedy, I. and Grubb, A. (2000). *Medical Law*, 3rd edn. London: Butterworths.

Mental Health Act Commission Guidance Note 3. (1999). *Guidance on the treatment of Anorexia Nervosa under the Mental Health Act 1983* (issued August 1997 and updated March 1999). Available on the Mental Health Act Commission website: www.mhac.org.uk

Mental Health Act Commission Guidance note GN1/2001. (2001). *Use of the Mental Health Act 1983 in General Hospitals without a Psychiatric Unit.* Available on the Mental Health Act Commission website: www.mhac.org.uk

Mental Capacity Act. (2005). HMSO.

Mental Health Act. (1983). HMSO.

R (on the application of B) v. *Ashworth Hospital Authority* 2003 EWCA Civ 547; Court of Appeal, 15 April 2003.

Re B (consent to treatment: capacity) 2002 1FLR 1090

Re C (adult: refusal of medical treatment) [1994] 1 All ER 891 (Fam Div)

Re KB 1993 19 BMLR 144 (Fam Div)

Re MB (an adult: medical treatment) 1997 38 BMLR 175 (CA)

Re S (adult patient's best interests) 2000 2FLR 389 at 400

Re T (adult: refusal of medical treatment) 1992 9 BMLR 46

St George's Healthcare NHS Trust v. *S* [1998] 3 All ER 673 CA at 702

4

Understanding psychological reactions to physical illness

Geoffrey Lloyd

People react to illness in a manner that reflects a complex and evolving interaction of several factors. These include their premorbid personality, previous experience of ill health, interpersonal relationships, perceived threat of the illness, the physical treatment required and their interaction with medical and nursing staff to whom they turn for treatment. Most illnesses, except the very trivial, require a period of adjustment and a reappraisal of lifestyle, ability to work and engagement in leisure activities.

Coping strategies

The great majority of people cope constructively with illness in the sense that they seek medical advice appropriately and co-operate with treatment in a manner which maximizes their chances of recovery. If an illness is chronic and associated with permanent disability, lifestyle changes are made which enable a realistic adjustment to take place. Coping is a dynamic process. Most people have a range of coping strategies which they can use flexibly, according to the particular problems that their illness creates at the time. Some cope by involving themselves closely with the treatment plan, seeking out information about their illness not only from their doctor but also from medical textbooks and websites. They may become involved in medical charities devoted to their illness and in the case of rare conditions some become so well informed that they know more about the illness than their doctor.

In sharp contrast to this strategy some people cope by distancing themselves from the emotional implications of their illness. They develop other interests and attempt to minimize any disability, ignoring, rejecting or making light of any

Handbook of Liaison Psychiatry, ed. Geoffrey Lloyd and Elspeth Guthrie. Published by Cambridge University Press. © Cambridge University Press 2007.

information which has a threatening content. This involves a certain degree of denial which protects people from emotional distress but which is maladaptive if it interferes with access to appropriate treatment and if it prevents them changing their lifestyles in a healthy manner. In extreme cases denial acquires a delusional intensity.

Although most people cope adaptively with illness, in a significant proportion the coping strategies are inadequate to prevent the development of a psychiatric disorder which fulfils the diagnostic criteria established by the Diagnostic and Statistical Manual (DSM-IV) or International Classification of Disease (ICD-10). The development of a psychiatric disorder makes it much more difficult to cope with physical and social restrictions (Dickens *et al.* 2006). Depression and anxiety are associated with increased healthcare costs and impaired health-related quality of life (Creed *et al.* 2002). Adherence to a treatment regime may be compromised and the prognosis worsened. Dementia, delirium and depression are all associated with increased mortality after hip fracture (Nightingale *et al.* 2001). It has also been shown that patients who are depressed following a myocardial infarction are known to have a greater risk of recurrent infarction and a higher mortality rate. This is discussed further in a subsequent section of this chapter.

Factors which influence psychological response

Personal factors

Individual characteristics play an important role in shaping the response to illness. They influence how an illness is perceived and how the patient copes with the adversity. An assessment of a patient's usual defence mechanisms and coping style is therefore essential if the psychological response is to be understood. It is also important to know whether there has been a history of serious illness in childhood or affecting close family members and, if so, how the individual coped with this.

People who are habitually anxious tend to worry more about their health and some of these people develop symptoms of anxiety to such a degree that the psychological response becomes a problem in its own right. The anxiety is focused on their health and on bodily sensations which are often interpreted in a morbid manner. A hypochondriacal pattern is established and this leads to excessive invalidism. Obsessional people react similarly. They have a desire to find out as much information about their illness as possible and become preoccupied with new and existing symptoms. The easy availability of medical information on the Internet will inevitably result in more people becoming better informed about their illnesses and doctors need to be prepared to enter into a more detailed discussion of symptoms, differential diagnosis and treatment options than was previously required of them. The concept of 'the expert patient' has evolved in recent years, particularly with regard to those coping with a long-term illness. Acquiring expertise gives people a greater sense of control over their illness and enables them to communicate more effectively with professionals. The combination of personal experience of an illness together with detailed information can also provide an invaluable source of advice and support to other patients.

People who deny or minimize the significance of their illness often have a life-long tendency to play down the importance of any adversity. This can be an adaptive mechanism in that it protects against anxiety and depression. However if carried to extreme lengths it prevents people seeking appropriate medical care or, if they have sought care, it often results in advice on treatment and lifestyle changes being ignored. This can have a major negative influence on prognosis.

People with paranoid traits are likely to blame their illness on others. The targets include close relatives, employers, doctors and other healthcare professionals. It is from this group of patients that complaints and litigation are most likely to arise. Not surprisingly doctors find them difficult to deal with. Consistency and openness of communication are vitally important to avoid breakdown of therapeutic relationships. In a few people of paranoid disposition an acute paranoid reaction develops following admission to hospital. Others develop a chronic delusional system which involves the belief that a particular doctor has permanently harmed them, deliberately or otherwise, as a result of a medical procedure. This is classified as delusional disorder (F22.0) by the International Classification of Disease.

The effects of ageing should also be considered. There is no clear distinction between elderly and younger adults with regard to their coping strategies. Ageing is a gradual process and any age criterion used to distinguish older and younger adults is essentially an arbitrary one, often based on the age at which people are entitled to receive state pensions. Nevertheless older people are more likely to develop multiple physical pathology; they are more vulnerable to bereavement, sensory loss due to hearing and visual impairment, financial hardship and loss of independence. They also have to cope with the decline in cognitive function which is characteristic of the ageing process. Comorbid physical and psychiatric disorders are therefore common in the elderly who are comprising an increasing proportion of patients in general hospitals. There is evidence that their psychiatric needs have been under-recognized, perhaps because of therapeutic nihilism and a failure to distinguish symptoms of psychiatric disorders from those of normal ageing. Comparative studies have shown that, when referred to a psychiatric service, elderly patients are more likely than younger patients to receive a diagnosis of cognitive impairment and less likely to be diagnosed as having a personality disorder (Unutzer *et al.* 2002). The number of elderly patients admitted to general hospitals is going to increase rapidly. It is important that their psychological needs are recognized and met. There should be easy pathways of referral to a liaison psychiatry service. This might be facilitated if there is a specific liaison psychiatry service for the elderly.

Nature of the illness

Potentially fatal and rapidly progressive disease might be expected to result in more severe psychological reactions but the evidence indicates that there is surprisingly little correlation between psychiatric morbidity and disease severity when this has been measured in a standardized manner. Some of the older studies suggested that certain categories of illness are more likely to be followed by distressing psychological symptoms. Cavanaugh (1983) found that highest scores for psychological symptoms were obtained by patients with cancer and autoimmune disorders together with diseases of the renal, haematological, genitourinary and gastrointestinal systems. Feldman *et al.* (1987) found that the highest rates of affective disorder were associated with haematological malignancy, ischaemic heart disease and chest disease. Malignant disease is still stigmatized by the general public, as are conditions such as tuberculosis, sexually transmitted disease and acquired immunodeficiency syndrome (AIDS).

The nature of the illness is perhaps best understood by considering its subjective significance, that is, the patient's perception of the condition. Lipowski (1969) was one of the first to emphasize the subjective importance of the part of the body affected by illness in determining the emotional response. The more highly valued the bodily part, the more intense will be the psychological reaction.

It can be very difficult for patients to adjust to terminal illness. Medical practice in this area has changed considerably during the last two or three decades in recognition of the fact that most patients wish to be informed that they have a terminal condition. Communication between professional staff and their patients has become more open. Terminally ill patients wish to know if death is coming and they need to be supported during the terminal phase. Emotional suffering can be reduced if patients are afforded dignity and privacy and if they are enabled to retain control over as many aspects of their lives as possible. These include choosing the location of treatment, having adequate control over pain and other symptoms and being able to make advance directives which ensure their wishes are respected. Terminally ill patients should have access to emotional and spiritual support and to hospice care if requested.

Treatment environment

The hospital environment is stressful for most patients. Its unfamiliarity and the presence of complex technology are frightening and bewildering. When inpatient treatment is necessary the patient has to cope with loss of privacy and independence as well as loss of usual sources of comfort such as cigarettes and alcohol. The most distressing areas of a hospital are those which involve complex machinery as found in intensive care and coronary care units. An environment of this type can easily be seen as threatening and some patients develop paranoid ideas about the unit and the staff treating them.

Isolation is another potent source of stress. Patients undergoing bone marrow transplantation and those infected with methicillin resistant *Staphylococcus aureus* (MRSA) may have to spend several weeks in an isolated room, with all staff and visitors having to wear protective clothing and facial masks. Tarzi *et al.* (2001) have shown that, among older adults, isolation for MRSA has a negative effect on mood in addition to that resulting from hospitalization.

Special procedures

Investigations such as colonoscopy, cardiac catheterization and imaging are potentially stressful and can lead to anxiety not only because they are intrinsically unpleasant but because their findings have crucial diagnostic implications which will determine the need for further treatment. Similar considerations apply to blood tests, for example for HIV infection, and tissue biopsies for suspected cancer, which the patient knows might convey bad news. Patients need to be specially prepared and counselled before investigations of this nature are undertaken and the significance of the results should be discussed with them as soon as possible.

Similarly, genetic screening can be stressful, particularly during the interval between the test being carried out and the result being available. Pretest screening and support following disclosure of the result do much to alleviate anxiety. Michie *et al.* (2001) observed that adults receiving a positive result following genetic testing for familial polyposis coli were more likely to become anxious if they were low on optimism or self-esteem and suggested that counselling should be targeted at those with poor psychological resources.

Drug treatment

Many drugs used in medical practice are known to have significant neuropsychiatric side-effects and therefore affect the patient's psychological response to becoming ill. The relationship between a drug and an adverse reaction can be established with varying degrees of confidence as recommended by Karch and Lasagna (1975). See Table 4.1.

Table 4.1. Assessing side-effects of medication.

Definite — a reaction that:

1. follows a temporal sequence from administration of the drug or the drug level has been established in body fluids or tissues;
2. follows a known response pattern to the drug;
3. improves on stopping the drug (dechallenge);
4. reappears on repeated exposure to the drug (rechallenge).

Probable — a reaction that:

1. follows a temporal sequence from administration of the drug;
2. follows a known response pattern to the drug;
3. improves with dechallenge;
4. could not reasonably be explained by the patient's underlying clinical condition.

Possible — a reaction that:

1. follows a temporal sequence from administration of the drug;
2. follows a known response pattern to the drug;
3. could be explained by the patient's underlying clinical condition or other administered drug.

Conditional — a reaction that:

1. follows a temporal sequence from administration of the drug;
2. does not follow a known response pattern to the drug;
3. could not follow a known response pattern to the drug.

Doubtful

Any reaction that does not meet the above criteria.

Depression, mania, anxiety, agitation, sedation, delirium and isolated psychotic symptoms have all been linked with various drugs. Corticosteroids, adrenergic antagonists, anticonvulsants and antiparkinsonian drugs are well established as potential precipitants of psychiatric symptoms. The antiretroviral drugs are also known to affect mental state. Efavirenz, a non-nucleoside reverse transcriptase inhibitor, is particularly associated with the onset of depression and with suicidal thoughts which may be disproportionately intense in relation to the severity of other symptoms of depression. (See Turjanski and Lloyd 2005 for a review of this topic.)

Other physical factors

Metabolic changes accentuate the emotional response to illness. Hypoxia, dehydration, electrolyte imbalance, endocrine changes and infections can all produce affective symptoms in their own right and make it more difficult for patients to adjust effectively.

Communication

Effective communication is an essential element of good clinical practice. Conversely, poor communication is a source of frustration for patients, leading to uncertainty, resentment, anxiety and depression. It increases the likelihood of a psychiatric disorder and is often the reason why patients make a written complaint or take legal action for compensation regarding their medical care. All healthcare professionals who interact with patients need to have communication skills commensurate with their clinical role, whether this be in a hospital, primary care or the community.

Dissatisfaction with communication relates to three separate areas:

- insufficient information
- lack of interest
- lack of involvement in decision making.

Most patients want more information about their illness than they are given. However there is much individual variation on this matter and doctors need to explore how much a particular patient wishes to know about the illness and its treatment. This takes time. Many consultations are hurried and conducted in situations which lack privacy, so patients often feel they have not had the opportunity to ask questions. Likewise doctors do not have time to evaluate the patient's level of understanding and need for information.

However, it is important to avoid information overload. If too much information is provided at once the patient is likely to feel perplexed, particularly if the information is expressed in technical terms or in medical jargon. Studies of clinical consultations have shown that no more than half the information provided is recalled subsequently. Even less may be recalled if the patient is anxious or depressed at the time of the interview. It is best to give information early during a consultation and to repeat this at the end. Written material, in the form of specially prepared leaflets, is a valuable aid which facilitates recall once the consultation has finished. In the UK the Department of Health has advised that patients should, as a matter of right, be sent copies of all correspondence between doctors concerning their illness. This is another useful source of information, one which has generally been well received by patients.

The essentials of good communication have been summarized as follows (Royal College of Physicians and Royal College of Psychiatrists 2003):

- expressing interest in the patient
- eliciting the patient's beliefs and concerns
- acknowledging and responding to the patient's distress
- avoiding jargon and overly complex information
- establishing a collaborative and empowering approach
- maintaining privacy and confidentiality.

Special issues arise when treating patients from a different cultural background. This is a common occurrence in a multicultural society and all clinicians need to have an understanding of the patient's beliefs about illness, medical and other treatments and the healthcare system. This can be achieved by asking patients to explain their understanding of how their symptoms developed, what has caused them and what treatment they think is appropriate. It is also important to be aware how cultural background influences the way people express emotional distress, often using somatic complaints rather than the psychological complaints expressed by people from Western cultures. If the patient's language ability does not permit adequate description of complaints an interpreter should be engaged to facilitate communication. It is preferable to involve a professional interpreter rather than a close relative.

Communication problems also arise with patients who have disabilities such as visual or hearing impairment, dysarthria, dysphasia or global cognitive difficulties, either congenital or acquired. Special provision needs to be made to help overcome these problems (Royal College of Physicians and Royal College of Psychiatrists 2003).

Involving patients in decisions concerning their illness is an element of practice which has only recently been given importance in medical training. Patients vary in the degree to which they wish to be involved in decision making. Some wish the doctor to take a paternalistic approach and prefer to leave all decisions about management to the professionals. On the other hand a growing number wish to be involved in deciding what investigations are required and what course of treatment should be adopted. It is important that the doctor establishes what the patient's attitudes are on this issue. Those who wish to be involved in decision making need accurate information. Many people now obtain knowledge about medical matters from various sources on the Internet and they may wish to discuss this with their doctor. The doctor needs to establish the patient's current level of understanding about the illness. Misunderstandings need to be corrected and gaps in knowledge filled in.

Stress and previous psychiatric illness

Stressful life events are known to increase the risk of developing a depressive illness. Adverse events affecting a person shortly before or after the onset of illness therefore make it more likely that a depressive illness will develop. Patients are also more likely to become depressed if they have had a previous psychiatric illness (Dickens *et al.* 2004; Feldman *et al.* 1987). Those who have been psychiatrically ill are also more likely to become physically ill. Harris and Barraclough (1998) have reviewed mortality studies of a wide range of psychiatric disorders. In the case of affective disorders they found that the mortality was increased from infections and from nervous, circulatory and respiratory disorders. It is not clear what the causal links might be but it is apparent that those who develop an affective disorder are more prone to become physically ill. Their affective illness is likely to recur or to be exacerbated following the onset of physical illness.

Psychiatric disorders following physical illness

Adjustment disorder

This is probably the most common emotional reaction to illness that satisfies the criteria for a psychiatric diagnosis. The symptoms involve a disturbance of mood, either depression or anxiety or a mixture of both. In severity they form a continuum, with no clear cut-off between a normal and a pathological reaction. Psychological symptoms should be regarded as pathological when they themselves are a source of distress or when they interfere with adjustment to the illness and the requirements of treatment.

By definition the symptoms of an adjustment disorder are transient, usually resolving within a few weeks, but they can be very distressing to the patient while they last. After the development of an acute physical illness the symptoms of an adjustment disorder become apparent within a few days and tend to remit with physical recovery or when the patient comes to terms with the implications of the illness and the limitations it involves. It is often difficult for the clinician to decide whether the symptoms of anxiety and depression represent an adjustment disorder, which can be expected to be self-limiting, or a more prolonged specific mood disorder. There is no clear distinction between the diagnostic categories. They merge imperceptibly with one another and adjustment disorders are often regarded as partial syndromes of a mood disorder. The passage of time usually clarifies the picture and indicates whether specific treatment is required. Anxiety tends to be the early response to illness, developing within a few days of the onset, while depression tends to be a later and more persistent reaction. The content of the psychological symptoms is characteristically centred on the implications of the illness and on the treatment that will be needed. Similar patterns of adjustment disorder are seen in a wide variety of illnesses and have been particularly described in relation to myocardial infarction, cancer and AIDS.

Anxiety disorders

Anxiety takes a number of different forms which have led to various diagnostic categories:
- generalized anxiety disorder
- panic disorder

- phobic anxiety disorder
- post-traumatic stress disorder.

All can be seen in patients following physical illness. Anxiety is a normal response to threat and uncertainty. In the context of new and unfamiliar medical symptoms anxiety can have a constructive function in that it motivates people to seek advice and commence whatever course of treatment is considered necessary. Excessive anxiety is distressing and counterproductive and can result in dysfunctional behaviour. Generalized anxiety is pervasive. It is not linked to specific objects or situations. In many cases it represents an exacerbation of a previous anxiety trait, amplified by the onset of illness.

Panic disorder, which is characterized by sudden episodic bouts of anxiety with very prominent somatic symptoms, gives rise to diagnostic difficulties when it accompanies physical illness. Episodes of panic may develop after a myocardial infarction if the patient is excessively worried about a recurrent heart attack. The somatic symptoms of sweating, palpitations and chest pain may convince the patient that another heart attack is imminent and medical help is sought urgently, often at an accident and emergency centre. Any diagnostic doubt on the part of the doctor serves to convince the patient that there is some serious cardiac pathology and a pattern of recurrent panics and medical presentations is established. Panic attacks may also cause diagnostic uncertainty in patients with neurological disease if the somatic symptoms are centred on the head. Dizziness, tension headaches and a sensation of faintness often lead to fears of a cerebral tumour or other sinister cerebral pathology.

Phobic anxiety disorders develop in response to some medical procedure which for some people may rekindle traumatic memories from childhood. Undergoing venepuncture, having a subcutaneous or intramuscular injection, receiving chemotherapy or being treated with large, modern equipment such as a linear accelerator can all induce a phobic anxiety response which may lead to complete avoidance of the procedure. Patients with insulin dependent diabetes avoid injecting themselves with insulin, thus resulting in poor glycaemic control and the early development of a range of diabetic complications. Patients with cancer may terminate chemotherapy or radiotherapy and worsen their prognosis unless their phobic condition is treated adequately.

Post-traumatic stress disorder (PTSD) is conventionally defined in ICD-10 as a delayed and/or protracted response to a stressful event or situation of an exceptionally threatening or catastrophic nature. The event or situation is likely to cause distress to almost anyone and they include serious accidents, natural or man-made disasters, and assaults. Witnessing a disaster or violent death also predisposes to PTSD. In general hospital practice most cases are seen following assaults or road traffic accidents. Given that the emergence of symptoms may be delayed for up to six months after the triggering event many who develop PTSD do so long after they have been discharged from hospital. Indeed, their physical injuries may have been relatively minor but at the time of the incident victims often perceive that their injuries are going to be fatal. Mayou and his colleagues have conducted several studies of victims of road traffic accidents and have found that 12 months after an accident 32% had at least one of four psychiatric conditions, namely PTSD, phobic travel anxiety, generalized anxiety or depression. There was considerable overlap between these conditions with many accident victims having more than one disorder (Mayou & Bryant 2001). There was a significant reduction in the number of cases of PTSD three years after the accident, although there were some cases of late-onset PTSD.

Post-traumatic stress disorder has also been described as a reaction to medical illness and treatment. It appears to develop when the illness is life-threatening or when the treatment is intensely frightening (Mayou and Smith 1997) and has been most commonly observed in patients treated in intensive care units and those with HIV infection (Tedstone and Tarrier 2003). Childbirth, when traumatic for the mother, can also be followed by PTSD (Ballard *et al.* 1995). Partial syndromes of PTSD are probably more common than the full-blown syndrome.

Depressive disorders

Depressive disorders are common following physical illness. Numerous studies have shown that the prevalence is significantly elevated, probably twice that of the general population.

Depression resulting from the emotional impact of an illness follows an appraisal of the implications that the illness has on relationships, lifestyle, work prospects, long-term disability and mortality. It represents a psychological reaction to the illness and reflects a sense of loss for those activities and ambitions that the illness has precluded, either temporarily or permanently. Depression can also result from the physical effects of the illness on cerebral anatomical pathways or physiological systems. This type of depression is classified as an organic mood disorder, defined by ICD-10 as being caused by a physical disorder which must be demonstrated independently. The mood disorder must follow the presumed organic factor and be judged not to represent an emotional response. Although the mood disorder follows the physical illness it may become manifest before the physical condition is diagnosed. Depression may, therefore, be the presenting symptom of an underlying condition which has yet to become clinically apparent. It is often associated with symptoms of anxiety which in some illnesses, for example hyperthyroidism, dominate the clinical picture. Suspicion of an

Table 4.2. Causes of organic depressive disorders.

Neurological

Stroke, multiple sclerosis, Parkinson's disease, head injury, tumours, degenerative disorders.

Endocrine

Cushing's disease, Addison's disease, hypothyroidism, hyperthyroidism, hypoparathyroidism, hyperparathyroidism.

Collagen diseases

Systemic lupus erythematosus, rheumatoid arthritis, polyarteritis nodosa.

Infections

Encephalitis, cerebral syphilis, extracerebral infections, e.g. pneumonia or urinary infection.

Malignant disease

Primary or secondary cerebral tumour, non-metastatic effects of distant tumours.

underlying physical condition should be considered particularly in the following circumstances:

- depression presents in middle or old age
- there is no previous history of mood disorder
- there is no family history of mood disorder
- the patient has a stable premorbid personality
- there is no apparent psychosocial precipitant.

Organic depressive disorders can result from many different conditions, the commonest of which are listed in Table 4.2.

Not all episodes of depression represent an emotional reaction to illness or a consequence of organic changes. Depression may also be a precursor of illness. There is strong evidence that depression is an independent risk factor for the development of ischaemic heart disease and cerebrovascular disease (Roose *et al.* 2001).

Depression in physically ill patients is often undiagnosed because symptoms are not volunteered or are not elicited by professional staff. Even when staff are aware of a patient's depressed mood the depression may be regarded as an inevitable and understandable consequence of being ill and therefore not amenable to treatment. The biological symptoms of depression cannot be given their usual significance when trying to establish a diagnosis of a depressive illness. Anorexia, weight loss, fatigue, reduced libido and sleep disturbance can all be directly caused by physical pathology so attention has to be focused on the psychological symptoms listed in Table 4.3.

These are similar to the core symptoms identified by Cavanaugh *et al.* (1983) who found that high and low ratings of depression were distinguished by feelings of failure, loss of interest in people, feeling punished, suicidal ideas, dissatisfaction,

Table 4.3. Key psychological symptoms of depression.

(Symptoms must be persistent and present for at least two weeks)
- Persistent lowering of mood.
- Diminished interest or pleasure in most activities.
- Reduced motivation.
- Guilt, worthlessness or self-blame.
- Hopelessness.
- Suicidal thoughts.

difficulty with decisions and crying. They may have to be elicited by direct questions if there is reason to suspect depression from the patient's appearance or behaviour.

Physically ill patients who are depressed are likely to be more functionally incapacitated (Pohjasvaara *et al.* 2001) and to consume more medical resources, including spending more time in hospital and having more outpatient visits (Koenig & Kuchibatla 1998). Depression also worsens the outcome of some conditions. Frasure-Smith *et al.* (1993) have shown that following a myocardial infarction cardiac mortality in the first six months is increased in patients who are depressed. In a subsequent, longer-term study the significance of other emotional factors such as anxiety, anger and social support was also investigated, but only depression predicted mortality when adjustment was made for severity of cardiac disease (Frasure-Smith & Lesperance 2003a). These observations led to a multicentre trial to establish whether psychological intervention, specifically cognitive behaviour therapy, and antidepressants where appropriate, could reduce cardiac mortality and recurrent myocardial infarction. The results were disappointing. Although there were small improvements in depression and social support in the intervention group there was no effect on mortality or recurrent infarction (ENRICHD Investigators 2003). Frasure-Smith and Lesperance (2003b) have concluded that depression remains an ischaemic heart disease risk factor in search of a treatment.

In view of the high levels of depression accompanying illness it is inevitable that the risk of suicide is increased. A literature review by Harris and Barraclough (1994) found that the suicide rate was increased for a wide range of illnesses including HIV/AIDS, malignant diseases, Huntington's disease, multiple sclerosis, peptic ulcer, renal disease, spinal cord injury and systemic lupus erythematosus. It is likely that depression, either untreated or unresponsive to treatment, is the connecting factor between illness and suicide but in a small number of cases suicide may occur in the absence of depression or any other psychiatric disorder.

In these cases suicide is considered a rational decision, occurring in the face of terminal illness and unbearable suffering.

In a few countries, notably the Netherlands, Belgium, Switzerland and the American state of Oregon, it is now legal for doctors to provide the means to facilitate suicide if these patients have expressed a consistent and competent wish to die when they are no longer prepared to suffer the untreatable symptoms of terminal illness. If the patient does not have the physical ability to commit suicide doctors may take an active role in ending the patient's life.

Psychotic reactions

An acute psychotic reaction may develop in some patients following admission to hospital, particularly when the admission involves an intensive care or coronary care unit or some other unfamiliar and frightening environment. The reaction takes the form of an acute delusional system, the delusions often having a paranoid content and involving the nursing and medical staff who the patient believes are deliberately trying to harm or even kill him. There are usually no hallucinations nor any thought disorder. The reaction is sometimes mistaken for an acute delirium but careful mental state examination reveals that there are no features of organic impairment. The patient is alert, correctly orientated and has no memory impairment. Antipsychotic medication alleviates the psychotic symptoms but complete resolution may not occur until the patient can be moved to an environment which is perceived as less threatening. Every effort should therefore be made to transfer the patient from an intensive care unit to a general ward or from a general ward to the home if adequate care can be provided there.

A chronic delusional system can also occur following medical or surgical treatment. These delusions are predominantly paranoid or hypochondriacal in nature and consist of a fixed belief that some damage has been deliberately inflicted by a particular member of the medical or nursing team. This type of disorder is classified as a persistent delusional disorder (F 22.0) by ICD-10.

Sexual dysfunction

Sexual dysfunction is greatly increased in prevalence in medical and surgical patients compared with the rest of the population. It can be caused by:
- the direct effects of the illness
- the psychological effect of the illness
- side-effects of prescribed medication
- a coexisting psychiatric disorder such as depression.

Loss of libido follows most physical illnesses. It is usually transient, resolving in tandem with recovery from the physical condition and most patients are reassured if this explanation is given. They should also be advised of the sexual side-effects of prescribed medications. Anticholinergic and ganglion-blocking drugs are particularly likely to cause impotence or ejaculatory failure while sedative drugs often lead to a loss of desire. Sexual problems may be increased if antidepressant drugs are used to treat a depressive reaction. The selective serotonin reuptake inhibitors are all associated with sexual problems. They can cause decreased sexual interest, diminished genital sensation, erectile dysfunction and delayed ejaculation and orgasm. Venlafaxine causes similar problems. These side-effects resolve once the medication can be withdrawn and many patients are content to wait until this can be achieved. However for some the sexual side-effects are so problematic that a change of antidepressant needs to be made. Mirtazapine is a useful alternative in that it has no appreciable sexual side-effects.

Sexual dysfunction is likely to be persistent if it follows chronic illness with structural changes in the vascular or neurological systems. Chronic renal failure and diabetes mellitus are often accompanied by microvascular changes and peripheral neuropathy which result in impotence or reduced arousal. Other neurological disorders such as multiple sclerosis, stroke and spinal cord trauma are also accompanied by a high prevalence of sexual difficulties. Prostatic surgery, especially for malignant disease, carries a high risk of permanent impotence.

Advice about overcoming sexual problems and adjusting to permanent disability can be given in the context of an outpatient appointment once the doctor has established a trusting relationship with the patient and partner (Royal College of Physicians and Royal College of Psychiatrists 2003). In addition to counselling the use of sildenafil or a similar drug should be considered for patients with decreased arousal, including impotence, due to chronic disease or to the side-effects of medication. For more complicated problems referral to a special sexual dysfunction clinic should be made if the patient wishes to have expert treatment. This topic is discussed in greater detail in Chapter 10.

Eating disorders

The commonest eating disorder encountered in medical practice is overeating but it receives less attention in the medical literature than anorexia or bulimia nervosa. The prevalence of obesity is rising in most Western countries and results from an excessive calorie intake in relation to energy expenditure. This often occurs in response to illnesses that result in reduced mobility. Physical exercise is greatly reduced but food intake remains unchanged or even increases as a way of coping with boredom. Weight gain is therefore inevitable. This greatly adds to the disability of most chronic diseases. Dietary advice, if followed, and an appropriate exercise regime should ensure that eating habits are modified and weight reduced.

There have been several reports that anorexia nervosa and bulimia nervosa can be triggered by the onset of a medical condition. Diabetes mellitus has been particularly implicated in this respect and eating disorders have been described in young, female, insulin-dependent diabetes patients, occurring soon after treatment for diabetes has been established (Steel *et al.* 1987). It has been proposed that the rapid weight gain which can follow insulin treatment causes a body image disturbance which then leads to a desire to lose weight. However the association has not been firmly established. This may be due to the fact that eating disorders in diabetics have an atypical presentation. Food intake may be relatively normal but weight loss is achieved by omission of insulin. Glycaemic control becomes erratic and complications of diabetes such as retinopathy and peripheral neuropathy may develop at an early age.

The physical changes associated with anorexia are essentially those of starvation and profound weight loss (Fairburn and Harrison 2003). They include dehydration, bradycardia, syncope, electrolyte disturbances, osteoporosis, osteopenia, anaemia and thrombocytopenia. In patients with electrolyte disturbances, particularly hypokalaemia, potentially fatal cardiac arrhythmias may develop. Most of these changes revert to normal with gradual restoration of weight.

Abnormal illness behaviour

When people become ill they expect to receive treatment appropriate to their condition and advice about changes in levels of activity, work, diet and personal habits such as smoking and alcohol consumption so that they can maximize their prospects of recovery and reduce the risks of complications. This is one of the main reasons why they consult their doctor. Broadly speaking medical advice is usually followed but some people find it impossible to adjust their lifestyles in keeping with conventional practice. They may ignore medical advice on the one hand or adopt an exaggerated level of disability which is out of keeping with the severity of the objective pathology. Both these patterns are sometimes referred to as abnormal illness behaviour.

Some rebel against the limitations imposed by their illness. Patients with ischaemic heart disease may not follow advice to reduce levels of stress in their lives; they may over-exert themselves physically or they may persist with smoking or overeating, all of which increase the likelihood of recurrent illness. Similar patterns of behaviour can be observed in some patients on haemodialysis for chronic renal failure and in diabetics who cannot come to terms with the demands of dietary control and regular insulin injections. Adjustment is most difficult for those who develop diabetes during adolescence. They resent having to behave differently to their peer group and prefer to follow the trend towards consuming chocolate, sweets and quickly prepared foods with a high calorie content. Glycaemic control is unstable. Episodes of hypoglycaemia and ketoacidosis are relatively common and vascular and neurological complications develop early.

The reverse pattern involves exaggerating the extent of functional disability or prolonging its duration beyond the time when recovery would be expected to have occurred. This has been referred to as illness deception. Halligan *et al.* (2003) have written a useful review of this topic, pointing out that any physical illness can be exaggerated or feigned. Exaggeration of symptoms sometimes occurs when a patient wishes to impress a doctor concerning the validity and severity of his condition. Much of this amplification occurs without full insight on the patient's part. Illness deception is defined as a conscious voluntary act which is intended to obtain personal advantage by securing the social, financial or legal benefits which society confers on the sick role. This may occur in the complete absence of physical pathology, but it can also be a reaction to illness when the patient is seeking to exaggerate symptoms and signs to obtain disability benefits, sickness absence from work, compensation for personal injury or medical negligence or early retirement on grounds of ill-health. Great care needs to be taken to distinguish those symptoms that can be confidently attributed to a disease process from those which are being consciously exaggerated. This is not an easy task nor is it always possible to determine whether the patient is deliberately or unconsciously exaggerating. In medicolegal cases covert videotaped evidence may be produced to help clarify this dilemma.

The most extreme example of abnormal illness behaviour is seen in patients with factitious disorders in which symptoms and signs of disease are deliberately fabricated. Motivation for this type of behaviour is difficult to establish. It often appears that the only gain the patient achieves is to receive medical attention and to create diagnostic confusion. Dermatitis artefacta is the best recognized of these disorders. Ulcerating skin lesions are produced surreptitiously and fail to heal even after treatment with occlusive dressings because of deliberate excoriation. Other examples include iron deficiency anaemia due to repeated self-induced bleeding, hyperthyroidism resulting from ingestion of thyroxine and hypoglycaemic episodes due to self-administered insulin. Any of these conditions may coexist with, and complicate, genuine physical pathology. This pattern of behaviour is seen most often in young women, many of whom are employed in nursing or other paramedical professions. They have been described as having unresolved dependency needs which are partially met by gaining unwarranted access to the sick role.

Munchausen's syndrome is a variant form of factitious disorder. Its clinical features include simulated disease with a dramatic presentation, pathological lying and a tendency to move from one hospital to another, often presenting with a different name and identity. The clinical presentations simulate clinical emergencies such as myocardial infarction, pulmonary embolism or acute intestinal problems. This behaviour is more likely to be seen in men from lower socioeconomic groups with a chronic pattern of social maladjustment. Once the nature of the condition is realized by medical staff the patient usually discharges himself from hospital, angrily protesting the validity of his symptoms. Attempts at psychiatric treatment are usually unrewarding. Munchausen's syndrome by proxy is seen in paediatric practice. Mothers repeatedly bring their children to medical attention, giving fraudulent histories or fabricating signs of disease in their children. Some of these mothers themselves have a history of fabricating their own symptoms. Further information on this condition should be sought in paediatric textbooks.

Implications for management

Understanding how people cope with becoming ill is a necessary step towards providing better management through improved communication, emotional support, recognition of emerging psychiatric symptoms and treating those who require specific psychological or pharmacological intervention. The treatments available are discussed in Part IV.

REFERENCES

Ballard, C.G., Stanley, A.K. and Brockington, I.F. (1995). Post-traumatic stress disorder (PTSD) after childbirth. *British Journal of Psychiatry*, **166**, 525−8.

Cavanaugh, S.V. (1983). The prevalence of emotional and cognitive dysfunctions in a general medical population: using the MMSE, GHQ and BDI. *General Hospital Psychiatry*, **14**, 28−34.

Cavanaugh, S.V., Clarke, D.C. and Gibbons, R.D. (1983). Diagnosing depression in the hospitalised medically ill. *Psychosomatics*, **84**, 809−15.

Creed, F., Morgan R., Fiddler, M., *et al.* (2002). Depression and anxiety impair health-related quality of life and are associated with increased costs in general medical inpatients. *Psychosomatics*, **43**, 302−9.

Dickens, C.M., Percival, C., McGowan, L., *et al.* (2004). The risk factors for depression in first myocardial infarction patients. *Psychological Medicine*, **34**, 1083−92.

Dickens, C.M., McGowan, L., Percival, C., *et al.* (2006). Contribution of depression and anxiety to impaired health-releated quality of life following first myocardial infarction. *British Journal of Psychiatry*, **189**, 367−72.

ENRICHD Investigators. (2003). Effects of treating depression and low perceived social support on clinical events after myocardial infarction: the Enhancing Recovery in Coronary Heart Disease Patients (ENRICHD) randomised trial. *Journal of the American Medical Association*, **289**, 3106−16.

Fairburn, C.G. and Harrison, P.J. (2003). Eating disorders. *Lancet*, **361**, 407−16.

Feldman, E., Mayou, R., Hawton, K., *et al.* (1987). Psychiatric disorder in medical inpatients. *Quarterly Journal of Medicine*, **63**, 405−12.

Frasure-Smith, N., Lesperance, F. and Talajic, M. (1993). Depression following myocardial infarction: impact on 6 month survival. *Journal of the American Medical Association*, **270**, 1819−25.

Frasure-Smith, N. and Lesperance, F. (2003a). Depression and other psychological risks following myocardial infarction. *Archives of General Psychiatry*, **60**, 627–36.

Frasure-Smith, N. and Lesperance, F. (2003b). Depression – a cardiac risk factor in search of a treatment. *Journal of the American Medical Association*, **289**, 3171–3.

Halligan, P. W., Bass, C. and Oakley, D. A. (2003). Wilful deception as illness behaviour. In *Malingering and Illness Deception*, ed. P. W. Halligan, C. Bass and D. A. Oakley. Oxford: Oxford Unversity Press, pp. 3–28.

Harris, E. C. and Barraclough, B. (1994). Suicide as an outcome for medical disorders. *Medicine (Baltimore)*, **73**, 281–96.

Harris, E. C. and Barraclough, B. (1998). Excess mortality of mental disorder. *British Journal of Psychiatry*, **173**, 11–53.

Karch, F. E. and Lasagna, L. (1975). Adverse drug reactions: a critical review. *Journal of the American Medical Association*, **234**, 1236–41.

Koenig, H. G. and Kuchibatla, M. (1998). Use of health services by hospitalised medically ill depressed elderly patients. *American Journal of Psychiatry*, **155**, 871–7.

Lipowski, Z. J. (1969). Psychosocial aspects of disease. *Annals of Internal Medicine*, **71**, 1197–206.

Mayou, R. and Bryant, B. (2001). Outcome in consecutive emergency department attenders following a road traffic accident. *British Journal of Psychiatry*, **179**, 528–34.

Mayou, R. A. and Smith, K. A. (1997). Post traumatic symptoms following medical illness and treatment. *Journal of Psychosomatic Research*, **43**, 121–3.

Michie, S., Bobrow, M. and Marteau, T. M. (2001). Predictive genetic testing in children and adults: a study of emotional impact. *Journal of Medical Genetics*, **38**, 519–26.

Nightingale, S., Holmes, J., Mason, J., *et al.* (2001). Psychiatric illness and mortality after hip fracture. *Lancet*, **357**, 1264–5.

Pohjasvaara, T., Vataja, R., Leppavuori, A., *et al.* (2001). Depression is an independent predictor of poor long-term functional outcome post-stroke. *European Journal of Neurology*, **8**, 315–19.

Roose, S., Glassman, A. H. and Seidman, S. N. (2001). Relationship between depression and other medical illnesses. *Journal of the American Medical Association*, **286**, 1687–90.

Royal College of Physicians and Royal College of Psychiatrists. (2003). *The Psychological Care of Medical Patients: a Practical Guide*. London: RCP and RCPsych.

Steel, J. M., Young, R. J., Lloyd, G. G., *et al.* (1987). Clinically apparent eating disorders in healthy young diabetic women: associations with painful neuropathy and other complications. *British Medical Journal*, **294**, 859–62.

Tarzi, S., Kennedy, P., Stone, S., *et al.* (2001). Methicillin-resistant *Staphylococcus aureus*: psychological impact of hospitalisation and isolation in an older adult population. *Journal of Hospital Infection*, **49**, 250–4.

Tedstone, J. E. and Tarrier, N. (2003). Posttraumatic stress disorder following medical illness and treatment. *Clinical Psychology Reviews*, **23**, 409–48.

Turjanski, N. and Lloyd, G. G. (2005). Psychiatric side-effects of medications: recent developments. *Advances in Psychiatric Treatment*, **11**, 58–70.

Unutzer, J., Small, G. and Gunay, I. (2002). Geriatric medicine. In *Textbook of Consultation-liaison Psychiatry*, 2nd edn, ed. M. G. Wise and J. R. Rundell. Washington: American Psychiatric Publishing, pp. 853–69.

5

Detection of psychiatric disorders in the general hospital: a practical guide

Damien Longson

Introduction

Trainees in liaison psychiatry are frequently surprised to find that the detection and management of psychiatric disorders in the general hospital is a complex and time-consuming process. Liaison psychiatrists need to integrate a broad range of skills — communication, clinical, diagnostic, medical, legal and pharmacological. Interviewing patients in challenging situations, for example on intensive care units or following maxillo-facial surgery, requires the development of unique clinical skills and a certain amount of improvisation. This chapter considers those aspects of psychiatric assessment that are unique to the general hospital, and offers guidance on the assessment of the most prevalent psychiatric symptoms. The supportive use of objective questionnaires is also considered.

Clinical skills

Information gathering

The assessment process starts as soon as the referral is received. Ideally, the referral should ask a specific question about a patient's psychological health, or ask for guidance on the psychological components of a more complex management problem (for example in situations where capacity to consent is a problem). Often, a telephone call to the referrer clarifies the nature of the clinical conundrum, and it helps establish whether the referral has been made with the agreement of both the patient and the patient's senior physician. Previous psychiatric notes should be obtained at this stage.

It is essential to telephone the ward prior to the consultation to establish a mutually convenient time for both the patient and the ward staff. Patients in the

Handbook of Liaison Psychiatry, ed. Geoffrey Lloyd and Elspeth Guthrie. Published by Cambridge University Press. © Cambridge University Press 2007.

general hospital frequently undergo procedures or investigations off the main ward, when they are not available for interview, and there may be times of the day when key informants (for example the nurses) are unavailable. It may be helpful to time the visit to the ward to coincide with a ward round or team review.

A face-to-face dialogue with the ward-based team starts the interview, when much information can be gained about the patient. Don't forget to talk to anyone who might have had therapeutic contact with the patient. Typical issues to consider might include:

- what question do the team think you have been asked to answer?
- what do they think is the matter?
- what have they observed about the patient and the patient's visitors?
- what is the management plan for the patient? When is the patient going home?
- are there any challenging behaviours?
- what is the attitude towards the patient?

This discussion may contribute significantly to a greater understanding of the referral, and it provides the first opportunity for an exchange of new knowledge, skills or attitudes (Guthrie and Creed (1996) examine the educational value of this informal educational process).

The patient's case notes are an equally important source of information. It is worth spending time on these, in particular thinking about some of the following:

- what is the patient's medical history?
- is there a history of previous contact with (liaison) psychiatry?
- have the team considered psychological or social issues already?
- have the necessary physical investigations been carried out? How many of these produced positive results?
- is there correlation between physical illness and psychosocial stressors?
- do the notes disclose any attitudinal issues which might be impacting on the patient's care?

Interviewing the patient

Completing a psychiatric assessment in the general hospital presents challenges not normally found in psychiatric units. Foremost is the need for privacy. In many cases, a side-room or office may not be available, necessitating an interview in the main ward, by the patient's bed. This may be particularly problematic on intensive or high-dependency care units, or in cases where patients are unable to move (for instance in orthopaedics). There is often little alternative to drawing curtains round the patient's bed, creating a false air of confidentiality.

Similarly, environmental noise is commonly a problem, either from other patients and staff, or from the movement of beds, trolleys, cleaning machines or clinical equipment. In many cases the only measure appears to be a raising of voices, leading to further problems with confidentiality, and increasing discomfort of the patient.

Interruptions are common, and largely not preventable. Although they are usually brief — for example the arrival of a food tray — they interrupt the flow of the interview, and disrupt exploration of sensitive issues.

Hospitalization may be stressful in itself, over and above the stress of the illness. This needs to be acknowledged, although its impact can be reduced by good communication

In many cases, the patient will not have had previous contact with mental health specialists, or indeed may not know that they had been referred to mental health at all. For this reason it is essential, whenever possible, to establish that the patient has consented to a psychiatric opinion. It is helpful to explore the patient's expectations at the beginning of the interview. Common misunderstanding arises when relationships between the patient and the medical team or nurses have become strained, leading the patient to believe that others see their symptoms as being 'all in the mind'. It may be helpful to explain to the patient that you have been asked to see them to evaluate the emotional impact of being physically ill, and that you are one of a team of specialists who routinely become involved in the management of patients on that unit.

The most extreme circumstance arises on the intensive care unit where the patient may still be intubated, although interviewing patients following maxillo-facial surgery may be similarly challenging. Often this causes considerable difficulty to the mental health specialist who is used to an open-question style of interviewing. Alternative strategies include the use of writing or picture boards. In many cases closed questions requiring a 'yes' or 'no' gesture can be used, having established that the patient can comprehend the nature and purpose of the interview. In all cases, the value of non-verbal cues is enhanced — these should be closely observed and carefully documented as a valuable part of the mental state examination. In some cases, it may be helpful to enlist the help of a speech therapist.

Problems frequently arise where a patient's first language is not English. This may lead to particularly severe problems in the general hospital if there has been a resulting poor level of communication between healthcare professionals and the patient. Language or communication difficulties should be identified early in the first visit and appropriate steps initiated, which will nearly always involve an interpreter, a professional in preference to asking the family to help. This may be the treating team's first opportunity of explaining to the patient what is going on.

Mental state examination

Patients on medical and surgical units may often be wearing nightwear, may be unwashed, unshaven and paying less attention to personal appearance. Assessment of appearance therefore needs to be standardized against that which could normally be expected in similar circumstances. Behaviours such as abnormal movements, neglect of one side of the body, or visible responses to imaginary cues are all important parts of the assessment, and should be documented.

Assessment of the patient's mood can usually be supplemented by the observations of ward-based staff, and it is helpful to observe and enquire about the patient's interactions with nurses and visitors wherever possible. Nurses should be asked about sleep, appetite and weight changes, although the relevance of these is diminished in the general hospital context.

Thought content and perception in general hospital patients is assessed in a similar fashion to other settings. As discussed elsewhere, illness beliefs, attitudes and expectations are particularly important in liaison psychiatry – this should be enquired of both the patient and the attending staff or family. Psychotic symptoms underlying illness beliefs, or other beliefs, should be established. Visual hallucinations are more typically associated with organic brain disease, and tactile hallucinations with limb amputations or substance misuse.

Assessment of cognitive abilities is often required, particularly as delirium is common in the general hospital even in patients who do not overtly appear to be very confused. Attention should be paid to the level of consciousness, including alertness and attention. A specific and standardized screening tool should be used whenever possible, particularly as cognitive impairments may not be picked up during a standard interview. The Mini Mental State Examination (MMSE) is widely used, because of its ease of administration and validity in the medical setting (Folstein *et al.* 1975).

Insight and motivation are key determinants for a successful intervention, both physical and psychiatric. The patient's understanding of the problem should be documented, as well as their views on how they can contribute to their own management. In some cases, it may be relevant to assess and document the patient's ability to understand the nature and purpose of the treatment being offered, as well as alternatives and consequences if not accepting treatment.

Common disorders

Many referrals to liaison psychiatry services are for patients in whom depression or anxiety are suspected. Sometimes, the declared reason for referral might be a failure to progress, poor compliance, or a breakdown in the relationship between the patient and the hospital staff, in which case clinical psychological symptoms may not have been detected.

In many more cases, psychological distress remains undetected. Three myths underpin this:

1. Depression or anxiety in physically ill people is 'understandable', and therefore not appropriate for treatment. This implies that all patients with serious diagnoses should be depressed whereas, in fact, less than half such patients meet diagnostic criteria for a psychiatric disorder.

2. Depression in the physically ill cannot be distinguished from normal sadness, or demoralization. It is normal for physically ill patients to have a period of adaptation to their illness. In many patients the change in mood or increase in anxiety is short-lived, and it tends to resolve. Either physical recovery progresses, or with the passage of time the patient adjusts to the limitations or consequences of their illness. However, an important minority of patients go on to develop an anxiety or depressive disorder in which symptoms have become persistent, extreme, disabling or psychotic.

3. Depression in the physically ill cannot be distinguished from the symptoms of physical illness. Whereas most biological symptoms of depression (e.g. weight loss, low energy, sleep disturbance) and some of anxiety (e.g. abdominal pain, headaches, sweating) are common in physical illness, many more cognitive and emotional symptoms are specific to psychological distress. Methods to identify psychiatric disorders in the physically ill are discussed below.

One outcome of these myths is that depression is underdiagnosed in patients with serious physical illnesses, and that even in those in whom it is identified, too little is done. Simple questions can be used to elicit depression and non-psychiatric staff can be trained to do this, provided that support and advice is available for them from a member of the liaison psychiatry team (Table 5.1). The following sections examine in more detail depression, anxiety and

Table 5.1. Questions to elicit symptoms of depression.

Patients may attribute symptoms of pathological mood states as being somatic features of, or an understandable response to, their neurological disease. It is therefore helpful to 'orientate' the enquiry accordingly. The following examples may be helpful.

• Have your symptoms got you down at all?
• Do you ever get the feeling that you can't be bothered to do things?
• Is there anything you look forward to (or does your illness stop you)?
• Has this illness affected your confidence?
• Do things ever get so bad you think about death?

psychosis, the first two being the most prevalent psychiatric disorders in the physically ill.

Depression

Numerous studies have measured depressive illness in physically ill individuals. Prevalence varies widely, reflecting variation in methodological approaches, diagnostic criteria and instruments used. Overall depressive disorder is at least twice as common in medically ill patients as in the general population, although prevalence in certain disorders may be as high as 50%. Some physical disorders have stronger association with depression, particularly when these are serious, life-threatening or chronic:

- neurological disorders (e.g. stroke, epilepsy, Parkinson's disease, multiple sclerosis)
- human immuno-deficiency (e.g. HIV disease)
- cancer
- disorders of chronic pain (e.g. rheumatoid arthritis).

Depression is also associated with some functional physical syndromes, such as chronic fatigue, fibromyalgia, irritable bowel syndrome and somatization disorder. Some pharmacological treatments are also linked to depression, especially steroids, several cancer chemotherapeutic agents, beta-interferon and cimetidine. (See Chapter 4.)

Not surprisingly, depression has an adverse effect on many aspects of a medical patient's life. Mortality is increased (both from the physical illness and from suicide), functional recovery is prolonged, quality of life is impaired, hospital attendances are increased, hospital stays are longer and motivation to comply with treatment is poorer. Biochemical changes associated with depression may be contributing to this poorer prognosis.

Depressed patients are associated with increased economic costs, not only for reasons outlined above, but also because they tend to have a poorer perception of their health, increased disability, and impaired occupational functioning.

Psychological symptoms commonly arise in the context of physical illness, so that a key task is to differentiate between different levels of psychological reaction. It is helpful to consider three types of relationship between depression and physical illness (Moffic & Paykel 1975). These are:

1. Depressive disorder that is a clear reaction to physical illness. This will have started after the onset of the physical illness, and its severity will fluctuate in accordance to the physical illness.

2. Depressive disorder that is aetiologically unrelated and that has clearly preceded the physical illness. This should be evident from the history, leading to a diagnosis of coincidental depressive and physical illness.

3. Depressive disorder that has caused the physical symptoms. This can either occur in somatization (the presentation of psychological distress as physical symptoms), or when depression causes the symptoms of a physical illness to become more severe.

Being medically ill and hospitalization are stressful events, leading many patients to feel tired, weak, anxious, and uncertain about the future. There may be a sense of loss of control, failure, isolation and stigma. In some patients, this amounts to an adjustment disorder, which is characterized by a state of subjective distress and emotional disturbance, often leading to social or functional impairment. Although a broad palette of symptoms may arise, depressed mood or anxiety symptoms are particularly common, associated with a feeling of inability to cope or plan ahead. Constitutional vulnerability plays an important part in determining whether an individual develops an adjustment, anxiety or depressive disorder as a consequence of physical illness.

In some individuals the symptoms become sufficiently severe or persistent to warrant a diagnosis of depressive disorder. Suspicion should particularly arise when symptoms of an adjustment disorder persist longer than six months.

In patients with physical illness, depression can be caused directly by the medical illness itself, or by medication used to treat that illness. Neurological disorders, such as stroke, Huntington's disease, epilepsy and multiple sclerosis are aetiologically related, as are endocrine disorders such as Addison's disease, Cushing's syndrome, or hyper/hypothyroidism. Infection with the human immunodeficiency virus (HIV) has also been associated with depression, although this may illustrate the difficulty of causality — both the International Classification of Diseases (ICD) 10 (WHO 1992), and the American Diagnostic and Statistical Manual IV (American Psychiatric Association 1994) require evidence that the psychiatric illness has arisen as a direct consequence of the physical illness, and that there is recovery or significant improvement once the cause has been removed.

Similarly, many medications are associated with the development of depressive symptoms, or a depressive disorder. This is particularly problematic with certain drug groups, including corticosteroids and other steroids (for example the oral contraceptive pill), beta-blockers, some antihistamines, cancer chemotherapy and drugs acting on the central nervous system (benzodiazepines and opiates). Because the list is large, it is always wise to check with a reference source (pharmacy, pharmacopoeia or drug manufacturer) if there is a coincidence between the onset of depressive symptoms and the start of a particular treatment. In contrast to many other side-effects, this may be particularly difficult with depressive symptoms where there might be a delay of several weeks between the start of treatment and the development of depressive symptoms.

Table 5.2. Diagnostic criteria for depressive disorder (ICD-10 F32).

At least two symptoms from List A, and enough from List B to make a total of at least four symptoms.

List A	List B
Depressed mood to a degree that is definitely abnormal for that individual	Loss of confidence or self-esteem
	Unreasonable self-reproach or guilt
	Recurrent suicidal thoughts
Loss of interest or pleasure in normally pleasurable activities	Decreased ability to concentrate, or indecisiveness
	Agitation or retardation, subjective or objective
Decreased energy or increased fatiguability	Sleep disturbance
	Increased or decreased appetite with corresponding weight change

Achieving a diagnosis of a functional depressive disorder in the physically ill presents difficulties, particularly if the diagnosis is to be made using the internationally recognized diagnostic criteria in ICD-10 (Table 5.2) or DSM-IV. This is because fatigue, sleep disturbance, weight changes, appetite loss and changes in libido – all part of the somatic syndrome in depression – are nearly universally present in physical illness, even in the absence of any psychological illness. Therefore, some combinations of symptoms, such as fatiguability, loss of interest in normally pleasurable activities, sleep disturbance and appetite change would be sufficient to reach a false positive diagnosis of mild depressive disorder in some physically ill patients.

A number of different solutions have been proposed, which include discounting symptoms that could clearly be attributed to physical illness, or excluding fatigue and anorexia from the list of depressive symptoms. However, it seems reasonable to adopt a method which maximizes sensitivity, even at the risk of treating the occasional false positive, which means counting all depressive symptoms present, regardless of aetiology. In the confusing situation where the patient has several somatic symptoms, it is worth remembering that anhedonia or persistent depressed mood also need to be present.

Some symptoms should open the possibility of a depressive disorder, or of a complicated adjustment disorder. These include:
- guilt
- feeling of worthlessness
- suicidal thoughts
- poor physical recovery
- anger or hostility at staff

- poor social interaction
- very severe and persistent distress.

A cognitive construct-based approach to assessing depression in medically ill patients may have particular validity in certain scenarios. There is some evidence that recently developed screening instruments, which focus upon cognitive processes in depression, perform well in discriminating clinically depressed medically ill patients from those who are not depressed (Parker *et al.* 2002).

Suicide risk assessment

Physical illness is a predictor of completed suicide, so that an assessment of risk should form part of every patient evaluation. The psychological impact of chronic or severe physical illness, and the increased prevalence of physical illness in severe and enduring mental disorder both contribute to this. Assessment of suicide risk is reviewed in more detail in the chapter on suicide and self-harm (Chapter 11).

Treatment

This is considered in more detail in Part IV. However it is worth noting here that treatment of the hospitalized patient requires particular attention for the following reasons:

1. The dose or type medication for treatment of physical illness may be changed frequently during a period of hospitalization. Doctors should therefore be continuously aware of the interaction between psychotropic and other treatments.
2. Identification of a safe psychotropic may be difficult during the phase of severe acute illness, thus requiring increased emphasis on psychosocial interventions. There is, in any case, good evidence for the efficacy of psychological treatments when compared to medication, which may be important in patients for whom psychotropics are relatively contraindicated.
3. As described above, hospitalization is a stressful event, characterized by both feeling ill, and the adjustment to 'bad news' of varying severity. During this time particular attention should be paid to good communication and supportive psychotherapy.

Anxiety

As in other settings, anxiety in the general hospital can range from an isolated psychological symptom such as worry or an isolated physical symptom such as tachycardia, to a full syndrome meeting diagnostic criteria (generalized anxiety disorder, panic disorder, adjustment disorder or post-traumatic stress disorder).

Table 5.3 lists the diagnostic criteria of generalized anxiety disorder as defined in ICD-10.

It is worth noting that many of the symptoms of anxiety could also present either as symptoms of physical illness (sweating, palpitations, chest pain, etc.) or as side-effects of medication (dry mouth, nausea, flushes). Questions to elicit anxiety states are suggested in Table 5.4.

Table 5.3. Diagnostic criteria for generalized anxiety disorder (ICD-10 F41.1).

Prominent tension, worry and apprehension
PLUS four symptoms including at least one from List A

List A	List B
Palpitations	Difficulty breathing
Sweating	Feeling of choking
Trembling	Chest pain
Dry mouth	Nausea or churning abdomen
	Dizzy/faint
	Derealization
	Depersonalization
	Irritability
	Fear of losing control
	Fear of dying
	Hot flushes
	Tingling
	Aches and pains
	Restlessness
	Feeling keyed-up
	Lump in throat
	Exaggerated startle
	Difficulty concentrating
	Sleep disturbance because of worry

Table 5.4. Questions to elicit symptoms of anxiety and panic.

- Do you ever worry about your symptoms?
- When you're worrying like this is it sometimes hard to stop yourself?
- Do you ever have attacks where you have a lot of symptoms all at once? What happened? Was it frightening?
- Did you do anything differently because of these attacks?

Symptoms of anxiety are a nearly universal component of serious medical illness and hospitalization. In any case, anxiety disorders are common. The National Comorbidity Survey (Judd *et al.* 1998) found that there was a 25% lifetime prevalence of anxiety disorder, greater in women (30%) than in men (19%). Estimates of the prevalence of anxiety disorders (panic or generalized anxiety disorder) in medically ill patients have varied widely, particularly as this has depended on the illness being studied. However, prevalence rates 50% higher than the normal population have been reported, with particularly high rates in patients with chest pain, abdominal symptoms, neurological disorders and pulmonary disease.

The aetiology of anxiety symptoms falls into two broad categories:
- symptoms secondary to an organic cause
- symptoms arising concurrently.

There are a very wide range of medical conditions associated with anxiety. Particularly common causes are listed below — this list is illustrative rather than exhaustive:
- cardiovascular: coronary insufficiency, arrhythmias, heart failure
- respiratory: pulmonary emboli and obstructive pulmonary disease
- neurological: epilepsy and post-concussion
- endocrine: thyroid disease, diabetes, Cushing's disease
- metabolic: hypoxia
- drugs: very many, particularly stimulating drugs.

Sometimes, anxiety (or depression) is the presenting symptom of an otherwise undiagnosed medical disorder. At other times, anxiety symptoms herald the onset of a more serious psychiatric disorder, such as depression, drug withdrawal or acute confusional state.

Alternatively, anxiety presenting in the general hospital setting may be the result of a personality disorder, a generalized anxiety disorder present before the physical illness, or one of the symptoms of a severe and enduring psychiatric disorder. Frequently, anxiety that has become apparent during medical illness is the consequence of the stressful effects of illness/hospitalization arising in the context of previous psychological vulnerability.

As in other disorders that occur in general hospital setting, the first task is to elicit a comprehensive history, particularly focusing on factors that might expose vulnerability to psychological distress, such as previous episodes of anxiety, a family history of anxiety or concomitant substance misuse. The history should also identify recent changes in pharmacotherapy, as well as other recent psychosocial stressors. However, the presence of obvious psychological predisposing factors should not exclude the possibility of an additional medical cause.

In assessing the predisposing, precipitating and maintaining factors for the patient's anxiety, it is also important to remember factors related specifically to the illness and hospitalization. These include anxiety about medical interventions, possibility of death or disfigurement, anxiety about prognosis, physical pain and the unfamiliarity of the hospital environment. It is easy to overestimate what the patient knows about their illness or disorder, or what they have been told about their treatment. Helpful topics to explore might include:

1. How much information has the patient been given? It is often incorrectly assumed that information sharing will increase the patient's distress. Does the patient believe what they have been told, or are they worried that they have been incorrectly reassured?
2. What does the patient know about the procedure? Have they read anything in books or on the Internet? Do they know someone with a similar illness, and what was the outcome?
3. What outcome is the patient expecting? Is there worry about loss of function or appearance, or is the patient worried about the possibility of death?
4. How much support is the patient expecting to need once out of hospital? What follow-up arrangements will be made?
5. How has the patient previously coped with psychosocial stressors?

Sometimes the liaison psychiatrist is asked to see a patient for whom no obvious physical pathology has been found. This is explored in greater detail in the chapter on functional somatic symptoms (Chapter 7). However, it may help the patient to understand that unexplained physical symptoms can sometimes be the expression of psychological distress, thus encouraging the patient to talk about emotional symptoms.

Assessment of a patient with anxiety symptoms cannot be complete without the use of diagnostic tests. These should include, as a minimum, measurement of electrolytes, liver and thyroid function, cardiac and pulmonary function as well as a general physical and neurological examination.

As discussed below, the use of an objective questionnaire such as the Hospital Anxiety and Depression scale (Zigmond & Snaith 1983) is helpful, not only in reaching a diagnosis, but also in demonstrating to the patient that a clinically relevant number of symptoms of anxiety are present.

Treatment

Pharmacological and psychological treatments are discussed elsewhere. Generally, management depends on whether the anxiety disorder is secondary to a medical condition or treatment, in which case removal or modification of the cause is required, or whether the anxiety has arisen as a psychological reaction to the illness or hospitalization. In the latter case, management will follow normal bio-psychosocial principles. However, supportive psychotherapy is so central to the role of the liaison psychiatrist that it merits further mention here. The therapeutic power of spending time with the patient to explore perceptions and concerns, facilitating or mediating contact between the patient and other members of staff, and ensuring that appropriate information is given should not be underestimated.

Often, patients may be reluctant to take medication for anxiety, particularly if they perceive that such treatment might be stigmatizing. In other cases, additional medication may be difficult to prescribe in the medically ill. In every case, therefore, well-established adjunctive treatments for anxiety should be considered, such as behaviour modification (for treatment phobias), relaxation and meditation.

Psychosis

Psychosis arising in the general hospital is often the source of great consternation amongst non-psychiatric doctors and nurses, and it frequently gives rise to urgent referrals. The psychotic symptoms may arise from:

1. An acute confusional state.
2. A brief psychotic episode may be produced by various drugs. However, sometimes a patient may develop psychotic symptoms in clear consciousness as a reaction to being in a strange, stressful or unfamiliar place, in which case there may be prominent paranoid delusions.
3. Admission of a patient with a previous diagnosis of severe and enduring mental illness (schizophrenia or bipolar affective disorder), in which case, admission may have arisen as a consequence of an overdose, or because of a coincidental medical or surgical illness.

Whereas establishing a diagnosis of psychosis may be straightforward in most cases, the management of such an illness in the general hospital presents certain challenges:

1. Care should be taken not to discontinue long-term psychotropic medication, particularly oral and depot antipsychotics, or for changes to be made carefully. Medication may be unexpectedly discontinued in intensive care units, or following an overdose.
2. Patients may have been transferred to the general hospital under a legally enforceable treatment order (Mental Health Act in England and Wales). General hospital staff will need guidance on the meaning of the order, including restrictions on the patient's ability to discharge themselves against medical advice, or take unprescribed leave.
3. Patients may behave in ways unfamiliar to general hospital staff, or say unusual things as a consequence of delusions or hallucinations. Staff may need support and education to help them effectively manage an unusual nursing and clinical situation.
4. Advice may also be needed about environmental issues, such as the possible inappropriateness of managing the patient away from the ground floor.

5. Questions may arise about the psychotic patient's ability to consent to invasive or non-invasive procedure. The role of the psychiatrist is to train and support those who will be doing the procedure to elicit whether the patient has capacity to consent. It is frequently assumed, incorrectly, that capacity is always absent in psychosis, or that consent is less important. Staff should be trained to check that the patient:
   - understands the nature of the intervention
   - understands the risks and consequences
   - understands the alternatives, and the consequences of the 'do nothing' option
   - can retain the information for long enough to make an informed choice
   - believes what is being said to them.
6. Consultation-liaison staff may play an important role in establishing links between the patient and services normally responsible for support of the patient in the community.

Questionnaires

Rating scales can supplement information obtained during clinical interviews, whilst assessing medically ill patients. Rating scales assist in the differentiation of major psychiatric disorders, measure a patient's quality of life, emotional wellbeing and social functioning, and evaluate the role of emotional factors in the patient's physical illness. Scales can provide the physically ill patient with an objective measure or 'number' which sometimes carries more weight than the verbal opinion of the mental health-care professional! Some scales have been developed to measure change over time, thus providing an objective measure of the patient's progress. Numerous scales have been developed, either for research or clinical use, and either self-rated or physician-administered.

The use of rating scales for general hospital inpatients is not straightforward. To be usable, the questionnaires need to be:

1. Easily available: usually not available on wards, although supplies could be left on wards where demand is high.
2. Rapid to complete: time constraints on the healthcare professional are often considerable, and the patient's ability to concentrate may be impaired. In practice, the questionnaire needs to be completed at one end of the interview so that results can be discussed with the patient, and be taken away at the end of the consultation.
3. Validated for inpatient use: as discussed above, the presence of biological symptoms such as weight loss, fatigue and sleep disturbance in organic disorders complicates the assessment of mood in general-hospital patients, leading to a high false-positive rate.

4. Straightforward: patients who are medically unwell may have difficulty understanding difficult questions.
5. Cross-culturally validated: to allow for the wide ethnic mix present in general hospitals.
6. Disease-specific: in the case of quality-of-life questionnaires.

Hospital Anxiety and Depression scale

The Hospital Anxiety and Depression scale (HAD) is a self-rated scale which is widely used in hospital inpatients (Zigmond & Snaith 1983). It measures both anxiety and depression, each on a 21-point scale, and it excludes biological symptoms of mood disorders (for example: sleep, energy, weight loss). Questions focus on cognitive symptoms, such as feelings of tension, enjoyment, humour, worry, cheerfulness. Scores of 11 or over on either scale indicate the presence of either depressive disorder or anxiety disorder, whereas a total score of 18 or more (for example 9 and 9) probably indicates significant psychological distress. The scale was not originally designed to measure change over time. The HAD has been well validated in several countries in a number of clinical settings (e.g. Bambauer et al. 2005; Barczak et al. 1988; Desmond et al. 2005; Johnston et al. 2000; Martin et al. 2000; Mirzamani et al. 2005; Vaeroy et al. 2005). The HAD is easy to understand, easy to interpret with the patient, and takes only 5 minutes to complete.

Beck Depression Inventory

This is the best-known depression inventory, widely used in general psychiatry. The Beck Depression Inventory (BDI) is a 21-question scale on which patients rate the severity of their depressive symptoms (Beck et al. 1961). It has been widely used for the assessment of depression in the medically ill (Furlanetto et al. 2005; Razavi et al. 1990; Waller et al. 2005). Although widespread, its use in medically ill patients has been criticized because of the inclusion of somatic symptoms which lead to high false-positive rates for depression. Results should therefore be interpreted with caution, taking into particular account the pattern of distribution of positive answers. The BDI is self-administered and takes about 5 minutes to complete.

Symptom Checklist 90 and Brief Symptom Inventory

The Symptom Checklist Revised (SCL-90-R; Derogatis 1992) and the Brief Symptom Inventory (BSI; Derogatis et al. 1983) are medical and psychiatric symptom checklists, as well as measures of general distress, both of which are self-rated, and completed within 10 (BSI) to 20 (SCL-90) minutes. Their utility in medically ill patients has been questioned, but their judicious use, particularly in the interpretation of cut-off values, probably contributes useful information on symptom severity during a comprehensive biopsychosocial assessment. Both measures have been used widely in the medically ill (Aslan *et al.* 2005; Endermann 2005; Franke *et al.* 1995; Moser *et al.* 2003).

Social Function scales

The SF-36 (Ware & Sherbourne 1992) and SF-12 (Jenkinson *et al.* 1997) are generic health instruments that tap into the following areas: physical functioning, performance in physical role, performance in emotional role, vitality, social functioning, bodily pain, general health perceptions, and mental health. The results are generally displayed as either eight scales or the two summary scales that capture physical and mental health. The questionnaires are widely used and have been found to be very useful in monitoring health outcomes in various disease and condition areas (Bennett *et al.* 2005; Claar *et al.* 2005; Davis *et al.* 2005; Iglesias *et al.* 2005; Moore *et al.* 2005).

Single-item screening interview

In a study of terminally ill cancer patients, the single item question 'are you depressed?' had significantly more diagnostic validity than either the Beck Depression Inventory, or a visual analogue scale (Chochinov 2001; Chochinov *et al.* 1997). This illustrates the value and importance of very simple screening tools which could be used by general hospital healthcare professionals in the detection of psychologically-distressed medically ill patients.

Using psychological questionnaires in the general hospital setting

It is possible to train general medical and nursing staff to use psychological questionnaires in the general hospital setting to aid detection of psychiatric disorder. Many nurses value the structure and focus that a questionnaire provides. Such initiatives, however, will only work if clear backup and support is provided for staff who are using the measures.

Improving the detection and management of psychiatric disorder in the general hospital setting should be a key performance target of liaison psychiatry services. Achieving this aim will require sufficient funding of liaison services, and an increased awareness of mental health issues by general hospital staff.

REFERENCES

American Psychiatric Association. (1994). *Diagnostic and Statistical Manual of Mental Disorders*, 4th edn. Washington, DC: APA.

Aslan, S., Ersoy, R., Kuruoglu, A. C., *et al.* (2005). Psychiatric symptoms and diagnoses in thyroid disorders: a cross-sectional study. *International Journal of Psychiatry in Clinical Practice*, **9**(3), 187–92.

Bambauer, K. Z., Locke, S. E, Aupont, O., *et al.* (2005). Using the Hospital Anxiety and Depression Scale to screen for depression in cardiac patients. *General Hospital Psychiatry*, **27**(4), 275–84.

Barczak, P., Kane, N., Andrews, S., *et al.* (1988). Patterns of psychiatric morbidity in a genito-urinary clinic: a validation of the Hospital Anxiety Depression scale (HAD). *British Journal of Psychiatry*, **152**, 698–700.

Beck, A. T., Ward, C. H., Mendelson, M., *et al.* (1961). An inventory for measuring depression. *Archives of General Psychiatry*, **4**, 561–71.

Bennett, R. M., Schein, J., Kosinski, M. R., *et al.* (2005). Impact of fibromyalgia pain on health-related quality of life before and after treatment with tramadol/acetaminophen. *Arthritis & Rheumatism: Arthritis Care & Research*, **53**(4), 519–27.

Chochinov, H. M. (2001). Depression in cancer patients. *Lancet*, **2**(8), 499–505.

Chochinov, H. M., Wilson, K. G., Enns, M., *et al.* (1997). 'Are you depressed?' Screening for depression in the terminally ill. *American Journal of Psychiatry*, **154**(5), 674–6.

Claar, R. L., Parekh, P. I., Palmer, S. M., *et al.* (2005). Emotional distress and quality of life in caregivers of patients awaiting lung transplant. *Journal of Psychosomatic Research*, **59**(1), 1–6.

Davis, J. C., van der Heijde, D., Dougados, M., *et al.* (2005). Reductions in health-related quality of life in patients with ankylosing spondylitis and improvements with etanercept therapy. *Arthritis & Rheumatism: Arthritis Care & Research*, **53**(4), 494–501.

Derogatis, L. R. (1992). *The SCL-90-R Manual-II: Scoring, Administration and Procedures for the SCL-90-R*, 2nd edn. Towson, MD: Clinical Psychometric Research.

Derogatis, L. R. and Melisaratos, N. (1983). The Brief Symptom Inventory: an introductory report. *Psychological Medicine*, **13**(3), 595–605.

Desmond, D. M. and MacLachlan, M. (2005). The factor structure of the Hospital Anxiety and Depression Scale in older individuals with acquired amputations: a comparison of four models using confirmatory factor analysis. *International Journal of Geriatric Psychiatry*, **20**(4), 344–9.

Endermann, M. (2005). The Brief Symptom Inventory (BSI) as a screening tool for psychological disorders in patients with epilepsy and mild intellectual disabilities in residential care. *Epilepsy & Behavior*, **7**(1), 85–94.

Folstein, M. F., Folstein, S. E. and McHugh, P. R. (1975). 'Mini-Mental Stak'. A practical method for grading the cognitive state of patients for the clinician. *Journal of Psychiatric Research*, **12**(3), 189–98.

Franke, G. H., Jager, H. and Stacker, K.-H. (1995). The Symptom Checklist (SCL-90–R): an application among patients with HIV infections. *Zeitschrift für Differentielle und Diagnostische Psychologie*, **16**(3), 195–208.

Furlanetto, L. M., Mendlowicz, M. V. and Bueno, J. R. (2005). The validity of the Beck Depression Inventory-Short Form as a screening and diagnostic instrument for moderate and severe depression in medical inpatients. *Journal of Affective Disorders*, **86**(1), 87–91.

Guthrie, E. and Creed, F. (1996). Basic skills. In *Seminars in Liaison Psychiatry*, ed. E. Guthrie, F. Creed and P. Gaskell. London: Gaskell Publications, Royal College of Psychiatrists, pp. 21–52.

Iglesias, C. P., Birks, Y., Nelson, E. A., *et al.* (2005). Quality of life of people with venous leg ulcers: a comparison of the discriminative and responsive characteristics of two generic and a disease specific instruments. *Quality of Life Research: An International Journal of Quality of Life Aspects of Treatment, Care & Rehabilitation*, 14(7), 1705–18.

Jenkinson, C., Layte, R., Jenkinson, D., *et al.* (1997). A shorter form health survey: can the SF-12 replicate results from the SF-36 in longitudinal studies? *Journal of Public Health Medicine*, **19**(2), 179–86.

Johnston, M., Pollard, B. and Hennessey, P. (2000). Construct validation of the hospital anxiety and depression scale with clinical populations. *Journal of Psychosomatic Research*, **48**(6), 579–84.

Judd, L. L., Kessler, R. C., Paulus, M. P., *et al.* (1998). Comorbidity as a fundamental feature of generalized anxiety disorders: results from the National Comorbidity Study (NCS). *Acta Psychiatrica Scandinavica, Supplementum*, **393**, 6–11.

Martin, C. R. and Thompson, D. R. (2000). A psychometric evaluation of the Hospital Anxiety and Depression Scale in coronary care patients following acute myocardial infarction. *Psychology, Health & Medicine*, **5**(2), 193–201.

Mirzamani, S. M., Sadidi, A., Sahrai, J., *et al.* (2005). Anxiety and depression in patients with lower back pain. *Psychological Reports*, **96**(3), 553–8.

Moffic, H. S. and Paykel, E. S. (1975). Depression in medical in-patients. *British Journal of Psychiatry*, **125**, 346–53.

Moore, R. K., Groves, D., Bateson, S., *et al.* (2005). Health related quality of life of patients with refractory angina before and one year after enrolment onto a refractory angina program. *European Journal of Pain*, **9**(3), 305–10.

Moser, D. K., Dracup, K., McKinley, S., *et al.* (2003). An international perspective on gender differences in anxiety early after acute myocardial infarction. *Psychosomatic Medicine*, **65**(4), 511–16.

Parker, G., Hilton, T., Bains, J., *et al.* (2002). Cognitive-based measures screening for depression in the medically ill: the DMI-10 and the DMI-18. *Acta Psychiatrica Scandinavica*, **105**(6), 419–26.

Razavi, D., Delvaux, N., Farvacques, C., *et al.* (1990). Screening for adjustment disorders and major depressive disorders in cancer in-patients. *British Journal of Psychiatry*, **156**, 79–83.

Vaeroy, H., Tanum, L., Bruaset, H., *et al.* (2005). Symptoms of depression and anxiety in functionally disabled rheumatic pain patients. *Nordic Journal of Psychiatry*, **59**(2), 109–13.

Waller, N. G., Compas, B. E., Hollon, S. D., *et al.* (2005). Measurement of depressive symptoms in women with breast cancer and women with clinical depression: a differential item functioning analysis. *Journal of Clinical Psychology in Medical Settings*, **12**(2), 127–41.

World Health Organization. (1992). *10th Revision of the International Statistical Classification of Diseases and Related Health Problems.* Geneva: World Health Organization.

Ware, J. E. and Sherbourne, C. D. (1992). The MOS 36-item short-form health survey (SF-36): 1. Conceptual framework and item selection. *Medical Care*, **30**, 473–83.

Zigmond, A. S. and Snaith, R. P. (1983). The Hospital Anxiety and Depression Scale. *Acta Psychiatrica Scandinavica*, **67**(6), 361–70.

6

The role of the nurse in liaison psychiatry

Anthony Harrison

Introduction

This chapter:
- outlines the development of mental health liaison nursing
- identifies the core skills and competencies required for effective practice within the liaison setting
- outlines the role of the mental health liaison nurse
- outlines the role of the mental health liaison nurse in the care and treatment of individuals with specific mental health needs in the general hospital.

The role of the nurse within liaison psychiatry developed significantly throughout the 1990s, with many health service trusts employing mental health nurses to practise within the general hospital. The nursing role is closely linked to that of doctors and psychologists practising in this area, and is primarily concerned with the provision of specialist mental health nursing assessment and intervention in the general hospital. Nurses working within liaison psychiatry use the skills of consultation, liaison and collaborative working, providing a service that transcends traditional professional, departmental and organizational boundaries. Mental health liaison nurses (MHLNs) can be seen as working at the interface between psychiatry and general hospital services. This chapter provides an overview of:
- the development of mental health liaison nursing
- core skills and competencies for MHLNs
- the role of the MHLN in relation to self-harm and the care of people with physical illness.

Handbook of Liaison Psychiatry, ed. Geoffrey Lloyd and Elspeth Guthrie. Published by Cambridge University Press. © Cambridge University Press 2007.

The development of mental health liaison nursing

The term 'liaison nursing' within the general hospital context is not new, having been used in the United States throughout the 1960s and 1970s (Jones 1989; Roberts 1997). The recognition that mental health nurses have a role in the care of individuals within the general hospital is also underpinned by the work of the nursing theorist, Peplau (1964). She maintained that at the heart of nursing is the need to understand the person in a holistic way, placing equal emphasis on the physical and psychological domains of care. Her theories are based on the fundamental interactions that occur within the nurse–patient relationship, and it is this that is pertinent to liaison nursing, with its emphasis on holisim and effective intra- and interpersonal communication. This predates current professional and service developments that have led to the expansion of mental health liaison within the general hospital (Roberts 1997).

The growth of mental health liaison nursing roles within the UK has been slow and somewhat haphazard, with little in the way of strategic professional, service or educational development to support it (Roberts & Whitehead 2002). This remains the case today, with a lack of national guidelines or consensus on standards for service delivery. The changing nature of mental health services, with the focus on the development of community-based care, has also meant that the general hospital has become less of a priority in terms of clinical practice and overall development for both community and specialist mental health providers. Psychiatrists, who traditionally provided mental health input into the general hospital, have become less focused in this area, something that has also supported the introduction of the growing number of ad-hoc nursing posts. Although this expansion of nursing roles has been positive, it is unfortunate that these developments have lacked any coherent professional or educational strategies to support them.

Despite increasing recognition of the need for general hospitals to have planned and co-ordinated mental health arrangements (Department of Health and Social Security 1984; Department of Health 1994, 2004), including developing the role of nurses, there remains a significant lack of strategic thinking as far as this area of service development is concerned. A survey by Tunmore (1994) of UK nurses working in mental health liaison demonstrated how varied these roles are, with marked differences in clinical grades, managerial arrangements, educational preparation and areas of practice. Another survey, by Roberts and Whitehead (2002) again showed that MHLNs were working in a wide variety of settings, with little consistency in terms of grade, professional focus and employment arrangements. More recently, there has been an attempt by some to address the dearth of specific policy in this area (Hart *et al.* 2003), with the development of guidance for the establishment of nursing teams that focus on mental health provision in the general hospital.

Current public health policy and central government nursing strategy, including the various *National Service Frameworks* (Department of Health 2001; National Institute for Clinical Excellence 2004), alongside the *Essence of Care* initiative (Department of Health 2003), continue to challenge professionals and health communities to address healthcare in a holistic way. There is increasing emphasis on service developments that ensure that individuals are able to access specialist mental health care, whatever setting they are in. This includes the general hospital, and provides a reminder that this is an environment where high rates of psychiatric morbidity are common, but paradoxically is also a setting that often has limited access to specialist mental health nursing input.

The other factor that influenced the development of mental health liaison nursing was the growth of specialist nursing roles during the 1980s and 1990s, as more nurses adopted a specialist focus to their practice. Many liaison roles have developed secondary to recognition of the importance of psychological assessment following self-harm, and a significant number of nurse-led liaison services throughout the UK were established as a result of the need to ensure that this specialist assessment was undertaken within the general hospital (Tunmore 1997a). The provision of a mental health assessment service is often a primary focus of the MHLN's work, with many practitioners describing assessment as the most common reason for referral (Loveridge & Carr 1996; Roberts & Taylor 1997). Assessments following self-harm, addressing suicide risk, screening for mental illness, and identification of follow-up and ongoing care needs, are some of the most common activities undertaken by the MHLN. MHLNs have a number of other core components to their role, including the provision of direct and indirect psychiatric nursing care, patient, carer and staff education, provision of clinical supervision, and input into service planning, development and evaluation (Figure 6.1).

The practice of mental health liaison nursing

Within the general hospital, MHLNs practise in a wide variety of settings focusing on a number of different clinical specialities. The overall aim is to make the skills of the mental health nurse available to patients who may be suffering from a variety of physical illnesses and somatic complaints. The specific aims of mental health liaison nursing can be summarized as:

• ensuring prompt access to specialist mental health nursing assessment and intervention

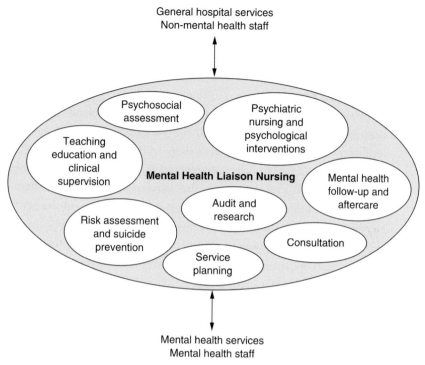

General hospital services
Non-mental health staff

Psychosocial
assessment

Psychiatric
nursing and
psychological
interventions

Teaching
education and
clinical
supervision

Mental Health Liaison Nursing

Mental health
follow-up and
aftercare

Audit and
research

Risk assessment
and suicide
prevention

Consultation

Service
planning

Mental health services
Mental health staff

Figure 6.1.   Overview of the core components of the MHLN role.

- ensuring access to expert mental health care in a setting where psychiatric needs are often unrecognized and untreated
- enabling non-mental health staff to recognize and participate in the assessment and management of psychiatric and psychological morbidity
- contributing to the provision of holistic care, which acknowledges biological, psychological, sociological and spiritual dimensions
- participating in the education and support of non-mental health staff, in order to increase their confidence when addressing patients' mental health needs.

Core skills and competencies

Many of the skills and competencies required for effective practice can be considered as generic to all mental health staff working in this setting. Skills and knowledge in risk assessment, mental state examination, psychopharmacology and the psychological consequences of physical illness are required by all staff involved in liaison. In the United States, MHLNs are educated to a minimum of Masters level, as well as having extensive experience within the speciality (Shahinpour *et al.* 1995). In the UK traditional educational programmes have been considered inadequate preparation for taking on the role (Regal & Davies

1995), and the general consensus is that there need to be improved post-registration educational opportunities for nurses working in this speciality (Brendon & Reet 2000). Some higher education institutes have responded to the growing educational needs of MHLNs however, recognizing that appropriate educational preparation is required to support practice. The University of Birmingham and the University of the West of England have both developed post-registration modules for MHLNs, one of which has been offered at Masters level (Loveridge & Carr 1996; University of the West of England 2004).

Although much of the clinical and professional activity undertaken by MHLNs is consistent with a model of specialist nursing practice, such as that identified by Castledine (2003), there is debate as to whether the generic nature of the liaison nursing role within the general hospital can be viewed as specialist practice (Torn & McNichol 1996). However, a number of elements of the MHLN's work can be considered as consistent with the specialist practitioner's role (Table 6.1) and are linked to the following core liaison activities:

• assessment
• consultation and advice
• treatment
• administration and management
• audit and research.

Table 6.1. Core domains of practice for the mental health liaison nurse.

Practice domain	Aspect of mental health liaison and consultation	Example
Assessment	Liaison assessment	Patient presenting with depression following admission for primary physical health problem, e.g. cardiac illness
Assessment	Assessment following self-harm	Patient attending the ED following a deliberate overdose of medication
Assessment	Crisis mental health assessment	Patient presenting to the ED with agitated behaviour and psychotic symptoms
Assessment/consultation and advice	Complex psychosocial and behavioural presentations	Patient admitted with multiple unexplained physical symptoms
Assessment/consultation and advice	Assessment of capacity and ability to consent to treatment	Patient refusing treatment following an overdose of medication
Assessment/consultation and advice, treatment	Risk assessment and management	Quantifying suicide risk and initiating a risk management plan

Table 6.1. (*cont.*)

Practice domain	Aspect of mental health liaison and consultation	Example
Consultation and advice	Substance misuse	Patient admitted to a medical ward who has a co-existing psychiatric and substance misuse problem.
Consultation and advice	Accepting and making referrals	Referral onto secondary mental health services following initial assessment at the general hospital
Consultation and advice	Medication and psychopharmacology	Advice regarding prescription of antidepressant medication
Consultation and advice	Management of behavioural problems	Advice regarding the management of an acute confusional episode of an older adult patient on an orthopaedic ward
Consultation and advice	Legal issues	Advice regarding the use of the Mental Health Act
Consultation and advice	Education and support to other clinicians	Provision of education to nursing staff regarding the recognition and management of depression associated with physical illness
Treatment consultation and advice	Working with patients with specific medical conditions	Accepting referral from nurse specialist in cardiology for a patient experiencing symptoms of anxiety and depression.
Treatment consultation and advice	Specific treatments used by mental health liaison nurses	Utilizing anxiety management interventions following traumatic injury Utilizing cognitive behavioural therapy skills in treating a patient with somatization.
Administration	Maintaining comprehensive documentation	Completing detailed assessment documentation for patients attending hospital following self-harm
Administration	Writing court and other statutory reports	Compiling reports to legal representatives, e.g. solicitor
Audit and research	Evaluating interventions and services	Auditing suicide risk profiles of patients attending hospital following self-harm

Source: Adapted, with permission, from Hart & Eales (2004).

Focus of clinical practice for the mental health liaison nurse

Self-harm and suicide prevention

Admissions to UK general hospitals following overdose account for approximately 11% of medical admissions, with hospital attendance following self-harm among the highest in Europe (House *et al.* 1998). Clinical guidelines reinforce the importance of a specialist psychosocial assessment for each patient prior to discharge from hospital (National Institute for Clinical Excellence 2004). Despite self-harm being such a common reason for hospital attendance, individuals frequently encounter negative attitudes from clinical staff (Hemmings 1999), who themselves often feel that they lack the skills to deal effectively with such patients. The way in which staff approach the patient, communication between staff and patient, and staff-to-staff dialogue are important issues for the MHLN, and are aspects of consultation work that are a major focus of practice. This is particularly so within areas that assess and treat relatively high numbers of individuals following self-harm, such as emergency departments (EDs) and medical assessment units.

Patients frequently report negative responses from staff in these settings (Anon 2001; Murray 1998), which may well be a reflection of the fact that clinicians struggle to understand the motivations and feelings that exist behind the presenting behaviour (Pembroke 1998). There is often a lack of differentiation by staff between the motivations behind the various behaviours associated with self-harm; for example, assuming that individuals who self-injure by cutting themselves are 'attention seeking' or attempting to end their life. Understanding the triggers and meanings behind this behaviour can be difficult, and this is something that can be compounded by a lack of education and clinical supervision, as well as the pressures caused by numerous other clinical and operational priorities within a busy physically-orientated healthcare environment.

Despite increasing recognition of the link between physical and mental health, staff in the general hospital frequently fail to address these areas in clinical practice (Teasdale & Mulraney 2000). The problem is often underpinned by dualistic notions of health and illness, or the mind–body split, which result in viewing the patient's problems as either physical or psychological, rather than in a holistic, or interdependent way. Caplan (1964) identified four main reasons why non-mental health staff may have difficulty in addressing mental health needs in their patients, namely lack of understanding of psychological problems, lack of skill, lack of objectivity and lack of confidence and self-esteem. Traditional approaches to the professional education of medical and nursing staff tend to reinforce this way of thinking, making it difficult for non-mental health staff to believe that they have a legitimate part to play in addressing a person's mental health needs.

The attitude can be 'we haven't got time', and, if the person is a regular in the department, 'stick them in the corner until the psychiatric team comes'. If people aren't trained in self-injury all they see is what's presented to them — the cut or burn. They can't see the emotional distress that underlies it. (Pacitti 1998)

It is vital for the MHLN to understand the factors that influence the ability of staff to respond to the mental health needs of patients, in particular the needs of those who attend following self-harm. The MHLN has a role both in direct client-centred work, as well as in consultee-centred work, and developing this knowledge base will assist the practitioner to decide upon the most appropriate focus in terms of liaison and consultation activity.

The reduction in suicide rates is a national public health priority in England, which is reflected in the publication of both suicide reduction targets (Department of Health 1999) and the English *National Suicide Prevention Strategy* (Department of Health 2002). A mental health liaison service, as part of a co-ordinated suicide prevention strategy, has an important role to play in achieving such targets. The relationship between self-harm and suicide has been demonstrated by the increased risk of suicide in individuals who have self-harmed (Hawton & Fagg 1988), and this is one of the main reasons for ensuring that all individuals who attend hospital following self-harm have access to a specialist psychosocial assessment (Department of Health and Social Security 1984; National Institute for Clinical Excellence 2004; see also Chapter 11).

Although psychiatrists largely undertook this task until the 1990s, it is now a role that is predominantly the domain of MHLNs, and forms one of the core functions for many mental health liaison nursing teams (Callaghan *et al.* 2003). The involvement of nurses and other professionals, such as social workers, in the assessment of patients following self-harm is supported by the evidence that appropriately trained and supervised individuals, other than doctors, are as effective in undertaking this work (Brooking & Minghella 1987; Catalan *et al.* 1980). MHLNs now form a core component of such services and are often engaged in the education of trainee psychiatrists, thereby helping to ensure that doctors gain the required experience in this aspect of psychiatric practice. The overall purpose of assessment following self-harm is to undertake a risk assessment aimed at maintaining the patient's safety, whilst providing the opportunity for the person to benefit psychologically from the interaction with the assessor (Roberts & Mackay 1999).

The areas of self-harm, risk assessment and suicide prevention provide valuable opportunities for MHLNs to engage in practice development and to support general hospital staff. Many mental health liaison services do not operate outside core hours, so it is important that general hospital staff are aware of the clinical management arrangements when immediate referral to the MHLN is not an option. For example, staff should be aware of how to access an urgent psychiatric assessment, which may involve contact with relevant crisis and intensive home treatment services. For individuals deemed not to be at immediate or short-term risk of repetition, discharge home with an urgent appointment for review by the

MHLN the following day may be an appropriate option. Joint operational policies, relevant clinical practice guidelines and appropriate training and supervision must support any such arrangements and discharge decisions. This is of particular importance when considering risk and in the management of individuals who attend hospital on a regular basis (Department of Health 2004).

Risk assessment

Risk assessment is a key competency for the MHLN and is closely linked to the practice of risk management, whereby a mutually agreed plan, or specific therapeutic strategies, aimed at reducing or managing the identified risks, is initiated with the full collaboration of the individual concerned. Although this is a core skill, such an assessment needs to occur within the multiprofessional context involving other relevant disciplines. The process is underpinned by the following core principles:

1. Risk cannot be eliminated, as there is no such thing as a completely risk-free situation or scenario. Untoward or undesirable outcomes (for example, self-injury or suicide) may still result following comprehensive risk assessment and management, but by the same token, untoward outcomes may not occur, even though staff failed to follow the key principles associated with the assessment of risk. The nursing goal following assessment is the reduction and minimization of risk and the prevention of harm or further harm.

2. Risk is not static; it is a dynamic process, influenced by any number of factors and variables within a given situation. Risk can fluctuate over very short periods of time and is context-dependent, in that it is influenced by the experiences, perceptions and interactions that the individual is subject to at any point in time. It therefore follows that risk management plans and strategies to reduce risk must be constantly evaluated and amended in the light of new information and any alteration in the individual's risk profile.

3. 'Risk factors' are based on population studies and do not necessarily allow practitioners to identify risks in a particular individual. For example, although males are statistically more likely to complete suicide, the individual man receiving care may not automatically be at increased risk of suicide simply because of his gender.

4. Engagement and emotional support are key nursing strategies that can reduce risk. For example, research suggests that individuals within mental health settings who are judged to be at high risk of suicide are less likely to engage in self-injurious behaviour when cared for by nurses who demonstrate empathy and acceptance, use active listening techniques, involve the person in the care planning process, and use meaningful activity as a therapeutic tool (Jones *et al.* 2000). The MHLN will generally have limited time during which to

provide such emotional support, so it is vital that they are able to form a rapport quickly by understanding the person's distress and facilitating psychological engagement.

5. It is not possible to state categorically that one particular risk factor is of more significance than another within a given risk situation. The 'relative weighting' given to each factor will vary from person to person, and will also be influenced by the skill, competence and confidence of the nurse under-taking the assessment.

6. Training, ongoing education and clinical supervision are all elements of effective clinical work and risk assessment practice is likely to be more effective in teams where these are in place.

Risk assessment should be underpinned by an empathic and non-judgemental attitude, as this will promote a sense of safety and of feeling valued. This in turn is likely to encourage the person to express information crucial to forming a judgement regarding the level of risk. The issue of confidentiality needs to be addressed early on, with the nurse explaining the limits of confidentiality and how he/she will use the information gained during the assessment. All potential sources of information should be utilized throughout the assessment process, including information from other key informants such as the person's partner, GP and friends. In order to obtain the necessary information, a thorough history should be taken, aimed at eliciting information about the current crisis or focus of the present problem. Focusing questions on the precipitants and triggers to the current presentation is a useful way of clarifying personal risk indicators, as is an understanding of how the person usually deals with stressful situations and interpersonal problems. The 48 hours immediately prior to the crisis is often a critical time, and information about this period can significantly assist in making judgements about the level of ongoing risk. Key personal, social and clinical information (Table 6.2) should be recorded systematically and shared with other members of the clinical team to pinpoint key risk areas, as well as factors that may decrease risk. Finally, it is essential to identify a timeframe within which risk is likely to be raised, for example, over the following 24 hours, 2-to-3 days, or weeks.

Certain individuals, often those who are already known to mental health services, may present to hospital either as a result of some form of crisis, or as a way of accessing services (Ryan *et al.* 1996). Some may attend so regularly that they become labelled as 'frequent attenders'. In order to ensure consistency in clinical management and as a means of clarifying management and discharge arrange-ments, the MHLN should be informed about those individuals who attend on a regular basis. The role of the liaison service is to facilitate effective communication between the general hospital and secondary mental health services. Care and

Table 6.2. Key information necessary when undertaking a suicide risk assessment (Harrison 2003).

Social	*Personal*
Accommodation and housing	Age
Occupation	Gender
Details of contacts with other health, social and criminal justice services	Key relationships and supports
	Alcohol and drug use
Historical	*Recent and present circumstances*
Physical health problems/illnesses	Precipitants to current problem or crisis
Relevant family history	Circumstances of self-harm or factors leading to contact with services
Previous/current contact with mental health services	Intent
Mental health/psychiatric history	Access to potentially lethal means, e.g. supplies of medication
Previous self-harm or attempts to end life	
Clinical	*Information from other sources*
Mental state examination – to include appearance, behaviour, rapport, speech, mood, perception, cognitive functioning, somatic or physical symptoms, attitude to recent events and future plans	Partner, family members, friends
	Professionals, e.g. GP, social worker
Risk summary	
Factors that may increase or decrease level of risk	
Likelihood of exposure or of experiencing events that may increase level of risk	
Actions taken to reduce or manage the level of assessed risk	

treatment plans should be accessible to staff within the ED (Department of Health 2004) and updated on a regular basis. A mental health care plan, in a summarized format, should contain the following information:

- essential biographical information
- details of relevant agencies and professionals involved in the person's mental health care
- the circumstances under which the individual is most likely to present requesting help
- the known or relevant personal risk factors
- the most appropriate response and helping strategies to a crisis presentation – this should be negotiated and agreed with the service user in advance
- the indications, if any, for an inpatient psychiatric admission
- other relevant personal or social information
- details of whom to contact following attendance at hospital.

This information should be easily accessible within the ED or medical unit, preferably via both the electronic patient record system and a paper-based mechanism. Such care plans should be updated regularly and liaison teams will need to ensure that there are effective communication systems in place between the general hospital and secondary mental health services to ensure that this happens.

Individuals with specific physical illness

Mental health problems and psychiatric illnesses are frequently seen within the general hospital (Arlott *et al.* 1997). The prevalence of psychiatric disorders is high, with 25% of patients experiencing adjustment and mood disorders; 10% of patients have delirium, and 25% of older medical patients have some degree of dementia (Bowler *et al.* 1994; Wattis & Curran 2001). Clinical staff are likely to come across individuals who are experiencing mental health problems, either as part of an existing medical condition such as cardiac disease, or as a consequence of coping with an illness that has major adjustment and lifestyle implications, such as following a stroke. Comorbid psychiatric illness is a frequent consequence of a range of illnesses, including common conditions such as cardiac illness, epilepsy, diabetes and respiratory disease (see Chapter 4). Common comorbid symptoms include depression, anxiety and psychosis, and psychiatric symptoms often occur as a direct result of the medications used to treat physical illness. Psychiatric problems have been shown to worsen the prognosis in a number of illnesses, including cardiac disease, neurological illnesses and gastrointestinal problems (Bauer & Whybrow 1999; Parker & Kalucy 1999).

Some MHLNs have developed a specialist focus in working with patients suffering from specific physical health problems. These include oncology, cardiology, neurology, gastroenterology and haematology. The focus of practice varies from speciality to speciality, and even within speciality, with examples of both direct liaison activity, such as Gardner's work with neuro-oncology patients and their families (1992), and consultee-centred work with nursing staff caring for cancer patients (Tunmore 1989).

Common consequences of a diagnosis of physical illness include:

1. Difficulty in accepting the diagnosis and prognosis.
2. Withdrawal and depression secondary to original diagnosis or as a result of prognosis.
3. Acute anxiety about forthcoming treatment or interventions – may manifest as an acute stress reaction in the early stages, or as symptoms of post-traumatic stress disorder in the later stages.

4. Adjustment difficulties — these may be as a result of the specific consequences of certain treatments — for example, changes in appearance, hair loss, amputation, loss of mobility.
5. Fear of a further episode of illness — for example, preoccupation with the possibility of suffering another 'heart attack' associated with cardiac illness.
6. Depression, secondary to diagnosis or as a consequence of specific treatments — for example, following the use of beta-blockers to control hypertension.
7. Changes in the patient's 'personality' and behaviour, which are unusual and inconsistent with premorbid personality traits — for example, intolerant of previously accepted situations, sudden outbursts of anger or 'loss of temper'. Some may demonstrate such changes through an exaggeration of pre-existing personality traits, such as excessive irritability, or marked emotional lability.
8. Expressing suicidal ideas and a potential increase in suicide risk — often linked to depressive symptoms, feelings of hopelessness and the adjustment process.
9. Interpersonal, communication and relationship difficulties — for example, role changes within the person's relationship, sexual dysfunction, loss of independence.
10. Stress, anxiety and increased risk of mental health problems among family members.

One of the potential problems for liaison staff is deciding at what point specialist mental health intervention is necessary. This is in part due to the fact that the experience of illness is unique for each individual, and will be influenced by personal health and illness beliefs, pre-existing psychological and psychiatric problems, and the idea that there is a period of 'normal' psychological adjustment to be gone through. The severity and duration of symptoms is therefore a key factor in deciding whether a referral to liaison staff is indicated. For instance, depressive symptoms may become more pronounced when the underlying illness becomes severe and disabling, or when there is some other social stressor or significant life event occurring at the same time. A balance needs to be achieved between the acknowledgement and acceptance of psychological responses as a normal part of the adjustment process, and the fact that persistent symptoms may be manifestations of co-existing psychiatric illness. However, the involvement of the MHLN should always be considered when individuals with a pre-existing psychiatric problem are admitted to a non-mental health unit. Such individuals are susceptible to worsening of their psychiatric symptoms (particularly if psychiatric medication regimens are altered or discontinued) and possibly to extended hospital stay (Gardner 2006).

MHLNs may become involved at an earlier stage in recovery and rehabilitation, such as within routine cardiac rehabilitation programmes

(Fisher & Tunmore 2002), although such input is likely to have resource and service delivery implications. There are few such dedicated joint working arrangements throughout the UK at present and it may be more cost-effective to exploit the potential for non-mental health staff to develop enhanced skills in this aspect of care.

A major role for the MHLN is to act as a resource for staff within the general hospital, offering both direct liaison and indirect consultation input (Edwards 1999). However, it is neither appropriate nor practical for the MHLN to be directly involved in the care of every patient within a specialist setting, so opportunities for joint working, group work, teaching, psycho-education, clinical supervision and practice (skills) development should be the focus for liaison work. Interventions can be divided into three tiers of liaison and consultation activity (Table 6.3) and specific skills utilized include cognitive behavioural interventions, problem-solving, motivational interviewing, advice on psychotropic medication and stress management.

In facilitating non-mental health staff to develop knowledge and skills in this area, the MHLN will need to assist them to identify a focus for assessment and intervention with their individual client group (Box 6.1). Aspects of care that staff will need to address include:

1. Assessment and understanding the problem, which may include the use of psychiatric screening tools, explicit assessment questions that address psychological needs, and the potential impact of medications on the patient's mental state. For example, certain medications used to treat physical illness, such as steroids and antihypertensives, can cause psychiatric symptoms. This is particularly so in neurological treatments, and other medication side-effects can include depression, elation, confusion and hallucinations.

2. The process of psychological adjustment following illness, trauma and hospitalization. Such difficulties are common, although these features can cause difficulty for staff when attempting to judge 'normal' and 'abnormal' responses to the underlying condition. Feelings of shock, grief, anger and hopelessness are common adjustment reactions, as are mood swings and depression (Livneh 1986).

3. The creation of time and space to respond to these needs will be influenced by the nurse's ability to incorporate the principles of psychological care into routine practice. Time should be set aside to discuss the patient's feelings, perceptions, fears and anxieties and doing this will allow the person 'to have a personal side to his illness and validating it by showing that it merits separate attention, but dealing with it as a normal part of care in the ward' (Nichols 1993).

Table 6.3. Aspects of mental health liaison and consultation input for patients experiencing physical illness.

Intervention	By whom
1. Communication and assessment	
• Information giving: clarifying expectations, being made aware of what to expect, likelihood of psychological complications. This information should be given verbally and in an appropriate non-verbal format, e.g. leaflets, audiotapes, etc.	• All members of the ward/department clinical team. • Specific responsibility for ensuring this input occurs lies with the patient's named or primary nurse.
• Interviewing and empathic listening: making available protected time to discuss person's fears, anxieties and concerns as a routine part of clinical practice.	
• Discussion of psychological needs or psychiatric problems within the multidisciplinary team.	
• Awareness of when to refer for specialist assessment or help.	
• Information and advice regarding psychological assessment and screening for psychiatric illness.	• MHLN
2. Preventive psychological care	
• Ability to deal with and respond positively to emotional distress.	• All members of the ward/department clinical team. • Specific responsibility for ensuring this input occurs lies with the patient's named or primary nurse.
• Establishing rapport.	
• Normalizing and dealing with psychological symptoms, e.g. sudden variations in mood, feelings of anxiety, fluctuating sense of despair or hopelessness.	
• Allowing time for emotional expression: use of protected time, access to a quiet and confidential environment.	
• Use of relaxation and distraction techniques.	
• Awareness of when to refer for specialist assessment or help.	
• Advice and information regarding screening and assessment.	• MHLN
• Risk assessment.	
• Clinical supervision, advice and support.	

Table 6.3. (*cont.*)

Intervention	By whom
3. Specific psychological or mental health nursing interventions	
• Psychosocial assessment.	• MHLN
• Monitoring effects and side-effects of psychotropic medication.	
• Specific psychological interventions, e.g. problem-solving, cognitive behavioural work, anxiety management.	
• Input into the development of care plans.	
• Referral to secondary mental health services.	
• Liaison and collaboration with specialist mental health staff, e.g. consultant psychiatrist, clinical psychologist.	

Source: Developed from Tunmore (1990) and Edwards (1999).

Conclusion

This chapter has explored the concepts and practice associated with mental health liaison nursing, illustrating the various approaches and settings in which MHLNs can provide input into the general hospital. Its focus is based on the principles of collaborative working and the belief that key therapeutic skills are transferable and can be adapted to specific clinical settings and to specific clinical problems. The overall aim of the role is to make mental health nursing skills available to individuals within this setting, as a way of preventing and treating mental health problems and psychiatric illness, as well as making such skills available to patients with a range of physical illnesses. Such nursing roles have proliferated since the 1990s and are now firmly established in the majority of district general hospitals, although it is disappointing that there are no national standards against which to benchmark service configurations and models of service delivery.

MHLNs have a significant contribution to make to overall healthcare delivery. Through direct liaison activity and indirect consultation work, they can have a positive effect on the health and well-being of specific groups of patients, as well as enabling general hospital practitioners to focus on psychological issues, and allowing them to make mental health care a routine part of

Box 6.1 Critical factors in the effective assessment and care of the psychological aspects of illness (Harrison 2000).

Assessment

- Explicit acknowledgement that all patients have psychological needs and that these are a legitimate area of nursing concern.
- Identify any limitations in current nursing practice, such as inadequate nursing documentation, that discourage the incorporation of psychological issues into the assessment process.
- Clarify the possible psychological consequences of the person's underlying condition.
- Be aware of the potential side-effects of medication used to treat physical illness, and the effect these may have on the person's mental state.
- Become familiar with the use of psychiatric screening instruments. Organize training and supervision from the MHLN in order to develop skills in the use of such tools.
- Observe and record relevant behaviour and symptoms that may indicate an alteration in mental state. Avoid non-specific statements such as, 'appears depressed'. Use descriptions of behaviour, or record the individual's self-report regarding their feelings or problems.

Intervention

- Provide 'protected time' with the patient in order to address specific psychological needs. Do not avoid the issue by seeing these needs as the exclusive responsibility of other professionals.
- Develop effective interpersonal skills, particularly active listening, use of empathic responses and the adoption of an open and receptive manner.
- Avoid separating the physical and psychological aspects of care; be aware of the impact of adjustment and adaptation on the person's treatment and rehabilitation.
- Involve the patient's partner or carers at an early stage; be aware that they will also require psychological support and advice.
- Provide reassurance in the form of explanation and information giving. Assisting the person to understand and accept that changes may be a normal consequence of the illness or injury can assist in recovery and adaptation.
- Arrange for referral to specialist staff, for example the MHLN or liaison psychiatrist, if symptoms persist or worsen.
- Be aware of your own needs and those of the whole team; arrange for regular clinical supervision and support, as well as ongoing training in aspects of psychological care.

their practice. Their role in education, practice development and clinical supervision has been identified and it can be seen that by adopting flexible and collaborative working arrangements they can have a positive impact on overall patient care.

REFERENCES

Anon. (2001). Self-harm keeps me alive. *Openmind*, **111**(Sep/Oct), 10.

Arlott, V., Driessen, M. and Dilliry, H. (1997). The Lubeck general hospital study 1: prevalence of psychiatric disorders in medical and surgical inpatients. *International Journal of Psychiatry in Clinical Practice*, **1**(3), 207–16.

Bauer, M. and Whybrow, P. C. (1999). Depression and other psychiatric illnesses associated with medical conditions. *Current Opinion in Psychiatry*, **12**, 325–9.

Bowler, C., Boyle, A., Branford, M., *et al.* (1994). Detection of psychiatric disorders in elderly medical inpatients. *Age and Ageing*, **23**, 307–11.

Brendon, S. and Reet, M. (2000). Establishing a mental health liaison nurse service: lessons for the future. *Nursing Standard*, **14**(17), 43–7.

Brooking, J. and Minghella, E. (1987). Parasuicide. *Nursing Times*, **83**(21), 40–4.

Callaghan, P., Eales, S., Coates, T., *et al.* (2003). A review of the structure, process and outcome of liaison mental health services. *Journal of Psychiatric and Mental Health Nursing*, **10**, 155–65.

Caplan, G. (1964). *Principles of Preventive Psychiatry*. New York: Basic Books.

Castledine, G. (2003). The development of advanced nursing practice in the UK. In *Advanced Nursing Practice*, 2nd edn, ed. P. McGee and G. Castledine. Oxford: Blackwell Publishing, pp. 8–16.

Catalan, J., Marsack, P., Hawton, K., *et al.* (1980). Comparison of doctors and nurses in the assessment of deliberate self-poisoning patients. *Psychological Medicine*, **10**, 483–91.

Department of Health. (1994). *Working in Partnership: the Report of the Mental Health Nursing Review Team.* London: HMSO.

Department of Health. (1999). *Saving Lives: Our Healthier Nation.* London: DoH.

Department of Health. (2001). *National Service Framework for Older People.* London: DoH.

Department of Health. (2002). *The National Suicide Prevention Strategy for England.* London: DoH.

Department of Health. (2003). *Essence of Care: Patient-focused Benchmarks for Clinical Governance.* London: DoH.

Department of Health. (2004). *Improving the Management of Patients with Mental Ill Health in Emergency Care Settings.* London: DoH.

Department of Health and Social Security. (1984). *The Management of Deliberate Self-Harm.* London: DHSS.

Edwards, M. J. (1999). Providing psychological support to cancer patients. *Professional Nurse*, **15**(1), 9–13.

Fisher, S. and Tunmore, R. (2002). Cardiac rehabilitation: assessment and intervention strategies. In *Mental Health Liaison*, ed. S. Regal and D. Roberts. Edinburgh: Baillière Tindall/Royal College of Nursing, pp. 181–22.

Gardner, R. (1992). Psychological care of neuro-oncology patients and their families. *British Journal of Nursing*, **1**(11), 553–6.

Gardner, B. (2006). Caring for the person with a serious mental illness. In *Mental Health Care for Nurses: Applying Mental Health Skills in the General Hospital*, ed. A. Harrison and C. Hart. Oxford: Blackwell Publishing, pp. 166–80.

Hart, C. and Eales, S. (2004). *A Competence Framework for Liaison Mental Health Nursing*. London: London Liaison Mental Health Nurses' Special Interest Group.

Hart, C., Harrison, A., Hegan, J., *et al.* (2003). Liaison Mental Health Services: a Briefing Paper for Professor Sir George Alberti. London: Unpublished briefing paper.

Harrison, A. (2000). Psychological problems in the neurology setting. *Professional Nurse*, **15**(11), 706–9.

Harrison, A. (2003). A guide to risk assessment. *Nursing Times*, **99**(9), 44–5.

Hawton, K. and Fagg, J. (1988). Suicide and other causes of death following attempted suicide. *British Journal of Psychiatry*, **152**, 359–66.

Hemmings, A. (1999). Attitudes to deliberate self-harm among staff in an accident and emergency team. *Mental Health Care*, **2**(9), 300–2.

House, A., Owens, D. and Patchett, L. (1998). *Effective Health Care: Deliberate Self-Harm*. York: NHS Centre for Reviews and Dissemination.

Jones, A. (1989). Liaison consultation psychiatry: the CPN as clinical nurse specialist. *Community Psychiatric Nursing Journal*, **9**(2), 7–14.

Jones, J., Ward, M., Wellman, N., *et al.* (2000). Psychiatric inpatients' experience of nursing observation. *Journal of Psychosocial Nursing*, **38**(12), 10–20.

Livneh, H. (1986). A unified approach to existing models of adaptation to disability: a model of adaptation. *Journal of Applied Rehabilitation Counselling*, **17**(6), 5–16.

Loveridge, L. and Carr, N. (1996). Advantageous liaisons. *Nursing Times*, **92**(50), 42–3.

Murray, I. (1998). At the cutting edge. *Nursing Times*, **94**(27), 36–7.

National Institute for Clinical Excellence. (2004). *Improving Supportive and Palliative Care for Adults with Cancer*. London: NICE.

Nichols, K. (1993). *Psychological Care in Physical Illness*, 2nd edn. London: Chapman and Hall.

Pacitti, R. (1998). Damage limitation. *Nursing Times*, **94**(27), 38–9.

Parker, G. and Kalucy, M. (1999). Depression comorbid with physical illness. *Current Opinion in Psychiatry*, **12**, 87–92.

Pembroke, L. (1998). Only scratching the surface. *Nursing Times*, **94**(27), 38–9.

Peplau, H. E. (1964). Psychiatric nursing skills and the general hospital patient. *Nursing Forum*, **3**(2), 28–37.

Regal, S. and Davies, J. (1995). The future of mental health nurses in liaison psychiatry. *British Journal of Nursing*, **4**(18), 1052–6.

Roberts, D. (1997). Liaison mental health nursing: origins, definitions and prospects. *Journal of Advanced Nursing*, **25**, 101–8.

Roberts, D. and Mackay, G. (1999). A nursing model of overdose assessment. *Nursing Times*, **95**(3), 58–60.

Roberts, M. and Taylor, B. (1997). Emergency action. *Nursing Times*, **93**(30), 30–2.

Roberts, D. and Whitehead, L. (2002). Liaison mental health nursing: an overview of its development and current practice. In *Mental Health Liaison*, ed. S. Regal and D. Roberts. Edinburgh: Baillière Tindall/Royal College of Nursing.

Ryan, J., Clemmett, C. and Perez-Avila, C. (1996). Managing patients with deliberate self-harm admitted to an accident and emergency observation ward. *Journal of Accident and Emergency Medicine*, **13**, 31–3.

Shahinpour, N., Hollinger-Smith, L. and Perlia, M. (1995). The medical-psychiatric consultation liaison nurse. *Nursing Clinics of North America*, **30**(1), 77–86.

Teasdale, K. and Mulraney, S. (2000). An analysis of the ability of nurses to identify the anxiety levels of patients in general medical and surgical wards. *NT Research*, **5**(5), 364–70.

Torn, A. and McNichol, E. (1996). Can a mental health nurse be a nurse practitioner? *Nursing Standard*, **11**(2), 39–44.

Tunmore, R. (1989). Liaison psychiatric nursing in oncology. *Nursing Times*, **85**(33), 54–6.

Tunmore, R. (1990). The consultation liaison nurse. *Nursing*, **4**(3), 31–4.

Tunmore, R. (1994). Encouraging collaboration. *Nursing Times*, **90**(20), 66–7.

Tunmore, R. (1997). Liaison mental health nursing and mental health consultation. In *Mental Health Nursing: Principles and Practice*, ed. B. Thomas, S. Hardy and P. Cutting. London: Mosby, pp. 207–22.

University of the West of England. (2004). Mental health liaison and consultation. *Post-Registration Prospectus*. Faculty of Health and Social Care, Bristol: UWE.

Wattis, J. P. and Curran, S. (2001). *Practical Psychiatry of Old Age*, 3rd edn. Oxford: Radcliffe Medical Press.

Part II

Common psychiatric problems across the general hospital

7

Functional somatic syndromes

Lisa Page and Simon Wessely

Definition and terminology

The 'functional somatic syndromes' (FSS) refer to a number of related syndromes that have been characterized by the reporting of somatic symptoms and resultant disability rather than on the evidence of underlying conventional disease processes. Many FSS have been described. Some of these, such as irritable bowel syndrome, are well recognized within mainstream medicine but some, such as sick-building syndrome are not; all however share the feature of a disconnection between subjective symptomatology and objective biomedical pathology. Most medical specialities have at least one FSS (see Table 7.1), whilst FSS on the periphery of mainstream medicine continue to capture public attention. The symptoms required for the diagnosis of a FSS are usually 'medically unexplained', that is physical symptoms for which there is no adequate organic explanation. Chronic fatigue syndrome, irritable bowel syndrome and fibromyalgia have been more extensively researched than most other FSS which has led to specific pathophysiological mechanisms being advanced for each. Nevertheless, as yet no specific explanation is convincing and it remains the case that the similarities between the different FSS are sufficiently striking for there to be a compelling case for considering them together (Barsky & Borus 1999; Wessely *et al.* 1999).

Conceptual issues

Whilst the diagnostic criteria for FSS (where they exist) have usually been produced by the medical specialities, the psychiatric classification systems of the International Classification of Disease (ICD-10) or Diagnostic and Statistical

Handbook of Liaison Psychiatry, ed. Geoffrey Lloyd and Elspeth Guthrie. Published by Cambridge University Press. © Cambridge University Press 2007.

Table 7.1. Functional somatic syndrome by speciality.

Gastroenterology	Irritable bowel syndrome
Rheumatology	Fibromyalgia
	Repetitive strain injury
Cardiology	Non-cardiac chest pain
Infectious disease	Chronic fatigue syndrome/myalgic encephalomyelitis (sero-negative) Lyme disease
Respiratory medicine	Hyperventilation syndrome
Dentistry	Atypical facial pain
	Temporomandibular joint dysfunction
	Burning mouth syndrome
Gynaecology	Chronic pelvic pain
	Pre-menstrual syndrome
Ear, nose and throat	Globus syndrome
Neurology	Tension headache
Non-allied FSS	Gulf War syndrome
	Chronic whiplash
	Sick-building syndrome
	Candidiasis hypersensitivity
	Organophosphate poisoning
	Multiple chemical hypersensitivity

Manual of Mental Disorders (DSM-IV) exist in parallel, although it might be fairer to say in conflict. The standard (medical) diagnostic criteria for FSS usually require specific symptoms to be present, whereas psychiatric classification (under the somatoform disorders) emphasizes the number of symptoms and alleged associated psychological disturbance. These parallel classification systems reflect a conceptual split between psychiatry and medicine which will need addressing as classification systems are updated (Mayou *et al.* 2003). At present the medical diagnostic criteria tend to sideline psychiatric features and the psychiatric classification system tends to ignore the role of comorbid physical disorder. The psychiatric classification is also, despite pleas to the contrary, not atheoretical and assumes the presence of psychopathological processes, often on dubious grounds. Liaison psychiatrists are in a unique position to bridge this gap both clinically and conceptually (Deary 1999; Sharpe & Carson 2001).

Many of the symptoms of FSS are non-specific, such as fatigue, sleep disturbance, muscle ache and abdominal discomfort, and are commonly experienced by the general population. Population surveys show that in any two-week period up to 30% of the population complain of muscle aches and pains, 38% of headache, 15% of eye problems and 14% of skin problems

(Dunnell & Cartwright 1972; Hannay 1978). Experiencing chronic symptoms is also extremely common, with headache and fatigue being the most prevalent long-term symptoms. A typical finding is that 30% of women and 20% of men will say that they have felt tired all the time, every day, for the previous month (Wessely 1995), whilst over a six-week period only 11% of men and 5% of women experience no symptoms at all (Verbrugge & Ascione 1987). The high prevalence of such symptoms in healthy populations calls into question whether these symptoms can be diagnostically specific.

Due to the high degree of overlap between the various FSS in terms of symptoms, epidemiology, non-symptom characteristics and management, it has been proposed that FSS are best considered together rather than separately (Barsky & Borus 1999; Wessely *et al.* 1999). The evidence to support this position is outlined below.

Symptomatic overlap

Simple comparisons of the case definitions of FSS demonstrate considerable overlap. For example, abdominal bloating and headache are each highlighted in 8 out of 12 published case definitions, whilst fatigue is mentioned in 6 (Wessely *et al.* 1999). In 2001, a review of 53 published studies concluded that there were high rates of comorbidity between different FSS, with percentage overlap ranging from 13 to 80% between chronic fatigue syndrome, irritable bowel syndrome, fibromyalgia, multiple chemical sensitivity and temporomandibular joint dysfunction (Aaron & Buchwald 2001). Certain FSS have consistently shown a greater degree of overlap than others; for example fibromyalgia and chronic fatigue syndrome may overlap by as much as 70% (Buchwald & Garrity 1994; Goldenberg *et al.* 1990).

Several studies have used latent class or factor analytic techniques in an attempt to clarify the nature of symptom overlap between various FSS. Confirmatory factor analysis was used in a study by Robbins *et al.* (1997) to assess the underlying relationship between the symptoms of irritable bowel syndrome, fibromyalgia and chronic fatigue syndrome. They concluded that a five-factor model best explained the pattern of variables, thereby giving support to the notion that these syndromes (as well as somatic anxiety and somatic depression) are discrete entities. However, when the data were re-analysed a large proportion of the variance could best be explained by a single general factor, thereby calling into question the original interpretation of the data (Deary 1999). Although support for the five-factor model was subsequently provided by a study of a community sample with chronic fatigue by Taylor *et al.* (2001), they found that the best fit for their data was explained by the following five factors: fibromyalgia factor, chronic fatigue factor, irritable bowel factor, depression factor and anxiety factor. Yet another study used latent class analysis on the symptoms of patients with chronic fatigue syndrome and/or fibromyalgia, revealing four classes which strongly suggested a continuum of symptoms and comorbidity; this was consistent with a single underlying dimension rather than distinct dimensions (Sullivan *et al.* 2002).

Acute infection with *Campylobacter* has been found to lead to greater odds of developing irritable bowel syndrome (IBS) than chronic fatigue syndrome (CFS), whilst the reverse pattern was true after infectious mononucleosis (Moss-Morris & Spence 2006). This finding represents some evidence that IBS and CFS have differing aetiological pathways.

A study that looked at the inter-relationship between 13 FSS amongst new patients attending general hospital outpatient clinics found that over 50% of patients with one FSS fulfilled criteria for at least one other (Nimnuan *et al.* 2001). Exploratory factor analysis suggested that a two-cluster model gave the best fit; with one cluster (termed 'fatigue—pain') encompassing irritable bowel syndrome, chronic fatigue syndrome, fibromyalgia, tension headache, atypical facial pain, non-ulcer dyspepsia and chronic pelvic pain; and a second cluster (termed 'cardiorespiratory') encompassing non-cardiac chest pain and hyperventilation.

A study by Ciccone and Natelson supported the idea that FSS may best be considered as part of a single syndrome. In a sample of women with chronic fatigue syndrome attending a tertiary referral centre, only 38% had 'pure' chronic fatigue syndrome whilst 43% met criteria for fibromyalgia, 35% for multiple chemical sensitivity and 16% for all three syndromes (no other FSS were assessed). The major differences between the groups were that, as the number of syndromes increased, so did the risk of psychiatric morbidity, whereby the lifetime prevalence of suffering from an Axis I disorder increased from 44% in the pure chronic fatigue group to 85% in the group suffering from all three syndromes (Ciccone & Natelson 2003). The authors showed that this effect on psychiatric morbidity was unlikely to be due to increased symptom burden nor did they find evidence of widespread differences in symptom severity between the groups, which they interpreted as evidence in support of the single syndrome hypothesis.

Several studies have highlighted the heterogeneity within a single FSS. In an international multicentre trial investigating chronic fatigue syndrome, the possibility of two subtypes emerged; the largest subtype (68% of the sample) consisted of younger patients who were less functionally impaired with less psychiatric comorbidity, whilst the profile of the smaller subtype seemed consistent withv typical somatoform illness, showing a greater number of symptoms and greater health service utilization (Wilson *et al.* 2001). These findings confirmed the results of a previous study in chronic fatigue syndrome (Hickie *et al.* 1995).

To summarize, most studies to have addressed the issue of symptomatic overlap have yielded results that do not support the concept that each FSS is discrete, although two studies have provided support for a five-factor model. These apparently disparate findings are likely to be due to differences in the study populations and differing statistical methods. In the only study to consider overlap between all (or nearly all) FSS, a two-cluster model of 'fatigue–pain' and 'cardiorespiratory' gave the best fit (Nimnuan *et al.* 2001). Therefore, on present evidence, it seems that the splitting of the various FSS may be misleading and a more useful approach would be to withhold judgement until pathophysiological and cognitive mechanisms are better elucidated (Wessely 2001). Additionally, studies within chronic fatigue syndrome highlight the heterogeneity within a single FSS. This does not imply that the solution is to further subclassify by symptoms, rather it may serve to emphasize the utility of a multi-axial approach (Wessely *et al.* 1999; Wilson *et al.* 2001). Overall it appears that the current labelling of the functional somatic syndromes is likely to be an artefact of specialization of physicians.

Epidemiology

Whilst the symptom of 'chronic fatigue' affects 20–30% of the population, the prevalence of chronic fatigue syndrome has been estimated to affect between 0.007 and 2.8% of the general adult population (Afari & Buchwald 2003), with the estimates of the latter varying due to differences in the study population and the study methodology used. Similarly, chronic pain is common in the general population with prevalence rates of 7.3–12.9%, whilst estimates of the prevalence of fibromyalgia range from 0.5 to 5% (Neumann & Buskila 2003; Wolfe *et al.* 1995). Bowel symptoms are amongst the most common symptoms reported in general population samples, with 60–70% reporting one or more troublesome gastrointestinal symptom, whilst estimates of the population prevalence of irritable bowel syndrome are also high and range from 3 to 20% depending on the criteria used (Brandt *et al.* 2002). Fewer data are available on the prevalence of the more controversial FSS, partly due to the lack of agreed operationally defined diagnostic criteria. However, it is likely that other FSS would be diagnosed in similar numbers in the general population; one review estimated the prevalence of multiple chemical sensitivity to be around 4–6% (Bell *et al.* 1998). These figures illustrate that not only are the symptoms that constitute these syndromes commonly experienced, but that the syndromes themselves are diagnosable in a substantial proportion of the general population. It is therefore not surprising that over half of new attendees in general medical clinics fulfil criteria for one or more FSS (Nimnuan *et al.* 2001). Where longitudinal data are available it seems that FSS are usually chronic conditions, with most patients still experiencing symptoms years later (Joyce *et al.* 1997; Kay *et al.* 1994; Potts & Bass 1993), although it must be conceded that most of this evidence comes from specialist care.

Attention has been drawn to the historical and epidemiological similarities between the FSS (Barsky & Borus 1999; Hazemeijer & Rasker 2003). Most FSS surfaced as medical entities towards the end of the last century, but given the probability that people's experience of ubiquitous symptoms such as pain and fatigue have not changed, it is likely that it is the labels that are new or different (Wessely 1990). Frequently the medical profession has been left behind when a new FSS has appeared in the public domain and lay ideas on causation and treatment have often been incorporated into the illness paradigm (Arksey 1994; Shorter 1995). Cultural factors are crucial when determining whether a FSS gains a following; for example the whiplash syndrome has been shown to be absent in countries that lack a compensation mechanism (Schrader *et al.* 1996) and chronic fatigue syndrome is curiously absent from paediatric practice in France (Mouterde 2001). Indeed the process by which FSS may actually be caused (or worsened) by factors within society has been termed 'social iatrogenesis' (Cleland 1987). This raises the question as to whether the use of FSS diagnostic labels serves any useful purpose. It appears that the conferring of a label on a cluster of symptoms is favoured by patients themselves, who often find that the giving of a name to disabling symptoms brings relief and empowerment (Reid *et al.* 1991; Woodward *et al.* 1995). Patients with multiple medically unexplained symptoms often feel stigmatized and a diagnosis can help reduce this sense of stigma (Asbring & Narvanen 2002). However, others have argued that the use of a label, such as fibromyalgia, is iatrogenic and represents the endpoint of an iatrogenic medical process (Hadler 1993).

Gender

Female patients are likely to be over-represented in the setting of the specialist clinic, as are white patients and those from higher socioeconomic backgrounds (Afari & Buchwald 2003). Population prevalence studies have confirmed that women are more likely to experience symptoms than men (Kroenke & Price 1993), even when menstrual complaints are excluded. Studies in primary care have confirmed this association both for symptoms in general and medically unexplained symptoms in particular (Kroenke & Spitzer 1998). Population-based studies have confirmed that women experience higher rates of chronic fatigue syndrome (Jason *et al.* 1999), fibromyalgia (Wolfe *et al.* 1995) and multiple chemical sensitivity (Bell *et al.* 1998) than men, although the gender difference is less pronounced in irritable bowel syndrome (Saito *et al.* 2000).

An increased prevalence of females with FSS is also seen in primary and secondary care where there may be an even greater gender discrepancy. In new patients attending general medical outpatient clinics, significantly more women than men (60% vs. 48%) fulfilled criteria for one of thirteen FSS (Nimnuan *et al.* 2001). The over-representation of women suffering from medically unexplained symptoms is only partly explained by increased rates of anxiety and depression in women (Kroenke & Spitzer 1998).

Comorbid psychiatric disorder

Much evidence suggests that the reporting of symptoms and psychological distress are closely inter-related. Individuals who score highly on measures of depression and anxiety consistently report more symptoms than those having low scores on such measures (Hotopf *et al.* 1998; Kroenke *et al.* 1994). Patients fulfilling criteria for FSS are more likely to have a psychiatric diagnosis than normal controls (Fiedler *et al.* 1996; Wessely *et al.* 1996), and also to have a history of psychiatric illness predating their current somatic symptoms (Wessely *et al.* 1996). Studies that have compared patients with FSS to medical illness control groups have found higher rates of psychiatric disorder, somatic symptomatology and familial psychiatric disorder in the FSS group (Gomborone *et al.* 1995; Hudson *et al.* 1992; Robbins & Kirmayer 1990; Walker *et al.* 1990), without necessarily showing evidence of increased disability (Robbins & Kirmayer 1990). The lifetime prevalence of somatization disorder is probably raised in patients with FSS (Manu *et al.* 1989; Walker *et al.* 1990), although rates are nearly always over-represented in studies set in specialist centres. In a prospective study, those who measured more highly on measures of anxiety, depression and neuroticism were more likely to go on to develop irritable bowel syndrome following an episode of acute gastroenteritis (Gwee *et al.* 1996). Against this some authors have emphasized caution, pointing out that the association with psychiatric morbidity (in for example irritable bowel syndrome) is much diminished when considering population, as opposed to clinic-based, samples (Talley & Spiller 2002). One possibility is that the greater the level of psychiatric distress, the more likely a symptomatic individual is to present to a doctor and obtain a FSS label. As regards the association between FSS and other somatoform disorders, it has been suggested that patients with FSS may have an underlying tendency to experience and report bodily distress, which explains the high level of somatic symptoms often experienced prior to the onset of an FSS (Barsky & Borus 1999).

Difficulties in the doctor–patient relationship

Patients with FSS have been rated as one of the three most common types of patients that are 'difficult to help' (Sharpe *et al.* 1994) and doctors are often uncertain about how best to care for these patients (Woodward *et al.* 1995). The number of physical (and somatoform) symptoms that a patient reports is correlated with the extent to which a doctor finds the patient difficult (Hahn 2001). Likewise patients with FSS are more likely to be dissatisfied by their medical care than general medical patients (Twemlow *et al.* 1997) and to feel stigmatized by their illness (Looper & Kirmayer 2004). Patients with medically unexplained symptoms in general and FSS in particular have been shown to be dissatisfied with the quality of care and interaction that they get from their doctor (Deale & Wessely 2001; Peters *et al.* 1998), finding that their own experience of symptoms provides them with an expert perspective on their condition that their doctor lacks (Peters *et al.* 1998).

Patients with medically unexplained symptoms often make their doctors feel helpless, which can lead to inappropriate investigations, treatments or referrals being instigated (Page & Wessely 2003). Qualitative studies from primary care have found that patients with medically unexplained symptoms tended not to overtly request physical interventions, but rather exerted pressure on the general practitioner by the use of criticism or emotive language (Ring *et al.* 2004). It may be that such patients are not actually looking for physical interventions, but doctors usually respond with them all the same (Ring *et al.* 2005). Data from secondary care indicates that, in this setting, patients with medically unexplained symptoms probably use more explicit requests for treatment (Salmon & Marchant-Haycox 2000). The tendency of those with FSS to turn to alternative medicines for treatment is likely to be not just due to a lack of confidence in traditional medicine, but also because alternative remedies often endorse the FSS patient's own physical illness attributions (Moss-Morris & Wrapson 2003).

Aetiology

There is limited data on the predisposing and precipitating factors in FSS. Many of the specific biological factors that have been proposed have not been replicated. There is better evidence for the factors that maintain both symptoms and functional impairment, particularly where illness beliefs impact on the condition (Moss-Morris & Wrapson 2003). A summary of the most salient aetiological evidence, organized within the biopsychosocial framework, is presented below.

Predisposing factors

Genetics

One twin study has shown that diffuse somatic distress (assumed not to be due to a discrete medical cause) is likely to be due to a combination of specific gene action and non-shared environmental influences and that these are independent of depression or anxiety (Gillespie *et al.* 2000). The FSS for which there is most genetic data is chronic fatigue syndrome, with research ongoing in this area; to date there is some evidence from family and twin studies for a genetic influence. In a family study by Walsh *et al.* (2001) relatives of people with chronic fatigue syndrome had higher rates of chronic fatigue syndrome than relatives of people with medical illness. Twin studies examining fatigue as a symptom (but not chronic fatigue syndrome) have shown that it is likely to be substantially heritable but that non-shared environmental effects are also important (Farmer *et al.* 1999; Hickie *et al.* 1999; Sullivan *et al.* 2005). The only twin study of (females with) chronic fatigue syndrome showed that concordance rates for the illness were higher between monozygotic than dizygotic twins (38% vs. 11%), and that additive genetic factors and environmental effects each accounted for greater than 40% of the variance in susceptibility (Buchwald *et al.* 2001). In the largest twin study to date, there was no evidence that stricter case definitions of chronic fatigue were more genetically mediated than less-refined definitions (Sullivan *et al.* 2005). Preliminary evidence is now emerging of differential gene expression in people with CFS for a number of potentially relevent genes — see the April 2006 issue of *Pharmacogenetics* for a collection of papers in this area (www.futuremedicine.com/loi/pgs). The picture is similar for irritable bowel syndrome, with twin studies showing that the condition is twice as frequent in monozygotic as compared to dizygotic twins, but that environmental factors remain important, with approximately half the liability for the disorder being attributable to genetic influence (Morris-Yates *et al.* 1998; Levy *et al.* 2001).

Childhood experiences

A history of childhood abuse is more common in those who suffer from irritable bowel syndrome (Reilly *et al.* 1999), chronic fatigue syndrome (Van-Houdenhove *et al.* 2001), fibromyalgia (Anderberg *et al.* 2000; Van-Houdenhove *et al.* 2001) and unexplained chronic pelvic pain (McGowan *et al.* 1998) than it is in control groups. Although all of the above studies are retrospective, the results are congruent with findings from the general somatization literature (Craig *et al.* 1993). Likewise in the general literature it is established that those who have childhood experience of illness or have experienced parental illness as a child are more vulnerable to the experience of medically unexplained symptoms in adulthood (Craig *et al.* 1993; Hotopf *et al.* 1999); as yet the data on this is limited in FSS apart from a few studies (Levy *et al.* 2000).

Precipitating factors

Infection or injury

The role of infection in precipitating conditions such as chronic fatigue syndrome has been much debated. It is now generally accepted that there is no single infective agent involved in the pathogenesis of chronic fatigue syndrome (Afari & Buchwald 2003) or irritable bowel syndrome (Talley & Spiller 2002), nor have specific infective agents been shown to be crucial to the onset of fibromyalgia or any of the other FSS. The Epstein–Barr virus has been shown to lead to chronic fatigue syndrome in a minority of cases (White *et al.* 1998) as have viral illnesses requiring hospitalization (Hotopf *et al.* 1996). However, psychiatric morbidity, female gender and prolonged convalescence are still the most important predictors of developing chronic fatigue syndrome following infection (Candy *et al.* 2003; Hotopf *et al.* 1996) and many patients with chronic fatigue syndrome do not recall experiencing a specific infective illness prior to onset of their symptoms. Although many potential abnormalities of the immune system have been suggested in chronic fatigue syndrome, a systematic review found little evidence of consistent immune abnormality (Lyall *et al.* 2003). In clinical practice patients often cite an injury as the precipitant to their unexplained musculoskeletal symptoms and this has some limited support in the literature (Al-Allaf *et al.* 2002).

Stress

Both acute and chronic stress have been implicated in the onset of FSS. A recent case control study showed that stressful life events occurred much more frequently prior to the onset of chronic fatigue syndrome than in matched controls; in particular 30% of chronic fatigue patients (and no controls) experienced 'dilemmas' in the months preceding onset (Hatcher & House 2003). Chronic stress (or life events) have also been shown to be important in the onset and maintenance of symptoms in irritable bowel syndrome (Bennett *et al.* 1998; Creed *et al.* 1988) and fibromyalgia (Anderberg *et al.* 2000). These findings are in keeping with the results of the South London Somatization Study, which found high rates of life events in the period leading up to an episode of somatization (Craig *et al.* 1994).

Maintaining factors

Many specific and complex biological mechanisms have been proposed by researchers in the various FSS to account for their patients' symptoms, but in most instances these mechanisms are either not generalizable across the syndrome or are likely to be secondary effects. One useful approach when considering biological mechanisms is to consider the manner in which normal physiological processes can become pathological, giving rise to distressing symptoms which then become chronic (Sharpe & Bass 1992). Therapeutically, cognitive behavioural techniques have been developed which address some of the biological and psychological maintaining factors discussed below.

Deconditioning

In the FSS for which rest and avoidance of physical activity are key features (e.g. fibromyalgia, chronic fatigue syndrome and chronic pain syndromes), physical deconditioning offers an appealing mechanism for the maintenance of symptoms. There is some evidence for reduced physical fitness in fibromyalgia (Valim *et al.* 2002) and reduced exercise capacity in chronic fatigue syndrome when compared to sedentary controls (Fulcher & White 2000). However, it is difficult to prove that physical deconditioning is a secondary phenomenon to prolonged inactivity and there is conflicting evidence that patients with chronic fatigue syndrome do not differ in overall fitness from sedentary controls, despite baseline physical activity levels being higher in controls (Bazelmans *et al.* 2001). Nonetheless the success of graded exercise and cognitive behavioural regimes in treating fibromyalgia and chronic fatigue syndrome is evidence of the importance of improving fitness and activity in the treatment of these conditions. Indeed, adequate and regular physical activity has been shown to be a positive outcome predictor in fibromyalgia (Wigers 1996).

Neuroendocrine changes

Changes within the neuroendocrine system offer an interesting explanation for some of the biological changes seen in the FSS, although studies so far have failed to provide a totally coherent story. Most intensive research in this field has been done in chronic fatigue syndrome and, less so, in fibromyalgia. There is some evidence of low circulating cortisol in chronic fatigue syndrome, which is in contrast to the pattern seen in depression (Parker *et al.* 2001). In addition the serotonergic system may be overactive in chronic fatigue syndrome (Parker *et al.* 2001). A reduction in the responsivity of the hypothalamic−pituitary−adrenal (HPA) axis has also been shown in fibromyalgia (Parker *et al.* 2001).

Neuroendocrine changes in irritable bowel syndrome have been examined less often, although there is some evidence of abnormal activity of the HPA axis and also that the gut may be overactivated by corticotrophin-releasing hormone in those with the condition (Fukudo *et al.* 1998). It is unclear whether the neuroendocrine abnormalities that have been observed are primary or secondary, and longitudinal studies of groups at risk of developing FSS will be needed to evaluate this further.

Central dysfunction

Some preliminary neuroimaging studies have been conducted in chronic fatigue syndrome, irritable bowel syndrome and pain syndromes, which suggest that central mechanisms may play a role in these disorders. At present, the usefulness of neuroimaging research in FSS is limited, but taken as a whole the evidence probably does support the idea of aberrant patterns of brain activation in these conditions (particularly in response to relevant probes such as experimentally induced pain).

In chronic fatigue syndrome, observations concerning structural brain changes have been inconsistent (Afari & Buchwald 2003) and will not be discussed further here. However functional studies have shown some interesting (albeit inconsistent) leads. Studies have often been confounded by the presence of comorbid depression in the chronic fatigue group, but one resting-state single photon emission computed tomography (SPECT) study which included only non-depressed chronic fatigue patients and which used depressed controls found few differences between the chronic fatigue group and the depressed group, although both differed from a normal control group by showing increased thalamic activation (MacHale *et al.* 2000). In a SPECT cognitive activation study (which again excluded chronic fatigue subjects who were depressed), the chronic fatigue group were found to have a pattern of unusually diffuse cerebral blood flow (consistent with some previous studies), with particular differences compared to controls in activation in the left anterior cingulate (Schmaling *et al.* 2003). Against these positive findings, however, a well-controlled SPECT study of twins who were discordant for chronic fatigue syndrome found no differences in cerebral perfusion between the groups (Lewis *et al.* 2001).

In irritable bowel syndrome, initial functional neuroimaging studies have used rectal distension as a perceptual challenge whilst monitoring brain activation (Mertz *et al.* 2000; Naliboff *et al.* 2001; Silverman *et al.* 1997). Differences have been highlighted in the pattern and intensity of frontal and brainstem activation in those with irritable bowel syndrome compared with those without the disorder, with the activation of the anterior cingulate cortex (a brain region consistently associated with the higher processing of pain in normal individuals) highlighted as abnormal across studies. Subjective ratings of discomfort to the procedure of rectal distension were also higher in those with irritable bowel syndrome (Mertz *et al.* 2000; Naliboff *et al.* 2001). One interpretation of these results is that although predominantly normal brain areas for pain processing seem to be activated in response to painful bowel stimulation in people with irritable bowel syndrome, the neural activation is excessive (or at least aberrant) and linked to the subjective appraisal of increased pain.

In fibromyalgia, a recent fMRI study demonstrated that not only are patients with fibromyalgia more sensitive to experimentally induced pain, but when given non-painful stimuli they exhibit areas of brain activation typically associated with pain perception and exhibit greater brain activation than controls to painful stimuli (Cook *et al.* 2004). Resting regional cerebral blood flow has also been found to be diminished in the thalamus of a group with fibromyalgia (Kwiatek *et al.* 2000), with the implication that brain areas known to be involved in the normal perception of pain are activated abnormally in the condition. Neuroimaging studies continue to try and elucidate more clearly the networks involved in the normal perception and experience of pain. These studies are important if future studies in groups with FSS are to be adequately interpreted.

Illness beliefs

Research has yet to specifically address how illness beliefs in different FSS may overlap, although there is indirect evidence that this is likely to be the case (Moss-Morris & Wrapson 2003). At present, chronic fatigue syndrome is the FSS for which there is most evidence that beliefs about the illness may impact on the course of the illness itself. Patients with chronic fatigue syndrome are more likely to make physical illness attributions (rather than normalizing or psychologizing attributions) for a selection of common symptoms compared to controls (Butler *et al.* 2001); and are more likely to believe their illness will be chronic and have serious consequences when compared with patients with chronic medical conditions (Weinman *et al.* 1996). In one study, physical illness attributions were found to be the most important risk factor for developing chronic fatigue syndrome after viral illness (Cope *et al.* 1994), implying a clear aetiological role. A systematic review of prognosis in chronic fatigue syndrome found that patients with physical illness attributions had a worse prognosis (Joyce *et al.* 1997), a conclusion that has been confirmed by subsequent studies. Illness worry was found to be strongly correlated with disability in fibromyalgia, but not in a control group with rheumatoid arthritis (Robbins & Kirmayer 1990). Likewise, those with irritable bowel syndrome were found to score more highly on hypochondriacal and bodily preoccupation scales than either a depressed group or a group with organic bowel disease (Gomborone *et al.* 1995). Buchwald and Garrity compared groups with chronic fatigue syndrome, multiple chemical sensitivity and fibromyalgia on a measure of 'locus of control' for their illness and found the results to be similar across diagnoses (Buchwald & Garrity 1994).

Barsky and Borus have used the term 'symptom amplification' to describe the manner in which innocuous symptoms become misattributed and then incorporated into an FSS label, which leads to further misattribution of other symptoms as they arise (Barsky & Borus 1999). These beliefs and attitudes about symptoms may act as a mechanism that then guides the patient to adopt avoidant behaviours, which leads to limitation of activity, which in turn leads to the secondary deconditioning and neuroendocrine effects outlined above. In fact, it is change to beliefs about avoidance, rather than changes to the causal attribution of symptoms that predicts good outcome from cognitive behavioural therapy in chronic fatigue syndrome (Deale *et al.* 1998), highlighting the need for more research into the way in which illness attributions maintain ill-health and may or may not be altered during successful treatment.

Social factors

Several of the FSS, including chronic fatigue syndrome, Gulf War syndrome and repetitive strain injury, have gained public credibility in spite of widespread medical scepticism as to their very existence. This phenomenon has been attributed to changes within society, including the erosion of the physician's traditional role, a resistance to perceived psychologization and the role of the media (Shorter 1995). Patient support groups, although undoubtedly valued by those suffering from a FSS and often providing much needed support, may have some negative consequences; for example membership of a chronic fatigue support group has been associated with poorer prognosis in longitudinal studies (Bentall *et al.* 2002; Sharpe *et al.* 1992). The availability and explosion in Internet sites has also meant that patients may inadvertently be exposed to information that is inaccurate or even harmful (Kisely 2002).

The media has often been highlighted as playing an important role in the genesis of FSS (Barsky & Borus 1999; Hazemeijer and Rasker 2003; Shorter 1995). Certainly, the coverage of the FSS by the media tends to reflect inaccurately the scientific debate of the moment and will usually amplify organic causation at the expense of a more balanced biopsychosocial perspective (MacLean & Wessely 1994).

The financial 'reward' to be gained from disability payments or litigation has been argued as playing a role in the maintenance of ill-health in those suffering from FSS (Malleson 2002). For example, being in receipt of sickness benefit or certification has been shown to be a poor prognostic sign in chronic fatigue syndrome (Bentall *et al.* 2002; Cope *et al.* 1994) and fibromyalgia (Wigers 1996), whilst the whiplash syndrome has not been reported in countries without an insurance and compensation culture (Schrader *et al.* 1996). Opinions vary on this topic – perhaps the only way to resolve the issue would be via a randomized controlled trial; somehow one doubts this will ever happen.

Treatment

Evidence-based treatments for FSS share striking similarities. The most robust evidence for efficacy is from psychosocial interventions and/or antidepressants with the syndrome-specific pharmacological interventions showing mixed and generally disappointing results. Psychosocial treatments, such as cognitive behavioural therapy, have been shown to be beneficial in a range of somatoform disorders (Kroenke & Swindle 2000), including the most intensively researched FSS (i.e. chronic fatigue syndrome, irritable bowel syndrome and fibromyalgia), although it is difficult to draw firm conclusions about how long-lasting or clinically meaningful the benefits are (Allen *et al*. 2002). A brief review of published systematic reviews of treatment in FSS follows.

Chronic fatigue syndrome

A recently updated systematic review has found evidence that cognitive behavioural therapy and graded excercise therapy are helpful in CFS, but for other interventions the evidence was inconclusive or lacking (Chambers *et al*. 2006). An older Cochrane Collaboration systematic review has concluded that individual cognitive behavioural therapy in adults was superior to both relaxation therapy and treatment as usual in chronic fatigue syndrome, with the 'number needed to treat' to prevent one unsatisfactory physical outcome being two (Price & Couper 1998). Cognitive behavioural therapy was shown to improve physical functioning, fatigue and quality of life; importantly it was also shown to be acceptable to patients (Price & Couper 1998). Generally, antidepressants have not been shown to be beneficial either alone or in combination with behavioural therapies, although monoamine oxidase inhibitors have demonstrated some promise (Whiting *et al*. 2001).

Fibromyalgia

A Cochrane Collaboration systematic review showed that exercise improves aerobic performance, tender points and global wellbeing and may or may not improve pain, fatigue and sleep in fibromyalgia (Busch *et al*. 2002). Although multidisciplinary rehabilitation for fibromyalgia is popular, another Cochrane systematic review found little evidence for its effectiveness (Karjalainen *et al*. 1999). Cognitive behavioural therapy has been investigated less often in fibromyalgia than in chronic fatigue syndrome and we could find no systematic reviews assessing its effectiveness. However, systematic reviews on 'non-pharmacological' (Sim & Adams 2002) and 'mind—body therapies' (Hadhazy *et al*. 2000) for fibromyalgia found the evidence to be inconclusive for the majority of treatments, with Sim and Adams highlighting the poor methodological quality of most studies in this field. Nevertheless a meta-analysis of pharmacological and non-pharmacological interventions in fibromyalgia found that non-pharmacological interventions appeared to be more efficacious in improving symptoms than pharmacological interventions (Rossy *et al.* 1999). In a systematic review and meta-analysis looking at the use of antidepressant medication in fibromyalgia, Arnold *et al.* found tricyclic antidepressants to have a moderate overall effect, with the largest effect on sleep quality, global functioning and pain (Arnold *et al.* 2000). There was little evidence for the efficacy of selective serotonin reuptake inhibitors (SSRIs; Arnold *et al.* 2000).

Irritable bowel syndrome

Despite the large number of pharmacological and non-pharmacological trials that have been conducted in irritable bowel syndrome, there are significant methodological drawbacks in the vast majority (Akehurst & Kaltenthaler 2001). At present it would seem that there is some evidence that psychotherapies in general (including behavioural therapy, cognitive behavioural therapy, hypnotherapy, relaxation therapy and biofeedback) are efficacious in treating irritable bowel syndrome (Brandt *et al.* 2002). Tricyclic antidepressants have been shown to be effective in relieving abdominal pain and may improve global symptoms (Jailwala *et al.* 2000), but there is insufficient evidence to be able to assess the effectiveness of SSRIs (Brandt *et al.* 2002). Tegaserod (a $5HT_4$ receptor agonist) has been shown to improve overall symptomatology with the 'number needed to treat' being 17 (Evans *et al.* 2004). Loperamide may be an effective treatment for diarrhoea related to the condition, whilst bulking agents are not effective and there is insufficient evidence to recommend the use of antispasmodics (Brandt *et al.* 2002).

Repetitive strain injury

A Cochrane review found the evidence for biopsychosocial rehabilitation in repetitive strain injury to be limited due to a paucity of high-quality trials, although there was some preliminary evidence that hypnosis may decrease pain in the short term (Karjalainen *et al.* 2004b). A second Cochrane review on 'upper extremity work-related disorders' found little evidence for the effectiveness of specially designed keyboards or other ergonomic interventions (Verhagen *et al.* 2004a).

Other functional somatic syndromes

A Cochrane review in burning mouth syndrome concluded that high quality treatment trials were needed but that vitamin tablets and cognitive behavioural treatment may be helpful (Zakrzewska *et al.* 2004), whilst another systematic review on a range of dental FSS found there to be insufficient evidence for the use of analgesics in these conditions (List *et al.* 2003). Another Cochrane review found little or no evidence for the use of dental splints in temporomandibular joint dysfunction (Al-Ani *et al.* 2004), whilst it is unclear whether active treatments are preferable to passive treatments in whiplash (Verhagen *et al.* 2004b). Psychological treatments have been shown to be effective in the treatment of non-cardiac chest pain (Kisely *et al.* 2005).

Conclusions

The FSS share many similarities in terms of symptomatic overlap and effective treatments as well as non-symptom characteristics; these observations imply that it may be unhelpful to regard each as a separate condition. The aetiology of all these conditions is multifactorial, with emerging evidence of the importance of genetic predisposition and stressful life events in both childhood and adulthood. Research has also helped to highlight the role of a number of biological and psychosocial factors that maintain the FSS once symptoms are established. Cognitive behavioural therapy and exercise therapy appear to lead to therapeutic change by tackling these maintaining factors, whilst centrally acting drugs such as anti-depressants can sometimes be helpful. For many of the less well recognized FSS, operationalized diagnostic criteria are lacking, as are high quality treatment trials.

REFERENCES

Aaron, L. and Buchwald, D. (2001). A review of the evidence for overlap among unexplained clinical conditions. *Annals of Internal Medicine*, **134**(9), 868–81.

Afari, N. and Buchwald, D. (2003). Chronic fatigue syndrome: a review. *American Journal of Psychiatry*, **160**, 221–36.

Akehurst, R. and Kaltenthaler, E. (2001). Treatment of irritable bowel syndrome: a review of randomised controlled trials. *Gut*, **48**, 272–82.

Al-Allaf, A. W., Dunbar, K. L., Hallum, N. S., *et al.* (2002). A case-control study examining the role of physical trauma in the onset of fibromyalgia syndrome. *Rheumatology*, **41**(4), 450–3.

Al-Ani, M., Davies, S., Gray, R. J., *et al.* (2004). Stabilisation splint therapy for temporo-mandibular pain dysfunction syndrome (Cochrane Review). *Cochrane Library*. Chichester: John Wiley & Sons Ltd.

Allen, L., Escobar, J., Lehrer, P. M., *et al.* (2002). Psychosocial treatments for multiple unexplained physical symptoms: a review of the literature. *Psychosomatic Medicine*, **64**(6), 939–50.

Anderberg, U., Marteinsdottir, I., Theorell, T., *et al.* (2000). The impact of life events in female patients with fibromyalgia and in female healthy controls. *European Psychiatry*, **15**, 295–301.

Arksey, H. (1994). Expert and lay participation in the construction of medical knowledge. *Sociology of Health and Illness*, **16**(4), 448–68.

Arnold, L. M., Keck, P. E. and Welge, J. A. (2000). Antidepressant treatment of fibromyalgia. A meta-analysis and review. *Psychosomatics*, **41**, 104–13.

Asbring, P. and Narvanen, A. (2002). Women's experiences of stigma in relation to chronic fatigue syndrome. *Qualitative Health Research*, **12**(2), 148–60.

Barsky, A. and Borus, J. (1999). Functional somatic syndromes. *Annals of Internal Medicine*, **130**, 910–21.

Bazelmans, E., Bleijenberg, G., Van Der Meer, J. N., *et al.* (2001). Is physical deconditioning a perpetuating factor in chronic fatigue syndrome? A controlled study on maximal exercise performance and relations with fatigue, impairment and physical activity. *Psychological Medicine*, **31**, 107–14.

Bell, I., Baldwin, C. and Schwartz, G. E. (1998). Illness from low levels of environmental chemicals: relevance to chronic fatigue syndrome and fibromyalgia. *American Journal of Medicine*, **105**, 74S–82S.

Bennett, E., Tennant, C., Piesse, C., *et al.* (1998). Level of chronic life stress predicts clinical outcome in irritable bowel syndrome. *Gut*, **43**, 256–61.

Bentall, R., Powell, P., Nye, F. J., *et al.* (2002). Predictors of response to treatment for chronic fatigue syndrome. *British Journal of Psychiatry*, **181**, 248–52.

Brandt, L., Bjorkman, D., Fennerty, M. B., *et al.* (2002). Systematic review on the management of irritable bowel syndrome in North America. *American Journal of Gastroenterology*, **97**(11), S7–26.

Buchwald, D. and Garrity, D. (1994). Comparison of patients with chronic fatigue syndrome, fibromyalgia and multiple chemical sensitivities. *Archives of Internal Medicine*, **154**, 2049–53.

Buchwald, D., Herrell, R., Ashton, S., *et al.* (2001). A twin study of chronic fatigue. *Psychosomatic Medicine*, **63**, 936–43.

Busch, A., Schachter, C., Peloso, P. M., *et al.* (2002). Exercise for treating fibromyalgia syndrome (Cochrane Review). *The Cochrane Database of Systematic Reviews*. Chichester: John Wiley & Sons Ltd.

Butler, J., Chalder, T. and Wessely, S. (2001). Causal attributions for somatic sensations in patients with chronic fatigue syndrome and their partners. *Psychological Medicine*, **31**, 97–105.

Candy, B., Chalder, T., Cleare, A. J., *et al.* (2003). Predictors of fatigue following the onset of infectious mononucleosis. *Psychological Medicine*, **33**, 847–55.

Chambers, D., Bagnall, A.-M., Hempel, S., *et al.* (2006). Interventions for the treatment, management and rehabilitation of patients with chronic fatigue syndrome/myalgic encephalomyelitis: an updated systematic review. *Journal of the Royal Society of Medicine*, **99**, 506–20.

Ciccone, D. and Natelson, B. (2003). Comorbid illness in women with chronic fatigue syndrome: a test of the single syndrome hypothesis. *Psychosomatic Medicine*, **65**, 268–75.

Cleland, L. (1987). 'RSI': a model of social iatrogenesis. *Medical Journal of Australia*, **147**(5), 236–9.

Cook, D., Lange, G., Ciccone, D. S., *et al.* (2004). Functional imaging of pain in patients with primary fibromyalgia. *Journal of Rheumatology*, **31**, 364–78.

Cope, H., David, A., Pelosi, A., *et al.* (1994). Predictors of chronic 'postviral' fatigue. *Lancet*, **344**, 864–8.

Craig, T., Boardman, A., Mills, K., *et al.* (1993). The South London somatisation study I: longitudinal course and the influence of early life experiences. *British Journal of Psychiatry,* **163**, 579–88.

Craig, T., Drake, H., Mills, K., *et al.* (1994). The South London somatisation study II: influence of stressful life events and secondary gain. *British Journal of Psychiatry,* **165**, 248–58.

Creed, F., Craig, T. and Farmer, R. (1988). Functional abdominal pain, psychiatric illness and life events. *Gut,* **29**, 235–42.

Deale, A., Chalder, T. and Wessely, S. (1998). Illness beliefs and treatment outcome in chronic fatigue syndrome. *Journal of Psychosomatic Research,* **45**(1), 77–83.

Deale, A. and Wessely, S. (2001). Patients' perceptions of medical care in chronic fatigue syndrome. *Social Science & Medicine,* **52**, 1859–64.

Deary, I. (1999). A taxonomy of medically explained symptoms. *Journal of Psychosomatic Research,* **47**(1), 51–9.

Dunnell, K. and Cartwright, A. (1972). *Medicine Takers, Prescribers and Hoarders.* London: Routledge, Kegan Paul.

Evans, B., Clark, W., Moore, D. J., *et al.* (2004). Tegaserod for the treatment of irritable bowel syndrome (Cochrane Review). *Cochrane Database of Systematic Reviews.* Chichester, John Wiley & Sons Ltd.

Farmer, A., Scourfield, J., Martin, N., *et al.* (1999). Is disabling fatigue in childhood influenced by genes? *Psychological Medicine,* **29**, 279–82.

Fiedler, N., Kipen, H., DeLuca, J., *et al.* (1996). A controlled comparison of multiple chemical sensitivities and chronic fatigue syndrome. *Psychosomatic Medicine,* **58**, 38–49.

Fukudo, S., Nomura, T. and Hongo, M. (1998). Impact of corticotropin-releasing hormone on gastrointestinal motility and adrenocorticotropic hormone in normal controls and patients with irritable bowel syndrome. *Gut,* **42**(6), 845–9.

Fulcher, K. Y. and White, P. D. (2000). Strength and physiological response to exercise in patients with chronic fatigue syndrome. *Journal of Neurology, Neurosurgery and Psychiatry,* **69**, 302–7.

Gillespie, N., Zhu, G., Heath, A. C., *et al.* (2000). The genetic aetiology of somatic distress. *Psychological Medicine,* **30**, 1051–61.

Goldenberg, D., Simms, R., Geiger, A., *et al.* (1990). High frequency of fibromyalgia in patients with chronic fatigue seen in a primary care practice. *Arthritis and Rheumatism,* **33**(3), 381–7.

Gomborone, J., Dewsnap, P., Libby, G., *et al.* (1995). Abnormal illness attitudes in patients with irritable bowel syndrome. *Journal of Psychosomatic Research,* **39**(2), 227–30.

Gwee, K. A., Graham, J. C., McKendrick, W., *et al.* (1996). Psychometric scores and persistence of irritable bowel after infectious diarrhoea. *Lancet,* **347**, 150–3.

Hadhazy, V., Ezzo, J., Creamer, P., *et al.* (2000). Mind-body therapies for the treatment of fibromyalgia. A systematic review. *Journal of Rheumatology,* **27**(12), 2911–18.

Hadler, N. (1993). The dangers of the diagnostic process: iatrogenic labeling as in the fibromyalgia paralogism. *Occupational Musculoskeletal Disorders.* New York: Raven Press, pp. 16–33.

Hahn, S. (2001). Physical symptoms and physician-experienced difficulty in the physician-patient relationship. *Annals of Internal Medicine,* **134**, 897–904.

Hannay, D. (1978). Symptom prevalence in the community. *Journal of the Royal College of General Practitioners,* **28**, 492–9.

Hatcher, S. and House, A. (2003). Life events, difficulties and dilemmas in the onset of chronic fatigue syndrome: a case-control study. *Psychological Medicine*, **33**, 1185–92.

Hazemeijer, I. and Rasker, J. (2003). Fibromyalgia and the therapeutic domain. A philosophical study on the origins of fibromyalgia in a specific social setting. *Rheumatology*, **42**, 507–15.

Hickie, I., Hadzi-Pavlovic, D., Parker, G., *et al.* (1995). Can the chronic fatigue syndrome be defined by distinct clinical features? *Psychological Medicine*, **25**, 925–35.

Hickie, I., Kirk, K. and Martin, N. (1999). Unique genetic and environmental determinants of prolonged fatigue: a twin study. *Psychological Medicine*, **29**, 259–68.

Hotopf, M., Noah, N. and Wessely, S. (1996). Chronic fatigue and minor psychiatric morbidity after viral meningitis: a controlled study. *Journal of Neurology, Neurosurgery and Psychiatry*, **60**(5), 504–9.

Hotopf, M., Mayou, R., Wadsworth, M., *et al.* (1998). Temporal relationships between physical symptoms and psychiatric disorder: results from a national birth cohort. *British Journal of Psychiatry*, **173**, 255–61.

Hotopf, M., Mayou, R., Wadsworth, M., *et al.* (1999). Childhood risk factors for adults with medically unexplained symptoms: results from a national birth cohort study. *American Journal of Psychiatry*, **156**(11), 1796–800.

Hudson, J., Goldenberg, D., Pope, H. G., Jr, *et al.* (1992). Comorbidity of fibromyalgia with medical and psychiatric disorders. *American Journal of Medicine*, **92**, 363–7.

Jailwala, J., Imperiale, T. and Kroenke, K. (2000). Pharmacologic treatment of the irritable bowel syndrome: a systematic review of randomized, controlled trials. *Annals of Internal Medicine*, **133**, 136–47.

Jason, L., Richman, J., Rademaker, A. W., *et al.* (1999). A community-based study of chronic fatigue syndrome. *Archives of Internal Medicine*, **159**, 2129–37.

Joyce, J., Hotopf, M. and Wessely, S. (1997). The prognosis of chronic fatigue and chronic fatigue syndrome: a systematic review. *Quarterly Journal of Medicine*, **90**, 223–33.

Karjalainen, K., Malmivaara, A., Van Tulder, M., *et al.* (1999). Multidisciplinary rehabilitation for fibromyalgia and musculoskeletal pain in working age adults (Cochrane Review). *Cochrane Database of Systematic Reviews*. Chichester, John Wiley & Sons Ltd.

Karjalainen, K., Malmivaara, A., Van Tulder, M., *et al.* (2000). Biopsychosocial rehabilitation for upper limb repetitive strain injuries in working age adults (Cochrane Review). *Cochrane Database of Systematic Reviews*. Chichester, John Wiley & Sons Ltd.

Kay, L., Jorgensen, T. and Jensen, K. H. (1994). The epidemiology of irritable bowel syndrome in a random population: prevalence, incidence, natural history and risk factors. *Journal of Internal Medicine*, **236**, 23–30.

Kisely, S. R. (2002). Treatments for chronic fatigue syndrome and the internet: a systematic survey of what your patients are reading. *Australian and New Zealand Journal of Psychiatry*, **36**, 240–5.

Kisely, S., Campbell, L. and Skerrit, P. (2005). Psychological interventions for symptomatic management of non-specific chest pain in patients with normal coronary anatomy. *Cochrane Database of Systematic Reviews*. Chichester, John Wiley & Sons Ltd.

Kroenke, K. and Price, R. (1993). Symptoms in the community: prevalence, classification and psychiatric comorbidity. *Archives of Internal Medicine*, **153**, 2474–80.

Kroenke, K. and Spitzer, R. (1998). Gender differences in the reporting of physical and somatoform symptoms. *Psychosomatic Medicine*, **60**(2), 150–5.

Kroenke, K. and Swindle, R. (2000). Cognitive-behavioural therapy for somatization and symptom syndromes: a critical review of controlled clinical trials. *Psychotherapy and Psychosomatics*, **69**, 205–15.

Kroenke, K., Spitzer, R., Williams, J. B., *et al.* (1994). Physical symptoms in primary care: predictors of psychiatric disorders and functional impairment. *Archives of Family Medicine*, **3**, 774–9.

Kwiatek, R., Barnden, L., Tedman, R., *et al.* (2000). Regional cerebral blood flow in fibromyalgia. *Arthritis and Rheumatism*, **43**(12), 2823–33.

Levy, R. L., Whitehead, W. E., Von Korff, M. R., *et al.* (2000). Intergenerational transmission of gastrointestinal illness behavior. *American Journal of Gastroenterology*, **95**(2), 451–6.

Levy, R. L., Jones, K. R., Whitehead, W. E., *et al.* (2001). Irritable bowel syndrome in twins: heredity and social learning both contribute to etiology. *Gastroenterology*, **121**(4), 799–804.

Lewis, D., Mayberg, H., Fishcher, M. E., *et al.* (2001). Monozygotic twins discordant for chronic fatigue syndrome: regional cerebral blood flow SPECT. *Radiology*, **219**, 766–73.

List, T., Axelsson, S. and Leijon, G. (2003). Pharmacologic interventions in the treatment of temporomandibular disorders, atypical facial pain and burning mouth syndrome. A qualitative systematic review. *Journal of Orofacial Pain*, **17**(4), 301–10.

Looper, K. and Kirmayer, L. (2004). Perceived stigma in functional somatic syndromes and comparable medical conditions. *Journal of Psychosomatic Research*, **57**, 373–8.

Lyall, M., Peakman, M. and Wessely, S. (2003). A systematic review and critical evaluation of the immunology of chronic fatigue syndrome. *Journal of Psychosomatic Research*, **55**, 79–90.

MacHale, S., Lawrie, S., Cavanagh, J. T., *et al.* (2000). Cerebral perfusion in chronic fatigue syndrome and depression. *British Journal of Psychiatry*, **176**, 550–6.

MacLean, G. and Wessely, S. (1994). Professional and popular representations of chronic fatigue syndrome. *British Medical Journal*, **308**, 776–7.

Malleson, A. (2002). *Whiplash and Other Useful Illnesses*. Toronto: McGill-Queen's University Press.

Manu, P., Lane, T. and Matthews, D. A. (1989). Somatization disorder in patients with chronic fatigue. *Psychosomatics*, **30**(4), 388–95.

Mayou, R., Levenson, J. and Sharpe, M. (2003). Somatoform disorders in DSM-V. *Psychosomatics*, **44**(6), 449–51.

McGowan, L., Clark-Carter, D., Pitts, M. K., *et al.* (1998). Chronic pelvic pain: a meta-analytic review. *Psychology and Health*, **13**, 937–51.

Mertz, H., Morgan, V., Tanner, G., *et al.* (2000). Regional cerebral activation in irritable bowel syndrome and control subjects with painful and non-painful rectal distension. *Gastroenterology*, **118**, 842–8.

Morris-Yates, A., Talley, N. J., Boyce, P. M., *et al.* (1998). Evidence of a genetic contribution to functional bowel disorder. *American Journal of Gastroenterology*, **93**(8), 1311–17.

Moss-Morris, R. and Spence, M. (2006). To 'lump' or 'split' the functional somatic syndromes: can infectious and emotional risk factors differentiate between the onset of chronic fatigue syndrome and irritable bowel syndrome? *Psychosomatic Medicine*, **68**, 463–9.

Moss-Morris, R. and Wrapson, W. (2003). Representational beliefs about functional somatic syndromes. In *The Self-regulation of Health and Illness Behaviour*, ed. L. Cameron and H. Leventhal. New York: Routledge, pp. 119–37.

Mouterde, O. (2001). Myalgic encephalomyelitis in children. *Lancet*, **357**(9255), 562.

Naliboff, B., Derbyshire, S., Munakata, J., *et al.* (2001). Cerebral activation in patients with irritable bowel syndrome and control subjects during rectosigmoid stimulation. *Psychosomatic Medicine*, **63**, 365–75.

Neumann, L. and Buskila, D. (2003). Epidemiology of fibromyalgia. *Current Pain & Headache Reports*, **7**, 362–8.

Nimnuan, C., Rabe-Hesketh, S., Wessely, S., *et al.* (2001). How many functional somatic syndromes? *Journal of Psychosomatic Research*, **51**(4), 549–57.

Page, L. and Wessely, S. (2003). Medically unexplained symptoms: exacerbating factors in the doctor-patient encounter. *Journal of the Royal Society of Medicine*, **96**, 223–7.

Parker, A., Wessely, S. and Cleare, A. J. (2001). The neuroendocrinology of chronic fatigue syndrome and fibromyalgia. *Psychological Medicine*, **31**, 1331–45.

Peters, S., Stanley, I., Rose, M., *et al.* (1998). Patients with medically unexplained symptoms: sources of patients' authority and implications for demands on medical care. *Social Science & Medicine*, **46**(4–5), 559–65.

Potts, S. and Bass, C. (1993). Psychosocial outcome and use of medical resources in patients with chest pain and normal or near-normal coronary arteries: a long term follow up study. *Quarterly Journal of Medicine*, **86**, 583–93.

Price, J. and Couper J. (1998). Cognitive behavioural therapy for chronic fatigue syndrome in adults (Cochrane Review). *The Cochrane Database of Systematic Reviews*. Chichester: John Wiley & Sons Ltd.

Reid, J., Ewan, C. and Lowy, E. (1991). Pilgrimage of pain: the illness experiences of women with repetition strain injury and the search for credibility. *Social Science & Medicine*, **32**(5), 601–12.

Reilly, J., Baker, G., Rhodes, J., *et al.* (1999). The association of sexual and physical abuse with somatization: characteristics of patients presenting with irritable bowel syndrome and non-epileptic attack disorder. *Psychological Medicine*, **29**, 399–406.

Ring, A., Dowrick, C., Humphris, G., *et al.* (2004). Do patients with unexplained physical symptoms pressurise general practitioners for somatic treatment? A qualitative study. *British Medical Journal*, **328**, 1057.

Ring, A., Dowrick, C., Humphris, G. M., *et al.* (2005). The somatising effect of clinical consultation: what patients and doctors say and do not say when patients present medically unexplained physical symptoms. *Social Science and Medicine*, **61**, 1505–15.

Robbins, J. and Kirmayer, L. (1990). Illness worry and disability in fibromyalgia syndrome. *International Journal of Psychiatry in Medicine*, **20**, 49–63.

Robbins, J., Kirmayer, L. and Hemani, S. (1997). Latent variable models of functional somatic distress. *The Journal of Nervous and Mental Disease*, **185**, 606–15.

Rossy, L., Buckelew, S., Dorr, N., *et al.* (1999). A meta-analysis of fibromyalgia treatment interventions. *Annals of Behavioral Medicine*, **21**(2), 180–91.

Saito, Y., Locke, R., Talley, N. J., *et al.* (2000). A comparison of the Rome and Manning criteria for case identification in epidemiological investigations of irritable bowel syndrome. *American Journal of Gastroenterology*, **95**, 2816–24.

Salmon, P. and Marchant-Haycox, S. (2000). Surgery in the absence of pathology. The relationship of patients' presentation to gynaecologists' decisions for hysterectomy. *Journal of Psychosomatic Research*, **49**, 119–24.

Schmaling, K., Lewis, D., Fiedelak, J. I., *et al.* (2003). Single-photon emission computerized tomography and neurocognitive function in patients with chronic fatigue syndrome. *Psychosomatic Medicine*, **65**, 129–36.

Schrader, H., Obelieniene, D., Bovim, G., *et al.* (1996). Natural evolution of late whiplash syndrome outside the medicolegal context. *Lancet*, **347**, 1207–11.

Sharpe, M. and Bass, C. (1992). Pathophysiological mechanisms in somatisation. *International Review of Psychiatry*, **4**, 81–97.

Sharpe, M. and Carson, A. (2001). 'Unexplained' somatic symptoms, functional syndromes and somatization: do we need a paradigm shift? *Annals of Internal Medicine*, **134**, 926–30.

Sharpe, M., Hawton, K., Seagroatt, V., *et al.* (1992). Follow up of patients presenting with fatigue to an infectious diseases clinic. *British Medical Journal*, **305**, 147–52.

Sharpe, M., Mayou, R., Seagroatt, V., *et al.* (1994). Why do doctors find some patients difficult to help? *Quarterly Journal of Medicine*, **87**, 187–93.

Shorter, E. (1995). Sucker-punched again! Physicians meet the disease-of-the-month syndrome. *Journal of Psychosomatic Research*, **39**(2), 115–18.

Silverman, D., Munakata, J., Ennes, H., *et al.* (1997). Regional cerebral activity in normal and pathological perception of visceral pain. *Gastroenterology*, **112**, 64–72.

Sim, J. and Adams, N. (2002). Systematic review of randomized controlled trials of non-pharmacological interventions for fibromyalgia. *The Clinical Journal of Pain*, **18**, 324–36.

Sullivan, P., Smith, W. and Buchwald, D. (2002). Latent class analysis of symptoms associated with chronic fatigue syndrome and fibromyalgia. *Psychological Medicine*, **32**, 881–8.

Sullivan, P., Evengard, B., Jacks, A., *et al.* (2005). Twin analyses of chronic fatigue in a Swedish national sample. *Psychological Medicine*, **35**, 1327–36.

Talley, N. and Spiller, R. (2002). Irritable bowel syndrome: a little understood organic bowel disease? *Lancet*, **360**, 555–64.

Taylor, R., Jason, L. and Schoeny, M. E. (2001). Evaluating latent variable models of functional somatic distress in a community-based sample. *Journal of Mental Health*, **10**(3), 335–49.

Twemlow, S., Bradshaw, Jr, S., Coyne, L., *et al.* (1997). Patterns of utilization of medical care and perceptions of the relationship between doctor and patient with chronic illness including chronic fatigue syndrome. *Psychological Reports*, **80**(2), 643–58.

Valim, V., Oliveira, L., Suda, A. L., *et al.* (2002). Peak oxygen uptake and ventilatory anaerobic threshold in fibromyalgia. *Journal of Rheumatology*, **29**, 353–7.

Van-Houdenhove, B., Neerinckx, E., Lysens, R., *et al.* (2001). Victimization in chronic fatigue syndrome and fibromyalgia in tertiary care. *Psychosomatics*, **42**, 21–8.

Verbrugge, L. and Ascione, F. (1987). Exploring the iceberg. Common symptoms and how people care for them. *Medical Care*, **25**(6), 539–69.

Verhagen, A., Bierma-Zeinstra, S., Feleus, A., *et al.* (2004a). Ergonomic and physiotherapeutic interventions for treating upper extremity work related disorders in adults (Cochrane Review). *Cochrane Database of Systematic Reviews.* Chichester: John Wiley & Sons Ltd.

Verhagen, A., Schotten-Peeters, G., de Bie, R., *et al.* (2004b). Conservative treatments for whiplash. *Cochrane Database of Systematic Reviews.* Chichester: John Wiley & Sons Ltd.

Walker, E., Roy-Byrne, P., Katon, W. J., *et al.* (1990). Psychiatric illness and irritable bowel syndrome: a comparison with inflammatory bowel syndrome. *American Journal of Psychiatry*, **147**, 1656–61.

Walsh, C., Zainal, N., Middleton, S. J., *et al.* (2001). A family history of chronic fatigue syndrome. *Psychiatric Genetics*, **11**, 123–8.

Weinman, J., Petrie, K., Moss-Morris, R., *et al.* (1996). The illness perception questionnaire: a new method for assessing the cognitive representation of illness. *Psychology and Health*, **11**, 431–45.

Wessely, S. (1990). Old wine in new bottles: neurasthenia and 'ME'. *Psychological Medicine*, **20**, 35–53.

Wessely, S. (1995). The epidemiology of chronic fatigue syndrome. *Epidemiologic Reviews*, **17**, 139–51.

Wessely, S. (2001). Chronic fatigue: symptom and syndrome. *Annals of Internal Medicine*, **134**, 838–43.

Wessely, S., Chalder, T., Hirsch, S., *et al.* (1996). Psychological symptoms, somatic symptoms and psychiatric disorder in chronic fatigue and chronic fatigue syndrome: a prospective study in the primary care setting. *American Journal of Psychiatry*, **153**, 1050–9.

Wessely, S., Nimnuan, C. and Sharpe, M. (1999). Functional somatic syndromes: one or many? *Lancet*, **354**, 936–9.

White, P., Thomas, J., Amess, J., *et al.* (1998). Incidence, risk and prognosis of acute and chronic fatigue syndromes and psychiatric disorders after glandular fever. *British Journal of Psychiatry*, **173**, 475–81.

Whiting, P., Bagnall, A.-M., Sowden, A. J., *et al.* (2001). Interventions for the treatment and management of chronic fatigue syndrome. A systematic review. *Journal of the American Medical Association*, **286**, 1360–8.

Wigers, S. (1996). Fibromyalgia outcome: the predictive values of symptom duration, physical activity, disability pension and critical life events – a 4.5 year prospective study. *Journal of Psychosomatic Research*, **41**(3), 235–43.

Wilson, A., Hickie, I., Hadzi-Pavlovic, D., *et al.* (2001). What is chronic fatigue syndrome? Heterogeneity within an international multicentre study. *Australian and New Zealand Journal of Psychiatry*, **35**, 520–7.

Wolfe, F., Ross, K., Anderson, J., *et al.* (1995). The prevalence and characteristics of fibromyalgia in the general population. *Arthritis and Rheumatism*, **38**(1), 19–28.

Woodward, R., Broom, D. and Legge, D. G. (1995). Diagnosis in chronic illness: disabling or enabling – the case of chronic fatigue syndrome. *Journal of the Royal Society of Medicine*, **88**, 325–9.

Zakrzewska, J., Forsell, H. and Glenny, A. (2004). Interventions for the treatment of burning mouth syndrome (Cochrane Review). *Cochrane Database of Systematic Reviews.* Chichester: John Wiley & Sons Ltd.

8

Alcohol problems in the general hospital

Jonathan Chick

Liaison psychiatrists may have misgivings when surgeons and physicians refer patients with alcohol problems. Psychiatrists have no monopoly in how to advise on lifestyle change. The professional background of those treating the problem drinker differs between cities and countries, and the available services vary greatly. That alcohol problems are seen in all departments of a general hospital is not in doubt, as will be seen in the first section of this chapter. What can then be done effectively, and by whom, follows later.

Alcohol-related diseases

Table 8.1 lists the conditions seen in the general hospital with an established association with alcohol consumption. Epidemiological overviews including meta-analyses have quantified the relationship of alcohol consumption to morbidity and mortality (English *et al.* 1995; Gutjahr & Gmel 2001; Single *et al.* 1999). Beyond lists of harm, these epidemiological reviews agree that for some disorders of middle age, namely coronary heart disease, ischaemic stroke, diabetes and cholelithiasis, consumption of alcohol up to four 'drinks' per day (40 g ethanol, or five UK 'units'; three 'drinks' per day for women) is associated with reduced morbidity and mortality.

Some non-fatal conditions appear in Table 8.1, e.g. nosebleed (McGarry *et al.* 1994), myopathy (Preedy & Peters 1994) and, known for centuries, secondary erectile impotence. Some admissions to medical wards that do not acquire a disease appellation have also been shown to be alcohol-related, such as 'non-specific chest pain' (Chick *et al.* 2000) or 'variant angina' (e.g. Matsuguchi *et al.* 1984). While weight loss with malnutrition occurs in severe alcohol

Handbook of Liaison Psychiatry, ed. Geoffrey Lloyd and Elspeth Guthrie. Published by Cambridge University Press. © Cambridge University Press 2007.

Table 8.1. Alcohol-related presentations to the general hospital.

Trauma
Multiple presentations to A&E with trauma and head injury
Assault
Falls and collapses in the elderly
Traffic accidents
Industrial injuries
Accidental hypothermia
Drowning
Fire injury

Poisoning
Overdose
Alcohol poisoning

Gastrointestinal
Dyspepsia, gastritis, haematemesis
Diarrhoea and malabsorption
Acute and chronic pancreatitis
Liver abnormalities from deranged LFTS, through hepatitis to fatty liver and cirrhosis

Cardiac
Cardiac arrhythmias
Hypertension and stroke
Cardiomyopathy with heart failure

Neurological
Peripheral neuropathy, cerebellar ataxia
Impotence and problems with libido
Withdrawal seizures and fits starting in middle age
Wernicke's encephalopathy
Dementia

Haematological
Bleeding disorders, including presentation as nosebleed
Thrombocytopaenia
Neutropaenias

Skin
Acne rosacea, discoid eczema, psoriasis, multiple bruising

Cancer
Cancers of mouth, lip, pharynx, larynx, oesophagus, breast, liver, colon

Musculo-skeletal
Gout
Acute and chronic myopathies
Osteoporosis

Table 8.1. (*cont.*)

Respiratory
Aspiration of vomitus
Rib fractures

Reproductive
Unexplained infertility
Spontaneous abortion; fetal damage; prematurity; low birth weight

---

dependence where there is gastritis or liver disorder, heavy drinking is a cause of obesity (Wannamethee & Shaper 2003).

Alcohol use disorders account for 1.4% of the total world burden of disease, and about 8% of disability, according to recent estimates of the World Health Organization (WHO 2002).

The prevalence of patients with an alcohol-related diagnosis in the beds of a general hospital varies depending on the location, e.g. downtown urban hospitals will have higher rates than rural hospitals. It may also vary according to the point in time of the survey, as rates change with social and cultural change. For example, through the 1980s and 1990s in North America, indices for alcohol-related liver disease declined (Smart *et al.* 1998) while during the same period in Scotland (Scottish Executive 2002) and England (Department of Health 2001) alcohol-related mortality rates increased, as did the admission rates for alcohol-related disorders. In Scotland alcohol-related admissions increased from 12 220 in 1990 to 32 925 in 2000. This does not include admissions where the primary diagnosis did not mention alcohol but alcohol may have contributed, e.g. pancreatitis or injuries. Butler *et al.* (2001) found that alcohol-related conditions (19%) and respiratory conditions (19%) were the two most common categories of acute medical admission.

In most general hospitals, the inpatient services addressing the highest rates of alcohol problems are toxicology (related to overdose), head injury (due to falls, assaults and road accidents), and gastrointestinal (haemorrhage and liver disorder; Gerke *et al.* 1997).

Reviews have attempted to quantify the considerable cost to health services of managing alcohol problems (Royal College of Physicians 2001; Scottish Executive 2002).

The concept of hazardous drinking

The above disorders are classified as harmful drinking (i.e. harm has been caused by consuming alcohol), or, if there has been repeated harm, as dependence on alcohol. The term 'hazardous drinking' does not appear in disease classifications, but has wide use. Hazardous drinking is sometimes used loosely for those who have experienced minor as opposed to serious harm. It is synonymous with 'at-risk drinking' and may be defined as the consumption of:

- over 40 g of pure ethanol (5 units) per day on average for men
- over 20 g of pure ethanol (2.5 units) per day on average for women.

These figures are based on epidemiological and clinical evidence of the point at which self-reported levels of drinking begin to show an increased risk of harm. The point on the risk curve deemed to merit a warning is arbitrary (Corrao et al. 1999; Greenfield 2001; Rydberg & Albeck 1998).

Men who admit to alcohol consumption of 40 g per day on average have double the risk for liver disease, hypertension and some cancers. This risk level also applies to the risk for trauma and death, because some drinkers whose *average* daily consumption of alcohol is 40 g per day might only drink once per week but consume seven times that amount on a single day and incur harm associated with acute intoxication. For women, 20 g per day average alcohol consumption puts them at greater risk of liver disease and breast cancer.

Detection

Detecting alcohol dependence and harmful drinking

Detection of active alcohol dependence by the admitting staff in general hospitals is extremely important (a) to prevent the emergence of delirium tremens on the second or third day of admission, (b) to detect Wernicke's syndrome and (c) to reduce unnecessary investigations. Psychiatrists should be aware that alcohol dependence can obscure psychiatric diagnosis.

Sometimes the liaison psychiatrist will be the first to make the diagnosis. These patients may not have been candid to the admitting staff about their consumption, because of shame, or because they fear that declaring their drinking will trigger hostile or critical reactions and an order to abstain from alcohol which they are not yet ready to contemplate.

The physical diagnosis will often be the alerting signal to the clinician. But even when the diagnosis is obvious, a sensitive interview to clarify contributants to the presentation will lay a foundation for a therapeutic alliance, which is an important predictor of outcome in the treatment of alcohol dependence (Connors et al. 1997).

Diagnosis as the first step in therapy

In clinical practice, where a behaviour change is implicated the diagnostic process is a first step in therapy. The interview should be empathic and non-judgemental.

- Start with the patient's current symptoms and concerns.
- Ask the patient about relieving and exacerbating factors, including, without premature closure on alcohol as the whole cause, how alcohol relates to the symptoms, e.g. while morning nausea and vomiting may be due to alcoholic gastritis or withdrawal, the patient may have perceived alcohol as relieving the discomfort.
- Elicit weekly total consumption, and recent maximum on an occasion.
- Enquire into any family, work or legal concerns, and the contribution, if any, of the drinking.
- Check for dependence symptoms (Box 8.1).

A spirit of collaborative enquiry helps patients reach their own conclusions about the role of alcohol in their troubles. Patients are more convinced by what they hear themselves say than by a recitation of medical advice.

Blood test markers should be obtained, to validate the self-report, to give motivating feedback and for monitoring future consumption. An interview with significant others adds information about the drinking and associated problems, as well as perhaps opening up possibilities for changing some of the social reinforcers of the drinking (see below).

For rapid detection, the CAGE screening questionnaire has survived the test of time because it is brief and easily remembered (Box 8.2). However, if introduced too bluntly, the CAGE questions can seem confrontational or intrusive. CAGE was not designed to detect 'hazardous drinking' and does not do so (McKenzie *et al.* 1996). Its purpose is to detect more severely affected alcohol-dependent patients.

Box 8.1 Clinically important dependence symptoms.

Morning tremor	*Indicate probable need for medication for*
Drinking to relieve withdrawal anxiety	*withdrawal*
or tremor	
Repeated difficulty in cutting down	*Indicates probable need for relapse*
	prevention assistance

Box 8.2 The CAGE questions for screening for alcohol dependence (Ewing 1984).

'Have you:

...attempted to Cut back on drinking

...been Annoyed at criticisms about your drinking

...felt Guilty about drinking

...used alcohol as an Eye-opener'

- Positive answers to 2 or more = probable alcohol dependence

In more recent research, it has been supplemented by adding one, or two, questions on consumption: maximum amount in any recent occasion and/or total week's consumption, in order to capture less severe cases.

Screening for hazardous drinking

AUDIT (Alcohol Use Disorders Inventory; Allen *et al.* 1997; Saunders *et al.* 1993) was designed to detect alcohol use disorders in general, including hazardous drinking. It evolved because of evidence that had emerged in the 1980s that drinkers who did not meet criteria of 'dependence' but were 'hazardous drinkers' were sometimes receptive to a discussion about their drinking with a health worker. The essential elements of AUDIT (10 questions) have been distilled to yield briefer tools, for situations when brevity compensates for slight loss of coverage (sensitivity). 'FAST' (Table 8.2; Hodgson *et al.* 2002) has been tested in a UK maxillofacial injury follow-up clinic and in primary care, and the Paddington Alcohol Test (PAT) in Accident and Emergency (A&E) departments (Wright *et al.* 1998).

Physical signs

Signs at physical examination suggesting heavy drinking are:

- tremor of the tongue and hands
- excessive capillarization of the facial skin and conjunctivae
- bruising and other injuries (including in the elderly) and/or healed rib fractures on X-ray
- alcohol on the breath, or positive breathalyser test
- heavily nicotine-stained fingers
- obesity
- hypertension
- enlarged liver.

Blood-test markers

Many studies have shown that the following are markers of heavy drinking in preceding weeks: mean red blood cell volume (MCV), serum gamma glutamyl transferase (GGT; and, with lower sensitivity, serum aspartate amino-transferase (AST)) and serum carbohydrate deficient transferrin (CDT; Dufour *et al.* 2000; Salaspuro 1999; Scouller *et al.* 2000). The difficulty in assessing their accuracy as diagnostic tests has been that the only available 'gold-standard' has been self-reported consumption. But it is, of course, possible that a biological marker may be more accurate than a self-report; which should be the gold standard?

False-positive results occur due to the other causes of elevation: for GGT, liver disease, obesity and several medications (e.g. statins, anticonvulsants and certain

Table 8.2. The Fast Alcohol Screening Test (FAST) for the detection of probable hazardous drinking.

For the following questions please circle the answer which best applies.
1 drink = 1 unit = 1/2 pint of beer or 1 glass of wine or 1 single spirits

1. MEN: How often do you have EIGHT or more drinks on one occasion?
WOMEN: How often do you have SIX or more drinks on one occasion?
Never   Less than monthly   Monthly   Weekly   Daily/almost daily

Only ask questions 2, 3 and 4 if the response to question 1 is 'Less than monthly' or 'Monthly'.

2. How often during the last year have you been unable to remember what happened the
night before because you had been drinking?
Never   Less than monthly   Monthly   Weekly   Daily/almost daily

3. How often during the last year have you failed to do what was normally expected of you
because of drink?
Never   Less than monthly   Monthly   Weekly   Daily/almost daily

4. In the last year has a relative or friend, or a doctor or other health worker been concerned
about your drinking or suggested you cut down?
No   Yes, on one occasion   Yes, on more than one occasion

Scoring is completed with a glance at the pattern of responses as follows

Stage 1
The first stage only involves question 1.
If the response to question 1 is Never then the patient is not misusing alcohol.
If the response to question 1 is Weekly/Daily or Almost daily then the patient is a hazardous, harmful or dependent drinker. Over 50% of people will be classified using just this one question. Only consider questions 2, 3 and 4 if the response to question 1 is Less than monthly or Monthly.

Stage 2
If the response to question 1 is Less than monthly or Monthly then each of the four questions is scored 0–4. These are then added resulting in a total score between 0 and 16. The person is misusing alcohol if the total score for all four questions is 3 or more.

Score questions 1, 2 and 3 as follows:	Score question 4 as follows:
Never = 0	No = 0
Less than monthly = 1	Yes, on one occasion = 2
Weekly = 3	Yes, on more than one occasion = 4
Daily or almost daily = 4	

In summary, score questions 1–3: 0,1,2,3,4. Score question 4: 0,2,4
The minimum score is 0; the maximum score is 16. The score for hazardous drinking is 3 or more.

Table 8.3. Blood test markers: accuracy in a working male drinking over 60 g per day.

	Sensitivity	False positives	Time to normalize with abstinence (approximate)[a]
MCV	30%	5%	6 weeks
GGT	60%	15%	3–4 weeks
CDT	50%	2%	2 weeks

Notes: MCV = Mean red blood cell volume; GGT = serum gamma glutamyl transferase; CDT = serum carbohydrate deficient transferrin.   [a]Depending on the magnitude of the initial elevation.

antidepressants, notably lofepramine); for MCV (which is the least sensitive and least specific of these markers), macrocytic anaemias, hypothyroidism, liver disease, or anticonvulsants. If elevated due to alcohol, GGT will fall with abstinence with a half-life of about three weeks. MCV remains elevated for several weeks after consumption has reduced and will not detect a recent relapse.

Measuring CDT may be a more accurate marker of very recent (past two weeks) drinking than GGT (Anton *et al.* 1998; Conigrave *et al.* 2002). CDT is normal in mild-to-moderate liver disease. It may be raised in severe liver disease, but otherwise gives few false positives. In most countries there are only selected laboratories routinely performing CDT analysis. It is useful in patients with abnormal liver enzymes suspected to be due to alcohol who may be minimizing the amount they are drinking.

Even though these tests have limited sensitivity and specificity, if elevated in a given patient, they are then useful in monitoring change in consumption.

Biological tests have their greatest role:
- where patients have a reason for minimizing their consumption
- in monitoring patients' progress in reducing their drinking.

Distinguishing primary anxiety and mood disorders

Liaison psychiatrists see many patients whose presenting physical symptoms have been attributed to depression or anxiety. Some are heavy drinkers. The co-existence of these disorders with alcohol dependencies is bi-directional. The evidence supports several mechanisms (Chick 1999a):
- depressed or anxious people may self-medicate with alcohol
- alcohol causes anxiety or depressive symptoms because of the social difficulties and losses which excessive drinkers incur
- in dependent drinkers, withdrawal causes anxiety
- alcohol has a depressive effect (in some individuals, in some settings)

> **Box 8.3 Patients frequently attribute withdrawal symptoms to other causes.**
>
> A teacher who had drunk heavily on holiday stopped drinking on the last day to be ready for work. She had a seizure at the Spanish airport. She believed it had been 'caused by the heat', until she had a second fit some months later, again on sudden cessation of drinking.
>
> A bank executive who drank a half litre of gin every evening woke one morning sweaty and fearful at 4 a.m., thinking he had had a heart attack, which he attributed to stress at work. For several weeks he noticed that his hands shook at morning meetings, which he had put down to 'stress'.

- there is some genetic overlap.

Some features of alcohol dependence mimic the symptoms of anxiety and depressive disorders:

- as alluded to already, mood may be low because of disharmony at home or marital separation, threats of dismissal from work or loss of employment and earning
- early-morning wakening occurs: the patient may have gone quickly to sleep after an evening's drinking, but wakes feeling uneasy when the effect of the alcohol wanes during the night
- the drinker expresses guilt at letting others down
- the drinker may feel a failure
- when drunk, people can be weepy and remorseful
- the drinker may complain of anxiety or even panic, because of an impending stress, e.g. a court appearance or disciplinary hearing at work
- anxiety symptoms occur in alcohol withdrawal (indeed, the first attack in a drinker's emerging panic disorder was usually experienced on a day when he abstained or tried to cut down, or had been unable to get a drink; see Box 8.3).

For correct treatment it is important to make the distinction between primary and secondary mood disorder. But it will almost always be more effective for the patient and therapist to attend to the alcohol problem first (see below).

Alcohol withdrawal syndrome

For the patient newly admitted to a general hospital bed, it is important for the physician to be alert to, and prevent, the emergence of severe alcohol withdrawal symptoms.

The alerting features are:

- At admission:
  - alcohol on the breath
  - the patient has been drinking over half a bottle of spirits a day, or equivalent (6−7 pints of beer, cider or lager; i.e. over 15 units per day)

- history of morning tremor or relief drinking
- elevated MCV and/or GGT
- history of previous severe withdrawal syndrome
- recent codependence on benzodiazepine or other sedative.
- First 24 hours:
  - apprehension
  - tremor
  - insomnia
  - nausea
  - vomiting
  - tachycardia.

High-risk cases

In Palmstierna's (2001) series of 334 patients admitted in alcohol withdrawal, 23 developed delirium despite benzodiazepine treatment. After multivariate analysis, five factors predicted the development of delirium: current infectious disease; heart rate above 120 beats per minute at admission; signs of alcohol withdrawal when the blood alcohol concentration was more than 1 g/litre (i.e. over 100 mg per cent); a history of epileptic seizures; and a previous history of delirium.

Management of alcohol withdrawal

The symptoms of minor withdrawal are those of autonomic arousal (Table 8.4). Patients feel anxious, irritable, restless and easily distracted. They may be reluctant

Table 8.4. Clinical features of alcohol withdrawal.

'Minor'	Intermediate 24–72 hours	Major (delirium tremens) 24–72 hours
Apprehension, anxiety	Clinical features as for minor withdrawal plus the symptoms listed below	Clinical features as for intermediate withdrawal plus the symptoms listed below
Irritability	Hypertension	Hallucinations (may provoke self-harm)
Restlessness	Illusions	Delusions
Weakness	Confusion	Seizures
Tachycardia	Agitation	Cardiac arrhythmias
Sweating	Disorientation	Circulatory collapse
Anorexia	Fear	
Insomnia		

to conform to the restrictions normally expected during hospitalization. It may therefore be preferable to accommodate them in a single room. Staff should be encouraged to talk to them, adopting a quiet, non-judgemental, attitude, to orientate them to the environment, and to give reassurance that the symptoms are temporary. Explaining calmly why they feel as they do, and providing information about the duration of the episode, may help to allay anxiety.

Medication

Early instigation of an oral benzodiazepine (Mayo-Smith 1997) in sufficient dose (e.g. diazepam 40 mg immediately followed by 20 mg 4–6-hourly for 24 hours, reducing to zero over four days) will usually prevent the full-blown syndrome. Protocols should be available so that nurses can monitor symptoms and use extra medication as required. An example would be the Alcohol Withdrawal Scale used by Foy *et al.* (1988), where a 2-hourly dose of diazepam is repeated until the symptoms score has diminished below 10. Giving excess benzodiazepine will result in an unsteady or sleepy patient, whereas not giving sufficient allows a withdrawal seizure or delirium to occur. If delusions and hallucinations are suspected, antipsychotic medication such as haloperidol should be used.

Intravenous diazepam (10–20 mg) is needed if the patient has already reached the point of confusion. Intramuscular haloperidol (10 mg) is added if agitation is severe. Restraint may be necessary.

Notes on type of medication for withdrawal

1. Clomethiazole. Some European medical and surgical units have a tradition of using clomethiazole infusion to control withdrawal symptoms. It is effective but its use has caused concern:
   a. fatal respiratory depression during infusion has been reported
   b. hospital use may have encouraged some general practitioners to prescribe it in oral form for alcohol withdrawal, with fatal respiratory depression in patients who took the drug with alcohol (McInnes 1987)
   c. fluid overload from the infusion (Payne 1986).
2. Which benzodiazepine?
   a. For general hospital use, diazepam is preferred because of ease of moving between oral and intravenous use if necessary. Also its rapid onset of action is suitable for the acute situation where the syndrome is already developing before treatment has been commenced.
   b. For outpatients and in the community, chlordiazepoxide is preferred: it is less likely to be abused than diazepam, or sold on the street, because its onset of action is slower and does not therefore cause a 'buzz' (SIGN 2003).

c. All benzodiazepines can cause temporary cognitive slowing and interfere with new learning and planning. This and the need to avoid benzodiazepine dependence are reasons for keeping the prescription as short as possible.

d. For patients with compromised hepatic metabolism, a benzodiazepine with a short or intermediate half-life and without intermediate metabolites is logical, such as lorazepam or oxazepam

3. Use of antipsychotics: theoretical reduction of seizure threshold is relatively unimportant when an anticonvulsant dose of benzodiazepine has already been given and there is an urgent need to control psychotic symptoms.

4. There appears to be no difference between alcohol withdrawal symptoms in the elderly, or the amount of benzodiazepine required for detoxification, as compared to younger patients. Some studies indicate an increased incidence of delirium in the elderly and this may be related to a greater incidence of acute physical illness (SIGN 2003).

Wernicke's syndrome

Wernicke's syndrome is believed to be due to critical deprivation of thiamine (vitamin B_1) in neurones in the midbrain or thalamus. It often has a rapid onset following weeks of heavy drinking which have interfered with the absorption of thiamine from the intestine; diet may have been deficient. Typically, the family doctor or police may have found the patient in a confused or near-collapsed state, and he is brought to the emergency department. An infection or accident may have led to hospital admission, at which time the consequent sudden cessation of alcohol intake seems to precipitate the condition. A first carbohydrate meal or a dextrose infusion, given with good intentions by admitting hospital staff, may have used up the body's remaining thiamine.

Wernicke's syndrome can be fatal, and if untreated, may be followed by permanent memory damage.

The signs

Any of the following signs in a heavy drinker point to the diagnosis:

- confusion
- unsteadiness
- squint or double vision due to eye muscle paralysis (ophthalmoplegia)
- nystagmus
- memory disturbance
- hypothermia
- hypotension
- coma.

The clinician should not wait for all or even several signs to show. A single sign is sufficient to make the diagnosis (Thomson *et al.* 2002).

Prophylaxis of Wernicke's syndrome

Patients at risk may have one or more of the following features:
- appear malnourished
- recent diarrhoea or vomiting
- drinking 20 units (14 'drinks') per day, or more.

Even without the clinical signs of Wernicke's syndrome, at-risk patients should be given, parenterally, thiamine or high-potency multivitamins daily for 3 days.

Treatment of established Wernicke's syndrome

It is not sufficient to give vitamin supplements by mouth, even in large doses, because small-intestine absorption in these patients is limited (Thomson *et al.* 2002). Thiamine or high-potency multivitamins should be given parenterally twice daily for two days. If no response is seen, this is discontinued and the diagnosis is reviewed. If symptoms respond, it is continued for a further three days.

The risk of an allergic reaction (anaphylaxis) due to parenteral thiamine is low, at least for the product used in the UK (Pabrinex); it has occurred at about one in one million doses (SIGN 2003). Nevertheless, resuscitation equipment and 1 in 1000 adrenaline injection should be available to treat the extremely rare instance of laryngospasm.

Effective interventions for alcohol problems

The systematic review by Miller and Willbourne (2002; Table 8.5) examined the published literature on treatment outcome studies for alcohol problems. They found 361 relevant studies, in which a total of over 60 000 patients had been followed. They devised a cumulative evidence score for each treatment. This score represented the consistency of the advantage to the treatment seen in the trials versus control, adjusted for the methodological quality of those trials, quality points being gained for adequate randomization, clearly defined treatment, clear outcome measures, high follow-up rate, evidence from collaterals and/or biological markers, blindness of the assessors, appropriate statistics, and being multicentre.

At the time of writing, the most up-to-date review of treatment efficacy is by Slattery *et al.* (2003). It dealt with relapse prevention for alcohol dependence following detoxification in treatment-seeking populations. It did not deal with

Table 8.5. Top seven treatments for alcohol problems in the ranking by Miller and Wilbourne (2002): summary scores of reviewed papers.

	% clinical[a]	n +ve[b]	n −ve[b]	CES[c]
Brief intervention	48	20	11	280
Motivational enhancement	53	12	5	173
Acamprosate	100	5	0	116
Naltrexone/nalmefene	100	4	1	100
Social skills training	88	17	8	85
Community reinforcement approach	100	4	0	80
Behaviour contracting	100	4	1	64
Behavioural−marital therapy	100	5	3	60
Case management	100	4	2	33

Notes: [a] % clinical = percentage of studies which were in treatment-seeking clinical populations;
[b] n +ve = number of studies included which were positive (n −ve = negative);
[c] CES = cumulative evidence score (see text).

opportunistic interventions in hazardous drinkers. It analysed published as well as unpublished trials. Studies of sufficient methodological quality, which reported data on outcomes, either specified as rates of abstinence or rates of controlled drinking (typically defined as fewer than five drinks per day or fewer than four per day for women), were meta-analysed so that rates of recovery could be compared. Table 8.6 shows those treatments for which data satisfied these requirements, and which were shown to be more effective than no-treatment-control or basic support.

Social skills training and coping skills training are specialist treatments often provided in group settings. These will not be described further. 'Case management' and 'community reinforcement therapy' have been tested when run by specialist teams, but aspects of each which might transfer to the work of the liaison psychiatry service are the co-ordination of housing applications, advice on benefits and whenever available, the bolstering of family or other supports for socially unsupported patients. A social work colleague knowledgeable about local services may be invaluable. Community reinforcement therapy usually includes prescribing supervised disulfiram (see below) and behavioural marital counselling, in which attention is paid to improving communication and helping couples to find more rewards in the relationship.

Behavioural self-control training, as tested, was conducted by specifically trained clinical psychologists, and has not been widely used by psychiatrists. It is for patients where reduction, rather than abstinence, is the agreed goal.

Table 8.6. Extracted findings of the meta-analyses of Slattery *et al.* (2003) of effectiveness of treatments to prevent relapse in alcohol dependence.

	Number of patients pooled for the meta-analysis	Number of positive studies	Number of negative studies	% patients successful (defined either as totally abstinent, or not drinking >5 drinks in a day, depending on the study's criteria)
Basic support (estimated from UK outcome studies)				15
Acamprosate	4529	14	3	23
Naltrexone	2112	12	5	21
Coping skills training	631	8	1	27
Behavioural self-control training	276	5	0	24
Motivational enhancement	154	2	0	25
Behavioural–marital therapy (including studies of the community reinforcement approach)	742	12	4	26

Notes: study lengths vary from three months to two years; to be included studies had to meet methodological quality criteria, be in alcohol-dependent treatment-seeking populations and report categorical data on drinking outcome specifying an abstinence/or controlled drinking definition.

'Brief intervention'

There is no evidence that 'brief intervention' (BI) is effective in alcohol dependence. In the meta-analyses by Moyer *et al.* (2002), most studies reviewed fell into one of two types: those comparing BI with control conditions in non-treatment-seeking samples ($n=34$) and those comparing BI with extended treatment in treatment-seeking samples ($n=20$). For studies of the first type, small-to-medium aggregate effect sizes in favour of brief interventions emerged across different follow-up points. After 3–6 months, the effect for brief interventions compared to control conditions was significantly greater when individuals with more severe alcohol problems were excluded. For studies of the second type, the effect sizes were largely not significantly different from zero.

Thus, BI is effective for hazardous or harmful drinking identified opportunistically in screening or in medical encounters.

Efficacy studies of BI in the general hospital have been less numerous than in primary care settings. For men admitted to a medical ward, screening for problem drinking followed by a motivating interview by a specialized nurse, in which advice was given, was associated with a reduction in problems and an advantage in GGT after one year (Chick *et al.* 1985). Extrapolated to the routine situation, it is suggested that the admitting nurse and/or physician should include questions about alcohol consumption and problems, and if indicated should have a further 10–20 minute dialogue to help the patient weigh up the pros and cons of his/her current pattern of drinking. BI is supposed to be within the scope of healthcare professionals who have received only limited training in this intervention, without specialist training in substance abuse (see Box 8.4: FRAMES).

Several trials have been conducted in trauma units. A randomized controlled study in men attending a clinic following jaw or facial injuries sustained in falls or fights showed a greater reduction in hazardous drinking 6 and 12 months later than in a control group of fellow-patients, if they had been counselled by the nurse (Smith *et al.* 2003). Likewise, patients admitted to a Seattle trauma unit who screened positive with GGT, a blood-alcohol concentration, or a brief screening interview were randomly allocated to control or BI, which if appropriate also offered addresses of community alcohol treatment agencies. There was a reduction after 12 months in self-reported consumption, and in trauma recidivism. This was clearer in those with a mild/moderate alcohol problem than a severe problem (Gentillelo *et al.* 1999).

Staff working in trauma services may be motivated to offer BI because alcohol is a common factor in repeat attenders. Rivara *et al.* (1993) found that attenders who

Box 8.4 The acronym FRAMES captures the essence of the interventions commonly tested under the rubric 'brief intervention' and 'motivational interviewing'.

- Feedback: about personal risk or impairment possibly linked to the drinking
- Responsibility: emphasis on personal responsibility for change
- Advice: to cut down, or abstain if indicated because of severe dependence or harm
- Menu: of alternative options for changing drinking pattern and, jointly with the patient, setting a target; intermediate goals of reduction can be a start. (Information on calculating how much alcohol the person drinks may be required.)
- Empathetic interviewing: listening reflectively without cajoling or confronting; exploring with patients the reasons for change as they see their situation
- Self-efficacy: an interviewing style which enhances people's belief in their ability to change.

After Bien *et al.* (1993).

were intoxicated were 2.5 times more likely to return in the same year as the average patient, and attenders with a raised GGT were 3.5 times more likely to return.

Intervention of this nature is unlikely to have even a short-term effect on the drinking of the patient with an established alcohol problem or dependence. Referral on to more specialized help will be needed (Elvy *et al.* 1988; Welte *et al.* 1998). However, what intervention is offered and the manner in which it is done, as well as the severity of the population treated, seem to affect the results from these studies. In a gastroenterological ward, Kuchipudi *et al.* (1990) found no benefit of a 'motivational intervention' in 'alcoholics' compared with a non-intervention control condition. Similarly, in a quasi-experimental trial among excessive drinkers on hospital wards, screening and feedback by computer with or without computer advice plus self-help manual showed there was no advantage of adding to the computer advice and manual.

Motivational interviewing

The style of approach used in the original brief intervention studies was already close to that which has become known as motivational interviewing (Miller & Rollnick 2002). Its elements are shown in Table 8.7. As a stand-alone therapy,

Table 8.7. Important elements of motivational interviewing.

Portraying empathy
• Use of open-ended questions and avoiding premature closure.
• Respect for individual differences.
• Reflective listening so that patients sense you are trying to 'get on their wavelength'.
• Expressing interest/concern.
• Acceptance that ambivalence is normal.

Developing discrepancy
• Patients are helped to see the gap between the drinking and its consequences and their own goals/values — the gap between 'where I see myself, and where I want to be'.
• Enhancing their awareness of consequences, perhaps adding feedback about medical symptoms and test results: 'How does this fit in?', 'Would you like the medical research information on this?'
• Weighing up the pros and cons of change and of not changing.
• Progressing the interview so that patients present their own reasons for change.

Avoiding argument ('rolling with resistance')
• Resistance, if it occurs (such as arguing, denial, interrupting, ignoring) is not dealt with head-on, but accepted as understandable, or side-stepped by shifting focus.
• Labelling, such as 'I think you have an alcohol problem' is unnecessary, and can lead to counter-productive arguing.

Table 8.7. (*cont.*)

Supporting self-efficacy
- Encouraging the belief that change is possible.
- Encouraging a collaborative approach (patients are the experts on how they think and feel, and can choose from a menu of possibilities).
- The patient is responsible for choosing and carrying out actions towards change.

Facilitating and reinforcing 'self-motivating statements', e.g.
- Recognizing that alcohol has caused adverse consequences.
- Expressing concern about effects of drinking.
- Expressing the intention to change.
- Being optimistic about change.
- 'People believe what they hear themselves say'.

Source: SIGN 2003, adapted from Miller and Rollnick 2002.

it was ranked eleventh in the evidence table of Miller and Willbourne (2002), but there has been little support for its effect in treating established alcohol dependence on its own, except that it was shown to be the most effective approach in patients who scored as 'angry' at their intake interview in the large US treatment outcome study, Project Match.

Motivational interviewing is, however, a useful skill for all those who interact with patients who are ambivalent about making a lifestyle change for health reasons.

Medications to prevent relapse

Acamprosate

It is possible that acamprosate (calcium homotaurinate) acts to stabilize glutamate receptors left 'oversensitive' in the newly abstinent alcohol-dependent patient. This oversensitivity may hypothetically persist for some months. Animals made dependent on alcohol reinstate their drinking rapidly after a period without alcohol, when alcohol is again made available. This phenomenon is attenuated in animals pretreated with acamprosate (Spanagel *et al.* 1996). Slattery *et al.* (2003) pooled data from all the 17 known randomized controlled trials (RCTs) of acamprosate (including some unpublished studies) — data from a total of 4529 patients. Of these trials, 14 were positive. The trials' duration varied from 3 to 12 months. The meta-analysis yielded an effectiveness odds ratio of 1.73, and a number needed to treat (NNT) of 13 (i.e. for one extra patient to achieve complete abstinence, the drug will need to be prescribed for 13 patients). This is a less impressive NNT than for some antidepressants in treating major depressive disorder, but compares favourably with other medical conditions where costly treatment is offered (SIGN 2000).

Acamprosate is given to dependent patients who have been detoxified (which was not the case in a large US study in which acamprosate was ineffective; Anton *et al.* 2006) and who intend to abstain from drinking. It should be started as soon as that step is clarified, and then its efficacy monitored fortnightly at a minimum at the outset, as only some patients will benefit from it.

Acamprosate is not a drug of abuse: there is no obvious mood-altering effect, no wish to escalate the dose, and no withdrawal syndrome. It is metabolized mainly in the kidney, and is safe in mild and moderate liver disorder.

Opiate antagonists

Naltrexone and nalmefene are antagonists of the brain's endorphin receptors, and have been shown to reduce heavy drinking in alcohol-dependent patients, and, in some studies, to increase rates of complete abstinence. The action by which these drugs reduce alcohol consumption is believed to be via reducing those euphoric effects of the first few alcoholic drinks that lead to 'losing control' during a drinking episode, and perhaps by reducing some of the conditioned positive response to other triggers to drinking before even the first drink is taken. Following the custom in the naltrexone studies to employ 'relapse', defined as drinking five or more drinks in a day (i.e. 8 UK units) as the primary outcome criterion, Slattery *et al.* (2003) combined data for meta-analysis on 2112 patients from 17 RCTs of naltrexone versus placebo where outcome data in the form of 'number not relapsed' were available. Of those studies, 12 were positive. This yielded an odds ratio of 1.46 and a NNT of 17. Naltrexone in the form of a monthly sustained-release preparation has been licensed in the USA.

The literature suggests that naltrexone may only be effective when the physician accepts that, for better or worse, the patient may still wish to drink occasionally, and is prepared to discuss strategies for limiting consumption as well as abstinence.

Disulfiram

Disulfiram's therapeutic function is to act as a deterrent to drinking alcohol. Evidence of efficacy is limited to studies in which the patient swallows the drug under the supervision of a person (e.g. the spouse, partner, a nurse at the workplace, a clinic nurse, or occasionally even an older child), agreed by the patient and the treating therapist. Marital behavioural therapy has been successful in conjunction with a disulfiram prescription, with an agreement that the spouse will monitor the patient taking the disulfiram (e.g. Azrin 1976). This approach is well supported by evidence (Brewer *et al.* 2000). It has been shown to be more effective in single-blind studies than either naltrexone or acamprosate (de Sousa & de Sousa 2004, 2005).

There are a number of unwanted effects (reviewed by Chick 1999b), of which tiredness is the most common. There are rare reports of idiosyncratic liver hypersensitivity, and liver failure, possibly related to drug interactions, that have been fatal on occasion (Chick 1999b; Masia *et al.* 2002). Disulfiram can mobilize nickel stored in the body, causing a 'recall' dermatitis in nickel-allergic individuals. This may clear in a few days. Disulfiram interacts with a number of medications that are metabolized in the liver, sometimes, as with some antidepressants, increasing the bioavailability of the antidepressant, but possibly altering the toxicity of disulfiram or its conversion to its active metabolite, which could weaken its efficacy as a deterrent.

Hypotension is the most dangerous aspect of the disulfiram-ethanol interaction, should the patient risk drinking after regularly taking disulfiram. Therefore, it is necessary to give extra warnings to a patient on hypotensive medication prescribed disulfiram. When a patient has another medical problem being treated by the referring physician, consultation before prescribing disulfiram is advised.

Special situations

Treating the anxious drinker

Anxiety symptoms are common in dependent drinkers but resolve within 6–8 weeks of abstinence (Allan *et al.* 2002; Driessen *et al.* 2001). If they persist, the prognosis is worse (Allan *et al.* 2002; Driessen *et al.* 2001; Willinger *et al.* 2002).

There is emerging evidence that offering at the outset cognitive behavioural therapy specifically for the anxiety disorder, be it social phobia or panic disorder, has no advantage, either for the prevention of relapse or the reduction of anxiety symptoms (Bowen *et al.* 2000; Thevos *et al.* 2000), or even that the outcome might be worse if treatment is initially directed at the anxiety disorder (Randall *et al.* 2001). Thus, priority should be given to treating the alcohol problem.

There is some evidence that buspirone might have a place in alcohol dependence where anxiety disorders persist (Garbutt *et al.* 1999). The advantages and disadvantages of serotonin-specific reuptake inhibitors (SSRIs) for these patients are being investigated.

Treating the depressed drinker

Antidepressants are not effective in preventing relapse in alcohol dependence. However, if major depressive disorder is diagnosed after alcohol withdrawal has been completed for 2–3 weeks, fluoxetine and tricyclics help both the mood and the drinking (Garbutt *et al.* 1999; Pettinati *et al.* 2000).

There is emerging concern that SSRIs might worsen drinking in some patients, specifically, those patients who report an onset of problem drinking before age 25 (who tend to have higher than average rates of social problems; Chick *et al.* 2004; Kranzler *et al.* 1996; Pettinati *et al.* 2000). They have been termed 'type B' (see Kranzler *et al.* 1996).

The liver service

The liaison psychiatrist's role in patients with alcoholic liver disease is reviewed in Chapter 17.

The head injury unit

Memory impairment after head injury is common and contributes to the difficulties in rehabilitating heavy drinkers who sustain an additional trauma due to covert Wernicke's disorder. It is possible that prophylactic parenteral thiamine, given to acutely head-injured drinkers, might reduce some of this disability. A study in a specialist neurosurgical unit found that fewer than half of very heavy drinking head-injured patients were given thiamine. Furthermore, when thiamine was given, it was usually administered orally rather than, as advised above, parenterally (Ferguson *et al.* 1997).

The family may not be able to cope with the aggressive behaviour or repeated drinking that can happen when such brain-damaged patients return to their home. There are a very few specialized residential centres for such patients. Supporting the family in limiting the money to which the patient has access sometimes helps.

The cardiovascular service

Referrals to the liaison psychiatrist of cardiology patients who drink can cause a dilemma. The relation between alcohol and heart disease is complex.

There is an increased rate of sudden cardiac deaths in heavy drinkers. Heavy smoking will be a factor and possibly an arrhythmia brought on by a heavy drinking session. Cardiomyopathy in association with chronic heavy alcohol abuse (see Lee & Regan 2002 for recent review) plays a part and can also lead to congestive cardiac failure.

In Scotland, where heavy session drinking is common, there is an excess of deaths from coronary heart disease on Mondays amongst people with no previous admission for coronary heart disease, particularly amongst men and women under 50 years of age. This has been partly attributed to binge drinking at weekends (Evans *et al.* 2000).

Angina may be brought on by large doses of alcohol (Matsuguchi *et al.* 1984). The clinical dilemma is that, given the epidemiological evidence that alcohol has a protective association for coronary and cerebral arteriosclerosis, abstinence will not appear to be the best advice for some cardiac patients (Chick 1998). However, if cardiac patients are unable to reduce drinking to moderate levels and risk continuing to drink in heavy sessions, then they are probably safer to abstain. Stopping smoking and losing weight, two other lifestyle changes, are found by some to be easier if they are abstinent.

There are similar dilemmas for advising diabetics. While drinking to drunkenness is associated with poor blood sugar control, light and moderate alcohol consumption is associated with reduced risk of diabetic complications and improved life expectancy (Tanescu & Hu 2001).

Liaison psychiatrists may be asked to see patients presenting with hyperventilation syndrome. Alcohol or marijuana was a factor in 17% of acute admissions with that syndrome (Saisch *et al.* 1996). Alcohol dependence should also be considered when the cardiologist refers patients with more classic panic disorder (see above).

The obstetric service

Some studies have found that without specific antenatal advice pregnant women stop or reduce their drinking. However, other services perform specific detection and intervention to reduce the fetal risks from heavy drinking. A short questionnaire, TWEAK, tested in the USA in antenatal clinics, uses two tolerance questions, e.g. 'How many drinks does it take before you feel the first effects of alcohol' (review by Bradley *et al.* 1998). TWEAK may be less stigmatizing and therefore more acceptable, especially in indigent populations than, for example, AUDIT, CAGE or variations. Patients answering 'more than two drinks' (equivalent to just over 3 UK units) are deemed 'at-risk drinkers' (and just 'two drinks' in later work of Chang *et al.* (1999a)). There is no evidence that offering counselling increases the number of antenatal patients who abstain, although one study found that those who are already abstinent tend to remain abstinent if they receive brief counselling (Chang *et al.* 1999b; SIGN 2003).

The emergency department

Intoxicated patients threatening violence to themselves or others

The liaison psychiatrist may be faced with a request to assess intoxicated patients who have attempted self-harm or state that they intend to harm themselves or others. (See Chapter 11 on assessing suicidal behaviour.)

There is ambivalence about performing this difficult task. In London, a third of psychiatrists and nurses answering a survey about managing alcohol problems thought that intoxicated patients presenting at A&E should 'often/always be sent away and asked to return when sober', and 44% of each discipline thought an assessment should 'never/rarely' be made; 55% thought it was not possible to apply the Mental Health Act for compulsory admission to an intoxicated person (Keaney *et al.* 2002).

Patients who are intoxicated are prone to being theatrical, uncooperative or abusive. The doctor should consider whether any injury, illness, or other prescribed or illicit substance is being masked by alcohol consumption. The risk of additional injury to him or herself, or violence to staff or nearby patients, should also be assessed. The doctor's manner should be non-threatening but confident. It might be best to remain seated and use slow measured movements, thereby reducing the risk of provoking aggressive behaviour. Acting calmly and quietly, giving precise instructions and requests, and according the patient the same respect as is given to others, helps achieve the co-operation of such patients who may be bewildered, and due to intoxication lack their normal ability to control their emotions and behaviour. More than one member of staff should be present if the patient is potentially violent. An escape route should be maintained. It may be necessary to have security staff or police on hand.

Requests for 'drying out'

Requests for 'help' (unspecified) or for admission or medication for withdrawal by the individual who is actively drinking are seldom best dealt with as emergencies if withdrawal symptoms are not objectively deemed significant. An assessment should be made of the individual's intentions for the period after he or she has been helped through the withdrawal phase, so that plans can be in place to optimize the chance of a full recovery from the alcohol problem. This is best done in a specialized service. It is important to choose the right timing for the patient to commence the journey of abstinence from alcohol, because that may involve considerable change in way of life. Otherwise, a cycle of repeated detoxifications occurs with only short-term benefits, which can increase patients' sense of hopelessness about their condition. It may even increase the risk of developing seizures in the future (Booth & Blow 1993; Lechtenberg & Worner 1990).

Brief interventions in the A&E setting

A few studies of brief interventions to non-admitted emergency department patients have been conducted. One involved the use of a routine follow-up letter to patients advising attendance at alcohol counselling services. The letter appeared to be useful in encouraging a significant minority of people to attend appropriate specialist services (Batel *et al.* 1995). Open studies have pointed also to some effect of a brief discussion, or an offer of an appointment the next day (Green *et al.* 1993), and Brooks (1987) found that 30% of patients with presumed alcohol problems who were simply handed an information card about local alcohol services subsequently attended those services. The use of follow-up correspondence may be a low-cost intervention that could produce positive results, but more research is needed in this area. Another study delivered an on-site intervention to adolescents presenting with alcohol problems and showed a positive effect of a single intervention (Monti *et al.* 1999).

A further study compared standard care, motivational interviewing or motivational interviewing plus a booster session 7−10 days later (Longabough *et al.* 2001). This study recruited injured patients who screened positive for harmful or hazardous drinking. At one-year follow-up, the 'motivational interviewing plus booster session' group reduced their alcohol-related injuries by 30% more than standard care. There was no difference between standard care and a motivational interview offered at the time without the booster session. The motivational interviewing was delivered by suitably trained research staff.

The evidence to date suggests that brief intervention in the emergency department is beneficial when conducted by specially trained and allocated staff offering and arranging follow up. There is insufficient evidence to recommend routine brief intervention without follow up in A&E (SIGN 2003). Furthermore, transferring research to the real world without specialized staff on site may cause demoralization and tensions (Peters *et al.* 1998).

Recommendation

Patients seen in the emergency department and not admitted who are noted to be drinking harmfully or alcohol dependent should be encouraged to seek advice from their GP or given information on how to contact another suitable agency.

A first seizure in adulthood

In Europe, a first seizure in adulthood has been found to be due to alcohol withdrawal in about a third of cases (Edmonstone 1995; Morrison & McAlpine 1997; Schoenenberger & Heim 1994). Although computerized tomography (CT) shows cerebral atrophy in half of those patients, this finding probably has little or no therapeutic or prognostic value, and a case has been made for omitting a request for a brain CT where a generalized seizure without focal or other neurological signs has occurred in undisputed alcohol withdrawal (Schoenenberger & Heim 1994). However, with the increasing availability of magnetic resonance imaging of the brain, some neurologists would now recommend this more precise investigation.

The elderly

While moderate alcohol consumption in postmenopausal women may protect against osteoporosis, heavy drinking reduces bone density. Helping older patients to use alcohol safely can help prevent disabling injuries.

In assessing confusion in newly admitted elderly patients, withdrawal from alcohol, or from benzodiazepines, may be missed. It was found in English hospitals in the early 1990s that elderly patients tended to report a higher consumption of alcohol if, as well as being asked direct questions about their consumption of alcohol, they were asked about adding spirits to their tea or coffee (Naik & Jones 1994). It is not known whether that was a generational idiosyncrasy or is still true.

The liaison psychiatrist should be aware of the emerging evidence that moderate alcohol consumption, possibly in the form of wine, is associated with lower risk of stroke and dementia than abstention in those over 65 years old, even after adjustments have been made for the other healthy lifestyle influences that are associated with moderate drinking (Chick 1999c; Truelsen *et al.* 2002).

Organizational issues

A delirious patient running amok in a general hospital ward can do serious harm to himself, other patients and staff. Compensation claims can be expected from the families of patients who die in an uncontrolled succession of withdrawal seizures, or fracture the spine jumping from a hospital window in a delirium, or who remain permanently impaired following a missed diagnosis of Wernicke's syndrome.

Less dramatically, alcohol problems can be costly to the general hospital in that these patients are often 'repeaters'. General hospitals are advised to:

- have protocols for the prevention and management of the alcohol withdrawal syndrome and Wernicke's syndrome.
- have an on-call team to assemble in emergencies to help ward staff deal with the aggressive or agitated patient.
- encourage intervention, and onward referral if necessary, for alcohol-dependent patients and hazardous drinkers, with a view to reducing repeat admission.
- employ alcohol specialist nurses, who train and support ward nurses and junior medical staff in detecting and managing alcohol problems, promulgate brief intervention for hazardous drinkers, and arrange appropriate onward referral for dependent drinkers (Hillman *et al.* 2001).

REFERENCES

Allan, C., Smith, I. and Mellin, M. (2002). Changes in psychological symptoms during ambulant detoxification. *Alcohol & Alcoholism*, **37**, 241–4.

Allen, J. P., Litten, R. Z., Fertig, J. B., *et al.* (1997). A review of research on the Alcohol Use Disorders Identification Test (AUDIT). *Alcoholism: Clinical & Experimental Research*, **21**, 613–19.

Anton, R. F., Stout, R. L., Roberts, J. S., *et al.* (1998). The effect of drinking intensity and frequency on serum carbohydrate-deficient transferrin and gamma-glutamyl transferase levels in outpatient alcoholics. *Alcoholism: Clinical & Experimental Research*, **22**, 1456–62.

Azrin, N. H. (1976). Improvements in the community reinforcement approach. *Behaviour Research & Therapy*, **14**, 339–48.

Batel, P., Pessione, F., Bouvier, A. M., *et al.* (1995). Prompting alcoholics to be referred to an alcohol clinic: the effectiveness of a simple letter. *Addiction*, **90**, 811–14.

Bien, T. H., Miller, W. R. and Tonigan, J. S. (1993). Brief interventions for alcohol problems: a review. *Addiction*, **88**, 315–36.

Booth, B. M. and Blow, F. C. (1993). The kindling hypothesis: further evidence from a US National study of alcoholic men. *Alcohol & Alcoholism*, **28**, 593–8.

Bowen, R. C., D'Arcy, C., Keegan, D., *et al.* (2000). A controlled trial of cognitive behavioural treatment of panic in alcoholic inpatients with comorbid panic disorder. *Addictive Behaviors*, **25**, 593–7.

Bradley, K. A., Boyd-Wickizer, J., Powell, S. H., *et al.* (1998). Alcohol screening questionnaires in women: a critical review. *Journal of the American Medical Association*, **280**, 166–71.

Brewer, C., Meyer, R. J. and Johnsen, J. (2000). Does disulfiram help to prevent relapse in alcohol abuse? *CNS Drugs*, **14**, 329–41.

Brooks, S. C. (1987). Use of cards to offer follow-up to patients seen in an Accident and Emergency Department with an alcohol related problem. *British Journal of Accident and Emergency Medicine*, **2**, 11.

Butler, S. R., Hislop, W. S., Fisher, B. M., *et al.* (2001). Consultants workload due to alcohol related conditions in acute medical receiving, gastroenterology and endocrinology. *Scottish Medical Journal*, **46**, 104–5.

Chang, G., Wilkins-Haug, L., Berman, S., *et al.* (1999a). The TWEAK: application in a prenatal setting. *Journal of Studies on Alcohol*, **60**, 306–9.

Chang, G., Wilkins-Haug, L., Berman, S., *et al.* (1999b). Brief intervention for alcohol use in pregnancy: a randomized trial. *Addiction*, **94**, 1499–508.

Chick, J. (1998). Alcohol, health and the heart: implications for clinicians. *Alcohol & Alcoholism*, **33**, 576–91.

Chick, J. (1999a). Alcohol dependence, anxiety and mood disorders. *Current Opinion in Psychiatry*, **12**, 297–301.

Chick, J. (1999b). Safety issues concerning the use of disulfiram in treating alcohol dependence. *Drug Safety*, **20**, 427–35.

Chick, J. (1999c). Can light or moderate drinking benefit mental health? *European Addiction Research*, **5**, 74–81.

Chick J., Lloyd, G. G. and Crombie, E. (1985). Counselling problems drinkers in medical wards: a controlled study. *British Medical Journal*, **290**, 965–7.

Chick, J., Morrell, J., Paterson, J., *et al.* (2000). A middle-aged professional man presents with a number of clinical features which are probably alcohol related. *Coronary Health Care*, **4**, 33–8.

Chick, J., Aschauer, H. and Hornik, K. (2004). Efficacy of fluvoxamine in preventing relapse in alcohol dependence: a one-year, double blind, placebo-controlled multicentre study with analysis by typology. *Drug & Alcohol Dependence*, **74**, 61–70.

Conigrave, K. M., Louisa, J., Degenhardt, L. J., *et al.* (2002). CDT, GGT, and AST as markers of alcohol use: the WHO/ISBRA Collaborative Project. *Alcoholism: Clinical & Experimental Research*, **26**, 332–9.

Connors, G. J., Carroll, K. M., DiClemente, C. C., *et al.* (1997). The therapeutic alliance and its relationship to alcoholism treatment participation and outcome. *Journal of Consulting & Clinical Psychology*, **65**, 588–98.

Corrao, G., Bagnardi, V., Zambon, A., *et al.* (1999). Exploring the dose-response relationship between alcohol consumption and the risk of several alcohol-related conditions: a meta-analysis. *Addiction*, **94**, 1551–73.

Department of Health (DoH). (2001). *The Annual Report of the Chief Medical Officer of the Department of Health 2001: On the State of the Public Health*. London: DoH.

De Sousa, A., and de Sousa, A. (2004). A one-year pragmatic trial of naltrexone vs disulfiram in the treatment of alchol dependence. *Alcohol & Alcoholism*, **39**, 528–31.

De Sousa, A., and de Sousa, A. (2005). An open randomized study comparing disulfiram and acamprosate in the treatment of alcohol dependence. *Alcohol & Alcoholism*, **40**, 545–8.

Driessen, M., Meier, S., Hill, A., *et al.* (2001). The course of anxiety, depression and drinking behaviours after completed detoxification in alcoholics with and without comorbid anxiety and depressive disorders. *Alcohol & Alcoholism*, **36**, 249–55.

Dufour, D. R., Lott, J. A., Nolte, F. S., *et al.* (2000). Diagnosis and monitoring of hepatic injury. II. Recommendations for use of laboratory tests in screening, diagnosis, and monitoring. *Clinical Chemistry*, **46**, 2050–68.

Edmonstone, W. M. (1995). How do we manage the first seizure in adults? *Journal of the Royal College of Physicians of London*, **29**, 289–94.

Elvy, G. A., Wells, J. E. and Baird, K. A. (1988). Attempted referral as intervention for problem drinking in the general hospital. *British Journal of Addiction*, **83**, 83–90.

English, D. R., Holman, C. D. J., Milne, E., *et al.* (1995). *The Quantification of Drug-caused Morbidity and Mortality in Australia 1995*. Canberra: Commonwealth Department of Human Services and Health.

Evans, C., Chalmers, J., Capewell, S., *et al.* (2000). 'I don't like Mondays' – day of the week of coronary heart disease deaths in Scotland: study of routinely collected data. *British Medical Journal*, **320**, 218–19.

Ewing, J. A. (1984). Detecting alcoholism: the CAGE questionnaire. *Journal of the American Medical Association*, **252**, 1905–7.

Ferguson, R. K., Soryal, I. N. and Pentland, B. (1997). Thiamine deficiency in head injury: a missed insult? *Alcohol & Alcoholism*, **32**, 493–500.

Foy, A., March, S. and Drinkwater, V. (1988). Use of an objective clinical scale in the assessment and management of alcohol withdrawal in a large general hospital. *Alcoholism: Clinical & Experimental Research*, **12**, 360–4.

Garbutt, J. C., West, S. L., Carey, T. S., *et al.* (1999). Pharmacological treatment of alcohol dependence – a review of the evidence. *Journal of the American Medical Association*, **281**, 1318–25.

Gentilello, L. M., Rivara, F. P., Donovan, D. M., *et al.* (1999). Alcohol interventions in a trauma center as a means of reducing the risk of injury recurrence. *Annals of Surgery*, **230**, 473–80; discussion 480–3.

Gerke, P., Hapke, U., Rumpf, H. J., *et al.* (1997). Alcohol-related diseases in general hospital patients. *Alcohol & Alcoholism*, **32**, 179–84.

Green, M., Setchell, J., Haines, P., *et al.* (1993). Management of alcohol abuse in accident and emergency departments. *Journal of the Royal Society of Medicine*, **86**, 393–5.

Greenfield, T. K. (2001). Individual risk of alcohol related disease and problems. In *International Handbook of Alcohol Dependence and Problems*, ed. N. Heath, T. Peters and T. Stockwell. London: Wiley, pp. 413–37.

Gutjahr, E. and Gmel, G. (2001). Defining alcohol-related fatal medical conditions for social-cost studies in western societies: an update of the epidemiological evidence. *Journal of Substance Abuse*, **13**, 239–64.

Hillman, A., McCann, B. and Walker, N. P. (2001). Specialist alcohol liaison nurses in general hospitals improve engagement in alcohol rehabilitation and treatment outcome. *Health Bulletin*, **58**, 420–3.

Hodgson, R., Alwyn, T., John, B., *et al.* (2002). The FAST Alcohol Screening Test. *Alcohol & Alcoholism*, **37**, 61–6.

Keaney, F., Boys, A., Jones, C. W., *et al.* (2002). Assessing alcohol-intoxicated patients. *Psychiatric Bulletin*, **26**, 468.

Kranzler, H. R., Burleson, J. A., Brown, J., *et al.* (1996). Fluoxetine treatment seems to reduce the beneficial effect of cognitive-behavioural therapy in Type B alcoholics. *Alcoholism: Clinical & Experimental Research*, **20**, 1534–41.

Kuchipudi, V., Holbein, K., Flickinger, A., *et al.* (1990). Failure of a 2-hour motivational intervention to alter recurrent drinking behaviour in alcoholics with gastrointestinal disease. *Journal of Studies on Alcohol*, **51**, 403–23.

Lee, W. K. and Regan, T. J. (2002). Alcoholic cardiomyopathy: is it dose-dependent? *Congestive Heart Failure*, **8**, 303–6.

Lechtenberg, R. and Worner, T. M. (1990). Seizure risk with recurrent alcohol detoxification. *Archives of Neurology*, **47**, 535–8.

Longabaugh, R., Woolard, R. E., Nirenberg, T. D., *et al.* (2001). Evaluating the effects of a brief motivational intervention for injured drinkers in the emergency department. *Journal of Studies on Alcohol*, **62**, 806–16.

Masia, M., Gutierrez, F., Jimeno, A., *et al.* (2002). Fulminant hepatitis and fatal toxic epidermal necrolysis (Lyell disease) coincident with clarithromycin administration in an alcoholic patient receiving disulfiram therapy. *Archives of Internal Medicine*, **162**, 474–6.

Matsuguchi, T., Araki, H., Anan, T., *et al.* (1984). Provocation of variant angina by alcohol ingestion. *European Heart Journal*, **5**, 906–12.

Mayo-Smith, M. F. (1997). Pharmacological management of alcohol withdrawal. A meta-analysis and evidence-based practice guideline. American Society of Addiction Medicine Working Group on Pharmacological Management of Alcohol Withdrawal see comments. *Journal of the American Medical Association*, **278**, 144–51.

McGarry, G. W. M., Gatehouse, S. and Hinnie, J. (1994). Relation between alcohol and nose bleeds. *British Medical Journal*, **309**, 640.

McInnes, G. T. (1987). Chlormethiazole and alcohol: a lethal cocktail. *British Medical Journal*, **314**, 592.

McKenzie, D. M., Lange, A. and Brown, T. M. (1996). Identifying hazardous or harmful alcohol use in medical admissions: a comparison of AUDIT, CAGE and Brief MAST. *Alcohol & Alcoholism*, **31**, 591–9.

Miller, W. R. and Rollnick, N. (2002). *Motivational Interviewing*, 2nd edn. New York and London: Guilford Press.

Miller, W. R. and Wilbourne, P. L. (2002). Mesa Grande: a methodological analysis of clinical trials of treatments for alcohol use disorders. *Addiction*, **97**, 265–77.

Monti, P. M., Colby, S. M., Barnett, N. P., *et al.* (1999). Brief intervention for harm reduction with alcohol-positive older adolescents in a hospital emergency department. *Journal of Consulting & Clinical Psychology*, **67**, 989–94.

Morrison, A. D. and McAlpine, C. H. (1997). The management of first seizures in adults in a district general hospital. *Scottish Medical Journal*, **42**, 73–5.

Moyer, A., Finney, J. W., Swearingen, C. E., *et al.* (2002). Brief interventions for alcohol problems: a meta-analytic review of controlled investigations in treatment-seeking and non-treatment-seeking populations. *Addiction*, **97**, 279–92.

Naik, P. C. and Jones, R. G. (1994). Alcohol histories taken from elderly people on admission. *British Medical Journal*, **308**, 248.

Palmstierna, T. (2001). A model for predicting alcohol withdrawal delirium. *Psychiatric Services*, **52**, 820–3.

Payne, J. P. (1986). Anaesthesia and the problem drinker. *Hospital Update*, **April**, 287–96.

Peters, J., Brooker, C., McCabe, C., *et al.* (1998). Problems encountered with opportunistic screening for alcohol-related problems in patients attending an Accident and Emergency department. *Addiction*, **93**, 589–94.

Pettinati, H. M., Oslin, D. and Decker, K. (2000). Role of serotonin and serotonin-selective pharmacotherapy in alcohol dependence. *CNS Spectrums*, **5**, 33–46.

Preedy, V. R. and Peters, T. J. (1994). Alcohol and muscle disease. *Journal of the Royal Society of Medicine*, **87**, 188–9.

Randall, C. L., Thomas, S. and Thevos, A. K. (2001). Concurrent alcoholism and social anxiety disorder: a first step toward developing effective treatments. *Alcohol: Clinical & Experimental Research*, **25**, 210–20.

Rivara, F. P., Koepsell, T. D., Jurkovich, G. J., *et al.* (1993). The effects of alcohol abuse on readmission for trauma. *Journal of the American Medical Association*, **270**, 1962–4.

Royal College of Physicians. (2001). *Alcohol – Can the NHS Afford It? Recommendations for a Coherent Strategy for Hospitals.* Report of a working party. London: Royal College of Physicians.

Rydberg, U. S. and Allebeck, P., ed. (1998). Proceedings: State of the Art Conference: risks and protective factors of alcohol on the individual. *Alcoholism: Clinical & Experimental Research*, **22**, 269S–373S.

Saisch, S. G., Wessely, S. and Gardner, W. N. (1996). Patients with acute hyperventilation presenting to an inner-city emergency department. *Chest*, **110**, 952–7.

Salaspuro, M. (1999). Carbohydrate-deficient transferrin as compared to other markers of alcoholism: a systematic review. *Alcohol*, **19**, 261–71.

Saunders, J. B., Aasland, O. G., Babor, T. F., *et al.* (1993). Development of the Alcohol Use Disorders Identification Test (AUDIT): WHO collaborative project on early detection of persons with harmful alcohol consumption – II. *Addiction*, **88**, 791–804.

Scottish Executive. (2002). *Plan for Action on Alcohol Problems.* Scottish Executive; available: www.scotland.gov.uk/health/alcoholproblems.

Scouller, K., Conigrave, K. M., Macaskill, P., *et al.* (2000). Should we use carbohydrate-deficient transferrin instead of gamma-glutamyltransferase for detecting problem drinkers? A systematic review and meta-analysis. *Clinical Chemistry*, **46**, 1894–902.

Schoenenberger, R. A. and Heim, S. M. (1994). Indication for computed tomography of the brain in patients with first uncomplicated generalised seizure. *British Medical Journal*, **309**, 986–9.

SIGN. (2000). *Secondary Prevention of Coronary Heart Disease Following Myocardial Infarction.* Edinburgh: Scottish Intercollegiate Guidelines Network SIGN; (SIGN publication no. 41). Available: www.sign.rcpe.ac.uk.

SIGN. (2003). *The Management of Harmful Drinking and Alcohol Dependence in Primary Care: a National Clinical Guideline.* Edinburgh: Scottish Intercollegiate Guidelines Network, Royal College of Physicians of Edinburgh. Available: www.sign.rcpe.ac.uk.

Single, E., Robson, L., Rehm, J., *et al.* (1999). Morbidity and mortality attributable to alcohol, tobacco, and illicit drug use in Canada. *American Journal of Public Health*, **89**, 385–90.

Slattery, J., Chick, J., Cochrane, M., *et al.* (2003). *Prevention of Relapse in Alcohol Dependence.* Glasgow: Health Technology Assessment Report 3, Health Technology Board of Scotland. Available: www.htbs.co.uk.

Smart, R. G., Mann, R. E. and Suurvali, H. (1998). Changes in liver cirrhosis death rates in different countries in relation to per capita alcohol consumption and Alcoholics Anonymous membership. *Journal of Studies on Alcohol*, **59**, 245–9.

Smith, A. J., Hodgson, R. J., Bridgeman, K., *et al.* (2003). A randomized controlled trial of a brief intervention after alcohol-related facial injury. *Addiction*, **98**, 43–53.

Spanagel, R., Holter, S. M., Allingham, K., *et al.* (1996). Acamprosate and alcohol: I. Effects on alcohol intake following alcohol deprivation in the rat. *European Journal of Pharmacology*, **305**, 39–44.

Tanescu, M. and Hu, F. B. (2001). Alcohol consumption and risk of coronary heart disease among individuals with type 2 diabetes. *Current Diabetic Reports*, **1**, 187–91.

Thevos, A. K., Roberts, J. S., Thomas, S. E., *et al.* (2000). Cognitive behavioral therapy delays relapse in female socially phobic alcoholics. *Addictive Behaviors*, **25**, 333–45.

Thomson, A. D., Cook, C. C., Touquet, R., *et al.* (2002). The Royal College of Physicians Report on Alcohol: guidelines for managing Wernicke's encephalopathy in the Accident and Emergency Department. *Alcohol & Alcoholism*, **37**, 513–21.

Truelsen, T., Thudium, D. and Gronbaek, M. (2002). Amount and type of alcohol and risk of dementia: the Copenhagen City Heart Study. *Neurology*, **59**, 1313–19.

Wannamethee, S. G. and Shaper, A. G. (2003). Alcohol, body weight and weight gain among middle-aged men. *American Journal of Clinical Nutrition*, **77**, 1312–17.

Welte, J., Perry, P., Longabaugh, R., *et al.* (1998). An outcome evaluation of a hospital-based early intervention program. *Addiction*, **93**, 573–81.

Willinger, U., Lenzinger, E., Hornik, K., *et al.* (2002). Anxiety as a predictor of relapse in detoxified alcohol-dependent patients. *Alcohol & Alcoholism*, **37**, 609–12.

World Health Organization. (2002). *The World Health Report 2002: Reducing Risks, Promoting Healthy Life*. Geneva: WHO.

Wright, S., Moran, L., Meyrick, M., *et al.* (1998). Intervention by an alcohol health worker in an accident and emergency department. *Alcohol & Alcoholism*, **33**, 651–6.

9

Drug misuse in medical patients

Ilana Crome and Hamid Ghodse

Introduction

There has been an increasing interest in and awareness of drug problems in the UK over the last decade. This has been reflected in a raft of policy initiatives which include:

- Purchasing Effective Treatment and Care for Drug Misusers (1996)
- Clinical Guidelines on the Management of Drug Misuse and Dependence (1999)
- Substance Misuse Detainees in Police Custody (2000)
- Safer Services (1999)
- Safety First (2001)
- Tackling Drugs to Build a Better Britain (1998)
- National Drugs Strategy (1999, 2000, 2001)
- Recommendations from the British Association of Psychopharmacology (2004).

Substance problems may present in a variety of different medical settings in both primary care and secondary care. Indeed, no speciality is exempt from drug misusers presenting; accident and emergency, paediatrics, geriatrics, cardiology, dermatology, neurology, gastroenterology, infectious disease, obstetrics, neonatology, trauma and orthopaedic surgery, and general surgery will all be seeing patients who are using, misusing or are dependent on drugs. All psychiatric specialities, including liaison psychiatry, will have their fair share; in particular those dealing with general psychiatry, child and adolescent psychiatry, old age psychiatry, forensic psychiatry, learning disability, and eating disorders, will be assessing and treating patients with substance problems. Thus, the liaison psychiatrist will undoubtedly come across patients with drug problems.

For the purposes of this chapter, we will concentrate on illicit drugs and the misuse of prescribed medication. Thus, we include central nervous system

Handbook of Liaison Psychiatry, ed. Geoffrey Lloyd and Elspeth Guthrie. Published by Cambridge University Press. © Cambridge University Press 2007.

depressants, e.g. benzodiazepines, solvents and gases, opiates and opioids, drugs that alter perception, e.g. LSD (lysergic acid diethylamide), hallucinogenic mushrooms, cannabis, khat, central nervous stimulants, e.g. amphetamines, cocaine, and ecstasy. Alcohol-related problems are reviewed in Chapter 8.

However, it should be noted that there is a growing trend, for young people especially, to use a combination of substances including alcohol and tobacco. Thus, patients may present with symptoms relating to the misuse of one or more substances.

Substances may cause intoxication, a withdrawal state with specific features, a psychotic state, or amnesia, as well as affective, anxiety and behavioural problems.

Even if the presentation is for a drug problem, this may not be the patient's main problem. In addition, patients may have other associated difficulties due to their social circumstances, e.g. homelessness, their age, i.e. very young or very old, pregnancy, associated criminal involvement due to drug taking, or a comorbid psychiatric and/or physical illness (Herring & Thom 1999).

It should be noted that there are many complex ways in which psychological and/or physical symptoms may be associated with a drug problem:

- a primary psychiatric and/or physical illness may precipitate or lead to a substance problem
- substance misuse may worsen or alter the course of a psychiatric and/or physical illness
- intoxication and/or substance dependence may lead to psychological and physical symptoms
- substance misuse and/or withdrawal may lead to psychiatric or physical symptoms or illnesses
- primary psychiatric disorder may precipitate substance use, which may lead to psychiatric and/or physical symptoms or syndromes.

Diagnosis and classification

The criteria for the diagnosis of substance problems are outlined in Tables 9.1 and 9.2 for both ICD-10 (International Classification of Diseases; World Health Organization 1992) and the DSM-IV (Diagnostic and Statistical Manual of the American Psychiatric Association; American Psychiatric Association 1994).

For the purposes of treatment it is helpful to distinguish non-dependent substance misuse from dependent use. Not surprisingly, the more serious the substance problem, the more likely there are to be associated psychological, physical and social problems, which require a more intensive level of treatment intervention

Table 9.1. Criteria for substance abuse (DSM-IV) and harmful use (ICD-10).

DSM-IV	ICD-10

A. A maladaptive pattern of substance use leading to clinically significant impairment or distress, as manifested by one (or more) of the following occurring within a 12-month period:
  1. Recurrent substance use resulting in a failure to fulfil major role obligations at work, school, or home.
  2. Recurrent substance abuse in situations that are physically hazardous.
  3. Recurrent substance-abuse-related legal problems.
  4. Continued substance abuse despite having persistent or recurrent social or interpersonal problems caused or exacerbated by the effects of the substance.
B. Has never met the criteria for substance dependence for this class of substance.
	A. A pattern of psychoactive substance use that is causing damage to health; the damage may be to physical or mental health.

Epidemiology

Mortality

Over the last decade the drug problem in the UK has increased dramatically. Drug misuse is responsible for approximately 3000 deaths each year (Ghodse *et al.* 1998; Lind *et al.* 1999). In the UK each year 120 000 deaths are a result of smoking-related disorders, 40 000 are due to alcohol-related disorders, and about 2000 are due to illicit drug use. The mortality of excessive drinkers is at least twice, and that of drug users up to 22 times, that of the general population.

Morbidity: health aspects

Substances impact on every organ of the body: the central nervous, gastro-intestinal, cardiovascular, respiratory, musculoskeletal and endocrine systems. Some problems, e.g. intoxication, withdrawal, deliberate overdose, injecting accidents, hypothermia and hyperthermia, dehydration and choking or suffocating may require urgent medical attention (Vidal-Trecan *et al.* 2003; Vuori *et al.* 2003).

Table 9.2. Criteria for dependence syndrome in DSM-IV and ICD-10.

DSM-IV	ICD-10
A. Diagnosis of dependence should be made if three (or more) of the following have been experienced or exhibited at any time in the same 12-month period:	A. Diagnosis of dependence should be made if three or more of the following have been experienced or exhibited at some time during the last year:
1. Tolerance defined by either need for markedly increased amount of substance to achieve intoxication or desired effect or markedly diminished effect with continued use of the same amount of the substance.	1. A strong desire or sense of compulsion to take the substance.
2. Withdrawal as evidenced by either of the following: the characteristic withdrawal syndrome for the substance or the same (or closely related) substance is taken to relieve or avoid withdrawal symptoms.	2. Difficulties in controlling substance-taking behaviour in terms of its onset, termination, or levels of use.
3. The substance is often taken in larger amounts over a longer period of time than was intended.	3. Physiological withdrawal state when substance use has ceased or been reduced, as evidenced by either of the following: the characteristic withdrawal syndrome for the substance or use of the same (or closely related) substance with the intention of relieving or avoiding withdrawal symptoms.
4. Persistent desire or repeated unsuccessful efforts to cut down or control substance use.	4. Evidence of tolerance, such that increased doses of the psychoactive substance are required in order to achieve effects originally produced by lower doses.
5. A great deal of time is spent in activities necessary to obtain the substance, use the substance, or recover from its effects.	5. Progressive neglect of alternative pleasures or interests because of psychoactive substance use and increased amount of time necessary to obtain or take the substance or to recover from its effects.
6. Important social, occupational, or recreational activities given up or reduced because of substance use.	6. Persisting with substance use despite clear evidence of overly harmful consequences (physical or mental).
7. Continued substance use despite knowledge of having had a persistent or recurrent physical or psychological problem that was likely to have been caused or exacerbated by the substance.	

Poor physical health is strongly correlated with poverty and social deprivation, including accidents, dietary neglect and failure to access primary care. Substance misuse must be viewed in the context of multiple social influences and associations. It is very difficult to attribute 'cause' directly, because many of the risk factors for adverse psychosocial consequences and the development of substance misuse are shared. However, clinical experience suggests that once substance misuse is established, further social problems accumulate. The implication is that removal of the substance will not necessarily reduce the social harm.

Substance users are vulnerable to exploitation, especially if they are homeless, mentally ill or have learning difficulties. Unsafe injecting behaviour, high-risk sexual activity, unwanted pregnancy and sexually transmitted infections, and accidental overdose compound drug-taking behaviour. Crack cocaine use – common in sex workers – is linked to hepatitis infection and termination of pregnancy.

Furthermore, pregnant teenage substance misusers are at increased risk not only due to chaotic patterns of use, but also due to physical and emotional violence. Substance misuse is associated with early, unplanned or undesired pregnancy and abortion. Since substance use is often accompanied by amenorrhoea, young women may not realize that there is a possibility of pregnancy, and may not be aware until an advanced stage. This can obviously lead to poor antenatal care (Ghodse 2002).

Substance use, sexual abuse and prostitution have common predisposing factors; poverty, homelessness, psychiatric illness and physical and emotional abuse are some. Indeed, the term 'childhood sexual abuse' is used to describe the involvement of young people in the sex industry in order to subsidize their drug use. Cocaine, alcohol and benzodiazepines are commonly used to cope with their totally unmanageable situation. Naturally, these young women are at risk of sexually transmitted infections, bloodborne viruses (gonorrhoea, syphilis, chlamydia) and bacterial infections, which may cause infertility and pelvic disease.

Psychiatric disorders such as depression, anxiety, psychosis, eating disorders, and post-traumatic stress disorders are associated with the direct intoxicating effects of acute and chronic substance misuse and withdrawal syndromes, often within an inhospitable social environment. Thus, for this group, outreach work, social care, and screening and treatment for sexually acquired infections are part of the spectrum of management. Risk of self-harm and suicide is greatly increased in substance misusers, and prevention of suicide is inextricably linked with reduction in substance misuse (Oyefeso *et al.* 1999).

Prevalence of illicit drug use in samples of hospital patients

Accident and Emergency units

There is an increased risk of traumatic injury resulting in hospitalization among substance users (Rosenberg 1995), and those who have sustained one traumatic injury are at greatly increased risk of re-injury. Cocaine, amphetamines and marijuana, especially in combination with alcohol, play a significant role in all types of injuries, especially in motor vehicle crashes. Brookoff *et al.* (1994) reported that when urine samples were tested, 59 out of 150 drivers tested positive for either cocaine (13%), or marijuana (33%), or for both drugs (12%).

Other international reports confirm these findings. Soderstrom *et al.* (1995, USA) reported positive tests for marijuana in 2.7% of automobile drivers and 32% of motorcyclists admitted to a shock trauma centre, 8% and 5% of automobile and motorcycle drivers respectively were positive for cocaine use, while 1.5% and 3.1% tested positive for phencyclidine (PCP). Sugrue *et al.* (1995, Australia) reported a detection rate of 15.2% for cannabinoids in a sample of 164 road trauma drivers and a small number of drivers had mixed alcohol and illicit drug use. In France, a nationwide case-controlled study among 18–35-year-old patients, carried out in the emergency departments of five hospitals, found cannabinoids in 13.9% of the sample of drivers and 7.5% in the sample of patients who were non-drivers, opiates were present in 10.5% of drivers and in 10.4% of non-drivers, cocaine metabolites were detected in 1.0% and 1.1% of the samples respectively, and amphetamines in 1.4% and 2.5% of the samples. The study demonstrates the presence of illicit drugs in a considerable number of patients attending hospitals (Marquet *et al.* 1998).

In Canada El Guebaly *et al.* (1998) reviewed six studies reporting on screening for drug (or drug and alcohol) use among patients attending emergency or trauma departments. These studies found varying rates of use for a range of different drugs, but overall indicated that about 40% of patients attending these departments were likely to test positive for the use of illicit drugs.

Patients in acute general medical settings

In the UK, Canning *et al.* (1999) reported the results of a study which identified drug use using a health and lifestyle questionnaire administered by the admitting doctor. The study found that 6% of patients (total $n = 609$) were drug dependent and 14% were positive on 'drug misuse'. Cannabis was the most commonly used illegal drug and the only one used in 79% of screened drug users. Other drugs used by this group included: amphetamines (11%), ecstasy (10%), cocaine (10%). Screening identified polydrug use in 46 patients (8%). Amongst these,

41 (89%) used cannabis in addition to alcohol, and 15 (32%) used alcohol and two or more illegal drugs. This indicates that it is important to detect drug misuse, since this may be related to the presenting health problems (Kouimtsidis *et al.* 2003).

In the USA, Brown *et al.* (1998) screened patients attending general medical services and general surgery. They found that 3% of patients were currently using one or more illicit drugs, current use of marijuana was reported by 2.8% of patients, use of cocaine by 1.9%, use of sedatives/tranquillizers by 0.6%, use of analgesics/opioids by 2.5% and use of inhalants by 0.3%. Prevalence of lifetime use of these drugs was higher. The study suggested that (including alcohol) there was a slightly greater than one-in-five prevalence of current substance use disorders among general medical, general surgical and orthopaedic inpatients aged 18–49 inclusive. Stein's (1996, USA) study found a higher percentage of drug use, with 7.6% of patients attending an acute care hospital reporting the use of illicit drugs in the previous month.

Psychiatric patients

It is now well recognized that patients with severe mental illness are especially at risk of substance misuse (Carey & Correia 1998). General population studies demonstrate that lifetime diagnoses of substance abuse or dependence occur in 47% of individuals with schizophrenia and 56% of individuals with bipolar disorder (Robins *et al.* 1988), while studies on psychiatric patients have demonstrated the frequent presence of illicit substance use (Cohen *et al.* 1999). Appleby *et al.* (1997) reported that 25% of their sample had a drug-related disorder, while 32% were abusing or dependent on more than one substance. Indeed, although substance dependence emerges as one of the most common mental health related disorders, it is one that is least likely to be treated (Wolff *et al.* 1999).

McCann *et al.* (2000, USA) cite studies indicating that approximately 50% of adults with attention-deficit hyperactivity disorder (ADHD) have a history of psychoactive substance use disorders; further they record that a history of childhood ADHD has been found in between 22% and 71% of substance-abusing patients. In their sample of patients attending an adult ADHD centre, 33.8% were found to have a positive screen for drug abuse. Clerici and Carta (1996) in their study of Italian opioid addicts review the international literature and confirm the close association between psychoactive substance use and personality disorders among drug-using samples.

Substance misuse is common in adolescents who have significant adjustment problems, disruptive behaviour disorders and conduct disorders, as well as depression. One study reported a figure as high as 50% of adolescents consecutively admitted into a psychiatric inpatient unit (studies 1990–1997 cited in

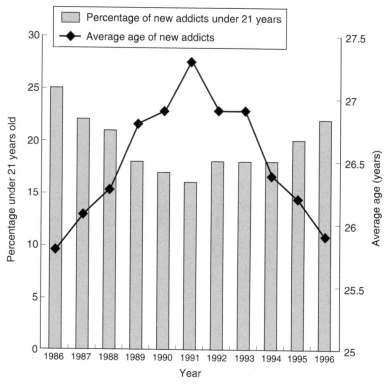

Figure 9.1.   UK Home Office Addicts Index (Ghodse 2002).

Martino *et al.* 2000). Furthermore, the number of young addicts overall is increasing (see Figure 9.1).

Failure to identify substance use disorders was also recorded in a study of 2347 patients referred consecutively to the consultation-liaison psychiatry services of four general teaching hospitals in Australia. While psychiatrists gave a diagnosis of substance use disorder in 14% of cases, 56% of those cases had been missed by the referring doctor (Smith *et al.* 1995). Substance use disorders are frequently undiagnosed in psychiatric settings, although about 50% of patients with a severe mental illness meet lifetime criteria for substance use disorder (Wolford *et al.* 1999). Carey and Correia (1998) offer a number of explanations for failure to detect cases, including ambiguity in the cause of some symptoms and the relative insensitivity of standard screening measures in detecting comorbidity. Above all, it is because screening and comprehensive history taking are not routinely undertaken.

Patients attending obstetric and paediatric units

Pregnant women and parents are another group to be considered. In Dublin, urine testing of 504 'first-visit' antenatal patients, and a separate sample of

Table 9.3. Framework for integration of epidemiological methods and provision of services.

Definitions	Estimates of consumption and/ or criteria for diagnosis	Population on which estimates likely to be based	Service framework
Use/misuse	Quantity/frequency	General population School surveys	Tier 1
Use/misuse	Quantity/frequency – 'regular' use	General population School surveys	Tier 2
Harmful use	Harmful use, dependence criteria according to ICD-10	General medical, criminal justice and social services	Tier 3 – specialist multidisciplinary services
Dependence	Dependence criteria according to ICD-10	Clinical treatment populations attending specialist services	Tier 4 – intensive very specialized services

Source: Frischer *et al.* 2004.

515 post-delivery patients, found a prevalence of 2.8%, the most frequently used drug being cannabis. The authors note that their figures are similar to the results from an earlier study in Birmingham, which found that 2% of women tested positive on a first antenatal visit, but lower than figures reported from studies in the USA in the late 1980s (Bosio *et al.* 1997). Kemper *et al.* (1993, USA) found a prevalence rate of 3% in a sample of mothers attending paediatric clinics. This suggests that paediatricians should screen for parental substance abuse.

Overall, these studies demonstrate that drug misusers are presenting to a wide range of services, that their problems are not detected, and that failure to recognize the problem may result in inappropriate treatment and recurrence of the health problems, since at least one associate factor, namely the drug misuse, is not being effectively treated, hence the importance of assessment (Table 9.3).

Assessment

Key issues

- An awareness of and a high index of suspicion about drug use must pervade all aspects of practice, especially assessment.
- Assessment should be conceptualized as part of treatment and thus is an ongoing and continuous process.

- Assessment must take account of developmental stage in children and adolescents, and age in adults and older people.
- The most important aspect is to *ask* about substance use, misuse and dependence.
- There should be a focus on the process, purpose and practicalities of assessment.
- Assessment must be communicated and co-ordinated between medical and other professionals.

Asking the right questions

A procedure for establishing key components of the person's past and current situation is necessary (see Table 9.4). It is recognized that there are certain impediments to assessment, and these are summarized in Table 9.5.

The key principles underlying assessment

Detection   Determine the nature and extent, and interaction of, substance use and psychological and physical symptomatology.

Table 9.4. Suggested outline for schedule of issues to be covered in assessment.

Demographic characteristics	Age
	Gender
	School, college or employment, retired, unemployment
	Nationality, religious affiliation, ethnicity and culture
	Living arrangements, e.g. with parent(s), spouse, relatives, friends, homeless, institutional care
	General environment, e.g. deprivation, affluence, violence
Presenting complaint(s) or problems	May or may not be a substance problem or mental health issue
Each substance should be discussed separately:	Age of initiation: 'first tried'
	Age of onset of weekend use
alcohol	Age of onset of weekly use
amphetamines	Age of onset of daily use
benzodiazepines	Pattern of use during each day
cannabis	Route of use, e.g. oral, smoking, snorting, intramuscular, intravenous
cocaine	
ecstasy	Age of onset of specific withdrawal symptoms and dependence syndrome features
heroin and other opiates	
methadone	Current use over previous day, week, month
nicotine	Current cost of use

Table 9.4. (*cont.*) Suggested outline for schedule of issues to be covered in assessment.

over-the-counter medication	Maximum use ever
prescribed medication	How is the substance use being funded?
	Periods of abstinence
	Triggers to relapse
	Preferred substance(s) and reasons
Treatment episodes	Dates, service, practitioner details, treatment
for substance problems	interventions, success or otherwise, triggers to relapse
Family history	Parents, siblings, grandparents, uncles, aunts
	History of substance misuse and related problems
	History of psychiatric problems, e.g. suicide, self-harm, depression, anxiety, psychotic illness
	History of physical illness
	Separation, divorce, death
	Family relationships, conflict, support
	Occupational history
Medical history	Episodes of acute or chronic illnesses: respiratory, infective, HIV, hepatitis, injury including accidents, surgery
	Admission to hospital, dates, problems, treatment and outcome
Psychiatric history	Assessment by general practitioner for any 'minor' complaints, e.g. anxiety, depression
	Treatment by general practitioner with any psychoactive drugs
	Referral to specialist psychiatric services: dates, diagnosis, treatment and outcome
	Mental Health Act assessments
Personal history	Developmental milestones, occupational, sexual, marital relationships and maturity
Educational background	Age started and left school, including truancy
	Achievements and aspirations
Vocational history	Ongoing activities and plans
Criminal activities	Involvement in criminal activities preceding or directly related to substance problems
	Cautions, charges, convictions
	Shoplifting, violence, prostitution
Social services	Child protection history
	Child abuse and neglect
	Other social service involvement
Social environment	Level of community support and network

Table 9.4. (*cont.*)

Social activities	Sports, hobbies, community work, religious affiliation and activities
Financial situation	Debt to finance substance problems
Useful information	Current address Phone number including mobile phone General practitioner's name, address and phone number Details of other professionals involved
Investigations	Biochemical, haematological, urinary, salivary, sweat, hair Special investigations
Collateral information	Family and friends School or occupational colleagues Social services Criminal justice agencies Health services Voluntary agencies
Consent and confidentiality	Particularly in under-18-year-olds
Current stressors	Bereavement, promotion, marriage, divorce, ongoing legal problems
How the client perceives the problems and what they want	Belief systems
Profile of strengths and risks	
Readiness to engage in treatment	
Mental state examination	
Physical examination	

Diagnosis	Determine and differentiate whether the substance use has led to misuse, dependence and psychosocial or medical problems and provide a balanced interpretation of the consistency between history, clinical status and investigations.
Risk assessment	Identify a hierarchy of need based on ensuring safety, accommodation, care and treatment.
Goals	Retention in treatment is vital, and goals need to be flexible and adaptive, within a framework of harm reduction and taking account of patient expectations.

Table 9.5. Some factors that can impact on dual diagnosis assessment.

Systems impediments	Clinical impediments	Process impediments
• **Parallel vs. sequential vs. integrated treatment approaches**	• **Understanding the nature of the symptoms and presentation**	• Setting
• Philosophy issues	• Assessment tools – reliability, validity and utility	• Confidentiality
• Lack of training		• Access
• Debate over focus of care (i.e. Responsible Medical Officer)	• Client's mental state – issue of stability, intoxicated/withdrawing, cognitive impairment	• Time-frame
• Transcultural issues	• Reliance of self-report	• Trust
• Protocols, procedures and policies	• Client's motivation/ preparedness, insight	• Poor previous experience (client and staff)
	• Perception of risk	• Protocols, procedures and policies
		• Interview skills
		• Consent
		• Collateral informants
		• Resources, e.g. laboratory tests

Source: Banerjee *et al.* (2002).

Delivery	Ensure that the appropriate type and intensity of intervention can be provided in the most suitable setting.
Management	Engage, liaise, negotiate and collaborate effectively with multidisciplinary colleagues and multi-agencies.
Monitoring	Provide a baseline against which progress is monitored.
Communication	With the person, their family, and carers, regarding the level of need and approaches to meeting this.

Consideration should be given to prejudice, stigma, groups with particular needs, e.g. learning disability, physically disabled, ethnic minorities, young people and older people, and issues of consent and confidentiality.

Assessment tools

There are a growing range of instruments available to assess both substance use and mental disorders separately, and coexisting mental health problems and substance misuse (De Las Cuevas *et al.* 2000; Hodgson *et al.* 2003; Kellogg *et al.* 2003; Knight *et al.* 1999; Raistrick *et al.* 1994; Topp & Mattick 1997).

Substance use

Assessment can be carried out by the following methods:

• by self-report questionnaires
• by interview

• from collateral informants, e.g. relatives, friends, colleagues, health professionals, other professionals.

Use of biochemical tests on blood, saliva, sweat, urine and hair are other methods (Wolff *et al.* 1999).

Apart from long-acting benzodiazepines, methadone and cannabis, it should be noted that drugs do not remain in the urine for longer than two to three days. It is also important to be sure that the sample provided is that of the patient whom you are treating.

There are a vast spectrum of instruments available for screening, for charting the pattern of drug use, for the estimation of problems (social, physical and psychological) associated with drug use, for the assessment of dependence and the degree of dependence, for the associated psychiatric illness, and for measuring motivation to change, expectations that treatment will help, and personal coping styles. All these issues are pertinent to clinical history taking. These are outlined below.

Screening

DAST: Drug Abuse Screening Test (Skinner 1982)

Problems

Patterns of use

Physical, psychological and social problems associated, e.g. Opiate Treatment Index

SAAQ: The Substance Abuse Assessment Questionnaire: a multidimensional structural assessment tool, appropriate for both clinical assessment and research (Ghodse 2002)

Dependence on alcohol or drugs, e.g. ASI (Addiction Severity Index) (McLellan *et al.* 1980)

Diagnosis of psychiatric illness, e.g. PRISM (Psychiatric Research Interview for Substance and Mental Disorder), DIS (Diagnostic Interview Schedule), SCAN (Schedules for Clinical Assessment in Neuropsychiatry), SCID (Structured Clinical Interview for DSM-IV-TR), CIDI (Composite International Diagnostic Interview)

Outcome expectancies

Coping styles

Relapse risk

Self-efficacy

Personal assessment, i.e. psychopathology, emotional state, general life function

Treatment-related factors, e.g. motivation to change substance use, barriers to treatment, reasons for seeking treatment, treatment goals and service utilization

Substance use and severe mental illness

There are four different instruments appropriate for substance misuse in comorbidity:

- Dartmouth Assessment of Lifestyle Instrument (DALI): an 18-item questionnaire, administered by interviewer (Rosenberg *et al.* 1998)
- Clinical use, abuse and dependency scale (CUAD): is a brief instrument for measuring substance misuse in dual diagnosis patients (McGovern & Morrison 1992)
- Substance Abuse Treatment Scale (SATS): measure of treatment progress or as an outcome measure (McHugo *et al.* 1995)
- SAAQ (Ghodse 2002).

The UK evidence base: outcome research

Over the last decade, the confidence with which we can assert that 'treatment works' has grown immeasurably. To date, about 300 randomized controlled trials (RCTs) have been carried out in the alcohol field, 100 in the tobacco field, and 60 in the opiate field. This indicates that cheap, brief interventions carried out by generalists are likely to reap benefits as first-line interventions. However, the more costly intensive psychological interventions (often combined with pharmacological treatment) are effective for those with more complex needs.

For instance, specialist smoking cessation, which costs £800 for six weeks, is the most cost-effective intervention in medicine. However, smoking-related illnesses cost £16 000 per patient per year. Alcoholics cost the health service two to three times more than the general population, and in alcoholics with comorbidity the cost is 60% more see Chapter 8.

Over the last decade there has been increasing interest in and emphasis on the implementation and evaluation of 'brief' or 'minimal' interventions for the treatment of alcohol problems (Bien *et al.* 1993). This seminal work was instigated in the UK in the early 1970s. The cumulative evidence demonstrated the effectiveness and cost effectiveness of such interventions and for this reason has had enormous impact on the way services are being configured and delivered to adults with alcohol problems in the UK and elsewhere (See Chapter 8).

Brief, minimal and short-term interventions include 'counselling' and motivational interviewing. There is good evidence of effectiveness and cost effectiveness in alcohol misusers in primary care settings, in Accident and Emergency departments, and in educational settings (Longabaugh *et al.* 2001).

This type of approach has also proven effective in cigarette smoking (Richmond & Anderson 1994). Research from the USA and Australia has produced some promising results when applied to young people (Aubrey 1998; Hulse *et al.* 2001; Monti *et al.* 1999; Senft *et al.* 1997). Even if the success rates are relatively modest, if widely and consistently applied, they could result in gains to public health.

More recently, recruitment of subjects in the UK Alcohol Treatment Trial (UKATT), which is the largest alcohol treatment trial ever launched in the UK, has now been completed. It has collected data from 720 alcohol-dependent clients who prescribed to alcohol treatment agencies from 1999–2001. It is similar in design to the American research, Project MATCH (1997a, b), where 1700 patients were allocated to three different interventions: CBT (cognitive behavioural therapy), MET (motivational enhancement therapy) and 12-Step programme (modelled on Alcoholics Anonymous).

In Project MATCH, by 36 months follow up, 90% of clients had reduced use or were abstinent, irrespective of allocation to particular treatment modalities (Project MATCH 1997a, b). UKATT has utilized MET and SNBT (social network behaviour therapy). Findings indicate that both interventions are effective.

The first relatively long-term, prospective, observational study on outcome in drug misusers in the UK, the National Treatment Outcome Research Study (NTORS), has been underway since 1995 (Gossop *et al.* 2000, 2003). This study follows up 1075 drug misusers in two types of residential services (inpatient and residential units), and two kinds of community services (methadone reduction and methadone maintenance). The age range is 16–58, half of whom are responsible for caring for children. The 16–18 age group has not been analysed or reported on separately.

Most important to note is that the specific nature of the treatment modalities provided has not been identified and described in any depth or in detail. Opiates, amphetamines, cocaine, non-prescription benzodiazepines and alcohol were assessed. The impact of treatment on psychological health, suicide, mortality and crime was evaluated. In summary, the study reports that drug use, as well as injecting and sharing needles, was reduced. Crime also decreased with concurrent improvement in physical and psychological health. However, 20% of the study population continued to use daily, and 40% continued to use once a week. Over the five-year period, 62 people died, alcohol use remained at a constantly high level, and 80 were using two or more illicit drugs and were long-term users. There was a history of treatment for psychiatric disorder in the two years prior to treatment, and in the three months prior to treatment 30% had suicidal ideation.

At five years, between 33.3% and 50% of users achieved abstinence in community and residential services respectively. However, 20% were still using daily. While 40% used illicit drugs regularly, this had reduced from 66% at intake in the residential services and 80% in community services.

In summary, daily and regular use was found in 20–40% respectively. Injecting reduced from 60 to 40% and criminal activity halved, but 25% were still drinking above safe limits. This evidence is encouraging despite the limitations in design described above. The study points to some value in the treatment programmes which are currently being implemented in the UK.

Pharmacotherapy for addiction

Over the last decade, the capacity to intervene pharmacologically has increased greatly. Pharmacotherapy is available for opiates, alcohol and nicotine (Lingford-Hughes *et al.* 2004). Pharmacological agents can be used:

- in emergency treatments for accidents, overdose, septicaemia, convulsions, hypothermia and dehydration
- to alleviate withdrawal symptoms so as to achieve abstinence, i.e. detoxification (e.g. lofexidine, methadone, buprenorphine)
- to substitute for the drug misused and thus reduce drug-related harm, i.e. stabilization, reduction, maintenance (e.g. methadone, buprenorphine)
- to prevent relapse through relapse prevention, e.g. by blocking pleasant opiate effects (e.g. naltrexone)
- in treatment of comorbid substance-use disorders, e.g. alcohol and nicotine
- in treatment of comorbid psychiatric conditions
- in treatment of the physical consequences of drug use, e.g. HIV/Hepatitis C
- in treatment of co-existing physical problems, e.g. diabetes.

Illicit drugs

Opiates

There are a range of medications available for detoxification, stabilization, and reduction. These include codeine, methadone, buprenorphine, clonidine, lofexidine, naltrexone and combinations, e.g. lofexidine/naltrexone, as well as 'accelerated' regimes, e.g. naltrexone or lofexidine. In young people it is mandatory that specialist support be enlisted at the earliest possible stage. This is likely to be the safest option for severely dependent adults as well.

Stimulants and cannabis

Since substitute medication is not available for cocaine and cannabis, and not commonly used for amphetamine administration, the implementation of general treatment measures is advised.

In stimulant withdrawal patients may become drowsy and depressed, and even suicidal. Thus, regular monitoring of mental state and physical examination are very important. Urine screens should be regularly and randomly taken.

Similarly, cannabis withdrawal may result in insomnia, and hypnotic sedatives should be prescribed cautiously.

Except for buprenorphine, all medication is not licensed for under-18-year-old age groups. Indeed, generalists should not prescribe for young people without prior assessment by a specialist addiction psychiatrist, and even specialists should work with a multidisciplinary team and not in isolation.

Psychiatric disorders and drug treatment (summarized from Andrews & Jenkins 1999; see also Chapter 33)

'Older' antipsychotics

Antipsychotic medication (neuroleptics or major tranquillizers) is the main form of medication. These drugs reduce relapse, the most common reason for which is non-compliance. 'Classical' antipsychotics, e.g. chlorpromazine, thioridazine, sulpiride, act on 'positive' symptoms. The long-acting depot injections available may be appropriate for substance misusers.

Atypical antipsychotics

These act on both the 'positive' acute symptoms and 'negative' symptoms. Examples of these drugs are clozapine, risperidone, olanzapine, quetiapine and amisulpride. These drugs do not have the anticholinergic and extrapyramidal side-effects of the 'older' drugs. However some, e.g. weight gain, seizures, sedation, dizziness and agranulocytosis, are common to both.

Antidepressant medication

There is a large range of antidepressant medication available. Despite this, and the commonness of depression in substance-use disorders, there is very little research on the treatment of depression in drug misuse and alcohol addiction. We should also draw attention to the work of Schuckit et al. (2000) who demonstrated that few patients presenting with alcohol and depression have a major depressive disorder.

Antidepressants fall into the following categories:

- Tricyclic, e.g. amitriptyline, clomipramine, dosulepin, doxepin, imipramine, lofepramine, nortriptyline, trimipramine. Imipramine has been demonstrated to be effective in methadone maintenance (Nunes et al. 1998).
- Tetracyclic, e.g. mianserin, maprotiline, amoxapine.

- Selective serotonin reuptake inhibitors (SSRIs), e.g. citalopram, sertraline, fluoxetine, fluvoxamine, paroxetine. Fluoxetine has been shown to be effective in reduction of marijuana, alcohol and depression (Cornelius *et al.* 1997).
- Monoamine oxidase inhibitors (MAOIs), e.g. isocarboxazid, phenelzine, tranylcypromine, moclobemide.
- Serotonin−noradrenaline reuptake inhibitors (SNRIs), e.g. venlafaxine.
- Post-synaptic serotonin receptor blockers and reuptake inhibitors, e.g. nefazodone, trazodone. Nefazodone (no longer available) leads to increased methadone in patients being treated in this way.
- Noradrenergic/specific serotonergic antidepressants (NaSSA), e.g. mirtazapine.
- Lithium, sodium valproate and carbamazepine are also used for the prophylaxis and treatment of mania and depression, alone or in combination.

Benzodiazepines

Benzodiazepines are used as hypnotics, sedatives or anxiolytics with different half-lives. It is important to recognize that they can produce a withdrawal syndrome, i.e. dependence, even if low doses have been prescribed (or misused). If taken in combination with other drugs and alcohol, this can result in overdose.

There are alternatives, e.g. buspirone, zolpidem and zopiclone, which can be used and do not appear to lead to dependence.

Drug withdrawal: abstinence syndromes

Drug-dependent individuals may seek urgent professional help, asking for immediate treatment of withdrawal symptoms often on the grounds that they claim to be unable to get to their usual treatment unit or that their prescribed supplies have been lost or stolen. In this situation, and regardless of manipulative threats that, if they are not given a prescription, they will have to resort to illegal activity, the governing principle is that nothing should be prescribed unless there are clear physical signs of the appropriate abstinence syndrome (Table 9.6). Rigid application of this rule is essential, otherwise there is a risk that hospital A&E departments or GP surgeries will be regularly used as supplementary sources of supply and that casual non-dependent users will be ovided with pharmaceutically pure preparations of dependence-producing drugs (on which they may overdose). It is therefore essential to take a careful history to establish that there is dependence and to carry out a thorough physical examination to establish the nature and severity of the abstinence syndrome.

Opiate abstinence syndrome

Although the opiate withdrawal syndrome is very distressing for the individual concerned, it is less dangerous because withdrawal fits do not occur. The physical

Table 9.6. Symptoms of intoxication and withdrawal.

Intoxication	Withdrawal
Benzodiazepine	
Euphoria, disinhibition, lability of mood	Confusion and convulsions
Apathy, sedation	Tremor, postural hypotension
Abusiveness and aggression	Nausea and vomiting
Impaired attention, amnesia	Agitation Paranoid ideation
Impaired psychomotor performance	Tachycardia
Unsteady gait, slurred speech, nystagmus	Rebound insomnia, tension
Decreased level of consciousness, hypothermia	
Opiate	
Apathy, sedation, disinhibition, psychomotor retardation, impaired attention, impaired judgement	Craving
	Sneezing, yawning, runny eyes
	Muscle aches, abdominal pains
Interference with personal functioning	Nausea, vomiting, diarrhoea
	Pupillary dilatation
Drowsiness, slurred speech, pupillary constriction	Goose-flesh, recurrent chills
Decreased level of consciousness	Restless sleep
Cannabis	
Euphoria and disinhibition	Anxiety
Anxiety and agitation	Irritability
Suspiciousness and paranoid ideation	Tremor
Impaired reaction time	Sweating
Impaired judgement and attention	Muscle aches
Hallucinations with preserved orientation	
Depersonalization and derealization	
Increased appetite	
Dry mouth	
Conjunctival injection	
Tachycardia	
Stimulant	
Euphoria and increased energy	Lethargy
Hypervigilance; repetitive stereotyped behaviours	Psychomotor retardation or agitation
Grandiose beliefs and actions	Craving
Paranoid ideation	Increased appetite
Abusiveness, aggression and argumentativeness	Insomnia or hypersomnia
Auditory, tactile and visual hallucinations	Bizarre and unpleasant dreams
Sweats, chills, muscular weakness	
Nausea or vomiting, weight loss	
Pupillary dilatation, convulsions	
Tachycardia, arrhythmias, chest pain, hypertension	
Agitation	

signs include: yawning, sweating, runny eyes and nose, dilated pupils, goose-flesh, muscle twitching and shivering, tachycardia, abdominal cramps and diarrhoea. If symptoms are mild, symptomatic treatment may be sufficient, for example a low dose of phenothiazine (chlorpromazine or haloperidol) and an antispasmodic, antidiarrhoeal preparation (co-phenotrope). More severe cases may be given methadone mixture 20 mg orally and must then be observed for one hour, when they should be feeling much better. Because methadone is long-acting, there is no need to prescribe take-home medication, but the patient should be referred for specialist advice.

Pregnant women presenting with the opiate abstinence syndrome should be admitted to hospital and stabilized on methadone before undertaking gradual withdrawal to avoid precipitating fetal distress or premature labour.

Sedative abstinence syndrome

Early signs of sedative withdrawal (barbiturates, benzodiazepines, alcohol) include tremor, agitation, tachycardia and postural hypotension. Despite a correct reluctance not to prescribe dependence-producing drugs unnecessarily, it is equally important not to miss these early signs, otherwise there is a risk of withdrawal fits. Those dependent on benzodiazepines or alcohol should be given diazepam 20 mg orally immediately. The rarer condition of barbiturate withdrawal is treated with phenobarbital 120 mg orally. The patient's condition should be reviewed one hour later, by which time they should be feeling less agitated. Although many are reluctant to be admitted to hospital, every effort should be made to persuade them to do so because of the risks of unsupervised sedative withdrawal. In the absence of any formal indication for detention under the 1983 Mental Health Act, they should be allowed to leave but, whenever possible, arrangements for their follow-up (GP, treatment services) should be made. In the interim they should be provided with an adequate supply of benzodiazepines to prevent the re-occurrence of the abstinence syndrome before they contact their GP or usual clinic. For example, they may need 20 mg diazepam orally 6-hourly as takeaway medication for a minimum period (e.g. overnight). Larger supplies should not be given because of the risk of overdose, injection or supply to another person.

Alcohol withdrawal syndromes

Alcohol withdrawal in an alcohol-dependent individual results in symptoms and signs very similar to those described under sedative abstinence. However, in severely dependent individuals, sudden withdrawal may lead to delirium tremens with clouding of consciousness, confusion, bizarre hallucinations and tremor; fits occur in about 5—15% of alcohol-dependent individuals when they stop drinking. Although these severe manifestations can usually be prevented by the careful management of alcohol withdrawal, some patients may present with delirium tremens following unsupervised withdrawal.

Patients with delirium tremens who are disturbed and confused should be cared for in a safe, well-lit environment by experienced staff who are able to remain calm. Physical restraint and parenteral sedatives may be necessary if there is severe agitation, e.g. intravenous diazepam 5—10 mg given over 1—2 minutes, or intramuscular droperidol 10 mg (not available in the UK). Wernicke's encephalopathy, characterized by ataxia and confusion, can arise suddenly and without warning and is easily missed because the signs may be attributed to drunkenness. It is therefore wise to give vitamin B_1 to all patients with a heavy alcohol intake because this will prevent the permanent brain damage that may follow untreated Wernicke's encephalopathy. Parenteral administration is preferable because heavy drinkers have impaired intestinal absorption, and Pabrinex High Potency should be given intravenously or intramuscularly for five days, followed by oral administration. Pabrinex should only be given in an inpatient setting because the small risk of an anaphylactic reaction requires the immediate availability of resuscitation facilities.

Convulsions

Convulsions may occur either in the course of sedative (including alcohol) withdrawal, or during intoxication with stimulant drugs such as amphetamine or cocaine. More rarely they occur after very high doses of opiates or LSD. Whatever the cause, the immediate management is the same. Single, brief fits do not necessarily require any treatment, but if they are repeated or prolonged they should be treated with intravenous diazepam (preferably in emulsion form to reduce thrombophlebitis), injected at a rate of 5 mg per minute until the convulsions are controlled. A dose of 10—20 mg is usually sufficient and may be repeated if necessary after 30—60 minutes. Prolonged recurrence can be managed by slow intravenous infusion of diazepam. Resuscitation equipment should be immediately available because of the risk of respiratory depression.

The acutely disturbed patient

The advice of liaison psychiatrists is often sought in relation to a patient with acutely disturbed behaviour under the influence of psychoactive substance(s). There is no clear-cut 'match' between a particular behaviour and a particular drug and, moreover, the picture may be complicated by polydrug abuse. However, friends or family members may be able to provide helpful information. A physical examination should be carried out if possible, but this may be very difficult or even impossible if the patient is very disturbed and/or hostile. The pulse rate, blood pressure and body temperature should be recorded and a sample of urine sent for toxicological analysis.

The patient's mental state should be assessed and recorded in a systematic fashion, covering the following areas: general behaviour, talk, mood, abnormal beliefs (e.g. delusions), abnormal experiences (e.g. hallucinations, illusions) and cognitive state. On the basis of these observations, it should be possible to decide whether the patient is suffering from a psychotic state, a panic reaction with fear as the overwhelming symptom, or an organic mental state, characterized by confusion and often accompanied by disorders of perception. Any of these reactions can occur with any drug and, in the absence of independent information, it may be impossible to decide which drug(s) caused the disturbed mental state.

However, regardless of the cause, the basic principles of management are the same: the patient should be cared for in a quiet environment that is safe for both the patient and the staff. It should be adequately lit, so that there are no shadows that might worry a confused or paranoid patient. Most importantly, the staff should be adequately trained so that they are confident when dealing with disturbed patients and remain calm. They will understand that they should not move too close to the patient, nor walk behind him/her, because this may seem very threatening to a paranoid individual. Similarly, while trying to avoid unnecessary noise and stimulation, talking should be quiet but not whispered so that patients do not misinterpret what is being said about them. Reassuring the patient that their symptoms are drug-related and will wear off gradually, explanation of everything that is being done, and re-orientation – telling the patient where he/she is, and what time it is – are all important.

Acutely disturbed patients are in a state of high sympathetic arousal; they may have raised body temperature and may be sweating profusely, leading to dehydration and an associated electrolyte imbalance which can exacerbate their abnormal mental state. It is therefore important to encourage them to rest and to drink enough. Although it may be difficult to achieve all of this in a busy A&E department, attention to such measures is positively therapeutic and reduces the likelihood of much more disruptive outbursts of violent behaviour. It may obviate the need for sedative medication which risks clouding an already confused clinical picture and adding to the problems of drug-induced changes in the mental state.

Although the best approach is undoubtedly to care for the patient conservatively, as outlined above, and to wait for the effects of the drug(s) to wear off, some patients are so disturbed that general supportive measures are inadequate. In the absence of a definitive diagnosis about the cause of the abnormal mental state, an empirical approach to treatment must be adopted. When psychotic symptoms are the most prominent features, chlorpromazine may be administered orally (100 mg) or intramuscularly (50–100 mg). However, it should not be given if intoxication with phencyclidine is suspected (see below). Diazepam is indicated for panic states and severe agitation, given in a dose of 10 mg either orally or by slow intravenous injection (with resuscitation facilities available because of the risk of respiratory depression). If an organic mental state is suspected it is best to avoid all psychoactive medication.

Differential diagnosis and drug-specific treatment

Cannabis

The combination of organic (confusion, impaired concentration and memory) and psychotic symptoms (delusions, hallucinations) is very suggestive of intoxication with cannabis and can occur when only a small dose has been used; the patient's eyes may be red (injected conjunctivae) (see Table 9.6).

Although 'talking down' by those who are familiar with these toxic effects may be sufficient, prolonged symptoms may require treatment with chlorpromazine (25–50 mg intramuscularly) which acts as a sedative and an antipsychotic drug; flashbacks may occur and can be treated in a similar way.

LSD and other hallucinogens

The abnormal perceptual experiences that are the desired effects of hallucinogens may sometimes be extremely unpleasant, leading to states of severe agitation and panic, alternating perhaps with periods of mute withdrawal when the patient is wholly preoccupied by inner experiences. Diazepam 10–30 mg orally may be helpful if the patient is excessively agitated.

Stimulants (amphetamine and cocaine)

Psychotic symptoms occurring in a setting of clear consciousness, with no confusion or disorientation, suggest abuse of stimulant drugs and may be accompanied by evidence of sympathomimetic stimulation (tachycardia, hypertension, sweating, dilated pupils, raised temperature). Stimulant psychosis usually occurs with chronic abuse but a single large dose may have a similar effect. It comes to medical attention more commonly when due to amphetamine rather than cocaine because the effects of cocaine wear off more quickly. An acutely disturbed patient may be treated with chlorpromazine (25–50 mg intramuscularly or 50–100 mg orally), repeated as necessary. Haloperidol is also effective and diazepam may be indicated if agitation and anxiety are prominent symptoms.

The physical side-effects of stimulant intoxication are potentially serious and must therefore be treated. Specifically, body temperature must be monitored regularly because hyperthermia may be the forerunner of convulsions. It should be treated by sponging with cold water, ice packs and fanning. Chlorpromazine (25–50 mg) can be given but may cause hypotension. Adequate hydration, to compensate for water loss through sweating, is important and will speed the excretion of amphetamine. Stimulant-induced hypertension increases the risk of cerebral haemorrhage and cardiovascular collapse and may require treatment with phentolamine.

Patients recovering from stimulant intoxication should be kept in a peaceful environment. As the effects of the drugs wear off they may sleep for many hours and may later become apathetic and depressed, sometimes suicidally. Antidepressant medication may be necessary, but not immediately.

Phencyclidine

Phencyclidine is often responsible for bizarre clinical states which are very challenging to manage. Characteristically there may be periods of intense agitation with panic and sudden outbursts of very violent behaviour alternating with periods of mutism, with severe muscle rigidity and gross ataxia and with the eyes held wide open. Pulse, respiration, blood pressure and temperature are usually increased and there may be episodes of nausea and vomiting.

Patients intoxicated with phencyclidine should ideally be cared for in isolation, on a cushioned floor and subjected to minimum verbal and physical stimulation. However, they require constant monitoring in case convulsions or unconsciousness occur. It is best not to give any psychoactive medication at all but to wait for the effects of phencyclidine to wear off, which will probably take 2–4 hours, although monitoring should continue for a further two hours. If necessary, diazepam 10–20 mg may be given to control excessively violent behaviour that threatens other people; haloperidol can also be used, but chlorpromazine is contraindicated because it may potentiate the anticholinergic effects of phencyclidine and cause severe and prolonged hypotension. If physical restraint is essential to protect the patient and staff, this is achieved more safely by using people rather than mechanical restraints.

Sedatives

Acutely disturbed behaviour associated with sedative abuse occurs in the context of both chronic intoxication and acute withdrawal. The management of the latter has been described above.

Patients who take sedatives regularly become tolerant to their effects and may then increase the dose until the ceiling of tolerance is reached. At this point they manifest the signs and symptoms of chronic intoxication, which include a confused mental state, slurred speech, staggering gait and nystagmus; they are often hostile, aggressive and unco-operative. Little can be done except to wait for the effects of the drug(s) to wear off and during this time the patient may be very disruptive and difficult to manage. However, they cannot be discharged at this time because they are in a state of intoxication, which requires regular monitoring of vital signs and appropriate intervention if they lapse into unconsciousness, as more drugs are absorbed into the bloodstream.

After recovery, patients should be admitted to hospital for supervised withdrawal of their drugs. Many refuse this option and discharge themselves to resume their drug abuse, only to present again in a similarly intoxicated state – much to the exasperation of the healthcare professionals who treat them. It requires a high degree of professionalism to maintain high standards of medical care each time the same patient presents in the same, drug-induced condition.

Solvents

Patients with solvent intoxication do not usually present for medical attention because the effects of the drug wear off quickly. They may appear to be drunk with an exhilarated mood and impulsivity of behaviour, but the smell of volatile inhalants confirms the diagnosis. The patient may also be confused and have slurred speech and staggering gait, and sometimes hallucinations and delusions. There is no specific treatment other than to wait for the effects of the solvents to wear off.

The management of pain

Drug-dependent patients may be admitted to hospital for the treatment of conditions unrelated to their dependence or for one of its complications. The staff on general wards are often very anxious about this and, specifically, often seek advice about the best way to provide adequate analgesia for patients who are already dependent on opioid analgesics. A useful rule of thumb is that the patient will require the usual analgesic dose in addition to their usual maintenance dose. Establishing the latter may require advice from a specialist drug and alcohol liaison team (see below). Only doctors with a special licence from the Home Office may prescribe heroin to addicts for the purpose of treating their addiction; however, if an addict requires heroin for analgesia, any doctor can prescribe it for this purpose.

Psychological interventions

The majority of interventions are based on learning theory models, but there is also the recognition that there are non-treatment routes to improvement (Ghodse 2002).

Information-based approaches, e.g. health education and information, are useful in situations that are less complicated. This might include education about harm minimization, immunization, vaccination and contraception.

In the addiction literature the term 'counselling' is used to incorporate brief or intensive interventions, be they supportive, directive or motivational counselling, individual, family or group behavioural treatments as well as social network behavioural therapy. Counselling may aim to reduce the use of alcohol and drugs, as well as the negative consequences or related problems, e.g. lifestyle issues such as housing, sexual health or careers.

The term may encompass assessment, engagement and support, together with the development of therapeutic relationships. The non-judgemental and empathic method of challenging decisions and assumptions in motivational interviewing is included in the gamut of techniques.

Important common objectives may include:

- problem solving: developing competence in dealing with a specific problem
- acquisition of social skills: mastery of social and interpersonal skills by assertiveness or anger control
- cognitive change: modification of irrational beliefs and maladaptive patterns of thought
- behaviour change: modification of maladaptive behaviour
- systemic change: introducing change into family systems.

Counselling is a widely used term and is a form of therapy or intervention that includes a wide range of theoretical models. There are many different definitions, each emphasizing specific aspects of the counselling role and processes practised in a multiplicity of settings. It embodies psychodynamics, cognitive behavioural and person-centred approaches.

The choice of options depends on the nature and extent of the problems and what approach may appear more appropriate and suitable for a particular drug user. These include counselling, motivational enhancement, cognitive behavioural therapy, family therapy and group therapy.

1. Non-directive counselling. The patient determines the content and direction of the counselling and explores conflict and emotions at the same time. While allowing empathic reflection, the counsellor does not offer advice and feedback.
2. Motivational interviewing aims to build motivation for change. The focus is on a non-judgemental approach, patient's concerns about, and choice regarding future drug use, and elicits strategies from the patient. Motivational enhancement directs the patient to motivation for change by offering empathic feedback, advice and information and selectively reinforces certain discrepancies that emerge between current behaviour and goals, in order to enhance motivation for change. Significant others play some role in the

treatment but not a central role. It is, by and large, an individual therapeutic situation where the individual's motivation is seen as central. It aims to alter the decisional balance so that patients themselves direct the process of change.

3. A cognitive behavioural approach assumes that the patient would like to change, and analyses situations that cause drug use, so that these can be altered. Problem-solving techniques, self-monitoring, anger management, relapse prevention, assertiveness training and the acquisition of social skills and modification of irrational beliefs or patterns of thought or behaviour are used. Individual, group and family therapies used in the treatment of addiction problems are often based along cognitive behavioural lines.

4. Social network behaviour therapy considers the social environment as being important in the development, maintenance and resolution of substance problems. It maximizes positive social support, which is central to the process. The therapist offers advice and feedback and thereby facilitates change in the patient's social world; behaviour is not interpreted; engagement with significant others is key in bringing about change and achieving goals.

5. Family therapy involves attempts to understand and interpret the family dynamics in order to change the psychopathology. Substance use is perceived as a symptom of family dysfunction and altering dynamics brings about change in the substance misuse. Family members are viewed as contributory to the problems. Behavioural techniques may be used in family therapy as well as psychodynamic techniques.

Group therapies and 12-step programmes

Participation in self-help groups is an important feature of many treatment programmes, where participants receive support from recovering members who often take members back to the negative consequences of substance misuse. A variant group therapy is the 12-step approach. Central to the 12 steps philosophy is the idea that recovery from addiction is possible only if the individual recognizes his or her problem, and admits that he/she is unable to use substances in moderation. Alcoholics Anonymous and Narcotics Anonymous are examples of the '12-step' philosophy where drug users have to abstain completely.

Residential rehabilitation and therapeutic communities

Residential treatments such as therapeutic communities offer long-term intensive psychological interventions. These have typically been used in the USA for those with substance-abuse and related problems who require treatment that is intensive, highly structured and of long duration. The relatively few studies have reported that long-term residential treatments are more effective than outpatient modalities, where length of stay and retention in treatment is related to long-term outcome. The most consistent outcome is that of improvement in criminal involvement.

Ancillary support

Evidence suggests that support with housing, other health and social services and family involvement produce a better outcome (McLellan *et al.* 1999). Thus inter-agency collaboration is not just of academic importance.

Special groups

When planning interventions, care must be taken of the special needs of women, young people, older people, ethnic minority groups, the homeless, professional groups (e.g. healthcare professionals), and those involved with the criminal justice system (e.g. on probation, in custody or on Drug Treatment and Testing Orders) with regard to availability and acceptability of interventions (Crome 1997; Crome & Day 1999; Crome *et al.* 2003; Day *et al.* 2003). In summary, one can say with a degree of confidence that treatment 'works well' for about 40% of patients, and that treatment helps another 30%. There is still a proportion for whom treatment is apparently not beneficial for reasons that are not clear. Thus, while overall evidence of effectiveness is substantial, and growing as the research base develops, not surprisingly, there is no one single approach that is universally effective for such a complex group of conditions.

Pregnant users

Care of the pregnant drug user is focused on giving the patient the best chance of delivering a healthy child and this is achieved by assisting the woman to come off drugs as early in pregnancy as possible. As a general principle, withdrawal should be gradual to avoid precipitating fetal distress or premature labour and, whenever possible, pregnant users should be encouraged to come into hospital for initial assessment and supervised withdrawal, ideally at least two months before the expected date of delivery. Hospital admission also facilitates liaison with all the professionals (obstetrician, paediatrician, social worker) involved in the care of the mother-to-be and her child.

Pain control in labour for women who have been using opiates may be more difficult than usual because the dose of opiate required to achieve adequate analgesia may be too high for the baby. In this situation, an epidural anaesthetic may be helpful and this, and other methods of pain control, should be discussed with the mother beforehand.

If drug withdrawal was not possible before delivery or if illicit drug use is likely to continue after discharge from hospital, the mother should be advised to bottle-feed her baby because many drugs that may cause toxicity in the infant enter breast milk in pharmacologically significant quantities (e.g. opiates, barbiturates, benzodiazepines).

Healthcare professionals

Healthcare professionals who abuse drugs (doctors, dentists, nurses, pharmacists) are different to other drug users because they have access to and usually take pharmaceutical preparations of drugs which they have obtained by deception (Ghodse *et al.* 2000). They suffer fewer infective complications of drug abuse but may become severely dependent very quickly because they can consume large quantities of pure drugs. In addition, they often manage to conceal their dependence for a long time and, when it does become apparent, they rationalize it as a consequence of recent stress, minimizing the quantity of drugs being consumed and the duration of the problem. Friends, family and colleagues, trying to act protectively, may tacitly collude with the drug-taking behaviour, making excuses for their fellow-professional and covering up for drug-related behaviour. However well meant, this merely prolongs drug abuse and delays the initiation of treatment. In addition, it completely ignores the hazards to which the patients of the drug-abusing professional are exposed.

In this situation the best approach is to discuss the problem with senior colleagues who are in a position to influence the drug-abusing professional and to encourage him/her to admit to the problem and to seek help for it. Any confrontation is best managed by two colleagues, one from the same speciality to offer support and friendship, and one with a knowledge of drug abuse to give expert practical advice on possible routes into treatment. Although the overriding message is one of genuine concern for the individual, there should be no doubt that refusal to seek help will have serious implications for his/her future career with involvement of the appropriate professional body if necessary. It must be emphasized that the safety of patients comes first at all times and that all healthcare professionals have an ethical responsibility to act if they feel that a colleague has a drug problem that impairs their ability to practise.

Children and young people

Children may be involved in drug abuse either directly (taking drugs themselves) or indirectly, if they are in close physical and/or emotional proximity to others who are abusing drugs.

Children who abuse drugs themselves may first come to medical attention via the police, having been taken into custody for a drug-related offence. They often have comorbid psychiatric disorders and there may be a preceding history of self-harming and/or excessive alcohol consumption; psychiatric assessment should specifically explore these topics. Although it is customary to seek the parent's consent, or that of a responsible adult, before examining or treating a child, it should be remembered that children have the right to be kept informed about what is happening to them, and why. Furthermore, some children are competent to make decisions for themselves and, if so, their decisions should be respected as far as possible.

Children growing up in homes where drugs are being abused may come to medical attention when their parent(s) seek(s) help for their drug problem. Although professional care may be focused on the parent, it is essential that the child is not overlooked and that specific attention is paid to his/her welfare. A thorough assessment should be made of their physical and emotional needs and of the risks to which they are exposed as a result of parental drug abuse. The assessment should cover the provision of basic necessities (accommodation, food, clothing, heating), the nature of the home environment and the direct health risks to the child. A management plan should be drawn up and a keyworker identified who will maintain contact with the family and who will assume special responsibility for the child, so that the most vulnerable members of what is often a very dysfunctional family unit are safeguarded.

Older people

It is easy to overlook drug abuse in older people because the necessary high index of suspicion, the need for which was emphasized earlier in this chapter, is often suspended when dealing with this generation (Crome & Day 1999; Gfroerer et al. 2003; McInnes & Powell 1994). However, a long history of drug abuse may be concealed within an apparently routine and orderly lifestyle, and this will only be elicited if assessment is as rigorous for this age group as for those who are much younger (Beckett et al. 2002; Ghodse 1997).

Among older people drug abuse may encompass the long-standing use of illicit drugs but may also involve both prescription and over-the-counter medications taken to treat a variety of symptoms. Age-related decline in hepatic or renal function, sometimes combined with the acute onset of a specific illness, may precipitate drug-related changes in mental function, even if there has been no change in drug consumption. The problem may be compounded by the prescription of a new drug to deal with a new condition, which then interacts with other medication of which the prescribing doctor may be unaware.

The patient is unlikely to recognize that the drugs themselves are now part of the problem and, indeed, may increase their dose in an attempt to alleviate new problems. It is therefore all the more important that the professionals who become involved recognize the need for a thorough, detailed drug history. As always, this includes exploration of alcohol intake.

Compulsory treatment

Drug abuse/dependence do not, alone, constitute grounds for compulsory admission to hospital. However, admission under a section of the 1983 Mental Health Act is appropriate if a patient is so severely disturbed as a result of taking drugs, that he/she is a danger to self or others (Tables 9.7 and 9.8).

Liaison with the police

Substance abusers are often detained by the police and may need to be transferred to hospital, sometimes to the A&E department, particularly if they are intoxicated or suffering drug-related injuries. Following treatment, a patient may be well enough to be discharged from hospital but may not be fit enough for detention in a police cell. The hospital doctor should take this into account when assessing the patient's fitness for discharge and, if necessary, recommend reassessment by the forensic physician at the police station.

Hospital doctors may be asked by the police for their opinion about the patient's fitness for interview. Before providing this advice they need to establish if the patient is currently under the influence of drugs/alcohol, whether there is evidence of the abstinence syndrome and whether the detainee is fully aware of his/her surroundings and is well enough to withstand potentially stressful questioning, to cope with the interview and, if necessary, to instruct a solicitor. The timing and duration of the interview will help to inform this advice, which is important because of the issue of the admissibility of confessions obtained when the individual's mental state is impaired or when they are in withdrawal and desperate for a 'fix'. If an individual is obviously intoxicated, it is customary to wait for the effects of the drug to wear off; however, the mental state may fluctuate markedly following the use of hallucinogenic drugs, making it difficult to ascertain when the patient is fit for interview (Association of Forensic Physicians and Royal College of Psychiatrists 2006).

Intimate searches for drugs must be carried out at a hospital or other medical premises and must be carried out by a registered medical practitioner or registered nurse. However, the responsibility for carrying out the examination lies with the forensic physician and not the hospital doctor.

Table 9.7. Summary of the Classes of the Misuse of Drugs Act, 1971.

Class	Main drugs in each class	Maximum penalties for possession	Maximum penalties for possession with intent to supply
A	Heroin, cocaine (and crack cocaine), ecstasy, LSD, methadone, methylamphetamine,[a] morphine, opium, dipipanone and pethidine Class B drugs when designed for injection become Class A	Six months or a fine of £5000 or both (in a magistrates' court) Or, in a trial by jury seven years or an unlimited fine or both	Six months or a fine of £5000 or both (in a magistrates' court) Or, in a trial by jury life or an unlimited fine or both
B	Amphetamines, barbiturates, codeine and dihydrocodeine	Three months or a fine of £2500 or both (in a magistrates' court) Or, in a trial by jury five years or an unlimited fine or both	Six months or a fine or of £ both (in a magistrates' court) Or, in a trial by jury 14 years or an unlimited fine or both
C	Benzodiazepines, buprenorphine, cannabinol and cannabinol derivatives, cannabis[b] (herbal and resin), diethylpropion and anabolic steroids	Three months or a fine of £1000 or both (in a magistrates' court) Or in a trial by jury two years or an unlimited fine or both	Three months or a fine of £ 2500 or both (in a magistrates' court) Or, in a trial by jury 14 years or an unlimited fine or both

Notes: [a]From 18 January 2007. [b]Cultivation of the cannabis plant carries a maximum penalty of six months or a fine of £5000 or both in a magistrates' court, or in a trial by jury, 14 years or an unlimited fine or both.

Table 9.8. Summary of schedules of the Misuse of Drugs Regulations, 2001.

Schedule	Main drugs included	Restrictions
1	LSD, ecstasy, raw opium, psilocin, cannabis (herbal and resin).	Import, export, production, possession and supply only permitted under Home Office licence for medical or scientific research. Cannot be prescribed by doctors or dispensed by pharmacists.
2	Heroin, cocaine, methadone, morphine, amphetamine, dexamphetamine, pethidine and quinalbarbitone.	May be prescribed and lawfully possessed when on prescription. Otherwise, supply, possession, import, export and production are offences except under Home Office licence. Particular controls on their prescription, storage and record keeping apply.
3	Barbiturates, temazepam, flunitrazepam, buprenorphine, pentazocine and diethylpropion.	May be prescribed and lawfully possessed when on prescription. Otherwise, supply, possession, import, export and production are offences except under Home Office licence. Particular controls on their prescription and storage apply. Temazepam prescription requirements are less stringent than those for the other drugs in this Schedule.
4 Part 1	Benzodiazepines (except flunitrazepam and temazepam), ketamine and pemoline.	May be prescribed and lawfully possessed when on prescription. Otherwise, supply, possession, import, export and production are offences except under Home Office licence.
4 Part 2	Anabolic steroids.	May be lawfully possessed by anyone even without a prescription, provided they are in the form of a medical product.
5	Compound preparations such as cough mixtures which contain small amounts of controlled drugs such as morphine. Some may be sold over-the-counter.	Authority needed for their production or supply but can be freely imported, exported or possessed (without a prescription).

Planning services: the role of a substance misuse liaison team

Drug and alcohol liaison team (Lind *et al*. 1999; Kouimtsidis *et al*. 2003)

The high medical morbidity rate associated with substance abuse results in the frequent attendance of drug abusers at A&E departments and in their admission to general medical and surgical wards. There they are often perceived by the staff as 'difficult' patients, although this verdict is likely to be based on anecdotal experience of a small number of challenging patients and probably reflects the staff's own lack of confidence, knowledge and skills. Whatever the cause, the consequence for patients is far from satisfactory because the threshold for their admission to hospital may be higher than for other patients and their management, whether in A&E, in the outpatient clinic or on a ward, may be impaired, as staff try to avoid becoming engaged in a situation that they fear may be too challenging.

A drug and alcohol liaison team (DALT), along the lines of that pioneered at St George's Healthcare NHS Trust and the SW London and St George's Mental Health Trust, may be helpful in supporting staff and in ensuring that patients' needs are met. It does this by liaising closely with professional colleagues (particularly medical and nursing colleagues) and providing specialist input to the care of patients with substance misuse problems. It also provides education and training to junior medical and nursing staff in the assessment and management of drug and alcohol misuse. All of this heightens awareness of substance misuse within the general hospital setting so that screening and early diagnosis and intervention occur more frequently and fewer cases go un-noticed.

The DALT service is primarily provided by doctors and nurses, but they are part of a wider multidisciplinary team that includes social work and psychology input. It accepts referrals of any patient currently receiving treatment in the hospital, either as an outpatient, in the A&E department or as an inpatient, and the service can be provided in a variety of clinical settings — on the ward, in the A&E department, or as a telephone response. A regular clinic is also held to accept referrals of patients attending other outpatient services, particularly those with a high proportion of substance misuse attendees (e.g. hepatitis and genito-urinary medicine (GUM) clinics). Patients who were initially seen on the ward can also be seen in this clinic if they require additional, short-term input.

Conclusion

Substance users are heterogeneous, no one approach is universally effective, and evaluation of treatment outcome should be multidimensional. However, it is acknowledged that the routes to 'natural recovery' are multiple and require further elucidation. Whatever the treatment 'label', new relationships and friends, success at school or work, emotional support from families, self-help and structured activities are important components. In the literature on adults, not only have cognitive and behavioural approaches, motivational enhancement therapy, relapse prevention therapy and community reinforcement approaches empirical support, but they have much in common with other cognitive behavioural interventions for children and youths with behaviour problems. In the child and adolescent substance misuse field, these therapies are just beginning to be systematically studied.

Treatment must take into account issues of age, gender, disability, ethnicity, cultural background, and stages of readiness to change. There must be sensitivity to the motivational barriers to change at the outset of treatment, and therapist empathy influences outcome. Where the evidence is lacking, there are a number of good-practice principles. These should include the unique developmental needs of patients, including delay in normal cognitive and socioemotional development. While not all drug users will be dependent, misusers may relapse, and many may have other comorbid disorders which must be recognized and treated.

There is a need for innovation in research specifically directed at this group of people in the UK. This can include careful descriptive studies, detailed evaluation of ongoing projects, and scrutiny of 'older' techniques in 'newer' settings and situations. Ingenuity may be required in identifying some of the settings where drinkers or drug users may be found. For it is not only in A&E departments, geriatric and paediatric wards, and obstetrics and gynaecology departments that prevalence of substance misuse is high, but also in sexual health clinics, primary care clinics and generic counselling services. Screening and assessment of these groups, in effect a captive audience, can foster a 'teachable moment' in which to deliver and evaluate brief interventions. Brief interventions must be adapted in form and content to the particular needs as they may work either alone or, in complex situations, synergistically with other prevention activities, policy measures and specialized treatment interventions. Thus, detection and management in general psychiatric and medical settings offers the potential for a significant public health impact in the short and longer term (Royal College of Physicians 2001). Duration of treatment is emerging as the key element in successful outcome (Moos & Moos 2003). General medical settings may offer that link in the process of securing continuity.

Acknowledgement

We would like to acknowledge Dr B. Thom for review of prevalence data in hospital setting.

REFERENCES

American Psychiatric Association. (1994). *Diagnostic and Statistical Manual of Mental Disorders IV*. Washington DC: American Psychiatric Association.

Andrews, G. and Jenkins, R. (1999). *Management of Mental Disorders*. Sydney: World Health Organization Collaborating Centre for Mental Health and Substance Abuse.

Appleby, L., Dysonk V., Luchinsk, D. J., *et al.* (1997). The impact of substance use screening on a public psychiatric inpatient population. *Psychiatric Services*, **48**, 1311–16.

Association of Forensic Physicians and Royal College of Psychiatrists. (2006). *Substance Misuse Detainees in Police Custody: Guidelines for Clinical Management*, 3rd edn. London: Royal College of Psychiatrists.

Aubrey, L. (1998). *Motivational Interviewing with Adolescents Presenting for Outpatient Substance Abuse Treatment: Doctoral Dissertation*. University of New Mexico Dissertation Abstracts DAI-B 59–03 1357.

Banerjee, S., Clancy, C. and Crome, I., eds (2002). *Co-existing Problems of Mental Disorder and Substance Misuse (Dual Diagnosis): an Information Manual*. London: Royal College of Physicians, College Research Unit.

Beckett, J., Kouimtsidis, C., Reynolds, R., *et al.* (2002). Substance misuse in elderly general hospital in-patients. *International Journal of Geriatric Psychiatry*, **17**, 193–6.

Bien, T. H., Miller, W. R. and Tonigan, J. S. (1993). Brief interventions for alcohol problems: a review. *Addiction*, **88**, 315–36.

Bosio, P., Keenan, E., Gleeson, R., *et al.* (1997). The prevalence of chemical substance and alcohol abuse in an obstetric population in Dublin. *Irish Medical Journal*, **90**, 149–50.

Brookoff, D., Cook, C. S., Williams, C., *et al.* (1994). Testing reckless drivers for cocaine and marijuana. *New England Journal of Medicine*, **331**, 518–22.

Brown, R. L., Leonard, T., Saunders, L. A., *et al.* (1998). The prevalence and detection of substance use disorders among inpatients ages 18 to 49: an opportunity for prevention. *Preventive Medicine*, **27**, 101–10.

Canning, U. P., Kennell-Webb, S. A., Marshall, E. J., *et al.* (1999). Substance misuse in acute general medical admissions. *Quarterly Journal of Medicine*, **92**, 319–26.

Carey, K. B. and Correia, C. J. (1998). Severe mental illness and addictions: assessment considerations. *Addictive Behaviours*, **23**, 735–48.

Clerici, M. and Carta, I. (1996). Personality disorders among psychoactive substance users: diagnostic and psychodynamic issues. *European Addiction Research*, **2**, 147–55.

Cohen, J., Runciman, R. and Williams, R. (1999). Substance use and misuse in psychiatric wards. *Drugs: education, prevention and policy*, **6**, 181–94.

Cornelius, J. R., Salloum, I. M., Ehler, J. G., *et al.* (1997). Fluoxetine in depressed alcoholics: a double-blind placebo controlled trial. *Archives of General Psychiatry*, **54**, 700–5.

Crome, I. B. (1997). Editorial: young people and substance problems – from image to imagination. *Drugs: Education, Prevention and Policy*, **4**, 107–16.

Crome, I. B. and Day, E. (1999). Substance misuse and dependence: older people deserve better services. *Reviews in Clinical Gerontology*, **9**, 327–42.

Crome, I. B., Ghodse, A.-H., Gilvarry, E., *et al.* (2003). *Young People and Substance Misuse.* London: Gaskell.

Day, E., Porter, L., Clarke, A., *et al.* (2003). Drug misuse in pregnancy: the impact of a specialist treatment service. *Psychiatric Bulletin*, **27**, 99–101.

De Las Cuevas, C., Sanz, E. J., De La Fuente, J. A., *et al.* (2000). The Severity of Dependence Scale (SDS) as screening test for benzodiazepine dependence: SDS validation study. *Addiction*, **95**, 245–50.

El-Guebaly, N., Armstrong, S. J. and Hodgins, D. C. (1998). Substance abuse and the emergency room: programmatic implications. *Journal of Addictive Diseases*, **17**, 21–40.

Frischer, M., McArdle, P. and Crome, I. B. (2004). The epidemiology of substance misuse in young people. In *Young People and Substance Misuse*, ed. I. B. Crome, H. Ghodse, E. Gilvarry, *et al.* London: Gaskell, pp. 35–50.

Gfroerer, J., Penne, M., Pemberton, M., *et al.* (2003). Substance abuse treatment need among older adults in 2020: the impact of the aging baby-boom cohort. *Drug and Alcohol Dependence*, **69**, 127–35.

Ghodse, A. H. (1997). Substance misuse by the elderly. *British Journal of Hospital Medicine*, **58**, 451–3.

Ghodse, A. H. (2002). *Drugs and Addictive Behaviour*, 3rd edn. Cambridge: Cambridge University Press.

Ghodse, A. H., Oyefeso, A. and Kilpatrick, B. (1998). Mortality of drug addicts in the United Kingdom 1967–1993. *International Journal of Epidemiology*, **27**, 273–8.

Ghodse, A. H., Mann, S. and Johnson, P. (2000). *Doctors and Their Health.* Surrey: Reed Business Information.

Gossop, M., Marsden, J. and Stewart, D. (2000). Treatment outcomes of stimulant misusers: one-year follow-up results from the National Treatment Outcome Research Study (NTORS). *Addictive Behaviors*, **25**, 509–22.

Gossop, M., Marsden, J., Stewart, D., *et al.* (2003). The National Treatment Outcome Research Study (NTORS): 4–5 year follow-up results. *Addiction*, **98**, 291–303.

Herring, R. and Thom, B. (1999). Resisting the gaze?: nurses' perceptions of the role of accident and emergency departments in responding to alcohol-related attendances. *Critical Public Health*, **9**, 135–48.

Hodgson, R., John, B., Abbasi, T., *et al.* (2003). Fast screening for alcohol misuse. *Addictive Behaviors*, **28**, 1453–63.

Hulse, G. K., Robertson, S. I. and Tait, R. J. (2001). Adolescent emergency department presentations with alcohol- or other drug-related problems in Perth, Western Australia. *Addiction*, **96**, 1059–67.

Kellogg, S. H., McHugh, P. F., Bell, K., *et al.* (2003). The Kreek-McHugh-Schluger-Kellogg scale: a new, rapid method for quantifying substance abuse and its possible applications. *Drug and Alcohol Dependence*, **69**, 137–50.

Kemper, K. J., Greteman, A., Bennett, E., *et al.* (1993). Screening mothers of young children for substance abuse. *Journal of Developmental and Behavioural Pediatrics*, **14**, 308–12.

Knight, J. R., Shrier, L. A., Bravender, T. D., *et al.* (1999). A new brief screen for adolescent substance abuse. *Archives of Pediatrics & Adolescent Medicine*, **153**, 591–6.

Kouimtsidis, C., Reynolds, M., Hunt, M., *et al.* (2003). Substance use in the general hospital: a survey of a large general hospital population. *Addictive Behaviours*, **183**, 15–21.

Lind, J., Oyefeso, A., Pollard, M., *et al.* (1999). Death rate from use of ecstasy or heroin (Letter). *The Lancet*, **354**, 277–82.

Lingford-Hughes, A., Welch, S. and Nutt, D. J. (2004). Evidence-based guidelines for the pharmacological management of substance misuse, addiction and comorbidity: recommendations from the British Association of Psychopharmacolgy. *Journal of Psychopharmacology*, **18**, 293–335.

Longabaugh, R., Woolard, R. F., Nirenberg, T. D. D., *et al.* (2001). Evaluating the effects of a brief motivational intervention for injured drinkers in the emergency department. *Journal of Studies on Alcohol*, **63**, 806–16.

Marquet, P., Delpla, P. A., Kerguelen, S., *et al.* (1998). Prevalence of drugs of abuse in urine of drivers involved in road accidents in France: a collaborative study. *Journal of Forensic Science*, **43**, 806–11.

Martino, S., Grilo, C. M. and Fehon, D. C. (2000). Development of the drug abuse screening test for adolescents (DAST-A). *Addictive Behaviours*, **25**, 57–70.

McCann, B., Simpson, T. L., Ries, R., *et al.* (2000). Reliability and validity of screening instrument for drug and alcohol abuse in adults seeking evaluation for attention-deficit/hyperactivity disorder. *The American Journal on Addictions*, **9**, 1–9.

McGovern, M. P. and Morrison, D. H. (1992). The Chemical Use, Abuse and Dependency Scale (CUAD): rationale, reliability and validity. *Journal of Substance Abuse Treatment*, **9**, 27–38.

McHugo, G. J., Drake, R. E., Burton, H. L., *et al.* (1995). A scale for assessing the stage of substance abuse treatment in persons with severe mental illness. *The Journal of Nervous and Mental Disease*, **183**, 762–7.

McInnes, E. and Powell, J. (1994). Drug and alcohol referrals: are elderly substance abuse diagnoses and referrals being missed? *British Medical Journal*, **308**, 444–6.

McLellan, A. T., Luborsky, L., Woody, G. E., *et al.* (1980). An improved diagnostic evaluation instrument for substance abuse patients: the Addiction Severity Index. *The Journal of Nervous and Mental Disease*, **168**, 26–33.

McLellan, A. T., Hagan, T. A., Levine, M., *et al.* (1999). Does clinical case management improve outpatient addiction treatment? *Drug and Alcohol Dependence*, **55**, 91–103.

Monti, P. M., Colby, S. M., Barnett, N. P., *et al.* (1999). Brief interventions for harm reduction with alcohol positive older adolescents in a hospital emergency department. *Journal of Consulting and Clinical Psychology*, **67**, 989–94.

Moos, R. H. and Moos, B. S. (2003). Long-term influence of duration and intensity of treatment on previously untreated individuals with alcohol use disorders. *Addiction*, **98**, 325–37.

Nunes, E., Weissman, M., Goldstein, R., *et al.* (1998). Psychopathology in children of parents with opiate dependence and/or major depression. *Journal of the American Academy of Child and Adolescent Psychiatry*, **37**, 1142–51.

Oyefeso, A., Ghodse, A. H., Clancy, C., *et al.* (1999). Suicide among drug addicts in the UK. *British Journal of Psychiatry*, **175**, 277–82.

Project MATCH Research Group. (1997a). Matching alcoholism treatments to client heterogeneity: project MATCH post treatment drinking outcomes. *Journal of Studies on Alcohol*, **58**, 7–29.

Project MATCH Research Group. (1997b). Project MATCH secondary a priori hypotheses. *Addiction*, **92**, 1671–98.

Raistrick, D., Bradshaw, J., Tober, G., *et al.* (1994). Development of the Leeds Dependence Questionnaire (LDQ): a questionnaire to measure alcohol and opiate dependence in the context of a treatment evaluation package. *Addiction*, **89**, 563–72.

Richmond, R. L. and Anderson, P. (1994). Lessons from conducting research in general practice for smokers and excessive drinkers: the experience in Australia and the United Kingdom: 1 Interpreting the results. *Addiction*, **89**, 35–40.

Robins, I. N., Helzer, J. E., Przybeck, T. R., *et al.* (1988). Alcohol disorders in the community: a report from the epidemiologic catchment area. In *Alcoholism Origins and Outcomes*, ed. R. Rose and J. Barret. New York: Raven, pp. 15–29.

Rosenberg, P. O. (1995). *Alcohol and Other Drug Screening of Hospitalized Trauma Patients.* (Treatment Improvement Protocol (TIP) Series 16.)

Rosenberg, S. D., Drake, R. E., Wolford, G. L., *et al.* (1998). Dartmouth Assessment of Lifestyle Instrument (DALI): a substance use disorder screen for people with severe mental illness. *The American Journal of Psychiatry*, **155**, 232–8.

Royal College of Physicians. (2001). *Alcohol – Can the NHS Afford It?* London: Royal College of Physicians.

Schuckit, M. A., Smith, T. L., Radziminski, S., *et al.* (2000). Behavioural symptoms and psychiatric diagnoses among 162 children in alcoholic and non alcoholic families. *American Journal of Psychiatry*, **157**, 1881–3.

Senft, R. A., Freeborn, D. K., Polen, M. R., *et al.* (1997). Brief intervention in a primary care setting for hazardous drinkers. *American Journal of Preventive Medicine*, **13**, 464–70.

Skinner, H. A. (1982). The Drug Abuse Screening Test. *Addictive Behaviours*, **7**, 363–71.

Smith, G. C., Clarke, D. M. and Handrinos, D. (1995). Recognising drug and alcohol problems in patients referred to consultation-liaison psychiatry. *The Medical Journal of Australia*, **163**, 307–12.

Soderstrom, C. A., Dischinger, P. C., Kerns, T. J., *et al.* (1995). Marijuana and other drug use among automobiles and motorcycle drivers treated at a trauma center. *Accident Analysis and Prevention*, **27**, 131–5.

Stein, M. D., Wilkinson, J., Berglas, N., *et al.* (1996). Prevalence and detection of illicit drug disorders among hospitalized patients. *American Journal of Drug and Alcohol Abuse*, **22**, 463–71.

Sugrue, M., Seger, M., Dredge, G., *et al.* (1995). Evaluation of the prevalence of drug and alcohol abuse in motor vehicle trauma in South Western Sydney. *Australia and New Zealand Journal of Surgery*, **65**, 853–6.

Topp, L. and Mattick, R. P. (1997). Choosing a cut-off on the Severity of Dependence Scale (SDS) for amphetamine users. *Addiction*, **92**, 839–45.

Vidal-Trecan, G., Varescon, I., Nabet, N., *et al.* (2003). Intravenous use of prescribed sublingual buprenorphine tablets by drug users receiving maintenance therapy in France. *Drug and Alcohol Dependence*, **69**, 175–81.

Vuori, E., Henry, J. A., Ojanpera, I., *et al.* (2003). Death following ingestion of MDMA (ecstasy) and moclobemide. *Addiction*, **98**, 365–8.

Wolff, K., Farrell, M., Marsden, J., *et al.* (1999). A review of biological indicators of illicit drug use, practical considerations and clinical usefulness. *Addiction*, **94**, 1279–98.

Wolford, G. L., Rosenberg, S. D., Drake, R. E., *et al.* (1999). Evaluation of methods for detecting substance use disorder in persons with severe mental illness. *Psychology of Addictive Behaviours*, **13**, 313–26.

World Health Organization. (1992). *International Classification of Diseases 10 (ICD-10)*. Geneva: World Health Organization.

10

Sexual problems in medical patients

Michael King

Introduction

Sexual dysfunction is a common consequence of medical illness and should be considered in any medical patient undergoing a psychological assessment. Even though sexual problems can be among the most demoralizing and disabling features of medical disorders, they are frequently overlooked or neglected by clinicians. Furthermore, there is uncertainty about how sexual problems should be defined, particularly in women. In order to make a complete assessment of sexual difficulties the clinician must have a working knowledge of the anatomy, physiology and psychology of sexual function. As in all areas of liaison psychiatry, psychiatrists can only assess the role of psychological factors if they are knowledgeable about the presenting medical problem.

The anatomy and physiology of sex

The penis is composed of two functional compartments, the dorsal, paired corpora cavernosa and the ventral, corpus spongiosum, surrounded by the tunica albuginea. The corpora cavernosa are complex structures composed of smooth muscle fibres, neurones, endothelial-lined vascular spaces, coiled arteries and arterioles. The blood supply arises from the paired cavernosal arteries, which are terminal branches of the internal pudendal artery. Branches of the cavernosal artery, the helicine arteries, open directly into the cavernosal spaces. Blood drains into post-cavernosal venules to reach larger veins that pass through the tunica albuginea and connect with the deep dorsal vein. Blood is retained in the penis during erection by passive compression of the cavernosal venules against the tunica albuginea. Innervation is by somatic and autonomic nervous systems. The somatic system supplies sensory innervation to the penis and perineal skeletal

Handbook of Liaison Psychiatry, ed. Geoffrey Lloyd and Elspeth Guthrie. Published by Cambridge University Press. © Cambridge University Press 2007.

muscle motor fibres. The sacral parasympathetic neurones are chiefly responsible for initiating and maintaining erection, while sympathetic supply co-ordinates detumescence and maintains the penis in a flaccid state. Sympathetic activity also predominates in the control of ejaculation. A potential 'ejaculation generator' has recently been discovered in the lumbar spinal cord in rats (Truitt & Coolen 2002). Several neurotransmitters are involved in erection, but the principal mediator is nitric oxide. Nitric oxide activates the enzyme guanil cyclase, which facilitates the production of guanosine monophosphate (GMP), a potent smooth muscle relaxant. Phosphodiesterases break down GMP, and thus blocking their action using phosphodiesterase inhibitors such as sildenafil facilitates and prolongs erection. Other active neurotransmitters in the pathway are vasoactive intestinal polypeptide, prostaglandin I_2 and prostaglandin E.

Our knowledge of the physiology of the female sexual response has lagged far behind that of the male. However, there is increasing evidence that the neurological and vascular changes occurring in sexual arousal in men have their counterparts in the clitoral engorgement, vaginal expansion and lubrication seen in women. If a woman is mentally responsive to her partner, but lacks appropriate increases in genital blood flow, it has been suggested that treatment with phosphodiesterase inhibitors may have a role (Basson 2001). However, sildenafil has had no obvious benefit in a number of randomized trials. Androgens appear to be important mediators of sexual desire in both sexes (Kandeel *et al.* 2001; Tuiten *et al.* 2000).

Common sexual problems

The classification of sexual problems in men was not controversial until recently, when the pharmaceutical industry took an increasing interest in the field. There is concern that epidemiological studies funded by pharmaceutical companies are reporting inflated prevalences of sexual disorders and therefore creating a 'need' for treatment (Akkus *et al.* 2002; Mirone *et al.* 2002; Tiefer 2000). This has led to claims that the pharmaceutical industry is 'building the science of female sexual dysfunction' (Moynihan 2003). The word dysfunction implies a state of dis-ease that requires treatment. A woman-centred definition of sexual problems has recently been suggested as an alternative to concepts of sickness and health (Tiefer 2000; Moynihan 2003) and the international classifications of sexual dysfunction are currently under review (Basson *et al.* 2000; Vroege *et al.* 1998). Some consider that a woman's sexual function is completely different to a man's, in being responsive rather than spontaneous and more influenced by emotional intimacy with her partner (Basson 2001). We need further evidence that the common complaints of lack or loss of sexual desire in men or women are obstacles to

Table 10.1. Difficulties of sexual function not explained by medical disorders (based on DSM-IV).

Problem area	Manifested as
Desire	• Hypoactive sexual desire disorder: persistently or recurrently deficient (or absent) sexual fantasies and desire for sexual activity. • Sexual aversion disorder: persistent or recurrent extreme aversion to, and avoidance of, all (or almost all) genital sexual contact with a partner.
Arousal	• Female sexual arousal disorder: persistent or recurrent inability to attain, or maintain until completion of sexual activity, an adequate lubrication-swelling response of sexual excitement. • Male erectile disorder: persistent or recurrent inability to attain, or maintain until completion of sexual activity, an adequate erection.
Orgasm	• Female orgasmic disorder: persistent or recurrent delay in, or absence of, orgasm following a normal sexual excitement phase. • Male orgasmic disorder: persistent or recurrent delay in, or absence of, orgasm following a normal sexual excitement phase. • Premature ejaculation (PE): persistent or recurrent ejaculation before, on, or shortly after penetration and before the person wishes it.
Pain	• Dyspareunia (not due to a medical condition): recurrent or persistent genital associated with sexual intercourse in men or women. • Vaginismus (not due to a medical condition): recurrent or persistent spasm of the musculature of the outer third of the vagina that interferes with sexual intercourse. There may be associated spasm of the internal adductor muscles of the thighs.

satisfactory sexual relations or that a medical solution is indicated. For many people, reduced sexual interest or response may be a normal adaptation to stress or an unsatisfactory relationship.

Sexual problems that are not due primarily to physical disorders can be divided into difficulties of desire, arousal and orgasm (Table 10.1).

Assessment of a sexual problem

Taking a sexual history is a sensitive task. The clinician must make an objective assessment of sexual behaviour, while taking account of the emotional issues and personal values that the patient brings to the interview. Sexual history taking should not be conducted in isolation but should be regarded as part of the medical or psychiatric history. What follows is an outline of the main features of a sexual history. However, in medical settings, time and other constraints may mean that only a part of it can be taken during any one consultation. Do not assume that because the patient has medical problems they are the cause of the sexual difficulty. Most sexual disorders arise from a combination of psychological and physical factors.

The presenting problem

It is important to identify and explore the presenting problem with regard to timing, the situation in which the problem occurs, whether the difficulty is primary or secondary, whether there is comorbidity and whether any precipitating or alleviating factors can be identified. For example, in a patient who presents with premature ejaculation, one would explore if this occurs in masturbation as well as sexual intercourse (situation), whether the man has always ejaculated early or whether the problem has appeared after a period of normal sexual function (primary or secondary) and whether drugs or alcohol alleviate or exacerbate the problem (precipitating, alleviating).

Current sexual relationship

If the patient has a sexual partner, a detailed assessment of this relationship should be made. This includes the quality of communication, dominance issues within the relationship, specific matters such as jealousy or resentment, the strengths and weaknesses of the relationship, and the detailed sexual nature of the partnership. The latter will include the nature of their sexual behaviour and the frequency of sexual intercourse, if this is occurring. Whether or not the partner can be interviewed depends on the setting and the wishes of the patient. An independent interview with the partner, however, may provide a useful, alternative perspective on the sexual difficulties.

Sexual development

The patient's developmental history is important. The following breakdown may be helpful:

1. Age at which erections, nocturnal emissions and masturbation first occurred.
2. Age at menarche and the responses of the patient and her family to these developmental changes.
3. Details of pubertal development, including the reaction of the patient and others to the physical and emotional changes.
4. History of dating and first sexual approaches.
5. Age at first sexual experience and nature and quality of this experience.
6. History of unwanted sexual experiences as a child or adult. This may take the form of a sensitive enquiry about 'unwelcome' sexual experiences. Great care is needed here as patients may discuss such experiences for the first time and such disclosures arouse considerable emotion.

Family environment, sexual education and knowledge

An assessment should be made of the attitude of the patient's family of origin to sexual matters. Was sex ever discussed and in what context? What was the nature of the parents' emotional and sexual relationship? What was the atmosphere in the home including the quality of the family life? An exploration of the patient's knowledge of sexual function and how he or she has acquired this knowledge is helpful. Many people with sexual problems lack knowledge of normal sexual behaviour and are often preoccupied with unreasonable expectations of themselves and their partners.

Past sexual relationships

The nature and duration of previous sexual relationships should be explored with attention to how they ended and the reactions of the patient to these breakdowns.

Current sexual preferences and practices

This part of the sexual history is the most sensitive and may be deferred beyond the first assessment. Much can be learned, however, from an exploration of patients' preferred sexual activities and fantasies. A tactful exploration of sexual orientation should be attempted. Although this information need not be collected during the first interview, it may be the cause of the sexual difficulty and people in heterosexual relationships may have particular trouble admitting (particularly if their partner is present) to same-sex desire, fantasy and behaviour. The types of clothing that are arousing, the time of day when sexual activity is most preferred and the sorts of sexual interaction that the patient fantasizes about (whether or not these are acted upon) should be explored. This would include activities such as fetishistic behaviour, sexual arousal to children and sadomasochism.

Contraceptive and obstetric history

Where it is appropriate, an assessment of the contraceptive, gynaecological and obstetric history may be made. Has the woman's sexual drive or enjoyment of sex changed following childbirth or gynaecological interventions? Is there resentment about issues such as contraception or infertility between her and her partner? Are there physical problems related to past obstetric or gynaecological surgery?

Medical history

Much will already be known about the patient's medical history. However, a careful review should be made with reference to disorders that may affect sexual function, such as peripheral vascular disease. Full documentation should be made of prescribed drugs taken. As described later in this chapter, medications with particular effects on sexual functioning should always be considered.

These include the antidepressant and antipsychotic drugs, beta-blockers, anti-hypertensive medication, and other drugs such as digoxin, cimetidine, metoclopramide, L-dopa, and anticonvulsant medication. A careful history of the patient's intake of alcohol and recreational drugs is important. The quantity and frequency of each substance consumed should be detailed. Particular attention should be paid to the patient's view of the effect of such substances on his or her sexual life.

Physical examination

No assessment of a sexual problem is complete without a physical examination. In several schools of psychosexual medicine, the physical examination forms the centrepiece of the psychosexual history, as it elicits clues as to the patient's feelings about sex and anxieties about their body shape and genitalia. It is important to conduct a brief assessment of the peripheral circulation and the blood pressure (lying and standing) as well as an assessment of secondary sexual characteristics such as development of breasts, body hair distribution and body shape. Finally it is important to examine the genitals. In men, look for a foreskin that will not retract fully and any lesions on the penis. The testes should be of firm consistency and non-tender. They should be readily palpable, free of masses and relatively mobile within the scrotum. Varicocele of the testicular veins are common and although not related to sexual dysfunction, may reduce fertility (Paduch & Niedzielski 1996). Each testis should be between 4.1 and 5.2 cm in length and 2.5–3.3 cm in width (Bondil *et al.* 1992). Normal penile length is greater than 4 cm in the unstretched, flaccid state or more than 7.5 cm in the stretched, flaccid state (this is roughly equivalent to the erect state; Wessells *et al.* 1996).

In women, secondary sexual characteristics and the shape and condition of the external labia are usually the focus of the examination. Sensitive vaginal examination is reserved for treatment settings where vaginismus, other sexual phobia or problems consequent to a sexual assault is the presenting problem. In both sexes it is important to note the patients' reactions to having their bodies and particularly genitalia examined and their view of their genitalia and body image. At this time men and women may make 'casual' remarks about the size or shape of their genitals or other bodily characteristics that can be a clue to a strong but hidden preoccupation with feelings of inferiority. Remember that the presence of a chaperone is advisable regardless of the sex of patient or examiner (Bignell 1999).

Mental state examination

Features of the mental state are often explored during the interview, paying particular attention to the possibility of depression. An assessment of the patient's previous personality will also be helpful in arriving at a formulation of the problem.

Prevalence of sexual problems

As already mentioned, there is debate about the classification of sexual dysfunction, particularly in women. The fourth edition of the Diagnostic and Statistical Manual of the American Psychiatric Association (DSM-IV) stipulates that dysfunction be accompanied by marked distress or interpersonal difficulty. However, this can be difficult to separate from the distress caused by physical disease or interpersonal strife with a partner. There have been a number of epidemiological studies in normal populations that show that sexual dysfunction is relatively common (Simons & Carey 2001). This high background prevalence of the disorder should be kept in mind in assessing a medical patient. However, many epidemiological studies are conducted using simple rating scales, do not provide a diagnostic classification according to international criteria and do not place the disorder within the context of medical help seeking. In a study using strict diagnostic criteria according to the tenth edition of the International Classification of Diseases (ICD-10), we found that prevalence of sexual problems in 1512 people attending their general practitioners in London was relatively high (Nazareth *et al.* 2003). Although general practice attendees might be expected to report higher rates of sexual problems than people recruited in the community, in fact our rates were somewhat lower than those reported in epidemiological studies (Simons & Carey 2001), particularly in men (Table 10.2).

Table 10.2. Prevalence of ICD-10 sexual dysfunction.

ICD-10 sexual dysfunction	Men[a]	Women[a]
Lack or loss of sexual desire F52.0	6.7 (4.6−9.4)	16.8 (14.6−19.1)
Sexual aversion F52.1	2.5 (1.2−4.4)	4.1 (3.0−5.5)
Failure of genital response F52.2		
F52.2 Male erectile dysfunction (failure at insertion during intercourse)	8.5 (6.1−11.5)	
F52.2 Female sexual arousal dysfunction		3.6 (2.5−4.9)
Orgasmic dysfunction F 52.3 & F 52.4		
Male orgasmic dysfunction F52.3 (inhibited orgasm during intercourse)	2.5 (1.2−4.4)	
Premature ejaculation F52.4 (at insertion during intercourse)	3.6 (2.1−5.7)	
Inhibited female orgasm F52.3 (during intercourse)		18.6 (16.3−20.9)
Non-organic vaginismus F52.5		4.5 (3.3−5.9)
Non-organic dyspareunia F52.6	1.1 (0.4−2.6)	2.9 (2.0−4.1)
At least one ICD-10 diagnosis	21.7 (17.9−25.5)	39.6 (36.7−42.6)

Note: [a]All figures are percentages; those in parentheses are 95% confidence intervals.

Standardized assessment of sexual problems

There are a number of brief, rating scales of sexual function that may be useful in clinical practice or research. A recent review established which among them were the best developed and most useful (Daker-White 2002). In men, these are the Brief Sexual Function Questionnaire for Men (Reynolds *et al.* 1988) which takes a broad view of sexual function and the International Index of Erectile Function (Rosen *et al.* 1997) which focuses mainly on erectile dysfunction. In women, the McCoy Female Sexuality Questionnaire assesses sexual interest and responsiveness (McCoy & Matyas 1998). However, it has only been validated in post-menopausal women. A close competitor is the Self Report Assessment of Female Sexual Function (Taylor *et al.* 1994), which is an adaptation of the Brief Sexual Function Questionnaire for Men. Although no substitute for careful clinical assessment, these pen-and-paper tests are well received by patients and can provide a reliable short-cut to establishing the nature of the problem.

Sexual problems in medical patients

Normal sexual function depends upon a complex system of vascular, neurological, endocrine and psychological factors and sexual disorders can occur at any stage in the complex cycle of fantasy and arousal, genital response, lubrication and orgasm. A large number of medical disorders is associated with sexual problems in men and women (Table 10.3). They can be loosely grouped into systemic and endocrine, neurological, vascular and (particularly in men) local genital disorders. What follows is a summary of the sorts of problems that might be encountered, but is by no means intended to be exhaustive. The clinician must keep in mind that sexual medicine is a fast-developing field and

Table 10.3. Medical disorders that affect sexual function.

Conditions that affect both sexes
Cardiovascular disease, diabetes, neurological disorders such as epilepsy and multiple sclerosis, endocrine disorders, cancer, brain or spinal injury, irritable bowel syndrome, urological problems/infections (including cystitis), sexually transmitted infections, side-effects of medication; infertility.
Conditions that affect women
Endometriosis, menstrual problems, menopause, hysterectomy, mastectomy, termination of pregnancy, pregnancy miscarriage, hormone replacement therapy, genital problems.
Conditions that affect men
Vasectomy, prostate problems, testicular or penile problems.

that as we increase our understanding of the cognitive and biological factors in sexual dysfunction, recognition of the pathways for disorder will expand.

Distinguishing medical from psychological aetiology

There has been considerable discussion over the years about how best to distinguish psychogenic from biological causes of sexual dysfunction, particularly in men. In the 1960s, when sexual therapies were developing, sexual problems were regarded as mainly psychological in origin and a psychotherapeutic or behavioural approach to treatment was advocated (Kaplan 1974; Masters & Johnson 1970). With the advent of effective pharmaceutical treatments for erectile disorder in the 1990s this has given way to a view that medical causes predominate. Although there are useful indicators that the disorder is primarily psychogenic or organic in origin (Table 10.4), most disorders are a complex combination of both. For example, men with peripheral vascular disease may develop intense anxiety about their inability to initiate a full erection, which increases autonomic (sympathetic) tone, inhibits erections and makes the dysfunction much worse. In general, regular morning erections are a sign of normal physical functioning in men. Absence of morning erections, however, does not mean the cause is physical, as decreased sexual arousal is common in

Table 10.4. Suggestions from the history as to the origin of the sexual disorder.

Possible psychological aetiology
Sudden onset
Loss of arousal during sexual activity
Complaints about genital size or appearance
Dysfunction in some situations but not in others
No difficulty in masturbation
Major life event or ongoing chronic stress
Psychological difficulties, particularly depression
Relationship difficulties
Age below 30

Possible organic aetiology
Gradual onset
Global loss of arousal
Medical risk factors such as endocrine or cardiovascular diseases
Recent surgery, particularly in genital or pelvic area
Use of prescribed drugs known to cause sexual dysfunction
Heavy consumption of alcohol and/or recreational drugs

major depression (Seidman & Roose 2000). A rating scale has been developed to help make the distinction between physical and organic causes (Speckens *et al.* 1993)

Cardiovascular disorders

Erectile dysfunction has been reported in 20–40% of men with hypertension or ischaemic heart disease. It is likely that vascular insufficiency leads to reduced clitoral engorgement and lubrication in women but the evidence for this is mixed. Furthermore, it is not at all clear that women need to experience congestion of their vulval or clitoral erectile tissues to have fulfilling sexual experiences (Basson 2001). Peripheral vascular disease reduces blood flow to the penis and is a potent cause of erectile dysfunction despite normal desire. In fact, presentation of erectile dysfunction in a middle-aged man may be the first sign of ischaemic heart disease (Jackson *et al.* 1999).

Smoking is a risk factor for erectile dysfunction in men and possibly arousal difficulties in women. The relative risk of developing arterial atherosclerosis in the penile arteries and subsequent erectile dysfunction is 1.3 for every 10 pack-years smoked, and 86% of smokers have an abnormal penile vascular state (Kandeel *et al.* 2001). This has led to the introduction of sexual health warnings on cigarette packets, a potentially more effective deterrent than other (more distant) health risks for adolescent men and women.

A British consensus statement on erectile dysfunction in the cardiovascular patient states that the cardiac risk of sexual activity in patients with cardiovascular diseases is minimal in properly assessed and advised patients and that sexual activity is no more stressful to the heart than walking one mile in 20 minutes. Patients are at 'intermediate' risk if they have had a myocardial infarction or cerebrovascular accident within the previous six weeks and thus careful assessment and advice on a return to sexual activity before that time is advisable (Jackson *et al.* 1999). Despite this sensible advice, many patients and their partners are hesitant to resume their sexual life after a cardiac event and may need careful assessment for anxiety or depression.

Diabetes

There is considerable overlap in sexual dysfunction due to diabetes and cardiovascular diseases as both affect the vascular status of patients. However, diabetes also has severe effects on the autonomic nervous system that may disrupt arousal and orgasm in both sexes. Erectile dysfunction occurs in one in two men with diabetes and increases with age from 25% at age 35 to more than 70% by age 60 (Kandeel *et al.* 2001) and (as for other complications) is undoubtedly affected by the degree of control of blood sugar. This excess in sexual difficulties is not accounted for by other psychological difficulties in diabetic patients (Schiavi *et al.* 1995a).

Neurological disorders and spinal injuries

Sexual dysfunction is such a common manifestation of disorders affecting the central or peripheral nervous systems that the brain has been called the principal sexual organ of the body (Frohman 2002). Multiple sclerosis and spinal cord injuries are the two neurological conditions most likely to result in sexual difficulty in men and women. Prevalence of arousal and orgasmic disorders in multiple sclerosis is between 60 and 80%, and up to 95% of people with spinal cord injuries (Frohman 2002).

Sexual dysfunction in multiple sclerosis gradually progresses as the neurological condition worsens (Zorzon *et al.* 2001). Despite this well-recognized link between multiple sclerosis and sexual problems, most patients with neurological disorders are never asked to discuss their sexuality by the clinicians caring for them (Hulter & Lundberg 1995).

Sexual dysfunction (arousal or orgasmic dysfunction) is also very common in Parkinson's disease, affecting up to 60% of patients. However prevalence of sexual dysfunction increases with normal ageing and it is important to estimate the role of age-related changes in each patient. Sexual function before the onset of Parkinson's is obviously the key to this assessment. Treatment with L-dopa may increase sexual drive (see below) and lead to a return of erections.

Although sexual dysfunction in men with spinal cord injuries is very common, men with partners are usually sexually active, engage in a variety of sexual behaviours and enjoy the sexual parts of their lives (Phelps *et al.* 2001). They seldom present to sexual dysfunction clinics.

Sexual dysfunction after stroke is also very common (59% of men and 44% of women), but is intimately related to depressive symptoms and impaired activities of daily living, and attention to psychological symptoms is paramount (Kimura *et al.* 2001).

Cancer

Sexual problems in the context of cancer are difficult to assess, as they may be the result of a depressive reaction to the diagnosis, pain and disfigurement following surgery, cachexia and weakness if the cancer progresses, or chemotherapy (Syrjala *et al.* 2000). Disfiguring and mutilating surgery to the face, breasts, genitals and reproductive organs often have deleterious effects on a person's self-image and sexual function. Although there has been considerable study of the impact of breast cancer on women's sexual function (Hordern 2000), there has been less examination of the impact of cancer in men and of surgery for cancers in men and women. We know little about patients' attitudes to their sexual life, particularly in the later, terminal stages of their illnesses. Nor do we understand how best to manage such difficulties. This arises partly from a popular conception that ill people are not interested in sex, but also from possible embarrassment and ignorance on the part of staff. We recently compared the nature and prevalence of sexual problems in people attending oncology services with those receiving palliative care and with well, general practice attendees (Ananth 2003). We found that many patients with cancer were willing to discuss their sex lives and the impact of disease on their sexual function. Sexual function was only slightly impaired in patients receiving oncology treatment compared to those in receipt of palliative care, suggesting that the debility associated with terminal illness may have greatest impact, rather than the cancer diagnosis per se.

Genital and reproductive organs

There has been a large number of studies examining whether disorders of the genital tract are associated with sexual dysfunction. This is exemplified by testicular cancer in men and by hysterectomy in women. Two recent reviews of the psychosexual consequences of testicular cancer indicate that although sexual sequelae, particularly ejaculatory dysfunction, are common, many studies have been poorly conducted and there has been little good, controlled evidence (Jonker-Pool et al. 2001; Nazareth et al. 2001). Changes in sexual function after hysterectomy are difficult to assess. Although retrospective reports of sexual dysfunction occur in up to 50% of cases, prospective studies have been equivocal in their results (Carlson 1997). At least eight studies have examined sexual function one or more years after hysterectomy. Although dyspareunia reduced or resolved, in two studies sexual interest and activity improved, in two there was no change and in two it declined (Carlson 1997).

Pregnancy and childbirth clearly have the potential to affect a couple's relationship through the physical changes of the pregnancy and parturition and the disruption in the household with the arrival of children. Up to half of first-time parents describe their sex life as not very good or poor eight months after the birth, and one in five would like help with the difficulty (Dixon et al. 2000). Dyspareunia, orgasmic dysfunction and loss of sexual enjoyment is common for women during pregnancy (Oruc et al. 1999). This may relate to myths about sexual activity in pregnancy, fears about the baby and delivery and changes in relationship with the partner (Read 1999). There may be prolonged loss of sexual desire in women and their partners following childbirth, which can be the result of many biological and psychological factors. When this persists for many years, it is almost always due to psychological or relationship difficulties.

The prostate gland has an important role in semen production and ejaculation. Relaxation of the voluntary post-prostatic sphincter, together with prostatic contractions, leads to ejaculation. Hence any disruption of this anatomy and physiology puts sexual function at risk. About half of men undergoing trans-urethral prostatectomy report a consequent reduction in orgasmic sensation and up to three-quarters report retrograde ejaculation. Many are very concerned about this side-effect, particularly if not warned about it before surgery (Dunsmuir *et al.* 1996). Although impaired erectile function is unusual after transurethral prostatectomy, it frequently follows radical prostatectomy for prostatic cancer (as well as other radical pelvic surgery for cancer), despite recent surgical techniques to spare the pelvic nerve, which lies immediately adjacent to the prostate. As with other cancers, however, depression and anxiety often complicate the picture and contribute to the sexual difficulties. Chronic prostatic inflammation may also alter sensation and the ejaculatory reflex. Prostatitis has been reported in over half of men with premature ejaculation. However, only one-third of such men have prostatic symptoms (Screponi *et al.* 2001). Premature ejaculation presenting after years of normal ejaculatory function suggests a particular need to investigate for prostatitis. Once again, however, psychological and personality factors are likely to be paramount in men with premature ejaculation, particularly those who have had the condition intermittently or constantly throughout their sexual life.

Local conditions of the genitals, such as Peyronie's disease of the penis and dyspareunia of gynaecological origin in women are generally seen in specific medical and surgical settings and are unlikely to enter the province of the liaison psychiatrist. Dyspareunia, however, is a particularly difficult syndrome that would possibly benefit from greater involvement by mental health specialists. Careful examination of this condition reveals that knowing whether the pain during intercourse is life-long or acquired and generalized or situational tells us very little about whether physical or psychological pathology, marital stress, sexual attitudes or a history of abuse have anything to do with its cause (Meana *et al.* 1997). It may be better to regard it as a pain syndrome resulting in sexual dysfunction rather than a sexual dysfunction per se. Dyspareunia in men is rare and is usually related to prostatic infection or other organic disorder of the genitals. Complaints of numbness or reduced genital sensation in men without neurological disease is almost always a sign of sexual anxieties.

Prescribed drugs

A large number of prescribed drugs causes sexual dysfunction and it is critical to evaluate all drugs the patient is taking (Crenshaw & Goldberg 1996; Table 10.5).

Table 10.5. Prescribed drugs affecting sexual function.

Drugs reducing sexual drive
Antihypertensives and other cardiovascular drugs such as digoxin
Antidepressants such as fluoxetine
Sedatives such as barbiturates
Anxiolytics such as benzodiazepines
Antipsychotic and other dopamine-blocking drugs
Oestrogens in men
Anabolic agents
Opioids and opioid analogues
Dopamine agonists (increase drive)
Antiandrogens
Drugs depressing arousal
H_2 antagonists
Metoclopramide
Antipsychotics
Thiazide diuretics
Antidepressants — serotonin reuptake inhibitors and tricyclic preparations
Trazodone (stimulating and may cause priapism)
Anticholinergics
Antiandrogens
Drugs impairing orgasm
Antidepressants such as fluoxetine or clomipramine
Antihypertensives including monoamine oxidase inhibitors
Antipsychotics
Antiandrogens

The commonest to impair sexual function are those that impact on dopamine and noradrenaline pathways in the brain, pathways that are intimately related to the sexual response. Other important prescribed drugs are those that affect endocrine function, particularly exogenous steroids (including the contraceptive pill — although evidence here is mixed), and on vascular competence.

Although antihypertensive drugs are frequently cited as causing sexual dysfunction, a careful meta-analysis of quality of life in clinical trials (including the older generation of drugs arising from 1970 onwards) found no effect for impact on sexual life (Beto & Bansal 1992). In similar vein, a recent systematic review of sexual dysfunction secondary to antidepressants was critical of the evidence and called for confirmation from randomized trials (Montgomery *et al.* 2002). In many depressed patients it is difficult to decide whether the drugs, as distinct from the depressed mood, are impairing sexual responsiveness. Whatever the reason, it is risky to reduce or withdraw antidepressants in order to reduce sexual dysfunction because of the possibility of self-harm or other adverse effects of the depressive illness (Montgomery *et al.* 2002). In other medical disorders, such as hypertension, judicious reduction in dosage of the offending drug may be worth a try, but this is not always possible without losing good control of blood pressure. Alternatives such as sildenafil may be useful in both situations.

Other medical conditions

HIV infection has attracted particular interest in terms of its effects on sexual function (Hijazi *et al.* 2001). All manner of sexual dysfunction is common with 60–90% of men and women with HIV infection complaining of dysfunction and dissatisfaction (Keane *et al.* 1997). The dysfunction does not appear to be a consequence of treatment with protease inhibitors (Catalan & Meadows 2000; Lallemand *et al.* 2002). Sexual dysfunction is sometimes due to shame and guilt about having a serious, sexually transmitted infection, preceding unresolved conflicts about sexuality in homosexual men and personality and psychiatric disturbance in intravenous drug users. However, distress about the life-threatening nature of the disorder, end organ insensitivity to testosterone and the debilitating effects of long-term physical illness and debility are likely to be much more common causes. Improvement in sexual function is possible, at least in gay and bisexual men with HIV who actively seek help (Catalan & Meadows 2000). See Chapter 20 for further discussion.

Sexually transmitted infections are also closely associated with sexual dysfunction. One-quarter of men and 40% of women attending clinics for sexually transmitted infections may report a sexual problem (Keane *et al.* 1997). See Chapter 31 for further discussion.

Transsexualism

Although transsexualism is relatively uncommon, it is discussed in this chapter because it involves assessments by psychiatrists and may entail a complex and invasive process of medical and surgical treatments. The term transsexualism describes the conviction that despite congruence of genotype and phenotype and an uneventful physical development, one's sex has been wrongly assigned by nature. It is distinguished from transvestism in which (usually) men dress in feminine attire to derive sexual satisfaction. The transsexual believes that he (or less commonly she) has been born in the wrong body and is unable to express his or her 'true' masculinity or femininity. Many people seeking gender reassignment have been convinced since childhood that their gender identity is at variance with their biological gender. For some, the conviction develops in adulthood after many years of transvestite behaviour when fetishistic excitement declines and the wish to live in the opposite gender role predominates.

Most transsexual people in Western countries regard themselves as heterosexual if given the chance to function as the opposite sex. However, some will become technically homosexual in their new role (Blanchard & Sheridan 1990; Coleman *et al.* 1992). It also seems that sexual orientation can change following surgical reassignment (Daskalos 1998). Reports from Eastern cultures, in which most male and female transsexuals are described as homosexual (Tsoi 1992), indicate that cultural factors are important in the way people in this predicament define their sexuality.

Cross-dressing in itself appears not be to be associated with psychopathology (Brown *et al.* 1996). In fact, dressing and behaving as a woman has a soothing and reassuring effect for a small proportion of men, no matter what their sexual orientation (Levine 1993). Although transsexualism is listed as a diagnosis in all international psychiatric diagnostic glossaries, psychiatrists do not regard it as a delusional disorder on the grounds that it is not accompanied by other serious psychopathology (Cohen *et al.* 1997; Cole *et al.* 1997). More importantly, the belief is not considered delusional, as it is not regarded as culturally discordant. Although people with such a belief may be distressed, this is regarded as in keeping with their dilemma. Transsexualism has come to be regarded as a mistake of nature that requires correction, rather than variation in the human phenotype. However, its cause is completely unknown.

People uncomfortable with their gender have been described since at least the 1890s (von Krafft-Ebing 1892; Schaefer & Wheeler 1995; Snaith & Hohberger 1994). However, by the mid twentieth century the view arose that transsexuals needed specific psychological and medical management in order to achieve 'gender reassignment' (Money 1955, 1994; Money & Gaskin 1970/71). Technological developments in medicine and surgery fuelled the establishment of centres for gender reassignment in the United States and Western Europe in the early 1960s. People seeking reassignment are required to 'pass' as a member of the opposite sex for at least one year before being considered for surgery and during this time they take oestrogen or testosterone to begin the process of remodelling the body into the desired gender (Blanchard & Steiner 1990). Psychiatrists are generally the gatekeepers of whether a candidate makes the grade in the opposite gender role and can be considered for surgery. Many outcome studies of gender reassignment surgery have also been published. Most claim that candidates achieve satisfactory adaptation to their assigned gender (Blanchard & Steiner 1990; Edlh *et al.* 1997; Snaith *et al.* 1993) and that only a small percentage regrets the surgery (Landen *et al.* 1998). However, outcome is said to be dependent on adequate assessment and preparation and may go wrong (Anonymous 1991).

Alcohol and recreational drugs

Alcohol has extensive and complex effects on sexual function. Although frequently used as a social lubricant to decrease social anxiety in sexual settings, alcohol depresses sexual function by inhibiting arousal and retarding orgasm. The acute effects that lead to difficulty initiating and maintaining an erection (a dilemma familiar to every young man who has had one too many) may not be as innocent as first thought. It may reflect autonomic nerve damage (Buus 1981) and it is possible that each episode is cumulative, eventually leading to the chronic erectile dysfunction that is so common in people who misuse alcohol (Schiavi 1990; Peugh & Belenko 2001). There is evidence that this impairment of sexual function may resolve, should the drinker become abstinent, as long as there is no substantial hepatic or gonadal failure (Schiavi *et al.* 1995b). However, sexual adjustment may not improve in the wives of alcoholic men even with marital therapy (O'Farrell *et al.* 1998)

Recreational drugs are almost all depressant in their effects on sexual function and frequently lead to sexual dysfunction (Peugh & Belenko 2001). Although they may cause perceptual changes, including an enhanced perception of sexual stimuli, generally such drugs impair sex. For example, opioid-dependent people do not have very much sex. Although popularly imagined to enhance the experience of sex, cannabis is probably also a depressant in its action.

Screening investigations

Useful tests to investigate underlying problems are available. In men, serum testosterone should be taken in the early morning at the peak of its diurnal rhythm. A serum testosterone anywhere within the normal range for the laboratory is acceptable. Sex-hormone-binding globulin transports testosterone in the bloodstream. In men, the normal range for total serum testosterone is 9.9–27.8 mMol/L and sex-hormone-binding globulin is 13–71 nMol/L. The free androgen index is a useful measure of free (and therefore active) testosterone. The index is the ratio of serum testosterone to sex hormone binding globulin and should be in excess of 30% for normal sexual function. Follicle-stimulating hormone and luteinizing hormone control sperm production and testosterone production respectively in the testes and their levels may be useful hints to whether the testicular dysfunction is testicular or hypothalamic in origin. A raised serum prolactin may be responsible for low sexual drive in men and women and erectile dysfunction in men, although interpretation of the result requires discussion with a pathologist. Persistent hyperprolactinaemia without symptoms may actually be due to macroprolactinaemia which has much less impact on sexual function and other pituitary hormones and is not associated with a pituitary adenoma (Olukoga *et al.* 1999). The rate of testosterone production in young women is about 300 μg per day, of which about half is produced by the ovaries and half by the adrenal glands. In women, the normal range for total serum testosterone is 14–54 ng/dL, free testosterone 1.3–6.8 pg/mL and sex-hormone-binding globulin 36–185 nMol/L (Shifren *et al.* 2000).

Treatments

Physical treatments

The phosphodiesterase-5 inhibitor sildenafil has revolutionized treatment of men with erectile difficulties of physical or psychological origin. By inhibiting breakdown of GMP in penile tissues, it prolongs smooth muscle relaxation and facilitates erection. Adverse effects relate to its action on other phosphodiesterase systems in the body. These include headache, flushing of the skin (particularly of the face and neck), stomach upsets and nasal stuffiness. However, in randomized controlled studies, only 1% of men ceased the drug because of adverse effects (Goldstein *et al.* 1998). The blue visual tinge that is very rarely reported is due to its weak action on phosphodiesterase-6 activity in the retina. Although initial trial reports indicated efficacy rates of 80–90%, success in clinical practice is closer to 50% (Morgentaler 1999). Efficacy in diabetes is about 50%, but is much lower after radical prostatectomy, particularly if nerve-sparing techniques have not been used. Nitrate drugs are the main contraindication, as in combination with sildenafil they may lead to profound and life-threatening hypotension. Tadalafil, a second phosphodiesterase-5 inhibitor with a half-life at least twice that of sildenafil, has recently been approved for prescription in Europe and others are in development. Unfortunately, easy availability of an oral treatment for erectile dysfunction may mean that major psychological factors are overlooked or by-passed. Although sildenafil is useful in men with primarily psychogenic erectile dysfunction, clinical impression suggests that psychological dependence on using the drug can quickly become established and simply compound the difficulties. Where performance anxiety is very high, however, sildenafil can reduce tension enough to re-establish a sense of relaxation, help the man to focus on his anxious cognitions and eventually return to normal sexual function. It can also be useful in sexual relationships that are unconsummated, particularly where the man loses his erection at the moment of penetration. Possibly its greatest role in men with psychological difficulties is that it gives hope that sexual function can return to normal and allows a breathing space for psychological work to proceed. As discussed above, phosphodiesterase-5 inhibitors appear to have no role in women with reduced arousal or orgasmic dysfunction.

Other physical treatments include oral apomorphine, which acts centrally on dopamine systems to promote erection. Its action on dopamine means that it may also increase sexual drive. This latter observation is now under investigation in women. Prostaglandin-E (alprostadil) injected into the corpora cavernosa will cause erections that are not mediated by sexual activity. Although running a low risk of priapism, penile pain and fibrosis if used frequently in the longer term, prostaglandin-E remains a useful alternative for men who do not respond to sildenafil, particularly after radical prostatectomy. Transurethral preparations of prostaglandin-E are less effective, particularly where there is vascular insufficiency (Porst 1997).

Testosterone replacement in men is beyond the scope of this chapter and is used mainly where hypogonadism is well established (Morgentaler 1999). There is no good evidence yet for an andropause (male menopause), although there is speculation that androgen insensitivity may occur in later life and respond to testosterone replacement (Gould *et al.* 2000).

Testosterone therapy in women with low sexual drive is currently under investigation and appears to have beneficial effects in women who have undergone oophorectomy and hysterectomy, although placebo response is high (Schifren *et al.* 2000). However, its use is fraught with the risk of masculinizing side-effects (Modelska & Cummings 2003). When a woman lacks sexual drive, it is well worth asking who is complaining? Hormone replacement therapy in menopausal women is the main physical treatment that will enhance sexual function through its action on the vaginal epithelium and the vulval and clitoral erectile tissues. Tibolone, a synthetic steroid that has oestrogenic, progestagenic and androgenic activity is used to treat menopausal symptoms and may have a place in enhancing sexual function in post-menopausal women (Modelska & Cummings 2003).

Psychological treatments

Although psychological treatments for sexual dysfunction have been established since the time of Masters and Johnson's pioneering work in the 1960s, few attempts were made to assess their efficacy. Masters and Johnson published recommendations for couple therapy and claimed very high success rates (Masters & Johnson 1970). Clinical practice eventually revealed that success rates were much lower but behavioural treatments established a place in this field that remains the case today. Cognitive behavioural treatments also have a definite role in sexual therapy where reactive anxiety and depression are so common and where dysfunctional beliefs play a prominent part in prolonging and compounding people's difficulties. However, once again the evidence base for cognitive behavioural treatments in sexual therapy is sparse (Roth & Fonagy 1996).

Cognitive approaches to the treatment of sexual dysfunction are based closely on cognitive methods established for other psychological problems. They are welcomed by patients and may work by reducing embarrassment about sexual topics, improving education, assisting communication between the patient and partner and providing opportunities for homework that will advance the couple's understanding of their difficulties. David Burns's paperback *Feeling Good — The New Mood Therapy* (1999) is a useful self-help manual to recommend to patients which is based firmly on Aaron Beck's model of cognitive therapy. Although not explicitly about sexual problems, its emphasis on the role of cognitions in psychological health is central to this work.

Understanding the role of medical factors in sexual disorders is essential and a judicious use of physical and psychological treatments is likely to have greatest acceptance to many patients. Clinical impression suggests that although sildenafil and related drugs may restore erectile function, many men are left dissatisfied and puzzled by their difficulties and eager to seek out psychological help. They may still lack sexual drive or encounter difficulties in their relationships with partners. Men with psychological problems are most likely to eventually stop using sildenafil if their psychological problems are also addressed. We urgently need more evidence in this field and for research councils to take the issue seriously. Unfortunately far less research monies are spent on evaluating psychological as averse to physical treatments for sexual dysfunction, particularly as the latter mean large profits for pharmaceutical companies.

REFERENCES

Akkus, E., Kadioglu, A., Esen, A., *et al.* (2002). Prevalence and correlates of erectile dysfunction in Turkey: a population based study. *European Urology*, **41**, 298—304.

Ananth, H., Jones, C. L., King, M. B., *et al.* (2003). The impact of cancer on sexual function: a controlled study. *Palliative Medicine*, **17**, 202—5.

Anonymous. (1991). Transsexualism. *Lancet*, **338**, 603—4.

Basson, R. (2001). Female sexual response: the role of drugs in the management of sexual dysfunction. *Obstetric and Gynecology*, **98**, 350—3.

Basson, R., Berman, J., Burnett, A., *et al.* (2000). Report on the international consensus development conference on female sexual dysfunction: definitions and classifications. *Journal of Urology*, **163**, 888—93.

Beto, J. A. and Bansal, V. K. (1992). Quality of life in treatment of hypertension. A meta-analysis of clinical trials. *American Journal of Hypertension*, **5**, 124—33.

Bignell, C. J. (1999). Chaperones for genital examination. *British Medical Journal*, **319**, 137—8.

Blanchard, R. and Sheridan, P. M. (1990). Gender reorientation and psychosocial adjustment. In *Clinical Management of Gender Identity Disorders in Children and Adults,* ed. R. Blanchard and B.W. Steiner. Washington DC: American Psychiatric Press, pp. 159–89.

Blanchard, R. and Steiner, B. W., eds. (1990). *Clinical Management of Gender Identity Disorders in Children and Adults.* Washington DC: American Psychiatric Press.

Bondil, P., Costa, P., Daures, J. P., *et al.* (1992). Clinical study of the longitudinal deformation of the flaccid penis and its variation with aging. *European Urology,* **21**, 284–6.

Brown, G. R., Wise, T. N., Costa, P. T., *et al.* (1996). Personality characteristics and sexual functioning of 188 cross-dressing men. *Journal of Nervous and Mental Disease,* B**184**, 265–73.

Burns, D. (1999). *Feeling Good – The New Mood Therapy.* New York: Avon.

Buus, J. S. (1981). Sexual dysfunction in male diabetics and alcoholics. *Sexuality and Disability,* **4**, 215–19.

Carlson, K. J. (1997). Outcomes of hysterectomy. *Clinical Obstetrics and Gynecology,* **40**, 939–46.

Catalan, J. and Meadows, J. (2000). Sexual dysfunction in gay and bisexual men with HIV infection: evaluation, treatment and implications. *AIDS Care,* **12**, 279–86.

Cohen, L., de Ruiter, C., Ringelberg, H., *et al.* (1997). Psychological functioning of adolescent transsexuals: personality and psychopathology. *Journal of Clinical Psychology,* **53**, 187–96.

Cole, C. M., O'Boyle, M., Emory, L. E., *et al.* (1997). Comorbidity of gender dysphoria and other major psychiatric diagnoses. *Archives of Sexual Behaviour,* **26**, 13–26.

Coleman, E., Colgan, P. and Gooren, L. (1992). Male cross-gender behaviour in Myanmar (Burma): a description of the acault. *Archives of Sexual Behaviour,* **21**, 313–21.

Crenshaw, T. L and Goldberg, J. P. (1996). *Sexual Pharmacology – Drugs that Affect Sexual Function.* New York: Norton.

Daker-White, G. (2002). Reliable and valid self-report outcome measures in sexual dysfunction: a systematic review. *Archives of Sexual Behaviour,* **31**, 197–209.

Daskalos, C. T. (1998). Changes in the sexual orientation of six heterosexual male-to-female transsexuals. *Archives of Sexual Behaviour,* **27**, 605–14.

Dixon, M., Booth, N. and Powell, R. (2000). Sex and relationships following childbirth: a first report from general practice of 131 couples. *British Journal of General Practice,* **50**, 223–4.

Dunsmuir, W. D., Emberton, M., Wood, C., *et al.*, on behalf of the steering group of the National Prostatectomy Audit. (1996). There is significant sexual dissatisfaction following TURP. *British Journal of Urology,* **77**, 161A.

Eldh, H., Berg, A. and Gustafsson, M. (1997). Long-term follow up after sex reassignment surgery. *Scandinavian Journal of Plastic and Reconstructive Surgery and Hand Surgery,* **31**, 39–45.

Frohman, E. M. (2002). Sexual dysfunction in neurologic disease. *Clinical Neuropharmacology,* **25**, 126–32.

Goldstein, I., Lue, T. F., Padma-Nathan, H., *et al.*, for the sildenafil study group. (1998). Oral sildenafil in the treatment of erectile dysfunction. *New England Journal of Medicine,* **338**, 1397–404.

Gould, D. S. C., Petty, R. and Jacobs, H. S. (2000). The male menopause – does it exist? *British Medical Journal,* **320**, 858–61.

Hijazi, L., Nandwani, R. and Kell, P. (2001). Medical management of sexual difficulties in HIV-positive individuals. *International Journal of STD AIDS*, **12**, 587–92.

Hordern, A. (2000). Intimacy and sexuality for the woman with breast cancer. *Cancer Nursing*, **23**, 230–6.

Hulter, B. and Lundberg, P. O. (1995). Sexual function in women with advanced multiple sclerosis. *Journal of Neurology, Neurosurgery and Psychiatry*, **59**, 83–6.

Jackson, G., Betteridge, J., Dean, J., *et al.* (1999). A systematic approach to erectile dysfunction in the cardiovascular patient: a consensus statement. *International Journal of Clinical Practice*, **53**, 445–51.

Jonker-Pool, G., Van de Wiel, H. B. M., Hoekstra, H. J., *et al.* (2001). Sexual functioning after treatment for testicular cancer – review and meta-analysis of 36 empirical studies between 1975–2000. *Archives of Sexual Behaviour*, **30**, 55–74.

Kandeel, F. R., Koussa, V. K. T. and Swerdloff, R. S. (2001). Male sexual function and its disorders: physiology, pathophysiology, clinical investigation and treatment. *Endocrine Reviews*, **22**, 342–88.

Kaplan, H. S. (1974). *The New Sex Therapy*. New York: Brunner/Mazel.

Keane, F. E. A., Carter, P., Goldmeier, D., *et al.* (1997). The provision of psychosexual services by genitourinary medicine physicians in the United Kingdom. *International Journal of STD AIDS*, **8**, 402–4.

Kimura, M., Murata, Y., Shimoda, K., *et al.* (2001). Sexual dysfunction following stroke. *Comprehensive Psychiatry*, **42**, 217–22.

Lallemande, F., Salhi, Y., Linard, F., *et al.* (2002). Sexual dysfunction in 156 ambulatory HIV-infected men receiving highly active antiretroviral therapy combinations with and without protease inhibitors. *Journal of Acquired Immune Deficiency Syndrome*, **30**, 187–90.

Landen, M., Walinder, J., Hambert, G., *et al.* (1998). Factors predictive of regret in sex reassignment. *Acta Psychiatrica Scandinavica*, **97**, 284–9.

Levine, S. B. (1993). Gender-disturbed males. *Journal of Sexual and Marital Therapy*, **19**, 131–41.

Masters, W. H. and Johnson, V. (1970). *Human Sexual Inadequacy*. Boston: Little Brown.

McCoy, N. L. and Matyas, J. R. (1998). McCoy Female Sexuality Questionnaire. In *Handbook of Sexuality-related Measures*, ed. C. M. Davis, W. L. Yarber, R. Bauserman, *et al.* London: Sage pp. 249–51.

Meana, M., Binik, Y. M., Khalifé, S., *et al.* (1997). Dyspareunia: sexual dysfunction or pain syndrome? *Journal of Nervous and Mental Disease*, **185**, 561–9.

Mirone, V., Imbimbo, C., Bortolotti, A., *et al.* (2002). Cigarette smoking as a risk factor for erectile dysfunction: results from an Italian epidemiological study. *European Urology*, **41**, 294–7.

Modelska, K. and Cummings, S. (2003). Female sexual dysfunction in postmenopausal women: systematic review of placebo-controlled trials. *American Journal of Obstetrics and Gynecology*, **188**, 286–93.

Money, J. (1955). An examination of some basic sexual concepts: the evidence of human hermaphroditism. *Bulletin of Johns Hopkins Hospital*, **97**, 301–19.

Money, J. (1994). The concept of gender identity disorder in childhood and adolescence after 39 years. *Journal of Sex and Marital Therapy*, **20**, 163–77.

Money, J. and Gaskin, R. (1970/71). Sex reassignment. *International Journal of Psychiatry*, **9**, 249–69.

Montgomery, S. A., Baldwin, D. S. and Riley, A. (2002). Antidepressant medications: a review of the evidence for drug-induced sexual dysfunction. *Journal of Affective Disorders*, **69**, 19–40.

Morgentaler, A. (1999). Male impotence. *Lancet*, **354**, 1713–18.

Moynihan, R. (2003). The making of a disease: female sexual dysfunction. *British Medical Journal*, **236**, 45–7.

Nazareth, I., King, M. and Lewin, J. (2001). Sexual dysfunction after treatment for testicular cancer. A systematic review. *Journal of Psychosomatic Research*, **51**, 735–43.

Nazareth, I., King, M. and Boynton, P. (2003). Problems with sexual function in people attending London general practitioners. *British Medical Journal*, **327**, 423.

O'Farrell, T. J., Kleinke, C. L. and Cutter, H. S. G. (1998). Sexual adjustment of male alcoholics: changes from before to after receiving alcoholism counselling with and without marital therapy. *Addictive Behaviours*, **23**, 419–25.

Olukuga, A. O., Dornan, T. L. and Kane, J. W. (1999). Three cases of macroprolactinaemia. *Journal of the Royal Society of Medicine*, **92**, 342–4.

Oruc, S., Esen, A., Lacin, S., *et al.* (1999). Sexual behaviour during pregnancy. *Australian and New Zealand Journal of Obstetrics and Gynecology*, **39**, 48–50.

Paduch, D. A. and Niedzielski, J. (1996). Semen analysis in young men with varicocele: a preliminary study. *Journal of Urology*, **156**(2S), 788–90.

Peugh, J. and Belenko, S. (2001). Alcohol, drugs and sexual function. *Journal of Psychoactive Drugs*, **33**, 223–32.

Phelps, J., Albo, M., Dunn, K., *et al.* (2001). Spinal cord injury and sexuality in married or partnered men: activities, function, needs and predictors of sexual adjustment. *Archives of Sexual Behaviour*, **30**, 591–602.

Porst, H. (1997). Transurethral alprostadil with MUSE (medication urethral system for erection) vs. intracavernosal alprostadil – a comparative study in 103 patients with erectile dysfunction. *International Journal of Impotence Research*, **9**, 187–92.

Read, J. (1999). Sexual problems associated with infertility, pregnancy, and ageing. *British Medical Journal*, **318**, 587–9.

Reynolds, C. F., Frank, E., Thase, M. E., *et al.* (1988). Assessment of sexual function in depressed, impotent, and healthy men: factor analysis of a brief sexual function questionnaire for men. *Psychiatry Research*, **24**, 231–50.

Rosen, R. C., Riley, A., Wagner, G., *et al.* (1997). The International Index of Erectile Dysfunction (ILEF). A multidimensional scale for assessment of erectile dysfunction. *Urology*, **49**, 822–30.

Roth, A. and Fonagy, P. (1996). *What Works for Whom? A Critical Review of Psychotherapy Research*. London: Guildford.

Schaefer, L. C. and Wheeler, C. C. (1995). Harry Benjamin's first ten cases (1938–1953): a clinical historical note. *Archives of Sexual Behaviour*, **24**, 73–93.

Schiavi, R. C. (1990). Chronic alcoholism and male sexual dysfunction. *Journal of Sexual and Marital Therapy*, **16**, 23–33.

Schiavi, R. C., Stimmel, B. B., Mandeli, J., *et al.* (1995a). Diabetes, psychological function and male sexuality. *Journal of Psychosomatic Research*, **39**, 305–14.

Schiavi, R. C., Stimmel, B. B., Mandeli, J., *et al.* (1995b). Chronic alcoholism and male sexual function. *American Journal of Psychiatry*, **152**, 1045–51.

Schifren, J. L., Braunstein, G. D., Simon, J. A., *et al.* (2000). Transdermal testosterone treatment in women with impaired sexual function after oophorectomy. *New England Journal of Medicine*, **343**, 682–8.

Screponi, E., Carosa, E., Di Stasi, S. M., *et al.* (2001). Prevalence of chronic prostatitis in men with premature ejaculation. *Urology*, **58**, 198–202.

Seidman, S. N. and Roose, S. P. (2000). The relationship between depression and erectile dysfunction. *Current Psychiatric Reports*, **2**, 201–5.

Simons, J. S. and Carey, M. P. (2001). Prevalence of sexual dysfunctions: results from a decade of research. *Archives of Sexual Behaviour*, **30**, 177–219.

Snaith, R. P. and Hohberger, A. D. (1994). Transsexualism and gender reassignment. *British Journal of Psychiatry*, **165**, 417–19.

Snaith, P., Tarsh, M. J. and Reid, R. (1993). Sex reassignment surgery. A study of 141 Dutch transsexuals. *British Journal of Psychiatry*, **162**, 681–5.

Speckens, A. E. M., Hengeveld, M. W., Lycklama à Nijeholt, G. A. B., *et al.* (1993). Discrimination between psychogenic and organic erectile disorder. *Journal of Psychosomatic Research*, **37**, 135–45.

Syrjala, K. L., Schroeder, T. C., Abrams, J. R., *et al.* (2000). Sexual function measurement and outcomes in cancer survivors and matched controls. *Journal of Sex Research*, **37**, 213–25.

Taylor, J. F., Rosen, R. C. and Leiblum, S. R. (1994). Self report assessment of female sexual function. *Archives of Sexual Behaviour*, **23**, 627–43.

Tiefer, L. (2000). Sexology and the pharmaceutical industry: the threat of co-optation. *The Journal of Sex Research*, **37**, 273–83.

Truitt, W. A. and Coolen, L. M. (2002). Identification of a potential ejaculation generator in the spinal cord. *Science*, **297**, 1566–9.

Tsoi, W. F. (1992). Male and female transsexuals: a comparison. *Singapore Medical Journal*, **33**, 182–5.

Tuiten, A., Van Honk, J., Koppeschaar, H., *et al.* (2000). Time course of effects of testosterone administration on sexual arousal in women. *Archives of General Psychiatry*, **57**, 149–53.

von Krafft-Ebing, R. (1892). *Psychopathia Sexualis*. London.

Vroege, J. A., Gijs, L. and Hengeveld, M. W. (1998). Classification sexual dysfunctions: towards DSM-V and ICD-11. *Comprehensive Psychiatry*, **39**, 333–7.

Wessells, H., Lue, T. F. and McAninch, J. W. (1996). Penile length in the flaccid and erect state guidelines for penile augmentation. *Journal of Urology*, **156**, 995–7.

Zorzon, M., Zivadinov, R., Monti Bragadin, L., *et al.* (2001). Sexual dysfunction in multiple sclerosis: a 2-year follow-up study. *Journal of Neurological Sciences*, **187**, 1–5.

11

Suicide and deliberate self-harm

Julia Sinclair and Keith Hawton

Introduction

The aims of this chapter are threefold. First, to give an overview of the multi-faceted context in which the management of those presenting following an episode of self-harm needs to be considered. Second, to consider the link between the spectrum of suicidal behaviours and completed suicide. Finally, to consider assessment and management procedures and review the evidence for effectiveness of current practices.

Throughout this chapter the term 'deliberate self-harm' will be used to denote 'an act of intentional self-poisoning or injury, irrespective of the apparent purpose of the act'. It describes a spectrum of behaviours from impulsive, superficial, self-cutting, which rarely presents to medical attention, through to premeditated and carefully planned suicide attempts which, for some reason, have not resulted in death. Whilst there is controversy concerning this definition (Van Heeringen 2001), it allows for the inclusion of the full range of self-harming behaviours, without drawing arbitrary distinctions based on perceived intent, which is often far from clear.

Suicide, as a term, appears easier to define, namely as 'a self-destructive behaviour with a fatal outcome'. It is classified within the International Classification of Diseases (ICD) as codes E950–959. However, major differences exist in the process of determining death, both within and between countries (Neeleman *et al.* 1997) and therefore cross-cultural epidemiological findings need to be considered with caution.

Handbook of Liaison Psychiatry, ed. Geoffrey Lloyd and Elspeth Guthrie. Published by Cambridge University Press. © Cambridge University Press 2007.

Epidemiology

Suicide

Despite the variations in the categorization of suicide, these can only in part explain the wide variations in suicide rates across countries and over time. What is certain is that internationally suicide is a major contributor to life years lost. The Global Burden of Disease Study (Murray & Lopez 1997) states that 'self-inflicted injuries' as a cause of death is likely to rise from 12th to 10th in the rank order of causes of death world-wide by 2020. World Health Organization (WHO) figures suggest that in Western countries the annual incidence of suicide varies from 10 to 30 per 100 000. The recent increase in young male suicides in many countries is also of great concern, and not fully explained, although theories relating to loss of religious and cultural identity and increasing urbanization have been suggested, especially in countries with a pioneering history (Cantor 2000).

Within Europe, suicide rates are significantly higher in former Eastern-bloc countries and the disparity continues as rates are still increasing in the East and reducing in the West (Chishti *et al.* 2003; Sartorius 1995). In England and Wales, suicide rates are considered together with 'undetermined deaths', as the latter has been shown to consist mainly of suicides (O'Donnell & Farmer 1995). Although rates in England and Wales continue to decline in both sexes (Kelly & Bunting 1998), data from the Office for National Statistics show that suicide is ranked third in life years lost in men and fifth in women, and is the major cause of death in young people, being more common than death in road traffic accidents.

Temporal patterns in suicide rates are determined at least in part by the availability and acceptability of a particular means of death. In the UK, prior to the change in the domestic gas supply from coal gas to natural gas, over 50% of all suicides used gassing as a means of suicide. Following the change, overall rates of suicides declined with little evidence of a relative increase in other methods (Kreitman 1976).

Public health measures designed at limiting the access to various means have had some success, as in the legislation restricting paracetamol sales (Hawton *et al.* 2001a, 2004), and the use of catalytic converters in cars (Kendell 1998). However, the relative increase in death by hanging and suffocation, which is now the most common method in men and second in women, is a more challenging public health problem.

Deliberate self-harm

Deliberate self-harm (DSH) has been recognized as an increasing public health problem in many contemporary societies for some time, but until relatively recently attempts to compare cross-sectional and longitudinal data on rates of

DSH have been hampered both by the variation in definition of the behaviour and lack of standardized data. One of the WHO targets for the European region is 'the continued reduction in the rising trends in suicide and attempted suicide'. As part of the implementation of this target the WHO/Euro Study of Suicidal Behaviour aimed to collect standardized data across a broad range of European countries (Platt *et al.* 1989). Sixteen centres in 13 different countries participated in the project to monitor hospital presentations following DSH. The data from the 1989–1992 period (Schmidtke *et al.* 1996) showed that rates varied considerably between centres. The age standardized rates for men varied sevenfold between Guipuzcoa in Spain (45/100 000) and Helsinki in Finland (314/100 000), and for women similar differences in rates were found. Of the 16 centres, 15 reported that the age-standardized rates for DSH was greater in women than in men, and in all centres the highest rates were found in the younger age groups, and in social categories associated with social destabilization and poverty.

Self-poisoning was the most common reason for presentation, accounting for 64% of cases in men and 80% in women, psychotropic medication being used in 71% of episodes (Michel *et al.* 2000). There were significant differences between centres in the substances used, especially in the 15–24 age group; Oxford (UK) had the highest rates of overdose in females, mainly due to frequent use of analgesics, whilst Szeged (Hungary) had exceptionally high rates of pesticide and solvent use.

Data from Oxford since the early 1990s have shown a continued rise in rates of DSH presentations to hospital in both males and females, which is more frequent in females at a younger age. Thus, in 12-year-olds in Oxford the ratio of male-to-female episode is about eight to one, but this declines to two to one by the age of 18 (Hawton *et al.* 2003a).

Not all episodes of DSH result in presentation for medical treatment. In a recent study of DSH in 15- and 16-year-old school pupils only 12.6% of those who reported DSH in the previous year said that they had been seen at a hospital (Hawton *et al.* 2002), suggesting that the problem of DSH is far greater than that recorded in hospital statistics.

Links between suicide and DSH

The link between DSH and suicide is a clear but complex one, with many of the factors associated with suicide also common to DSH. There is a significant association between episodes of DSH and suicide, with 15–25% of those who die by suicide having presented with an episode of DSH in the year prior to their death (Appleby *et al.* 1999a; Gairin *et al.* 2003), and between one-third and two-thirds of those who ultimately commit suicide having a lifetime history of DSH (Sakinofsky 2000). Conversely, 0.7–1.0% of DSH patients die within a year by suicide, which is approximately 66 times the annual risk of suicide in the general population in the UK (Hawton *et al.* 2003b). A recent UK study traced deaths following self-harm over a 16-year period and found an overall death rate of 17% and a suicide rate of 3.5% (Owens *et al.* 2005). There appears to be marked variability between different groups, with rates of suicide following DSH increasing markedly with age at initial presentation, living alone, and in those with multiple episodes of DSH. Males have almost twice the risk of females of committing suicide following an episode of DSH, especially in the following year (Hawton & Fagg 1988; Hawton *et al.* 2003b; Nordentoft *et al.* 1993).

National suicide prevention strategies

Both the WHO (World Health Organization 1990) and the United Nations (United Nations 1996) identified suicide as a major area of public health policy that required comprehensive national and international strategies to combat suicide as a significant cause of death globally. As suicide is an intentional behaviour of diverse causality and method, rather than a disease, it does not neatly fit into the established public health model of prevention and intervention. Therefore the UN also advocated the development of a conceptual framework to identify suitable targets for intervention and suggested five key elements that should guide any national strategy. These were:
- an overt government policy
- a coherent model for suicide behaviour and therefore prevention
- general aims and goals
- measurable objectives
- monitoring and evaluation.

Several countries have implemented national suicide prevention strategies based on this model, including, for example, Finland, Norway, Australia, the USA and England (Department of Health 2002). The strategy in England was developed to help meet the national target for suicide reduction in England, which aims to reduce the level of suicides (and open verdicts) by 20% by the year 2010, from its baseline level of 11 per 100 000 in 1997. A key element of this strategy is the improved management of DSH patients presenting to general hospitals. This will be discussed later, after consideration of the aetiology of suicide and DSH.

Aetiology

Despite the burgeoning of studies attempting to examine and quantify the specific risk factors involved in the suicidal process, the prediction of suicidal behaviour remains an inexact science. The complex interactions between state and trait characteristics, well-known risk and lesser-known protective factors, and their differential effects at varying time points in the causal pathway, all add to the low sensitivity and specificity of individual factors in the prediction of risk. Add to this the low base rate of the occurrence of suicide within the general population and the difficulty of attempting to develop meaningful aetiological pathways becomes apparent. However, the recognition of these factors has been important in driving research to develop integrated models of suicidal behaviour as a biopsychosocial process which has implications for targeting intervention at the level of both populations and high-risk groups.

We will first briefly review some of the actuarial risk factors for suicide and DSH prior to a consideration of how these may fit into more complex models that need to be considered in the assessment and management of those presenting following an episode of DSH.

Risk factors for suicide

General population

Within the general population, suicide is a relatively rare event and as such risk factors identified as being associated with it will have high levels of false-positives. As already mentioned, in most Western countries suicide is more common in men than women and despite the increase in suicides in young men, the elderly are at greatest risk. Unemployment (Platt & Hawton 2000), lower social class (Kelly et al. 1995), and substance misuse (Harris & Barraclough 1997) are all associated with greater risk. Marriage is a protective factor for both sexes, although being widowed or divorced is a greater risk factor for suicide in men (Cantor & Slater 1995).

A recent study of 21 169 suicides in Denmark (Qin et al. 2003) suggested that the effect, size and even direction of many risk factors differed significantly by gender. The population-attributable risk, a measure of how much a particular factor influences the total population rate of an outcome (in this case suicide), was highest for a lifetime history of psychiatric admission (40.3%), single marital status (25.8%) and old-age retirement (10.2%).

Psychiatric disorders

Suicide rates are increased in all psychiatric disorders, except dementia (Harris & Barraclough 1997). An early psychological autopsy study of 100 suicides in Wessex in England gave a primary diagnosis of depression to 64% and of alcoholism in 15% of those studied (Barraclough et al. 1974). A later study in Northern Ireland using similar methodology gave a primary Axis I diagnosis to 86% of suicides, most commonly unipolar depression (31%) and alcohol dependence (24%). Suicides over 75 years were much more likely to have a depressive illness as their

Table 11.1. Risk factors for suicide in patients with schizophrenia.

Increased risk is associated with:
- previous depressive disorder
- previous self-harm
- drug misuse
- agitation
- fear of mental disintegration
- poor adherence to treatment
- recent loss

Reduced risk is associated with:
- hallucinations

principal diagnosis (77%). In many cases there is comorbidity of personality disorder with Axis I disorder. The same study found comorbid personality disorder in 41% of suicides (Foster *et al.* 1997, 1999). However, in a case-control study of psychiatric inpatients, those who went on to commit suicide within a year of discharge from hospital were no more likely to have a comorbid diagnosis of personality disorder than their controls, matched for diagnosis (King *et al.* 2001). Suicide risk is greatly increased in schizophrenia and the risk is heightened by a variety of factors, including a history of previous self-harm and depression (Table 11.1; Hawton *et al.* 2005a). Recent work has suggested that suicides amongst those with psychiatric illness may cluster together, providing evidence that imitative suicide occurs in this population, and it may account for about 10% of those who are or have been psychiatric inpatients (McKenzie *et al.* 2005).

Almost 25% of suicides in the UK have been in contact with mental health services in the 12 months prior to death and the times of highest risk are following discharge from inpatient care (Appleby *et al.* 1999b; Goldacre *et al.* 1993). A large case-control study of 234 psychiatric inpatients who committed suicide within one year of discharge found that 34% did so within 28 days of discharge from hospital and 86% by six months (King *et al.* 2001). Across diagnoses a history of DSH was a significant risk factor for suicide; OR 4.1 (95% CI 2.6–6.5).

Risk factors for deliberate self-harm

General population risk factors

Rates of DSH are highest in young people, especially teenage females and young adult males, two-thirds of patients being under 35 years of age. Females have higher rates than males, although in the UK the gender ratio has narrowed in recent years. Rates are highest in the lowest social class group and are associated with socioeconomic deprivation and social isolation (Hawton *et al.* 2001b; Schmidtke *et al.* 1996).

Whilst there are numerous difficulties in conducting methodologically robust studies in the area of sexuality and its relationship to DSH, studies which have attempted to do so are limited to more liberal Western societies. Several studies have shown that homosexual men and women have higher lifetime rates of DSH than heterosexuals, but the relative risks of DSH in gay men and lesbians is less consistent (Catalan 2000).

Immigrant populations have been shown to have higher rates of DSH. Studies in young Asian women in the UK have shown significantly higher rates than in the indigenous population (Bhugra *et al.* 1999). Cultural differences, the stigma attached to academic and social failure, and the overriding authority of community elders, are thought to be important factors.

Adolescents

Rates of DSH increase steadily in girls from age 12, reaching a peak in the late teens. For boys the rates rise more slowly, peaking in the twenties. The mean proportion of adolescents who report that they have attempted suicide at some point in their lives is 9.7% (95% CI, 8.5–10.9) and nearly one-third (29.9%; 95% CI, 26.1–33.8) report experiencing suicidal ideas (Evans *et al.* 2005). In a recent systematic review of psychosocial and psychological risk factors for adolescent DSH (Webb 2002) focusing on UK-relevant studies, the key psychological factors identified were depression and hopelessness, which became more significant in those who repeated self-harm.

In a study of 12–18-year-olds presenting following DSH, an association with school stress was found, with fewer presentations during holiday periods. Higher levels of drug misuse and violence were found amongst boys, which increased during the study period. Suicide intent was also higher in boys (Hawton *et al.* 2003c).

Aetiological models of risk for DSH

A central issue in attempting to identify those at greatest risk of DSH is the consideration of the complex interaction between biological, psychological and social characteristics. There is now overwhelming evidence that both genetic and environmental factors impact on the aetiology of emotional and behavioural disorders.

The stress-diathesis model proposed by Mann and colleagues (1999) postulates an underlying, stable trait of aggression or impulsivity associated with hyposerotonergic functioning (the diathesis). This diathesis, it is suggested, interacts causally with various stressors, such as adverse life events and mental disorders, to lead to suicidal behaviours. Other diatheses, both biological and psychological, may also independently exert a protective effect on an individual. These complex interactions may help explain the low sensitivity and specificity of individual risk factors when considered in isolation.

Biological aspects of suicidal behaviour

Research into the biological markers of suicidality seems to suggest associations which are independent of any specific underlying psychiatric pathology, such as depression. The role of the serotonergic system in suicidal behaviour has been the most researched, although studies investigating alterations in the hypothalamic–pituitary–adrenal (HPA) axis, serum cholesterol, as well as dopamine and noradrenaline, have also been undertaken, often with conflicting results.

The relationship between low levels of the serotonin metabolite 5-HIAA in the cerebrospinal fluid (CSF) and suicidality was first demonstrated in 1976 (Asberg et al. 1976) and has been replicated many times since. A summary of 33 of these studies (Asberg & Forslund 2000) found that 28 demonstrated an association between low CSF 5-HIAA and various estimates of suicidal behaviour, especially when the attempt involved a violent means or had a high intended lethality.

Results of studies investigating peripheral markers of serotonergic function in relation to suicidal behaviour have been less consistent, and no reliable link between CSF serotonin levels and any of the peripheral receptor indices has been delineated (Asberg & Forslund 2000).

Social characteristics of suicidal behaviour

The work of Durkheim (1897) was a pivotal driving force in the sociological study of suicidal behaviour in the nineteenth and twentieth centuries, particularly the concept of 'anomie'. This term was used to describe a situation in which the norms and values of society change so fast that old structures are rejected prior to new ones becoming established, such that individuals are unable to internalize any reliable frames of support, and have little sense of a communal belonging. This has an effect on the way in which social crises are perceived and negotiated. DSH frequently follows life events (Paykel et al. 1975), which often occur against the background of more long-term coping difficulties (Bancroft et al. 1977). The links between suicidal behaviour and unemployment have also been extensively researched. In a systematic review of the effect of labour market changes and suicidal behaviour from 1984 onwards (Platt & Hawton 2000), three aspects of change were considered: female labour force participation (FLFP); occupational status and risk. The results showed that DSH was inversely related to social class, but that there was little evidence for an effect of FLFP on suicidal behaviour.

Psychological models of suicidal behaviour

The psychological theories for DSH integrate individual risk factors into models which attempt to describe a person's response to the situation in which they find themselves. Several studies comparing DSH patients and healthy controls have found important quantitative differences in problem-solving capacity (Pollock & Williams 1998, 2001). It has been suggested that lack of problem-solving ability is an end result of other more fundamental difficulties in memory recall, specifically autobiographical memories. This theory posits that those who are less able to retrieve personal memories of specific events have a less functional database for solving current problems, and are consequently more likely to feel 'trapped' in an insoluble situation (Williams & Broadbent 1986). It is suggested that those who have suffered early trauma are more likely to stop the recall of events at a more general level in order to protect themselves from the pain of a more specific memory. On the autobiographical memory test, in which subjects are asked to recall memories in response to key words, DSH patients tend to recall fewer specific memories than either psychiatric patients without a history of DSH, or normal controls. This difference in specific memories is associated with poorer problem solving (Pollock & Williams 2001), the latter particularly affecting interpersonal problem solving (Evans *et al.* 1992; Sidley *et al.* 1997).

The concepts of dichotomous 'black-and-white' thinking and cognitive rigidity (Neuringer 1968) both contribute to feelings of hopelessness, which have long been thought by psychologists to be one of the key factors in the final common pathway to suicidal behaviour (Weishaar & Beck 1992). Feelings of hopelessness can occur in the absence of a depressive episode. However, in suicidal individuals, where hopelessness presents as part of a depressive syndrome, it often appears proportionally greater than other depressive features (Mann *et al.* 1999). Whether feelings of hopelessness lead to suicidal behaviour depends on the presence of other protective or risk factors.

Impulsive and aggressive personality features, together with an oversensitivity to apparently minor life events is another constellation of psychological characteristics which have been shown to be associated with an increased risk of DSH. There is a debate about whether this is primarily a state phenomenon associated with stress and low mood, or more a trait phenomenon, possibly linked to a genetically determined vulnerability. Evidence increasingly points to this representing a trait disorder, with manifestation of certain behaviours such as DSH when other state factors (e.g. low mood) are present (Van Heeringen 2003).

Assessment

The assessment of a patient presenting following an episode of DSH has several purposes. First and foremost it is necessary to detect those at high risk of suicide or repetition of DSH; second, to identify those with significant mental health problems requiring treatment; third, to determine what aftercare may be required; and finally as a therapeutic process in its own right, which is little researched, but may be particularly important in affecting the uptake of future interventions which could be of benefit.

Unless there are pressing reasons to the contrary, a psychosocial assessment should be conducted after the patient has fully recovered from any medical complications or toxic effects of DSH. The assessment should be conducted in a private setting, out of hearing of other patients. Where at all possible additional information should be gathered from close informants and any key professionals already involved in the patient's care (Hawton & Catalan 1987). The topics that should be covered in the assessment are shown in Table 11.2.

A semi-structured assessment procedure is most likely to ensure that all the relevant topics are covered with a patient whilst allowing space and flexibility for issues specific to the individual patient to be discussed. The use of scales within the assessment is likely to be of most benefit in supplementing this procedure, as a screening tool for underlying psychiatric disorder, and collecting standardized data for research purposes. A number of scales have been developed for use in this population, but should be interpreted with care when they are used as a screening tool for who should be referred for psychiatric assessment, due to the poor sensitivity and specificity of individual risk factors, discussed above, and the variable way in which responses are elicited and interpreted.

Table 11.2. Topics to be covered in the assessment of patients who have self-harmed.

- Events and difficulties preceding DSH
- Suicidal intent and other motives involved
- Current and ongoing difficulties
- Alcohol and other substance use
- Evidence of psychiatric disorder, and past psychiatric history
- Personality traits and disorder
- Family and personal history
- Previous DSH and consequences
- Risk of suicide
- Coping resources and available supports
- Available aftercare and patient's wish to engage

Suicidal intent (i.e. the extent to which the patient wished to die at the time of the attempt) can usefully be assessed by means of the Beck Suicidal Intent Scale (Beck *et al.* 1974; Harriss *et al.* 2005), which includes the items listed in Table 11.3. It is extremely important to recognize that the actual medical dangerousness of an overdose is a poor and potentially misleading measure of the extent to which a patient may have wanted to die (Beck *et al.* 1975). Many patients are extremely ignorant of the relative dangers of substances taken in overdose, and so it is important to ensure that the patient's understanding of the effect of the overdose is taken into account.

However, suicide is not the only motive for DSH (see Table 11.4), and assessment of motives is important in identifying areas that may be amenable to intervention. Assessment of motives should be based on the precedents and circumstances of the acts, both from the patient's own account and that of any informants (Bancroft *et al.* 1976; Hjelmeland *et al.* 2002).

Risk of repetition of DSH has been found to occur more commonly in those with certain sociodemographic and clinical characteristics (summarized

Table 11.3. Factors indicating higher suicidal intent after DSH.

- Act of DSH planned long in advance
- Suicide note written
- Actions in anticipation of death (e.g. will writing, sorting personal effects)
- Alone at time of DSH
- Attempts to avoid discovery
- Did not seek help following the act
- Stated wish to die
- Thought act would prove fatal
- Sorry or angry that the act failed
- Ongoing suicidal intent

Table 11.4. Motives or reasons for DSH.

- To die
- To escape from unbearable anguish
- To get relief
- To escape from a situation
- To show desperation to others
- To change the behaviour of others
- To get back at other people or make them feel guilty
- To get help

Table 11.5. Factors associated with risk of repetition of DSH.

- Previous attempt(s) of DSH
- Personality disorder
- Alcohol or drug misuse
- Previous psychiatric treatment
- Unemployment
- Lower social class
- Criminal record
- History of violence
- Age 25–54 years
- Single, divorced or separated

in Table 11.5), which form the basis of the scales to assess risk of repetition that were developed by Buglass and Horton (1974) and Kreitman and Foster (1991). Again whilst useful as an *aide memoire* in covering areas of risk, their ability to predict who will repeat DSH is limited (Hawton & Fagg 1995; Kapur & House 1998).

Rating scales to assess levels of depression may have a role in assessment of DSH patients. The Hamilton Depression Rating Scale (Hamilton 1967) is one example and the Beck Depression Inventory (Beck *et al.* 1961), whilst not validated in the diagnosis of depression, may provide a useful subjective rating of a patient's feeling of low mood (Malone *et al.* 2000).

Special groups

Adolescents

Adolescents will often require clinical input from child and adolescent psychiatric services. Admission to a general hospital bed is usually recommended (Royal College of Psychiatrists 1982). Very young patients should be admitted to a paediatric bed. Admission allows time for adequate assessment, including interviews with families and, where appropriate, close friends.

Mentally ill

Deliberate self-harm may be the presenting occurrence in any psychiatric disorder and acts of DSH are often associated with anxiety symptoms and alcohol misuse. The most common psychiatric diagnoses found in DSH patients are depression, personality disorder, and alcohol abuse or dependence (Haw *et al.* 2001a). Alcohol dependence is more frequent amongst males than females and comorbidity is common (Beautrais *et al.* 1996; Hawton *et al.* 2003c; Suominen *et al.* 1996).

In assessing those known to psychiatric services it is important to consider the episode of DSH both within the context of the patients' psychiatric history and also their current social situation. Close liaison with the team involved in their longer-term care is essential.

Frequent repeaters

Approximately 5–10% of DSH patients have a history of five or more episodes of self-harm, with a small proportion engaging in a very large number of episodes. They form a heterogeneous group, whose suicidal intent is highly variable between individuals and episodes. Comorbidity of affective symptoms with substance misuse and personality disorder is common and patients often have limited ability to engage constructively with services. This, combined with an often hostile attitude from medical staff, makes assessment and management difficult. However, the long-term risk of eventual suicide is high in such patients, and there is a need for clear communication between the (often multiple) agencies involved in their care.

The elderly

In the WHO/Euro Multicentre Study of Suicidal Behaviour, the ratio of DSH to suicide in the over-65-year-old age group was approximately 2:1 (De Leo et al. 2001), considerably lower than that in younger adults, and the profile of those who self-harm in this age group is much nearer that of completed suicides. A full psychosocial assessment is therefore recommended for all older DSH patients. Deliberate self-harm is less common in older people but more often associated with significant suicidal intent. The risk of completed suicide is particularly high in older DSH patients (Hawton et al. 2003b).

Deliberate self-harm services

Deliberate self-harm is an increasing problem in many countries. In the UK, rates have risen significantly over the last 20 years, and it is now estimated that there are over 170 000 presentations to hospitals each year (Kapur et al. 1998), representing a significant challenge in terms of service delivery and secondary prevention. Across Europe the rates of presentation to hospitals vary widely, and there is little consistency in how best to manage patients either on an individual level or within a service framework (Kapur et al. 2002; Rancans et al. 2001; Runeson et al. 2000). Evaluation of services in Australia suggests a similarly ad-hoc basis for managing DSH, with psychiatric services commonly reserved for those with more medically severe overdoses requiring admission to a medical facility (Whyte et al. 1997).

In 1994, the Royal College of Psychiatrists published guidelines advising on levels of service provision (Royal College of Psychiatrists 1994). However, without an adequate implementation strategy or sufficient resources, changes have been slow and a baseline level of under-provision remains (Hughes *et al.* 1998). A comparison of practices in four teaching hospitals within the UK suggested that general hospital services were disorganized, with inequitable access to specialist assessment and aftercare (Kapur *et al.* 1999). Only 53% of patients studied received a specialist assessment. Patients discharged directly from the emergency departments were less likely to receive a specialist assessment, and also less likely to be offered aftercare. A recent study (Gunnell *et al.* 2002) investigated the contacts with general practitioners following DSH and found that in a study of 968 consecutive admissions in the west of England 31% and 53% contacted their GP's within one and four weeks after the episode respectively, this being more likely in those discharged directly from the emergency department.

Recommendations of who should assess DSH patients have changed significantly over the last 30 years. In the UK, official guidelines in the 1960s specified that all such patients should be assessed by a psychiatrist (Ministry of Health 1961). Changes in the role of nurses and social workers since then, and the development of multidisciplinary teams and working styles have enabled a major change in the pattern of DSH services. In the UK it has been demonstrated that nurses, social workers and other clinicians can assess these patients reliably, make effective aftercare arrangements and provide effective therapy (Catalan *et al.* 1980; Gardner *et al.* 1978; Newson-Smith & Hirsch 1979) guidelines reflect this change (Department of Health 2002; Royal College of Psychiatrists 2004).

Hospital management

Most of the studies on the epidemiology and outcome of DSH are based on the population of patients who present to hospital and who receive some form of medical assessment. However there is a group of patients who do not stay for assessment and our knowledge about the characteristics and outcomes of this group is sparse. Several attempts have been made to quantify in what way this group may be different from those who do stay for a full assessment. The proportions of those who presented to hospital but then left prior to a full assessment varied between 11% and 15% of all presentations in two UK studies (Crawford & Wessely 1998; Hickey *et al.* 2001) and 29% in a Swedish study (Runeson 2001). Patients who left without a full assessment were more likely to have exhibited 'difficult' behaviour and presented out of hours. They also more often repeated self-harm in the follow-up period.

The attitude of health service staff towards patients who self-harm, particularly those who frequently repeat the behaviour, is often one of hostility and frustration. They are often seen as undeserving and detracting from the clinical care of others, whose illnesses are not perceived as self-inflicted, as well as posing often complex management problems. DSH patients are frequently aware of the negative attitudes of staff, and their consequent hostility towards staff can make management all the more difficult. Empathic efforts to understand the patients' difficulties in the context of their life experience may improve management. The attitude of front-line staff to patients may in part be due to their feelings of inadequacy in being able to offer any help. An educational intervention in one region of the UK found that training in suicide risk assessment and management was well received and improved feeling of competency among staff (Appleby *et al.* 2000).

Hospital management of DSH patients needs to be well co-ordinated at a service level to ensure that all patients have some form of assessment and patients can then be directed towards appropriate aftercare and follow up. Deliberate self-harm patients are prone to low rates of compliance with aftercare (Crawford & Wessely 2000) and many are returned to the care of their general practitioner, without any additional specialist psychiatric service input (Crawford and Wessely 1998; Van Heeringen *et al.* 1995). It is also important that patients receive access to prompt and efficient medical treatment, as a small but significant proportion of patients die in hospital from the consequences of their self-poisoning (about 6%). These patients are more likely to be female than male and to have ingested paracetamol. Improved medical management of this group of patients may contribute to future suicide prevention (Kapur *et al.* 2005).

Treatment interventions

The evidence for the effectiveness of treatment interventions to prevent repetition of DSH is at present somewhat disappointing. A systematic review of psychological and pharmacological treatment trials (Hawton *et al.* 1998, 2000) showed that the majority of studies did not show greater efficacy for particular treatment approaches. However, the results were not all negative. Dialectical behaviour therapy (an intensive form of cognitive behaviour therapy) had a substantial initial impact on the repetition of self-harm in female patients with borderline personality disorder, although this did not persist in the longer term (Linehan *et al.* 1993). A study of low-dose depot flupentixol also showed a significant reduction in repetition in frequent self-harmers (Montgomery *et al.* 1979).

A subsequent meta-analysis of the trials of problem-solving therapy suggested there may be beneficial effects for depression, hopelessness and specific problems (Townsend *et al.* 2001). Also, in a recent trial, brief problem-orientated psychotherapy was more effective than treatment as usual (TAU) in reducing repetition of DSH after six months (Guthrie *et al.* 2001). In a randomized controlled trial of recurrent suicide attempters without a major psychiatric DSM-IV Axis I disorder, in a subgroup of patients who had a history of less than five episodes of DSH the antidepressant paroxetine appeared to reduce repetition over one year, whereas those with higher ratings for cluster B personality disorder (e.g. dissocial, borderline and histrionic traits) and more than five previous episodes derived little or no benefit (Verkes *et al.* 1998). However, the subgroup analysis was conducted *post hoc*.

Following a promising pilot study (Evans *et al.* 1999), Tyrer and colleagues conducted a large UK multicentre trial, which compared a treatment combining a brief form of cognitive therapy (CBT) and a manual (manual assisted cognitive therapy – MACT) with treatment as usual in 480 patients with a history of recurrent (at least two episodes) DSH (Tyrer *et al.* 2003a, b). The main outcome measure, the proportion of those repeating DSH within 12 months, showed no significant difference between MACT and TAU. There were also no significant differences between the treatments on any of the secondary outcome measures.

There are several difficulties in conducting treatment studies in DSH patients that need to be considered in evaluating these results. First, DSH patients constitute such a heterogeneous group that those designing treatment studies must either select a specific subgroup in which to evaluate the efficacy of a treatment, but which will have limited generalizability, or include a broadly representative sample, which have such diverse characteristics that no one intervention is likely to be effective for all patients. Second, due to clinical and ethical concerns about control groups in high-risk populations, TAU comparison groups have been proposed as an ethically defensible alternative, and given the diverse range of services and therapies this includes is likely to have a significant influence on the results (Spirito *et al.* 2002). Third, the need for good outcome data and low attrition rates in clinical trials means that those patients at highest risk of repetition and ultimately suicide, for instance those with substance dependency (Inskip 1998), are often excluded, thus preventing the development and evaluation of potentially effective treatments in these groups. Nevertheless, there is a need for further large-scale treatment evaluations.

Long-term outcome

A systematic review of outcome studies in DSH, focusing on the rates of fatal and non-fatal repetition after at least one year (Owens *et al.* 2002), found that of the 90 studies included 80% had been carried out within Europe. Non-fatal repetition occurred in a median of 16% (interquartile range (IQR) 12–25%) of patients by one year, rising to 23% (IQR 11–32%) in studies lasting more than four years. The median suicide rate was 1.8% (IQR 0.8–2.6) by one year, increasing to 6.7% (IQR 5–11%) after nine years. In a subgroup analysis, the UK studies showed a median suicide rate at one year nearly five times lower than in the rest of the studies. The reasons for this include the much larger proportion of young DSH patients (who have a relatively low rate of suicide) in the UK samples, the greater prevalence of people with severe mental disorder in DSH patients in some other countries, and the generally low background rate of suicide in the UK.

There have been few follow-up studies of DSH patients which measure outcome of psychopathology. Those which have been conducted have shown that patients with comorbid psychiatric and personality disorders have greater levels of depression, impulsivity and aggression, and poorer problem-solving skills. They are also more likely to repeat DSH (Curran *et al.* 1999; Haw *et al.* 2001b, 2002).

Costs

To date there has been no comprehensive study estimating the cost burden of DSH on the individual, the health service or society. However, several attempts have been made at calculating some of the component costs involved in the management of DSH patients. Early studies have generally been of uncertain quality (Rodger & Scott 1995; Yeo 1993) One English study estimated the average cost of the hospital care following an episode of DSH at £425 in 1991 (Yeo 1993). In an Irish study measuring the overall costs of hospital attendance in the year prior to and after DSH, O'Sullivan and colleagues (O'Sullivan *et al.* 1999) found that there was a 50% increase in the uptake of hospital services in the year after DSH, resulting in almost a doubling of expenditure. Several studies have compared the relative costs of treating overdoses of serotonin-specific reuptake inhibitors (SSRIs) with the more sedating tricyclic antidepressants (D'Mello *et al.* 1995; Kapur *et al.* 2001; Ramchandani *et al.* 2000; Revicki *et al.* 1997). All have found that hospital stay and time spent in intensive care beds are significantly less for those taking an overdose of SSRI, with an associated reduction in the cost of treatment per episode (Sinclair 2006).

A recent analysis of the factors influencing the cost of DSH management in children and adolescents (Byford *et al.* 2001) found no significant relationship between costs and measures of illness severity, such as levels of depression, hopelessness and suicidal ideation. Service provision was highest in those who showed greatest immediate practical need, poorer parental wellbeing, being in foster care, current problems, and intent to die, although there was some evidence that particular high-risk groups (e.g. those with a diagnosis of conduct disorder), were poorly compliant with treatment despite persisting difficulties. The cost-effectiveness analysis of the recent intervention study comparing a manual and CBT intervention with TAU (Byford *et al.* 2003), using a decision-making approach highlights the complexity of the factors which drive the provision and uptake of services for self-harm (Hawton & Sinclair 2003).

Summary

Deliberate self-harm and suicide include a wide range of behaviours and motivations, the aetiology of which need to be considered within a multi-faceted context of individual and societal factors. Deliberate self-harm is also a significant public health problem requiring adequate clinical provision. It represents one of the most common reasons for presentation to general hospitals, especially in young people, often signifies significant psychopathology, is frequently repeated and is the most consistent risk factor for suicide.

However, the quality of clinical services for DSH patients is highly variable, and sometimes extremely rudimentary. Good standards for services are required, although different models need to be evaluated. Large-scale studies of specific treatments for DSH patients are necessary to identify which approaches are most effective.

All DSH patients should receive at least a brief psychosocial assessment, aimed at identifying those with severe mental illness, as well as those at risk of suicide or immediate repetition of DSH. A more extensive psychosocial assessment should be conducted in most cases. Certain subgroups of patients, especially the very young, older patients, those who misuse substances and those who engage in frequent repetition of DSH, will require assessment and management tailored to their needs.

REFERENCES

Appleby, L., Cooper, J. and Amos, T. (1999a). A psychological autopsy study of suicides by people aged under 35 years. *British Journal of Psychiatry*, **175**, 168–74.

Appleby, L., Shaw, J., Amos, T., *et al.* (1999b). Suicide within 12 months of contact with mental health services: national clinical survey. *British Medical Journal*, **318**, 1235–9.

Appleby, L., Morriss, R., Gask, L., *et al.* (2000). An educational intervention for front-line health professionals in the assessment and management of suicidal patients (The STORM Project). *Psychological Medicine*, **30**(4), 805–12.

Asberg, M. and Forslund, K. (2000). Neurobiological aspects of suicidal behaviour. *International Review of Psychiatry*, **12**, 62–74.

Asberg, M., Traskman, L. and Thoren, P. (1976). 5-HIAA in the cerebrospinal fluid. A biochemical suicide predictor? *Archives of General Psychiatry*, **33**, 1193–7.

Bancroft, J. H. J., Skrimshire, A. M. and Simkin, S. (1976). The reasons people give for taking overdoses. *British Journal of Psychiatry*, **128**, 538–48.

Bancroft, J., Skrimshire, A., Casson, J., *et al.* (1977). People who deliberately poison or injure themselves: their problems and their contacts with helping agencies. *Psychological Medicine*, **7**, 289–303.

Barraclough, B. M., Bunch, J., Nelson, B., *et al.* (1974). A hundred cases of suicide: clinical aspects. *British Journal of Psychiatry*, **12**, 355–73.

Beautrais, A., Joyce, P., Mulder, R., *et al.* (1996). Prevalence and comorbidity of mental disorders in persons making serious suicide attempts: a case control study. *American Journal of Psychiatry*, **153**, 1009–14.

Beck, A., Ward, C., Mendelson, M., *et al.* (1961). An inventory for measuring depression. *Archives of General Psychiatry*, **4**, 561–71.

Beck, A. T., Schuyler, D. and Herman, I. (1974). Development of suicidal intent scales. In *The Prediction of Suicide*, ed. A. T. Beck, M. L. P. Resnik and I. J. Lettieri. Philadelphia, PA: Charles Press, pp. 45–56.

Beck, A. T., Beck, R. and Kovacs, M. (1975). Classification of suicidal behaviors: I. Quantifying intent and medical lethality. *American Journal of Psychiatry*, **132**, 285–7.

Bhugra, D., Desai, M. and Baldwin, D. S. (1999). Attempted suicide in West London, I. Rates across ethnic communities. *Psychological Medicine*, **29**, 1125–30.

Buglass, D. and Horton, J. (1974). A scale for predicting subsequent suicidal behaviour. *British Journal of Psychiatry*, **124**, 573–8.

Byford, S., Barber, J. A. and Harrington, R. (2001). Factors that influence the cost of deliberate self-poisoning in children and adolescents. *Journal of Mental Health Policy and Economics*, **4**, 113–21.

Byford, S., Knapp, M., Greenshields, J., *et al.* (2003). Cost-effectiveness of brief cognitive behaviour therapy versus treatment as usual in recurrent deliberate self-harm: a decision-making approach. *Psychological Medicine*, **33**, 977–86.

Cantor, C. H. (2000). Suicide in the Western world. In *The International Handbook of Suicide and Attempted Suicide*, ed. K. Hawton and K. Van Heeringen. Chichester: Wiley, pp. 9–28.

Cantor, C. and Slater, P. J. (1995). Marital breakdown, parenthood and suicide. *Journal of Family Studies*, **1**, 91–102.

Catalan, J. (2000). Sexuality, reproductive cycle and suicidal behaviour. In *The International Handbook of Suicide and Attempted Suicide*, ed. K. Hawton and K. Van Heeringen. Chichester: Wiley, pp. 293–308.

Catalan, J., Marsack, P., Hawton, K. E., *et al.* (1980). Comparison of doctors and nurses in the assessment of deliberate self-poisoning patients. *Psychological Medicine*, **10**, 483–91.

Chishti, P., Stone, D. H., Corcoran, P., *et al.* (2003). Suicide mortality in the European Union. *European Journal of Public Health*, **13**, 108–14.

Crawford, M. J. and Wessely, S. (1998). Does initial management affect the rate of repetition of deliberate self-harm? Cohort study. *British Medical Journal*, **317**, 985.

Crawford, M. J. and Wessely, S. (2000). The management of patients following deliberate self harm – what happens to those discharged from hospital to GP care? *Primary Care Psychiatry*, **6**, 61–5.

Curran, S., Fitzgerald, M. and Greene, V. T. (1999). Psychopathology 8½ years post parasuicide. *Crisis*, **20**, 115–20.

De Leo, D., Padoani, W., Scocco, P., *et al.* (2001). Attempted and completed suicide in older subjects: results from the WHO/EURO Multicentre Study of Suicidal Behaviour. *International Journal of Geriatric Psychiatry*, **16**, 300–10.

Department of Health. (2002). *National Suicide Prevention Strategy for England*. London: Department of Health.

D'Mello, D. A., Finkbeiner, D. S. and Kocher, K. N. (1995). The cost of antidepressant overdose. *General Hospital Psychiatry*, **17**, 454–5.

Evans, J., Williams, J. M., O'Loughlin, S., *et al.* (1992). Autobiographical memory and problem-solving strategies of parasuicide patients. *Psychological Medicine*, **22**, 399–405.

Evans, K., Tyrer, P., Catalan, J., *et al.* (1999). Manual-assisted cognitive-behaviour therapy (MACT): a randomized controlled trial of a brief intervention with bibliotherapy in the treatment of recurrent deliberate self-harm. *Psychological Medicine*, **29**, 19–25.

Evans, E., Hawton, K., Rodham, K., *et al.* (2005). The prevalence of suicidal phenomena in adolescents: a systematic review of population-based studies. *Suicide & Life-Threatening Behavior*, **35**, 239–50.

Foster, T., Gillespie, K. and McClelland, R. (1997). Mental disorders and suicide in Northern Ireland. *British Journal of Psychiatry*, **170**, 447–52.

Foster, T., Gillespie, K., McClelland, R., *et al.* (1999). Risk factors for suicide independent of DSM-III-R Axis I disorder. *British Journal of Psychiatry*, **175**, 175–9.

Gairin, I., House, A. and Owens, D. (2003). Attendance at the accident and emergency department in the year before suicide: retrospective study. *British Journal of Psychiatry*, **183**, 28–33.

Gardner, R., Hanka, R., Evison, B., *et al.* (1978). Consultation-liaison scheme for self-poisoned patients in a general hospital. *British Medical Journal*, **2**, 1392–4.

Goldacre, M., Seagroatt, V. and Hawton, K. (1993). Suicide after discharge from psychiatric inpatient care; see comments. *The Lancet*, **342**, 283–6.

Gunnell, D., Bennewith, O., Peters, T. J., *et al.* (2002). Do patients who self-harm consult their general practitioner soon after hospital discharge? A cohort study. *Social Psychiatry and Psychiatric Epidemiology*, **37**, 599–602.

Guthrie, E., Kapur, N., Mackway-Jones, K., *et al.* (2001). Randomised controlled trial of brief psychological intervention after deliberate self poisoning. *British Medical Journal*, **323**, 135–7.

Hamilton, M. (1967). Development of a rating scale for primary depressive illness. *British Journal of Social and Clinical Psychology*, **6**, 278–96.

Harris, E. C. and Barraclough, B. (1997). Suicide as an outcome for mental disorders. A meta-analysis. *British Journal of Psychiatry*, **170**, 205–28.

Harriss, L., Hawton, K. and Zahl, D. (2005). Value of measuring suicidal intent in the assessment of people attending hospital following self-poisoning or self-injury. *British Journal of Psychiatry*, **186**, 60–6.

Haw, C., Hawton, K., Houston, K., *et al.* (2001a). Psychiatric and personality disorders in deliberate self-harm patients. *British Journal of Psychiatry*, **178**, 48–54.

Haw, C., Houston, K., Townsend, E., *et al.* (2001b). Deliberate self harm patients with alcohol disorders: characteristics, treatment and outcome. *Crisis*, **22**, 93–101.

Haw, C., Houston, K., Townsend, E., *et al.* (2002). Deliberate self-harm patients with depressive disorders: treatment and outcome. *Journal of Affective Disorders*, **70**, 57–65.

Hawton, K. and Catalan, J. (1987). *Attempted Suicide: a Practical Guide to its Nature and Management.* Oxford: Oxford University Press.

Hawton, K. and Fagg, J. (1988). Suicide, and other causes of death, following attempted suicide. *British Journal of Psychiatry*, **152**, 359–66.

Hawton, K. and Fagg, J. (1995). Repetition of attempted suicide: the performance of the Edinburgh predictive scales in patients in Oxford. *Archives of Suicide Research*, **1**, 261–72.

Hawton, K. and Sinclair, J. M. A. (2003). The challenge of evaluating the effectiveness of treatments for deliberate self-harm. *Psychological Medicine*, **33**, 955–8.

Hawton, K., Arensman, E., Townsend, E., *et al.* (1998). Deliberate self-harm: systematic review of efficacy of psychosocial and pharmacological treatments in preventing repetition. *British Medical Journal*, **317**, 441–7.

Hawton, K., Townsend, E., Arensman, E., *et al.* (2000). Psychosocial and pharmacological treatments for deliberate self-harm. In *The Cochrane Review, Library Issue 3*. Oxford: Update Software.

Hawton, K., Harriss, L., Simkin, S., *et al.* (2001a). Social class and suicidal behaviour: the associations between social class and the characteristics of deliberate self-harm patients and the treatment they are offered. *Social Psychiatry and Psychiatric Epidemiology*, **36**, 437–43.

Hawton, K., Townsend, E., Deeks, J. J., *et al.* (2001b). Effects of legislation restricting pack sizes of paracetamol and salicylates on self poisoning in the United Kingdom: before and after study. *British Medical Journal*, **322**, 1203–7.

Hawton, K., Rodham, K., Evans, E., *et al.* (2002). Deliberate self-harm in adolescents: self report survey in schools in England. *British Medical Journal*, **325**, 1207–11.

Hawton, K., Hall, S., Simkin, S., *et al.* (2003a). Deliberate self-harm in adolescents: a study of characteristics and trends in Oxford, 1990–2000. *Journal of Child Psychology & Psychiatry & Allied Disciplines*, **44**, 1191–8.

Hawton, K., Zahl, D. and Weatherall, R. (2003b). Suicide following deliberate self-harm: long term follow-up study of patients who presented to a general hospital. *British Journal of Psychiatry*, **182**, 537–42.

Hawton, K., Houston, K., Haw, C., *et al.* (2003c). Comorbidity of Axis I and Axis II disorders in patients who attempt suicide. *American Journal of Psychiatry*, **160**, 1494–500.

Hawton, K., Simkin, S., Deeks, J., *et al.* (2004). UK legislation on analgesic packs: before and after study of long term effect on poisonings. *British Medical Journal*, **329**, 1076.

Hawton, K., Sutton, L., Haw, C., *et al.* (2005a). Schizophrenia and suicide: systematic review of risk factors. *British Journal of Psychiatry*, **187**, 9–20.

Hawton, K., Simkin, S., Gunnell, D., *et al.* (2005b). A multicentre study of coproxamol poisoning suicides based on coroners' records in England. *British Journal of Clinical Pharmacology*, **59**, 207–12.

Hickey, L., Hawton, K., Fagg, J., *et al.* (2001). Deliberate self-harm patients who leave the accident and emergency department without a psychiatric assessment. A neglected population at risk of suicide. *Journal of Psychosomatic Research*, **50**, 87–93.

Hjelmeland, H., Hawton, K., Nordvik, H., *et al.* (2002). Why people engage in parasuicide: a cross-cultural study of intentions. *Suicide and Life-Threatening Behavior*, **32**, 380–93.

Hughes, T., Hampshaw, S., Renvoize, E., *et al.* (1998). General hospital services for those who carry out deliberate self-harm. *Psychiatric Bulletin*, **22**, 88–91.

Inskip, H. M., Harris, E. C. and Barraclough, B. (1998). Lifetime risk of suicide for affective disorder, alcoholism and schizophrenia. *British Journal of Psychiatry*, **172**, 35–7.

Kapur, N. and House, A. (1998). Against a high-risk strategy in the prevention of suicide. *Psychiatric Bulletin*, **22**, 534–6.

Kapur, N., House, A., Creed, F., *et al.* (1998). Management of deliberate self poisoning in adults in four teaching hospitals: descriptive study. *British Medical Journal*, **316**, 831–2.

Kapur, N., House, A., Creed, F., *et al.* (1999). General hospital services for deliberate self-poisoning: an expensive road to nowhere? *Postgraduate Medical Journal*, **75**, 599–602.

Kapur, N., House, A., Dodgson, K., *et al.* (2001). Hospital management and costs of antidepressant overdose: multicentre comparison of tricyclic antidepressants and selective serotonin reuptake inhibitors. *Journal of Medical Economics*, **4**, 193–7.

Kapur, N., House, A., Dodgson, K., *et al.* (2002). Management and costs of deliberate self-poisoning in the general hospital: a multi-centre study. *Journal of Mental Health UK*, **11**, 223–30.

Kapur, N., Turnbull, P., Hawton, K., *et al.* (2005). Self-poisoning suicides in England: a multicentre study. *Quarterly Journal of Medicine*, **98**, 589–97.

Kelly, S. and Bunting, J. (1998). Trends in suicide in England and Wales, 1982–96. *Population Trends*, **92**, 29–41.

Kelly, S., Charlton, J. and Jenkins, R. (1995). Suicide deaths in England and Wales, 1982–92: the contribution of occupation and geography. *Population Trends*, **80**, 16–25.

Kendell, R. E. (1998). Catalytic converters and prevention of suicides. *The Lancet*, **352**, 1525.

King, E. A., Baldwin, D. S., Sinclair, J. M., *et al.* (2001). The Wessex Recent In-patient Suicide Study, 1. Case-control study of 234 recently discharged psychiatric patient suicides. *British Journal of Psychiatry*, **178**, 531–6.

Kreitman, N. (1976). The coal gas story: United Kingdom suicide rates 1960–1971. *British Journal of Preventive and Social Medicine*, **30**, 86–93.

Kreitman, N. and Foster, J. (1991). The construction and selection of predictive scales, with special reference to parasuicide. *British Journal of Psychiatry*, **159**, 185–92.

Linehan, M. M., Heard, H. L. and Armstrong, H. E. (1993). Naturalistic follow-up of a behavioral treatment for chronically parasuicidal borderline patients. *Archives of General Psychiatry*, **50**, 971–4.

Malone, K. M., Oquendo, M. A., Haas, G. L., *et al.* (2000). Protective factors against suicidal acts in major depression: reasons for living. *American Journal of Psychiatry*, **157**, 1084–8.

Mann, J. J., Waternaux, C., Haas, G. L., *et al.* (1999). Toward a clinical model of suicidal behavior in psychiatric patients. *American Journal of Psychiatry*, **156**, 181–9.

McKenzie, N., Landau, S., Kapur, N., *et al.* (2005). Clustering of suicides among people with mental illness. *British Journal of Psychiatry*, **187**, 476–80.

Michel, K., Ballinari, P., Bille-Brahe, U., *et al.* (2000). Methods used for parasuicide: results of the WHO/EURO Multicentre Study on Parasuicide. *Social Psychiatry and Psychiatric Epidemiology*, **35**, 156–63.

Ministry of Health. (1961). *HM Circular* (61), 94, London.

Montgomery, S. A., Montgomery, D. B., Jayanthi-Rani, S., *et al.* (1979). Maintenance therapy in repeat suicidal behaviour: a placebo controlled trial. *Proceedings of the 10th International Congress for Suicide Prevention and Crisis Intervention*, pp. 227–9.

Murray, C. J. and Lopez, A. D. (1997). Alternative projections of mortality and disability by cause 1990–2020: Global Burden of Disease Study. *Lancet*, **349**, 1498–504.

Neeleman, J., Mak, V. and Wessely, S. (1997). Suicide by age, ethnic group, coroners' verdicts and country of birth. *British Journal of Psychiatry*, **171**, 463–7.

Neuringer, C. (1968). Divergences between attitudes toward life and death among suicidal, psychosomatic and normal hospitalised patients. *Journal of Consulting and Clinical Psychology*, **32**, 59–63.

Newson-Smith, J. G. B. and Hirsch, S. (1979). A comparison of social workers and psychiatrists in evaluating parasuicide. *British Journal of Psychiatry*, **134**, 335–42.

Nordentoft, M., Breum, L., Munck, L. K., *et al.* (1993). High mortality by natural and unnatural causes: a 10 year follow up study of patients admitted to a poisoning treatment centre after suicide attempts. *British Medical Journal*, **306**, 1637–41.

O'Donnell, I. and Farmer, R. (1995). The limitations of official suicide statistics. *British Journal of Psychiatry*, **166**, 458–61.

O'Sullivan, M., Lawlor, M., Corcoran, P., *et al.* (1999). The cost of hospital care in the year before and after parasuicide. *Crisis*, **20**, 178–83.

Owens, D., Horrocks, J. and House, A. (2002). Fatal and non-fatal repetition of self-harm. *British Journal of Psychiatry*, **181**, 193–9.

Owens, D., Wood, C., Greenwood, D. C., *et al.* (2005). Mortality and suicide after non-fatal self-poisoning: 16-year outcome study. *British Journal of Psychiatry*, **187**, 470–5.

Paykel, E. S., Prusoff, B. A. and Myers, J. K. (1975). Suicide attempts and recent life events: a controlled comparison. *Archives of General Psychiatry*, **32**, 327–33.

Platt, S. and Hawton, K. (2000). Suicidal behaviour and the labour market. In *The International Handbook of Suicide and Attempted Suicide*, ed. K. Hawton and K. Van Heeringen. Chichester: Wiley, pp. 303–78.

Platt, S., Bille-Brahe, U., Kerkhof, A., *et al.* (1989). Parasuicide in Europe: the WHO/EU multicentre study on parasuicide. I. Introduction and preliminary analysis for 1989. *Acta Psychiatrica Scandinavica*, **85**, 97–104.

Pollock, L. R. and Williams, J. M. G. (1998). Problem solving and suicidal behavior. *Suicide and Life-Threatening Behavior*, **28**, 375–87.

Pollock, L. R. and Williams, J. M. G. (2001). Effective problem solving in suicide attempters depends on specific autobiographical recall. *Suicide and Life-Threatening Behavior*, **31**, 386–96.

Qin, P., Agerbo, E. and Mortensen, P. B. (2003). Suicide risk in relation to socioeconomic, demographic, psychiatric, and familial factors: a national register-based study of all suicides in Denmark, 1981–1997. *American Journal of Psychiatry*, **160**, 765–72.

Ramchandani, P., Murray, B., Hawton, K., *et al.* (2000). Deliberate self-poisoning with antidepressant drugs: a comparison of the relative hospital costs of cases of overdose of tricyclics with those of selective-serotonin re-uptake inhibitors. *Journal of Affective Disorders*, **60**, 97–100.

Rancans, E., Alka, I., Renberg, E. S., *et al.* (2001). Suicide attempts and serious suicide threats in the city of Riga and resulting contacts with medical services. *Nordic Journal of Psychiatry*, **55**, 279–86.

Revicki, D. A., Palmer, C. S., Phillips, S. D., *et al.* (1997). Acute medical costs of fluoxetine versus tricyclic antidepressants. A prospective multicentre study of antidepressant drug overdoses. *PharmacoEconomics*, **11**, 48–55.

Rodger, C. R. and Scott, A. I. (1995). Frequent deliberate self-harm: repetition, suicide and cost after three or more years. *Scottish Medical Journal*, **40**, 10–12.

Royal College of Psychiatrists. (1982). The management of parasuicide in young people under sixteen. *Bulletin of the Royal College of Psychiatrists*, **6**, 182–5.

Royal College of Psychiatrists. (1994). *The General Hospital Management of Adult Deliberate Self-Harm.* Council Report CR32. 1–2. London: Royal College of Psychiatrists.

Royal College of Psychiatrists. (2004). *Assessment Following Self-Harm in Adults.* Council Report CR122. London: Royal College of Psychiatrists.

Runeson, B. (2001). Parasuicides without follow-up. *Nordic Journal of Psychiatry*, **55**, 319–23.

Runeson, B., Scocco, P., DeLeo, D., *et al.* (2000). Management of suicide attempts in Italy and Sweden: a comparison of services offered to consecutive samples of suicide attempters. *General Hospital Psychiatry*, **22**, 432–6.

Sakinofsky, I. (2000). Repetition of suicidal behaviour. In *The International Handbook of Suicide and Attempted Suicide*, ed. K. Hawton and K. Van Heeringen. Chichester: Wiley, pp. 385–404.

Sartorius, N. (1995). Recent changes in suicide rates in selected eastern European and other European countries. *International Psychogeriatrics*, **7**, 301–8.

Schmidtke, A., Bille Brahe, U., De Leo, D., *et al.* (1996). Attempted suicide in Europe: rates, trends and sociodemographic characteristics of suicide attempters during the period 1989–1992. Results of the WHO/EURO Multicentre Study on Parasuicide. *Acta Psychiatrica Scandinavica*, **93**, 327–38.

Sidley, G. L., Whitaker, K., Calam, R. M., *et al.* (1997). The relationship between problem-solving and autobiographical memory in parasuicide patients. *Behavioural and Cognitive Psychotherapy*, **25**, 195–202.

Sinclair, J. M. A., Gray, A. and Hawton, K. (2006). Systematic review of resource utilisation in the short term management of deliberate self-harm. *Psychological Medicine*, **36**, 1681−94.

Spirito, A., Stanton, C., Donaldson, D., *et al.* (2002). Treatment-as-usual for adolescent suicide attempters: implications for the choice of comparison groups in psychotherapy research. *Journal of Clinical Child and Adolescent Psychology*, **31**, 41−7.

Suominen, K., Henriksson, M., Suokas, J., *et al.* (1996). Mental disorders and comorbidity in attempted suicide. *Acta Psychiatrica Scandinavica*, **94**, 234−40.

Townsend, E., Hawton, K., Altman, D. G., *et al.* (2001). The efficacy of problem-solving treatments after deliberate self-harm: meta-analysis of randomised controlled t'rials with respect to depression, hopelessness and improvement in problems. *Psychological Medicine*, **31**, 979−88.

Tyrer, P., Jones, V., Thompson, S., *et al.* (2003a). Service variation in baseline variables and prediction of risk in a randomised controlled trial of psychological treatment in repeated parasuicide: the POPMACT study. *International Journal of Social Psychiatry*, **49**, 58−69.

Tyrer, P., Thompson, S., Schmidt, U., *et al.* (2003b). Randomized controlled trial of brief cognitive behaviour therapy versus treatment as usual in recurrent deliberate-harm: the POPMACT study. *Psychological Medicine*, **33**, 969−76.

United Nations. (1996). *Prevention of Suicide: Guidelines for the Formulation and Implementation of National Strategies*. New York: United Nations.

Van Heeringen, K. (2001). The suicidal process and related concepts. In *Understanding Suicidal Behaviour: The Suicidal Process Approach to Research, Treatment and Prevention*, ed. K. Van Heeringen. Chichester: Wiley, pp. 3−14.

Van Heeringen, C. (2003). The neurobiology of suicide and suicidality. *Canadian Journal of Psychiatry*, **48**, 292−300.

Van Heeringen, C., Jannes, S., Buylaert, W., *et al.* (1995). The management of non-compliance with referral to out-patient after-care among attempted suicide patients: a controlled intervention study. *Psychological Medicine*, **25**, 963−70.

Verkes, R. J., Van-der-Mast, R. C., Hengeveld, M. W., *et al.* (1998). Reduction by paroxetine of suicidal behavior in patients with repeated suicide attempts but not major depression. *American Journal of Psychiatry*, **155**, 543−7.

Webb, L. (2002). Deliberate self-harm in adolescence: a systematic review of psychological and psychosocial factors. *Journal of Advanced Nursing*, **38**, 235−44.

Weishaar, M. E. and Beck, A. T. (1992). Hopelessness and suicide. *International Review of Psychiatry*, **4**, 177−84.

Whyte, I. M., Dawson, A. H., Buckley, N. A., *et al.* (1997). Health care. A model for the management of self-poisoning. *Medical Journal of Australia*, **167**, 142−6.

Williams, J. M. and Broadbent, K. (1986). Autobiographical memory in suicide attempters. *Journal of Abnormal Psychology*, **95**, 144−9.

World Health Organization. (1990). *Consultation on Strategies for Reducing Suicidal Behaviour in the European Region*. Geneva: WHO.

Yeo, H. M. (1993). The cost of treatment of deliberate self-harm. *Archives of Emergency Medicine*, **10**, 8−14.

12

Delirium

Paul Gill, Marco Rigatelli and Silvia Ferrari

A short history of the concept of delirium

The term 'delirium' comes from the Latin expression *de lira*, literally 'out of the furrow', and was introduced by Celso (first century AD) to define an acute pathological state with alterations of consciousness, behavioural anomalies and fever. From the beginning, the relationship of delirium to intoxication and other conditions has been widely recognized (Fele *et al.* 1999; Lipowski 1980). Delirium was, in fact, one of the first psychiatric syndromes to be described.

In the nineteenth century, French psychiatrists introduced the concept of mental confusion as an acute psychotic state, independent of the cause (Chaslin 1892, 1895). Bonhoeffer noted that psychopathological phenomenology is not specific of organic aetiology (Bleuler 1967). Bonhoeffer, in 1909, defined delirium as a stereotypic manifestation of an acute cerebral disturbance, whilst Régis, in the same period, referred to toxic or infective causes.

Engel and Romano (1958), described typical electroencephalogram (EEG) pathological slow waves and considered the finding as distinctive of 'cerebral insufficiency', or 'acute brain failure'; latterly, Lipowski contributed greatly to research on delirium and its diagnostic definition in the Diagnostic and Statistical Manual (DSM; 1980, 1990).

Epidemiology and risk factors

Delirium is frequent among medical and surgical patients and is one of the most common psychiatric complications, affecting 10–30% of patients in the general hospital (GH) (Cohen-Cole *et al.* 1998; Rigatelli & Ferrari 1999; Wise *et al.* 2002). It is one of the main diagnostic groups referred for psychiatric consultation (Huyse *et al.* 2000), although the prevalence varies widely due to differences in

Handbook of Liaison Psychiatry, ed. Geoffrey Lloyd and Elspeth Guthrie. Published by Cambridge University Press. © Cambridge University Press 2007.

patient populations. The reported prevalence is as high as 80% in certain populations of patients, with significant risk and/or aetiological factors such as older age, patients who have had major surgery, those with pre-existing CNS lesions (e.g. dementia, Parkinson's disease, stroke), debilitation (e.g. a terminal condition, burns, renal dialysis), those with cancer, HIV infection, or substance abuse. Such factors establish a 'vulnerability at baseline', the higher this vulnerability, the greater the likelihood of delirium, even if exposure to trigger factors is minimal (Inouye & Charpentier 1996; Meagher 2001). The epidemiology of delirium in primary care and in the community is not known but, with the shortening of hospital stay and the increase of day-surgery, an increase in its presentation in the community and in residential institutes is to be expected (Brown & Boyle 2002).

Age is by far the most relevant risk factor, and with the progressive ageing of Western populations, there is likely to be an increase in the incidence and prevalence of delirium in the next 20 years. Jacobson (1997) calculated a 15–56% frequency of delirium in general medical elderly patients, in comparison with 10–40% prevalence reported in non-elderly patients (Brown & Boyle 2002). Ageing is both a direct and indirect risk factor for delirium, as ageing is associated with a higher frequency of other conditions that may complicate delirium. Male gender also adds to risk in elderly populations (American Psychiatric Association 2000). Recent reviews on the risk factors associated with delirium in older adults have identified significant methodological problems with published studies, so caution is required when discussing any of the data about delirium (Britton & Russell 2003; Elie *et al.* 1998).

Delirium is common after major surgery, and usually starts on the second or third post-operative day; estimates of frequency vary between 32% and 37% (Dyer *et al.* 1995; Mast & Roest 1996; Tune 1991). There is a reported high incidence following cardiotomy, aortic surgery, hip surgery and transplantation. Delirium occurs commonly after surgery because of a variety of factors including the stress of general anaesthesia, pain, insomnia, fever, haemorrhage, and multiple drug treatments in the post-operative phase. Surgery-specific and disease-specific factors have been found to play a role, such as duration of surgery, the degree and complexity of the surgical procedure, critical limb ischaemia, pre-existing dementia, and preoperative factors such as hypertension, cerebrovascular disease or chronic obstructive lung disease (Schneider *et al.* 2002). Delirium is also common in critically-ill medical and surgical patients admitted to intensive care units, who are challenged by great physical and emotional stress (Kishi *et al.* 1995; Rincon *et al.* 2001).

A pre-existing brain condition is an important risk factor for delirium, with a higher incidence in patients with stroke, Parkinson's disease, and dementia;

delirium may sometimes be the first sign of an underlying dementia (Rahkonen *et al.* 2000).

HIV-related diseases are associated with an increased incidence of delirium, due both to direct brain damage (HIV–dementia complex), to systemic illness or opportunistic infections and the necessary treatment regimes. Delirium has been found to be the most frequent neuropsychiatric complication of AIDS (Fernandez *et al.* 1989), with a prevalence of 30–40% among hospitalized AIDS patients (Brown & Boyle 2002).

Aetiology of delirium

Research into the pathophysiology of delirium has recently developed. Attention has focused upon neurotransmission (serotonin and acetylcholine) (Trzepacz 2000), neuroendocrine mechanisms (Robertsson *et al.* 2001) and possible immunological factors (e.g. the role of IGF-I and somatostatin) (Broadhurst & Wilson 2001). For many hospitalized patients, particularly if elderly or terminally ill, multiple causal factors are almost always identifiable (Brauer *et al.* 2000; Francis *et al.* 1990; Meagher 2001; Rudberg *et al.* 1997; Trzepacz *et al.* 1985).

We propose a reasoned approach to the aetiology of delirium according to where the primary cause is located (Table 12.1).

Identification of the cause(s) of delirium requires a thorough medical history and examination combined with appropriate laboratory tests or investigations. A collateral history from a relative or the patient's general practitioner is often helpful, particularly in relation to identifying previous problems with alcohol. Careful evaluation of the patient's past history, recent events in the patient's life, plus diligent study of the case notes all may contribute to diagnosis.

Sometimes no evident cause is found. This has led to the hypothesis of a setting-induced delirium, such as the 'ICU psychosis' or the idea that hospitalization alone can precipitate delirium in elderly patients, but no support from literature exists, and Koponen *et al.* (1989) found a specific organic aetiology in 87% of cases of delirium, if investigations were thorough.

Clinical features, differential diagnosis, prognosis

The clinical presentation of delirium is defined by psychopathology and temporal course: the latter may be crucial in differential diagnosis. Moreover, delirium is often a medical emergency, making time management a significant factor.

The main features are:
• disturbance of consciousness affecting orientation and ability to focus and maintaining attention,

Table 12.1. Causes of delirium.

Endogenous (from inside the body); further distinction in:

Intracranial	Extracranial
• Degenerative	• Metabolic disturbance: hypoxia,
• Inflammatory-infective: meningo-	hypoglycaemia, dehydration,
encephalitis, syphilis, vasculitis, HIV	disturbance, acidosis, alkalosis, anaemia,
and related disorders, etc.	hypoalbuminaemia, etc.
• Traumatic	• Endocrine disturbance: hypo- and
• Vascular: stroke, transient ischaemic	hyperthyroidism/parathyroidism,
attacks (TIA), haemorrhage, aneurysm,	Cushing's, Addison's, pituitary dysfunctions
atrioventricular malformation	• Hypovitaminosis: vitamin B_{12}, folate,
• Neoplastic (and pseudo-tumour cerebri)	niacin, thiamine; hypervitaminosis:
• Epilepsy (and post-ictal syndromes)	vitamin A
• Sensory deprivation: visual/hearing	• Heart-, lung-, liver-, kidney failure, shock
impairment (con-causal), sleep	• Systemic infections: sepsis, pneumonia,
deprivation (con-causal)	peritonitis

Exogenous (from outside the body)

- Medications (40% of cases):
  - psychoactive: sedative-hypnotics, anticonvulsants, antiparkinsonian medications, lithium, anaesthetics, antidepressive, disulfiram,
  - others: anticholinergics, digital, steroids, cimetidine, analgesics, antihistamines, antibiotics, antihypertensives, interferon, immunosuppressives, insulin, salicylates, muscle relaxants
- Substances of abuse (intoxication and withdrawal): alcohol, opiates, cocaine, amphetamines, LSD, phencyclidine, cannabis
- Toxins: organophosphates, carbon monoxide/dioxide, fuel, pesticides, solvents, heavy metals (lead, mercury)
- Withdrawal of psychoactive substances: alcohol (very common in the general hospital), benzodiazepines, barbiturates, opiates etc.

- disturbance in cognition,
- perceptual disturbances.

Patients are disorientated in time and/or space, more rarely to persons (though false recognition is common) and almost never to self. Disorientation to time is often the first warning sign of delirium (American Psychiatric Association 2000). Attention is poor and the patient is easily distractable, looking either apathetic or intensely focused upon something. Confusion is commonly defined as the main symptom of delirium (Fele *et al.* 1999).

Higher-level cognitive functions including abstraction, verbal fluency, memory and consequentiality are greatly affected, resulting in perseverance, concrete thinking, circumstantiality, loose associations, impaired recent memory, misinterpretations and associated disorders of language and behaviour (confabulation up to fluent aphasia; dysgraphia; paraphasia; dysnomia; stereotypical movements; Fele *et al.* 1999).

Common perceptual disturbances include illusions, pseudo-hallucinations and hallucinations. Hallucinations are typically visual (67.9%), more rarely in other sensory modalities (auditory 41.5% (Webster & Holroyd 2000; Wolff & Curran 1935)). Visual dysperceptions are commonly considered pathognomonic of organic aetiology. Visual hallucinations are particularly common, vivid and typical in delirium tremens (e.g. microzoopsia).

The onset is usually abrupt and acute; only in a few cases has a prodrome been described. Symptoms are typically fluctuating over the course of 24 hours, the patient undergoing alternating periods of awareness and lucidity with relapse of symptoms (though cognitive disturbances tend to persist despite reorientation). Agitation and disorientation may be worse at night, but such features should not be mistaken for sundowning, the darkness-related agitation of Alzheimer's and Parkinson's patients.

Associated clinical features include the following:

1. Psychomotor disturbances — either apathy, or agitation, or a combination of the two, so that the distinction between hyperactive, hypoactive and mixed variants of delirium has been proposed (Lipowski 1990; Philpott 1989); agitated delirium is that most frequently described, though a prompt and correct diagnosis of hypoactive delirium is more difficult (it is often mistaken for depression), so that its lower incidence could depend also on missed diagnosis; 'mixed' delirium, with alternation of agitation and apathy, seems to be the most frequent clinical presentation (Liptzin & Levkoff 1992); psychomotor activity typically fluctuates over the course of the day.

2. Disturbances of the sleep—wake cycle — patients may present with insomnia of growing severity, fragmentation of night sleep, day sleepiness, sometimes leading to a complete disruption and reversal of the sleep—wake cycle throughout the 24 hours.

3. Delusions — disorganized delusions, often persecutory in content and accompanied by a strong emotive involvement, are sometimes present (20—40% of cases), and may sometimes persist ('residual delusions'; Cutting 1987; Webster & Holroyd 2000); delirium tremens is often and typically accompanied by 'professional delusions', the patient believing to be and acting as if he/she was at work.

4. Mood disturbances — generally dysphoria and affective lability (rapid and incoherent changes in the emotional states). When prominent, and particularly in hypoactive delirium, these features may lead to a misdiagnosis of

depression or personality disorder (Farrell & Ganzini 1995). It is important to distinguish these two conditions, as many antidepressants have anticholinergic side-effects and delirium symptoms worsen if they are prescribed.

5. Neurovegetative symptoms — hyperthermia, hypertension, tachycardia, nausea, diarrhoea, constipation; in delirium tremens, fever is often the alerting signal of inhalation pneumonia, which is lethal if not properly addressed.

6. Neurological symptoms — a wide range of neurological abnormalities have been described: motor symptoms (tremors, myoclonus, reflex alterations, asterixis); nystagmus; ataxia; cerebellar signs; cranial nerve palsy; dysarthria; none of these is specific of delirium, but some may be indicative of its aetiology (e.g. liver flap).

7. EEG abnormalities — Engel's and Romano's findings have been subsequently clarified and specified: the EEG slowing with theta and delta waves reported by the two authors has been more specifically associated with encephalopathy of metabolic-toxic origin (e.g. liver failure); EEG changes in the opposite direction of quickening, with low-voltage beta waves, are associated with delirium due to alcohol or benzodiazepine withdrawal (Jacobson 1997). The EEG can nevertheless be normal or only slightly altered, the sensitivity of this investigation being not higher than 65% (Brenner 1991).

Diagnosis of delirium is based on the recognition of the symptoms listed above ('diagnosis of state') and their causal correlation to one or more underlying organic conditions. The mental state examination should first of all assess orientation, short-term memory, attention and high-level cognitive functioning (abstraction, judgement, criticism, verbal and written expression and comprehension, visuo-constructional abilities). The Mini-Mental State Examination (MMSE; Folstein *et al.* 1975) is an effective tool, suited for a consultation setting, but cannot discriminate delirium from dementia, and is also affected by educational level. A thorough collateral history should therefore be conducted as well, from whomever possible (patient, relatives, ward staff, GP, roommates), with reference both to present symptoms and previous mental state. An EEG is useful, though not mandatory. It is preferable to rely on good clinical diagnosis than to wait for an EEG if there is likely to be any delay. Several quantitative delirium-specific instruments have been developed, which may contribute to diagnosis and monitoring, such as the Delirium Rating Scale (Trzepacz 1999; Trzepacz *et al.* 1988) and the Confusion Assessment Method (CAM; Inouye *et al.* 1990).

Differential diagnosis of delirium requires exclusion of the following conditions:

1. Dementia: the differential diagnosis is based over the temporal course of the syndrome, together with medical and psychiatric past and present history and

other information from family members: acute and rapid onset in contrast to progressive, insidious onset; fluctuation of symptoms in the 24 hours in contrast to stability of impairment. In dementia, the patient is alert and disturbances of consciousness appear only at very advanced stages of the condition. Some variants of dementia are more difficult to rule out, such as Creutzfeldt—Jakob (more rapid onset, though not yet acute) and Lewy body (symptoms may fluctuate over the course of the day, recurrent visual hallucinations, transient confusional state (Robinson 2002)). Delirium is a potentially reversible condition, in contrast to the chronic progression of dementia. Of course delirium and dementia may coexist, either because of direct or indirect causality (dementia is a risk factor for delirium), or independently affecting the same patient. The reader is referred to Table 14.5 in Chapter 14 which summarizes the differences between delirium and dementia.

2. Aphasia, due to cerebrovascular accidents: distinction is based on the features of aphasia, the presence of focal neurological symptoms and the more limited impairment of cerebral functioning (orientation, attention, memory are usually normal).

3. Acute psychotic states, due to schizophrenia, depression or mania: thought disturbances are better organized; no significant alterations of consciousness or cognitive impairment are observed; hallucinations, if present, are more typically auditory than visual; in maniacal states, mood abnormalities are more definite and persistent; the patient's past and present pathological history are different.

Five possible outcomes of delirium have been described:

- complete remission
- progression to a chronic organic cerebral syndrome
- progression towards functional psychosis
- remission of an acute episode superimposed on pre-existing dementia
- death (Fele *et al.* 1999).

The first outcome is the most commonly observed of the five, as long as appropriate diagnosis and treatment are provided: delirium is conceptualized as a transient and reversible alteration of cerebral functioning; a mean course of 10—12 days has been described, though full recovery may take longer than the duration of hospital stay (Lipowski 1990). Cognitive impairment is the commonest residual symptom of delirium, especially in AIDS patients and, of course, patients with dementia (American Psychiatric Association 1999).

Delirium remains often undiagnosed: non-detection rates of 50—60% have been calculated (Brown & Boyle 2002; Francis *et al.* 1990; Inouye 1994; Rincon *et al.* 2001) and, despite its high frequency, psychiatric referral rate is low (1.4%; Huyse *et al.* 2000); low detection rates may also depend on fluctuation of symptoms and inadequate documentation (Dyer *et al.* 1995). As delirium could be the single indicator of worsening of patient's clinical status, an acute change in mental status in a medically ill patient without a psychiatric history should be presumed to be delirium until proven otherwise (Meagher 2001).

If not recognized or not adequately treated, the syndrome may persist and may worsen; the patient may die, depending on the underlying aetiology. The risk of dying during a hospital stay is 5.5 times higher in patients developing delirium, both as a direct consequence of delirium and of delirium being a significant sign of clinical severity (Rabins & Folstein 1982). Death rates remain higher among patients who have suffered from delirium even months following discharge (Wise *et al.* 2002): a recent study by McCusker *et al.* (2002) demonstrated delirium as being an independent risk factor for increased mortality in the 12 months after discharge, particularly among non-demented patients. Moreover, the rate of relapse is high, especially in elderly or debilitated patients; previous episodes of delirium are a significant risk factor for subsequent episodes.

Delirium not only independently affects mortality, but morbidity as well: it accounts for longer hospital stays, worse and slower recoveries, more complicated post-surgical courses, increased utilization of healthcare services, increased risk for admission to residential care, increased subsequent functional decline, and increased long-term disability (American Psychiatric Association 2000; Francis *et al.* 1990; Franco *et al.* 2001; Inouye *et al.* 1998; Marcantonio *et al.* 1994, 2000), with consequent high impact on healthcare costs.

Diagnostic DSM and ICD definitions

Delirium is defined in the Diagnostic and Statistical Manual of the American Psychiatric Association (DSM-IV) as a disorder 'characterized by a disturbance of consciousness and change in cognition that develops over a short period of time' (American Psychiatric Association 2000) and classified in a common section together with dementia, and amnestic and other cognitive disorders.

The DSM classification of delirium has explicitly aetiologically-based criteria: delirium due to a general medical condition, substance-induced delirium (included medication side-effects − iatrogenic delirium − and delirium due to substance withdrawal) and delirium due to multiple aetiologies, with a conclusive National Academy of Sciences (NAS) sub-category. The DSM-IV diagnostic criteria for the three aetiologic subcategories of delirium are summarized in Table 12.2.

The corresponding category of the International Classification of Diseases (ICD-10; 1992) is that identified by the code F05 as delirium, not induced by alcohol and other psychoactive substances; therefore, in the ICD-10, other

Table 12.2. DSM-IV diagnostic criteria for delirium.

Clinical features	Delirium due to general medical condition	Substance-induced delirium	Delirium due to multiple aetiologies
Common to all subcategories	• Disturbance of consciousness with reduced ability to focus, sustain or shift attention. • Change in cognition or development of a perceptual disturbance not better accounted for by a pre-existing, established, or evolving dementia. • The disturbance develops over a short period of time (usually hours to days) and tends to fluctuate during the course of the day.		
Distinguishing subcategories	Disturbance caused by the direct physiological consequences of a general medical condition	• Symptoms developed during substance intoxication or a withdrawal syndrome or a toxic exposure. • Medication use aetiologically related to the disturbance.	The delirium has more than one aetiology (either one or more general medical conditions or substance intoxication or withdrawal syndromes or a combination).
Notes	• If delirium is superimposed on a pre-existing vascular dementia, code it as 290.41, vascular dementia, with delirium. Include the name of the general medical condition	• Diagnosis possible only if the cognitive symptoms are excessive of those usually associated with the intoxication or the withdrawal syndrome and severe enough to warrant independent clinical attention.	

categories regarding delirium are to be found in the chapter 'Alcohol/substance abuse' (F10–19), with the codes F1x.03 (acute intoxication with delirium) and F1x.4 (withdrawal state with delirium) (World Health Organization 1992); this structure of classification recognizes no autonomy to the syndrome when it is a consequence of substance abuse, but intermixes it with several other syndromes due to the pathological effects of psychoactive substances. No aetiological criterion is explicitly fixed by the ICD-10, though the cited distinction in separate chapters is in itself an indirect reference to different causes. The ICD also differentiates delirium with or without a pre-existing dementia (F05.0 – not superimposed on dementia, and F05.1 – superimposed on dementia); a residual category of 'other delirium', including delirium of mixed origin and subacute confusional state, is also present in ICD-10 with the code F05.8.

Clinical management and therapeutic issues

Prevention

Primary prevention (aimed at preventing the onset of delirium) and secondary prevention (prevention of worsening) require taking into account data on risk and precipitating factors, previously reported. There is a distinct lack of research, and clinical trials on delirium prevention are still sparse: the few that are published are mainly focused on prevention of surgery-related delirium (Cole *et al.* 1996; Kornfeld *et al.* 1974; Weissman & Hackett 1958). It has been shown that preoperative psychiatric intervention significantly reduces the occurrence of subsequent delirium (Smith & Dimsdale 1989) and a recent randomized controlled trial by Inouye *et al.* (1999), involving a multicomponent intervention, obtained a decrease in the number of delirium episodes by screening and management of six identified risk factors. Inouye (2000) also proposed specific intervention strategies for elderly patients.

Given the high frequency of misdiagnosis or missed recognition, many authors discuss the need for routine screening at admission for high-risk populations of patients such as the elderly, surgical patients, those with cancer, AIDS, etc. (Franco *et al.* 2001; Strain *et al.* 1994). There is a need to define and quantify specific patient and hospital risk factors in particular populations, who differ from each other on a range of demographic and physiological features, and for care plans in the general hospital (Britton & Russell 2003; Zeleznik 2001).

Find the cause

This is the absolute priority in the management of delirium. Some of the possible causes of delirium are in themselves medical emergencies (e.g. electrolyte alterations, hypo-/hyperglycaemia), or could rapidly develop into emergencies. Psychiatric symptoms are rarely seen in isolation (other non-psychiatric symptoms and signs are present), but may be the most striking and disorientating for the medical staff, potentially delaying a prompt and proper medical diagnosis and misleading the physician towards considering the case to be of a 'pure' psychiatric nature (Rigatelli *et al.* 2003).

Delirium is one of the very few psychiatric conditions to be not only treatable, but also reversible: recognition and adequate correction of its cause is the greater part of treatment. Because of the frequent multiple aetiology, the investigation of causes, as well as the subsequent management and treatment, requires a combination of different skills: those of the physician, the nurse, the psychiatrist and the psychiatric nurse.

Delirium is a common reason for psychiatric referral in the general hospital (although, as already stated, delirium frequently goes unrecognized, and many cases will not be referred), and in our experience delirium is one of the most frequent reasons for urgent referral. The typical situation is that of a very agitated patient, shouting, hallucinating, aggressive, annoying other patients and possibly endangering him/herself. Implicit or explicit request for the patient to be transferred to the psychiatric ward is common. The consultation-liaison (C-L) psychiatrist has to resist such a request and advise that the patient stays in the medical ward, under strict combined medical-psychiatric observation. Moreover, the C-L psychiatrist should not take for granted that the medical therapeutic needs of the patient (hydration, monitoring of vital signs) will be properly addressed, as the disturbance of the patient may confound such routine monitoring. The psychiatrist has a responsibility for checking what investigations have already been performed, what the results are, and to advise regarding further investigation. It is not sufficient to assume that investigation of physical causes is the province of medical or surgical colleagues, and will therefore have been conducted.

Medication is responsible for 40% of cases of delirium: therefore a careful review of medication is necessary, non-essential medications should be discontinued and all should be kept at the lowest doses possible (American Psychiatric Association 1999). A common mistake is only to check on regular medication given to the patient. It is important that the psychiatrist also checks 'as-required' and single-dose medication. It is also vital to confirm that the patient has not regularly been taking medication prior to admission to hospital, which has subsequently been overlooked: inadvertent drug withdrawal is common in hospital settings.

Psychopharmacological intervention

The aim of giving psychotropic drugs to the patient with delirium is sedation, combined with correction of psychiatric (mainly psychotic) symptoms, therefore a consensus that high-potency antipsychotics are the treatment of choice in delirium is well documented, with haloperidol by far the commonest.

Haloperidol has a quick and effective antipsychotic action, a discrete sedative effect, can be administered either orally or parenterally and is safe and generally well tolerated even at high doses. A starting dose of 0.5–1 mg three times a day, possibly increased up to 10 mg per day, is usually effective, adjusting the distribution over 24 hours according to the level of sleep—wake disturbance. Very rarely higher doses are needed, though haloperidol has been used safely up to 100—1000 mg per day (Levenson 1995). Extrapyramidal side-effects are relatively rare and usually precipitated by other risk factors, particularly HIV dementia and Lewy body dementia. Intravenous administration has been associated with electrocardiogram (ECG) modifications (prolonged QT interval; Sharma *et al.* 1998), but also with less severe extrapyramidal side-effects (Menza *et al.* 1987). An oral and regular administration (not on an 'as-needed' basis) is preferable and should be continued at the same dose for some days after complete remission of symptoms; only then should it be gradually decreased (Lobo 2001).

Phenothiazines are generally avoided because of their low potency and higher toxicity (anticholinergic, hepatic and cardiovascular side-effects). Many atypical antipsychotics have recently been studied (Breitbart *et al.* 2002a; Leso & Schwartz 2002; Sipahimalani & Masand 1998; Sipahimalani *et al.* 1997; Torres *et al.* 2001) and the review by Schwartz and Masand (2002) concludes that their use is a 'reasonable first-line approach', though stating that further research is needed. Atypical antipsychotics have potential advantages, as they are generally associated with a lower risk of side-effects, and there is little doubt that many clinicians have developed considerable personal experience in their use in delirium. However, the limited availability of parenteral forms of atypicals restricts their use in delirium, although the use of dispersible tablets can be helpful. Recently, however, there have been major warnings regarding their use in patients with dementias, following reports of an increased risk of stroke associated with their use (Smith & Beier 2004; Wooltorton 2002, 2004). Because of the association between dementias and the risk of delirium, caution has to be advised regarding the use of atypical antipsychotics in delirium, until there is greater clarification of the risks involved.

Benzodiazepines are used for the treatment of alcohol or benzodiazepine withdrawal syndrome. In other cases, and especially in the elderly patient, benzodiazepines may worsen confusional symptoms and should be avoided or only used at very low doses to increase sedation and to lower the antipsychotic dose. Diazepam, chlordiazepoxide, or lorazepam (lower risk of accumulation) are the most commonly used for the treatment of delirium tremens. Lorazepam is safer when there is concern about hepatic function. The patient may require up to 12 mg per day of lorazepam, or 100 mg per day of diazepam. It is important that the dose is given regularly, and that a gradual reduction regime, over 5—10 days, is ensured. The route of administration is generally oral, but in acutely disturbed patients rectal or slow intravenous administration may be necessary. The intramuscular route should be avoided because of unpredictable systemic release of benzodiazepines from muscular tissue.

In delirium tremens, benzodiazepines are usually combined with vitamins of the B-complex and sometimes tiapride (100 mg three times a day), carbamazepine or valproate (Fele *et al.* 1999). Thiamine should be given in high dose to any patient suffering from delirium tremens. There has been concern about the possibility of anaphylaxis, but parental administration is more effective in reducing the risks of Wernicke's encephalopathy, and should be used rather than oral thiamine, provided there are full resuscitation facilities available.

Other treatments have been reported in the literature but are less common in clinical practice:

- clonidine for delirium due to opiate withdrawal (Fele *et al.* 1999)
- physostigmine for anticholinergic delirium (Stern 1983; American Psychiatric Association 1999)
- donepezil (Wengel *et al.* 1998)
- ECT (American Psychiatric Association 1999; Levin *et al.* 2002)
- immunology: IGF-I and somatostatin secretion has been found to be a neuroprotective response to brain injury (Broadhurst & Wilson 2001).

Non-pharmacological and environmental interventions

These aspects of treatment are often neglected or considered less important than drug prescription in the flurry of an emergency, whereas a considerable amount of literature supports evidence of their relevance (Cole *et al.* 1994; Inouye *et al.* 1999; Lobo 2001; Meagher 2001; Meagher *et al.* 1996).

Environmental intervention is important, and effective approaches include the following:

1. Protect the patient and other people: remove potentially dangerous objects, make the bed safe, use one-to-one nursing if possible; restraints should be a measure of last resort, when no real alternative is possible (and are not acceptable in the UK; Inouye & Charpentier 1996). The patient should be placed in a room near the nursing station, so that quick and continuous monitoring is possible.
2. Both excessive sensory stimuli (lights, noises, voices) and isolation of the patient's room should be avoided.
3. The light should be natural during the day (choose a room with wide windows), with artificial attenuated light during the night (enough to reduce misperceptions).
4. An attenuated light source above the patient's head prevents approaching staff appearing in silhouette from the patient's perspective.
5. A clock and a calendar should be visible to the patient.
6. If the patient usually wears glasses or hearing aids, return them as quickly as possible to recreate good sensory input.

7. Relatives should be given a clear explanation at an early stage, and be reassured that the condition is generally reversible, and is not indicative of impending madness; this explanation is sufficiently important that it should form part of the care plan, and should be recorded in the casenotes.

8. Ward staff and relatives should be encouraged to give the patient frequent re-orientation cues (tell him/her where he/she is, why, what time and date is, who they are) both to correct what the patient says and spontaneously (in hypoactive delirium); they should also be specifically advised to maintain a calm and reassuring attitude towards the patient.

9. Relatives could also bring some personal objects of the patient from home (pictures in frame, a blanket, a mug).

10. The patient should maintain good activity levels, either by accompanied walks or exercises in bed.

11. In approaching the patient, ward staff should always give their names and briefly explain what they are going to do, avoiding talking to each other in medical jargon which may encourage paranoia.

12. If feasible, a designated group of staff members should attend the patient so that the patient is not constantly dealing with new faces.

13. A rota of family members, or friends recognizable to the patient, who can sit with the patient can be of great assistance.

14. During remission of symptoms, ward staff and relatives should constantly reassure the patient that he/she 'is not going crazy', and has not to feel guilty or ashamed for his/her behaviour; that delirium is a temporary and totally reversible condition.

Constant monitoring of the patient and reassessment of his/her condition is crucial in dealing with delirium; the C-L team should programme regular follow-up, instead of simple 'as-needed' visits. The ward staff (doctors and nurses) should be instructed regularly to check vital signs and any changes in the patient's general medical condition, and to ensure appropriate fluid input and output and oxygen. Many authors have addressed the pivotal role of nurses (medical and psychiatric; Lobo 2001; Milisen *et al.* 2001; Morency 1990). Diagnostic tools such as the CAM can also be used to monitor delirium, to help with assessment of the clinical evolution of the condition, and the adjustment of treatment. Good management of delirium goes far beyond simple control of florid psychiatric symptoms (Brown & Boyle 2002).

Liaison issues

Delirium is a medical-psychiatric emergency: once a diagnosis has been established, procedures already described should be followed. The C-L psychiatrist is responsible for educating hospital staff, helping to develop guidelines and protocols, and working with the other clinicians in the management of the delirious patient (Rigatelli *et al.* 2003). Delirium is so frequent in the general hospital that a single C-L service cannot be involved directly with all cases, leaving the less problematic ones to ward physicians. Therefore liaison, education of medical and nursing staff, and good working relationships and alliances with physicians (American Psychiatric Association 1999), are particularly important in the management and prevention of delirium.

Formal liaison activities should take place on the initiative of the C-L psychiatry team, and directed to those concerned: physicians, surgeons, nurses, doctors in training (in psychiatry and other specialities), medical and nursing students. Formal teaching, seminars, and more interactive modalities such as case discussions, work-groups and consensus conferences are of great benefit. Moreover, day-to-day, person-to-person informal liaison is essential, based on mutual acquaintance and professional esteem; this should also address the distressing effects of dealing with the delirious patient (Breitbart *et al.* 2002b). Detailed and direct consultation letters addressed to primary care physicians, to co-ordinate post-discharge care and increase awareness in the event of future re-hospitalization are a vital, but easily overlooked, component of the service.

Relevant themes that should be covered in educational activities include primary and secondary prevention of delirium; delirium as a medical-psychiatric emergency, with high morbidity and mortality; the medical aetiology of delirium despite the florid psychiatric symptoms; the risks of misdiagnosis (especially hypoactive delirium mistaken for depression); the integrated management between psychiatric and non-psychiatric teams; and the development of shared guidelines. Emphasis should be placed on a problem-solving, simple and pragmatic approach.

Liaison interventions should also be addressed to relatives: interviewing the patient's family members or caregivers is essential to confirm the diagnosis of delirium. Relatives should also be closely involved in the care of the patient during hospital stay and after discharge. Clear communication, explanations and reassurance are important (Breitbart *et al.* 2002b).

Although improvement of knowledge and skills of individual healthcare providers is important, the greatest impact can be achieved by changes in institutional systems of care, such as hospital architecture and environment, nursing procedures, flexibility in the organization of wards and integration of care (Francis 1997; Kornfeld 2002). The creation of medical-psychiatric units or joint care units (Kathol 1998; Summergrad 1994), especially designed for patients with medical-psychiatric comorbidity (delirium, attempted suicide) can be extremely useful.

REFERENCES

American Psychiatric Association. (1999). *Practice Guideline for the Treatment of Patients with Delirium.* Washington DC: APA.

American Psychiatric Association. (2000). *Diagnostic and Statistical Manual of Mental Disorders, IV edition, Text Revision.* Washington DC: American Psychiatric Association, pp. 135–47.

Bleuler, E. (1967). *Trattato di Psichiatria*, X edizione. Milano: Feltrinelli.

Brauer, C., Morrison, R. S., Silberzweig, S. B., *et al.* (2000). The cause of delirium in patients with hip fracture. *Archives of Internal Medicine*, **160**, 1856–60.

Breitbart, W., Tremblay, A. and Gibson, C. (2002a). An open trial of olanzapine for the treatment of delirium in hospitalized cancer patients. *Psychosomatics*, **43**, 175–82.

Breitbart, W., Gibson, C. and Tremblay, A. (2002b). The delirium experience: delirium recall and delirium-related distress in hospitalized patients with cancer, their spouses/caregivers, and their nurses. *Psychosomatics*, **43**, 183–94.

Brenner, R. P. (1991). Utility of EEG in delirium: past views and current practice. *International Psychogeriatrics*, **3**, 211–29.

Britton, A. and Russell, R. (2003). Multidisciplinary team interventions for delirium in patients with chronic cognitive impairment (Cochrane Review). In *The Cochrane Library*, Issue 1. Oxford: Update Software.

Broadhurst, C. and Wilson, K. (2001). Immunology of delirium: new opportunities for treatment and research. *British Journal of Psychiatry*, **179**, 288–9.

Brown, T. M. and Boyle, M. F. (2002). ABC of psychological medicine. Delirium. *British Medical Journal*, **325**, 644–7.

Chaslin, P. (1892). La confusion mentale primitive. *Annales Medico-Psychologiques*, **16**, 225–73.

Chaslin, P. (1895). *La Confusion Mental Primitive. Stupidité, Démence, Aiguë, Stupeur Primitive.* Paris: Asselin et Houzeau.

Cohen-Cole, S. A., Saravay, S. M., Hall, R. C. W., *et al.* (1998). *Mental Disorders in General Medical Practice. Adding Value to Healthcare Through Consultation-liaison Psychiatry.* Taskforce on Healthcare Value Enhancement. Academy of Psychosomatic Medicine.

Cole, M. G., Primeau, F., Bailey, R. F., *et al.* (1994). Systematic intervention for elderly inpatients with delirium: a randomised trial. *Canadian Medical Association Journal*, **151**, 965–70.

Cole, M. G., Primeau, F. and McCusker, J. (1996). Effectiveness of interventions to prevent delirium in hospitalized patients: a systematic review. *Canadian Medical Association Journal*, **155**, 1263–8.

Cutting, J. (1987). The phenomenology of acute organic psychosis. *British Journal of Psychiatry*, **151**, 324–32.

Dyer, C. B., Ashton, C. M. and Teasdale, T. A. (1995). Postoperative delirium. *Archives of Internal Medicine*, **155**, 461–5.

Elie, M., Cole, M. G., Primeau, F. J., *et al.* (1998). *Journal of General Internal Medicine*, **13**, 204–12.

Engel, G. L. and Romano, J. (1958). Delirium, a syndrome of cerebral insufficiency. *Journal of Chronic Disease*, **9**, 260–77.

Farrell, K. R. and Ganzini, L. (1995). Misdiagnosing delirium as depression in medically ill elderly patients. *Archives of Internal Medicine*, **155**, 2459–64.

Fele, P., Fornaro, P., Mungo, S., *et al.* (1999). Delirium. In *Trattato Italiano di Psichiatria*, 2nd edn., ed. P. Pancheri and G. B. Cassano. Milano: Masson, pp. 1171–85.

Fernandez, F., Levy, J. and Mansell, P. (1989). Management of delirium in terminally ill AIDS patients. *International Journal of Psychiatry in Medicine*, **19**, 165–72.

Folstein, M. F., Folstein, S. E. and McHugh, P. R. (1975). Mini-Mental State Examination: a practical method for grading the cognitive state of patients for clinicians. *Journal of Psychosomatic Research*, **11**, 189–98.

Francis, J. (1997). Outcomes of delirium: can systems of care make a difference. *American Geriatric Society*, **45**, 247–8.

Francis, J., Martin, D. and Kapoor, W. (1990). A prospective study of delirium in hospitalised elderly. *Journal of the American Medical Association*, **263**, 1097–101.

Franco, K., Litaker, D., Locala, J., *et al.* (2001). The cost of delirium in the surgical patient. *Psychosomatics*, **42**, 68–73.

Huyse, F. J., Herzog, T., Lobo, A., *et al.* (2000). European C-L service and their user populations. The ECLW collaborative study. *Psychosomatics*, **41**, 330–8.

Inouye, S. K. (1994). The dilemma of delirium: clinical and research controversies regarding diagnosis and evaluation of delirium in hospitalised elderly medical patients. *American Journal of Medicine*, **97**, 278–88.

Inouye, S. K. (2000). Prevention of delirium in hospitalised older patients: risk factors and targeted intervention strategies. *Annals of Medicine*, **32**, 257–63.

Inouye, S. K. and Charpentier, P. A. (1996). Precipitating factors for delirium in hospitalised elderly persons: predictive model and interrelationships with baseline vulnerability. *Journal of American Medical Association*, **275**, 852–7.

Inouye, S. K., van Dyck, C. H., Alessi, C. A., *et al.* (1990). Clarifying confusion: the confusion assessment method. A new method for detection of delirium. *Annals of Internal Medicine*, **113**, 941–8.

Inouye, S. K., Rushing, J., Foreman, M., *et al.* (1998). Does delirium contribute to poor hospital outcomes? A three-site epidemiologic study. *Journal of General Internal Medicine*, **13**, 234–42.

Inouye, S. K., Bogardus, S. T., Charpentier, P. A., *et al.* (1999). A multicomponent intervention to prevent delirium in hospitalized older patients. *New England Journal of Medicine*, **340**, 669–76.

Jacobson, S. A. (1997). Delirium in the elderly. *The Psychiatric Clinics of North America*, **1**, 91–110.

Kathol, R. (1998). Integrated medicine and psychiatry treatment programs. *Medicine and Psychiatry*, **1**, 10–16.

Kishi, Y., Iwasaki, Y., Takezawa, K., *et al.* (1995). Delirium in critical care unit patients admitted through an emergency room. *General Hospital Psychiatry*, **17**, 371–9.

Koponen, H., Stenback, U. and Mattila, E. (1989). Delirium among elderly persons admitted to a psychiatric hospital: clinical course during the acute stage and one-year follow-up. *Acta Psychiatrica Scandinavica*, **79**, 579–85.

Kornfeld, D. S. (2002). Consultation-liaison psychiatry: contributions to medical practice. *American Journal of Psychiatry*, **159**, 1964–72.

Kornfeld, D. S., Heller, S. S., Frank, K. A., *et al.* (1974). Personality and psychological factors in postcardiotomy delirium. *Archives of General Psychiatry*, **31**, 249–53.

Leso, L. and Schwartz, T. L. (2002). Ziprasidone treatment of delirium. *Psychosomatics*, **43**, 61–2.

Levenson, J. L. (1995). High-dose intravenous haloperidol for agitated delirium following lung transplantation. *Psychosomatics*, **36**, 66–8.

Levin, T., Petrides, G., Weiner, J., *et al.* (2002). Intractable delirium associated with ziconotide successfully treated with electroconvulsive therapy. *Psychosomatics*, **43**, 63–6.

Lipowski, Z. J. (1980). *Delirium. Acute Brain Failure in Man.* Springfield: Charles C. Thomas Publisher.

Lipowski, Z. J. (1990). *Delirium; Acute Confusional States.* New York: Oxford University Press.

Liptzin, B. and Levkoff, S. E. (1992). An empirical study of delirium subtypes. *British Journal of Psychiatry*, **161**, 843–5.

Lobo, A. (2001). Psichiatria di consultazione: i temi scottanti della clinica. *Noos*, **7**, 281–304 (in Italian).

Marcantonio, E. R., Goldman, L., Mangione, C. M., *et al.* (1994). A clinical prediction rule for delirium after elective noncardiac surgery. *Journal of the American Medical Association*, **271**, 134–9.

Marcantonio, E. R., Flacker, J. M., Michaels, M., *et al.* (2000). Delirium is independently associated with poor functional recovery after hip fracture. *Journal of the American Geriatrics Society*, **48**, 618–24.

Mast, R. C. and van der Roest, F. H. J. (1996). Delirium after cardiac surgery: a critical review. *Journal of Psychosomatic Research*, **41**, 13–30.

McCusker, J., Cole, M., Abrahamowicz, M., *et al.* (2002). Delirium predicts 12-month mortality. *Archives of Internal Medicine*, **162**, 457–63.

Meagher, D. J. (2001). Delirium: optimising management. *British Medical Journal*, **322**, 144–9.

Meagher, D. J., O'Hanlon, D., O'Mahony, E., *et al.* (1996). The use of environmental strategies and psychotropic medication in the management of delirium. *British Journal of Psychiatry*, **168**, 512–15.

Menza, M. A., Murray, G. B., Holmes, V. F., *et al.* (1987). Decreased extrapyramidal symptoms with intravenous haloperidol. *Journal of Clinical Psychiatry*, **48**, 278–80.

Milisen, K., Foreman, M. D., Godderis, J., *et al.* (2001). Delirium in the hospitalized elderly: nursing assessment and management. *The Nursing Clinics of North America*, **33**, 417–39.

Morency, C. R. (1990). Mental status change in the elderly: recognizing and treating delirium. *Journal of Professional Nursing*, **6**, 356–65.

Philpott, R. (1989). Recurrent acute confusional states. In *The Clinical Neurology of Old Age*, ed. R. Tallis. New York: John Wiley & Sons, pp. 453–66.

Rabins, P. V. and Folstein, M. F. (1982). Delirium and dementia: diagnostic criteria and fatality rates. *British Journal of Psychiatry*, **140**, 149–53.

Rahkonen, T., Luukkainen-Markkula, R., Paanil, S., *et al.* (2000). Delirium episode as a sign of undetected dementia among community dwelling elderly subjects: a 2 year follow-up study. *Journal of Neurology, Neurosurgery and Psychiatry*, **69**, 519–21.

Rigatelli, M. and Ferrari, S. (1999). Differences and analogies in consultation-liaison activity to primary care and general hospital physicians: one or two services? *XV World Congress of Psychosomatic Medicine* (proceedings). Athens.

Rigatelli, M., Ferrari, S., Bertoncelli, B., *et al.* (2003). Tre tipi particolari di urgenze in psichiatria di consultazione. In *Psichiatria e Medicina. Dialogo e Confini*, ed. C. Gala, C. Bressi and M. Rigatelli. Roma: CIC Edizioni Internazionali, pp. 48–53 (in Italian).

Rincon, H. G., Granados, M., Unutzer, J., *et al.* (2001). Prevalence, detection and treatment of anxiety, depression and delirium in the adult critical care unit. *Psychosomatics*, **42**, 391–6.

Robertsson, B., Blennow, K., Brane, G., *et al.* (2001). Hyperactivity in the hypothalamic-pituitary-adrenal axis in demented patients with delirium. *International Clinical Psychopharmacology*, **16**, 39–47.

Robinson, M. J. (2002). Probable Lewy body dementia presenting as 'delirium'. *Psychosomatics*, **43**, 84–5.

Rudberg, M. A., Pompei, P., Foreman, M. D., *et al.* (1997). The natural history of delirium in older hospitalised patients: a syndrome of heterogeneity. *Age and Ageing*, **26**, 169–75.

Schneider, F., Böhner, H., Habel, U., *et al.* (2002). Risk factors for postoperative delirium in vascular surgery. *General Hospital Psychiatry*, **24**, 28–34.

Schwartz, T. L. and Masand, P. S. (2002). The role of atypical antipsychotics in the treatment of delirium. *Psychosomatics*, **43**, 171–4.

Sharma, N. D., Rosman, H. S., Padhi, D., *et al.* (1998). Torsades de pointes associated with intravenous haloperidol in critically ill patients. *American Journal of Cardiology*, **81**, 238–40.

Sipahimalani, A. and Masand, P. S. (1998). Olanzapine in the treatment of delirium. *Psychosomatics*, **39**, 422–30.

Sipahimalani, A., Sime, R. M. and Masand, P. S. (1997). Treatment of delirium with risperidone. *International Journal of Geriatric Psychopharmacology*, **1**, 24–6.

Smith, D. A. and Beier, M. J. (2004). Association between risperidone treatment and cerebrovascular adverse events: examining the evidence and postulating hypotheses for an underlying mechanism. *Journal of the American Medical Directors Association*, **5**(2), 129–32.

Smith, L. and Dimsdale, J. (1989). Postcardiotomy delirium: conclusions after 25 years? *American Journal of Psychiatry*, **146**, 452–8.

Stern, T. (1983). Continuous infusion of physostigmine in anticholinergic delirium: a case report. *Journal of Clinical Psychiatry*, **44**, 463–4.

Strain, J. J., Hammer, J. S. and Fulop, G. (1994). AMP Task Force on psychosocial interventions in the general hospital inpatient setting: a review of cost-offset studies. *Psychosomatics*, **25**, 253–62.

Summergrad, P. (1994). Medical psychiatry units and the roles of the inpatient psychiatric service in the general hospital. *General Hospital Psychiatry*, **16**, 20–31.

Torres, R., Mittal, D. and Kennedy, R. (2001). Use of quietiapine in delirium. *Psychosomatics*, **42**, 347–9.

Trzepacz, P. T. (1999). The delirium rating scale. Its use in consultation-liaison research. *Psychosomatics*, **40**, 193–204.

Trzepacz, P. T. (2000). Is there a final common neural pathway in delirium? Focus on acetylcholine and dopamine. *Seminars in Clinical Neuropsychiatry*, **5**, 132–48.

Trzepacz, P. T., Teague, G. B. and Lipowski, Z. J. (1985). Delirium and other organic mental disorders in a general hospital. *General Hospital Psychiatry*, **7**, 101–6.

Trzepacz, P. T., Baker, R. W. and Greenhouse, J. (1988). A symptom rating scale for delirium. *Psychiatry Research*, **23**, 89–97.

Tune, L. E. (1991). Post-operative delirium. *International Psychogeriatrics*, **3**, 325–32.

Webster, R. and Holroyd, S. (2000). Prevalence of psychotic symptoms in delirium. *Psychosomatics*, **41**, 519–22.

Weissman, A. D. and Hackett, T. P. (1958). Psychosis after eye surgery – establishment of a specific doctor-patient relationship in prevention and treatment of black patch delirium. *New England Journal of Medicine*, **258**, 1284–9.

Wengel, S. P., Roccaforte, W. H. and Burke, W. J. (1998). Donepezil improves symptoms of delirium in dementia: implications for future research. *Journal of Geriatric Psychiatry and Neurology*, **11**, 159–61.

Wise, M. G., Hilty, D. M., Cerda, G. M., *et al.* (2002). Delirium (confusional states). In *The American Psychiatric Publishing Textbook of Consultation-liaison Psychiatry. Psychiatry in the Medically Ill*, 2nd edn., ed. M. G. Wise and J. R. Rundell. Washington DC: American Psychiatric Publishing Inc, pp. 257–72.

Wolff, H. G. and Curran, D. (1935). Nature of delirium and allied states. *Archives of Neurology and Psychiatry*, **33**, 1175–215.

Wooltorton, E. (2002). Risperidone (Risperdal): increased rate of cerebrovascular events in dementia trials. *Canadian Medical Association Journal*, **167**(11).

Wooltorton, E. (2004). Olanzapine (Zyprexa): increased incidence of cerebrovascular events in dementia trials. *Canadian Medical Association Journal*, **170**(9).

World Health Organization. (1992). *The ICD-10 Classification of Mental and Behavioural Disorders*. Geneva: WHO.

Zeleznik, J. (2001). Delirium: still searching for risk factors and effective preventive measures. *Journal of the American Geriatrics Society*, **49**, 1729–32.

13

Childhood experiences

Mark Berelowitz

Experiences in childhood can have a tremendous influence on wellbeing in adulthood, and on the ways in which illness presents in adulthood. Conversely, illness in a parent, and the way the illness is managed, can have a great impact on the children in the family. This chapter will examine these two areas, examining the knowledge base and the implications for practice in adult liaison psychiatry. It will not attempt to cover every aspect of the field. The influences on children's health and development are manifold, and not all of those influences are relevant to liaison psychiatry. The chapter will therefore focus on those areas which have been best researched, and which have the greatest potential significance for the adult liaison psychiatrist.

Adult psychiatrists might also wish to bear in mind that the pathways into child psychiatric disorder are complex, as will be seen from the research quoted below. When a parent suffers from a particular condition, physical or psychological, that condition might have a direct effect on the parent's behaviour with the child, or on the child's thoughts and anxieties about the parent. However, the effects on the child might be influenced by other factors, such as the impact of parental illness on the marriage, the level of functioning of the healthy parent, and the child's relationship with that parent. Illness and bereavement may result in financial difficulties, so that the children need to be looked after by other carers. The way in which the child is told about the parental illness can also influence adjustment. Some confiding relationships may be protective.

Comorbidity is a particularly useful concept in child psychiatry. If a child has one disorder, they are far more likely than the average to have another psychiatric disorder.

Children's symptoms and presentations change with age and with gender. Boys are more likely to respond with behavioural disturbance and girls with depression

Handbook of Liaison Psychiatry, ed. Geoffrey Lloyd and Elspeth Guthrie. Published by Cambridge University Press. © Cambridge University Press 2007.

when faced with the same adversity. Depression occurs in all ages, but self-harm is rare until adolescence.

Childhood influences

Child abuse

Child abuse, and in particular child sexual abuse, is the environmental factor which has the greatest influence on those areas of adult functioning which are of interest to the liaison psychiatrist. The empirical research into the origins of borderline personality disorder (BPD) provides some of the most valuable information. Ogata *et al.* (1990), in a comparison of borderline and depressed inpatients, found that more than 70% of the borderline patients reported sexual abuse in childhood. Zanarini *et al.* (1998) found that 90% of borderline patients reported having been abused in childhood, and having been neglected. In a later study, patients with BPD reported particularly severe and unpleasant abuse, including penetration and the use of force and violence (Zanarini *et al.* 2002). Furthermore, the extent of self-harm in adulthood may be related to the extent of abuse in childhood, and may also explain the dissociation that is so commonly seen in these patients, especially in those who harm themselves (Brodsky *et al.* 1995; Dubo *et al.* 1997). More recently (and alarmingly), the odds of a sexually-abused borderline patient attempting suicide in adulthood was found to be over 10 times that of a patient who was never sexually abused (Soloff *et al.* 2002).

Much of the above research is based on patient samples. However, similar results are to be found in community samples. A community study in New York State found that personality disorders were four times as common in young adults who had been abused or neglected in childhood than for those who had not suffered such experiences (Johnson *et al.* 1999). The same group found that abuse and neglect in childhood were strongly associated with suicide attempts in late adolescence and early adulthood (Johnson *et al.* 2002).

Child abuse and neglect manifests in other predictable ways in adulthood. For example, women who have been sexually abused in childhood have higher healthcare costs. They have more consultations in primary care and hospital outpatients, and also attend the accident and emergency department (A&E) more frequently (Walker *et al.* 1999).

Research supports an association between childhood abuse and neglect and the development of somatization and dissociative symptoms in adulthood. Patients with conversion (dissociative) disorder report chronic and severe abuse more frequently than controls (Roelofs *et al.* 2002). Pribor *et al.* (1993) found a significant association between Briquet's syndrome, dissociation, and child abuse. Others have found strong links between dissociation and somatizating disorders (Saxe *et al.* 1994). There are strong links between child abuse and somatization. For example associations have been found for pelvic pain (Walker *et al.* 1997), chronic pain (Walling *et al.* 1994), irritable bowel syndrome (Walker *et al.* 1993), and for somatization in general (Springs & Friedrich 1992). The vast majority of the research has been conducted on women, but the findings with men are probably similar.

These findings have significant implications for the liaison psychiatrist. They affect the way consultations and examinations should be conducted, and are also informative about the dependency and volatility that characterize some clinical relationships. Sensitivity is required with patients who are reluctant to be interviewed alone, who are anxious about internal examinations, or indeed are excessively compliant and uncomplaining.

It should also be remembered that while much of the literature deals with child sexual abuse specifically, physical abuse and neglect are also extremely important.

Child psychiatric disorder

Mental health problems in childhood are common. Some of these conditions are shortlived. However, many conditions persist, in varying form, into adulthood, including anxiety, depression, eating disorders and conduct disorder. Occasionally minor symptoms in childhood will turn out to be the precursors of severe mental illness in adulthood.

Eating disorders

There is a strong association between eating disorders in adolescence and a variety of physical and mental health difficulties in adulthood (Johnson *et al.* 2002). Adolescents with eating disorders are at a substantially elevated risk for developing anxiety disorders, cardiovascular symptoms, chronic fatigue, chronic pain, depressive disorders, limitations in activities due to poor health, infectious diseases, insomnia, neurological symptoms, and suicide attempts during early adulthood. They are also at risk for osteoporosis and fertility problems.

Seventy per cent of patients with eating disorders in childhood and adolescence recover from their eating disorder. But only 50% have a good overall level of functioning in adulthood (Steinhousen *et al.* 2003). A 10-year follow-up study of teenagers with anorexia nervosa found high rates of obsessive compulsive disorder, depression and interpersonal difficulties. Furthermore, the sample had high rates of physical illness and physical complaints. The liaison psychiatrist will need to take a careful history and may also need to alert the medical team to investigations that they might not have considered, such as assessment of bone density.

Anxiety disorders and depression

For most children with depression, the condition remits by adulthood. However, these disorders in adulthood are almost invariably preceded by the same or a similar condition in childhood and adolescence. Persistence into adulthood is associated with severity of the underlying condition, and with adversity (Goodyer *et al.* 1997). Furthermore, even if the depression remits, previously depressed adolescents are at risk for poor social functioning and suicide in adulthood.

Most children who develop anxiety disorders in childhood do not have anxiety disorders in adulthood. However, anxiety disorders in childhood increase the risk for depressive disorders in adulthood. Also, most adults with anxiety and a mood disorder will have suffered from anxiety in childhood. Some attachment disorders will persist into adulthood.

In October 1988 a cruise ship with 400 schoolchildren on board was struck by another ship and sank. Almost all of the children on board were rescued, but many underwent terrifying experiences. Fifty-one per cent of the surviving children developed post-traumatic stress disorder (PTSD). A substantial number still had PTSD as young adults. There were also high rates of anxiety disorders and affective disorders in the group with persistent PTSD. The sample is unique, because of the unusual nature of the traumatic event. Nevertheless, the results are impressive (Bolton *et al.* 2000; Yule *et al.* 2000). Adult psychiatrists should remember that anyone who has suffered from PTSD for much of their adolescent years will have missed out on a good deal of their educational and social opportunities.

Children with adjustment disorders are vulnerable to the development of depression, anxiety and conduct problems in late adolescence (Kovacs *et al.* 1994). It is not clear whether these problems persist into adulthood.

Physical illness, adjustment and somatization

Many adult patients seen in a liaison psychiatry service will have been, or should have been, liaison patients in childhood. This will be true for many of the persistent chronic illnesses, including asthma, inflammatory bowel disease and chronic renal failure, to name but a few. A small but troubling group will have been victims of Munchausen by proxy abuse. The impact of the physical illness in childhood, and the adjustment to that illness, will have a great impact on their presentation in adulthood. A detailed review (Gledhill *et al.* 2000) indicates that school and work attainment, self-esteem, mood, socialization and marriage prospects may be affected in children and adolescents with a range of serious chronic illnesses. There may be problems with physical appearance and with sexual functioning.

The physical illness may have brought the child patient very much closer to one parent, usually the mother, sometimes with adverse consequences for the rest of family life. The style of paediatric care, and indeed of paediatric liaison psychiatry, may be very different from adult care, and the adolescent may find the transition difficult. On the other hand, the move to adult care may give the patient opportunities to address issues which they did not feel comfortable about in a paediatric setting, such as disclosing sexual problems.

Drug and alcohol abuse

The use of drugs other than inhalants is low in the pre-adolescent group. Drug use increases dramatically in adolescence, with well over half of all adolescents experimenting with illicit drugs, and about a quarter having tried more than one drug. However, only about 7% of these adolescents are heavy drug users. Overall, use of illicit drugs has probably increased over the last decade.

Occasional drug use is clearly remarkably common, and is usually without any lasting consequence. Information about why a small group progresses to sustained and harmful drug use is lacking. Violence, abuse and neglect at home, parental affective illness and drug use, affective illness in the child and failure to detect problems at school all seem to play a part.

Teenagers who use drugs heavily have poor outcomes. They are at high risk for suicide, accidental death, delinquency and depression. One study showed mortality within the teenage years to be 11 times the average for teenage boys, and 21 times the average for girls (Oyefoso *et al.* 1999). The majority of these deaths were the result of accidental overdoses. Among drug users who inject, there is substantially increased risk of hepatitis C and HIV. Poorer outcome is associated with drug use started at an early age.

More recently, studies have demonstrated greater risks associated with cannabis than was previously thought. Adolescent girls who use cannabis regularly are at greatly increased risk for depression and anxiety. Self-medication as treatment for affective disorder was thought unlikely to be the explanation (Patton *et al.* 2002).

There are also fresh concerns about cannabis and schizophrenia. An extensive study of Swedish conscripts found significantly increased levels of schizophrenia in cannabis users, with increased risk being associated with increased frequency of use of cannabis. The authors postulate a causal link (Zammit *et al.* 2002).

Unfortunately, the literature on prevention is dispiriting. There are probably benefits in treating affective illness in parents and carers, especially if they are also drug users. Affective illness in children and adolescents should also be identified early and treated. In adolescents, greater morbidity is associated with crack cocaine and heroin than with alcohol, cannabis and tobacco. Therefore, where primary prevention has failed, efforts should go into trying to prevent progression to these more damaging drugs.

HIV/AIDS

More and more HIV-infected children are surviving into adulthood. Some will be orphaned, and some of those orphans will have become street children. Indeed, in the USA many HIV-infected adolescents are homeless or living in the streets. Some will have been working in the sex industry for several years before they reach adulthood. The literature on psychiatric aspects of HIV disease in adolescents is limited. Not surprisingly, high rates of anxiety and affective illness have been reported, as have substance abuse and a history of sexual abuse (Hoffman *et al.* 1999; Pao *et al.* 2000).

Perinatally infected children who survive into adulthood face huge adversity. A wide range of psychiatric symptoms in childhood has been reported. However, factors associated with the parents, including prenatal drug exposure, prematurity and inherited parental psychopathology may indeed have the larger causative role (Havens *et al.* 1994; Mellins *et al.* 2003). Symptoms of encephalopathy may be helped by methylphenidate.

Parental influences

In the first part of this chapter the childhood influences that affect adjustment in adulthood were considered. Factors in the parents will now be considered, with particular focus on those conditions that will be likely to bring parents into contact with adult liaison psychiatrists, followed by consideration of some of the wider ramifications of illness in the parents that can also have consequences for children.

Parental physical illness

The research in this area is limited, but has nevertheless produced some compelling findings. Almost all the research has been done with mothers, mostly focusing on breast cancer. More research will need to be done before we can be confident on whether the current data can be generalized to other conditions affecting mothers and fathers.

When mothers have cancer, adolescent daughters may be the most vulnerable (Compass *et al.* 1994). In keeping with general research on children with emotional problems, it has been shown that parents with cancer are likely to under-report psychological distress in their children. Indeed, in some situations where children, especially adolescent girls, reported high levels of distress, their parents were quite unaware of this (Welch *et al.* 1996). This clearly poses a problem for the liaison psychiatrist who enquires about the children's welfare but does not actually get to meet the children on their own.

Many parents are reluctant to discuss the diagnosis explicitly with their children. However, it has been found that in families where a parent has cancer, the anxiety levels are lower in children who have been told about the diagnosis than in those who have not (Rosenheim & Reicher 1985). This has led to helpful research on communication to the children about the diagnosis. Parents may be keen to tell the children, but are also apprehensive about doing so. They would welcome expert advice about how and when to tell them (Barnes *et al.* 2000). Older children are likely to be told more than their younger siblings, and sooner. In a subsequent study it was found that not all children who were told that mother was ill were informed about the diagnosis. Children of more highly educated mothers were told less (Barnes *et al.* 2002). A description of the oncology service at Massachusetts General Hospital provides useful guidance for clinicians (Rauch *et al.* 2002).

Moving away from cancer, a small study has looked at the impact of parental inflammatory bowel disease on children (Mukherjee *et al.* 2002). The parental illness had the positive effect of increasing closeness in the parent–child relationship. Children became anxious when their parents were hospitalized, and reacted with anger and frustration to the inevitable restriction upon their own social activities.

Parents with mental health difficulties

Once again the research has concentrated on mothers, and on depression and eating disorders in particular. These two areas are discussed in detail below, after first making some general points.

Parental alcoholism, antisocial behaviour, schizophrenia and affective disorders are all associated with poorer child development and mental health. The problems in children are mediated through genetics, abuse and neglect, marital discord, poverty, and poor educational attainment. Marital discord continues to be one of the most important environmental factors impacting upon the mental health of children.

Maternal depression

A very large number of studies have shown that exposure to maternal depression in the early post-partum months may have an enduring influence on child psychological adjustment. These effects can include the child's behaviour with the mother, the presence of behavioural disturbance at home, and the content and social patterning of play at school (Murray *et al.* 1999). Post-natal and current maternal depression can also have persistent effects on children's functioning at school, both in terms of behaviour and intellectual development. Indeed boys of mothers depressed in the first year post-partum scored approximately one standard deviation lower on standardized tests of intellectual attainment than boys whose mothers were well during that year (Sharp *et al.* 1995; Sinclair & Murray 1998). Depressed mothers are less well attuned to their infants, and these effects can be evident in the way mothers read to infants (Reissland *et al.* 2003).

These persistent and powerful findings point to the need to identify and treat maternal depression actively. The impact of the depression on the marriage needs to be faced. There is some evidence that fathers may be helpful in preventing some of the consequences for the children (Tannenbaum & Forehand 1994).

Maternal eating disorders

The consequences of maternal eating disorders have been well studied, and have produced compelling results.

There is a strong association between maternal eating disorders and childhood feeding problems (Whelan & Cooper 2000). Mothers with eating disorders have difficulty in responding to the cues of their infants at feeding time, leading to conflict between mother and child (Stein *et al.* 1999). They have difficulty in maintaining breastfeeding, and give their children less encouragement to eat. The problems for mothers can begin antenatally, and can result in low birthweight (Waugh & Bulik 1999). There is evidence of delayed growth and inadequate weight gain in the infants and toddlers. These effects are probably related to the mothers' concerns about their own body shape, and the amount of conflict at mealtimes (Stein *et al.* 1994). These problems can have very serious consequences. Mothers of children with non-organic failure to thrive were found to be restricting their own food intake, and to be reluctant to give their children foods that would result in weight gain, even though the children were seriously underweight (McCann *et al.* 1994).

Unfortunately it is not yet clear how best to intervene in these cases. Treatment of the primary disorder in the mother, and efforts to help mothers and their partners understand how the parental disorder impacts on the child, should be attempted until further clear evidence emerges about the effectiveness of treatment.

Childhood bereavement

Children bereaved of a parent have higher rates of morbidity, and substantial numbers meet diagnostic criteria for major depressive disorder in the first year after parental death. Family history of depression and previous child psychiatric disorders are risk factors (Weller *et al.* 1991). A study of bereaved three- to six-year-olds showed high rates of anxiety and depression. Depression in the surviving parent was a powerful predictor of symptoms in the child (Kranzler *et al.* 1990). Attending the funeral does not have adverse consequences unless the child is forced to go. Economic adversity is an added stress for children. For those children unfortunate enough to be members of a family in which several people die, say because of a genetic condition, the consequences will be particularly problematic.

When dealing with a dying parent, liaison psychiatrists should be particularly attentive to the mental health of the surviving parent, and should try to ensure that the surviving parent is adequately supported and monitored.

Implications for the adult liaison psychiatrist

When faced with a seriously-ill patient who is also a parent, the liaison psychiatrist will need to address a number of factors if the wellbeing of the children of the family is to be promoted.

First, at an appropriate point in the consultation, the patient needs to be asked about his/her children. The patient may be afraid of addressing the subject, and will need the doctor's help in doing so. Our own experience is that oncologists do not mention the children at all, and nor do adult general psychiatrists.

Second, the spouse needs to be involved. The parents should be encouraged to keep the children well informed about the parent's illness, and to seek professional help in doing so if required. Close attention needs to be paid to the mental health of the spouse, as this will be a key determinant of the wellbeing of the children.

Third, the nature of the children's anxieties and difficulties will not be sufficiently clear unless the children themselves are interviewed directly. It will not usually be the responsibility of the liaison psychiatrist to carry out those interviews. However, the psychiatrist must ensure that the parents understand why the children need to be seen on their own, and arrange for the appropriate professional to carry out the work.

Fourth, specific problems will require specific attention. For mothers with eating disorders, and with depression, a paediatrician must take responsibility for monitoring the children's growth, weight gain and social and educational development. When the parental illness has produced marital discord, or depression in the spouse, the children will benefit enormously from active treatment for one or both parents.

Fifth, for adults who have chronic illnesses going back into childhood, attention needs to be paid to the problems of making the transition from children's services to adult services. This may entail not only the loss of familiar clinicians, but also of the peer group. Young adults with chronic illnesses may also be faced with the increasingly bitter realization that they are not growing out of their problems.

Sixth, for such adults who themselves have or are trying to have children, all of the above considerations apply, and the patient will need gentle assistance in beginning to think about the implications of their own illness for the wellbeing of their current or future children.

Last, but by no means least, the links between parental and child health, both physical and mental, point to the need for close working relationships between adult and child liaison psychiatry services. The adult and paediatric team clearly have ample scope for communicating about individual families, and for sharing information about contemporary research.

REFERENCES

Barnes, J., Kroll, L., Burke, O., *et al.* (2000). Qualitative interview study of communication between parents and children about maternal breast cancer. *British Medical Journal,* **321**, 479–82.

Barnes, J., Kroll, L., Lee, J., *et al.* (2002). Factors predicting communication about the diagnosis of maternal breast cancer to children. *Journal of Psychosomatic Research,* **52**(4), 209–14.

Bolton, D., O'Ryan, D., Udwin, O., *et al.* (2000). The long-term psychological effects of a disaster experienced in adolescence: II: General psychopathology. *Journal of Child Psychology and Psychiatry,* **41**(4), 513–23.

Brodsky, B. S., Cloitre, M. and Dulit, R. A. (1995). Relationship of dissociation to self-mutilation and childhood abuse in borderline personality disorder. *American Journal of Psychiatry,* **152**(12), 1788–92.

Compas, B. E., Worsham, N. L., Epping-Jordan, J. E., *et al.* (1994). When mom or dad has cancer: markers of psychological distress in cancer patients, spouses, and children. *Health Psychology,* **13**(6), 507–15.

Dubo, E. D., Zanarini, M. C., Lewis, R. E., *et al.* (1997). Childhood antecedents of self-destructiveness in borderline personality disorder. *Canadian Journal of Psychiatry,* **42**(1), 63–9.

Gledhill, J., Rangel, L. and Garralda, E. (2000). Surviving chronic physical illness: psychosocial outcome in adult life. *Archives of Disease in Childhood,* **83**(2), 104–10.

Goodyer, I. M., Herbert, J., Tamplin, A., *et al.* (1997). Short-term outcome of major depression: II. Life events, family dysfunction, and friendship difficulties as predictors of persistent disorder. *Journal of the American Academy of Child and Adolescent Psychiatry,* **36**(4), 474–80.

Havens, J. F., Whitaker, A. H., Feldman, J. F., *et al.* (1994). Psychiatric morbidity in school-age children with congenital human immunodeficiency virus infection: a pilot study. *Journal of Development and Behavioral Pediatrics*, **15**(3), S18−25.

Hoffman, N. D., Futterman, D. and Myerson, A. (1999). Treatment issues for HIV-positive adolescents. *AIDS Clinical Care*, **11**(3), 21−4.

Johnson, J. G., Cohen, P., Brown, J., *et al.* (1999). Childhood maltreatment increases risk for personality disorders during early adulthood. *Archives of General Psychiatry*, **56**(7), 600−6.

Johnson, J. G., Cohen, P., Gould, M. S., *et al.* (2002). Childhood adversities, interpersonal difficulties, and risk for suicide attempts during late adolescence and early adulthood. *Archives of General Psychiatry*, **59**(8), 741−9.

Kovacs, M., Gatsonis, C., Pollock, M., *et al.* (1994). A controlled prospective study of DSM-III adjustment disorder in childhood. Short-term prognosis and long-term predictive validity. *Archives of General Psychiatry*, **51**(7), 535−41.

Kranzler, E. M., Shaffer, D., Wasserman, G., *et al.* (1990). Early childhood bereavement. *Journal of the American Academy of Child and Adolescent Psychiatry*, **29**(4), 513−20.

McCann, J. B., Stein, A., Fairburn, C. G., *et al.* (1994). Eating habits and attitudes of mothers of children with non-organic failure to thrive. *Archives of Disease in Childhood*, **70**(3), 234−6.

Mellins, C. A., Smith, R., O'Driscoll, P., *et al.*, NIH NIAID/NICHD/NIDA-Sponsored Women & Infant Transmission Study Group. (2003). High rates of behavioral problems in perinatally HIV-infected children are not linked to HIV disease. *Pediatrics*, **111**(2), 384−93.

Mukherjee, S., Sloper, P. and Turnbull, A. (2002). An insight into the experiences of parents with inflammatory bowel disease. *Journal of Advanced Nursing*, **37**(4), 355−63.

Murray, L., Sinclair, D., Cooper, P., *et al.* (1999). The socioemotional development of 5-year-old children of postnatally depressed mothers. *Journal of Child Psychology and Psychiatry*, **40**(8), 1259−71.

Ogata, S. N., Silk, K. R., Goodrich, S., *et al.* (1990). Childhood sexual and physical abuse in adult patients with borderline personality disorder. *American Journal of Psychiatry*, **147**(8), 1008−13.

Oyefeso, A., Ghodse, H., Clancy, C., *et al.* (1999). Drug abuse-related mortality: a study of teenage addicts over a 20-year period. *Social Psychiatry and Psychiatric Epidemiology*, **34**(8), 437−41.

Pao, M., Lyon, M., D'Angelo, L. J., *et al.* (2000). Psychiatric diagnoses in adolescents seropositive for the human immunodeficiency virus. *Archives of Pediatric and Adolescent Medicine*, **154**(3), 240−4.

Patton, G., Coffey, C., Carlin, J., *et al.* (2002). Cannabis use and mental health in young people: cohort study. *British Medical Journal*, **325**, 1195−8.

Pribor, E. F., Yutzy, S. H., Dean, J. T., *et al.* (1993). Briquet's syndrome, dissociation, and abuse. *American Journal of Psychiatry*, **150**(10), 1507−11.

Rauch, P. K., Muriel, A. C. and Cassem, N. H. (2002). Parents with cancer: who's looking after the children? *Journal of Clinical Oncology*, **20**(21), 4399–402.

Reissland, N., Shepherd, J. and Herrera, E. (2003). The pitch of maternal voice: a comparison of mothers suffering from depressed mood and non-depressed mothers reading books to their infants. *Journal of Child Psychology and Psychiatry*, **44**(2), 255–61.

Roelofs, K., Keijsers, G. P., Hoogduin, K. A., *et al.* (2002). Childhood abuse in patients with conversion disorder. *American Journal of Psychiatry*, **159**(11), 1908–13.

Rosenheim, E. and Reicher, R. (1985). Informing children about a parent's terminal illness. *Journal of Child Psychology and Psychiatry*, **26**(6), 995–8.

Saxe, G. N., Chinman, G., Berkowitz, R., *et al.* (1994). Somatization in patients with dissociative disorders. *American Journal of Psychiatry*, **151**(9), 1329–34.

Sharp, D., Hay, D. F., Pawlby, S., *et al.* (1995). The impact of postnatal depression on boys' intellectual development. *Journal of Child Psychology and Psychiatry*, **36**(8), 1315–36.

Sinclair, D. and Murray, L. (1998). Effects of postnatal depression on children's adjustment to school. Teacher's reports. *British Journal of Psychiatry*, **172**, 58–63.

Soloff, P. H., Lynch, K. G. and Kelly, T. M. (2002). Childhood abuse as a risk factor for suicidal behavior in borderline personality disorder. *Journal of Personality Disorders*, **16**(3), 201–14.

Springs, F. E. and Friedrich, W. N. (1992). Health risk behaviors and medical sequelae of childhood sexual abuse. *Mayo Clinic Proceedings*, **67**(6), 527–32.

Stein, A., Woolley, H., Cooper, S. D., *et al.* (1994). An observational study of mothers with eating disorders and their infants. *Journal of Childhood Psychology and Psychiatry*, **35**(4), 733–48.

Stein, A., Woolley, H. and McPherson, K. (1999). Conflict between mothers with eating disorders and their infants during mealtimes. *British Journal of Psychiatry*, **175**, 455–61.

Steinhausen, H. C., Boyadjieva, S., Griogoroiu-Serbanescu, M., *et al.* (2003). The outcome of adolescent eating disorders. Findings from an international collaborative study. *European Child and Adolescent Psychiatry*, **12** (Suppl. 1), I91–8.

Tannenbaum, L. and Forehand, R. (1994). Maternal depressive mood: the role of the father in preventing adolescent problem behaviors. *Behavior Research and Therapy*, **32**(3), 321–5.

Walker, E. A., Katon, W. J., Roy-Byrne, P. P., *et al.* (1993). Histories of sexual victimization in patients with irritable bowel syndrome or inflammatory bowel disease. *American Journal of Psychiatry*, **150**(10), 1502–6.

Walker, E. A., Katon, W. J., Hansom, J., *et al.* (1997). Psychiatric diagnoses and sexual victimization in women with chronic pelvic pain. *Psychosomatics*, **36**(6), 531–40.

Walker, E. A., Unutzer, J., Rutter, C., *et al.* (1999). Costs of health care use by women HMO members with a history of childhood abuse and neglect. *Archives of General Psychiatry*, **56**(7), 609–13.

Walling, M. K., O'Hara, M. W., Reiter, R. C., *et al.* (1994). Abuse history and chronic pain in women: II. A multivariate analysis of abuse and psychological morbidity. *Obstetrics and Gynecology*, **84**(2), 200–6.

Waugh, E. and Bulik, C. M. (1999). Offspring of women with eating disorders. *International Journal of Eating Disorder*, **25**(2), 123–33.

Welch, A. S., Wadsworth, M. E. and Compas, B. E. (1996). Adjustment of children and adolescents to parental cancer. Parents' and children's perspectives. *Cancer*, **77**(7), 1409–18.

Weller, R. A., Weller, E. B., Fristad, M. A., *et al.* (1991). Depression in recently bereaved prepubertal children. *American Journal of Psychiatry*, **148**(11), 1536–40.

Wentz, E., Gillberg, C., Gillberg, I. C., *et al.* (2001). Ten-year follow-up of adolescent-onset anorexia nervosa: psychiatric disorders and overall functioning scales. *Journal of Child Psychology and Psychiatry*, **42**(5), 613–22.

Whelan, E. and Cooper, P. J. (2000). The association between childhood feeding problems and maternal eating disorder: a community study. *Psychological Medicine*, **30**(1), 69–77.

Yule, W., Bolton, D., Udwin, O., *et al.* (2000). The long-term psychological effects of a disaster experienced in adolescence: I: The incidence and course of PTSD. *Journal of Child Psychology and Psychiatry*, **41**(4), 503–11.

Zammit, S., Allebeck, P., Andreasson, S., *et al.* (2002). Self reported cannabis use as a risk factor for schizophrenia in Swedish conscripts of 1969: historical cohort study. *British Medical Journal*, **325**, 1199.

Zanarini, M. C., Williams, A. A., Lewis, R. E., *et al.* (1998). Reported pathological childhood experiences associated with the development of borderline personality disorder. *American Journal of Psychiatry*, **154**(8), 1101–6.

Zanarini, M. C., Yong, L., Frankenburg, F. R., *et al.* (2002). Severity of reported childhood sexual abuse and its relationship to severity of borderline psychopathology and psychosocial impairment among borderline inpatients. *The Journal of Nervous and Mental Disease*, **190**(6), 381–7.

Part III

Working with specific units

14

Neurological disorders

Alan Carson, Adam Zeman, Lynn Myles and Michael Sharpe

Introduction

In practice the psychiatrist working in a clinical neurosciences centre is likely to have to address three main categories of clinical problems on a daily basis:

- patients with cognitive impairment either as a primary presentation or as a secondary complication of a known condition, such as multiple sclerosis
- patients who present with neurological disease but in whom there is emotional disturbance in excess of the clinical norm
- patients who present with physical symptoms which do not correspond to any recognized pattern of neurological disease.

The approach to such cases should include a neuropsychiatric as well as a standard psychiatric assessment. The neuropsychiatric assessment depends upon the observation that predictable patterns of symptoms will result from damage to specific brain areas. The summary of the clinical assessment should include not only a 'headline' diagnosis but also a clinical problem list of the impairments and consequent disabilities that the patient suffers (Table 14.1). It is often the latter that will dictate the management of the individual patient. For example, a psychiatrist will seldom make the diagnosis of multiple sclerosis (MS) but will be frequently asked to assess patients with MS and to comment on their cognitive impairment, depressive and other emotional disorders and maladaptive coping strategies.

Treatments, and in particular psychological treatments, are not discussed in detail as they are covered in other chapters. Whilst we have described specific drug therapies the reader should be aware that in many neuropsychiatric conditions the mainstays of patient management are behavioural and environmental manipulation. Similarly, we have concentrated on the medical aspects of psychiatry but we hope the reader will understand that both assessment and management will benefit

Handbook of Liaison Psychiatry, ed. Geoffrey Lloyd and Elspeth Guthrie. Published by Cambridge University Press. © Cambridge University Press 2007.

Table 14.1. Definitions of impairment, disability and handicap according to the World Health Organization.

Impairment	Loss or abnormality of structure or function
Disability	A restriction or lack of ability to perform an activity in the manner or within the range considered normal for a human being
Handicap	The disadvantage for an individual that prevents or limits the performance of a role that is normal for that individual

from appropriate multidisciplinary contribution. Delirium is covered in a separate chapter in this book (Chapter 12). Finally, we have omitted descriptions of numerous less common brain diseases, which have marked cognitive and psychological consequences; indeed there is no such thing as a brain disease that does not. We have chosen instead to concentrate on commonly encountered conditions and to describe them in detail. The principles of assessment that we introduce in the context of these disorders can be applied to other rarer disorders.

Clinical assessment

Careful clinical assessment reveals the diagnosis in the majority of patients. It should include:

- taking a history from the patient, which both supplies relevant factual information and also provides an early opportunity to appraise the patient's cognitive function
- taking a history from an informant, a key part of the clinical assessment of patients with cognitive problems
- the mental state, cognitive, neurological and general medical examination.

The total assessment should be expected to take around 90 minutes. Three key questions need to be answered by the clinical assessment:

1. Are the symptoms suggestive of a structural deficit in the brain? (This will usually be indicated by cognitive impairment or neurological signs.) And if so, do the symptoms displayed match the deficit when its extent becomes known?
2. Is there evidence to suggest additional and significant psychiatric problems, in particular mood or anxiety disorders? The presence of depression, for example, does not rule out concomitant dementia, but its early recognition is important for management.
3. Is the patient's behavioural response to their symptoms adaptive or maladaptive?

History-taking

Table 14.2 highlights those symptoms that deserve particular attention when taking a history from the patient and/or informant. As well as documenting the details of the disorder, it is important to obtain a good background medical and psychiatric history including medical conditions such as a history of vascular disease as well as previous episodes of affective illness or the consumption of prescribed or recreational drugs. Both patient and informant should each be interviewed alone.

The cognitive examination (CE) will be introduced by way of the capacities that it aims to assess.

Table 14.2. Factors for consideration in a neuropsychiatric history.

Physical
- Smell
- Vision
- Hearing
- Speech/intelligibility
- Swallowing (choking)
- Pain:
  - neck and back symptoms
  - headaches
  - other
- Gait
- Weakness/spasticity
- Dizziness/balance
- Epilepsy (type and frequency)
- Other disturbances of consciousness
- Adverse effects of medication
- Movement disorder
- Skin/autonomic

Cognitive
- Conscious level (?fluctuating)
- Addenbrooke's Cognitive Examination (ACE)
- Perceptual neglect
- Dysexecutive – organizational ability
- Mental capacity (consent to treatment/management of property and affairs)

Communication/thinking
- Verbal, non-verbal and social skills
- Confabulation
- Perseveration

Table 14.2. (*cont.*) Factors for consideration in a neuropsychiatric history.

Behavioural
- Drive/motivation/fatigue
- Compliance
- Disinhibition
- Perseverative behaviour
- Wandering/absconding
- Irritability/aggression
- Disruptive/noisy
- Response to pain
- Use of aids/down-time

Emotional
- Dysphoria
- Lability/emotionalism
- Catastrophic reaction
- PTSD symptoms
- Depression
- Generalized anxiety
- Phobic anxiety
- Health-related anxiety

Activities of daily living

Personal
- Mobility
- Eating and drinking
- Continence
- Washing and dressing

Community
- Ability to use transport
- Fitness to drive
- Leisure

Domestic
- Cooking
- Laundry
- Shopping
- Money management

Available support
- Relatives/friends
- Day centres
- Social worker/benefits/legal representation

Table 14.2. (*cont.*)

Risk identification
- Self-harm
- Assault/violence/threat to others
- Criminal behaviour/fire risk
- Sexually inappropriate behaviour
- Alcohol/drug misuse
- Potential for exploitation by others
- Wandering, falling or choking
- Awareness of danger/road safety
- Family cohesion
- Able to self-medicate

Source: Adapted from Royal College of Psychiatrists Brain Injury Special Interest Group.

Wakefulness

Wakefulness depends on normal cerebral arousal by the brain stem and thalamic ascending activating system. A subject whose conscious level is impaired will inevitably perform poorly on cognitive testing. In patients with an impaired conscious level, the Glasgow Coma Scale (GCS) (Table 14.3) provides a widely used assessment tool. The GCS uses three parameters: eye opening, verbal responses and motor behaviour. Despite its undoubted value as a yardstick for consciousness, the GCS is a relatively blunt instrument, primarily designed to describe conscious level after acquired brain injury. The description of other parameters of consciousness may be more appropriate in certain cases particularly when metabolic disorders are suspected.

Orientation

Orientation in place and time depends on several psychological functions. However, a finding of disorientation does imply cognitive failure in one or several domains, and it is helpful to test orientation near the start of the cognitive assessment.

Attention

Attention can be 'sustained', 'selective', 'divided' or 'preparatory' or classified in terms of its object, for example 'spatial' and 'non-spatial'. The form most relevant to the clinical CE is the sustained attention that allows us to concentrate on cognitive tasks. This depends on the concerted functioning of a number of brain regions, including subcortical arousal centres, frontal 'executive' regions and posterior sensory or language areas. Disruption of attention – often by factors that

Table 14.3. Glasgow coma scale.

	Feature	Scale responses	Score
Eye opening	Spontaneous	4	
	To speech	3	
	To pain	2	
	None	1	
Verbal response	Orientated	5	
	Confused conversation	4	
	Words (inappropriate)	3	
	Sounds (incomprehensible)	2	
	None	1	
Best motor response	Obey commands	6	
	Localize pain	5	
	Flexion (normal)	4	
	Flexion (abnormal)	3	
	Extend	2	
	None	1	
	Total coma 'score'		3/15—15/15

disturb brain function in a diffuse way such as drugs, infection or organ failure — is the neuropsychological hallmark of a confusional state or 'delirium'. Sustained attention is best tested using moderately demanding, non-automatic tasks like reciting the months backwards or, as described in the Mini Mental State Examination (MMSE) (Folstein *et al.* 1975), spelling 'world' backwards or subtracting seven serially from 100.

Memory

Declarative memories can be articulated; procedural memories are enacted, as when, for example you ride a bike. Working (or 'short-term') memory allows you to keep information in mind while you use it: for example, carrying a phone number in your head from looking it up in the directory to the time of dialling. Long-term declarative memory is divided into episodic, the memory for unique events like your last holiday, and semantic, the data base of knowledge about language and the world which we constantly use to interpret what we perceive. These distinctions have a neurobiological basis. Working memory depends on frontal executive structures which direct attention, and posterior areas relevant to the material being rehearsed. The acquisition of new long-term declarative memories requires the integrity of limbic regions connected in the circuit of Papez, particularly the hippocampus and adjacent structures in the medial temporal lobes, the fornix and the anteromedial thalamus, damage to which underlies the classical 'amnestic syndrome'. Procedural memory is substantially independent of declarative memory, drawing, for example, on the cerebellum, which mediates classical conditioning, and on the basal ganglia.

In the clinic, memory is usually tested by asking the patient to register some information, such as a name and address or three words (working memory), and to recall the same information after an interval of at least one minute, whilst performing other mental tasks to prevent rehearsal (long-term memory). Some general-knowledge questions are often asked to tap semantic memory (which is also probed by questions requiring visual recognition and naming).

Executive function

'Executive function' refers to the complex of abilities which allows us to plan, initiate, organize and monitor our thoughts and behaviour. These abilities, which localize broadly to the frontal lobes, are essential for normal social performance, but are notoriously difficult to test. Functional subdivisions are recognized within the frontal lobes. Motor and premotor areas in and adjacent to Brodmann Area 4 more or less directly govern movement. The dorsolateral prefrontal cortex, lying anterior to motor and premotor cortex, is particularly involved in attention, working memory and organization of thought and behaviour; the orbitofrontal cortex is concerned with regulation of social behaviour; the medial frontal cortex, including the anterior cingulate gyrus, is closely connected to the limbic system and helps to mediate motivation and arousal.

Frontal-lobe disorders often make themselves apparent in social interaction with a patient. You should suspect one, for example, in a patient who sits very close to you or dismantles your pen. Tasks which can be used to clarify deficits in frontal lobe function include: verbal fluency, for example listing as many animals as possible in one minute; motor sequencing, for example asking a patient to copy a sequence of three hand positions; the go-no go task, requiring the patient to tap the desk once if the examiner taps once, but not to tap if the examiner taps twice; and tests of abstraction ('what do a tree and a snail have in common?'). The Frontal Assessment Battery is a reasonable bedside tool.

Language

The left hemisphere is dominant for language in almost all right-handers and most left-handers. The brain areas critical for language cluster around the Sylvian fissure ('perisylvian'), and include Broca's area in the inferior frontal lobe, required for fluent language production; Wernicke's area, in the posterior superior temporal lobe, required for language comprehension, and the arcuate fasciculus, the white matter tract that connects them. Damage to Broca's area causes a dysphasia characterized by effortful, dysfluent speech with reduced use of 'function words' (prepositions, articles, etc.) and 'phonemic paraphasias' (incorrect words approximating to the correct one in sound), with well preserved comprehension; Wernicke's dysphasia is characterized by fluent speech with both phonemic and semantic paraphasias (incorrect words approximating to the correct one in meaning) and poor comprehension. The stream of incoherent speech and lack of insight in patients with Wernicke's dysphasia sometimes leads to misdiagnosis of a primary thought disorder and consequently to a general psychiatric referral. The clue to the diagnosis of a language disorder is the severity of the comprehension deficit. Global dysphasia combines features of Broca's and Wernicke's dysphasias. The non-dominant hemisphere plays a part in appreciating the emotional overtones of language.

In assessing dysphasia (Table 14.4), first listen to the characteristics of the patient's speech (is it dysfluent or paraphasic?), then assess their comprehension. Naming is impaired in both major varieties of dysphasia and 'anomia' can be the clue to mild dysphasia. Selective impairment of repetition characterizes 'conduction aphasia' due to damage in or around the arcuate fasciculus. In 'transcortical' dysphasia, repetition is spared but damage closely adjacent to Broca's or Wernicke's area causes patterns of deficit otherwise typical of Broca's or Wernicke's dysphasia. Reading and writing should also be assessed. The main dysphasic syndromes are described in Table 14.4.

Arithmetic

Arithmetical skills localize to the dominant hemisphere, particularly the region of the angular gyrus, in the inferior parietal lobe. Damage to the angular gyrus can

Table 14.4. Classification of dysphasic syndromes.

Aphasia type	Fluency	Comprehension	Repetition	Naming
Global	+	+	+	+
Broca's	+	−	+	+
Wernicke's	−	+	+	+
Conduction	−	−	+	+
Transcortical sensory	−	+	−	+
Transcortical motor	+	−	−	+
Anomic	−	−	−	+

Note: + = affected; − = relatively spared.
Source: Adapted from Table 2.2 in Hodges (1994).

give rise to Gerstmann's syndrome of dyscalculia, dysgraphia (difficulty with writing), confusion of left and right and 'finger agnosia' (difficulty in identifying individual fingers).

Praxis

'Praxis' refers to the ability to perform skilled actions, dyspraxia to inability to perform skilled actions despite intact basic motor and sensory abilities. Knowledge of how to do such things as use a screwdriver or brush teeth, and of how to mime these actions, depends on areas in the frontal and parietal lobes of the dominant hemisphere. Dysphasia and dyspraxia often co-occur, but can dissociate. These abilities can be tested by asking a subject to mime actions, and by asking him or her to copy unfamiliar hand positions. 'Gait apraxia' is difficulty in initiating and maintaining gait despite intact basic motor functions in the legs, and is associated with bilateral medial frontal pathology, caused, for example, by hydrocephalus. 'Dressing apraxia' is difficulty in dressing caused by inability to puzzle out the spatial arrangement of clothes in relation to the body: it is a perceptual rather than a motor problem.

Perception

The right hemisphere is the 'dominant' one in tasks requiring an appreciation of spatial relationships. The syndrome of 'neglect' involves a failure to attend to or act towards the side of space contralateral to a brain lesion — as this is usually in the right hemisphere, it is usually the left side of space that is neglected. The right hemisphere is also the dominant partner in some other perceptual tasks: 'prosopagnosia', for example, selective difficulty in recognizing familiar faces, is more common after right than left hemisphere damage.

Where basic sensory functions are intact, difficulty in recognizing objects is described as 'agnosia'. Agnosia can be 'apperceptive', if relatively 'early' processes of percept formation are involved, or 'associative' if the failure lies in perceptual memory. Associative agnosias merge into deficits of semantic memory.

Perception is tested using naming tasks, which depend on recognition as well as name finding, and copying tasks, which tap perceptual as well as motor processes.

Standard instruments

The Mini-Mental State Examination (MMSE) (Folstein *et al.* 1975) is the most widely used brief instrument for CE. It should be remembered that the MMSE is insensitive to early cognitive decline in people with high IQ, and also insensitive to impairment in some cognitive domains, for example praxis and executive function. The Addenbrooke's Cognitive Examination (Mathuranath *et al.* 2000) is a more extensive 'bedside' battery. It incorporates the MMSE, supplementing it with a more demanding test of anterograde memory (the name and address), some 'current events' questions, tests of verbal fluency, and more extensive tests of language and perception than the MMSE provides. We use this in our memory clinic, in combination with some additional tests of motor sequencing and praxis.

The threshold of impairment at which 'dementia' is diagnosed is somewhat arbitrary, given the variability in baseline cognitive performance in health and the gradually falling scores seen in dementia: studies using MMSE scores of 25–27 to diagnose dementia have reported sensitivities of 78–90% and specificities of 70–87%. Using a score of 83/100 on the ACE as the cut-off for the diagnosis of dementia conferred a sensitivity of 82% and a specificity of 96% (Mathuranath *et al.* 2000).

Neurological examination

Psychiatrists should be able to perform a competent basic neurological examination as this often provides the crucial clues to a neuropsychiatric diagnosis. A scheme for this examination is suggested below, with some comments on the interpretation of key findings.

General observation	Look for involuntary movements, muscle wasting or fasciculations, abnormalities of limb or body posture
Gait	Is there abnormality of posture, stride length, stride base, pace, arm swing, stability?
	Cranial nerves (No):
	sense of smell (I)
	visual acuities and fields (II)
	fundi and pupillary responses (II, III)
	eye movements: pursuit and saccadic (III, IV, VI)
	facial sensation and jaw movement (V)
	muscles of facial expression (VII)
	hearing (VIII)
	palatal movement +/− gag reflex, phonation and cough (IX, X)
	shoulder shrug, neck rotation (XI)
	tongue movements (XII)
Limbs	Examine the arms and then the legs in turn:
	Is muscle bulk normal and are there fasciculations?
	Is tone normal, reduced, increased (if so is it rigid, spastic, or shows a failure to relax)?
	Power (work from proximal movements to distal)

Reflexes (tendon reflexes + plantar responses +
where relevant 'primitive' reflexes: pout, grasp
and palmo-mental)

Sensation: pin-prick and joint position sense

Co-ordination: 'finger to nose' and 'heel to shin'
manoeuvres; rapid alternating movements

Interpreting the findings

Dyskinesias

Involuntary — or semi-voluntary — movements of face, trunk or limbs are known
as 'dyskinesias'. The family of dyskinesias includes several types:

1. Tics are habitual, usually jerky, movements which can be voluntarily
   suppressed for a time.
2. Myoclonus is rapid, 'shock-like', muscle contractions which can be focal or
   generalized (we all experience generalized myoclonus from time to time as we
   drop off to sleep).
3. Tremor, rhythmic alternating contraction of agonist and antagonist muscles,
   occurring with the arms outstretched in 'postural tremor', often due to benign
   familial tremor, or at rest in the pill-rolling tremor of Parkinson's disease, or
   when nearing a target in the 'intention tremor' of cerebellar disease.
4. Chorea, the fidgety, changeful, distal movements which accompany some
   disorders of the basal ganglia (athetosis is the proximal equivalent of chorea,
   hemiballismus its pathological extreme).
5. Dystonia, relatively sustained abnormalities of posture, occurring focally in
   writer's cramp or torticollis, globally in generalized dystonia, also thought to
   reflect basal ganglia dysfunction. The 'tardive' orofacial dyskinesia sometimes
   induced by antipsychotics is particularly familiar to psychiatrists.

Abnormalities of gait

Observation of gait is often particularly revealing. Typical 'gestalts' include the
flexed, unsteady, small-stepping gait of Parkinson's disease with diminished arm
swing; the broad-based, unsteady gait of cerebellar disease; the lurching, chaotic
gait of Huntington's chorea; the stiff-legged, scissoring gait of upper motor
neurone dysfunction ('spasticity'); the failure of 'gait ignition' in gait apraxia, due
for example to hydrocephalus; the high-stepping gait accompanying foot drop.

Abnormalities of visual fields and eye movements

Markedly reduced acuity of recent onset should raise suspicion of a central
scotoma linked to optic nerve disease, for example in multiple sclerosis;

a hemianopia to left or to right present in both eyes' fields ('homonymous') points to pathology behind the optic chiasm, probably within the hemispheres; a hemianopia affecting the temporal field in each eye (bitemporal) suggests pathology at the chiasm, most often due to compression by a pituitary tumour.

Abnormalities of eye movement often mirror more widespread disturbances of motor function, for example in the 'cogging' of eye movement seen in Parkinson's disease. Isolated failures of eye movement, for example inability to abduct one eye, point to a lesion of a specific cranial nerve or its brainstem nucleus, in this case the sixth or abducent nerve. Palsies of gaze, for example inability to direct either eye to one side, indicate pathology in the brainstem or in tracts descending to the brainstem from the hemispheres. Inability to trigger rapid voluntary vertical eye movements ('saccadic' movements) is an early feature of progressive supranuclear palsy.

Pyramidal signs

Dysfunction of the pyramidal tracts, the direct descending pathway from motor cortex to the brainstem and spinal cord, gives rise to 'upper motor neurone signs': increased tone in the limbs with a 'clasp-knife' or 'catch-and-give' quality, weakness particularly affecting extensor muscles in the arms and flexors in the legs, excessively brisk reflexes, extensor plantar reflexes. Such signs are commonly seen, for example, after stroke and in multiple sclerosis. Pyramidal signs in the limbs may be associated with 'pyramidal' dysfunction of bulbar muscles (a 'pseudo-bulbar palsy', giving rise to dysphagia and dysarthria), and with lability of emotional expression or 'pseudo-bulbar affect' (e.g. easily-provoked 'pathological' crying).

Frontal release signs

Certain 'primitive' reflexes can be released by processes which impair frontal lobe function. These include the pout reflex (a pouting movement stimulated by stroking the upper lip or tapping the lips), the grasp reflex (flexion of the patient's hand around the examiner's finger despite a request 'not to grip'), and the palmo-mental reflex (puckering of the ipsilateral chin in response to drawing an orange stick briskly across the thenar eminence). These reflexes are usually significant in young adult patients, but can return with advancing age in normal subjects. They are associated with certain behavioural abnormalities seen in association with disorders of the frontal lobes or their connections: 'utilization behaviour' is the automatic utilization of objects, for example the downing of a proffered (but unwished-for) glass of water without comment; imitation behaviour is self-explanatory.

Extrapyramidal signs

Dysfunction of the basal ganglia (caudate, putamen, globus pallidus and linked subcortical regions) can cause either a 'negative' or a 'positive' neurological syndrome. The negative syndrome is typified by Parkinson's disease, with difficulty in initiating and slowness in performing movements (bradykinesia), reduction of automatic movements such as facial expression and arm swing, increased limb tone with a 'lead-pipe' or cogwheeling quality (rigidity), rest tremor and postural instability. The positive syndrome, typified by Huntington's disease, or over-treated Parkinson's disease, involves an excess of movement with choreo-athetosis. The neurological signs of basal ganglia disease are often accompanied by neuropsychiatric features, such as slowing of cognition in Parkinson's disease and impulsivity in Huntington's chorea.

Cerebellar signs

Cerebellar dysfunction impairs the co-ordination of movement. Signs include nystagmus, dysarthria, gait ataxia, incoordination of limb movements (e.g. 'finger-nose') and impairment of rapid alternating movements (e.g. tapping with one hand on the upper and lower surface of the other hand alternately). The idea that the cerebellum may play a part in co-ordinating thought and emotion as well as movement is a focus of current research.

Lower motor neurone signs

These result from disorders affecting the brainstem, spinal cord or peripheral nerves, for example in patients with peripheral neuropathies. The signs are muscle wasting and fasciculation, muscle weakness which is often generalized and loss of reflexes. Disorders causing lower motor neurone signs that can also be associated with neuropsychiatric features, such as dementia, include motor neurone disease, leucodystrophies and HIV infection.

Sensory signs

Sensory signs are generally the least reliable or helpful neurological findings. They can occasionally give useful clues to neuropsychiatric disorders – for example, loss of joint position and vibration sense in a patient with dementia would raise the possibility of vitamin B_{12} deficiency.

It is worth bearing in mind that more or less every 'neurological' finding can have a 'functional' ('psychogenic'/'hysterical') explanation.

Like the neurological examination, a careful general medical examination should be a routine part of the assessment of neuropsychiatric disorders. The cause of dementia, for example, may come to light when, for instance, pallor (due to the anaemia of vitamin B$_{12}$ deficiency), lymphadenopathy (associated with HIV infection), the slow pulse (of hypothyroidism), hypertension (causing subcortical ischaemia), or the testicular tumour (associated with paraneoplastic limbic encephalitis) is detected.

The dementias

Dementia is defined as a syndrome due to disease of the brain, usually of chronic or progressive nature, in which there is disturbance of multiple higher cortical functions but no clouding of consciousness.

Diagnosis

It is helpful to bear in mind two broad distinctions during the clinical assessment of patients with possible dementia. The first is the distinction between delirium (or 'confusion') and dementia (see Table 14.5). The presence of dementia is a risk factor for delirium, and some dementing illnesses, notably Lewy body disease, incorporate elements of delirium. However, the causes and management of delirium and dementia are largely separate, and the distinction is therefore useful. Delirium is covered in a separate chapter (Chapter 12).

Table 14.5. Delirium versus dementia.

Feature	Delirium	Dementia
Onset	Acute or subacute	Insidious
Course	Fluctuating	Slowly progressive
Duration	Hours—weeks	Months—years
Alertness	Abnormally low or high	Typically normal
Sleep—wake cycle	Disrupted	Typically normal
Attention	Impaired	Relatively normal
Orientation	Impaired	Intact in early dementia
Working (short-term) memory	Impaired	Intact in early dementia
Episodic (long-term) memory	Impaired	Impaired
Thinking	Disorganized, delusional	Impoverished
Speech	Slow or rapid, incoherent	Word-finding difficulty
Perception	Illusions, hallucinations common	Typically unimpaired in early dementia (Lewy body dementia is an exception)
Behaviour	Withdrawn or agitated	Varies with type of dementia but often intact in early stages

Source: Adapted from Table 1.4 in Hodges (1994).

The second distinction is between cortical and subcortical dementias (see Table 14.6). Cortical dementias, such as Alzheimer's disease, and some cases of cerebrovascular dementia, disrupt the 'modules' of cognitive function identified in the first section of this chapter – language, praxis, perception, etc. The classical syndromes of dysphasia, dyspraxia, agnosia ensue. In subcortical dementias these cortical functions remain more or less intact, but their subcortical activation and interaction are impaired: the cardinal feature of the resulting cognitive impairment is slowness, often accompanied by behavioural change reminiscent of the apathy and inertia that can follow damage to the frontal lobes. Subcortical cognitive impairment of this kind is seen in disorders as varied as 'small vessel' cerebrovascular disease, multiple sclerosis, HIV infection, Huntington's disease and progressive supranuclear palsy. The distinction between 'cortical' and 'subcortical' dementias can be helpfully refined by recognizing that some 'cortico-subcortical' disorders combine features of both (for example Lewy body dementia and prion dementia). Causes of dementia are listed in Table 14.7.

Investigations

Where the clinical assessment suggests that a dementia is likely, most patients will be suffering from one of the three most common causes: Alzheimer's disease, cerebrovascular dementia or Lewy body disease. If the clinical features are in keeping with one of these diagnoses, a set of 'standard' investigations (see Table 14.8) will generally suffice to support the diagnosis and exclude several of the more readily treatable causes of dementia (see Table 14.9). These relatively

Table 14.6. Cortical vs. subcortical dementia.

Function	Cortical dementia, e.g. Alzheimer's disease	Subcortical dementia, e.g. Huntington's disease
Alertness	Normal	'Slowed up'
Attention	Normal in early stages	Impaired
Executive function	Normal in early stages	Impaired
Episodic (long-term) memory	Amnesia	Forgetfulness (improves with cueing)
Language	Aphasic features	Normal except for reduced output
Praxis	Apraxia	Normal
Perception, visuospatial abilities	Impaired	Impaired
Personality	Preserved (unless frontal type)	Apathetic, inert

Source: Adapted from Table 1.6 in Hodges (1994).

Table 14.7. Causes of dementia.

This rough-and-ready classification of the causes of dementia assumes a broad understanding of dementia as significant cognitive impairment affecting more than one cognitive domain which is not primarily due to delirium. The list is not comprehensive, but the great majority of the causes of dementia fall under the categories listed. All dementias can be palliated: this list also includes causes which are potentially reversible, for example hydrocephalus, Wilson's disease and sleep apnoea. Rarely, some of the 'acquired' dementias listed here can be inherited (e.g. dominantly inherited Alzheimer's disease, inherited frontotemporal dementia and some prionopathies: see text).

Inherited
   Huntington's disease
   Wilson's disease
   Leucodystrophies

Acquired
Primary degenerative dementias
   Alzheimer's disease
   Dementia with Lewy bodies
   Frontotemporal lobar degeneration (including Pick's disease)
   Progressive supranuclear palsy
   Corticobasal degeneration

Vascular
   Multi-infarct
   Subcortical
   Strategic infarction

Infective
   HIV
   Transmissible spongiform encephalopathies (prion dementias)
   Herpes simplex encephalitis
   Whipple's disease
   Subacute sclerosing panencephalitis (SSPE)

Inflammatory
   Multiple sclerosis
   Vasculitis
   Hashimoto's encephalopathy

Neoplastic
   Primary and metastatic CNS tumours
   Paraneoplastic: limbic encephalitis

Traumatic
   Post-head-injury

Table 14.7. (*cont.*)

Structural
  Hydrocephalus
  Chronic subdural haematomas

Metabolic/endocrine
  Hypothyroidism

Deficiency disorders
  Vitamin B_{12}/folate deficiency

Sleep-related
  Obstructive sleep apnoea

Substance- or-drug induced
  Alcohol
  Anticholinergics, antiepileptics, neuroleptics, hypnotics, etc.

Psychiatric
  Depression ('pseudodementia')

Table 14.8. 'Standard' investigations in dementia.

Neuroimaging
Computerized tomography or magnetic resonance imaging

Blood screen
Full blood count (FBC), erythrocyte sedimentation rate (ESR)
Urea and electrolyte (U&E), liver function tests (LFTs), calcium
Glucose, cholesterol
Vitamin B_{12} and folate
Thyroid function
Syphilis serology

---

inexpensive tests should always be performed unless there is a good reason not to. It is a moot point whether formal neuropsychology should always be requested: careful 'bedside' cognitive assessment is usually sufficient.

More intensive investigation will generally be required if an unusual cause is suspected. The clinical features that should excite suspicion of an unusual cause include:

- early onset (under the age of 65)
- rapid progression (beyond the approximate three-point annual decrement on the MMSE expected in Alzheimer's disease)
- a family history, the presence of systemic or neurological features other than those associated with the three common dementias

• the presence of certain distinctive combinations of features, for example limb apraxia, myoclonus and alien limb phenomena in corticobasal degeneration, or dysarthria, dysphagia and personality change in the frontal lobe dementia linked with motor neurone disease.

Table 14.9. Reversible causes of dementia.

Wilson's disease

Whipple's disease

Hashimoto's encephalopathy

Vasculitis

Hydrocephalus, chronic subdurals, benign CNS tumours

Hypothyroidism

Vitamin deficiencies, e.g. vitamin B_{12} deficiency

Prescribed and recreational drugs

Obstructive sleep apnoea

Depression

Note: This list highlights causes that can sometimes be reversed: several other causes of dementia can be treated medically with some success, e.g. Alzheimer's disease, Lewy body disease and HIV-related dementia.

Table 14.10. Additional investigations which may be helpful in atypical dementia.

Formal neuropsychometric assessment

Neuroimaging: magnetic resonance imaging (MRI), single photon-emission computed tomography (SPECT)

Other imaging, e.g. chest X-ray

Specialized blood tests:

    Genetic testing, e.g. Huntington's, cerebral autosomal dominant arteriopathy with subcortical infarcts and leucoencephalopathy (CADASIL), mitochondrial disorders, familial Alzheimer's disease, familial prion dementia

    White cell enzyme studies in leucodystrophy

    HIV test

    Connective tissue serology in suspected CNS inflammation, e.g. erythrocyte sedimentation rate (ESR), anti-nuclear factor (ANF), anti-cardiolipin antibodies, anti-neutrophil cytoplasmic antibodies (ANCA), antibodies to extractable nuclear antigens (ENA), rheumatoid factors, complement fractions

    Anti-thyroid antibodies in suspected Hashimoto's encephalopathy

    Caeruloplasmin in suspected Wilson's disease

Electroencephalogram (EEG)

Cerebrospinal fluid (CSF) examination

Brain biopsy

Where an atypical cause is suspected but its nature is unclear a range of further tests is worth considering (see Table 14.10). The individual features of the case will determine how many of these should be performed: the decision is best taken by a neuropsychiatric team with expertise in the diagnosis of dementia.

Inherited dementias

Huntington's disease

Huntington's disease (HD), also known as Huntington's chorea, was first described in Long Island in 1872 by George Huntington. This dominantly inherited disorder, which causes a combination of progressive motor, cognitive, psychiatric and behavioural dysfunction results from an abnormality in the IT-15 gene on chromosome 4 encoding the protein Huntingtin.

Huntington's disease occurs with a prevalence of 5–7/100 000 in the USA with wide regional variations. The sexes are affected equally. Onset can occur at any age, but most commonly in young or middle adulthood. The disorder exhibits 'anticipation', the age of onset tending to decrease through the generations, especially with paternal transmission (see below).

Chorea, involuntary fidgety movements of the face and limbs, is the characteristic motor disorder. As the disease progresses, other extrapyramidal features, including rigidity, dystonia and bradykinesia, can develop, with associated dysphagia, dysarthria and pyramidal signs. Childhood-onset HD can be dominated by rigidity and myoclonus (the 'Westphal variant'). Epilepsy can occur. Cognitive dysfunction goes hand in hand with the motor disorder. The dementia of HD is predominantly 'subcortical', with impairment of attention, executive function, speed of processing, and memory. Psychiatric symptoms and behavioural change are the norm: depression, apathy and aggressivity occur very commonly, with psychosis, obsessional behaviour and suicide in a significant minority. Progression to a state of immobility and dementia typically occurs over 15–20 years. Cognitive and behavioural change may predate the clear-cut emergence of symptomatic HD.

The epicentre of the pathology of HD lies in the striatum, the caudate and putamen. The loss of small neurones in the striatum is accompanied by loss of neurones in the cerebral cortex, cerebral atrophy, ventricular dilatation and, eventually, neuronal depletion throughout the basal ganglia.

The underlying genetic abnormality is expansion of a base triplet repeat within the Huntington gene. 10–35 CAG (cytosine–adenine–guanine) repeats are present in the normal gene: repeat lengths beyond 39 give rise to symptomatic HD over the course of a normal lifespan. Repeats between 36 and 39 can cause disease.

Repeats in the 27–35 range appear to be unstable, and liable to increase into the pathological range in the next generation (Duyao *et al.* 1993). The tendency for pathologically expanded repeats to increase in length between generations, especially in paternal transmission, underlies the clinical phenomenon of anticipation.

A number of disorders can cause the combination of chorea and cognitive change, including other inherited disorders such as neuroacanthocytosis and dentato–rubro–pallido–luysian atrophy (DRPLA), and acquired disorders such as systemic lupus erythematosus (SLE). The diagnosis of HD can now be made with confidence by DNA analysis. Counselling by a clinical geneticist is mandatory before pre-symptomatic testing and should be considered in other circumstances.

Chorea may require treatment but this is often best avoided, given the psychological and extrapyramidal side-effects of the agents required – neuroleptics, dopamine-depletors such as tetrabenazine or benzodiazepines. Other psychological and behavioural symptoms should be treated along standard lines.

Wilson's disease (hepatolenticular degeneration)

First described by Wilson in 1912, Wilson's disease is a rare, autosomal recessive, progressive but eminently treatable disorder of copper metabolism, causing personality change, cognitive decline, an extrapyramidal disorder and cirrhosis of the liver.

The onset of Wilson's disease is most common in childhood or adolescence but can be as late as the fifth decade. It can present to psychiatrists with personality change, behavioural disturbance including psychosis, or dementia, and to neurologists with a variety of extrapyramidal features: these include tremor, dysarthria and drooling, rigidity, bradykinesia and dystonia. Examination reveals these features and also, in virtually all symptomatic cases, the presence of 'Kayser–Fleischer rings', rings of greenish-brown copper pigment at the edge of the cornea (in suspected cases an ophthalmologist should be asked to look for this with a slit lamp). Liver failure and the neuropsychiatric syndrome can occur together or independently.

The causative mutation is in the copper transporting P-type ATPase coded on chromosome 13. The result is excessive copper deposition in brain, cornea, liver and kidneys and increased copper excretion in urine. The globus pallidus and putamen (together known as the lenticular nucleus) are most severely affected, but the other basal ganglia and the cerebral cortex are affected. The serum of 95% of patients contains low levels of the copper binding protein, caeruloplasmin. Several copper-chelating agents are available to treat Wilson's disease to good effect, but with risk of significant side-effects (Brewer & Askari 2005).

Leucodystrophies

Leucodystrophies, recessively inherited or X-linked disorders of myelination, can present with neuropsychiatric syndromes, usually with associated neurological features. Metachromatic leucodystrophy, caused by a deficiency of the enzyme arylsulfatase A, and adrenoleucodystrophy, an X-linked disorder associated with abnormalities of very long chain fatty acids, are the most commonly encountered types.

Primary degenerative dementias

Frontotemporal lobar degeneration (including Pick's disease)

This complex group of disorders is of importance to psychiatrists as personality change and behavioural disturbance may be the presenting features. The frontotemporal dementias (FTDs) are a clinically and pathologically diverse group of focal dementias presenting with either features of frontal lobe dysfunction or features of temporal lobe dysfunction or both.

Although a rare cause of dementia overall, frontotemporal dementia (FTD) accounts for about 10–15% of cases of dementia occurring before the age of 65. Some cases are familial.

Dementia of frontal type, or 'frontal variant FTD', is characterized by the features listed in Table 14.11. The temporal lobe variant of FTD presents most commonly with semantic dementia, a syndrome of progressive word-finding difficulty, loss of language comprehension, depletion of conceptual knowledge (apparent on non-verbal as well as verbal tests) and impairment of object recognition. These features reflect left temporal lobe dysfunction. If the right temporal lobe is more severely affected, prosopagnosia (impaired face recognition) and loss

Table 14.11. Criteria for a diagnosis of dementia of frontal type.

A	Presentation with an insidious disorder of personality and behaviour.
B	The presence of two or more of the following features:
	loss of insight, disinhibition, restlessness, distractibility, emotional lability, reduced empathy or unconcern for others, lack of foresight, poor planning or judgement, impulsivity, social withdrawal, apathy or lack of spontaneity, poor self-care, reduced verbal output, verbal stereotypes or echolalia, perseveration, features of Kluver–Bucy syndrome (gluttony, pica, sexual hyperactivity).
C	Relative preservation of day-to-day (episodic) memory.
D	Psychiatric phenomena may be present (mood disorder, paranoia).
E	Absence of past history of head injury, stroke, alcohol abuse or major psychiatric illness.

Source: Gregory & Hodges (1993).

of knowledge about people may be especially prominent. Two other clinical varieties of FTD are recognized: 'progressive non-fluent aphasia' occurs in patients with degeneration of peri-Sylvian structures, including the insula, inferior frontal and superior temporal lobes; 'FTD with motor neurone disease' is the combination of frontal variant FTD or progressive aphasia with features of motor neurone disease, usually particularly affecting speech and swallowing ('bulbar' type).

Neuropsychological examination is particularly helpful in identifying these clinical syndromes. Imaging should reveal corresponding focal atrophy. A younger person presenting with an atypical dementia will clearly require full neuropsychiatric assessment. There is no proven specific treatment for these conditions (with the possible exception of riluzole for motor neurone disease).

Progressive supranuclear palsy

Progressive supranuclear palsy (PSP) is characterized by supranuclear gaze palsy (inability to direct eye movements voluntarily, especially vertical eye movements, in the presence of normal reflex eye movements); truncal rigidity, akinesia, postural instability and early falls; bulbar features, with dysarthria and dysphagia; subcortical dementia; alteration of mood, personality and behaviour. Neurofibrillary tangles, consisting of tau protein, are found in neurones of the basal ganglia and brain stem. Midbrain atrophy may be apparent on magnetic resonance imaging (MRI) scan.

Corticobasal degeneration

Corticobasal degeneration (CBD) typically presents with a combination of limb apraxia, usually asymmetric at onset, alien limb phenomena, limb myoclonus, parkinsonism and cognitive decline. The pathology involves neuronal loss in both the basal ganglia and the frontal and parietal cortex, with intraneuronal accumulations of tau protein resembling those seen in PSP. MRI usually reveals frontoparietal atrophy.

Infective dementias

Dementia associated with HIV-1 infection is discussed in Chapter 20. Other rare causes of infective dementia such as Whipple's disease are not discussed. This section focuses on the transmissible spongiform encephalopathies (TSEs; prion dementias).

These are a group of rare dementias caused by an accumulation of abnormal prion protein within the brain. Related illnesses occur in animals: indeed, one recently described disorder, variant Creutzfeldt–Jakob disease (vCJD) is thought to result from infection of humans by consumption of beef products from cattle with bovine spongiform encephalopathy (BSE). The term 'prion', coined by Stanley Prusiner, stands for 'a proteinaceous infectious pathogen'.

All the TSEs are rare. Sporadic Creutzfeldt–Jakob disease (spCJD), the most common human TSE, occurs with an annual incidence of one per million population, usually affecting people between the ages of 55 and 70. Variant CJD has been diagnosed in approximately 150 individuals at the time of writing, almost all in the UK. It usually develops in younger subjects than spCJD: most cases have occurred in the second to fourth decades of life (Irani 2003).

Sporadic CJD typically causes a rapidly progressive dementia, with early changes in behaviour, visual symptoms and cerebellar signs. Within weeks to months, marked cognitive impairment develops, often progressing to mutism, with pyramidal, extrapyramidal and cerebellar signs and myoclonus. The median duration of symptoms to death is only four months, although rarely the disorder evolves over several years.

Variant CJD differs markedly from spCJD (Spencer et al. 2002). The initial symptoms are usually psychiatric, in particular anxiety or depression, often sufficiently severe to lead to psychiatric referral. Limb pain or tingling is moderately common early in the course of the illness. After some months cognitive symptoms typically develop, causing difficulty at school or work, together with varied neurological features including pyramidal, extrapyramidal and cerebellar signs and myoclonus. The disorder evolves more slowly than spCJD, with an average duration, to death, of 14 months.

The light microscope reveals 'spongiform change' in the brain of patients with TSEs associated with neuronal loss, gliosis and deposition of 'amyloid'. Immunocytochemistry and direct biochemical analysis indicate that the amyloid is composed of a protease resistant form of prion protein (PrP).

The CJD Surveillance Unit, based in Edinburgh, can help to mobilize the substantial package of support that is now available for patients with CJD, and, in the interests of accurate diseased surveillance, it is vital that all cases should be reported to the Unit. However, at present, there is no proven remedy for the disease.

Inflammatory dementias

A number of inflammatory conditions affecting the central nervous system (CNS) can cause dementia. The diagnosis will generally be suggested by the presence of features atypical for other common causes. These may be systemic, such as the butterfly rash, arthralgia and renal impairment often associated with SLE, or the oral and genital ulcers and iritis of Behçet's syndrome, or neurological, such as the headache and fluctuating confusion of cerebral vasculitis, or the upper motor neurone signs which usually occur in multiple sclerosis. Features like these — or unexplained dementia in a younger person — call for some of the 'additional investigations' listed in Table 14.10, in particular serological tests for inflammatory disorders, neuroimaging with MRI and cerebrospinal fluid (CSF) examination.

Neoplastic dementias

While primary and metastatic CNS tumours typically present with headache, focal neurological signs or seizures, they can cause cognitive impairment, and occasionally their presentation mimics a dementing illness. Computed tomography (CT) scanning should reveal their presence in such cases, although occasionally diffusely infiltrating tumours are missed in the early stages.

Traumatic dementias

Trauma is one of the few causes of abrupt-onset dementia: it is discussed further under acquired brain injury.

Structural dementias

Hydrocephalus can cause a wide range of neurological and neuropsychiatric symptoms and signs: enlargement of the head (if present in infancy), headache, sudden death due to 'hydrocephalic attacks' with acute elevation of intracranial pressure, progressive visual failure, gait disturbance (often 'gait apraxia'), incontinence and subcortical cognitive impairment progressing to dementia. 'Normal-pressure hydrocephalus' in older people is classically associated with the triad of gait apraxia, incontinence and cognitive decline.

Subdural haematomas are accumulations of blood and blood products in the space between the fibrous dura mater and the more delicate arachnoid membrane which encloses the brain. Acute subdural haematomas accumulate rapidly following head injury; chronic subdural haematomas can sometimes, but not always, be traced back to a head injury.

Chronic subdural haematomas give rise to more gradually evolving symptoms and signs. While they, also, can cause headache, depressed consciousness and focal signs, they sometimes result in predominantly cognitive features, including confusion and dementia. Marked variability of the mental state, and sometimes also of the neurological features, is often a clue to the diagnosis. Seizures can occur.

Miscellaneous

Other causes of dementia include endocrine causes, and thyroid function tests should always be performed in patients with cognitive decline, as hypothyroidism can present with cognitive symptoms, progressing to dementia, and is readily treated. Deficiency of B vitamins, especially B_1 (thiamine) and B_{12} (cobalamin compounds), and of folic acid, are important organic causes of neuropsychiatric syndromes. Vitamin B_1 deficiency, causing Wernicke's encephalopathy in the acute phase, and Korsakoff's psychosis if untreated, is discussed under amnestic syndromes. Vitamin B_{12} and folate deficiency are relatively rare but highly treatable causes of dementia, and the concentration of these vitamins in the blood should be checked in patients with cognitive decline.

Obstructive sleep apnoea (OSA) typically presents with excessive daytime sleepiness (EDS) on a background of snoring and intermittent apnoea due to upper airways obstruction in sleep, most often in middle-aged men. OSA is a serious and treatable condition which should be considered in patients with cognitive symptoms who are excessively sleepy by day.

The question of whether excessive alcohol intake per se damages the brain — as against associated thiamine deficiency, head injury, secondary hypoglycaemia, etc. — has been much debated. The balance of evidence suggests that alcohol itself can cause cognitive impairment and cerebral atrophy, although its effects are often compounded by other factors.

Occasionally prescribed medication causes or contributes to cognitive impairment. Drugs which can be responsible include anticholinergics, anticonvulsants (especially barbiturates), hypnotics and neuroleptics.

'Pseudodementia'

In 'pseudodementia', a functional psychiatric disorder — or, very rarely, deliberate simulation — gives rise to a clinical picture that might be mistaken for an organic dementia. In depressive pseudodementia cognitive impairment occurs on the background of a depressive illness, sometimes in the absence of classical symptoms of depression. The term 'pseudodementia' may be misleading — as well as pejorative — as there is growing evidence that the cognitive impairment associated with depression has a distinctive biological basis. Hysterical pseudodementia is cognitive impairment mimicking organic dementia that proves not to be due to any definite organic pathology, but rather to be the outcome of predisposing, provoking and perpetuating factors, which are currently best understood at a psychological level. 'Functional dementia' might be a more appropriate term for both depressive and hysterical pseudodementia.

Simulated dementia is cognitive impairment that has been feigned deliberately in the pursuit of some form of gain. The 'Ganser symptom' describes the repeated occurrence of 'approximate answers' in the course of the questioning (for example, day, date and year all incorrect by one), suggesting that in some sense the respondent must know and be deliberately distorting the correct answer; the Ganser syndrome involves approximate answering, with additional hallucinations and a fluctuating level of consciousness. Both symptom and syndrome have been described in association with a wide variety of psychiatric disorders, with a particularly strong association with hysteria.

Depression is the most common potentially reversible cause of cognitive impairment encountered in memory clinics. Where cognitive impairment occurs in someone who is overtly depressed the diagnosis will be immediately suspected. But when loss of interest in the environment is coupled with slowing of thought and behaviour, in the absence of overt sadness, an organic cause, such as a subcortical dementia, might well be the first diagnostic consideration. The features of 'depressive pseudodementia' on cognitive examination are likely to include slowed responses, paucity of speech and impaired concentration in the absence of 'cortical' features such as dysphasia or agnosia (Kales *et al.* 2003).

Hysterical pseudodementia is suggested by unexpectedly severe and inconsistent impairment of cognitive function, especially in the context of other 'functional' symptoms and signs. Some cases occur on a background of dramatic psychological precipitants, and, in our experience, others occur following episodes of the somatic symptoms of panic coupled with depersonalization.

A number of cognitive mechanisms, including a tendency to retrieve distressing memories, and an over-general retrieval style, help to explain the cognitive deficits associated with depression. There is also recent evidence, from a combination of animal and human studies, that both depression and stress affect structure and function in the hippocampus by modulation of circulating glucocorticoids, mineralocorticoids and monoaminergic inputs. Research along these lines promises to illuminate the complex interrelationships between stress, mood, ageing and cognitive impairment.

The most commonly encountered clinical dilemma is the distinction between a primary depressive illness causing cognitive impairment and the onset of an organic dementia with associated mood disturbance: the diagnoses of dementia and depression are not, of course, mutually exclusive. Features which may point towards primary depression include the recent occurrence of negative life events, a relatively abrupt onset and variability of cognitive function. Psychometric testing can be helpful, but sometimes it is only possible to reach a definite conclusion in retrospect, after an adequate trial of treatment for depression and the passage of time.

Amnestic syndromes

The amnestic or amnesic syndrome is an abnormal mental state in which learning and memory are affected out of all proportion to other cognitive functions in an otherwise alert and responsive patient. The most common cause is Wernicke–Korsakoff syndrome (WKS) as a result of nutritional depletion, particularly thiamine deficiency. Other causes include carbon monoxide poisoning, herpes simplex encephalitis and other CNS infections, hypoxic and other acquired brain injuries, stroke, deep midline cerebral tumours, and surgical resections, particularly for epilepsy. In the vast majority of cases the pathology lies in midline or medial temporal structures but there are case reports of amnestic disorder following frontal lobe lesions.

Wernicke–Korsakoff syndrome is the result of thiamine depletion and any cause can lead to the syndrome. However, the overwhelming majority of cases arise secondary to alcohol abuse as a result of decreased intake and absorption. A genetic defect for thiamine metabolism has been described in a proportion of patients.

The syndrome presents acutely with Wernicke's encephalopathy, characterized by confusion, ataxia, nystagmus and ophthalmoplegia. There can also be peripheral neuropathy. Parenteral administration of high-dose B vitamins is a medical emergency. The majority of cases of Korsakoff's syndrome occur following a Wernicke's encephalopathy but this is not invariable; the possibility that the latter has just gone undetected must be considered.

On clinical examination, amnestic patients perform well on standard tasks of attention and working memory (serial sevens and reverse digit span), but may struggle on more complex tasks involving shifting and dividing attention. Memory impairments involve both anterograde and retrograde deficits. Defective encoding of new information has been implicated as the core component of this memory disorder. This results in a dense anterograde amnesia affecting declarative functions, and inconsistent, poorly organized retrieval of retrograde memories with a temporal gradient (more impairment for relatively recent than more remote memories). The retrograde amnesia is more pronounced in diencephalic amnestic syndromes like Korsakoff's than those of hippocampal origins, where it will be present, but with a deficit measured in months not years. Some learning may be possible, particularly if patients are given a strategy to follow. Confabulation commonly occurs particularly early in the disorder. Procedural memory is relatively intact.

Other cognitive impairments and behavioural sequelae may accompany the amnesia. Executive functions are commonly mildly affected but this may be secondary to chronic alcoholism rather than a specific deficit. Disorientation and apathy, often with utter lack of curiosity about the past, are common. Yet, such disengaged patients frequently demonstrate labile irritability.

The pathology consists of neuronal loss, microhaemorrhages, and gliosis in the paraventricular and paraqueductal grey matter. The mamillary bodies, mamillothalamic tract, and the anterior thalamus appear to be key structures affected. There is also likely to be a degree of generalized cortical atrophy, more marked in the frontal lobes. This may be non-specific, secondary to the years of alcohol abuse. MRI indicates specific atrophy in diencephalic structures.

With vitamin replacement and abstinence from alcohol, the prognosis is recovery for one-quarter of patients, improvement with persistent impairment for half, and no change for the final quarter. High-dose B vitamins should be given to all patients acutely but there are no data guiding how long to continue them. Recently the benefits of anticholinesterase drugs in Korskoff's syndrome have been explored (Angunawela & Barker 2001).

Transient amnesia can occur in several contexts: transient global amnesia (TGA) is a distinctive benign disorder affecting middle aged or elderly subjects who become amnestic for recent events, and unable to lay down new memories, for a period of around four hours. Repetitive questioning by patients of their companions is a characteristic feature. Episodes can be provoked by physical or emotional stress and are usually isolated (the medium-term recurrence rate is approximately 3% per year). There is good evidence that TGA results from reversible medial temporal lobe dysfunction, but the aetiology is uncertain. Other causes of transient amnesia include transient cerebral ischaemia (usually accompanied by other neurological symptoms and signs), migraine, drug ingestion, temporal lobe epilepsy and head injury.

Acquired brain injury

In the industrialized countries survivors of acquired brain injury (ABI) are creating an inconspicuous epidemic of neurological and neuropsychiatric disability. Modern advanced trauma and life support techniques have led to dramatic reduction in mortality rates, but this has resulted in an ever-increasing number of survivors, the majority young adult males, who although physically fit have severely damaged brains and multiple cognitive and emotional disabilities.

Estimates of incidence in Scotland are 330 per 100 000 and in the United States are 180−220 per 100 000 of population. Approximately 80% of cases are mild, 10% moderate and 10% severe (Kraus & Chu 2005). There is considerable geographical variation. The mortality associated with severe brain injury has dramatically reduced since the 1960s and is now around 10 per 100 000. However, post-injury life expectancy, although reduced, is measured in decades and as a result the prevalence of ABI associated disability is increasing annually (Table 14.12).

The neuropsychiatric effects of ABI will be dependent upon both the severity and the nature of the injury, as well as the pre-morbid state of the patient. This latter issue is of considerable importance as ABI is more likely to effect people who have problems with substance or alcohol abuse, violent tendencies or risk-taking traits in their personalities.

There is no single definitive marker of severity of brain injury. The Glasgow Coma Scale has been a major advance in documenting the severity of coma (Tables 14.3 and 14.13). It is highly predictive of both mortality and need for surgical intervention. However, it is less useful in predicting long-term outcomes, particularly when coma duration has been brief.

The length of post-traumatic amnesia (PTA) is the other main predictor of severity of injury (Table 14.14). Whilst most consider it to be the single best measure of severity, it does have significant problems with measurement error and it lacks the reliability of the GCS. Many experienced clinicians do not think precise measurement of PTA is essential and that for routine clinical work broad time-frames of hours, days or weeks will suffice.

In general, the two measures of severity are usually in agreement. However, formal comparison studies show correlations of the order of 0.7, indicating a significant number of cases where the measures are discrepant.

Post-traumatic amnesia is defined as the time from the moment of injury to the time of resumption of normal continuous memory. The termination of PTA

Table 14.12. Disability one year after head injury.

Initial injury	Severe disability	Moderate disability	Good outcome
Mild	20%	28%	45%
Moderate	22%	24%	38%
Severe	29%	19%	14%

Source: Thornhill et al. (2000).

Table 14.13. Assessment of outcome after acquired brain injury: Glasgow coma scale (GCS).

GCS score	Injury
13–15	Mild
9–12	Moderate
3–8	Severe

Table 14.14. Assessment of outcome after acquired brain injury: length of post-traumatic amnesia (PTA).

Length of PTA	Level of injury
<10 min	Very mild injury
10–60 min	Mild injury
1–24 hours	Moderate injury
1–7 days	Severe injury
>7 days	Very severe injury

is often abrupt, except in cases where enduring memory difficulties supervene. Brief islands of memory can punctuate the period of PTA. Behaviour while still within the period of PTA can be normal, but more commonly there is obvious difficulty with memory and mental confusion. Some degree of temporal disorientation can almost always be found if tested with care. Studies of cognitive function during PTA are rare but illustrate that some procedural memory functions remain intact whilst episodic memory is impaired. This retrograde impairment often shows a marked temporal gradient with differential forgetting of the more recent past.

Retrograde amnesia is defined as the time between the moment of injury and the last clear memory from before the injury that the patient can recall. It can usually be indicated with reasonable precision. It is usually dense and much shorter than PTA. It is of less predictive value.

Coup and contrecoup lesions result in direct impairment of cortical function at the site of the lesion. In injuries where there is bruising due to deceleration patients present with problems in the regulation and control of behaviour, in conceptual thinking and problem solving and with various memory and learning tasks. There are also likely to be changes to personality and social adjustment, and although these are often subtle, they can have a devastating effect on recovery. This is because the frontal and temporal parts of the brain are often involved.

Diffuse damage tends to compromise speed of processing, attentional functions, cognitive efficiency and high-level concept formation and complex reasoning. This can be seen directly or as irritability, fatigue and a general inability to do things as well as before the accident. Tasks requiring selective or divided attention tend to be particularly sensitive to diffuse effects and patients will perform poorly on tests of oral or sequential arithmetic. Patients will frequently perceive their slow processing and attentional difficulties as memory problems and complain of poor memory. They tend to avoid overly challenging situations such as parties, large family gatherings and supermarkets and become socially withdrawn.

Few patients with moderate or severe ABI demonstrate only one pattern of impairment and generally there is a combination of all three.

Special consideration should be given to sensory impairment, including loss of the sense of smell, visual disturbance, tinnitus and balance problems as it is a common complication of ABI and often underlies difficult or disturbed behaviour.

Mild head injury will involve short duration of loss of consciousness (<30 minutes) and PTA measured in hours not days. Around 80% of injuries are mild. Patients generally describe a triad of attention deficits, impaired verbal retrieval and emotional distress. Headache, dizziness and photophobia are also common accompaniments. This usually appears within a few days of the injury, but can be delayed for days and weeks.

Emotional distress is often accompanied by marked fatigue and concern over perceived cognitive deficits. The effort needed to overcome attentional deficits is particularly distressing. Frank depressive illness itself however, tends to be a later complication of injury not occurring until some three to six months after the event.

In general terms a GCS of 9–12 and a PTA of under 24 hours will be classed as a moderate head injury. Headaches, memory problems and difficulties with everyday life are the most common complaints. Two-thirds of patients will not return to work. Most patients exhibit some evidence of frontal or temporal contusions. Impulsivity, diminished initiative, affective muting and temper outbursts are all common. Temporal lobe damage is displayed as a true learning disorder with lateralization for verbal and non-verbal material.

Although severe head injury accounts for less than 10% of ABI, the differential costs to health services in terms of complex rehabilitation and long-term care are such that severe ABI is a major problem and growing annually. The associated impairments are generally categorized in three areas: cognitive, emotional and executive.

1. Cognitive deficits are usually multiple, but individual patterns tend to be unique, with some neural functions being severely impaired and others functioning at near normal levels.
2. Emotional disorders generally involve the exaggeration or muting of affective responses but, as well as reflecting the nature of the organic damage, will also be influenced by pre-morbid personality and mental state. Frontal lobe damage is associated with both an excitable (impulsive and labile) and an apathetic (flat, uninterested and non-initiating) response. Damage to temporal limbic structures tend to result in emotionalism with sudden temper outbursts or pathological crying. Social isolation is a common consequence of all mood disturbances.

3. Executive dysfunction involves impairment of self-determination, self-direction and self-control and regulation. This involves not just the cognitive ability itself but the ability to express it. Such patients frequently need external cues for activity and perseveration is commonplace.

Both psychotic symptoms and major depressive disorders occur at a greater than expected rate. Early psychosis usually involves delusions of misidentification and reduplicative paramnesias are particularly associated with ABI. In this striking disorder, the patient believes himself to be in a different place despite all evidence to the contrary. The majority remit spontaneously. Late presentations of psychotic illness also occur, with a two-fold increase in risk of a schizophreniform psychosis although some controversy exists as to whether this is a population at increased risk of schizophrenia anyway. More non-specific paranoid states, frequently related to memory impairment, also occur and can be hidden by communication difficulties. Treatment follows normal management but with increased caution regarding unwanted drug effects. Depressive disorders are commonplace. Their presentation and management is discussed under stroke.

Agitation and aggression cause clinically significant problems in around 10% of brain-injured patients acutely. In the chronic phase, such behaviours can be a major cause of disability and are one of the most frequent causes of complaint for relatives and carers. Cognitive impairments, and in particular communication disorders, are more frequently the cause of aggression than psychotic disorders or depression. Particular attention must be paid to the pre-morbid personality, which can be antisocial. Drug treatment is complicated and almost always needs to be supplemented with behavioural interventions.

In relation to prognosis

1. Age is a strong independent predictor of mortality with higher rates in children under 5 and the over-65s. Older adults also tend to have less functional and cognitive improvement after brain injury.
2. Gender. Although ABI occurs with increased frequency in men it is unclear if gender affects outcome.
3. Substance abuse is commonly associated with ABI and is associated with poorer outcome across all functions.
4. Mechanism of injury. Penetrating injuries are associated with significantly increased mortality rates but not necessarily poorer outcomes in survivors.
5. Severity of injury is the strongest predictor of mortality.

Compensation claims are frequent after ABI and often involve considerable sums as a result of loss of earnings and the need for care costs. In such cases, it is essential that examinations are conducted by clinicians experienced in head trauma as many of the conventional symptoms and signs of psychiatric and cognitive dysfunction will be normal after ABI. This also applies to prepacked neuropsychological test batteries; for instance some patients with ABI can score within normal range on the Wechsler Adult Intelligence Scale despite having severe difficulties with frontal apathy, memory deficits and slow processing that leave them unfit for work.

Formal studies have shown little difference between patients who do and do not seek compensation with the possible exception that claimants may complain more of their impairments. This can be exaggerated by anything up to 25% when employees blame their employer. Most authors have concluded that organic factors lead to enduring disability and enduring disability leads to an increased likelihood to sue.

Stroke

A cerebrovascular accident or stroke is 'a rapidly developed clinical sign of a focal disturbance of cerebral function of presumed vascular origin and of more than 24 hours duration'. Two main pathological processes are responsible – cerebral infarction or haemorrhage. Infarction may result from thrombosis of vessels or emboli lodged within them. Haemorrhage can be into either brain tissue directly or into the subarachnoid space. Infarctions are four times more common than haemorrhages and, as a result of a lower immediate fatality rate, a much greater source of enduring disability with approximately 75% survival compared to one-third survival at one year after haemorrhage. Strokes are the third commonest cause of death in the Western world. The Oxford Community Stroke Project reported a population incidence of 2 per 1000 for first-ever stroke (Bamford *et al.* 1988). Age is the major risk factor, although one-quarter of those affected are under 65 years, and there is an excess in men.

Psychiatrists are not usually involved in the diagnosis of acute stroke but are occasionally when alterations in cognition, affect, or behaviour dominate the clinical picture.

Delirium affects 30–40% of patients in the week after stroke with a marked increase following haemorrhagic stroke. It is important to distinguish delirium from focal cognitive deficits affecting declarative memory. Although this can often be complicated by the presence of agitation, the disturbance of attention and fluctuating pattern of impairment that accompany delirium are often absent in the latter. The presence of delirium after stroke is associated with poorer prognosis, longer duration of hospitalization and increased risk of dementia.

Dementia following stroke is common with approximately one-quarter of patients demented three months after a stroke. This figure rises significantly if focal impairments are also considered.

The diverse behavioural changes following stroke are not unique, but they do serve as a helpful model for understanding the clinical consequences of focal cerebral lesions of other causes (Bogousslavsky & Cummings 2000).

Aphasia

Global aphasia leads to the abolition of all linguistic faculties and the physician must draw inferences regarding mental state from behaviour and non-verbal communication.

Anosognosia

This refers to partial or complete unawareness of a deficit. It may coexist with depression (Starkstein *et al.* 1990), suggesting separate neural systems for different aspects of emotions (Damasio 1994), and that depression after stroke cannot be explained solely by psychological reaction to disability (Ramasubbu 1994).

Affective dysprosodia

This is the impairment of the production and comprehension of language components that allow the communication of inner emotional states in speech, such as stresses, pauses, cadence, accent, melody and intonation.

Apathy

Patients with apathy show little spontaneous action or speech, and have delayed, short, slow or absent responses. Apathy is frequently associated with hypophonia, perseveration, grasp reflex, compulsive motor manipulations, cognitive and functional impairment, and older age. Hypoactivity of frontal and anterior temporal regions has been observed (Starkstein *et al.* 1993a).

Depression

Although generally the presence of post-stroke depression is defined according to Diagnostic and Statistical Manual (DSM-IV) or International Classification of Diseases (ICD-10) criteria (Starkstein & Robinson 1989), the imposition of these categorical diagnoses on patients after stroke is problematic. It is often unclear to what extent symptoms are secondary to the stroke itself or to comorbid depressive illness (Gainotti *et al.* 1997). It is attractive to consider looking only at the cognitive symptoms of depression, and scales such as the Hospital Anxiety and Depression Scale have been designed to do this. However, it is almost certainly an erroneous approach in the neurologically ill, as the neurobehavioural consequences of cerebral lesions such as aphasia, indifference, denial, cognitive impairment and dissociation of subjective from displayed emotion can all lead to misleading results. Most clinicians take a pragmatic approach and will treat depression in patients who have symptoms suggestive of low mood or anhedonia accompanied by some somatic symptoms (e.g. insomnia, anorexia) and signs of lack of engagement with their environment such as poor participation in physiotherapy.

Most epidemiological studies have suggested an association between increased disability (Herrmann *et al.* 1995; Pohjasvaara *et al.* 2001), and possibly mortality (House *et al.* 2001), after stroke and increased rates of depression, but the direction of causality is unclear and most probably circular. Some, but not all, pharmacological treatment studies have suggested that effective treatment of the depression leads to a reduction in overall disability (Andersen *et al.* 1994a; Lipsey *et al.* 1984).

There has been a lot of speculation over the aetiological mechanisms of depression after stroke and much emphasis has been placed on the site of the stroke lesion, in particular the hypothesis that left frontal lesions are associated with an increased rate of depressive illness (Starkstein & Robinson 1989). There are several objections to this model. It has been consistently shown that patients with pre-morbid histories of depression are at higher risk of developing depression after stroke (Andersen *et al.* 1995), Second, it has proved impossible to clinically distinguish left frontal depression from depression associated with lesions in other brain regions (Gainotti *et al.* 1997). Finally, a recent, well-constructed meta-analysis showed that the available scientific literature does not support the left frontal hypothesis (Carson *et al.* 2000a).

It is generally recommended, but has not been conclusively demonstrated, that treatment should be started early, when depression is first suspected, in order to maximize functional outcome. There are disappointingly few randomized controlled trials (RCTs) in the field. Most studies suggest an improved outcome in mood variables but the effects of treatment on other general functional measures have shown contradictory results to date (Andersen *et al.* 1994a; Chemerinski *et al.* 2001; Gainotti *et al.* 2001; Lipsey *et al.* 1984; Robinson *et al.* 2000; Wiart *et al.* 2000). Both serotonin-specific reuptake inhibitors (SSRIs) and tricyclics have been shown to be effective and the side-effect profile of the SSRI drugs is probably preferable, particularly if cognitive or cardiac function is compromised. However, this must be balanced against the finding that nortriptyline was more effective than fluoxetine in the only head-to-head (small) trial that has been conducted (Robinson *et al.* 2000). What is clear is that all stroke patients on antidepressants should be closely monitored for both treatment effectiveness and adverse drug effects. Psychological treatment, in particular cognitive behavioural therapy, potentially offers a solution to this problem but unfortunately trials, to date, have not demonstrated effectiveness (Kneebone & Dunmore 2000), and only a minority of depressed patients have been suitable (Lincoln *et al.* 1997).

Anxiety

Anxiety disorders are a common occurrence after stroke and probably share the same risk factors as depression (Astrom 1996). Estimates of prevalence vary markedly depending upon whether investigators diagnose a separate anxiety disorder or subsume anxiety symptoms within the concept of major depressive disorder. Thus reports of the prevalence of a generalized anxiety disorder vary from 4% to 28% (Astrom 1996), but the actual number of patients suffering anxiety symptoms appears to be consistently around 25–30% (Burvill *et al.* 1995). Additionally, stroke is a sudden and unpredictable life-threatening stressor and not surprisingly is a highly aversive experience (McEwen 1996). Post-stroke anxiety states often include post-traumatic stress symptoms with compulsive and intrusive revisiting of the event, as well as health worries, with checking and reassurance-seeking behaviour regarding future recurrence (Lindesay 1991). This can lead to agoraphobia and the misinterpretation of somatic anxiety symptoms as evidence of recurrence, particularly with headache and dizziness. Estimates of phobic states suggest a prevalence of 5–10% with an excess in women (Burvill *et al.* 1995). Although there is a paucity of controlled trial evidence our experience is that symptoms seem to respond to standard drug and behavioural therapies.

Emotionalism

Emotionalism or lability with an increase in laughing or crying with little or no warning signals is frequent in acute stroke but can occur with delayed onset (Berthier *et al.* 1996). The displayed emotions are not related to the patient's general mental state. Whether there is an association with depression is a moot point but the two can exist independently (House *et al.* 1989; Robinson *et al.* 1993). It has been suggested that the abnormality is serotonergic and that there is a specific response to SSRIs (Andersen *et al.* 1994a), although the evidence is contradictory with reports of response to tricyclics (Robinson *et al.* 1993). There is no consistent evidence relating to a corresponding lesion location with pontine, subcortical and frontal lesions all being suggested (Andersen *et al.* 1994b; Derex *et al.* 1997; Morris *et al.* 1993).

Catastrophic reactions

These manifest as disruptive emotional behaviour when a patient finds a task unsolvable (Goldstein 1939). The sudden, dramatic appearance of such marked self-directed and stereotypical anger or frustration can be startling for staff and relatives. It is often associated with aphasia and it has been suggested that damage to language areas is a critical part of the aetiology (Carota *et al.* 2001). It generally exists independently of depression in acute strokes but many patients showing catastrophic reactions will over time develop depression (Starkstein *et al.* 1993b).

Psychosis

Psychoses, in particular mania, have been reported following acute stroke. Their true incidence is unknown although a rate of 1% for manic illness has been reported (Starkstein *et al.* 1987). Psychotic symptoms have generally been associated with right-sided lesions (Cummings & Mendez 1984), although the lessons from the depression story should lead to very cautious interpretation of such claims. Old age and pre-existing degenerative disease seem to increase the risk (Starkstein 1998). Reduplicative paramnesias can occur; one memorable patient believed he was being treated in a cruise liner and on looking out of the window and seeing hospital porters delivering goods he surmised that it must be in 'dry dock'.

Obsessive-compulsive disorder

Obsessive-compulsive disorder (OCD) symptoms have been reported after infarcts particularly affecting the basal ganglia (Maraganore *et al.* 1991; Rodrigo *et al.* 1997).

Hyposexuality

This is a common complaint in both men and women after stroke. The symptoms are generally non-specific although health worries concerning body image and fear of recurrence may be relevant. It has also been suggested that there is a relationship between reduced libido and emotionalism, suggesting serotonin dysfunction (Kim & Choi-Kwon 2000).

Executive function

The systems regulating executive function are complex and relatively resistant to damage after stroke. Isolated damage is unusual (Carota *et al.* 2002) although executive function is commonly impaired as part of a wider dementia.

Deficit of inhibition control

Such behaviours are impulsive, compulsive and only slightly limited by command. Most striking are grasp reflexes but utilization behaviour (a tendency to utilize automatically objects present in the environment), hyperphasia, and hypergraphia are all described. Such behaviour tends to improve in the first few months after stroke (Carota *et al.* 2002).

Loss of empathy

Loss of empathy has been reported after bilateral orbito-frontal lesions (Stone *et al.* 1998). It has been suggested that this difficulty in understanding and adapting to the needs of others may be at the origin of many of the personality difficulties associated with frontal lesions including lack of tact, inappropriate familiarity, lack of initiative and spontaneity, childish behaviour, sexual disinhibition and poverty of emotional expression (Carota *et al.* 2002).

Parkinson's disease

Parkinson's disease (PD) is of considerable interest to neuropsychiatrists as a result of the range of cognitive, psychotic and emotional sequelae that are commonly encountered in patients with this degenerative condition. Parkinson's disease highlights the close relationship between cognitive impairment, disease process and drug side-effects when considering the aetiology of psychotic symptoms in a patient with brain disease.

Approximately 17 per 100 000 people are affected by Parkinson's disease. There is a slight excess in men and the incidence of PD rises with age. The cause of PD remains unknown.

The core features of PD are the triad of tremor, rigidity and bradykinesia. Bradykinesia is the most common first sign, usually of insidious onset and easily misdiagnosed as depression or boredom, and ultimately the most disabling feature. Resting tremor is the most characteristic feature of PD and is found in over 70% of patients. In the early stages of disease it is described as 'pill-rolling'. The rigidity is detectable in terms of fixed abnormalities of posture and resistance to passive movement throughout the range of motion. Concurrent tremor creates a 'cogwheel' sensation. Postural instability is a common additional feature, giving rise to an increasing liability to falls as the disorder progresses. Abnormal involuntary movements are a result both of the disease process and dopaminergic therapy. Freezing of gait is very disturbing to patients and one of the most poorly understood features of PD. The response of freezing to visual cues (particularly freezing during 'off' periods) can lead to misdiagnosis in psychiatric settings as wilful behaviour.

The clinical diagnosis of Parkinson's disease may seem simple but several clinicopathological studies have suggested a significant false-positive rate, with only three-quarters of clinical diagnoses supported at autopsy.

Dementia with Lewy bodies (DLB), PD and PD with dementia share common neuropsychiatric features, motor symptoms and responses to treatment. The boundaries between these disorders may be less distinct than originally thought. Hallucinations and delusions occur in 57–76% of DLB cases, 29–54% in PD with dementia and 7–14% in PD without dementia. Delusions are often paranoid in type and mainly involve persecution and jealousy. Hallucinations usually occur with intact insight and are frequently visual and phenomenologically similar to those of Charles Bonnet syndrome.

In the early days of L-dopa treatment, about 40% of patients could not tolerate it because of psychotic side-effects. The addition of carbidopa to L-dopa made this less common. Some more recent studies have suggested that dopaminomimetic medication is a significant risk factor for psychosis but the effect is not dose related. Other studies have shown correlations between psychotic symptoms and higher rates of cognitive dysfunction and depression, but not dose or length of exposure to dopaminomimetic medication. Most likely, a combination of cortical PD pathology and age-related loss of central cholinergic integrity is the major psychotogenic factor. This is corroborated by the fact that psychotic symptoms in PD are often part of non-dopaminomimetic induced toxic (i.e. delirious) states and that psychosis was commonly reported in the pre-levodopa era. Cognitive impairment and sleep disruption are predictive of the development of psychosis.

Clinically, one should distinguish between a delirium with an acute onset with disorientation, impaired attention, perceptive and cognitive disturbance, and alteration to the sleep–wake cycle from true dopaminomimetic psychosis; a sub-acute, gradually progressive psychotic state without a primary deficit of attention. The former state may be induced by drugs such as selegiline or anticholinergic medication used in the treatment of PD. For the latter condition active treatment is recommended only if symptoms start to interfere with daily life. Dose reduction of dopaminomimetic drugs can be considered, but it is seldom a successful strategy. The role of cholinesterase inhibitors has become increasingly important in recent years.

Depression is a common occurrence with most studies citing a prevalence of around 40–50%. There is a bimodal distribution with peaks at early and late stages of disease. Several large-scale studies have demonstrated that depression is one of the major determinants of quality of life in PD. Its biochemical basis is unknown and the question remains as to whether it is an endogenous phenomenon reflecting a pathological substrate of PD or simply a response to motor disability.

Diagnosis is difficult as many depressive symptoms overlap with core features of PD — motor retardation, attention deficit, sleep disturbance, hypophonia, impotence, weight loss, fatigue, preoccupation with health, and reduced facial expression. The interpretation of diagnostic criteria and standardized rating scales is problematic, and more often one tends to be swayed by presence of anhedonia and sustained sadness, particularly if out of proportion to motor signs.

Mood swings can accompany the late-stage fluctuations in response to L-dopa, known as on-off phenomena, and some patients fulfil criteria for major depressive disorder during the off phase but not during the on phase. Bipolar mood change reflecting the on-off phases has also been described. There is currently insufficient evidence to make definitive recommendations for treatment of depression in PD. While SSRIs are popular, there have been concerns of exacerbation of motor symptoms with SSRIs (Gony *et al.* 2003). In recent small-scale trials, tricyclic drugs have shown better motor outcomes, but those with marked anticholinergic effects such as amitriptyline should be used with caution as a result of effects on cognition and autonomic function. It may be that newer drugs such as mirtazepine will offer a good compromise. The non-ergot dopamine agonist pramipexole has been found to improve both mood and motivation in PD. Case report data suggest that both electro-convulsive therapy and transcranial magnetic stimulation can be used to treat depression in PD, although the latter is associated with short-lived effects and seizures.

Anxiety phenomena are also common and tend to occur later than depression in the disease process and are more closely associated with the severity of motor symptoms. In particular, marked anticipatory anxiety about freezing of gait is common. Treatment with antidepressant drugs and cognitive behavioural therapy, particularly if delivered in conjunction with an active physiotherapy programme, can be helpful.

Multiple sclerosis

Multiple sclerosis (MS) can occur at any age but median age of onset is about 24, with a tendency for relapsing remitting disease to present earlier than primary progressive MS. It is more common in women, like all autoimmune disorders. Epidemiologic studies suggest that an exogenous or environmental factor plays a part, possibly viral infection, although its nature remains unclear. There is a marked geographical distribution, with the prevalence of the disorder rising with distance from the equator. Genetic factors clearly also influence susceptibility. A family history in a first-degree relative increases the risk some

30–50-fold: the sibling risk is usually quoted at 3–5%; for children of patients it is slightly lower.

Pathologically the disorder is characterized by multifocal areas of demyelination with relative preservation of axons, loss of oligodendrocytes and astroglial scarring.

Patients with unsuspected MS may first present to psychiatrists with changes in cognitive function, mood state or personality, but more often psychiatrists are involved in the treatment of established cases. MS demonstrates the interactive nature of many of the common symptoms of diffuse neurological disease, in particular the 'vicious circle' of mood symptoms, pain and fatigue, necessitating intervention across the spectrum of complaints in order to improve outcome.

Cognitive impairment affects at least half of all patients with MS. It is generally described as a subcortical dementia characterized by problems with memory, speed of processing and executive functions. Disorders of working memory may be prominent, particularly verbal but sometimes visuo-spatial memory.

Mood disorders are common with over half of patients reporting depressive symptoms but mania and emotional lability are also commonly reported. It is important to distinguish depression from primary MS fatigue and also pain disorders (see below). Similar to stroke there has been an attempt to separate out a 'biological' depression and a 'psychological reactive' depression and to link symptoms to the site of lesions. The results are inconsistent and hampered by small samples. It appears more productive to consider depression as a multifactorial complication of MS. There are few randomized controlled studies of treatment of depression but they show modest efficacy, as with treatment of depression in neurologic illness in general.

Beta-interferon therapy has been reported to cause depression (and fatigue) as a significant side-effect by some 40% of MS patients failing to tolerate the drug. However, depression is highly prevalent in MS and a number of studies have found no increase in depression following beta-interferon (Patten & Metz 2001; Zephir *et al.* 2003). In one prospective study, the rate of depression actually fell with beta-interferon treatment (Feinstein *et al.* 2002).

Fatigue is the most common symptom in multiple sclerosis, affecting 80% of sufferers. It is generally a disabling and aversive experience and affects motivation as well as physical strength. There should be an attempt to separate it from depression, adverse medication side-effects, or pure physical exhaustion secondary to gait abnormalities. The mechanism is poorly understood and almost certainly multifactorial. Amantadine 100 mg twice daily has some suggested benefits in RCTs (Krupp *et al.* 1995); pemoline has also been suggested, but trial results are less convincing (Krupp *et al.* 1995). A number of other agents have been suggested including 4-aminopyridine (Polman *et al.* 1994), 3,4-diaminopyridine (Sheean *et al.* 1997) and modafinil (Rammohan *et al.* 2002), but results to date are inconclusive. Some patients respond to SSRIs, and cognitive behavioural treatments, using the chronic fatigue syndrome model, have been used with success on occasion.

Pain, both acute and chronic, is a common complication of MS and a highly disabling one. A recent study found that a quarter of a large community-based sample of persons with MS had severe chronic pain (Ehde *et al.* 2003). Mechanisms may include dysaesthesia, altered cognitive function influencing symptom experience and pain secondary to other complications such as spasticity. Of the acute pain syndromes, trigeminal neuralgia is commonest and usually responds to carbamazepine. Chronic pain is more common and harder to manage. Dysaesthetic limb pain is particularly troublesome and treatment is usually with amitriptyline or gabapentin. Pain in the lumbar area by contrast usually tends to respond better to physiotherapy rather than analgesia.

Epilepsy

A seizure is a transient cerebral dysfunction resulting from an excessive abnormal electrical discharge of neurones. The clinical manifestations are numerous. As a result psychiatrists commonly encounter epilepsy, both when considering whether epilepsy is the primary cause of paroxysmal psychiatric symptoms and when treating its significant psychiatric complications.

Problems with case definition and ascertainment complicate epidemiological comparisons in epilepsy. However, incidence rates of between 40–70 per 100 000 in developed countries and 100–190 per 100 000 in developing countries are generally accepted. The prevalence of active epilepsy is around 7 per 1000 in the developed world. The reasons for the higher incidence in developing nations are believed to include increased rates of birth trauma and head injury and lack of health services to manage them, poor sanitation leading to high rates of CNS infection, and poverty and illiteracy leading to increased rates of social problems such as alcohol and substance misuse. Most studies show a bimodal distribution of the incidence with increased rates below 10 years and above 60 years old. Men have increased rates of between 1 and 2.4 compared to women. There have been suggestions of an increased rate among Black Africans although compounding social factors complicate the interpretation of studies.

In less than one-third of cases is an aetiological cause identified. These commonly include perinatal disorders, learning disabilities, cerebral palsy, head trauma, CNS infection, cerebrovascular disease, brain tumours,

Alzheimer's disease and substance misuse. Many idiopathic seizures are likely to have a genetic basis.

Epilepsy is a heterogeneous group of disorders with multiple causes and manifestations, and its clinical features reflect this diversity. The key clinical distinction is between seizures with a focal or a generalized cerebral origin. The former are more likely to be associated with a detectable and potentially remediable cerebral lesion; the latter more likely to start in childhood or adolescence and to be familial. Despite the wide variety of possible seizure manifestations, an individual patient's seizures are usually stereotyped. Their clinical features result from a recurrent pattern of cortical hyperactivity during the ictal event followed by hypoactivity in the same area post-ictally. This gives rise to a predictable set of symptoms dependent upon the brain region affected.

Tonic-clonic seizures are the most dramatic manifestation of epilepsy and are characterized by motor activity and sudden loss of consciousness. In a typical seizure a patient has no warning; with the possible exception of a couple of myoclonic jerks. The seizure begins with sudden loss of consciousness and a tonic phase during which there is sustained muscle contraction lasting 10–20 seconds. This is followed by a clonic phase of repetitive muscle contraction that lasts approximately 30 seconds. A number of autonomic changes may also occur, including an increase in blood pressure and pulse rate, apnoea, mydriaisis, incontinence, piloerection, cyanosis and perspiration. In the post-ictal period the patient is drowsy and confused. Abnormal neurological signs are often elicited.

Partial seizures are categorized according to whether they are simple (without impairment in consciousness), or complex (with impairment of consciousness). This classification is problematic in clinical practice and it may be abandoned.

Simple partial seizures depend on the brain region activated. Although the initial area is relatively localized, it is common for the abnormal activity to spread to adjacent areas producing a progression of seizure pattern. If the activity originates in the motor cortex there will be jerking movements in the contralateral body part. This can cause progressive jerking in contiguous regions known as a jacksonian march. Activity in the supplementary motor cortex causes head turning with arm extension on the same side – the classic 'fencer's posture'.

Seizures originating in the parietal lobe can cause tingling or numbness in a bodily region or more complex sensory experiences such as sense of absence on one side of the body, asomatognosia. Seizures in the inferior regions of the parietal lobe can cause severe vertigo and disorientation in space. Dominant hemisphere parietal lobe seizures can cause language disturbance.

Seizures of the occipital lobe are associated with visual symptoms which are usually elementary, such as simple flashing lights. However, if the seizure occurs at the border with the temporal lobe more complex experiences can occur including micropsia, macropsia and metamorphosia as well as visual hallucinations of previously experienced imagery.

Seizures affecting the temporal lobe can be the most difficult to diagnose, but it is also the most common site of onset, accounting for 80% of partial seizures. Symptoms may include auditory hallucinations ranging from simple sounds to complex language. Olfactory hallucinations, usually involving unpleasant odours, follow discharge in the mesial temporal-lobe. Seizures in the sylvian fissure or operculum will cause gustatory sensations, and ictal epigastric sensations such as nausea or emptiness generally have a temporal-lobe origin. The well-known emotional and psychic phenomena of temporal lobe seizure activity can occur in simple seizures but are more common in complex partial seizures

In a complex partial seizure the patient frequently experiences an aura at the onset of the seizure. The aura is a simple partial seizure lasting seconds to minutes. It should be distinguished from a prodrome, which is not an ictal event, and can last for hours or even days before a seizure. Prodromes usually consist of a sense of nervousness or irritability. The content of the aura will depend on the location of the abnormal discharge within the brain. Thus it may consist of motor, sensory, visceral or psychic elements. This can include hallucinations; intense affective symptoms such as fear, depression, panic or depersonalization; and cognitive symptoms such as aphasia. Distortions of memory can include dreamy states, flashbacks and distortions of familiarity with events (déjà vu or jamais vu). Occasionally rapid recollection of episodes from earlier life experiences occurs (panoramic vision). Rage is rare but when it does occur it is characterized by lack of provocation and abrupt abatement. This is then followed by impairment of consciousness and a seizure usually lasting 60–90 seconds, which may generalize into a tonic-clonic seizure. Automatisms may be present and can involve an extension of the patient's actions prior to seizure onset. They commonly include chewing or swallowing, lip smacking, grimacing, or automatisms in the extremities including fumbling with objects, walking or trying to stand up. Post-ictal confusion is usually significant and typically lasts 10 minutes or longer.

Complex partial seizures of a frontal lobe origin tend to begin and end abruptly with minimal post-ictal confusion and often occur in clusters. The attacks are usually bizarre with motor automatisms such as bicycling, or sexual automatisms and vocalizations.

Absence seizures are well defined clinical and EEG events. The essential feature is an abrupt, brief episode of decreased awareness without any warning, aura or post-ictal symptoms. At the onset there is a disruption of activity and a simple absence seizure is characterized by only an alteration in consciousness. The patient remains mobile, breathing is unaffected, there is no cyanosis or pallor and no loss of postural tone or motor activity. The ending is abrupt and the patient resumes previous activity immediately, often unaware that a seizure has taken place. An attack usually lasts around 15 seconds. A complex absence seizure displays additional symptoms such as loss or increase of postural tone, minor clonic movements of face or extremities, minor automatisms, or autonomic symptoms such as pallor, flushing, tachycardia, piloerection, mydriaisis or urinary incontinence.

Epilepsy, particularly when involving the temporal lobe, may cause emotional symptoms and this can very occasionally result in undirected violent behaviour. However, in the overwhelming majority of cases this is in response to being restrained during a seizure. One should be very cautious before attributing other violent assaults to a seizure.

The differential diagnosis of epilepsy from non-epileptic attack disorder (psychogenic or pseudoseizures) and syncope can be difficult (Table 14.15). Other paroxysmal disorders should also be considered including transient ischaemic attacks, hypoglycaemia, migraine, transient global amnesia, cataplexy, paroxysmal movement disorders, and paroxysmal symptoms in multiple sclerosis. Attacks during sleep can pose particular difficulties as informant reports are less useful.

Non-epileptic attack disorder (NEAD) also referred to as 'pseudo-seizures' or 'psychogenic epilepsy' is the most common alternative diagnosis, accounting for around 30% of patients attending clinics with suspected epilepsy. The terminology is confused and it is a moot point whether or not it is a diagnosis per se, or a collective term for a number of psychiatric diagnoses or symptoms that may cause seizure-like spells, including conversion, panic attacks, hyperventilation syndrome, post-traumatic stress disorder, and catatonia. We personally favour the view that it is a variant of panic disorder without the expression of fear (Vein *et al.* 1994). Some patients have both epilepsy and non-epileptic attacks, but

Table 14.15. Distinguishing non-epileptiform attack disorder (NEAD) and epilepsy.

	NEAD	Epilepsy
Female	75%	50%
Age of onset	23	15
Child abuse	50%	25%
Epilepsy	10—15%	—
Personality disorder	25—40%	10%
Educational level	Same	Same
Depression and anxiety	High	Almost as high

Table 14.16. Helpful signs in distinguishing non-epileptiform attack disorder (NEAD) from epilepsy.

	NEAD	Epilepsy
Resistance to eye opening	60%	0%
Eyes shut during attack	33%	5%
Patient who is responsive during generalized shaking attack (or where you can interrupt seizure)	84%	20%
Memory of seizure	50%	10%
Weeping during or after a seizure	10%	1%
A generalized attack lasting longer than two or three minutes	Yes	No

Table 14.17. Features unhelpful to a diagnosis of non-epileptiform attack disorder (NEAD).

- Presence of an aura or post-ictal confusion
- Tongue biting — no good evidence that lateral tongue biting occurs more commonly than tongue tip biting in epilepsy
- Injury — carpet burns may indicate pseudoseizure, fractured bones
- Faecal or urinary incontinence
- Pelvic thrusting
- Attack appearing from 'sleep'
- A presentation in 'status epilepticus'
- The patient was alone during a seizure
- Post-ictal prolactin — may be elevated in syncope, and in practice often not measured at the right time or without a baseline

probably only around 10% of those with NEAD fall into this category. Many of these patients are learning disabled and at increased risk of both epilepsy and psychiatric disorders. The diagnosis of NEAD can often be made on the basis of a careful history and examination. Clinical clues include the presence of prior or current psychiatric disorders, including somatoform disorders; atypical varieties of seizure, especially the occurrence of frequent and prolonged seizures in the face of normal inter-ictal intellectual function and electroencephalogram (EEG); a preponderance of seizures in public places, especially in clinics and hospitals; behaviour during an apparently generalized seizure which suggests preservation of awareness (e.g. resistance to attempted eye opening and persistent aversion of gaze from the examiner). See Tables 14.16 and 14.17. Previous childhood sexual abuse is very common but not always present. Where doubt remains after careful clinical assessment and standard investigations, the gold standard for diagnosis is observation of attacks during videotelemetry. A normal EEG during or immediately after an apparently generalized seizure provides strong evidence for NEAD.

Epilepsy is above all a clinical diagnosis and the use and interpretation of tests should reflect this. Routine blood tests should include a complete blood count (CBC) and routine chemistries including serum calcium and magnesium. An electrocardiogram (ECG) should always be performed. An EEG is helpful if there is doubt about the diagnosis, or to clarify the type of epilepsy (generalized or focal – this distinction is particularly relevant to children and adolescents). However, the EEG is insensitive: a single inter-ictal EEG will detect clearly epileptiform abnormalities in only about 30% of patients with epilepsy (Chabolla & Cascino 1997). Therefore a normal EEG does not exclude epilepsy just as minor non-specific abnormalities do not confirm it. Serial recordings, including sleep-deprived recordings, increase the diagnostic yield to about 80% (Chabolla & Cascino 1997). EEG can be supplemented with video recording to allow the correlation between clinical symptoms and EEG abnormality to be examined (videotelemetry). Twenty-four-hour ambulatory monitoring is sometimes helpful.

Some form of neuroimaging should be performed in all patients with epilepsy unless EEG has clearly demonstrated a syndrome of primary generalized epilepsy in a young patient. Computerized tomography (CT) is adequate to exclude tumours and major structural abnormalities and has the benefit of ease of access in most developed countries. However it will miss many subtle pathologies. Magnetic resonance imaging (MRI) is undoubtedly the imaging modality of choice, detecting pathological abnormalities in up to 90% of patients with intractable epilepsy, including mesial temporal sclerosis. It can however be difficult to access in some regions.

Measurement of serum prolactin after seizures has a limited role in diagnosis of NEAD. Prolactin will rise following a generalized seizure, but not as a rule after a non-epileptic attack. However the interpretation of the test requires knowledge of the basal prolactin and concurrent drug treatment (e.g. neuroleptics). Partial seizures and syncope can also elevate prolactin.

Additional cardiac investigations that may be helpful in selected cases include 24-hour ambulatory ECG to identify cardiac dysrhythmias; echocardiography, to identify structural cardiac abnormalities; and tilt-table testing to help confirm orthostatic syncope.

Psychiatric aspects of epilepsy

Recent record linkage studies have shown an increase in psychotic symptoms, particularly schizophreniform and paranoid psychoses in men, but not women with epilepsy. They have also shown a fourfold increase in the overall rates of psychiatric disorder, in both men and women with epilepsy, compared to random controls, but not when compared to controls with significant physical illness. This suggests that for 'neurotic-spectrum' disorders it is having a neurological illness and associated disability that is aversive rather than the pathological effects of epilepsy itself.

In describing the neuropsychiatry of epilepsy it is normal to relate symptoms temporally to seizure events. Psychotic symptoms generally divide into transient post-ictal psychoses and chronic inter-ictal psychoses. The former often present with manic grandiosity, religious and mystical features. A number of small studies have suggested that such patients are more likely to have psychic auras, bilateral inter-ictal spikes and nocturnal secondarily generalized seizures than other epilepsy patients. In general psychotic episodes do not start immediately after a seizure but follow a lucid interval of 2–72 hours. Patients with chronic inter-ictal psychoses had a higher frequency of perceptual delusions and auditory hallucinations than patients with post-ictal psychoses.

Transient psychosis has also been reported in 1% of patients following temporal lobotomy for epilepsy, particularly men with right-sided foci who were not seizure-free after surgery. There may be an increased risk of post-ictal psychoses in patients with temporal lobe epilepsy (TLE) and hippocampal sclerosis versus those with TLE and no sclerosis. How mesial temporal sclerosis relates to psychosis is unclear.

Anti-epileptic drugs (AEDs) may also contribute to the development of psychotic symptoms. Several of the newer drugs have significant neuropsychiatric effects. Vigabatrin, an irreversible inhibitor of GABA-transaminase, has been shown to precipitate psychotic and affective symptoms in between 3 and 10% of patients. This occurs more commonly in patients with significant past psychiatric histories.

Depressive and anxiety disorders affect approximately one-third of patients with epilepsy. Neurobiological, psychological, social and iatrogenic factors have all been suggested and probably all are relevant. Links have been suggested between complex partial seizures and concominant frontal lobe dysregulation in the genesis of depression; however, studies are small and the possibility of confounding variables large. Negative cognitions around 'external locus of control' have been of interest in the genesis of depressive disorders, and this form of learned helplessness may be significant in patients with epilepsy. Socially, living with a chronic illness and its effects on all aspects of patients' and their families' daily life, coupled with the still relevant effects of stigma in creating handicap and disadvantage are all relevant. Finally the treatment of epilepsy with AEDs can be a cause of depression in itself. The relationship between depression and epilepsy is bi-directional (i.e. each is a risk factor for the other) and there is increasing evidence that depression is an independent risk factor for unprovoked seizures increasing the risk fourfold, even when other medical therapies are controlled for. This effect seems to be particularly marked for partial-onset seizures.

Similarly, anxiety in epilepsy can have a complex aetiology. Anticipatory anxiety about having a seizure, in the absence of a warning, can lead to considerable secondary disability in the form of agoraphobic-like symptoms and behavioural responses.

The treatment of depressive and anxiety disorders follows the normal principles of treatment of anxiety and depression in the medically ill. The seizure risks associated with most psychiatric drugs need to be carefully considered before determining the best treatment options for the patient.

Tic disorders

Gilles de la Tourette's syndrome (GTS) is characterized by a combination of multiple waxing and waning motor and vocal tics. These vary from simple twitches and grunts to complex stereotypies. Premonitory sensory sensations in body parts that 'need to tic' are a common feature and complicate the picture as their temporary suppressibility lends them a voluntary component. Other features are echolalia and coprophasia, particularly in severe cases. GTS is strongly associated with obsessive-compulsive disorder (OCD) but many claim that it is qualitatively different from pure OCD, with greater concern with symmetry, aggressive thoughts, forced touching, fear of harming self in OCD-GTS compared to more frequent focus on hygiene and cleanliness in pure OCD. Depressive symptoms are commonplace.

The prevalence of GTS is around 5 per 10 000 with a 4:1 ratio of males to females. A debate exists as to whether OCD alone is a specific comorbid psychopathology with GTS, or whether diverse pathologies including attention-deficit hyperactivity disorder (ADHD), eating disorders, anxiety and substance misuse should also be considered part of the phenotype. This clearly has implications for genetic studies, which have suggested a strong hereditary component to the disorder, but the model is unclear. Similarly the neurobiology remains elusive with evidence supporting dysfunctional dopaminergic basal ganglia circuitry receiving most attention. Structural imaging is usually normal and functional imaging data are contradictory at the current time.

A syndrome known as paediatric autoimmune neuropsychiatric disorders associated with streptococcal infection (PANDAS) has been defined, consisting of OCD accompanied by tics with abrupt onset or exacerbation associated with β-haemolytic streptococcal infection. PANDAS may lie on the same clinical spectrum as Sydenham's chorea in which OCD and vocal tics have also been reported, and may cast light on the aetiology of Tourette's. Some pre-liminary studies have suggested a B-cell antigen D8/17, an immunological marker of susceptibility to rheumatic fever, may be associated with both PANDAS and Tourette's. This offers the attractive possibility of immune-mediated treatments as well as an explanation for the occurrence and subsequent successful treatment of Tourette's as a complication of both Lyme disease and oral herpes simplex.

Management is multidisciplinary with clear need to address the educational, social and family consequences of the disorder. Dopamine antagonists remain the mainstay of pharmacological management with haloperidol the most widely used. Pimozide has been shown to be superior in one of the few RCTs conducted but the potential cardiac side-effects generally prohibit its use. The D2 selective agent sulpiride is potentially attractive. Of the newer antipsychotic agents risperidone has attracted interest but so far has looked more effective in the treatment of related OCD phenomena than tics themselves (Robotson *et al.* 1996; Stein *et al.* 1997). Tetrabenazine, a presynaptic monoamine depleter with post-synaptic blockade has shown considerable efficacy in case-series studies, without the risk of dystonia or tardive dyskinesia, but with a high risk of depression. In patients with comorbid restless leg syndrome, the dopamine agonist pergolide has been effective in helping the Tourette's, despite the fact one might have predicted the opposite effect. Clonidine is used widely in the USA but in the UK is generally restricted to patients with comorbid ADHD symptoms. When setting treatment priorities, it should be remembered that associated OCD and ADHD symptoms probably cause more functional and educational disability than the tics themselves.

Dystonias

The dystonias are a group of movement disorders characterized by involuntary twisting and repetitive movements and abnormal postures. The traditional clinical categorization is based on age at onset, distribution of symptoms, and site of onset. Early onset dystonia often starts in a limb, tends to generalize and frequently has a genetic origin. In contrast, adult-onset dystonias usually spare the lower limbs and frequently involve the cervical or cranial muscles with a tendency to remain focal. They appear sporadic in most cases. Dystonias tend to improve with relaxation, hypnosis and sleep. With the exception of cervical dystonia, pain is uncommon. Erroneous attribution to a psychogenic cause is common because of the fluctuating nature of the symptoms, their often dramatic appearance, the ability to use 'tricks' to suppress them, and their association with task-specific symptoms (e.g. writer's cramp). However, uncommonly, dystonia may occur as the presentation of a conversion disorder. Medical treatment involves oral drugs and botulinum injections. Comorbid psychiatric disorders are commonly associated with dystonias, particularly OCD, panic disorder and depression. Their presence does not necessarily indicate that the dystonia is psychogenic and they should be actively treated in their own right.

Headache

Severe prolonged headache of abrupt onset can be due to subarachnoid haemorrhage (SAH), usually from a ruptured berry aneurysm, or to migraine, meningitis or other cranial infection such as otitis media or sinusitis. The diagnosis of SAH is suggested by the rapidity of onset ('thunderclap' headache, at its worst within 1 minute or so), and associated loss of consciousness, photophobia, vomiting and neck stiffness: headache with these features should trigger immediate neurological referral for assessment with CT scan (which reveals subarachnoid blood in the majority of cases) and lumbar puncture, when CT is negative, to examine for xanthochromia (which is present reliably from 12 hours after SAH). Psychiatrists are predominantly involved in the management of the associated brain injury following SAH, the principles of which are described in the section on stroke above.

Migraine can mimic SAH: the diagnosis is usually suggested by a past history of more typical migrainous headaches with prodromal visual (or other focal neurological) disturbance, and a gradually evolving hemicranial throbbing headache with photophobia and nausea or vomiting. Meningitis is suggested by severe headache, usually worsening over hours, with photophobia, nausea and neck stiffness, in association with fever and other features of infection.

Chronic headache is common. 'Tension-type headache' is familiar to most of us: a global headache, usually of mild-moderate severity, sometimes with a 'band-like' or pressing quality, often worsening as the day goes on or following stress, with few associated symptoms. 'Chronic daily headache' (CDH) is usually of tension type and there are well-described associations with depression or persisting stressors (Holroyd et al. 1993; Mitsikostas & Thomas 1999; Rasmussen 1992) but this does not indicate a causal mechanism. This is indicative of the need for more sophistication in our approach to understanding the complex interactions between biology of the brain, psychological processes and behavioural responses. The majority of cases of CDH have a prior history of migraine (Bahra et al. 2000; Lance et al. 1988) but it would appear that prolonged exposure to analgesics (opiate, ergotamine derivatives and non-steroidal anti-inflammatory drugs (NSAIDs)) may be a necessary contribution for transformation to CDH to take place. Certainly failure to withdraw from such analgesics usually results in failed treatment (Kudrow 1982). Treatment of comorbid mood disorders and cognitive behavioural therapy for symptom management can also be helpful interventions (Kroenke and Swindle 2000). The role of the specialist in psychosomatic medicine is to help manage the complexity and promote behaviour change without resort to excessive biological or psychological reductionism.

Classical migraine has the features described above; common migraine causes 'migrainous' throbbing hemicranial headache, nausea and photophobia in the absence of focal neurological symptoms such as visual disturbance (Cutrer 2003). Patients with chronic migraine headaches have often been described as having a 'typical' personality characterized as conscientious, perfectionistic, ambitious, rigid, tense, and resentful, but controlled studies have not supported any consistent conclusion. Specific personality traits in migraine appear more likely to be a consequence rather than a cause of suffering from recurrent headaches (Stronks *et al.* 1999) A community-based survey found more personality disturbance and 2.5 times more psychological distress in migraine sufferers than in matched control subjects, but there was no relationship between headache frequency and the severity of psychological distress or personality abnormality (Brandt *et al.* 1990). An association with both depression and bipolar disorder is recognized (Lipton *et al.* 2000; Merikangas 1994) and there are interesting genetic studies linking migraine with dopamine DRD2 gene (Peroutka *et al.* 1997). The role for psychiatric management is as with CDH.

'Cervicogenic headache' is headache originating in the neck, usually associated with neck pain and limitation of movement, radiating forward from the neck or occiput. Temporal arteritis is a disorder of older people — very rare under the age 55 — causing scalp pain and tenderness, jaw claudication, malaise and an elevated erythrocyte sedimentation rate (ESR), usually to >50 mm per hour: treatment with corticosteroids should be started immediately and arrangements made for confirmatory temporal artery biopsy. Raised intracranial pressure typically gives rise to a headache which is worse on lying, disturbing sleep and present in the mornings, relieved by standing, and eventually causing nausea and vomiting and, if brainstem compression occurs, progressive reduction of consciousness: it can result from space-occupying lesions such as tumours and subdural haematomas, hydrocephalus, and idiopathic intracranial hypertension.

Certain 'headaches' are felt mainly in the face. Cluster headache gives rise to severe retro-orbital pain, commonly in young men, occurring in bursts of an hour or so, recurrently for a period of days to weeks (the 'cluster'), often waking the patient in the middle of the night: the pain usually makes the sufferer extremely restless, in contrast to migraine which sends sufferers to their beds (May & Goadsby 1998). Trigeminal neuralgia causes stabs of lancinating pain in one of the three divisions of the trigeminal nerve (Graff-Radford 2000). Atypical facial pain is a diagnosis of exclusion, the facial equivalent of chronic daily headache.

Somatoform and conversion disorders in neurology

Physical symptoms that are unexplained by neurological disease are common in neurological practice, variably referred to as medically unexplained symptoms, somatoform disorders, psychogenic and functional disorders. DSM-IV uses the term somatoform disorders although patients express a clear preference for the term 'functional' (Stone *et al.* 2002). However, a subgroup of somatoform disorders, the conversion disorders, frequently present to neurological services. In DSM-IV, conversion disorder is defined as a condition in which there are one or more motor or sensory symptoms or deficits that suggest a neurological or other general medical condition. Psychological factors are judged to be associated with the symptoms because their initiation or exacerbation is preceded by conflicts or other stressors. Diagnosis is not facile, both because such conflicts or stressors cannot be identified in many patients with conversion, and because many patients who do have 'organic' neurological disease may also have coincidental emotional conflicts and traumatic experiences. Common conversion symptoms include paralysis, weakness, seizures, anaesthesia, aphonia, blindness, amnesia, and stupor. Neurological symptoms in the absence of neurological disease or grossly disproportionate to disease affect approximately one-third of patients attending neurological clinics (Carson *et al.* 2000b). Functional weakness and paralysis, a subgroup of these disorders, has an incidence of at least 4 per 100 000 (Binzer & Kullgren 1998), an approximately similar rate to multiple sclerosis. In less than half of patients do the symptoms remit spontaneously (Carson *et al.* 2003).

A careful history is essential to diagnosis, first concentrating on the physical symptoms, and then exploring psychological and social factors. Pain is the most common clinical feature (Carson *et al.* 2000b) and care must be taken around the patient's attribution of mood symptoms as they are often reported as secondary to loss of physical function. For making the diagnosis particular attention should be paid to the following: the presence of multiple somatic symptoms, depression or anxiety (particularly panic), a history of previous functional symptoms or of operations in the absence of organic pathology (Barsky & Borus 1999). Childhood aversive experiences, personality factors, recent life events, secondary gain (financial or otherwise) and illness beliefs may all be relevant, but their presence does not allow one to infer a diagnosis of conversion disorder (Stone *et al.* 2002).

The history of the onset of the symptoms can be particularly helpful. Patients with conversion weakness will often describe symptoms suggestive of depersonalization/derealization at the time of onset. This will often occur in combination with a panic attack, physical trauma (often minor), or unexpected physiological events (e.g. post-micturitional syncope or sleep paralysis). In this context patients will describe 'the leg felt as if it was not connected to me', 'I felt far away', or 'I was in a place of my own' (Stone *et al.* 2002).

However, paradoxically, the neurological exam is essential to diagnosis in functional disorders more than in any other area of neuropsychiatry. Helpful signs include inconsistency, Hoover's sign (Ziv *et al.* 1998), collapsing ('giveaway'), weakness (Gould *et al.* 1986), and co-contraction (Knutsson & Martensson 1985). Tone and reflexes should be normal although may be mildly asymmetrical. Mild temperature and colour changes in the affected limb are commonplace in conversion disorder (Stone *et al.* 2002). These signs should be demonstrated to patients in a collaborative, not confrontational, fashion.

The aetiology remains unknown and there is value in remaining neutral about the relative contributions of biological, psychological and social factors (Kroenke 2002). In particular, although Freudian theory relates conversion disorder as a mechanism for dealing with unconscious conflict and traumatic experience, this model only fits some patients. Further, epidemiological studies consistently demonstrate a linear association between increasing severity of conversion symptoms and overt (i.e. not unconscious) distress (Wessley *et al.* 1999). Early functional imaging studies show intriguing results (Vuilleumier *et al.* 2001) and numerous, although often inconsistent, biochemical abnormalities have been described (Clauw & Chrousos 1997). The psychological and social risk factors are similar to other somatoform disorders as described in Chapter 7.

Diagnostic accuracy is high with an error rate of 5–10%, which compares favourably with most common neurological conditions (Carson *et al.* 2003). Misdiagnosis may be more common when there is known psychiatric comorbidity such as schizophrenia or learning disability, particularly when this interferes with history taking. Further imaging or neurophysiological testing may be required dependent on the symptoms presented. As a general rule, further investigations tend to discredit putative 'organic' diagnoses rather than overturn conversion disorder (Crimlisk *et al.* 1998). Although generally doctors (including psychiatrists) predominantly worry about missing 'organic' disease and are therefore often very conservative in making a diagnosis of conversion disorder, the available evidence suggests the reverse is more of a problem, leading to iatrogenic complications of unneeded treatment and invalidism (Fink 1992; Nimnuan *et al.* 2000).

Patients are best managed within the context of a psychologically sophisticated medical model (Sharpe & Carson 2000). A key step is a clear, non-stigmatizing explanation of the diagnosis, followed by appropriate reassurance. Appropriate reassurance communicates that a full, but gradual recovery may be possible and that dreaded diseases (e.g. stroke or MS) have been ruled out. Proving to the patient that there is 'nothing wrong' is usually ineffective at amelioration, and may antagonize or humiliate the patient. There is a good evidence base for treatment with antidepressant drugs particularly tricyclics with an odds ratio for improvement of 3.4 compared to placebo (O'Malley *et al.* 1999). Interestingly this does not depend on the presence of depressive symptoms. Clinical experience suggests a role for gabapentin, particularly when pain symptoms are prominent, but controlled trials are lacking. Cognitive behavioural therapy is effective in 70% of cases (Kroenke & Swindle 2000). We find that physical therapy can be helpful in aiding a return to full function and in some patients with longstanding disuse due to conversion disorder, physical therapy is required to restore normal function.

Summary

Psychiatry in a neurology/neurosurgery setting can be both rewarding and challenging. The reward comes from working with colleagues who share an interest in disorders of the brain. The challenge is the sometimes bewildering array of problems that appear far removed from general psychiatric practice. In this chapter we have attempted to outline the principles of assessment and management particularly in relation to commonly encountered conditions. However, the same rules of assessment apply whether it is the everyday work of assessing mood in a patient with MS or the rarely encountered assessment of a teenager with mitochondrial encephalomyopathy, lactic acidosis, and stroke-like episodes (MELAS). New developments in neuroscience are bringing an understanding of the mechanisms of interaction between biological, psychological and social aspects of illness, making this one of the most intellectually fascinating areas of work for a psychiatrist.

REFERENCES

Andersen, G., Vestergaard, K. and Lauritzen, L. (1994a). Effective treatment of post-stroke depression with the selective reuptake inhibitor citalopram. *Stroke*, **25**, 1099–104.

Andersen, G., Ingemann-Nielsen, M., Vestergaard, K., *et al.* (1994b). Pathoanatomic correlation between poststroke pathological crying and damage to brain areas involved in serotoninergic neurotransmission. *Stroke*, **25**, 1050–2.

Andersen, G., Vestergaard, K., Ingemann-Nielsen, M., *et al.* (1995). Risk factors for post-stroke depression. *Acta Psychiatrica Scandinavica*, **92**, 193–8.

Angunawela, I. I. and Barker, A. (2001). Anticholinesterase drugs for alcoholic Korsakoff syndrome. *International Journal of Geriatric Psychiatry*, **16**, 338–9.

Astrom, M. (1996). Generalised anxiety disorder in stroke patients: a 3-year longitudinal study. *Stroke*, **27**, 270–5.

Bahra, A., Walsh, M., Menon, S., *et al.* (2000). Does chronic daily headache arise de novo in association with regular analgesic use? *Cephalagia*, **20**, 294.

Bamford, J., Sandercock, P., Dennis, M., *et al.* (1988). A prospective study of acute cerebrovascular disease in the community: the Oxfordshire Community Stroke Project 1981–86, I: methodology, demography and incident cases of first-ever stroke. *Journal of Neurology, Neurosurgery and Psychiatry*, **51**, 1373–80.

Barsky, A. J. and Borus, J. F. (1999). Functional somatic syndromes. *Annals of Internal Medicine*, **130**, 910–21.

Berthier, M. L., Kulisevsky, J., Gironell, A., *et al.* (1996). Poststroke bipolar affective disorder: clinical subtypes, concurrent movement disorders, and anatomical correlates. *Journal of Neuropsychiatry and Clinical Neuroscience*, **8**, 160–70.

Brewer, G. J. and Askari, F. K. (2005). Wilson's disease: clinical management and therapy. *Journal of Hepatology*, **42**(Suppl. 1), S13–21.

Binzer, M. and Kullgren, G. (1998). Motor conversion disorder: a prospective 2–5 year follow-up study. *Psychosomatics*, **39**, 519–27.

Bogousslavsky, J. and Cummings, J. L. (2000). *Behavior and Mood Disorders in Focal Brain Lesions.* New York: Cambridge University Press.

Brandt, J., Celentano, D., Stewart, W., *et al.* (1990). Personality and emotional disorder in a community sample of migraine headache patients. *Cephalagia*, **19**, 566–74.

Burvill, P. W., Johnson, G. A., Jamrozik, K. D., *et al.* (1995). Anxiety disorders after stroke: results from the Perth Community Stroke Study. *British Journal of Psychiatry*, **166**, 328–32.

Carota, A., Rossetti, O. A., Karapanayiotides, T., *et al.* (2001). Catastrophic reaction in acute stroke: a reflex behaviour in aphasic patients. *Neurology*, **57**, 1902–6.

Carota, A., Staub, F. and Bogousslavsky, J. (2002). Emotions, behaviours and mood changes in stroke. *Current Opinion in Neurology*, **15**, 57–9.

Carson, A. J., Machale, S., Allen, K., *et al.* (2000a). Depression after stroke and lesion location: a systematic review. *Lancet*, **356**, 122–6.

Carson, A. J., Ringbauer, B., Stone, J., *et al.* (2000b). Do medically unexplained symptoms matter? A study of 300 consecutive new referrals to neurology outpatient clinics. *Journal of Neurology, Neurosurgery and Psychiatry*, **68**, 207–10.

Carson, A. J., Postmas, K., Stone, J., *et al.* (2003). The outcome of neurology patients with medically unexplained symptoms: a prospective cohort study. *Journal of Neurology, Neurosurgery and Psychiatry*, **74**, 897–900.

Chabolla, D. R. and Cascino, G. D. (1997). Interpretation of extracranial EEG. In *The Treatment of Epilepsy: Principles and Practice*, 2nd edn., ed. E. Wylie. Baltimore, MD: Williams & Wilkins, pp. 264–79.

Chemerinski, E., Robinson, R. G. and Kosier, J. T. (2001). Improved recovery in activities of daily living associated with remission of PSD. *Stroke*, **32**, 113–17.

Clauw, D. J. and Chrousos, G. P. (1997). Chronic pain and fatigue syndromes: overlapping clinical and neuroendocrine features and potential pathogenic mechanisms. *Neuroimmunomodulation*, **4**, 134–53.

Crimlisk, H., Bhatia, K., Cope, H., *et al.* (1998). Slater revisited: 6 year follow up study of patients with medically unexplained motor symptoms. *British Medical Journal*, **316**, 582–6.

Cummings, J. L. and Mendez, M. F. (1984). Secondary mania with focal cerebrovascular lesions. *American Journal of Psychiatry*, **141**, 1084–7.

Cutrer, F. M. (2003). Migraine: does one size fit all? *Current Opinion in Neurology*, **16**, 315–17.

Damasio, A. R. (1994). *Emotion, Reason and the Human Brain.* New York: GP Putman & Sons.

Derex, L., Ostrowsky, K., Nighoghossian, N., *et al.* (1997). Severe pathological crying after left anterior choroidal artery infarct: reversibility with paroxetine treatment. *Stroke*, **28**, 1464–9.

Duyao, M., Ambrose, C., Myers, R., *et al.* (1993). Trinucleotide repeat length: instability and age of onset of Huntington's disease. *Nature Genetics*, **4**, 387–92.

Ehde, D. M., Gibbons, L. E., Chwastiak, L., *et al.* (2003). Chronic pain in a large community sample of persons with multiple sclerosis. *Multiple Sclerosis*, **9**, 605–11.

Feinstein, A., O'Connor, P. and Feinstein, K. (2002). Multiple sclerosis, interferon beta-1b and depression: a prospective investigation. *Journal of Neurology*, **249**, 815–20.

Fink, P. (1992). Surgery and medical treatment in persistent somatizing patients. *Journal of Psychosomatic Research*, **36**, 439–47.

Folstein, M. F., Folstein, S. E. and McHugh, P. R. (1975). Mini-Mental State Examination: a practical method for grading the cognitive state of patients for clinicians. *Journal of Psychosomatic Research*, **11**, 189–98.

Gainotti, G., Azzoni, A., Razzano, C., *et al.* (1997). The Post-Stoke Depression Scale: a test specifically devised to investigate affective disorders of stroke patients. *Journal of Clinical and Experimental Neuropsychology*, **19**, 340–56.

Gainotti, G., Antonucci, G., Marra, C., *et al.* (2001). Relation between depression after stroke, antidepressant therapy and functional recovery. *Journal of Neurology, Neurosurgery & Psychiatry*, **71**(2), 258–61.

Goldstein, K. (1939). *The Organism: a Holistic Approach to Biology Derived from Pathological Data in Man.* New York: American Books.

Gony, M., Lapeyre-Mestre, M. and Montastruc, J.-L. (2003). Risk of serious extrapyramidal symptoms in patients with Parkinson's disease receiving antidepressant drugs: a pharmaco-epidemiologic study comparing serotonin reuptake inhibitors and other antidepressant drugs. *Clinical Neuropharmacology*, **26**(3), 142–5.

Gould, R., Miller, B. L., Goldberg, M. A., *et al.* (1986). The validity of hysterical signs and symptoms. *Journal of Nervous and Mental Disorders*, **174**, 593–7.

Graff-Radford, S. B. (2000). Facial pain. *Current Opinion in Neurobiology*, **13**, 291–6.

Herrmann, M., Bartels, C., Schumacher, M., *et al.* (1995). Poststroke depression: is there a pathoanatomic correlate for depression in the postacute stage of stroke? *Stroke*, **26**, 850–6.

Hodges, J. R. (1994). *Cognitive Assessment for Clinicians.* Oxford: Oxford University Press.

Holroyd, K. A., France, J. L., Nash, J. M., *et al.* (1993). Pain state as artifact in the psychological assessment of recurrent headache sufferers. *Pain*, **53**, 229–35.

House, A., Dennis, M., Molyneux, A., *et al.* (1989). Emotionalism after stroke. *British Medical Journal*, **298**, 991–4.

House, A., Knapp, P., Bamford, J., *et al.* (2001). Mortality at 12 and 24 months after stroke may be associated with depressive symptoms at 1 month. *Stroke*, **32**, 696–701.

Irani, D. N. (2003). The classic and variant forms of Creutzfeldt–Jakob disease. *Seminars in Clinical Neuropsychiatry*, **8**(1), 71–9.

Kales, H. C. and Mellow, A. M. (2003). Psychiatric assessment and treatment of depression in dementia. In *Handbook of Dementia: Psychological, Neurological, and Psychiatric Perspectives*, ed. P. A. Lichtenberg, D. L. Murman and A. M. Mellow. Hoboken, NJ: John Wiley & Sons, Inc, pp. 269–307.

Kim, J. S. and Choi-Kwon, S. (2000). Poststroke depression and emotional incontinence: correlation with lesion location. *Neurology*, **54**, 1805–10.

Kneebone, I. I. and Dunmore, E. (2000). Psychological management of post-stroke depression. *British Journal of Clinical Psychology*, **39**, 53–65.

Knutsson, E. and Martensson, A. (1985). Isokinetic measurements of muscle strength in hysterical paresis. *Electroencephalography and Clinical Neurophysiology*, **61**, 370–4.

Kraus, J. F. and Chu, L. D. (2005). Epidemiology. In *Textbook of Traumatic Brain Injury*, ed. J. M. Silver, T. W. McAllister and S. C. Yudofsky. American Psychiatric Publishing, pp. 3–26.

Kroenke, K. (2002). Integrating psychological care into general medical practice. *British Medical Journal*, **324**, 1536–7.

Kroenke, K. and Swindle, R. (2000). Cognitive behavioural therapy for somatization and symptom syndromes: a critical review of controlled clinical trials. *Psychotherapy and Psychosomatics*, **69**, 205–15.

Krupp, L. B., Coyle, P. K., Doscher, C., *et al.* (1995). Fatigue therapy in multiple sclerosis: results of a double-blind, randomized, parallel trial of amantadine, permoline and placebo. *Neurology*, **45**, 1956–61.

Kudrow, L. (1982). Paradoxical effects of frequent analgesic use. *Advances in Neurology*, **33**, 335–41.

Lance, F., Parkes, C. and Wilkinson, M. (1988). Does analgesic abuse cause headaches de novo? *Headache*, **28**, 61–2.

Lincoln, N. B., Flannagan, T., Sutcliff, L., *et al.* (1997). Evaluation of cognitive behavioural treatment for depression after stroke: a pilot study. *Clinical Rehabilitation*, **11**, 114–22.

Lindesay, J. (1991). Phobic disorders in the elderly. *British Journal of Psychiatry*, **159**, 531–41.

Lipsey, J. R., Robinson, R. G., Pearlson, G. D., *et al.* (1984). Nortriptyline treatment of post-stroke depression: a double blind treatment trial. *Lancet*, **S2**, 297–300.

Lipton, R. B., Hamelsky, S. W., Kolodner, K. B., *et al.* (2000). Migraine, quality of life, and depression: a population-based case-control study. *Neurology*, **55**, 629–35.

Maraganore, D. M., Lees, A. J. and Marsden, C. D. (1991). Complex stereotypies after right putaminal infarction: a case report. *Movement Disorders*, **6**, 358–61.

Mathuranath, P. S., Nestor, P., Berrios, G. E., *et al.* (2000). A brief cognitive test battery to differentiate Alzheimer's disease and frontotemporal dementia. *Neurology*, **55**, 1613–20.

May, A. and Goadsby, P. J. (1998). Cluster headache: imaging and other developments. *Headache*, **11**, 199–203.

McEwen, B. (1996). Stressful experience, brain and emotions: developmental genetic and hormonal influences. In *The Cognitive Neurosciences*, ed. M. S. Gazzaniga. Cambridge, MA: MIT Press, pp. 1117–35.

Merikangas, K. R. (1994). Psychopathology and headache syndromes in the community. *Headache*, **34**, S17–22.

Mitsikostas, D. D. and Thomas, A. M. (1999). Comorbidity of headache and depressive disorders. *Cephalagia*, **19**, 211–17.

Morris, P. L., Robinson, R. G. and Raphael, B. (1993). Emotional lability after stroke. *Australian and New Zealand Journal of Psychiatry*, **27**, 601–5.

Nimnuan, C., Hotopf, M. and Wessely, S. (2000). Medically unexplained symptoms: how often and why are they missed? *Quarterly Journal of Medicine*, **93**, 21–8.

O'Malley, P. G., Jackson, J. L., Santoro, J., *et al.* (1999). Antidepressant therapy for unexplained symptoms and symptom syndromes. *Journal of Family Practice*, **48**, 980–90.

Patten, S. B. and Metz, L. M. (2001). Interferon beta-1 and depression in relapsing-remitting multiple sclerosis: an analysis of depression data from the PRISMS clinical trial. *Multiple Sclerosis*, **7**, 243–8.

Peroutka, S. J., Wilhoit, T. and Jones, K. (1997). Clinical susceptibility to migraine with aura is modified by dopamine D2 receptor (DRD2) NcoI alleles. *Neurology*, **49**, 201–6.

Pohjasvaara, T., Vataja, R., Leppavuori, A., *et al.* (2001). Depression is an independent predictor of poor long-term functional outcome poststroke. *European Journal of Neurology*, **8**, 315–19.

Polman, C. H., Bertelsmann, E. W., Van Loenen, A. C., *et al.* (1994). 4-Aminopyridine in the treatment of patients with multiple slerosis: long-term efficacy and safety. *Archives of Neurology*, **51**, 292–6.

Ramasubbu, R. (1994). Denial of illness and depression in stroke (letter). *Stroke*, **25**, 226–7.

Rammohan, K. W., Rosenburgh, J. H., Lynn, D. J., *et al.* (2002). Efficacy and safety of modafinil (Provigil) for the treatment of fatigue in multiple sclerosis: a two centre phase 2 study. *Journal of Neurology, Neurosurgery and Psychiatry*, **72**, 179–83.

Rasmussen, B. K. (1992). Migraine and tension-type headache in a general population: psychosocial factors. *International Journal of Epidemiology*, **21**, 1138–43.

Robertson, M. M., Schull, D. A., Eapen, V., *et al.* (1996). Risperidone in the treatment of Tourette syndrome: a retrospective case note study. *Journal of Psychopharmacology*, **10**, 317–20.

Robinson, R. G., Parikh, R. M., Lipsey, J. R., *et al.* (1993). Pathological laughing and crying following stroke: validation of a measurement scale and a double-blind treatment study. *American Journal of Psychiatry*, **150**, 286–93.

Robinson, R. G., Schultz, S. K., Castillo, C., *et al.* (2000). Nortriptyline versus fluoxetine in the treatment of depression and in short-term recovery after stroke: a placebo-controlled, double-blind investigation. *American Journal of Psychiatry*, **157**, 351–9.

Rodrigo, E. P., Adair, J. C., Roberts, B. B., *et al.* (1997). Obsessive-compulsive disorder following bilateral globus pallidus infarction. *Biological Psychiatry*, **42**, 410–12.

Sharpe, M. and Carson, A. (2000). Unexplained somatic symptoms, functional syndromes and somatization: do we need a paradigm shift? *Annals of Internal Medicine*, **134**, 926–30.

Sheean, G. L., Murray, N. M., Rothwell, J. C., *et al.* (1997). An electrophysiological study of the mechanism of fatigue in multiple sclerosis. *Brain*, **120**, 299–315.

Spencer, M. D., Knight, R. S. G. and Will, R. G. (2002). First hundred cases of variant Creutzfeldt–Jakob disease: retrospective case note review of early psychiatric and neurological features. *British Medical Journal*, **324**, 1479–82.

Starkstein, S. E. (1998). Mood disorders after stroke. In *Cerebrovascular Disease*, ed. M. Grinsberg and J. Bogousslavsky. Oxford: Blackwell Science, pp. 131–8.

Starkstein, S. E. and Robinson, R. G. (1989). Affective disorders and cerebral vascular disease. *British Journal of Psychiatry*, **154**, 170–82.

Starkstein, S. E., Pearlson, G. D., Boston, J., *et al.* (1987). Mania after brain injury: a controlled study of causative factors. *Archives of Neurology*, **44**, 1069–73.

Starkstein, S. E., Berthier, M. I., Fedoroff, P., *et al.* (1990). Anosognosia and major depression in 2 patients with cerebrovascular lesions. *Neurology*, **40**, 1380–2.

Starkstein, S. E., Fedoroff, J. P., Price, T. R., *et al.* (1993a). Apathy following cerebrovascular lesions. *Stroke*, **24**, 1625–30.

Starkstein, S. E., Fedoroff, J. P., Price, T. R., *et al.* (1993b). Catastrophic reaction after cerebrovascular lesions: frequency, correlates, and validation of a scale. *Journal of Neuropsychiatry and Clinical Neuroscience*, **5**, 189–94.

Stein, D. J., Bouwer, C., Hawkridge, S., *et al.* (1997). Risperidone augmentation of serotonin reuptake inhibitors in obsessive-compulsive and related disorders. *Journal of Clinical Psychiatry*, **58**, 119–22.

Stone, V. E., Baron-Cohen, S. and Knight, R. T. (1998). Frontal lobe contributions to theory of mind. *Journal of Cognitive Neuroscience*, **10**, 640–56.

Stone, J., Zeman, A. and Sharpe, M. (2002). Physical signs: functional weakness and sensory disturbance. *Journal of Neurology, Neurosurgery and Psychiatry*, **73**, 241–5.

Stronks, D. L., Tulen, J. H., Pepplinkhuizen, L., *et al.* (1999). Personality sufferers. *American Journal of Psychiatry*, **147**, 303–8.

Thornhill, S., Teasdale, G. M., Murray, G. D., *et al.* (2000). Disability in young people and adults one year after head injury: perspective cohort study. *British Medical Journal*, **320**, 1631.

Vein, A. M., Djukova, G. M. and Vorobieva, O. V. (1994). Is panic attack a mask of psychogenic seizures? A comparative analysis of phenomenology of psychogenic seizures and panic attacks. *Functional Neurology*, **9**, 153–9.

Vuilleumier, P., Chicherio, C., Assal, F., *et al.* (2001). Functional neuroanatomical correlates of hysterical sensorimotor loss. *Brain*, **124**, 1077–90.

Wessely, S., Nimnuan, C. and Sharpe, M. (1999). Functional somatic syndromes: one or many? *Lancet*, **354**(9182), 936–9.

Wiart, L., Petit, H., Joseph, P. A., *et al.* (2000). Fluoxetine in early poststroke depression: a double-blind placebo-controlled study. *Stroke*, **31**(8), 1829–32.

Zephir, H., De Seze, J., Stojkovic, T., *et al.* (2003). Multiple sclerosis and depression: influence of interferon beta therapy. *Multiple Sclerosis*, **9**(3), 284–8.

Ziv, I., Djaldetti, R., Zoldan, Y., *et al.* (1998). Diagnosis of 'non-organic' limb paresis by a novel objective motor assessment: the quantitative Hoover's test. *Journal of Neurology*, **245**(12), 797–802.

15

Cardiorespiratory disorders

Christopher Bass

Introduction

This chapter attempts to describe how psychosocial factors influence both cardiovascular and respiratory diseases. This will include an exploration of not only the ways in which psychosocial factors contribute to 'disease risk', but also the psychological consequences of disorders such as coronary heart disease (CHD) and chronic obstructive pulmonary disease (COPD). Psychosocial aspects of the transplantation of major organs will also be described. Only brief mention will be made of other topics such as non-cardiac chest pain and hyperventilation, which will be dealt with elsewhere (Chapter 7).

Cardiovascular disorders

Coronary heart disease

Around one-quarter of all deaths among men and one-fifth of all deaths of women in Britain are due to CHD. Among women the proportion is relatively stable throughout the adult years, whilst in men it peaks among 55–64-year-olds, for whom CHD accounts for a third of all deaths. The National Health Service in England deals with around 200 000 inpatient episodes due to CHD for men and 100 000 for women each year, representing around 5% of all hospital inpatient episodes for men and 3% for women. In addition, there are about 30 million work days lost due to certified incapacity for CHD among men and over 4 million among women each year in Britain (Ness & Davey-Smith 2003).

Coronary heart disease rates in Britain increased from the beginning of the century until the 1980s for men, but since the late 1970s CHD mortality has

Handbook of Liaison Psychiatry, ed. Geoffrey Lloyd and Elspeth Guthrie. Published by Cambridge University Press. © Cambridge University Press 2007.

declined steadily in both men and women. This fall in death rate due to CHD suggests that environmental factors are important and points to a role for prevention. It is also worth noting that in recent years there has been a change in the social distribution of CHD. In many European countries, as in the USA, the social distribution has changed to the now familiar pattern of an inverse social gradient: higher rates as the social hierarchy is descended (Marmot & Bartley 2002).

There is increasing evidence that psychological factors cannot only contribute to the cause but also influence survival among patients with CHD. Psychosocial factors may act alone or combine in clusters, and can exert influence at different stages of the life course (Kuh *et al.* 1997). In a recent review, Hemingway and Marmot (1999) suggested three inter-related pathways. First, psychosocial factors may affect health-related behaviours such as smoking, diet, alcohol consumption, or physical activity, which in turn may influence the risk of CHD. Second, psychosocial factors may cause direct acute or chronic pathophysiological changes, possibly by their effect on neuroendocrine or immune systems. Third, access to and content of medical care may be influenced by social factors. This model is shown in Figure 15.1.

Evidence for specific psychosocial risk factors

In a systematic review of prospective cohort studies, Hemingway and Marmot (1999) identified four groups of psychosocial factors using a predefined quality filter:
- psychological traits (type A behaviour, hostility)
- psychological states (depression, anxiety)
- psychological work characteristics (job control; demands; support)
- social networks and social supports.

Each of these will be considered in turn.

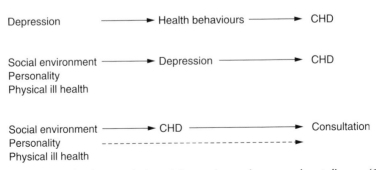

Figure 15.1. Mechanisms for the association of depression and coronary heart disease (CHD).

Hostility and type A behaviour

Type-A behaviour (TAB) is characterized by hard driving and competitive behaviour, a potential for hostility, pronounced impatience, and vigorous speech characteristics. Early reports of a link between TAB and CHD published in the 1970s and 1980s have not been borne out by subsequent work, and the evidence of TAB as an independent risk factor in relation to prognosis among patients with CHD has not been confirmed. As Williams has pointed out, however, just as a Medline search comparing the late 1990s with the late 1970s would show a decline in type A citations, a similar search using 'hostility' as the keyword would reveal a striking increase in the number of citations (Williams 2002). But a meta-analysis of research on the physical health consequences of hostility concluded that the psychological trait of hostility – cynical mistrust, anger, and aggression – is a risk factor for not only CHD but also for virtually any physical illness (Miller *et al.* 1996).

Anger, however, remains as potent a risk for ischaemic events as strenuous physical exertion during ambulatory electrocardiogram (ECG) monitoring of CHD patients (Gabbay *et al.* 1996). The risk of suffering a myocardial infarction (MI) is doubled during the two hours following an episode of intense anger (Mittelman *et al.* 1995), and trebled in people of low educational attainment, suggesting the compounding of acute risk by the combination of psychosocial risk factors. It has been established that episodes of intense anger are responsible for triggering 36 000 acute MIs in the USA each year (Verrier & Mittelman 1996).

Depression and anxiety

A number of longitudinal studies of depressive illness and depressive symptoms have provided strong evidence for depression as an antecedent of CHD. In one American study in which 1190 medical students were followed-up for a median period of 37 years, depressive illness was associated with an almost doubled risk of CHD in men (MI, angina pectoris, chronic ischaemic heart disease (IHD), requirement for angioplasty or by-pass surgery). The risk was also markedly increased in women (Ford & Mead 1998). In a UK-based case-control study carried out in primary care (Hippisley-Cox *et al.* 1998) men with a diagnosis of depression were three times more likely to develop CHD than control subjects, the risk persisting after adjusting for smoking, diabetes, hypertension and deprivation score. This finding did not hold for depressed women.

In contrast to the US study, there was evidence in this UK-based study that the recency of depression was associated with increased CHD risk. A longer latent period would suggest however that depression is influencing long-term patho-logical processes leading to CHD: this might mean chronic sympatho-adrenal hyperactivity, metabolic disturbance influencing the development of atherosclerosis, or hypothalamic-pituitary-adrenal (HPA) axis stimulation leading to chronically elevated cortisol levels (Checkley 1996). Patients with chronic depression would appear to be at most risk of subsequent CHD (see later). Another possible biological explanation for the association is that deficiencies in the central neurotransmitter serotonin may contribute to the development of not only psychiatric morbidity but also hypertension and cardiovascular risk (Davies *et al.* 2004; see later).

Depression in patients after MI seems to be of prognostic importance beyond severity of CHD (Rumsfeld *et al.* 2005). Intriguingly, there is some evidence that patients with phobic anxiety are at increased risk of sudden cardiac death, possibly mediated by a heightened susceptibility to arrhythmias (Haines *et al.* 1987).

Psychosocial work characteristics

There is good evidence that psychosocial factors at work are related to risk of CHD and may play an important part in contributing to the social gradient in CHD. Although the lay notion of 'executive stress' is widespread, with its connotations of high-achieving type-A behaviour, the Whitehall Study has revealed that the highest risk for CHD is among junior grade civil servants. This has prompted an observer to remark, 'it is not the bosses but the people that are bossed about who suffer most from work stress' (Whitehead 1995).

There is evidence that people in jobs characterized by low control over work and high conflicting demands appear to be at increased risk. For example, in the Whitehall II Study, both men and women with low job control, either self-reported or independently assessed, had a higher risk of new self-reported CHD during a mean follow-up period of five years (Bosma *et al.* 1997). A high plasma fibrinogen level may be the biological mechanism underpinning this association between job strain and risk of MI.

Furthermore, there is evidence that an imbalance between the effort of work and rewards is detrimental (Bosma *et al.* 1998). In addition to these adverse occupational characteristics, it is important to consider the health burden of long-term unemployment (Martikainen & Valkonen 1996). Moreover, stressful life events in an individual's personal life, such as marital problems and lack of social support, can exacerbate the burden of work-related stress and may increase a person's disposition towards developing disease (Brown & Harris 1999).

Social network structure and quality of social support

Social supports and networks relate to both the number of a person's social contacts and their quality (including emotional support and confiding support). There is now considerable evidence that high levels of social support are protective against CHD, while social isolation is related to increased mortality risk. It has been proposed that social supports may act to buffer the effect of various environmental stressors and hence increase susceptibility to disease (Alloway 1987), but most of the evidence supports a direct role.

What are the implications of these findings for clinical practice? Because randomized controlled trials of social supports after MI show a decrease in cardiac death or re-infarction rates (Bucher 1994), a patient's social circumstances should be elicited as part of the history, and the doctor may have a role in mobilizing social support.

Depression following myocardial infarction

Between 13 and 19% of survivors of MI suffer from major depressive illness (Creed 1999), although it is important to differentiate between those patients who were psychologically unwell before the infarction and those whose depression was precipitated by infarction (Lloyd & Cawley 1983). Lesperance *et al.* (1996) found a prior history of depression in 28% of patients, which increased the risk of depression following infarction. One-quarter of patients with depression after an MI have persistent psychopathology one year later (Mayou 1984).

Prognostic implications of depression following MI

Depression in the early period following MI has prognostic implications (Ladwig *et al.* 1994). Patients with severe depression, compared with the patients with moderate or low levels of depression, have higher levels of angina pectoris subsequently, continuing levels of emotional instability, lower levels of return to work, and higher maintenance of smoking. More than that, patients with high levels of depression or anxiety following MI are more likely to die of cardiac causes over the subsequent five years than other patients; in one study there was a 3.5-fold increase in mortality of depressed patients compared with non-depressed patients within six months of myocardial infarction (Frasure Smith *et al.* 1995).

What is the explanation for this increased mortality associated with depression following MI? The following factors are likely to be involved and this area has recently been reviewed by Shimbo *et al.* (2005):

1. Depressed patients are less likely to adhere to treatment.
2. Depressed patients are less likely to adhere to healthy behaviour, e.g. stop smoking, than patients who are not depressed.
3. Depression may lead to decreased heart rate variability, with a greater risk of fatal arrhythmias in a heart already sensitized by MI (Frasure Smith *et al.* (1995) found premature ventricular contractions predicted mortality over 18 months in patients with depression following MI).

4. Depression has been associated with heightened susceptibility to platelet activation and changes in platelet aggregatabilty, leading to greater risk of thrombosis (Musselman *et al.* 1998).

5. Depression has been associated with inflammatory markers in coronary heart disease (Empana *et al.* 2005).

Recent research also suggests that patients' pre-infarction mental state may also be significant. Patients who are depressed in the weeks preceding MI are more likely to have poorer cardiac function post-MI, which may be another mechanism whereby psychosocial factors influence mortality (Dickens *et al.* 2005). Although depression pre-MI is not associated with an increased mortality, lack of a confidant, pre-MI, appears to predict further cardiac events (Dickens *et al.* 2004a). What's more, the depression that follows MI has different risk factors associated with it than depression which precedes MI (Dickens *et al.* 2004b). Further work needs to be done to clarify the role of both pre- and post-MI depression, interpersonal relationships and their association to mortality.

Psychosocial interventions in coronary heart disease

It is evident that MI is a major cause of mortality and morbidity and often causes distress and impairment of quality of life for patients and their relatives. As a consequence many investigators have developed interventions (often referred to as rehabilitation), and some of these will be described.

Several studies have reported that psychosocial interventions reduce mortality in MI patients by up to 40%, possibly because of the beneficial effects on mood. On the other hand, two studies of psychosocial rehabilitation have produced negative results, one in Wales (Jones & West 1996) and another in Canada (Frasure Smith *et al.* 1991). In neither trial, however, was there a significant reduction of depression. In the Welsh study the depression scores remained identical in the experimental and the control groups — 19% in each were depressed at the end of the trial. In the Canadian Study the Beck Depression Inventory Score only dropped slightly from 8.1 to 6.9 in the intervention group, similar to the control group (8.4 to 7.6).

A major recent study, the Enhancing Recovery in CHD (ENRICHD) study, a multicentre, randomized controlled clinical trial, which has recently been completed in the United States, targeted patients post-MI who were at high psychosocial risk (those who were depressed and socially isolated), and enrolled large numbers of women and ethnic minorities (Berkman *et al.* 2003). Over 2400 patients were entered into the study and randomized to either receiving 11 sessions of cognitive therapy, enhanced by an antidepressant where appropriate, or usual care. There were small but significant improvements in depression and social function in the intervention group in comparison with the usual care group but no difference in overall long-term survival at follow-up.

White men, but not other subgroups, may have benefited from the ENRICHD intervention, suggesting that future studies need to attend to issues of treatment design and delivery that may have prevented benefit among sex and ethnic subgroups other than white men (Schneiderman *et al.* 2004).

It is important to note, however, that there is a small group of patients with chronic depression whose depression does not improve even when they are in a successful rehabilitation programme. This small group with chronic and persistent depression may be the group responsible for the association between depression and increased deaths, and because of this increased risk they should become the target of future intervention studies.

The importance of health beliefs after myocardial infarction

In the last 10 years it has become evident that patients' beliefs and perceptions of their illness are critically important in the recovery phase of MI. Patients who hold negative beliefs about their illness are less likely to return to work and to have lower levels of functioning regardless of the severity of the MI. The patients' view of their MI is an important factor in both rehabilitation attendance and in how quickly they return to work (Cooper *et al.* 1999; Petrie *et al.* 1996). For example, if a patient believes that his job nearly killed him he will be reluctant to return. Damaging beliefs can be reinforced by the media, friends and family as well as inadvertently from healthcare professionals. This was illustrated recently in a study in the non-cohabiting friends of patients with angina; the friends were more likely than their peers with heart disease to believe that angina was a) caused by a worn-out heart, b) a small heart attack, c) caused permanent damage to the heart, and d) people with angina should take life easy, avoid exercise and excitement. In a recent attempt to address these issues, Petrie *et al.* (2002) showed that an in-hospital intervention designed to alter patients' illness beliefs and perceptions about their MI resulted in improved functional outcome after MI. This is clearly a key area for future research in cardiac rehabilitation.

Practical advice on managing psychological factors

Structured advice and discussion of the factors known to effect recovery is important. The advice should be realistic, practical, and concrete, e.g. 'eat five portions of fresh fruit or vegetables every day'. The resumption of small amounts of activity should be encouraged from the first full day home. Partners should be advised to alter the family routines as little as possible except for lifestyle changes, such as smoking or diet, which should begin immediately. The patient and partner's understanding of the advice should be checked during the course and at the end of each session by asking them to summarize the advice imparted. As half of the advice in a five-minute consultation is forgotten within a further five minutes, it is helpful if written or tape-recorded advice is provided. A useful resource for patients with depression after a heart attack is http://familydoctor.org/handouts/702.html.

Cardiac rehabilitation

Cardiac rehabilitation (CR) is a multidisciplinary and multifactorial intervention that aims to restore wellbeing and retard disease progression in patients with heart disease. Although there is some scepticism regarding its effectiveness (Lewin *et al.* 2000), meta-analyses have suggested a significant reduction in total and cardiac mortality of at least 20% (Thompson & Lewin 2000).

It has been recommended that every district hospital that treats patients with heart disease should provide a CR service, and that individual programmes should evaluate their outcome, and a standard format of audit should be agreed nationally to allow comparison (Thompson *et al.* 1997). The new NSF for coronary heart disease (Department of Health 2000), developed to improve the quality and consistency of services in terms of prevention and treatment, should be helpful in implementing change. See Boxes 15.1, 15.2 and 15.3.

A six-week, home-based rehabilitation programme, the Heart Manual, delivered by a specially trained nurse has been found to be effective in reducing anxiety and depression, visits to the general practitioner and hospital readmissions up to six months after MI (Lewin *et al.* 1992). In a more recent study Mayou *et al.* (2002) showed that individualized educational behavioural treatment delivered by a cardiac nurse in hospital had substantial benefits compared to usual care in patients following acute MI.

Box 15.1 Cardiac rehabilitation: general points.

- For the majority of patients the best predictors of rehabilitation outcome are psychosocial not physiological.
- Psychological findings about adjustment to MI and lifestyle change must be integrated with routine care.
- Family members, especially the partner, should be included in the rehabilitation process.
- The greater part of any verbal interaction is quickly forgotten, and should be backed up with carefully constructed and empirically evaluated written and taped material.

> **Box 15.2 Early phase of rehabilitation.**
>
> • Immediately after diagnosis of MI, or as soon as is practical, patients should have their beliefs and knowledge about the MI and their lifestyle assessed and, where necessary, receive counselling.
> • Patients should be assessed for psychological problems using validated instruments, such as the Hospital Anxiety and Depression Scale, and if necessary have access to appropriate counselling/treatment and to follow up assessment.
> • Counselling should be concrete, with clearly defined and measurable goals, and must take into account the patient's own beliefs about what has happened and what should be done.
> • Patients should be prepared for the common physical and emotional sequelae which often only become problematic after discharge from hospital.

> **Box 15.3 Cardiac rehabilitation: early post-discharge.**
>
> • Support should be continued and need only consist of brief meetings or even telephone calls to go through the goals, reinforce progress, and help the patient solve any practical difficulties that may have arisen.
> • Care should be taken to ensure that congruent advice is given by primary care staff.
> • Patients should be formally assessed at 6–12 weeks post-MI to ascertain their success in making lifestyle changes and psychological adjustment.

Evidence is also accumulating that the success of rehabilitation may depend to a large extent upon the involvement of the patient's family, particularly the partner. Partners are likely to benefit from the support, information and enhanced feeling of control that they are likely to experience by being included in rehabilitation (Johnson *et al.* 1999).

If a patient has a depressive disorder an attempt should be made to treat this over and above any treatment of depression in cardiac rehabilitation programmes. A self-administered questionnaire to detect depression can be used, followed where appropriate, with treatment with antidepressant medication, cognitive therapy, or both. The selective serotonin reuptake inhibitors (SSRIs) appear to be safe for the treatment of depression in patients with cardiac disease (Creed 1999).

Hypertension

Hypertension constitutes one of the major risk factors for coronary heart disease, stroke, renal insufficiency and cardiac failure. In a recent British study of adults aged 16 years or more in 1994, 19% of men and 20% of women had a blood pressure of 160/95 mmHg or higher or were receiving antihypertensive drug treatment (Isles 2003). It is the third most common chronic disorder affecting the adult population in the USA, accounting for as many as 50 million cases of chronic illness (Mosterd *et al.* 1999). However, it is worth noting that the increasing use of antihypertensive medication has resulted in a decline in the prevalence of hypertension in the USA.

There is increasing evidence of an association between hypertension and panic attacks (and panic disorder). In a case-control study carried out in primary care, Davies *et al.* (1999) found a greater prevalence of panic attacks in patients with hypertension than normotensive controls. Furthermore, the reported diagnosis of hypertension antedated the onset of panic attacks in a large majority of patients. Possible pathophysiological mechanisms that may explain this association include autonomic dysregulation of cardiac activity and smooth muscle tone, and dynamic abnormalities of the coronary vasculature (Zaubler & Katon 1998).

Perhaps these findings should not be unexpected, given the reports that the detection and treatment of hypertension can result in adverse psychological and behavioural consequences (MacDonald *et al.* 1984). In a key paper Haynes *et al.* (1978) found that 'labelling' of patients as hypertensive increased their absenteeism rate from work: after screening and referral, absenteeism rose 80% compared to 9% in the general employee population during this period. The main factors associated with this absenteeism were becoming aware of the condition and low compliance with treatment. Significantly, absenteeism rose among those previously unaware of their condition, regardless of whether antihypertensive therapy was begun. These studies, like those in cardiac rehabilitation, emphasize the power of health beliefs in medicine, and their impact on a variety of health outcomes

Drug treatment in cardiovascular disease

Among the antidepressants the tricyclics (TCAs) have been demonstrated to be reasonably safe in patients with chronic stable heart disease, although their quinidine-like effects may cause (or aggravate) prolongation of the Q-T and QRS intervals. Orthostatic hypertension is another important side-effect, especially in the elderly. Based on our current state of knowledge, TCAs generally should be avoided following myocardial infarction.

Most of the newer antidepressants such as the SSRIs, venlafaxine, or mirtazapine do not have quinidine-like properties nor have they been associated with increases in heart rate, and most do not cause orthostasis. The SSRIs therefore present fewer concerns over cardiotoxicity: sertraline and citalopram have considerably less potential to inhibit metabolizing enzymes than do paroxetine and fluoxetine (Davies *et al.* 2004). These drugs are unequivocally safer from the cardiac standpoint after overdoses (Barbey & Roose 1998).

The serotonin and noradrenaline reuptake inhibitor venlafaxine may be used in patients with CHD. Caution is needed at high doses (>300 mg daily) as the drug shows a dose-dependent increase in blood pressure averaging 7 mmHg diastolic at the highest dose.

Psychiatric aspects of heart transplantation

There is now widespread agreement that heart transplantation improves life expectancy in the majority of recipients and permits an adequate quality of life in those subjects who survive surgery. The literature also shows that at every point in the procedure, from the time the patient is first evaluated for surgery until the period of post-operative rehabilitation, psychiatric and psychosocial problems may affect the patient's adjustment and influence surgical outcome (Mai 1993).

The literature on outcome supports the conclusion that the majority of recipients do well, both physically and psychologically. However, there is evidence that a substantial minority of patients experience family conflicts and sexual dysfunction after surgery. In a study of 76 patients who were undergoing heart, heart and lung, or lung transplantation, 39% were suffering from psychiatric disorder and 58% reported sexual dysfunction. Clinically significant psychiatric morbidity pre-operatively was associated with a history of treatment for mental disorder, unemployment, and length of physical illness. Patients with psychiatric disorder reported poorer quality of life on the SF36, with lower scores on subscales for general health perception, social functioning, and energy vitality (Trumper & Appleby 2001).

Respiratory disorders

Chronic obstructive pulmonary disease (COPD) and asthma produce considerable morbidity and mortality, and both will be discussed in this section. COPD is the sixth commonest cause of death worldwide, and set to become the third commonest by the year 2020. It is a slowly progressive condition characterized by airflow limitation that is largely irreversible. In clinical practice a diagnosis of COPD is usually associated with:

- a history of chronic progressive symptoms (cough, wheeze, and/or breathlessness), with little variation
- usually a cigarette-smoking history of more than 20 pack years (1 pack year is 20 cigarettes per day for 1 year) and
- objective evidence of airways obstruction, ideally by spirometry, that does not return to normal with treatment.

The differentiation of COPD from asthma remains a problem, particularly as a large proportion of patients with COPD show some reversibility of their airflow obstruction with bronchodilators (MacNee 2003).

Patients react emotionally to the discomfort of dyspnoea, the sensation of suffocation and threat of death, while hypoxia, hypocapnia, hyperventilation, respiratory failure and many pulmonary medications all have different effects on the brain. Among adults in the US population Goodwin and Pine (2002) found a specific association between self-reported respiratory disease, i.e. asthma, chronic bronchitis, or emphysema and panic attacks. Using the same data set from the Midlife Development in the US Survey ($n = 3032$) Goodwin and Hamilton (2002) found that panic attacks were associated with a greater risk of cigarette smoking and provided evidence that neuroticism may play an essential role in this relationship. The authors suggested that neuroticism may reflect a shared vulnerability for the co-occurrence of cigarette smoking and panic attacks. The relationship between psychological illness and lung disease is reviewed below, along with a brief description of hyperventilation and 'dysfunctional breathing' and its clinical relevance and management.

Psychological illness and COPD

There have been many studies of psychiatric morbidity in patients with COPD.

Rutter (1977) reported that, compared with non-bronchitic controls, patients with chronic bronchitis were not only more neurotic in personality but also had high levels of psychiatric disorder (48%) compared with 13% in the controls (measured with the GHQ-30). Furthermore, psychological factors such as attitudes to returning to work, beliefs about bronchitis and the value of exercise were more strongly related to outcome at one year than were a variety of physiological measures of disease severity (Rutter 1979).

In another early study of the mental health of chronic bronchitics using psychiatric interviews (DSM-II), Yellowlees *et al.* (1987) found high rates of psychiatric morbidity (50%), with panic and anxiety disorders (34%) being particularly prevalent. Yellowlees noted that all the patients who suffered from anxiety disorders hyperventilated at times, and many reported phobic avoidance of certain situations such as eating alone, lifts or travelling outside home without company or an inhaler. Fear, hyperventilation and panic tended to recur in situations whether the patient was alone, enclosed, or had worsening further airways obstruction. Phobic avoidance of these situations led to further anxiety and the development of a vicious circle of fear, hyperventilation, panic and avoidance. This behaviour often led to significant handicaps, with social and functional restrictions.

Using more rigorous methods of detecting psychiatric morbidity (the structured clinical interview for DSM-III; Spitzer *et al.* 1997), Karajgi *et al.* (1990) studied 50 consecutive patients with stable COPD. Although they reported lower rates of psychiatric disorder than Yellowlees (the overall prevalence of psychiatric disorder was 16%), panic disorder was found in 8%, which is 5.3 times higher than the 1.5% found in the general population (Robins *et al.* 1984).

What is the explanation for this high rate of anxiety disorders in patients with COPD? Porzelius *et al.* (1992), found that COPD patients with a history of panic did not differ from those who had not experienced panic on demographic, physiological or activity variables. However, patients who experienced panic reported significantly more agoraphobic cognitions and greater concern with bodily sensations than patients who did not experience panic. These are particularly important findings for COPD patients who must continue to be subjected to the physiological symptoms associated with this disorder. Since these patients suffer from chronically compromised respiratory function, the cognitive appraisal factors have a uniquely significant role. The physiological sensations associated with COPD are generally chronic, often progressive and may trigger more severe problems. Catastrophic interpretations of dyspnoeic body sensations cannot necessarily be termed 'misinterpretations', since the hyperventilation and panic that can result from these cognitions can indeed produce the health risk suggested by the catastrophic thoughts. Since the physiological sensations are not likely to be eliminated, cognitive modification is an important treatment option for these patients (see later).

A more recent survey of the contribution of coping and illness perceptions to outcome in patients with COPD using the Illness Perception Questionnaire (IPQ) found that first-time illness perceptions and coping significantly contributed to the prediction of social functioning, mental health, health perceptions, total functioning score, and prediction of visits to the outpatient clinic and prescribed medication one year later (Scharloo *et al.* 2000). These findings are consistent with an earlier study of health beliefs in chronic bronchitis. Morgan *et al.* (1983) found that disability in chronic bronchitics (measured by the 12-minute walking test) was significantly related to patients' belief about treatment and treatment outcome. That is to say, the more the subjects believed that their treatment would be successful, that it would require them to make a personal effort and that it would be new, the further they walked in 12 minutes relevant to their forced vital capacity (FVC). This is further evidence for the fundamental role of health beliefs in the functioning of patients with chronic medical disorders. Clinicians would be well advised therefore to assess health beliefs as well as physical variables. The use of the IPQ in the outpatient clinic may provide useful information in the management of these patients.

Depression in chronic lung disease

The diagnosis of depression may be difficult in patients with symptoms of chronic respiratory disease, since many depressive and pulmonary symptoms overlap, including fatigue, lassitude, weight loss, anorexia, and loss of interest in usual activities. Sleep disturbance may be caused by episodes of sleep apnoea or nocturnal coughing, as well as by nocturnal asthma attacks. Depression may be closely associated with the multiple significant losses sustained by an individual with chronic respiratory disease. These may include loss of occupation and earning capacity as well as loss of physical strength and changes in appearance. Some of these losses are due to physical wasting caused by chronic illness or to impairment of pulmonary function, and others are attributable to the side-effects of medications, especially corticosteroids. The diagnosis of depression in the medically ill is often difficult, and useful questions are shown in Box 15.4.

Spinhoven *et al.* (1994) have attempted to explain the association between lung disease and psychological distress as follows: anxiety may be more closely related to intermittent respiratory problems (such as asthma), whilst depression is more strongly associated with continuous lung obstruction (such as bronchitis). It is conceivable therefore that disturbed respiratory physiology may have differential effects depending on (a) the nature of the underlying lung disorder and (b) the appraisal by the patient.

Box 15.4 Useful criteria for diagnosing patients with a physical illness suspected of having depression.

- Depressed mood: objective or observed
- Marked diminished interest or pleasure in most activities, most of the day
- Fearful or depressed appearance
- Psychomotor retardation or agitation
- Social withdrawal or decreased talkativeness
- Feelings of worthlessness or excessive or inappropriate guilt
- Brooding, self-pity or pessimism
- Recurrent thoughts of death or suicide
- Mood is non-reactive

The following symptoms are not always good discriminators:
- Significant weight loss or gain (0.5% of body weight per month)
- Insomnia or hypersomnia
- Fatigue or loss of memory
- Diminished ability to think or concentrate, or indecisiveness
  Source: Endicott (1984).

Psychological illness and asthma

Asthma was long regarded as a 'psychosomatic disorder', although there are no major differences in the psychopathology of asthmatics and non-asthmatic controls defined in terms of overt mental illness, symptoms, signs and neurotic traits.

There is however evidence that in patients with severe difficult-to-treat asthma high levels of psychopathology (measured by GHQ-12 scores) are associated with frequent visits to the GP, frequent emergency visits, frequent exacerbations, and frequent hospitalizations as compared with the non-psychiatric patients (ten Brinke *et al.* 2001).

The association of panic and asthma

Patients with asthma frequently suffer from anxiety symptoms or disorders. The anxiety may stimulate or simulate an asthma attack, or may result from medications used to treat asthma. Studies have shown that both agoraphobia and panic disorder are more prevalent in patients with asthma than in the general population (Carr 1998; Goodwin & Pine 2002), and a 23% lifetime prevalence of spontaneous panic attacks has been reported in patients with asthma (Carr *et al.* 1994). The symptoms of panic attacks and pulmonary disease overlap, so that panic anxiety can reflect underlying cardiopulmonary disease and dyspnoea can reflect an underlying anxiety disorder.

The pathogenesis of panic may be related to respiratory physiology by several mechanisms:

- the anxiogenic effects of hyperventilation
- the catastrophic misinterpretation of episodic respiratory symptoms
- increased sensitivity of medullary chemoreceptors to carbon dioxide, lactate, or other signals of suffocation
- the possibility that patients with panic disorder have 'subclinical obstruction of lung airways' mediated through the airway's smooth muscle tone
- dysfunction of the autonomic nervous system, which regulates smooth muscle tone, may be responsible for both respiratory and panic symptoms with patients with panic disorder.

The theory that intermittent hypercapnia with obstructive pulmonary diseases may lead to increased locus ceruleus activity, causing panic and hyperventilation, is supported by the finding that exogenous CO_2 has been found to precipitate or worsen panic symptoms in most patients with panic disorder. But biological factors alone cannot be the sole cause; patients with panic disorder may be predisposed to catastrophize somatic sensations associated with respiratory illnesses and, consequently, may be much more concerned about the consequences of the respiratory symptoms, regardless of their severity, than patients without panic disorder (Carr 1998). A conditioning effect may occur in patients with panic disorder who experience frightening physical sensations during childhood respiratory illnesses. These patients may become conditioned to become anxious in response to the similar respiratory symptoms experienced as an adult. In support of this theory, the prevalence of childhood respiratory illnesses (40%) among patients with panic disorder is much higher than among patients with other psychiatric disorders.

Sleep-related disorders of breathing

Obstructive sleep apnoea (OSA) and its variants are now thought to impair the functioning of about 0.5–1% of the population. This is a sleep disruption syndrome that is due to a respiratory problem engendered by sleep itself. The main symptom is daytime sleepiness which can interfere with driving, work performance and home life. All psychiatrists should be familiar with this disorder, which often presents in middle-aged men complaining of increased daytime sleepinesss, worsening snoring with apnoeas. There may be a history of weight gain and fairly high alcohol intake and smoking. The possibility of OSA should be considered in any patient with hypertension and depression or unexplained fatigue who is receiving antihypertensive and antidepressant medication (Farney *et al.* 2004). Diagnosis is important because there is an effective treatment – nasal continuous positive airway pressure (NCPAP).

Dysfunctional breathing and hyperventilation

Abnormal breathing patterns have been recognized in medicine for many years (Baker 1934). A symptom complex characterized by unexplained breathlessness, chest pain and/or tightness, light-headedness, paraesthesiae and anxiety has been described in a variety of clinical situations and has been referred to as the hyperventilation syndrome (Bass 1997). Hyperventilation means breathing in excess of metabolic requirements, but there is disagreement whether hypocapnia is an essential diagnostic criterion, and some maintain that a normal $paCO_2$ does not exclude the syndrome (Howell 1997).

There has been considerable controversy over the last decade about the 'validity' of the hyperventilation syndrome, and some have suggested that the term be abolished (Hornsfled *et al.* 1997). However, others have challenged this and alternative terms have been suggested for the disorder, including behavioural breathlessness (Howell 1990), and more recently dysfunctional breathing (DB; Thomas *et al.* 2001).

Other abnormalities have been shown in patients with DB. These include unsteadiness of breathing in response to stimuli such as exercise and a period of voluntary over-breathing (Han *et al.* 1997), increased respiratory rate, abnormal orthostatic increases of respiratory gas exchange (Malmberg *et al.* 2000), predominantly intercostal respiratory effort, and frequent sighing (Thomas *et al.* 2001). The over-breathing aspect of the symptom complex may, however, be episodic and difficult to show with prolonged measurement of the end tidal or arterial carbon dioxide tension (Gardner *et al.* 1986). Furthermore, some symptoms associated with this syndrome have been shown to be unrelated to hypocapnia and may be mediated by other mechanisms (Howell 1997).

Diagnosis of DB can therefore be difficult; the characteristic symptoms are common to other diseases and there is no standard diagnostic test. This may lead to under-recognition of the effects of abnormal breathing patterns, and symptoms may be wrongly attributed to other causes, resulting in inappropriate investigations and ineffective treatment, specially in patients with coexisting lung disease (Thomas *et al.* 2001).

The significance of dysfunctional breathing in clinical practice

Dysfunctional breathing (which may include clinically significant hyperventilation) occurs in a wide variety of both physical and psychological disorders. These include not only lung diseases such as asthma (Demeter & Cordasco 1986) but also patients with chronic bronchitis whose breathlessness is disproportionate to their lung disease (Burns & Howell 1969).

Not surprisingly, DB has also been identified in patients with anxiety disorders (Abelson *et al.* 2001) and it is probable that a substantial proportion of patients with dysfunctional breathing have panic attacks (Davies *et al.* 2001). Dysfunctional breathing has also been identified in patients with functional cardiovascular syndromes (Gardner & Bass 1989) and chronic pain (Glynn *et al.* 1981; Wilhelm *et al.* 2001). It is important to identify DB because it can add to the 'symptom load' as well as contribute to disability in a wide variety of clinical situations. Another specific example is patients admitted to hospital (often under the care of neurology services) with unilateral physical symptoms with suspected cerebrovascular disease who are subsequently found to have symptoms attributable to over-breathing or hyperventilation (Blau *et al.* 1989; O'Sullivan *et al.* 1992).

Breathing retraining

Breathing retraining (BR) has been used for many years as a component for treatment not only for patients with anxiety disorders but also for those with lung disease such as asthma or COPD who have disproportionate symptoms and disability (Burns & Howell 1969). In a randomized controlled trial of outpatient pulmonary rehabilitation for patients with COPD, patients randomized to three months of outpatient breathing retraining and chest physiotherapy had a much better outcome in terms of perception of dyspnea, six-minute walking test and symptoms of dyspnoea and fatigue compared to patients receiving standard treatment. The authors concluded that an outpatient rehabilitation programme could achieve worthwhile benefits that persist for a period of two years (Guell *et al.* 2000).

De Guire *et al.* (1992) showed that BR was effective in patients with functional cardiovascular syndromes, and in a three-year follow-up study the same authors concluded that the treatment had lasting effects on respiratory physiology and was highly correlated with the reduction of reported functional cardiac symptoms (De Guire *et al.* 1996). In another study of breathing therapy in patients with hyperventilation syndrome (HVS) — most of the patients met criteria for an anxiety disorder — Han *et al.* (1996) showed that the improvement of the complaints was correlated mainly with the slowing down of breathing frequency. The favourable influence of breathing retraining on complaints appeared to be a consequence of its influence primarily on breathing frequency, rather than on levels of end-tidal CO_2.

Thomas *et al.* (2001) reported that one-third of women and one-fifth of men treated for asthma in a single general practice had symptoms suggestive of dysfunctional breathing. They hypothesized that these patients would show clinically relevant improvements in their quality of life as a result of breathing retraining. The authors carried out a randomized controlled trial comparing BR with asthma education (to control for non-specific effects of health professional attention) for asthmatic subjects in the community with symptoms suggestive of dysfunctional breathing. They found that over half the patients treated for asthma in the community who had symptoms suggestive of dysfunctional breathing showed a clinically relevant improvement in quality of life following a brief physiotherapy intervention, and that this improvement was maintained in over 25% six months after the intervention (Thomas *et al.* 2003).

If these findings are confirmed, breathing retraining may provide an opportunity to improve the well-being of a proportion of people treated for asthma in the community, although it may have implications for the provision of community physiotherapy services.

The utility of BR as a key therapeutic component of treatment in patients with panic disorder has been questioned however; rather, it has been suggested that the 'interoceptive exposure', i.e. repeated exposure to bodily sensations connected to the fear response, is relatively more potent compared with breathing control exercises aimed at slowing the respiratory rate (Craske *et al.* 1997; de Ruiter *et al.* 1989; Schmidt *et al.* 2000). Interoceptive exposure and training in cognitive reappraisal appear therefore to be the key therapeutic components of cognitive behavioural theory (CBT) in the treatment of panic disorder. Details about treatments for dysfunctional breathing, with and without panic attacks, can be found on the following websites: www.physiohypervent.org and www.nopanic.org.

Drug treatment in patients with lung disease

Buspirone should be considered as a first-line drug in respiratory patients with chronic anxiety. Several studies have shown buspirone to be as effective as benzodiazepines, such as diazepam, in relieving anxiety, although the onset may take two to four weeks. Benzodiazepine respiratory suppression occurs when subjects are awake as well as asleep; the latter may prolong sleep apnoeic episodes and may be dangerous. In general, in respiratory patients with acute anxiety, it is better to use a benzodiazepine with a short half-life, such as oxazepam, lorazepam, or temazepam, if buspirone is not the drug of choice, ineffective, or too slow to act. Respiratory depression may be less likely to resolve with these agents, and, if it does, the adverse effects can be reversed in a shorter interval. Zolpidem does not seem to have a negative impact on respiratory drive or pulmonary function tests in patients with COPD. Propranolol should be avoided in patients with COPD because it causes bronchoconstriction.

Antidepressants are frequently used to treat patients with chronic respiratory disease in lower doses for anxiety and standard doses for depression. Patients with compromised pulmonary function, especially COPD or sleep apnoea, should generally receive the less sedating antidepressants such as the tricyclic desipramine or the newer drug venlafaxine, which has a licence for the treatment of generalized anxiety disorder and is generally safe and well tolerated in most medically ill patients. Fluoxetine has been found to be a generally safe and effective antidepressant, and there have been no reports of adverse interactions with it and pulmonary medications. Sertraline surprisingly appears to have some antidyspnoeic effects (Smoller *et al.* 1998).

Protriptyline and tricyclic antidepressants are often used in patients with sleep apnoea because of their effect in suppressing rapid eye movement (REM) sleep.

REFERENCES

Abelson, J., Weg, J., Nesse, R., *et al.* (2001). Persistent respiratory irregularity in patients with panic disorder. *Biological Psychiatry*, **49**, 588–95.

Alloway, R. (1987). The buffer theory of social support; a review of the literature. *Psychological Medicine*, **17**, 91–108.

Baker, D. (1934). Sighing respiratory as a symptom. *Lancet*, **i**, 174–7.

Bass, C. (1997). Hyperventilation syndrome: a chimera? *Journal of Psychosomatic Research*, **42**, 421–6.

Barbey, J. and Roose, S. (1998). SSRI safety in overdose. *Journal of Clinical Psychiatry*, **59**(Suppl. 15), 42–8.

Berkman, L. F., Blumenthal, J., Burg, M., *et al.* (2003). Enhancing Recovery in Coronary Heart Disease Patients Investigators (ENRICHD). Effects of treating depression and low perceived social support on clinical events after myocardial infarction: the Enhancing Recovery in Coronary Heart Disease Patients (ENRICHD). *Journal of the American Medical Association*, **289**, 3106–16.

Blau, J., Wiles, C. and Solomon, F. (1989). Unilateral somatic symptoms due to hyperventilation. *British Medical Journal*, **286**, 1108.

Bosma, H., Marmot, M., Hemingway, H., *et al.* (1997). Low job control and risk of coronary heart disease in the Whitehall II (prospective cohort) study. *British Medical Journal*, **314**, 588–65.

Bosma, H., Peter, R., Siegrist, J., *et al.* (1998). Alternative job stress models and the risk of coronary heart disease: the effort–reward imbalance model and the job strain model. *American Journal of Public Health*, **88**, 68–74.

Brown, G. and Harris, T. (1999). *Life Events and Illness*. London: Guildford Press.

Bucher, H. C. (1994). Social support and prognosis following first angiocardial infarction. *Journal of General Internal Medicine*, **9**, 409–17.

Burns, B. and Howell, J. (1969). Disproportionately severe breathlessness in chronic bronchitis. *Quarterly Journal of Medicine*, **38**, 277–94.

Carr, R. (1998). Panic disorder and asthma: causes, effects and research implications. *Journal of Psychosomatic Research*, **44**, 43–52.

Carr, R. E., Lehrer, P., Rausch, L., *et al.* (1994). Anxiety sensitivity and panic attack in an asthmatic population. *Behaviour Research and Therapy*, **32**, 411–18.

Checkley, S. (1996). The neuroendocrinology of depression and chronic stress. *British Medical Bulletin*, **52**, 597–617.

Cooper, A., Lloyd, G., Weinman, J., *et al.* (1999). Why patients do not attend rehabilitation: role of intentions and illness beliefs. *Heart*, **82**, 234–6.

Craske, M., Rowe, M., Lewin, M., *et al.* (1997). Interoceptive exposure versus breathing retraining within cognitive behavioural therapy for panic disorder with agoraphobia. *British Journal of Clinical Psychology*, **36**, 85–99.

Creed, F. (1999). The importance of depression following myocardial infarction. *Heart*, **82**, 406–8.

Davies, S. J., Ghahramani, P., Jackson, P., *et al.* (1999). Association of panic disorder and panic attacks with hypertension. *American Journal of Medicine*, **107**, 310–16.

Davies, S., Jackson, P. and Ramsey, L. (2001). Dysfunctional breathing and asthma. Panic disorder needs to be considered. *British Medical Journal*, **323**, 631.

Davies, S., Jackson, P., Potokar, J., *et al.* (2004). Treatment of anxiety and depressive disorders in patients with cardiovascular disease. *British Medical Journal*, **328**, 939–43.

De Guire, S., Gervitz, R., Kawahara, Y., *et al.* (1992). Hyperventilation syndrome and the assessment of treatment for functional cardiac symptoms. *American Journal of Cardiology,* **70**, 673–7.

De Guire, S., Gervitz, R., Hawkinson, D., *et al.* (1996). Breathing retraining: a three year follow up study of treatment for hyperventilation syndrome and associated functional cardiac symptoms. *Biofeedback and Self Regulation,* **21**, 191–8.

de Ruiter, C., Ryken, H., Barssen, B., *et al.* (1989). Breathing retraining, exposure and a combination of both in the treatment of panic disorder with agoraphobia. *Behaviour Research and Therapy,* **27**, 647–55.

Demeter, S. and Cordasco, E. (1986). Hyperventilation syndrome and asthma. *American Journal of Medicine,* **81**, 989–94.

Department of Health. (2000). *National Service Framework for Coronary Heart Disease.* London: Department of Health.

Dickens, C. M., Percival, C., McGowan, L., *et al.* (2004a). The risk factors for depression in first myocardial infarction patients. *Psychological Medicine,* **34**, 1083–92.

Dickens, C. M., McGowan, L., Percival, C., *et al.* (2004b). Lack of a close confidant, but not depression, predicts further cardiac events after myocardial infarction. *Heart,* **90**, 518–22.

Dickens, C., McGowan, L., Percival, C., *et al.* (2005). Association between depressive episode before first myocardial infarction and worse cardiac failure following infarction. *Psychosomatics,* **46**, 523–8.

Empana, J. P., Sykes, D. H., Luc, G., *et al.*, PRIME Study Group. (2005). Contributions of depressive mood and circulating inflammatory markers to coronary heart disease in healthy European men: the Prospective Epidemiological Study of Myocardial Infarction (PRIME). *Circulation,* **111**, 2299–305.

Endicott, J. (1984). Measurement of depression in patients with cancer. *Cancer,* **53**, 2243–9.

Farney, R., Lugo, A., Jensen, R., *et al.* (2004). Simultaneous use of antidepressant and hypertensive medications increase the likelihood of diagnosis of obstructive sleep apnea syndrome. *Chest,* **125**, 1279–85.

Ford, D. E. and Mead, L. A. (1998). Depression is a risk factor for coronary artery disease in men: the precursors study. *Archives of Internal Medicine,* **158**, 1422–6.

Frasure-Smith, N., Lesperance, F., Prince, R., *et al.* (1991). Randomised trial of home-based psychological nursing intervention for patients recovering from myocardial infarction. *Lancet,* **350**, 473–9.

Frasure-Smith, N., Lesperance, F. and Talajic, M. (1995). Depression and 18 month prognosis after myocardial infarction. *Circulation,* **91**, 999–1005.

Gabbay, F. H., Krantz, D. S., Kop, W. J., *et al.* (1996). Triggers of myocardial ischaemia during daily life in patients with coronary artery disease: physical and mental activities, anger, and smoking. *Journal of the American College of Cardiology,* **27**, 585–92.

Gardner, W. N. and Bass, C. (1986). Hyperventilation in clinical practice. *British Journal of Hospital Medicine,* **41**, 73–81.

Gardner, W. N., Meah, M. and Bass, C. (1986). Controlled study of respiratory responses during prolonged measurement in patients with chronic hyperventilation. *Lancet,* **8511**, 826–30.

Glynn, C., Lloyd, J. and Folkhard, S. (1981). Ventilatory response to chronic pain. *Pain*, **11**, 201–11.

Goodwin, R. D. and Hamilton, S. P. (2002). Cigarette smoking and panic: the role of neuroticism. *American Journal of Psychiatry*, **159**, 1208–13.

Goodwin, R. D. and Pine, D. S. (2002). Respiratory disease and panic attacks among adults in the United States. *Chest*, **122**, 645–50.

Guell, R., Casan, P., Belda, J., *et al.* (2000). Long-term effects of out-patient rehabilitation of COPD: a randomised trial. *Chest*, **117**, 976–83.

Haines, A. P., Imeson, J. D. and Meade, T. W. (1987). Phobic anxiety and ischaemic heart disease. *British Medical Journal*, **295**, 297–9.

Han, J., Stegen, K., de Valck, C., *et al.* (1996). Influence of breathing therapy on complaints, anxiety and breathing pattern in patients with hyperventilation syndrome. *Journal of Psychosomatic Research*, **41**, 481–93.

Han, J., Stegen, K., Simkens, K., *et al.* (1997). Unsteadiness of breathing in patients with hyperventilation syndrome and anxiety disorders. *European Respiratory Journal*, **10**, 167–76.

Haynes, R., Sackett, D., Taylor, D., *et al.* (1978). Increased absenteeism from work after detection and labelling of hypertensive patients. *New England Journal of Medicine*, **299**, 741–4.

Hemingway, H. and Marmot, M. (1999). Psychosocial factors in the aetiology and prognosis of coronary heart disease: a systematic review of prospective studies. *British Medical Journal*, **318**, 1460–7.

Hippisley-Cox, J., Fielding, K. and Pringle, M. (1998). Depression as a risk factor for ischaemic heart disease in men: population based case-control study. *British Medical Journal*, **316**, 1714–18.

Hornsfeld, H., Garssen, B., Dop, M., *et al.* (1996). Double-blind placebo-controlled study of the hyperventilation provocation test and live validity of the hyperventilation syndrome. *Lancet*, **348**, 154–8.

Howell, J. B. (1990). Behavioural breathlessness. *Thorax*, **45**, 287–9

Howell, J. B. (1997). The hyperventilation syndrome: a syndrome under threat? *Thorax*, **52** (Suppl. 3), 530–4.

Isles, C. (2003). Prevalence, epidemiology, and pathophysiology of hypertension. In *Oxford Textbook of Medicine*, ed. D. Warrell, T. Cox, J. Firth, *et al.*, 4th edn. Oxford: Oxford University Press, pp. 1151–60.

Johnson, M., Foulkes, J., Johnson, D., *et al.* (1999). Impact on patients and partners of inpatient and extended cardiac counselling and rehabilitation: a controlled trial. *Psychosomatic Medicine*, **61**, 225–33.

Jones, D. and West, R. (1996). Psychological rehabilitation after myocardial infarction, multicentre randomised controlled trial. *British Medical Journal*, **313**, 1517–21.

Karajgi, B., Rifkin, A., Doddi, S., *et al.* (1990). The prevalence of anxiety disorders in patients with chronic obstructive pulmonary disease. *American Journal of Psychiatry*, **147**, 200–1.

Kuh, D. and Ben-Shlomo, Y. ed. (1997). *A Life-Course Approach to Chronic Disease Epidemiology*. Oxford: Oxford University Press.

Ladwig, K., Roll, G., Breithardt, G., *et al.* (1994). Post-infarction depression and incomplete recovery 6 months after acute myocardial infarction. *Lancet*, **343**, 20−3.

Lesperance, F. and Frasure-Smith, N. (1996). Negative emotions and coronary heart disease: getting to the heart of the matter. *Lancet*, **347**, 415−16.

Lewin, R., Roberson, I. H., Cay, E., *et al.* (1992). Effects of self-help post-myocardial infarction rehabilitation on psychological adjustment and use of health services. *Lancet*, **316**, 1036−40.

Lewin, R., Thompson, D. and Taylor, R. (2000). Cardiac rehabilitation. *European Heart Journal*, **21**, 860−1.

Lloyd, G. and Cawley, R. (1983). Distress or illness? A study of psychological symptoms after myocardial infarction. *British Journal of Psychiatry*, **142**, 120−5.

MacDonald, L., Sackett, D., Haynes, R., *et al.* (1984). Labelling in hypertension: a review of the behavioural and psychological consequences. *Journal of Chronic Disease*, **37**, 933−42.

MacNee, W. (2003). Chronic obstructive pulmonary disease. In *Oxford Textbook of Medicine*, ed. D. Warrell, T. Cox, J. Firth, *et al.*, 4th edn. Oxford: Oxford University Press, pp. 1377−96.

Mai, F. (1993). Psychiatric aspects of heart transplantation. *British Journal of Psychiatry*, **163**, 285−92.

Malmberg, L. P., Tamminen, K. and Sovijarvi, A. R. (2000). Orthostatic increase of respiratory gas exchange in hyperventilation syndrome. *Thorax*, **55**, 295−301.

Marmot, M. and Batley, M. (2002). Social class and coronary heart disease. In *Stress and the Heart*, ed. S. Stansfeld and M. Marmot. London: BMJ Books, pp. 5−19.

Martikainen, P. T. and Valkonen, T. (1996). Excess mortality of unemployed men and women during a period of rapidly increasing unemployment. *Lancet*, **348**, 909−12.

Mayou, R. (1984). Prediction of social and emotional outcome after heart attack. *Journal of Psychosomatic Research*, **28**, 17−25.

Mayou, R., Thompson, D., Clements, A., *et al.* (2002). Guideline-based early rehabilitation after myocardial infarction: a pragmatic randomised controlled trial. *Journal of Psychosomatic Research*, **52**, 89−95.

Miller, T. Q., Smith, T. W., Turner, C. W., *et al.* (1996). A meta-analytic review of research on hostility and physical health. *Psychological Bulletin*, **119**, 322−48.

Mittelman, M. A., McClure, M., Sherwood, J. B., *et al.* (1995). Triggering of acute myocardial infarction onset by episodes of anger. *Circulation*, **92**, 1720−5.

Morgan, A., Peck, D., Buchanan, D., *et al.* (1983). Psychological factors contributing to disproportionate disability in chronic bronchitis. *Journal of Psychosomatic Research*, **27**, 259−63.

Mosterd, A., Agestine, R. B., Silbershatz, H., *et al.* (1999). Trends in the prevalence of hypertension, antihypertensive therapy and left ventricular hypertrophy from 1950−1989. *New England Journal of Medicine*, **340**, 1221−7.

Musselman, D., Evans, D. and Nemeroff, C. (1998). The relationship of depression to cardiovascular disease. *Archives of General Psychiatry*, **55**, 580−92.

Ness, A. and Davey-Smith, G. (2003). The epidemiology of ischaemic heart disease. In *Oxford Textbook of Medicine*, ed. D. Warrell, T. Cox, J. Firth, *et al.*, 4th edn. Oxford: Oxford University Press, pp. 909−20.

O'Sullivan, G., Harvey, I., Bass, C., *et al.* (1992). Psychophysiological investigations of patients with unilateral symptoms in the hyperventilation syndrome. *British Journal of Psychiatry*, **161**, 664–7.

Petrie, K., Weinman, J., Sharpe, N., *et al.* (1996). Role of patients' view of their illness in predicting return to work and functioning after myocardial infarction: longitudinal study. *British Medical Journal*, **3112**, 1191–4.

Petrie, K., Cameron, L., Ellis, C., *et al.* (2002). Changing illness perceptions following myocardial infarction, an early intervention randomised controlled trial. *Psychosomatic Medicine*, **64**, 580–6.

Porzelius, J., Vest, M. and Nochomovitz, M. (1992). Respiratory function, cognitions, and panic in chronic obstructive pulmonary patients. *Behaviour Research and Therapy*, **30**, 75–7.

Rumsfeld, J. S., Jones, P. G., Whooley, M. A., *et al.* (2005). Depression predicts mortality and hospitalization in patients with myocardial infarction complicated by heart failure. *American Heart Journal*, **150**, 961–7.

Rutter, B. (1977). Some psychological concomitants of chronic bronchitis. *Psychological Medicine*, **7**, 459–64.

Rutter, B. (1979). The prognostic significance of psychological factors in the management of chronic bronchitis. *Psychological Medicine*, **9**, 63–70.

Scharloo, M., Kaptein, A., Weinman, J., *et al.* (2000). Physical and psychological correlates of functioning in patients with chronic obstructive pulmonary disease. *Journal of Asthma*, **37**, 17–29.

Schmidt, N., Woolaway-Bictel, K., Trakowski, J., *et al.* (2000). Dismantling cognitive behavioural treatment for panic disorder: questioning the utility of breathing retraining. *Journal of Consulting and Clinical Psychology*, **68**, 417–24.

Schneiderman, N., Saab, P. G., Catellier, D. J., *et al.* ENRICHD. (2004). Psychosocial treatment within sex by ethnicity subgroups in the Enhancing Recovery in Coronary Heart Disease clinical trial. *Psychosomatic Medicine*, **66**, 475–83.

Shimbo, D., Davidson, K. W., Haas, D. C., *et al.* (2005). Negative impact of depression on outcomes in patients with coronary artery disease: mechanisms, treatment considerations, and future directions. *Journal of Thrombosis & Haemostasis*, **3**, 897–908.

Smoller, J., Pollack, M., Systrom, D., *et al.* (1998). Sertraline effect on dyspnoea in patient with obstructive airway disease. *Psychosomatics*, **39**, 24–9.

Spinhoven, P., Ros, M., Westgeest, A., *et al.* (1994). The prevalence of respiratory disorders in panic disorder, major depressive disorder and V-code patients. *Behaviour Research and Therapy*, **32**, 647–9.

Spitzer, R., Williams, J., Sibbon, M., *et al.* (1992). The Structured Clinical Interview for DSM-III-R(SCID): history, rationale, and description. *Archives of General Psychiatry*, **49**, 624–9.

ten Brinke, A., Ouwerkerk, M., Zwinderman, A., *et al.* (2001). Psychopathology in patients with severe asthma is associated with increased heath care utilization. *American Journal of Respiratory Critical Care Medicine*, **163**, 1093–6.

Thomas, M., McKinley, R., Freeman, E., *et al.* (2001). Prevalence of dysfunctional breathing in patients treated for asthma in primary care; a cross sectional survey. *British Medical Journal*, **322**, 1098–100.

Thomas, M., McKinley, R., Freeman, E., *et al.* (2003). Breathing remaining for dysfunctional breathing in asthma; a randomised controlled trial. *Thorax*, **58**, 110–15.

Thompson, D. and Lewin, R. (2000). Coronary disease. Management of the post myocardial infarction patient: rehabilitation and cardiac neurosis. *Heart*, **84**, 101–5.

Thompson, D. R., Bowman, G. S., de Bono, D. P., *et al.* (1997). *Cardiac Rehabilitation: Guidelines and Audit Standards*. London: Royal College of Physicians.

Trumper, A. and Appleby, L. (2001). Psychiatric morbidity in patients undergoing heart, heart and lung, or lung transplantation. *Journal of Psychosomatic Research*, **50**, 103–5.

Verrier, R. L. and Mittelman, M. A. (1996). Life-threatening cardiovascular consequences of anger in patients with coronary artery disease. *Cardiology Clinics*, **14**, 289–307.

Whitehead, M. (1995). Tackling inequalities: a review of policy initiatives. In *Tackling Inequalities in Health: An Agenda for Action*, ed. M. Benzeval, K. Judge and M. Whitehead. London: Kings Fund.

Wihelm, F., Gevitz, R. and Rotts, W. (2001). Respiratory dysregulaton in anxiety, functional cardiac, and pain disorders. Assessment, phenomenology and treatment. *Behavior Modification*, **25**, 513–45.

Williams, R. (2002). Hostility, psychosocial risk factors, changes in brain serotonergic function, and heart disease. In *Stress and the Heart. Psychosocial Pathways to Coronary Heart Disease*, ed. S. Stansfeld and M. Marmot. London: BMJ Books, pp. 86–100.

Yellowlees, P., Alpers, J., Bowden, J., *et al.* (1987). Psychiatric morbidity in patients with chronic airflow obstruction. *Medical Journal of Australia*, **146**, 305–7.

Zaubler, T. and Katon, W. (1998). Panic disorder in the general medical setting. *Journal of Psychosomatic Research*, **44**, 25–42.

16

Gastrointestinal disorders

Elspeth Guthrie

Introduction

This chapter covers psychological issues and psychiatric morbidity in relation to diseases and conditions associated with the gastrointestinal (GI) tract. Both organic and so-called functional gastrointestinal disease states are considered. Chapter 17 covers psychiatric conditions associated with diseases of the liver.

Peptic ulcer disease

The term peptic ulcer refers to both gastric and duodenal ulcers. The epidemiology of peptic ulcer disease has changed dramatically over the last 20 years. Duodenal ulcer used to be 10 times as common in men as women and gastric ulcer had a male preponderance of 3:2. Now the difference in frequency between men and women is much less, largely because of *Helicobacter pylori* eradication. The annual age-standardized period prevalence of peptic ulceration in the UK decreased from 3.3 per 1000 in 1994 to 1.5 per 1000 in 1998 for men, and from 1.8 per 1000 to 0.9 per 1000 for women (Kang *et al.* 2002). Current trends are for a decreasing incidence in young men, with a rise in older women.

Important aetiological factors include *H. pylori*, non-steroidal anti-inflammatory drugs (NSAIDs), acid and pepsin. Other important factors include smoking, alcohol, bile acids, aspirin, steroids and stress.

The symptoms of peptic ulceration are very non-specific and diagnosis is unreliable on history alone. In uncomplicated cases there is often very little to find on examination. Treatment involves lifestyle changes including cessation of smoking and withdrawal of medication which may have caused the ulceration.

Handbook of Liaison Psychiatry, ed. Geoffrey Lloyd and Elspeth Guthrie. Published by Cambridge University Press. © Cambridge University Press 2007.

Helicobacter pylori eradication is implemented and acid suppression, using a proton pump inhibitor, is usually successful (69% of cases). Further management is outlined in the National Institute of Health and Clinical Excellence (NICE) guidelines (NICE 2005)

Prognosis is generally good if the underlying cause like *H. pylori* infection or drugs can be addressed, and the eradication of *H. pylori* has led to a very substantial decrease in the rate of recurrence of ulcers. However, peptic ulcers occur in 25% of patients who do not have *H. pylori*, and eradication with antibiotics does not always clear symptoms.

Peptic ulceration and psychological factors

Since the discovery that peptic ulceration was an infective disorder, there has been a decline in interest over the last 20 years in psychosocial aspects of the disease (Levenstein 2000). However, despite the obvious importance of *H. pylori*, psychosocial factors still play a role in the susceptibility of individuals to develop ulcers.

There is a clear association between peptic ulceration and anxiety (Rogers *et al.* 1994). Data from the National Comorbidity Survey (Kessler *et al.* 1994), a representative household survey of the adult population of the United States ($n = 8098$), have shown that generalized anxiety disorder (GAD) is associated with a significantly increased risk of self-reported peptic ulcer disease (PUD; odds ratio $= 2.8$, 95% confidence interval $= 1.4-5.7$; $p = 0.0002$), and there is a dose–response relationship between number of GAD symptoms (odds ratio $= 1.2$, 95% confidence interval $= 1.1-1.4$; $p = 0.001$) and increased risk of self-reported PUD (Goodwin *et al.* 2002). These associations remain after controlling for differences in sociodemographic characteristics and psychiatric and medical comorbidity between subjects.

Animal models have shown that stress induced in laboratory mammals can result in ulcer formation (Weiner 1991), and disturbances in attachment (early separation of the animal from its mother) alter the vulnerability of the animal's stomach to physical stress (Ackerman *et al.* 1975).

Longitudinal prospective studies have shown that depression and anxiety at baseline increase the risk of ulcer development over the next 9–15 years (Levenstein *et al.* 1995, 1997). Childhood physical abuse, sexual abuse and neglect are also associated with a statistically increased risk of peptic ulceration ($OR = 1.5$ (1.03, 2.2)), in addition to other physical conditions (Goodwin & Stein 2004). Acute severe stress in human beings, provoked by wars or earthquakes, can precipitate ulceration in susceptible individuals (Lam *et al.* 1995;

Aoyama *et al.* 1998). Once formed, psychosocial factors can impede recovery times in ulcer healing (Holtmann *et al.* 1992; Levenstein *et al.* 1996a) and contribute to a worse prognosis over several years (Levenstein *et al.* 1996b).

A biopsychosocial model is required to understand the relationship between psychological factors and stress. Central to the model is the idea that factors within the model can interact with each other, which in turn can then impact on another part of the causal pathway. For example, patients with a history of childhood abuse may develop an anxious and hypervigilant attitude to life. They may feel more stressed than others and as a result of this use alcohol, nicotine or other drugs to control anxiety. They are more susceptible to developing or experiencing painful symptoms than others, and may well use NSAIDs to control such symptoms. As adults they are more prone to develop stressful and violent relationships with partners which may (if animal models are to be believed) create a vulnerability to peptic ulceration via acute stress. The more alcohol they drink the greater the likelihood of peptic ulceration, and liver disease, which itself can cause peptic ulceration. Patients who drink or abuse other drugs are less likely to be compliant with any medication they may be given to treat the ulcer, or may continue to drink alcohol and smoke, increasing the risk of recurrence. Thus, psychosocial factors play a complex role in the development and maintenance of peptic ulceration.

In many cases, the risk factors for peptic ulceration (Box 16.1), have a behavioural component and are potential mediators in the aetiological matrix between stress and ulcer (Levenstein 2000).

There is little evidence, at present, that psychological treatments make a significant difference in patients with peptic ulcer disease although a small number of individual studies have explored the value of stress reduction (Han 2002). Treatment of any comorbid psychiatric conditions such as anxiety and depression should be carried out in those patients with peptic ulceration who report psychological symptoms.

Box 16.1 Risk factors for peptic ulcer which have a behavioural component.

Cigarette smoking

Heavy alcohol consumption

Lack of sleep

Not eating breakfast

Non-steroidal anti-inflammatory drugs

Hard on-the-job labour

Low socioeconomic status

Inflammatory bowel disease

The two main forms of inflammatory bowel disease are Crohn's disease and ulcerative colitis. Crohn's disease is a chronic inflammatory disorder that can affect the small intestine and/or the large intestine. Inflammation, which may or may not be accompanied by non-caseating granulomas, extends through all layers of the gut wall to involve adjacent mesentery and lymph nodes. The inflammatory process is frequently discontinuous, with normal bowel separating portions of diseased bowel.

Ulcerative colitis affects the colonic mucosa from the rectum to the cecum. It is a chronic disease characterized by rectal bleeding and diarrhoea, and given to remissions and exacerbations. Most of the histological features of the disease may be seen in other inflammatory states of the colon, such as those caused by bacteria or parasites. Since the inflammatory process in ulcerative colitis is confined to the mucosa (unlike Crohn's disease), sharp localized abdominal pain, perforation and fistula formation are uncommon in ulcerative colitis, whereas they are frequent features of Crohn's disease. Bleeding per rectum, however, is common in ulcerative colitis but not in Crohn's.

Prevalence

Crohn's disease occurs throughout the world, with a prevalence of 10–100 cases per 100 000 people. Ulcerative colitis is slightly more common with a prevalence of 35–100 per 100 000 people. In recent years, there has been an unexplained, dramatic increase in the incidence of Crohn's disease in North America and Europe, whereas the incidence rates of ulcerative colitis have remained fairly stable in the West. Inflammatory bowel disease was traditionally considered rare in the Asian Pacific region, but recent evidence suggests that both Crohn's disease and ulcerative colitis are becoming increasingly common in this region. Each year 5000 people develop ulcerative colitis in the UK and in total inflammatory bowel diseases affect approximately 1 in 500 people in the UK.

Psychological factors

There is a long history and, by now, a large amount of research regarding a connection between psychological and somatic factors and chronic inflammatory bowel disease (IBD). The prevalence of psychological problems in IBD varies between 21 and 35%. This is three to four times higher than comparable rates in the general population but lower than that found in patients with functional gastrointestinal disease (Walker *et al.* 1996). The prevalence of anxiety and depression in IBD is comparable to levels of morbidity found in other chronic physical disease states, and there is substantial evidence that the stress of the disease itself results in psychological distress. Higher disease activity in IBD is associated with more severe depressive symptoms (North *et al.* 1991), and more severe anxiety symptoms (Porcelli *et al.* 1994). Greater disease activity is associated with a greater experience of stress (Duffy *et al.* 1991) and poorer quality of life (Guthrie *et al.* 2002).

There is also, however, some evidence that psychosocial factors can affect the disease process in IBD. In the last 15 years there have been seven prospective studies which have examined the relationship between stress and IBD (Bitton *et al.* 2003; Duffy *et al.* 1991; Garrett *et al.* 1991; Levenstein *et al.* 2000; Mardini *et al.* 2004; Mittermaier *et al.* 2004; North *et al.* 1991; Table 16.1).

Three of these studies found that depression scores at baseline or perceived stress were predictive of relapse or worsening of disease, several months later (Levenstein *et al.* 2000; Mardini *et al.* 2004; Mittermaier *et al.* 2004). In the study by Mittermaier and colleagues (2004), 28% of patients were depressed at baseline and 59% experienced at least one relapse in their IBD during a period of 18 months of follow-up. Depression at baseline was significantly correlated with the time to a recurrence of IBD. In the study by Levenstein and colleagues (2000) baseline depression did not predict subsequent relapse but being in the high tertile for stress, at baseline, tripled the rate of subsequent exacerbation of colitis both in the medium term (six to eight months) and the long term (up to five years).

The four other studies found no evidence of an association between psychosocial factors at baseline and subsequent disease relapse (Bitton *et al.* 2003; Duffy *et al.* 1991; Garrett *et al.* 1991; North *et al.* 1991).

Table 16.1. Longitudinal, prospective cohort studies of psychosocial factors and disease process in IBD.

Study	Population	*n*	Duration of study period (months)	Association between baseline stress and subsequent relapse or disease activity
Garrett *et al.* (1991)	Crohn's	10	1	Nil
North *et al.* (1991)	IBD	85	3	Nil
Duffy *et al.* (1991)	IBD	130	3	Nil
Levenstein *et al.* (2000)	Ulcerative colitis	62	6 and <45	Positive for perceived stress
Bitton *et al.* (2003)	Ulcerative colitis	60	18	Minor association with stressful event
Mardini *et al.* (2004)	Crohn's	18		Positive for depression
Mittermaier *et al.* (2004)	IBD	60		Positive for depression

There are methodological problems with all the studies discussed above, but this is a difficult area to research and there are many confounding factors. Relapse is difficult to define in IBD, and Crohn's disease and ulcerative colitis are separate conditions, although they are often studied together. Both conditions have a varied presentation, so the experience of illness even within the same condition (either Crohn's disease or ulcerative colitis) may be very different. Most of the studies are relatively small and are underpowered. Finally causal relationships are difficult to disentangle because of the complex way different factors may interact with each other (e.g. smoking and stress). Thus, the evidence at present that stress actually affects the disease process in IBD is equivocal.

In recent years, there has been increased interest in the role of attachment and its developmental contribution to stress and disease. Abnormal attachment styles have been identified in patients who present with medically unexplained symptoms and have been implicated in the mechanisms that underlie poor control of chronic disease states (Ciechanowski *et al.* 2004).

Maunder (2005) has developed a model which describes paths by which problems with attachment may contribute to the disease process. He postulates that insecure attachment may be associated with disturbances of stress regulation, the use of external regulators of affect (e.g. alcohol use, eating behaviour, etc.) and non-use of protective behaviours (e.g. help-seeking, social support, treatment adherence and symptom attention). These mechanisms may be of particular relevance in patients with chronic illness and influence the management and outcome of the condition.

In relation to ulcerative colitis, a recent study suggests that those patients who are most likely to suffer from depression, when the disease becomes active, are ones that report greatest degrees of attachment anxiety. Thus attachment style appears to act as a moderator of the relationship between disease activity and depressive symptoms (Maunder *et al.* 2005). It is likely that more work in relation to attachment styles and their role in chronic illness will be carried out in the next few years.

Psychological treatment and self management

There have been eight randomized controlled trials of psychological interventions in inflammatory bowel disease (Milne *et al.* 1986; Shaw & Ehrlich 1987; Schwarz & Blanchard 1991; Larsson *et al.* 2003; Garcia-Vega & Fernandez-Rodriguez 2004; Keller *et al.* 2004; Bregenzer *et al.* 2005 and Elsenbruch *et al.* 2005). The studies are difficult to compare as they have focused on different populations of patients. Four have included mixed groups of Crohn's and ulcerative colitis patients in the same study; two focused on patients with Crohn's disease and two focused on patients with ulcerative colitis. The main results of the studies are summarized in Table 16.2.

Although some of the smaller studies showed some evidence of benefit for psychological treatments (Milne *et al.* 1986; Shaw & Ehrlich 1987), the larger studies with better methodology reported no major effects for psychological therapies either on the outcome of the disease process itself in IBD or on stress or emotional symptoms (Keller *et al.* 2004; Bregenzer *et al.* 2005).

A further open trial of psychological therapy for persons with inflammatory bowel disease by a respected group of researchers in North America showed no major effects of the treatment on either IBD or anxiety or depression (Maunder & Esplen 2001).

Table 16.2. Randomized controlled trials in which the effects of psychological interventions have been evaluated in inflammatory bowel disease (IBD).

Study	n	Type of IBD	Active intervention	Outcome
Milne *et al.* (1986)	40	IBD	Stress management	Improvement in IBD symptoms and stress
Shaw & Ehrlich (1987)	40	Ulcerative colitis	Relaxation training vs. attention	Reduction in pain in relaxation group
Schwarz & Blanchard (1991)	20	IBD	Cognitive behavioural therapy (CBT) vs. symptom monitoring	CBT group worse in both IBD symptoms and stress
Larsson *et al.* (2003)	49	Anxious IBD patients	Group-based education	No difference between groups
Garcia-Vega & Fernandez-Roderiguez (2004)	45	Crohn's disease	Stress management vs. self-directed stress management	Both intervention groups reported reduced tiredness and abdominal pain
Keller *et al.* (2004)	108	Crohn's disease	Psychotherapy	Trend for fewer surgeries in psychotherapy group post-treatment but no major differences in outcome
Bregenzer *et al.* (2005)	145	IBD	Education including stress management	No difference between groups either in knowledge, stress or outcome
Elsenbruch *et al.* (2005)	30	Ulcerative colitis	Stress management and self-care	Better quality-of-life scores for intervention group compared to controls

Only one of the above studies targeted patients with IBD who also had comorbid psychological symptoms (Larsson *et al.* 2003), but despite this, there was no evidence of any particular benefit for patients with psychological symptoms from a psychological intervention. It must be concluded that the generalized use of psychological treatments in IBD is not supported by the research findings. It remains to be established whether psychological treatments are of benefit in the treatment of IBD patients with comorbid psychiatric illness.

There is some recent evidence that self-management may be a cost-effective intervention for patients with inflammatory bowel disease (Kennedy *et al.* 2004), although this does not involve any specific psychological interventions.

Gastro-oesophageal reflux disease

Gastro-oesophageal reflux disease (GORD) is associated with a range of symptoms including heartburn, acid regurgitation and dysphagia which may or may not be accompanied by evident oesophagitis. Health-related quality of life in GORD is lower than in the general population regardless of evidence of oesophagitis (Wiklund 2004). Many patients report disturbed sleep, reduced energy, generalized body pain, impaired sexual dysfunction and anxiety about the underlying cause of their symptoms.

There is some evidence to support a psychosocial link to GORD although it is relatively weak. This area has been authoritatively reviewed by Olden (2004). There is evidence that there is a link between non-cardiac chest pain and panic disorder, and patients who seek treatment for GORD symptoms may have greater evidence of psychiatric disturbance than those who do not.

Gastro-oesophageal reflux disease is treated using proton pump inhibitors which are successful in the majority of cases. Further research is required to identify whether psychosocial factors play a mediating role in predicting response to treatment.

Functional gastrointestinal disorders

Gastrointestinal symptoms which have no underlying structural cause have been termed 'functional' symptoms. A range of functional gastrointestinal disorders have been defined and delineated by an international group of experts. The different disorders are shown in Table 16.3 according to 'Rome II' criteria, which were published in 1999 (Drossman *et al.* 1999a). A new updated revision of the Rome criteria is due to be published in the near future (Rome III).

Table 16.3. Functional gastrointestinal disorders.

Oesophageal disorders	Globus
	Rumination syndrome
	Functional chest pain or presumed oesophageal origin
	Functional heartburn
	Functional dysphagia
	Unspecified functional oesophageal disorder
Gastroduodenal disorders	Functional dyspepsia
	Ulcer-like dyspepsia
	Dysmotility-like dyspepsia
	Unspecified (non-specific) dyspepsia
	Aerophagia
	Functional vomiting
Bowel disorders	Irritable bowel syndrome
	Functional abdominal bloating
	Functional constipation
	Functional diarrhoea
	Unspecified functional abdominal disorder
	Functional abdominal pain syndrome
	Unspecified functional abdominal pain
Biliary disorders	Gall-bladder dysfunction
	Sphincter of Oddi dysfunction
Anorectal disorders	Functional faecal incontinence
	Functional anorectal pain
	Pelvic floor dyssynergia

In relation to most of the conditions, to make a diagnosis, symptoms must be present for at least 12 weeks out of the previous year. By definition, the aetiology of these syndromes is unknown but it is best conceptualized by a biopsychosocial model (Figure 16.1), in which biological, physiological, psychological and environmental factors each make a contribution to the development and persistence of symptoms in an individual. There is much overlap between some of these conditions (e.g. irritable bowel syndrome) and other functional somatic syndromes such as chronic fatigue syndrome, fibromyalgia, and chronic pelvic pain, and their validity as discrete disorders with aetiologies located in the gastrointestinal tract is unproven. However, the diagnostic groupings have aided consistency and standardization in research.

The two most common functional gastrointestinal disorders are irritable bowel syndrome and functional dyspepsia, and most work in relation to psychological factors has been carried out on individuals with these two conditions.

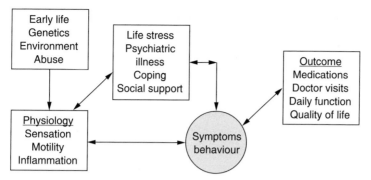

Figure 16.1. A biopsychosocial model for functional bowel disease (adapted from Drossman *et al.* 1999b).

Table 16.4. Diagnostic criteria for irritable bowel syndrome and functional dyspepsia.

Irritable bowel syndrome

At least 12 weeks, which need not be consecutive, in the preceding 12 months, of abdominal
   discomfort or pain that has two of three features:

• relieved with defaecation

• onset associated with a change in frequency of stool; and/or

• onset associated with a change in form of stool

Functional dyspepsia

At least 12 weeks, which need not be consecutive, in the preceding 12 months, of:

• persistent or recurrent dyspepsia (pain or discomfort in the upper abdomen)

• no evidence of organic disease that is likely to explain the symptoms

• no evidence that dyspepsia is exclusively relieved by defaecation or associated with the onset of
   a change in stool frequency or stool form (i.e. not irritable bowel).

Source: Adapted from Drossman *et al.* (1999a).

The diagnostic criteria (according to Rome II) for irritable bowel syndrome and functional dyspepsia are shown in Table 16.4. Individuals with irritable bowel syndrome complain of abdominal pain, bloating and altered bowel habit and individuals with functional dyspepsia complain of upper abdominal pain. There is much overlap between the conditions and patients can switch from one condition to the other over time.

Prevalence

A systematic review of dyspepsia in the community found that the prevalence is between 11.5 and 14.7% (El-Serag & Talley 2004). However, of 22 studies reviewed, only 2 provided sufficient information to calculate the prevalence of functional dyspepsia. The prevalence of uninvestigated dyspepsia was 10–40%.

Of those individuals with dyspepsia who receive an endoscopy, about 40% have functional or non-ulcer dyspepsia, 40% have gastro-oesophageal reflux and 13% have ulcer disease. Gastric cancer is found in just 2% with oesophageal cancer in a further 1%.

El-Serag and Talley (2004) found 13 studies which examined the clinical course of the condition. There was wide variation in the duration of follow-up (1.5–10 years for prospective studies and 5–27 years for retrospective studies). At least half the patients in 10 out of 13 studies, and two-thirds of patients in 6 studies, reported that they recovered (i.e. became asymptomatic).

Using Rome II criteria, the prevalence of irritable bowel syndrome has been estimated to be about 12% (Thompson *et al.* 2002). Approximately twice as many women than men report symptoms of either IBS or functional dyspepsia.

Two well-conducted epidemiologic surveys have been published on American samples in the last 10 years: the Olmsted County Study, by Talley *et al.* (1991a), and the US Householder Survey of Functional Gastrointestinal Disorders, by Drossman *et al.* (1993).

In the Olmsted County Study, an age- and sex-stratified sample ($n = 1021$) of the residents of Olmsted County, Minnesota, between the ages of 30 and 64 were sent a validated self-report questionnaire that identified GI symptoms experienced over the past year, thus leading to valid diagnoses of functional GI disorders. Altogether, 835 individuals (82%) returned usable surveys. Of these, 26% reported abdominal pain more than six times in the past year, 17.9% reported chronic diarrhoea, and 17.4% chronic constipation. Talley *et al.* (1991a) found an overall prevalence of IBS of 17.0% (range $= 14.4–19.6$; 95% confidence interval), with women outnumbering men 1.15 to 1.0. Of the 329 individuals with functional GI disorders, only 14% ($n = 46$) had seen a physician in the past year because of GI symptoms. In a second, larger study ($n = 4108$) with a larger age range (20–95) that tapped the same geographical area, Talley *et al.* (1995) found a prevalence rate of IBS of 17.7%, with women outnumbering men 1.44 to 1.0. Using available data, they estimated the medical costs of IBS to be $8 billion a year in the United States.

In the US Householder Survey, Drossman *et al.* (1993) surveyed by questionnaire 8250 US households, stratified to be similar to the makeup of the United States on geographic region, age, and household size. The return rate was 65.8% (51% female, 96% white). Overall, 69.3% of respondents acknowledged one or more functional GI disorders. According to Rome criteria, IBS was diagnosed in 606 individuals (11.2%), leading to a national estimate of prevalence of 9.4%. The sex ratio was 1.88 to 1 (female:male). It is interesting to note that IBS sufferers had missed an average of 13.4 days of work or school in the past year owing to IBS and other causes.

Health-related quality of life

A systematic review of health-related quality of life in IBS concluded that there is evidence of decreased health-related quality of life in patients with moderate to severe irritable bowel syndrome (El-Serag *et al.* 2002). The degree of severity is comparable to other chronic disorders such as GORD and depression. Both abdominal pain and psychological symptoms are independently associated with impaired health related quality of life in patients with severe IBS (Creed *et al.* 2001). In the Drossman and colleagues study (1993) it was established that IBS affects 19–34 million American adults, and costs almost $10 billion in medical care and leads to possibly 250 million lost work or school days per year. Even in primary care, the costs of IBS can be considerable (Akehurst *et al.* 2002).

Proposed pathophysiological mechanisms

A variety of different pathophysiological mechanisms have been explored including abnormal gut motility, visceral hypersensitivity, inflammation and brain–gut interactions. Stress appears to play a role in several of these different mechanisms (Monnikes *et al.* 2001). Many, but not all, patients with irritable bowel syndrome have an increased gut sensitivity to pain, which in turn is correlated with emotional status (Guthrie *et al.* 2004). The mechanism which underlies rectal hypersensitivity is unclear but could relate to altered receptor activity in the gut itself, or increased excitability of the spinal cord neurones, or altered central modulation of sensation in the brain. Women who have been sexually abused appear to have particular sensitivity to rectal distension (Whitehead *et al.* 1997). Inflammation appears to play a role in the development of some gastrointestinal functional disorders by peripheral sensitization. Approximately one-third of patients who present with an acute enteric infection will go on to develop irritable bowel syndrome-like symptoms (Gwee *et al.* 1999). The role of the central nervous system (CNS) in modulating gut activity and pain response has received specific attention in recent years with the development of positron emission tomography and other methods of imaging the brain and its function. There is some evidence to suggest that CNS response to rectal distension is altered in patients with IBS compared to controls (Mayer 2000).

Psychological factors

Severe life events have been shown to precipitate the onset of functional bowel disorders (Drossman *et al.* 1999b) and chronic life stress and difficulties impede the chances of recovery in patients with chronic irritable bowel syndrome (Bennett *et al.* 1998) and heartburn (Naliboff *et al.* 2004). In a recent well-conducted nested case-control study, psychosocial factors were clearly linked to individuals with functional gastrointestinal symptoms in the community (Locke *et al.* 2004).

The exact relationship between psychological symptoms and functional gastrointestinal disorders is unclear. In patients who develop an enteric infection, those with raised levels of anxiety and depression are more likely to develop irritable bowel syndrome in the subsequent weeks than those who are not psychologically distressed (Gwee *et al.* 1999). In addition, patients who develop functional gastrointestinal disorders are more likely to have a past history of psychiatric disorder than patients with organic gastrointestinal disorder. Thus, psychological factors play an important role in the development of certain functional gastrointestinal disorders, together with other physiological factors, and, as yet, other unidentified mechanisms.

Psychiatric disorder has been consistently found to be raised in patients with functional gastrointestinal disease in comparison with organic controls. The prevalence of psychiatric disorder in outpatients with irritable bowel syndrome varies from approximately 40 to 60%, whereas the rates of psychiatric disorder in organic controls is approximately 25%. Treatment-seeking appears to be linked to both the severity of an individual's physical symptoms and to associated psychological factors.

The most common forms of psychiatric disorder that occur in relation to functional abdominal disorders are mood disorders (major depression and dysthymic disorder), anxiety disorders (generalized anxiety disorder and panic disorder), and somatoform disorders (hypochondriasis and somatization disorder). No specific disorder has been uniquely associated with functional gastrointestinal disease. The presence of certain psychiatric disorders such as depression, panic disorder and neurasthenia predicts a poor outcome (Creed *et al.* 2005).

In a systematic review, Henningsen and colleagues (2003) identified 25 studies of irritable bowel syndrome in which patients with IBS had been compared to a healthy control group in terms of either symptoms of anxiety or depression. Patients with IBS were found to be significantly more depressed and anxious than healthy controls (effect size 0.8; confidence interval 0.56–1.04; $p < 0.0001$).

Even within the group of patients who have severe IBS, it is possible that there are different symptom clusters. Guthrie and colleagues (2003) found three distinct subgroups of patients with severe IBS: a group who had low distension thresholds, complex psychiatric problems, a history of abuse and frequent visits to the doctor; a group with high distension thresholds and low levels of psychiatric morbidity; and a third group with low distension thresholds, moderate levels of psychiatric disorder but low rates of abuse and low-to-moderate doctor consultation. The marked differences between the groups suggest that each may have a different pathogenesis and respond to different treatment approaches.

Patients with irritable bowel syndrome report high rates of childhood physical and sexual abuse (30–56%) (Drossman *et al.* 1995). Although initial studies were carried out in tertiary referral centres in the USA, other studies from Europe and Australia, carried out in different settings, have reported similar findings. The highest rates of sexual abuse are found in patients attending tertiary referral centres. High rates of sexual abuse have also been reported in other chronic pain syndromes, so the findings are not specific to functional gastrointestinal disease. See Figure 16.2.

Patients with functional gastrointestinal disease and an abuse history report more severe pain, greater psychological distress, poorer quality of life and more doctor visits than people without such a history. It is possible that some forms of childhood abuse may actually result in altered physiological gut function, but in general the impact of childhood sexual abuse appears to have most effect on the outcome of the disorder. This may be mediated by a variety of other factors including concurrent psychiatric disorder, poor coping strategies, lack of social support, impaired adult relationships (Biggs *et al.* 2004), and a tendency to catastrophize relationships.

Raised levels of neuroticism and anxiety traits have been reported in patients with functional gastrointestinal disorders compared to controls, but there is no specific personality profile. Recent work from two separate research groups suggests that patients with irritable bowel syndrome may have problems with assertiveness (Ali *et al.* 2000; Lackner & Gurtman 2005).

Intergenerational transmission of irritable bowel syndrome and other functional gastrointestinal disorders has been reported (Levy *et al.* 2000). The evidence

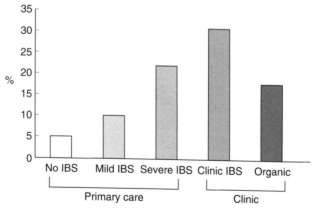

Figure 16.2. Prevalence of abuse history in functional GI disorders.

for a strong genetic component is relatively weak although there is a modest contribution (Levy *et al.* 2001). Children of adult IBS patients make more healthcare visits per year than children of parents who do not have IBS (Levy *et al.* 2004). Social reinforcement and modelling play an important role in the development and maintenance of symptoms in children. There is some evidence that reinforcement and modelling of bowel illness behaviour during childhood is higher in parents with IBS than in asymptomatic parent groups (Whitehead *et al.* 1994).

Treatment

Treatment issues are covered in detail in Chapter 34. However, both psychological interventions and antidepressants are helpful in IBS and other functional disorders. The evidence is stronger for IBS than other functional gastrointestinal disorders, as there have been far fewer treatment trials of psychological or psychotropic drugs involving the other functional gastrointestinal disorders. There have been five systematic reviews in IBS and one in functional dyspepsia. They are listed in Table 16.5. The evidence suggests that both psychological treatments and tricyclic antidepressants are of value in IBS. Two recent large studies of psychological treatment and antidepressant treatment in patients with chronic and severe IBS have recently been published (Creed *et al.* 2003; Drossman *et al.* 2003). Both showed little evidence of a major impact on patients' symptoms but there was evidence that the psychological treatments that were evaluated (cognitive behavioural therapy (CBT) in the Drossman *et al.* study; and psychodynamic-interpersonal therapy in the Creed *et al.* 2003 study) resulted in a major improvement in quality of life. Antidepressant treatment (a tricyclic antidepressant in the Drossman *et al.* study; and an SSRI in the Creed *et al.* study) also produced improved quality of life. There is evidence from the Creed *et al.* study that the psychotherapy was particularly helpful for patients with a history of abuse and it resulted in significant cost savings. Psychological treatment also improved rectal distension tolerance thresholds and this improvement was mediated by improvements in depression but not abdominal pain (Guthrie *et al.* 2004).

When treating depression with antidepressants it is important to remember that therapeutic effects can be delayed, and when using antidepressants to treat pain syndromes a similar delay can be expected. There is as yet insufficient evidence to conclude that selective serotonin reuptake inhibitors (SSRIs) are as effective as tricyclic antidepressants in treating pain syndromes associated with IBS. This may reflect the relatively small number of studies evaluating SSRIs in IBS that have been conducted, in comparison to those in which tricyclic antidepressants have been evaluated.

Table 16.5. Systematic reviews regarding psychological and psychotropic interventions in functional gastrointestinal disorders.

Study	Condition	Intervention	Number of studies	Conclusions
Brandt *et al.* (2002)	IBS	Antidepressants	32 RCTs	Bowel symptoms improved with most tricyclic antidepressants but not amitriptyline
El-Serag *et al.* (2002)	IBS	CBT	1 RCT	Significant positive changes in quality of life
Soo *et al.* (2004)	Functional dyspepsia	Psychological therapies	3 RCTs	All interventions improved bowel symptoms
Akehurst (2002)	IBS	Psychotropic medication	2 RCTs	Amineptine improved depressed mood
Jailwala *et al.* (2000)	IBS	Psychotropic medication	7 RCTs	Amitriptyline, nortriptyline and desipramine of benefit for bowel symptoms
Talley *et al.* (1991b)	IBS	Psychological treatments	14 studies	Psychological therapy superior to control for bowel symptoms in eight studies

Some studies report improvement in individual bowel symptoms whereas others report global change. The doses used have been smaller than those used to treat depression and benefit has been demonstrated in patients who are not depressed. Because of the antimuscarinic receptor effects of tricyclic antidepressants, they seem to be most effective in patients with diarrhoea-predominant IBS; however, it does not preclude their use in patients with constipation (Wald 2002). There is some evidence that tricyclic antidepressants raise visceral pain thresholds in IBS (Riberdy-Poitras *et al.* 2000).

In a useful review of the role of antidepressants in IBS, Wald (2002) has recommended that for IBS with predominant diarrhoea and pain, tricyclic antidepressants be considered (provided there is no evidence of a risk of self-harm). Doses should be started as low as 10 mg and increased as tolerated. For patients with constipation predominant IBS, an SSRI may be started in low doses and increased.

Chronic pancreatitis

The four cardinal manifestations of chronic pancreatitis (CP) are recurrent or protracted abdominal pain, diabetes, steatorrhea, and pancreatic calculi. Pain is the initial manifestation of CP and is the major reason for patients with CP to seek medical attention. The intractable pain associated with the condition is quite debilitating and disrupts lifestyle. It can lead to functional incapacity, drug and alcohol dependency, and a drug-seeking behaviour, as the patient becomes addicted to opiates and their pain relieving effect diminishes (Pitchumoni 1998). There is however very little research into the long-term psychosocial sequelae of chronic pancreatitis.

It is unusual for patients with CP not to have pain, with only about 5–10% of patients actually pain free. Lack of pain is a feature of the late-onset idiopathic CP, and painless CP may also be a stage late in the natural history of alcoholic pancreatitis after years of painful disease when the pancreas is 'burned-out' and not functional.

The onset of the persistent abdominal pain 12–48 hours after a drinking bout or 'on the afternoon after the night before' is said to be characteristic of alcoholic pancreatitis, but exacerbation of pain may occur even during abstinence from alcohol with no identifiable cause.

Management of pain in CP is a team approach. The gastroenterologist, a surgeon, a radiologist, and a psychiatrist should work together to achieve success. The aims should be treatment and management of the condition itself; control of pain; and treatment of any associated alcohol or drug addiction, depression or anxiety. The psychiatrist is unlikely to be involved in the first of these aims but can make an important contribution to the latter two aims.

The rate of pain relief is usually higher in patients who are abstinent from alcohol, and deterioration of pancreatic function is slower. The importance of alcohol abstention thus cannot be overemphasized. Considerable time should be spent in discussing with the patient and making him or her understand the inevitable progression of disease if alcohol use is continued. The help of a psychiatrist or other alcohol agencies or a hospital-based alcohol counsellor is often necessary.

Cigarette smoking is noted to be an associated factor in the pathogenesis of CP; it is prudent to advise against smoking. Most alcoholics who develop CP are heavy cigarette smokers.

The severity of pain is variable in CP and it can be difficult to assess the degree of pain in patients with this condition, as many have a prior history of addiction to alcohol and/or narcotics. Dependency upon opioids is of major concern, and some patients may show elements of drug-seeking behaviour in the form of exaggerated complaints of pain. However, in patients with a previous addiction to narcotics, tolerance to the analgesic effects of these drugs may occur, so that they require higher doses than would normally be expected. A liaison psychiatrist can help with the assessment of such patients and provide advice about withdrawal regimes in patients who are dependent upon opioids.

Stomas

Approximately 13 500 people undergo stoma formation every year in the UK (Baxter & Salter 2000). The most common underlying conditions resulting in the need for stoma surgery are colorectal (bowel) cancer, bladder cancer, ulcerative colitis and Crohn's disease. Inflammatory bowel diseases are the most common reasons for ileostomy formation.

Stoma formation can result in psychological morbidity (Nugent *et al.* 1999), although most people will adapt positively to their stoma. Brown and Randle (2005) recently conducted a systematic review of the psychosocial consequences of 'living with a stoma'. Stoma formation usually has a negative impact on quality of life and lifestyle in a number of ways. Nugent and colleagues (1999) conducted a postal questionnaire on 542 stoma patients (72% response rate). Twenty per cent of colostomists and 15% of ileostomists reported problems with work due to their stoma, 10% reported problems with diet and over 40% of both colostomists and ileostomists reported problems with sexual function.

A quality study by Persson and Hellstrom (2002) involving Swedish men and women 6–12 weeks post-surgery after ostomy described a variety of psychological issues. These included a sense of alienation from their bodies, lower self-confidence and self-respect, feelings of disgust and shock, altered body image and a negative effect on sexual life. Other important, non-psychological issues were physical problems to do with the stoma itself; influence on sport and leisure activities, and influence on social life.

Other emotional reactions to a stoma include hate, repulsion, embarrassment, devastation and unacceptance. Sexual problems appear to be common and nearly all stomatists report that they view themselves as less sexually attractive following formation of the stoma. This view does not appear to be shared by their partners.

Bekkers and colleagues (1997) conducted a four-year follow-up study comparing the psychosocial adjustment of stoma patients with bowel-resected non-stoma patients. The researchers found that both groups reported a similar level of psychosocial adjustment four years post-surgery. Higher income was associated with a better adjustment for both groups of patients.

The evidence suggests that patients may require help with their initial emotional responses to stoma formation and that long-term sexual problems and body image problems may need addressing.

Specialist stoma nurses play an important role and can help patients adjust cognitively and emotionally to their stomas (O'Connor 2005). Specialist stoma nurses are also best placed to identify persistent psychosocial problems which may need referral to liaison psychiatry services.

Gastrointestinal cancer

Many different forms of cancer can affect the gastrointestinal tract. However, in comparison to the large amount of research which has been carried out on the psychological sequelae of breast cancer, there is relatively much less information about the psychological sequelae of GI cancer. Psychological issues in relation to cancer are discussed in Chapter 23. Many of the issues and themes raised in that chapter can be extrapolated to patients with GI cancer. Only studies that have specifically focused upon GI cancer are discussed below.

In comparison with breast cancer, a recent four-year prospective study has shown that patients with rectal cancer report a better long-term outcome in terms of quality of life than breast cancer patients, even though breast cancer patients have a better prognosis (Engel *et al.* 2003). Breast cancer patients reported worse emotional functioning, fatigue, pain and sleeplessness than rectal cancer patients. Gender, age and therapy did not explain the differences.

A further study which compared the severity of psychological symptoms in patients with different forms of GI cancer found that the rates were higher for pancreatic/biliary cancer patients and stomach cancer patients compared with colorectal cancer patients (Nordin & Glimelius 1997). The prevalence of anxiety and depression was also higher in non-cured patients in comparison with those who had a good prognosis, and approximately 20% of the non-cured patients had symptoms of depression. The long term, psychological outcome following resection for oesophageal cancer also appears to be good (Hallas *et al.* 2001), with only a small number of patients reporting symptoms of anxiety five years post-surgery.

Although small in number, these studies suggest that different GI cancers are associated with different rates of psychological distress, and those individuals with colorectal cancer may have quite low levels of depression in comparison to other groups.

Colorectal cancer patients, however, have high rates of sexual dysfunction following their surgery. While a number of studies have examined rates of sexual dysfunction and quality-of-life (QOL) scores after surgery for rectal cancer, the primary focus has been on the male sexual issues of erectile dysfunction and retrograde ejaculation. Female sexual dysfunction after surgery for rectal cancer has been relatively ignored, due in part to the reluctance of women with rectal

Table 16.6. Prevalence of sexual dysfunction in males and females post-surgery for rectal cancer.

Type of sexual dysfunction	Males ($n = 99$)	Females ($n = 81$)
Decreased libido	47%	41%
Arousal	–	29%
Impotence	32%	–
Partial impotence	52%	–
Lubrication	–	56%
Orgasm	41%	35%
Ejaculation	43%	–
Dyspareunia	–	46%

Source: Data from Hendren *et al.* (2005).

cancer to respond to questions about their sexuality. Where sexual issues in women have been studied, the focus has usually been on dyspareunia. Validated instruments for measuring sexual functioning have seldom been used in studies of sexual changes after rectal cancer surgery.

A study which investigated the prevalence of male and female sexual dysfunction following surgery for rectal cancer found approximately one-third of the women were sexually active post-surgery in comparison with two-thirds prior to surgery and that 50% of the men were sexually active post-surgery prior to 91% prior to surgery (Hendren *et al.* 2005). This study employed validated instruments for measuring sexual function and obtained a response rate of over 80%. The rates of specific sexual problems for men and women are shown in Table 16.6.

Few patients reported that sexual problems had been raised by their doctors as a potential problem prior to surgery. The authors concluded that the potential for sexual dysfunction should be discussed with rectal cancer patients, and efforts should be made to identify problems and treat them.

Palliative care

It is very important that patients who are terminally ill receive appropriate palliative care and support and this is discussed in Chapters 23 and 25. In a study of patients with terminal colorectal cancer, Maguire and colleagues (1999) found that patients and their carers often have different views regarding illness concerns. They found that there was general agreement about physical symptoms such as nausea or pain, but there was little agreement between patients' concerns about their illness and their carers' perceptions of the patients' major concerns. Twenty per cent of the patients who took part in the study were suffering from an affective disorder, but this had only been recognized by the GP in 25% of the cases. Of the carers, one-third had recently suffered from a major depressive disorder or some other psychiatric condition. The findings of this study suggest that both patients and carers require help and support when the illness becomes terminal. Carers however may not accurately be aware of their loved ones' major concerns and efforts should always be made to elicit these direct from the patient.

Summary

Psychological and psychiatric conditions are common in patients with gastro-intestinal conditions. Psychological treatments and psychopharmacological agents are helpful in patients with moderate to severe functional gastrointestinal disease. Psychiatric conditions such as depression and anxiety should be treated if associated with physical disease as failure to treat results in poor quality of life and greater distress for the patient.

REFERENCES

Ackerman, S. H., Hofer, M. A. and Weiner, H. (1975). Age at maternal separation and gastric erosion susceptibility in the rat. *Psychosomatic Medicine*, **37**, 180−4.

Akehurst, R. L., Brazier, J. E., Mathers, N., *et al.* (2002). Health-related quality of life and cost impact of irritable bowel syndrome in a UK primary care setting. *Pharmacoeconomics*, **20**, 455−62.

Ali, A., Toner, B. B., Stuckless, N., *et al.* (2000). Emotional abuse, self-blame and self-silencing in women with irritable bowel syndrome. *Psychosomatic Medicine*, **62**, 76−82.

Aoyama, N., Kinoshita, Y., Fujimoto, S., *et al.* (1998). Peptic ulcers after the Hanshin-Awaji earthquake: increased incidence of bleeding gastric ulcers. *American Journal of Gastroenterology*, **93**, 311−16.

Baxter, A. and Salter, M. (2000). Stoma care nursing. *Nursing Standard*, **14**, 59.

Bekkers, M., van Knippenburg, F., van Dulmen, A., *et al.* (1997). Survival and psychosocial adjustment to stoma surgery and non-stoma bowel resection: a four-year follow-up. *Journal of Psychosomatic Research*, **42**, 235−44.

Bennett, E. J., Tennant, C. C., Piesse, C., *et al.* (1998). Level of chronic life stress predicts clinical outcome in irritable bowel syndrome. *Gut*, **43**, 256−61.

Biggs, A. M., Aziz, Q., Tomenson, B., *et al.* (2004). Effect of childhood adversity on health related quality of life in patients with upper abdominal or chest pain. *Gut*, **53**, 180−6.

Bitton, A., Sewitch, M. J., Peppercorn, M. A., *et al.* (2003). Psychosocial determinants of relapse in ulcerative colitis: a longitudinal study. *American Journal of Gastroenterology*, **98**, 2203−8.

Brandt, L., Locke, G. R., Olden, K., *et al.* (2002). An evidence-based approach to the management of irritable bowel syndrome in North America. *American Journal of Gastroenterology*, **97**(Suppl. 11), S1−26.

Bregenzer, N., Lange, A., Furst, A., *et al.* (2005). Patient education in inflammatory bowel disease does not influence patients knowledge and long-term psychosocial well-being. *Zeitschrift fur Gastroenterologie*, **43**(4), 367−71.

Brown, H. and Randle, J. (2005). Living with a stoma: a review of the literature. *Journal of Clinical Nursing*, **14**(1), 74−81.

Ciechanowski, P., Russo, J., Katon, W., *et al.* (2004). Influence of patient attachment style on self-care and outcomes in diabetes. *Psychosomatic Medicine*, **66**(5), 720−8.

Creed, F., Ratcliffe, J., Fernandez, L., *et al.* (2001). Health-related quality of life and health care costs in severe, refractory irritable bowel syndrome. *Annals of Internal Medicine*, **134**(2), 860−8.

Creed, F., Fernandes, L., Guthrie, E., *et al.* (2003). The cost-effectiveness of psychotherapy and paroxetine for severe irritable bowel syndrome. *Gastroenterology*, **124**, 303−17.

Creed, F. H., Ratcliffe, J., Fernandes, L., *et al.* (2005). Depressive, panic and neurasthenic disorders predict poor outcome in severe irritable bowel syndrome unless suitably treated. *British Journal of Psychiatry*, **186**, 507−15.

Drossman, D. A., Li, Z., Andruzzi, E., *et al.* (1993). U.S. householder survey of functional gastrointestinal disorders. Prevalence, sociodemography, and health impact. *Digestive Diseases & Sciences*, **38**(9), 1569−80.

Drossman, D. A., Talley, N. J., Olden, K. W., *et al.* (1995). Sexual and physical abuse and gastrointestinal illness: review and recommendations. *Annals of Internal Medicine*, **123**, 782−94.

Drossman, D. A., Corazzioari, E., Talley, N. J., *et al.* (1999a). *The Functional Gastrointestinal Disorders*, 2nd edn. McLean, VA: Degnon Associates.

Drossman, D. A., Creed, F. H., Olden, K. W., *et al.* (1999b). Psychosocial aspects of the functional gastrointestinal disorders. *Gut*, **45**(Suppl. II), II25−30.

Drossman, D. A., Toner, B. B., Whitehead, W. E., *et al.* (2003). Cognitive-behavioral therapy versus education and desipramine versus placebo for moderate to severe functional bowel disorders. *Gastroenterology*, **125**(1), 19−31.

Duffy, L. C., Zielezny, M. A., Marshall, J. R., *et al.* (1991). Relevance of major stress events as an indicator of disease activity prevalence in inflammatory bowel disease. *Behavioural Medicine*, **17**, 101−10.

Elsenbruch, S., Langhorst, J., Popkirowa, K., *et al.* (2005). Effects of mind-body therapy on quality of life and neuroendocrine and cellular immune functions in patients with ulcerative colitis. *Psychotherapy & Psychosomatics*, **74**(5), 277−87.

El-Serag, H. B., Olden, K. and Bjorkman, D. (2002). Health-related quality of life among persons with irritable bowel syndrome: a systematic review. *Alimentary Pharmacology and Therapeutics*, **16**, 1171−85.

El-Serag, H. B. and Talley, N. J. (2004). Systemic review: the prevalence and clinical course of functional dyspepsia. *Alimentary Pharmacology & Therapeutics*, **19**(6), 643−54.

Engel, J., Kerr, J., Schlesinger-Raab, A., *et al.* (2003). Comparison of breast and rectal cancer patients' quality of life: results of a four year prospective field study. *European Journal of Cancer Care*, 12(3), 215–23.

Garcia-Vega, E. and Fernandez-Rodriguez, C. (2004). A stress management programme for Crohn's disease. *Behaviour Research & Therapy*, 42(4), 367–83.

Garrett, V. D., Brantley, P. J., Jones, G. N., *et al.* (1991). The relation between daily stress and Crohn's disease. *Journal of Behavioural Medicine*, 14, 87–96.

Goodwin, R. D. and Stein, M. B. (2002). Generalized anxiety disorder and peptic ulcer disease among adults in the United States. *Psychosomatic Medicine*, 64(6), 862–6.

Goodwin, R. D. and Stein, M. B. (2004). Association between childhood trauma and physical disorders among adults in the United States. *Psychological Medicine*, 34(3), 509–20.

Guthrie, E., Jackson, J., Shaffer, J., *et al.* (2002). Psychological disorder and severity of inflammatory bowel disease predict health-related quality of life in ulcerative colitis and Crohn's disease. *American Journal of Gastroenterology*, 97, 1994–9.

Guthrie, E., Creed, F., Fernandes, L., *et al.* (2003). Cluster analysis of symptoms and health seeking behaviour differentiates subgroups of patients with severe irritable bowel syndrome. *Gut*, 52(11), 1616–22.

Guthrie, E., Barlow, J., Fernandes, L., *et al.* North of England IBS Research Group. (2004). Changes in tolerance to rectal distension correlate with changes in psychological state in patients with severe irritable bowel syndrome. *Psychosomatic Medicine*, 66, 578–82.

Gwee, K. A., Leong, Y. L., Graham, C., *et al.* (1999). The role of psychological and biological factors in postinfective gut dysfunction. *Gut*, 44(3), 400–6.

Hallas, C. N., Patel, N., Oo, A., *et al.* (2001). Five-year survival following oesophageal cancer resection: psychosocial functioning and quality of life. *Psychology, Health & Medicine*, 6(1), 85–94.

Han, K. S. (2002). The effect of an integrated stress management program on the psychologic and physiologic stress reactions of peptic ulcer in Korea. *Journal of Holistic Nursing*, 20(1), 61–80.

Hendren, S. K., O'Connor, B. I., Liu, M., *et al.* (2005). Prevalence of male and female sexual dysfunction is high following surgery for rectal cancer. *Annals of Surgery*, 242(2), 212–23.

Henningsen, P., Zimmerman, T. and Sattel, H. (2003). Medically unexplained physical symptoms, anxiety, and depression: a meta-analytic review. *Psychosomatic Medicine*, 65, 528–33.

Holtmann, G., Armstrong, D., Bauerfeind, A., *et al.* (1992). Members of the RUDER Study Group. Influence of stress on the healing and relapse of duodenal ulcers. *Scandinavian Journal of Gastroenterology*, 27, 917–23.

Jailwala, J., Imperiale, T. F. and Kroencke, K. (2000). Pharmacologic treatment of the irritable bowel syndrome: a systematic review of randomised controlled trials. *Annals of Internal Medicine*, 133, 136–47.

Kang, J. Y., Tinto, A., Higham, J., *et al.* (2002). Peptic ulceration in general practice in England and Wales 1994–98: period prevalence and drug management. *Alimentary Pharmacology & Therapeutics*, 16(6), 1067–74.

Keller, W., Pritsch, M., Von Wietersheim, J., *et al.* (2004). The German Study Group on Psychosocial Intervention in Crohn's Disease. Effect of psychotherapy and relaxation on the psychosocial and somatic course of Crohn's disease: main results of the German Prospective Multicenter Psychotherapy Treatment study on Crohn's Disease. Multicenter Study. *Journal of Psychosomatic Research*, **56**(6), 687–96.

Kennedy, A. P., Nelson, E., Reeves, D., *et al.* (2004). A randomised controlled trial to assess the effectiveness and cost of a patient orientated self management approach to chronic inflammatory bowel disease. *Gut*, **53**(11), 1639–45.

Kessler, R. C., McGonagle, K. A., Zhao, S., *et al.* (1994). Lifetime and 12-month prevalence of DSM-III-R psychiatric disorders in the United States: results from the National Comorbidity Survey. *Archives of General Psychiatry*, **51**, 8–19.

Lackner, J. and Gurtman, M. B. (2005). Patterns of interpersonal problems in irritable bowel syndrome patients: a circumplex analysis. *Journal of Psychosomatic Research*, **58**, 523–32.

Lam, S. K., Hui, W. M., Shiu, L. P., *et al.* (1995). Society stress and peptic ulcer perforation. *Journal of Gastroenterology and Hepatology*, **10**, 570–6.

Larsson, K., Sundberg Hjelm, M., Karlbom, U., *et al.* (2003). A group-based patient education programme for high-anxiety patients with Crohn disease or ulcerative colitis. *Scandinavian Journal of Gastroenterology*, **38**(7), 763–9.

Levenstein, S. (2000). The very model of a modern etiology: a biopsychosocial view of peptic ulcer. *Psychosomatic Medicine*, **62**, 176–85.

Levenstein, S., Kaplan, G. A. and Smith, M. (1995). Sociodemographic characteristics, life stressors, and peptic ulcer: a prospective study. *Journal of Clinical Gastroenterology*, **21**, 185–92.

Levenstein, S., Prantera, C., Scribano, M. L., *et al.* (1996a). Psychologic predictors of duodenal ulcer healing. *Journal of Clinical Gastroenterology*, **22**, 84–9.

Levenstein, S., Prantera, C., Varvo, V., *et al.* (1996b). Long-term symptom patterns in duodenal ulcer: psychosocial factors. *Journal of Psychosomatic Research*, **41**, 465–72.

Levenstein, S., Kaplan, G. A. and Smith, M. W. (1997). Psychological predictors of peptic ulcer incidence in the Alameda County Study. *Journal of Clinical Gastroenterology*, **24**, 140–6.

Levenstein, S., Prantera, C., Varvo, V., *et al.* (2000). Stress and exacerbation in ulcerative colitis: a prospective study of patients enrolled in remission. *American Journal of Gastroenterology*, **95**, 1213–20.

Levy, R. L., Whitehead, W. E., Von Korff, M. R., *et al.* (2000). Intergenerational transmission of gastrointestinal illness behavior. *American Journal of Gastroenterology*, **95**, 451–6.

Levy, R. L., Jones, K. R., Whitehead, W. E., *et al.* (2001). Irritable bowel syndrome in twins: heredity and social learning both contribute to etiology. *Gastroenterology*, **121**, 799–804.

Levy, R. L., Whitehead, W. E., Walker, L. S., *et al.* (2004). Increased somatic complaints and health-care utilization in children: effects of parent IBS status and parent response to gastrointestinal symptoms. *American Journal of Gastroenterology*, **99**, 2442–51.

Locke, G. R., III, Weaver, A. L., Melton, L. J., III, *et al.* (2004). Psychosocial factors are linked to functional gastrointestinal disorders: a population based nested case-control study. *American Journal of Gastroenterology*, **99**, 350–7.

Maguire, P., Walsh, S., Jeacock, J., *et al.* (1999). Physical and psychological needs of patients dying from colo-rectal cancer. *Palliative Medicine*, **13**(1), 45–50.

Mardini, H. E., Kip, K. E. and Wilson, J. W. (2004). Crohn's disease: a two-year prospective study of the association between psychological distress and disease activity. *Digestive Diseases and Sciences*, **49**, 492–7.

Maunder, R. G. (2005). Evidence that stress contributes to inflammatory bowel disease: evaluation, synthesis, and future directions. *Inflammatory Bowel Diseases*, **11**(6), 600–8.

Maunder, R. G. and Esplen, M. J. (2001). Supportive-expressive group psychotherapy for persons with inflammatory bowel disease. *Canadian Journal of Psychiatry – Revue Canadienne de Psychiatrie*, **46**(7), 622–6.

Maunder, R. G., Lancee, W. J., Hunter, J. J., *et al.* (2005). Attachment insecurity moderates the relationship between disease activity and depressive symptoms in ulcerative colitis. *Inflammatory Bowel Diseases*, **11**(10), 919–26.

Mayer, E. A. (2000). The neurobiology of stress and gastrointestinal disease. *Gut*, **47**, 861–9.

Milne, B., Joachin, G. and Niehardt, J. (1986). A stern management programme for inflammatory bowel disease patients. *Journal of Advanced Nursing*, **11**, 561–7.

Mittermaier, C., Dejaco, C., Waldhoer, T., *et al.* (2004). Impact of depressive mood on relapse in patients with inflammatory bowel disease: a prospective 18-month follow-up study. *Psychosomatic Medicine*, **66**, 79–84.

Monnikes, H., Tebbe, J. J., Hildebrandt, M., *et al.* (2001). Role of stress in functional gastrointestinal disorders. Evidence for stress-induced alterations in gastrointestinal motility and sensitivity. *Digestive Diseases*, **19**, 201–11.

Naliboff, B. D., Mayer, M., Fass, R., *et al.* (2004). The effect of life stress on symptoms of heartburn. *Psychosomatic Medicine*, **66**, 426–34.

NICE. (2005). *Guidelines on Peptic Ulcer*. London: Department of Health.

Nordin, K. and Glimelius, B. (1997). Psychological reactions in newly diagnosed gastrointestinal cancer patients. *Acta Oncologica*, **36**(8), 803–10.

North, C. S., Alpers, D. H., Helzer, J. E., *et al.* (1991). Do life events or depression exacerbate inflammatory bowel disease? *Annals of Internal Medicine*, **114**, 381–6.

Nugent, K., Daniels, P., Stewart, B., *et al.* (1999). Quality of life in stoma patients. *Diseases of the Colon and Rectum*, **42**, 1569–74.

O'Connor, G. (2005). Teaching stoma-management skills: the importance of self-care. *British Journal of Nursing*, **14**(6), 320–4.

Olden, K. W. (2004). The psychological aspects of noncardiac chest pain. *Gastroenterology Clinics of North America*, **33**(1), 61–7.

Persson, E. and Hellstrom, A. L. (2002). Experiences of Swedish men and women 6 to 12 weeks after ostomy surgery. *Journal of Wound, Ostomy and Continence Nursing*, **29**, 103–8.

Pitchumoni, C. S. (1998). Chronic pancreatitis: pathogenesis and management of pain. *Journal of Clinical Gastroenterology*, **27**(2), 101–7.

Porcelli, P., Zaka, S., Centonze, S., *et al.* (1994). Psychological distress and levels of disease activity in inflammatory bowel disease. *Italian Journal of Gastroenterology*, **26**, 111–15.

Riberdy-Poitras, M., Verner, P., Plourde, V., *et al.* (2000). Amitriptyline for the treatment of IBS (Abstract). *Gastroenterology*, A617.

Rogers, M. P., White, K., Warshaw, M. G., *et al.* (1994). Prevalence of medical illness in patients with anxiety disorders. *International Journal of Psychiatry and Medicine*, **24**, 83–96.

Schwarz, S. P. and Blanchard, E. B. (1991). Evaluation of a psychological treatment for inflammatory bowel disease. *Behaviour Research & Therapy*, **29**(2), 167–77.

Shaw, L. and Ehrlich, A. (1987). Relaxation training as a treatment for chronic pain caused by ulcerative colitis. *Pain*, **29**(3), 287–93.

Soo, S., Moayyedi, P., Deeks, J., *et al.* (2004). Psychological interventions for non-ulcer dyspepsia. *Update of Cochrane Database Systematic Review*, **3**.

Talley, N. J., Zinsmeister, A. R., Van Dyke, C., *et al.* (1991a). Epidemiology of colonic symptoms and the irritable bowel syndrome. *Gastroenterology*, **101**(4), 927–34.

Talley, N. J., Owen, B. K. and Boyce, P. (1991b). Psychological treatments for the irritable bowel syndrome. *American Journal of Gastroenterology*, **91**, 277–86.

Talley, N. J., Gabriel, S. E., Harmsen, W. S., *et al.* (1995). Medical costs in community subjects with irritable bowel syndrome. *Gastroenterology*, **109**(6), 1736–41.

Thompson, W. G., Irvine, E. J., Pare, P., *et al.* (2002). Functional gastrointestinal disorders in Canada: first population-based survey using Rome II criteria with suggestions for improving the questionnaire. *Digestive Diseases & Sciences*, **47**(1), 225–35.

Wald, A. (2002). Psychotropic agents in irritable bowel syndrome. *Journal of Clinical Gastroenterology*, **35**(Suppl.), S53–7.

Walker, E. A., Gelfand, M. D., Gelfand, A. N., *et al.* (1996). The relationship of current psychiatric disorder to functional disability and distress in patients with inflammatory bowel disease. *General Hospital Psychiatry*, **18**, 220–9.

Weiner, H. (1991). From simplicity to complexity (1950–1990): the case of peptic ulceration. II. Animal studies. *Psychosomatic Medicine*, **53**, 491–516.

Whitehead, W. E., Crowell, M. D., Heller, B. R., *et al.* (1994). Modeling and reinforcement of the sick role during childhood predicts adult illness behavior. *Psychosomatic Medicine*, **6**, 541–50.

Whitehead, W. E., Crowell, M. D., Davidoff, A. L., *et al.* (1997). Pain from rectal distension in women with irritable bowel syndrome: relationship to sexual abuse. *Digestive Diseases and Sciences*, **42**, 796–804.

Wiklund, I. (2004). Review of the quality of life and burden of illness in gastroesophageal reflux disease. *Digestive Diseases*, **22**(2), 108–14.

17

Liver disorders

Geoffrey Lloyd

The association between diseases of the liver and psychiatric disturbance has been a neglected area of clinical research despite the observations of ancient Greek physicians, notably Galen and Hippocrates, who had no doubt of the importance of the liver's influence on the mind. The term melancholia was derived from Galen's hypothesis that the disorder resulted from an excess of black bile while Hippocrates described behavioural changes in people whose madness he considered to be the result of bile (Chadwick & Mann 1950). Clinical reports of the neuropsychiatric consequences of liver failure began to appear in the 1950s following the emergence of hepatology as a distinct medical speciality and the development of units specifically designated for the treatment of liver disorders (Sherlock *et al.* 1954; Sumerskill *et al.* 1956). These reports were essentially descriptions of organic mental disorders consequent to the severe metabolic disturbance accompanying portal-systemic collateral circulation. Little attention was given to the affective disturbances and other so-called functional symptoms but this has changed in response to the increased prevalence of chronic hepatitis and the widespread establishment of successful liver transplant programmes (Collis & Lloyd 1992).

Psychiatric symptoms of liver disease

The pattern of psychiatric symptoms of liver disease is greatly influenced by whether the liver disease is acute or chronic in nature. In acute liver failure such as fulminating hepatitis, drug-induced necrosis or an acute deterioration in chronic liver disease, the clinical picture is dominated by overt signs of hepatic dysfunction. The patient will probably be jaundiced with a hyperdynamic circulation, fever, septicaemia, foetor hepaticus and disordered blood coagulation.

Handbook of Liaison Psychiatry, ed. Geoffrey Lloyd and Elspeth Guthrie. Published by Cambridge University Press. © Cambridge University Press 2007.

The mental state shows evidence of the characteristic features of delirium and is conventionally referred to as hepatic encephalopathy. In chronic liver disease the main psychological symptoms are fatigue, depression and gradual cognitive impairment.

Hepatic encephalopathy

Neuropsychiatric features are common. The clinical manifestations are those of delirium with impairment of consciousness, increased sleep, disorientation, impaired learning ability, hallucinations usually in the visual modality and retrograde amnesia. These are similar to the mental changes seen in other metabolic disorders, such as uraemia or hypoglycaemia; there are no psychological symptoms that are specific for liver disease. The level of consciousness tends to fluctuate and the other symptoms also vary in intensity. In severe cases consciousness becomes progressively impaired and the patient lapses into coma. Mood changes, particularly anxiety and depression, are common and in the early stages a diagnosis of a functional neurotic disorder may be made.

Neurological signs are also part of the clinical picture. There may be a mild tremor accompanied by exaggerated tendon reflexes but as the condition progresses a characteristic flapping tremor of the hands becomes apparent. This takes the form of a series of rapid flexion and extension movements at the wrist and metacarpo-phalangeal joints. It is absent at rest but is most easily demonstrated when the arms are held outstretched and the wrists hyperextended. It is aggravated by fatigue and anxiety. Other signs develop with clinical progression. These include dysarthria, ataxia, constructional apraxia and muscular rigidity. If episodes of hepatic encephalopathy are repeated there may be enduring changes of personality indicative of frontal lobe dysfunction and intellectual changes of dementia.

The electroencephalogram shows bilateral slow waves with a frequency of four cycles per second, in contrast to the normal eight to thirteen cycles per second. These changes, which are non-specific, occur early, before any biochemical or mental state abnormalities become apparent. Computerized tomography (CT) and magnetic resonance imaging (MRI) brain scans are normal in acute cases but show evidence of diffuse cortical atrophy in patients with chronic or recurrent encephalopathy.

Hepatic encephalopathy results from a shunting of blood from the portal into the systemic circulation. Blood therefore reaches the brain without being metabolized by the liver. In hepatocellular failure there is a functional shunt through the liver which cannot metabolize portal-vein contents absorbed from the gut. In cirrhosis there is an anatomical shunt through collateral veins which have become established due to portal hypertension. Blood also enters the systemic circulation after a surgical porto-systemic shunt has been established to relieve portal hypertension. Theses patients are therefore highly susceptible to the sedative effects of psychotropic drugs which can precipitate coma even in small doses. They should be avoided if at all possible. The encephalopathy can also be precipitated or exacerbated by infection, electrolyte depletion, a high protein diet, hypoglycaemia, hypoxia or acid—base abnormalities. Treatment of hepatic encephalopathy is best conducted by a specialist hepatologist. The essential principles consist of severe restriction of dietary protein and administration of enemas to clear the bowel of protein. Oral antibiotics are useful to reduce ammonia formation by gut bacteria.

Fatigue

Fatigue has become recognized as being one of the most debilitating symptoms of chronic liver disease. It has both psychological and physical components. Central to any definition of fatigue is a reduced capacity for sustained work and a prolonged time to recover from any form of activity. It has an unpleasant quality and usually leads to an aversion to take on any work which might bring on fatigue. This causes reduced drive and lack of initiative. Mental fatigue results in reduced concentration, impaired judgement and inability to make decisions. Errors are therefore more likely to be made on tasks which require mental effort. Physical fatigue is likewise associated with reduced exercise capacity, subjective weakness and a tendency to seek prolonged rest after even mild physical exertion.

It is not yet clear whether fatigue has a specific association with liver disease. It has been described in numerous reports of patients with hepatitis, particularly hepatitis C (Wessely & Pariante 2002) and those with biliary cirrhosis (Goldblatt *et al.* 2002) and other forms of cholestasis (Kumar & Tandon 2002). However fatigue is common in a wide variety of chronic medical conditions including malignancy, cardiac disease, respiratory disease and rheumatological conditions. It is often a source of major complaint but has been underestimated by doctors, perhaps because the patient's subjective complaints do not correlate closely with objective markers of disease activity.

Depression

Depression is closely linked to fatigue. Although they are separate complaints with different nosological constructs there is a great deal of overlap between them. When a mental state assessment is carried out many patients with fatigue will be found to suffer from depression. Conversely nearly all patients diagnosed as depressed will experience mental or physical fatigue or both. Depression associated with liver disease probably represents an emotional reaction to the debilitating effects of chronic illness. Many patients are unable to work, their income is reduced, they cannot enjoy leisure activities and their quality of life is markedly impaired. Family relationships become strained and the patient is in danger of becoming marginalized within the family. All these factors contribute to the onset of depression. In the case of patients with alcohol misuse there are often major family and financial problems predating the onset of liver disease. Morbid thoughts and attempts at self-harm increase the risk of suicide.

Chronic hepatocerebral degeneration

The symptoms of hepatic encephalopathy are usually reversible with appropriate treatment but in some patients symptoms persist following recovery from an acute episode. The risk of this happening is increased if acute episodes are recurrent or prolonged. The clinical picture is that of dementia. Patients are often apathetic and disinterested in their surroundings. Their results on neuropsychological testing show global deficits, with particular impairment on tests measuring visual and verbal abstraction. Chronic neurological signs are common, including tremor, extrapyramidal rigidity, increased reflexes, extensor plantar responses, orofacial dyskinesia and dysarthria. Structural changes are found in the brain on autopsy. There may be cerebral softening and cortical atrophy. Histology shows astrocytic proliferation and enlargement in the cortex, cerebellum, putamen and globus pallidus.

Specific liver disorders

Acute and chronic hepatitis

The liver can be affected by a number of viruses, some of which specifically attack the organ. In clinical practice the two most important are hepatitis B and hepatitis C. Hepatitis B is spread by infected blood or blood products. Thus it can be acquired through injections with contaminated needles, a mechanism which is particularly common among intravenous drug users who share needles. It was formerly transmitted through transfusions of blood and blood products and was a major problem for haemophiliacs and others who needed repeated transfusions. This mode of transmission has been virtually eliminated by testing blood pretransfusion and by the use of synthetic Factor VIII to control bleeds in haemophiliacs. Hepatitis B can also be transmitted in bodily secretions such as saliva, urine, semen and vaginal secretions. Intimate bodily contact is necessary for transmission. Sexual intercourse, particularly between male homosexuals, is an important route of infection. Vertical transmission from mother to child also occurs. During the prodromal phase of the acute illness, before the onset of jaundice, the patient may complain of a variety of non-specific symptoms including general malaise, anorexia, nausea and vomiting. If these are accompanied by a lowering of mood an erroneous diagnosis of a depressive illness may be made. Most patients make a full recovery but up to 20% go on to develop chronic hepatitis.

Chronic infection is much commoner following infection with hepatitis C, also transmitted via blood products. Parenteral drug users are therefore a high-risk group but sporadic cases occur in which the mode of transmission is never established. In some patients there is no history of an acute infection. Up to 80% of people infected with hepatitis C develop chronic hepatitis and these are at risk of developing cirrhosis. Because of its chronicity hepatitis C infection is a major health problem and it is estimated that 170 million people are affected throughout the world (Hoofnagle 2002). Fatigue is one of the most debilitating symptoms and has a considerable influence on the patient's quality of life and ability to work. Several studies have reported a strong association with depression. Dwight *et al.* (2000) diagnosed depression in 28% of a series of patients with hepatitis C and found that severity of depression correlated highly with severity of fatigue but not with other measures of disease severity.

Interferon-alpha has become established as an effective treatment for chronic hepatitis C but many studies have shown that its use leads to the development of depression; up to 50% of cases being reported in some series. Acute delirium and mania are less common complications (Raison *et al.* 2005). The development of depression is more likely if there is a history of depression before interferon treatment is initiated. Its high incidence has led to the practice in some centres for psychiatric screening to be arranged for all potential recipients of the drug. Those at high risk should be monitored with particular vigilance during the early stages of treatment. Fortunately there is good evidence that interferon-induced depression responds well to   selective serotonin reuptake inhibitors (SSRIs). Depression is not therefore an indication to discontinue interferon but the drug should be stopped, if only temporarily, if delirium or mania develop.

Primary biliary cirrhosis

Primary biliary cirrhosis is caused by destruction of the intrahepatic bile ducts and characteristically affects women in middle age. Typical presenting symptoms are fatigue, pruritis and abdominal pain. Its aetiology is unknown but autoimmune mechanisms are thought to be responsible in some cases. Fatigue is a prominent and debilitating symptom (Huet *et al.* 2000) and is a major factor impairing a patient's quality of life so much so that it is one of the factors taken into account when evaluating patients for transplantation.

It may be associated with sleep disturbance and depression, so it is important to evaluate whether antidepressant drugs should be prescribed before a decision to transplant is made.

Alcoholic liver disease

Alcohol is metabolized predominantly in the liver, which is very sensitive to the effects of excess consumption. Increased levels of liver enzymes are indicative of liver cell damage and are used clinically as screening tests and markers of progress in response to treatment. Aspartate transaminase is increased more than alanine transaminase. Serum gamma glutamyl transpeptidase is also elevated and is considered to be the most sensitive laboratory marker of liver damage. Macrocytosis, with a mean corpuscular volume greater than 95 fl, is another laboratory marker of pathological consumption. Detection is improved if clinicians maintain a high level of awareness of the possibility of heavy drinking and ask leading questions in a sensitive manner. The use of screening questionnaires (see Chapter 8) can improve the detection rate.

The risk of liver damage increases with the amount of alcohol consumed and with the duration of heavy drinking. So close is the link that a country's death rate from cirrhosis is often taken to be an indicator of the national consumption of alcohol. Deaths from cirrhosis in the UK have been increasing steadily in tandem with greater consumption of alcohol (Leon & McCambridge 2006). However, other factors also influence the development of alcoholic liver disease. The pattern of drinking is probably important, with liver disease being more likely when drinking occurs outside meal times, with multiple drinks and with daily as opposed to weekend drinking (Neuberger *et al.* 2002). Women are more susceptible, developing alcoholic liver disease at lower levels of consumption than men. Obesity is another major risk factor, possibly because of its association with steatosis. There is also a link with concomitant liver disease, especially infection with one of the hepatitis viruses. Twin studies have demonstrated a genetic effect, the concordance rate for alcoholic liver disease being two or three times higher in monozygotic than in dizygotic twins.

Clinical syndromes of alcoholic liver disease

Fatty liver

This represents the early stage of liver damage. Patients may be asymptomatic and be detected only as a result of screening tests. Others may present with general malaise, epigastric or right upper quadrant abdominal pain, anorexia, poor concentration and other non-specific symptoms and signs of habitual heavy drinking. The liver is found to be enlarged and smooth on clinical examination.

Liver function tests are normal or slightly elevated. The characteristic histological changes are seen on liver biopsy.

Acute alcoholic hepatitis

In mild cases this presents with fatigue, anorexia and weight loss while in more severe cases there is fever, jaundice, vomiting and diarrhoea. The liver is enlarged and tender on palpation.

Cirrhosis

Alcoholic cirrhosis develops gradually. Patients have usually been drinking heavily for at least 5 years and usually more than 10 years before cirrhosis becomes established. It presents either with features of progressive hepatocellular failure or with the consequences of portal hypertension such as ascites or massive gastrointestinal haemorrhage from oesophageal varices. Patients may have had previous episodes of alcoholic hepatitis but many have no history of acute illness. Once cirrhosis develops there is a greatly increased risk of hepatocellular cancer. It is estimated that there is a four-fold increase in the incidence of liver cancer in problem drinkers.

Cholestatic syndromes

These present with deep jaundice and hepatomegaly. Serum alkaline phosphatase, transaminases, triglycerides and cholesterol are raised. The definitive diagnosis is made on liver biopsy.

Management of alcoholic liver disease

Medical management predominates during the phase of acute illness. Once the patient's physical state has stabilized there should be a concerted attempt to help the patient stop drinking. For someone who has sustained serious liver pathology complete abstinence should be the goal. Brief intervention in the form of counselling supplemented by an information leaflet has been shown to be effective, the effect of the intervention being maintained over a 12-month period (Chick *et al.* 1985). In some cases counselling may need to be accompanied by drug treatment with acamprosate which can reduce craving for alcohol. For those who are physically dependent on alcohol referral to a specialist alcohol treatment service is advisable. Some patients find an inpatient treatment programme to be effective.

There may be a previous history of psychiatric disorder which needs to be considered when planning treatment. Ewusi-Mensah *et al.* (1983) found that two-thirds of inpatients with alcoholic liver disease had suffered from psychiatric disorder, this being significantly greater than in a control group with non-alcoholic liver disease. Anxiety disorders, including panic attacks, and depression are the commonest conditions. They may be secondary to the consequences of chronic alcohol abuse but in some cases the psychiatric disorder is the primary condition and heavy drinking has evolved in an attempt to cope with the psychological symptoms.

Liver transplantation has transformed the prognosis of patients with end-stage liver disease. Patients with alcoholic liver disease should not be excluded from consideration for transplantation. Their outcome is just as good as that of patients transplanted for non-alcoholic liver disease (Gledhill *et al.* 1999). The policy in most transplant centres requires the patient to have been abstinent for at least six months before the operation. Transplantation is further discussed later in this chapter.

Wilson's disease

This is a rare, genetically determined condition which results in abnormal copper metabolism. It has a prevalence of approximately 1 in 30 000 and has an autosomal recessive mode of inheritance. There are low levels or even complete absence of caeruloplasmin, the globulin fraction of the plasma proteins to which nearly all copper is bound. It is believed that the basic defect involves diminished synthesis of caeruloplasmin resulting in high plasma levels of unbound copper. Increased copper is excreted in the urine and deposited in the liver, brain, kidney and other organs including the periphery of the cornea which gives rise to the characteristic greenish-brown Kayser–Fleischer rings. The liver pathology ranges from a periportal fibrosis to a coarse macronodular cirrhosis and psychiatric symptoms may develop with liver failure. However, most of the psychopathology results from copper deposition in the brain, particularly in the basal ganglia and frontal cortex.

Psychiatric symptoms have been recognized as common manifestations of Wilson's disease. Indeed they were described by Wilson in his original paper and he considered them to be a fundamental component of the clinical picture (Wilson 1912). The largest series reported in the literature is that of Dening and Berrios (1989), who reviewed the case-notes of 195 patients with Wilson's disease, 60 of whom were assessed psychiatrically. Half had shown evidence of psychiatric disorder at some time. A fifth had been seen by a psychiatrist before the diagnosis of Wilson's disease had been made. The commonest psychiatric symptoms were personality changes involving disinhibited, incongruous or impulsive behaviour, irritability, aggression, depression and cognitive impairment. Psychotic symptoms were rare, occurring in only 1%. Substance misuse was also uncommon.

Neurological signs occur in at least 40% of cases. These include a flapping tremor at the wrists, dysarthria, fluctuating rigidity in the limbs, choreiform movements and dystonia. There is a strong association between the presence of psychiatric and neurological symptoms.

Dening and Berrios (1989) suggested that psychiatrists have two roles in managing patients with Wilson's disease, although, given the rarity of the condition, most psychiatrists will see very few cases during the course of their careers. The first is diagnostic and essentially depends on the recognition of signs of organic brain disease when the patient is initially referred. In particular the presence of neurological signs such as tremor, dysarthria, rigidity or drooling of saliva should lead to further investigations and neurological assessment. Dening and Berrios commented that a diagnosis of depression or hysteria in such cases can prove to be a recipe for disaster and a basis for potential litigation.

The second role for the psychiatrist is managing the behavioural, affective and cognitive symptoms once the diagnosis is established. This should be undertaken in collaboration with a neurologist and, in some cases, a hepatologist. Psychiatric symptoms should be treated appropriately. Antidepressant and antipsychotic drugs are not contraindicated, but their doses should be reduced considerably in view of the risk of incapacitating side-effects, particularly in those who already have evidence of extrapyramidal dysfunction. The fundamental treatment of the disease relies on chelating agents to increase copper excretion in the urine, thereby removing it from the liver, brain and other organs. Penicillamine is still the drug of first choice. Trientene can be used for patients intolerant of penicillamine. Liver transplantation is required for the fulminating form (which is otherwise usually fatal) or for chronic cases that do not respond to chelating agents.

Liver transplantation

The first human liver transplant was carried out in 1963. The survival rates were extremely low in the early years but improvements in surgical technique and immunosuppressive therapy have greatly improved the outcome. Consequently the indications for transplantation have broadened and the contraindications have decreased (Neuberger 2004). This has led to a greater demand for donor livers and to an increased gap between the number of potential recipients and the number of available donor livers. Various measures have been taken to improve the supply, including using split grafts and taking lobes from living donors, but the number of patients waiting for livers has continued to grow. Results from live donor transplantation are encouraging, indicating that resection and transplantation of the right lobe of the liver provide sufficient functioning liver mass for most adult recipients (Marcos 2000). There is low post-operative morbidity for donors. At present the use of xenografts is not a practical option.

> **Box 17.1 Guidelines for liver transplantation.**
> - Guidelines should be drawn up to indicate the selection criteria; they should be publicized and followed by all designated centres.
> - The main selection criteria should be based on the quality of life and anticipated life expectancy.
> - Patients should be offered transplantation if there is a 50% chance of their being alive five years after transplantation with a quality of life acceptable to them.
> - Livers should be allocated to give a maximum outcome in preference to allowing every potential recipient to have a chance to receive an available organ.

The implication of the shortage of organs is that there has to be some selection process to determine the priority of patients waiting for a transplant. Selection criteria have caused considerable controversy and a questionnaire survey of three separate groups – family doctors, gastroenterologists and members of the general public – showed that there were considerable differences between the groups in the selection of recipients. In particular, the views of the general public differed from those of clinicians, although patients with alcoholic liver disease and antisocial behaviour received low priority from all three groups (Neuberger *et al.* 1998). Following a colloquium attended by healthcare professionals, lay representatives and experts in medical ethics, a number of principles have been agreed for practice in UK liver centres (Neuberger & James 1999). See Box 17.1.

Selection criteria for transplantation

There are no absolute psychiatric containdications to transplantation. Levenson and Olbrisch (1993) conducted a survey of 72 liver transplant centres in the United States and asked what criteria might be considered absolute contra-indications to surgery. The following were listed by at least 50% of centres:

- active schizophrenia
- current suicidal ideation
- dementia
- current alcohol abuse
- current addictive drug abuse.

However, they found that selection criteria varied widely between different centres and they emphasized that the validity of selection criteria had not been established. In practice very few patients were turned down on psychosocial grounds. Evaluation was refused on psychosocial grounds in only 1.2% of cases and of those evaluated surgery was refused in only 2.8%.

Alcoholic liver disease has generated much debate on the grounds that it is considered a self-inflicted condition and that there is a risk of recurrent heavy drinking, resulting in damage and eventually loss of the transplanted liver

(Webb & Neuberger 2004). Patients with alcoholic liver disease have therefore been considered less worthy than some other potential recipients and well-publicized cases of relapse tend to reinforce this attitude. However follow-up studies have shown that, when carefully selected, patients transplanted for alcoholic liver disease do as well, at least in the short term as those transplanted for other conditions (Gledhill *et al.* 1999) and alcoholic liver disease is now one of the commonest indications for transplantation (Neuberger *et al.* 2002). It has been estimated that fewer than 10% return to drinking more than 21 units of alcohol weekly (Pageaux *et al.* 2003), while fewer than 5% of grafts are lost within five years as a result of alcohol misuse (Lucey *et al.* 1997). Psychiatric and social assessment preoperatively may help identify those who are likely to adhere to follow-up treatment and not return to a harmful pattern of drinking (Masterton 2000). Most transplant centres require that a patient should have been abstinent for a period of time, usually six months, before surgery is undertaken but this requirement has been questioned. There is no clear rationale for this rule and many centres do not follow their own guidelines on this criterion (Neuberger *et al.* 2002). However a period of abstinence enables some patients to recover sufficient liver function so that transplantation becomes unnecessary. Regular sessions with a counsellor experienced in treating patients with problem drinking may reduce the risk of relapse but this requires further evaluation before counselling services are established in all centres. Those who cannot achieve stable abstinence should be referred to a specialized alcohol treatment service. Transplantation is not indicated for those who are likely to resume a pattern of heavy drinking. Although the ability to identify those at risk of relapse is still poorly developed, some helpful information has been provided by Gish *et al.* (2001) who found that non-compliance with medication or clinic attendance and a diagnosis of personality disorder both predicted subsequent recidivism which the authors defined as any alcohol use once the patient engaged in the evaluation process, either before or after transplantation.

Similarly, previous illegal drug use is not a contraindication, provided the patient is likely to adhere to long-term immunosuppressive therapy. Abstinence from drugs has been considered important before transplantation is contemplated but there have been reports of successful outcomes in patients on current methadone maintenance treatment as part of their treatment for heroin addiction (Kanchana *et al.* 2002; Liu *et al.* 2003).

Patients who have sustained acute hepatic necrosis after deliberate overdose of paracetamol (acetaminophen) are also considered appropriate recipients (Makin *et al.* 1995). These patients usually present in coma or with severe hepatic encephalopathy. Unless transplantation is undertaken urgently the prognosis is poor. Decisions have to be made quickly. As much psychosocial information should be collected as it is possible to do in the circumstances but a full psychiatric assessment is usually not feasible. Self-poisoning with paracetamol is often impulsive and not always associated with serious suicidal intent, despite the inherent lethality of the method. Many people who take overdoses of paracetamol do so in the context of a situational crisis or a relatively minor depressive illness, both of which are amenable to resolution once physical recovery has occurred. Patients who have undergone transplantation in these circumstances should be referred to a liaison psychiatrist as soon as possible after surgery. The potential lethality of paracetamol overdose has led to legislation in the UK to limit the size of packs of the drug available for purchase over the counter in pharmacists' shops. This legislation has been followed by a significant reduction in the size of overdoses with a consequent reduction in morbidity and mortality and fewer admissions to liver units (Hawton *et al.* 2004).

Follow-up studies show that the recipients of liver transplantation have an improved quality of life post-operatively. Psychiatric problems are not frequent and can be treated with conventional measures. Particular attention should be paid to those with a previous psychiatric history, especially patients for whom psychiatric factors have been involved in the need for transplantation such as deliberate self-harm and chronic alcohol or drug misuse.

With the development of live donor transplantation careful consideration needs to be given to the selection of donors. Almost all potential donors have a close emotional relationship with the recipient. It is important to establish that there is no psychological pressure on the donor from the recipient or from other family members and that there is no financial inducement. Until more is known about the outcome of live donor transplants it is probably best to exclude donors with a significant current or previous psychiatric illness.

Psychotropic drugs and liver disease

Many psychotropic drugs are metabolized by the liver. Drugs that have a high rate of hepatic clearance are largely cleared during their first passage through the liver, a phenomenon known as the 'first-pass effect'. This is very important for drugs taken orally because liver damage increases the amount of drug which remains unmetabolized after oral administration. Doses of drugs taken orally, but not intravenously, therefore need to be reduced. Drug metabolism is also affected if blood albumin levels are reduced, as is often the case in chronic liver disease. This results in reduced plasma binding and high blood levels of drugs and therefore a greater risk of side-effects. As a general rule great caution should be exercised when prescribing psychotropic drugs for patients with liver disease, bearing in mind that the liver has a large functional capacity and liver damage has to be advanced before prescribing has to be modified. The following principles should be adopted:

- the greater the degree of hepatic impairment the lower should be the starting dose and maximum dose
- liver function tests provide a reasonable indication of hepatic impairment but do not necessarily correlate well with the impairment
- special care is required with drugs which have a first-pass clearance effect
- drugs which cause sedation and constipation should be avoided in severe liver disease
- start with low doses, increase the dose slowly and monitor liver function tests weekly.

Antidepressants

Antidepressant drugs are potentially hepatotoxic, their side-effects covering a spectrum from a transient increase in liver enzymes to, in rare cases, extensive necrosis and fulminant liver failure. Monoamine oxidase inhibitors and tricyclics are more likely to produce liver damage than the newer antidepressants although the hepatotoxicity associated with nefazodone led to its withdrawal by the manufacturers (Lucena *et al.* 2003). Most tricyclics have a high first-pass clearance and side-effects, particularly drowsiness, are common in patients with established liver disease. Selective serotonin reuptake inhibitors are easier to use. Alternate-day dosage of fluoxetine has been recommended while doses in the lower therapeutic range have been recommended for citalopram and paroxetine. There have been claims that paroxetine is the safest option, but this needs to be balanced against the risk of a discontinuation syndrome. Venlafaxine, mirtazapine and reboxetine appear to be safe if the starting dose is no more than 50% of the usual dose. Monoamine oxidase inhibitors are hepatotoxic and may precipitate coma. They are generally contraindicated. If a monoamine oxidase inhibitor is necessary on clinical grounds moclobemide should be used, the initial dose being reduced by a third or half.

Antipsychotics

The phenothiazines, particularly chlorpromazine, are well recognized as having the potential to cause intrahepatic cholestasis, and they should be used with caution. Several other antipsychotics are safer. Sulpiride and amisulpiride are almost unmetabolized by the liver and the incidence of liver toxicity appears to be very low. Transient asymptomatic rises in liver enzymes have been reported with olanzapine so monitoring of liver function tests should be undertaken if the drug is prescribed to patients with liver impairment. Risperidone and quetiapine can be used if the initial doses are reduced. Haloperidol is also safe if used cautiously;

it has the advantage of being able to be administered by intramuscular injection and is therefore useful if rapid control of psychotic symptoms is required. Severe liver disease is a contraindication to clozapine. If the drug needs to be used for chronic, resistant schizophrenia, lower doses and regular plasma monitoring are necessary. A toxic hepatitis has been reported with daily doses of clozapine in the range of 300–400 mg, with eosinophilia and a rapid rise in aspartate amino-transferase, both of which returned to normal within five weeks of stopping the drug.

Anxiolytics and hypnotics

Liver disease interferes with the metabolism of diazepam and chlordiazepoxide, with considerable prolongation of the half-lives of their metabolites. They can precipitate hepatic encephalopathy and coma. The benzodiazepines of choice are lorazepam, temazepam and oxazepam in low doses; their metabolism appears to be unchanged. The elimination of zopiclone is reduced. A dose of 3.75 mg can be used with caution; the total dose should not exceed 7.5 mg. Similarly zolpidem should be used in reduced doses. It is contraindicated in severe hepatic insufficiency.

REFERENCES

Chadwick, J. and Mann, W. (1950). The sacred disease. In *The Medical Works of Hippocrates*. Oxford: Blackwell Scientific Publications, p. 191.

Chick, J., Lloyd, G. and Crombie, E. (1985). Counselling problem drinkers in medical wards: a controlled study. *British Medical Journal*, **290**, 965–7.

Collis, I. and Lloyd, G. (1992). Psychiatric aspects of liver disease. *British Journal of Psychiatry*, **161**, 12–21.

Dening, T. R. and Berrios, G. E. (1989). Wilson's disease: psychiatric symptoms in 195 cases. *Archives of General Psychiatry*, **46**, 1126–34.

Dwight, M. M., Kowdley, K. V., Russo, J. E., *et al.* (2000). Depression, fatigue and functional disability in patients with chronic hepatitis C. *Journal of Psychosomatic Research*, **49**, 311–17.

Ewusi-Mensah, I., Saunders, J. C., Wodack, A. D., *et al.* (1983). Psychatric morbidity in patients with alcoholic liver disease. *British Medical Journal*, **287**, 1417–19.

Gish, R. G., Lee, A., Brooks, L., *et al.* (2001). Long-term follow-up of patients diagnosed with alcohol dependence or alcohol abuse who were evaluated for liver transplantation. *Liver Transplantation*, **7**, 581–7.

Gledhill, J., Burroughs, A., Rolles, K., *et al.* (1999). Psychiatric and social outcomes following liver transplantation for alcoholic liver disease: a controlled study. *Journal of Psychosomatic Research*, **46**, 359–68.

Goldblatt, J., Taylor, P. J. S., Lipman, T., *et al.* (2002). The true impact of fatigue in primary biliary cirrhosis: a population study. *Gastroenterology*, **122**, 1235–41.

Hawton, K., Simkin, S., Deeks, J., *et al.* (2004). UK legislation on analgesic packs: before and after study of long term effect on poisonings. *British Medical Journal*, **329**, 1076–9.

Hoofnagle, J. M. (2002). Course and outcome of hepatitis C. *Hepatology*, **36**(Suppl. 1), 21–9.

Huet, P. M., Deslauriers, J., Tran, A., *et al.* (2000). Impact of fatigue on the quality of life of patients with primary biliary cirrhosis. *American Journal of Gastroenterology*, **95**, 760–7.

Kanchana, T. P., Kaul, V., Manzarbeitia, C., *et al.* (2002). Liver transplantation for patients on methadone maintenance. *Liver Transplantation*, **8**, 778–82.

Kumar, D. and Tandon, R. K. (2002). Fatigue in cholestatic liver disease – a perplexing symptom. *Postgraduate Medical Journal*, **78**, 404–7.

Leon, D. A. and McCambridge, J. (2006). Liver cirrhosis mortality rates in Britain from 1950 to 2002: an analysis of routine data. *Lancet*, **367**, 52–6.

Levenson, J. L. and Olbrisch, M. E. (1993). Psychosocial evaluation of organ transplant candidates. A comparative survey of process, criteria and outcomes in heart, liver and kidney transplantation. *Psychosomatics*, **34**, 314–23.

Liu, L. U., Schiano, T. D., Lau, N., *et al.* (2003). Survival and risk of recidivism in methadone-dependent patients undergoing liver transplantation. *American Journal of Transplantation*, **3**, 1273–7.

Lucena, M. I., Carvajal, A., Andrade, R. J., *et al.* (2003). Antidepressant induced hepatotoxicity. *Expert Opinion on Drug Safety*, **2**, 249–62.

Lucey, M. R., Carr, K., Beresford, T. P., *et al.* (1997). Alcohol use after liver transplantation in alcoholics: a clinical cohort follow-up study. *Hepatology*, **25**, 1223–7.

Makin, A. J., Wendon, J. and Williams, R. (1995). A 7-year experience of severe acetaminophen-induced hepatotoxicity (1987–1993). *Gastroenterology*, **109**, 1907–16.

Marcos, A. (2000). Right lobe donor liver transplantation: a review. *Liver Transplantation*, **6**, 3–30.

Masterton, G. (2000). Psychosocial factors in selection for liver transplantation. *British Medical Journal*, **320**, 263–4.

Neuberger, J. (2004). Developments in liver transplantation. *Gut*, **53**, 759–68.

Neuberger, J. and James, O. (1999). Guidelines for selection of patients for liver transplantation in the era of donor-organ shortage. *Lancet*, **354**, 1636–9.

Neuberger, J., Adams, D., MacMaster, P., *et al.* (1998). Assessing priorities for allocation of donor liver grafts: survey of public and clinicians. *British Medical Journal*, **317**, 172–5.

Neuberger, J., Schulz, K. H., Day, C., *et al.* (2002). Transplantation for alcoholic liver disease. *Journal of Hepatology*, **36**, 130–7.

Pageaux, G. P., Bismuth, M., Perney, P., *et al.* (2003). Alcohol relapse after liver transplantation for alcoholic disease: does it matter? *Journal of Hepatology*, **38**, 629–34.

Raison, C. L., Demetrashvili, M., Capuron, L., *et al.* (2005). Neuropsychiatric adverse effects of interferon-alpha: recognition and management. *CNS Drugs*, **19**, 105–23.

Sherlock, S., Summerskill, W. H. J., White, L. P., *et al.* (1954). Portal-systemic encephalopathy. Neurological complications of liver disease. *Lancet*, **ii**, 453–7.

Summerskill, W. H. J., Davidson, E. A., Sherlock, S., *et al.* (1956). The neuropsychiatric syndrome associated with chronic liver disease and an extensive portal-systemic collateral circulation. *Quarterly Journal of Medicine*, **25**, 245–66.

Webb, K. and Neuberger, J. (2004). Transplantation for alcoholic liver disease. *British Medical Journal*, **329**, 63–64.

Wessely, S. and Pariante, C. (2002). Fatigue, depression and chronic hepatitis C infection. *Psychological Medicine*, **32**, 1–10.

Wilson, S. A. K. (1912). Progressive lenticular degeneration: a familial nervous disease associated with cirrhosis of the liver. *Brain*, **34**, 295–509.

18

Endocrine disorders

Antonio Lobo, M. Jesús Pérez-Echeverría and Antonio Campayo

Introduction

The relationships between endocrine disturbances and psychiatric conditions have stirred considerable interest for several reasons (Lishman 1998). Historically, several authors have speculated about the role of hormones and endocrine disorders in relation to psychiatric conditions, and attention has been devoted to the role of hormones in relation to control and feedback processes in neural structures (Carroll *et al.* 1981). Psychiatric syndromes have consistently been described or documented in endocrine diseases (Kathol 2002; Lishman 1998) and may pose a real clinical challenge for the liaison psychiatrist, but the evidence in the literature to support his or her intervention is limited. This chapter reviews available data in relation to the characteristics and frequency of specific psychiatric syndromes in primary endocrine disturbances; issues of diagnosis and differential diagnosis; mechanisms of production of psychiatric symptomatology; and treatment issues, including response of psychiatric syndromes to treatment of the endocrinopathy and to psychotropic medication.

Epidemiology

Some experts have suggested that the most severe psychiatric syndromes are not as prevalent as in the past, due to improvements in diagnosis and treatment of endocrine diseases (Kathol 2002). Still, a high prevalence of psychiatric disturbances has been reported in most endocrine conditions, depression and anxiety being the most common presentations (Tables 18.1 and 18.2). As expected, lifetime prevalence is even higher in several reports (Eiber *et al.* 1997). Cognitive impairment is rather frequent in conditions such as hyperparathyroidism, particularly among the elderly, and dementia can develop; delirium, but also

Handbook of Liaison Psychiatry, ed. Geoffrey Lloyd and Elspeth Guthrie. Published by Cambridge University Press. © Cambridge University Press 2007.

psychosis in clear consciousness, including paranoid psychosis and mania may be seen in severe endocrinopathies. Methodological issues limit the value of the available data. Case studies and case reports abound in the literature, research diagnostic criteria have rarely been used and comparison between studies is difficult due to wide differences in the samples selected and methods of assessment used. However, standardized research interviews were used in some studies reviewed here and standardized instruments in most. The general picture emerging suggests the clinical relevance of the documented psychopathology, including the depressive and anxiety syndromes, which may be very severe in diseases such as Cushing's or hyperthyroidism (Table 18.2).

We have also completed a study in 100 consecutive patients admitted to the endocrine unit in our University hospital (Lobo *et al.* 1988; Pérez-Echeverría 1985). Patients hospitalized in the internal medicine ward were used as a comparison group, as well as outpatients groups of both the internal medicine and the endocrine departments. Standardized instruments, including a standardized interview, were used throughout the study. In support of the relevance of psychiatric syndromes in these patients, the prevalence of disorder at the time of admission (first three days) was significantly higher in the endocrine inpatients than in all the comparison groups (Table 18.2). Similarly, according to standardized criteria, the severity of disorder was significantly higher in the endocrine inpatients (68% had 'moderate' or 'severe' syndromes) than in the control groups (26.6%, 16% and 40%, respectively).

General clinical aspects

This epidemiological documentation may be important in identifying the individuals at risk for specific psychiatric syndromes in liaison services with endocrine departments; or searching for the syndromes when consulting in specific endocrine patients. Screening instruments such as the Hospital Anxiety and Depression Scale (HADS) (Lloyd *et al.* 2000) or the General Health Questionnaire-28 Items (Lobo *et al.* 1988) are considered to be appropriate in endocrine patients. The sections dedicated to specific endocrine diseases suggest when the search may be mandatory, such as in cases of Cushing's disease, where depressive syndromes may be severe and accompanied by suicidal ideation. Table 18.1 also summarizes the authors' judgement about the clinical relevance (+ to +++) of the psychiatric syndromes in specific endocrine conditions, according to their frequency, severity and/or special characteristics.

Non-biological hypotheses have been formulated to explain depressive or anxiety syndromes when there is considerable stress and psychosocial difficulties associated with conditions such as diabetes mellitus. However, the authors suggest

Table 18.1. Psychiatric syndromes in endocrine disorders: prevalence and clinical relevance.

	Any disorder	Depression	Anxiety	Apathy	Delirium	Impaired cognition	Dementia	Others
Diabetes	15–59%[a,b]	++ 11–28%[c,d,e]	+ 10–59%[b,c]		+ 0–25%[b,f] Complication, progression to coma	++ Doubtful[g] When poorly controlled	+ Risk factor DAT?	• Abnormal illness behaviour
Hypothyroidism		++	+	+	+	+++ Cretinism	++	• Slowing/lethargy • Mania (treatment induced)
Hyperthyroidism	53–100%[f,h,i]	++ 30–70%[h,i]	+++ 45–61%[h,i]	'Apathetic hyperthyroidism'	+	++	Risk factor DAT?	• Overactivity • Irritability • Organic personality in the elderly
Hyperparathyroidism	23–66%[j,k]	++ 16–36%[l,m]	+ 12–16%[k,m]	+	++ 2–5%[k,l]	++ 3–12%[k,l]	+	• Fatigue • Violent behaviour?

Hypoparathyroidism	+	++		+/−	• Social withdrawal • 'Neurotic' behaviour
Hyperprolactinaemia	+ 37%[n]	++ 56%[n]		+	• Sexual dysfunction • Hostility
Cushing's syndrome	+++ 67–81%[o,p]	+ 51–86%[o,p,q] 18–66%[r,s]	+	+ 50–83%[r,t]	• Suicidal ideation • Retardation in Cushing's disease
Addison's disease	++	++	+++	+	• Fatigue +++ • Lethargy • Fluctuations of mood

Notes: DAT: Dementia, Alzheimer type; +/+++: clinical relevance; [a]Mayou *et al.* 1991; [b]Wilkinson *et al.* 1988; [c]Jalenques *et al.* 1993; [d]Eiber *et al.* 1997; [e]Lloyd *et al.* 2000; [f]Pérez-Echevarría 1985; [g]Deary & Frier 1996; [h]Trzepacz *et al.* 1988; [i]Kathol & Delahunt 1986; [j]Brown *et al.* 1987; [k]Joborn *et al.* 1986; [l]Petersen 1968; [m]White *et al.* 1996; [n]Oliveira *et al.* 2000; [o]Dorn *et al.* 1995; [p]Kelly *et al.* 1996; [q]Cohen 1980; [r]Starkman *et al.* 1981; [s]Hudson *et al.* 1987; [t]Mauri *et al.* 1993.

Table 18.2. Psychiatric disorders in endocrine inpatients: prevalence and correlations with biochemical variables.

	Prevalence of any disorder (%)		Correlations	Comments
	Admission	Discharge		
All patients (n = 100)	91	54		Severity of psychiatric disorders is significantly higher in endocrine inpatients (++); and decreases significantly at discharge (+++)
Controls				
Internal medicine inpatients (n = 30)	53.3			
Internal medicine outpatients (n = 100)	38			
Endocrine outpatients (n = 100)	70			
Diabetes (n = 25)	84 (25 delirium)	25	• Glycaemia dispersion/depression ++ • Glycaemia dispersion/global CIS^a ++ • Ketonic bodies/depression ++ • Ketonic bodies/global CIS ++	• Maximal improvement at discharge • Correlations biochemical variables (any)/ irritability, psychasthenia, GHQ^b
Hyperthyroidism (n = 22)	100	86	• T$_3$^{c}/anxiety ++ • T$_4$^{d}/anxiety ++ • Free T$_4$/anxiety ++	• Correlations biochemical variables (any)/ irritability, psychasthenia

Cushing's syndrome (n = 14)	92.9	60	• ACTH[e]/depression + • ACTH/psychomotor retardation ++ • ACTH/obsessions ++ • ACTH/global CIS +	• Maximal severity of depression and psychomotor retardation • Suicidal ideation in some patients • Correlations cortisol/anxiety
Addison's disease (n = 12)	91.7	45.4	• Cortisol/depression + • Cortisol/global CIS + • ACTH/depression + • ACTH/global CIS + • 17-OH[f]/depression + • 17-OH/global CIS +	• Correlations biochemical variables (any)/anxiety, GHQ
Hyperprolactinaemia (n = 18)	94.4	73.3	• Prolactin/depression ++	• Correlations prolactin/anxiety, obsessions, psychasthenia.

Notes: [a]CIS = clinical interview schedule; [b]GHQ = General Health Questionnaire-28 items; [c]T_3 = triiodothyronine; [d]T_4 = thyroxine;
[e]ACTH = adrenocorticotropic hormone; [f]17-OH = 17-hydroxycorticosteroids.   Significance: + $p < 0.05$; ++ $p < 0.01$; +++ $p < 0.001$.
Source: Pérez-Echeverría 1985; Lobo *et al.* 1988.

that the 'organic', endocrine origin of the psychiatric syndromes in these patients is most important. The following data support this contention: studies documenting a higher prevalence of psychiatric disturbance than in comparable general population samples (Mayou *et al.* 1991) and, in particular, in medical samples of comparable severity of the medical disorder (Pérez-Echeverría 1985); both clinical practice and studies documenting that the prevalence of psychiatric disorder and/or its severity decreases after successful treatment of the endocrine condition (Pérez-Echeverría 1985; Starkman *et al.* 1986). Although some reports are discrepant (Joborn *et al.* 1988), special support comes from studies documenting statistically significant correlations between severity of psychiatric symptoms/syndromes and hormonal levels or biological parameters (Table 18.2; Linder *et al.* 1988; Pérez-Echeverría 1985; Starkman *et al.* 1986).

In relation to diagnosis, the dictum of experienced liaison psychiatrists seems quite appropriate here: 'In the general hospital, every psychiatric symptom is "organic"... unless you can document otherwise'. In taking the history of rather atypical psychiatric presentations, the clinical psychiatrist should include questions related to the endocrine disorder, particularly when there are signs and/or symptoms suggesting an endocrine abnormality (Table 18.3). If the suggestions are well founded, he or she should also perform at least focal physical examinations to document the presence or absence of endocrine signs. In these cases, but not routinely, he or she should also indicate tests of endocrine function.

The diagnosis of an 'organic' psychiatric syndrome of endocrine origin (World Health Organization 1992) in a given patient should be considered when the presenting syndrome is known to be associated with a specific endocrine disease, and is supported by the absence of suggestive evidence of an alternative cause of the mental syndrome, namely:

- the psychiatric symptoms, the course of illness and/or the age of presentation are atypical for a primary psychiatric disorder
- there is no family or personal history of the psychiatric condition
- no precipitating stress is known
- there is a temporal relationship between the onset of the psychiatric and the endocrine symptoms.

The challenge for the consulting psychiatrist is to make explicit the diagnosis of the endocrine origin of the psychiatric syndrome early in the procedure, before his or her diagnosis is confirmed after observing that the syndrome disappears following the removal or improvement of the underlying endocrine disorder.

Most psychiatric syndromes in endocrine patients resolve with standard treatment of the endocrine disease. However, when symptoms are particularly

Table 18.3. Somatic symptoms and signs suggesting an endocrine disease.

Endocrinopathy	Symptoms	Signs
Hypothyroidism	Cold intolerance Menorrhagia	Goitre Slow relaxing reflexes Myxoedema
Hyperthyroidism	Diaphoresis Heat intolerance Oligomenorrhoea	Exophthalmos Tachycardia Arrythmia (in elderly) Tremor
Hyperparathyroidism	Nausea Muscular weakness (proximal) Abdominal pain	Hypertension
Hypoparathyroidism	Muscle spasms Paraesthesias	Choreiform movements Chvostek's sign Trousseau's sign
Hyperprolactinaemia	Galactorrhoea Amenorrhoea (in females) Impotence (in males)	Gynecomastia Osteoporosis
Cushing's syndrome	Menstrual dysfunction Muscular weakness (proximal)	Hirsutism Moon facies Hypertension Purplish stretch marks (striae)

Addison's disease	Gastrointestinal symptoms
	Weakness
		Hypotension
		Hyperpigmentation
		Loss of skin turgor
		Loose skin like damp leather
		Association with
		  autoimmune disease
		  (vitiligo)

severe or life-threatening, or when they last longer than reasonably expected, good clinical sense suggests the importance of psychiatric treatment. Well-controlled studies are lacking, but syndrome specific medication is usually recommended, as well as supportive psychotherapy and, recently, cognitive-behavioural psychotherapy in cases of abnormal illness behaviour. Relevant clinical factors, and exceptions to these general norms will now be discussed for specific endocrine diseases. Psychiatric disorders in relation to diabetes are discussed separately in Chapter 19.

Hypothyroidism

While no good prevalence studies of psychiatric disturbance have been completed in hypothyroid patients, different types of psychiatric syndromes have been described (Baumgartner 1993), and the greatest concern is the cognitive deficit as a result of changes in metabolic activity in the central nervous system. Congenital hypothyroidism results in profound intellectual and developmental deficits (cretinism), which were seen in Western countries before hormone levels were routinely tested in newborns, and treatment instituted early. In adults, common symptoms include lethargy, progressive slowing with diminished initiative and impaired memory and concentration. Ultimately the patient becomes indifferent. Longstanding disease may induce a marked dementia syndrome.

Depression, and to a lesser extent anxiety, also occur frequently, even with moderate hormonal deficits, and can be seen as early as three weeks after onset of hypothyroidism, before cognitive functions are altered. Patients with previous history of affective illness seem more vulnerable. Marked irritability, lability of mood and insomnia have been described, but the syndromes can closely mimic primary psychiatric disorders and need the checking of hormonal levels for the differential diagnosis, particularly in older women. The severity ranges from mild depression to psychotic depression with suicidal thoughts in cases of severe hypothyroidism. Delirium is seen in approximately 10% of people with severe hypothyroidism, and only rarely have 'organic' delusional syndromes been described.

Present knowledge on the effects of thyroid hormones in the central nervous system suggests that they critically influence the development of brain and probably play a direct role in adult brain homeostasis. Multiple isolated effects have been described, including a modulation of noradrenergic, serotonergic, and dopaminergic receptor function, and an influence on second messengers, calcium homeostasis, axonal transport mechanisms, and morphology. However, both the biochemical mechanisms and their physiological importance are poorly understood.

Even minor changes in thyroid hormone may induce important affective changes (Bauer & Whybrow 1990). However, the connections between this hormone and primary affective disorder remain controversial. Some authors conclude that depressed patients are basically euthyroid (Baumgartner 1993). However, thyroid autoimmunity has been reported in bipolar disorder (Kupka et al. 2002) and a high prevalence of thyroid dysfunction in patients with general anxiety disorder or panic disorder has been described (Simon et al. 2002). Hypothyroidism develops in 10% of patients treated with long-term lithium, particularly in vulnerable individuals such as women or rapid cyclers. The presence of thyroid antibodies is a predisposing factor.

The neuropsychiatric symptoms may be the first to recover, probably in a few days, with adequate hormonal replacement. Slow correction is usually recommended, particularly in the elderly, because of the risk of cardiac or psychiatric decompensation. Short periods of mania or hypomania may occur during treatment, but will typically subside during the replacement. Moderate doses of neuroleptics are usually well tolerated in cases of psychosis, but these cases may not recover totally. The treatment of hypothyroidism in patients with dementia does not necessarily reverse the memory deficits.

Hyperthyroidism

Psychological disturbance of some degree is universal in hyperthyroidism, and may delay the diagnosis of the endocrine disorder (Stern *et al.* 1996). Anxiety, and to a lesser extent depression, syndromes are most frequently reported, and they are usually accompanied by restlessness, overactivity and irritability, sometimes with hyperacuity of perception and over-reaction to noise. States of extreme anxiety and irritability may arise, with heightened tension leading to impatience and intolerance of frustration. Emotional lability may develop, accompanied by histrionic behaviour. Depression can be prominent and include fatigue, weakness and somatic symptoms. Retardation is rare, but 'apathetic hyperthyroidism' has been described, leading to stupor or coma.

In the past it used to be said that up to 20% of cases of hyperthyroidism had psychoses of some type, including those heralding fatal thyroid storms, but there probably was a selective reporting bias (Lishman 1998). Acute organic reactions with typical delirium are now rare; they should be considered medical emergencies and warrant urgent intervention. Psychoses with blurred margins between schizophrenic and affective disorders have been described, and paranoid features are common. Organic personality syndromes are seen in elderly patients, who are often apathetic. Over-arousal and distractibility, leading to cognitive impairment have also been reported, and may continue even once patients are believed to be euthyroid (Stern *et al.* 1996). The first prospective study to suggest that subclinical hyperthyroidism in the elderly increases the risk of dementia and Alzheimer's disease has been reported (Kalmijn *et al.* 2000).

The presenting symptoms of hyperthyroidism may be identical to anxiety disorders, but the diagnosis of the former is supported by signs and symptoms such as sensitivity to heat and preference for cold, increased appetite but loss of weight and dyspnoea on effort. The medical history and the search for these and other typical signs of hyperthyroidism (Table 18.3) are crucial in difficult cases;

the laboratory examinations give unequivocal results in the great majority of cases. Transient, mild hormonal elevations of thyroid hormones occur in 10% of psychiatric inpatients, and should not lead to misdiagnosis. In the elderly, the occasional case of 'apathetic hyperthyroidism' may pose a difficult distinction with depression. Acute drug intoxications by agents such as psychostimulants may mimic hyperthyroidism before the clinical and laboratory work-up is completed. On the contrary, alcoholism may wrongly be blamed for the tremulousness and emotional lability of hyperthyroidism.

Acute organic reactions seem to occur mainly at the peak of thyrotoxicosis. In less severe cases, increased hormonal levels and subsequent metabolic derangements in the central nervous system, including sympathetic hyperactivity and increased sensitivity to beta-adrenergic receptors, are considered to be the probable mechanisms for the affective signs and symptoms, particularly anxiety. Anxiety tends to subside in direct relation to hormonal levels, but depressive symptoms seem to be less closely related. Thyroid abnormalities have been documented in some studies in primary affective disorders (Oomen *et al.* 1996), but others were discrepant (Engum *et al.* 2002) and intervening variables or the effects of antidepressant medication make the interpretation of findings difficult. There is no good evidence to support the psychogenic, stress or personality theories about the origin of hyperthyroidism (Lishman 1998). The results of a cross-national, European study describing clinical practice in liaison psychiatry showed that physicians and endocrinologists do not request consultations based on the psychogenic hypothesis in this condition (Lobo *et al.* 1992).

In general, there is a good resolution of anxiety and depression with antithyroid treatment alone, unless there is previous psychiatric history (Kathol *et al.* 1986). However, recovery may be slow and reduced psychological well-being has been reported in a considerable proportion of patients with hyperthyroidism in remission (Pérez-Echeverría 1985). Psychosis may occur or be exacerbated by antithyroid medication. Low-potency neuroleptics are usually well tolerated in psychotic cases, but exacerbation of psychosis by neuroleptics such as haloperidol and perphenazine has been reported, including symptoms resembling thyroid storm and malignant neuroleptic syndrome. There is a limited clinical experience with the new generation of neuroleptics.

Hyperparathyroidism

Neuropsychiatric symptoms are considered to be very frequent in hyperparathyroidism (Brown *et al.* 1987), but the number of published reports is quite limited, samples studied are small and standardized methods have been rarely used (White *et al.* 1996). Depressive and anxiety disorders are the commonest syndromes observed (Joborn *et al.* 1986; Linder *et al.* 1988), and include symptoms of fatigue, apathy, irritability, decreased appetite and sleep and concentration difficulties. With the exception of elderly patients, symptoms are usually not as severe as in primary affective disorder (Linder *et al.* 1988). Cognitive dysfunction has also been observed, is frequent in the elderly (Joborn *et al.* 1986), and may lead to dementing syndromes. Florid delirium is also considered to be frequent when hypercalcaemia is high (above 16 mg/dl) and coma has been reported with serum levels above 19 mg/dl (Petersen 1968). Psychosis with hallucinations and paranoid ideas were found in one study (Joborn *et al.* 1986), and some case reports suggest violent behaviour, including attempted mass murder (Bresler *et al.* 2000), related to paranoid delusions in a clear sensorium. In chronic cases, personality changes have been described, leading to an isolated and reclusive behaviour.

Primary hyperparathyroidism may be asymptomatic and only appear as a laboratory finding. Therefore, the determination of serum calcium levels might be considered in the work-up of atypical psychiatric presentations of depressive syndromes or cognitive difficulties. Calcium levels should also be monitored in patients treated with lithium, since hypercalcaemia as a secondary effect of lithium therapy is also well known and may lead to a misdiagnosis of relapse of affective symptoms (Pieri-Balandraud *et al.* 2001). An electroencephalogram (EEG), which tends to show slowing of electrical activity and may be accompanied by frontal delta-paroxysms in hypercalcaemia, may be an important diagnostic tool.

In relation to pathogenesis, hypercalcaemia itself may be the main cause of the psychiatric syndromes, since it has been shown to produce similar symptoms independent of the aetiology. Calcium ions are considered to be fundamental in neurotransmission processes. They might influence the abnormal concentrations of monoamine metabolites in cerebrospinal fluid (CSF), in particular 5-hydroxy-indoleacetic acid (5-HIAA), found in patients with primary hyperparathyroidism, correlated with depressive symptoms and reversed to normal after successful parathyroid surgery (Joborn *et al.* 1988). Depressive symptoms in primary hyperparathyroidism have also been found to correlate with alterations in serum cortisol and melatonin, all improving after successful surgery (Linder *et al.* 1988). Similar findings have been observed in primary affective disorders. However, some studies could not document a direct correlation of psychopathology and level of calcium (Joborn *et al.* 1988; White *et al.* 1996). Vitamin D and parathormone itself, as well as hypomagnesaemia and hypophosphoraemia (frequently found in these patients) have also been implicated in the pathogenesis of the psychiatric symptoms.

Most reports conclude that psychiatric symptoms tend to resolve or significantly improve after successful surgical treatment, particularly if the endocrine disorder has not become chronic. The improvement may be evident within a few days and appears to plateau a few months later (Joborn *et al.* 1986). However, some studies suggest depressive symptoms improve more completely than cognitive symptoms (Brown *et al.* 1987). In view of the conflicting results the recommendation is a conservative treatment of hyperparathyroidism in asymptomatic cases or cases with mild symptoms.

Hypoparathyroidism

The removal of, or interference with, blood supply to the parathyroid glands during neck surgery is the commonest cause of hypoparathyroidism. Almost any kind of psychiatric disorder has been described in this condition (Table 18.1), but there has been very little systematic study in the last decades. Reviews of the subject estimated that half the cases due to surgery had psychiatric symptoms, and the prevalence might be even higher in idiopathic cases (Lishman 1998). Delirium is also frequent as a post-operative complication, probably due to abrupt biochemical changes. In more insidious cases, such as idiopathic hypoparathyroidism, patients may show cognitive difficulties leading to dementia, but also emotional lability, anxiety syndromes and, less frequently, depressive syndromes. Fluctuating symptoms and behavioural changes have also been described, including nervousness, irritability and social withdrawal. Psychotic syndromes are only rarely seen.

Hypocalcaemia is considered to be the fundamental cause of the psychological symptoms. In asymptomatic patients with calcium levels at the lower limit of normal ('partial parathyroid insufficiency'), anxiety, depression and related symptoms may be episodic, precipitated by calcium deprivation. A double-blind trial of calcium vs. placebo in these patients was effective in reducing symptomatology (Fourman *et al.* 1967).

There is considerable documentation in the literature regarding the difficulties detecting this condition. Special consideration merits the case of anxiety resistant to treatment. Anxiety can provoke hyperventilation and tetany in hypoparathyroid patients (Fourman *et al.* 1967). Calcium and phosphorus levels should be considered in doubtful cases, particularly in patients operated upon in the neck. Epileptic crisis or an abnormal EEG may be the only signs of hypoparathyroidism.

In general, the psychiatric syndromes due to hypoparathyroidism are considered to be remediable with calcium supplements and vitamin D. The response is good when affective syndromes are not severe. Even cognitive deterioration may improve in a substantial proportion of patients, with the exception of the severe and chronic dementing syndromes. Symptomatic treatment of anxiety with benzodiazepines is usually effective. Susceptibility of these patients to the parkinsonian side-effects of neuroleptics has also been suggested, but could not always be confirmed (Pratty et al. 1986).

Hyperprolactinaemia

Hyperprolactinaemia is a frequent disturbance in clinical endocrinology, mostly due to prolactinomas in women. Psychiatric syndromes, especially anxiety and depression (Pérez-Echeverría 1985), and hostility in some studies, have been reported in this condition (Fava et al. 1982). The hyperprolactinaemia was considered to represent an increased risk of 3.52 for depression, 3.32 for anxiety and 3.84 for other psychiatric symptoms, but no correlations were found between prolactin levels and the severity of psychiatric symptoms (Oliveira et al. 2000).

Neuroleptic treatment is the most frequent cause of prolactin elevation in psychiatric patients and may be induced even with low doses. It is frequently underdiagnosed, but can induce relevant clinical problems, such as galactorrhoea, sexual dysfunction and depression in the short-term, and poor compliance with treatment as a result and relapse of psychosis in the long-term (Maguire 2002). Therefore, enquiry about these symptoms is recommended when patients are taking antipsychotic medications for long periods of time. On the contrary, prolactin elevation is infrequent as a side-effect of antidepressants and very rare with other psychotropic medication.

Some studies document that both amantadine (Correa et al. 1987) and bromocriptine (Buckman & Kellner 1985) improve depressive syndromes induced by the hyperprolactinaemia. The treatment of choice when this is related to antipsychotic use is reduction of the dosage or discontinuation of therapy; if this fails to resolve the symptoms, bromocriptine or amantadine may be tried.

Cushing's syndrome

Psychiatric presentations in Cushing's syndrome are well substantiated. Depression has been documented in most studies (Cohen 1980), and clinical experience suggests that its assessment may be critical. While some reports found that 'neurotic' depression was the most common type (Kelly et al. 1996), the majority conclude that it is frequently severe. Dorn et al. (1995) found major depressions in 50% of cases and suicidal ideation has also been reported (Pérez-Echeverría 1985). Atypical features, including 'organic' symptoms are also commonly described (Dorn et al. 1995), and Pérez-Echeverría (1985) found severe psychomotor retardation in cases due to primary disturbance of pituitary or hypothalamus (Cushing's disease). Psychotic features, which may take the form of florid delusions and hallucinations, are relatively frequent when compared with primary affective disorder or depression associated with other medical illnesses (Lishman 1998). On the contrary, manic syndromes are rare, in contrast to what has been documented when steroids are administered for therapeutic purposes (Dorn *et al.* 1995).

Anxiety, somatic symptoms, and high neuroticism scores have also been documented in some studies (Kelly *et al.* 1996; Pérez-Echeverría 1985). Cognitive dysfunction (Belanoff *et al.* 2001) or more selective memory disturbances (Mauri *et al.* 1993) have been described, particularly in patients with chronic hypercortisolaemia, and delirium occurs in cases of metabolic complications such as electrolytic disturbances.

Psychiatric syndromes may lead to misdiagnosis, particularly in Cushing's patients without physical signs, because hypothalamic-pituitary-adrenal (HPA) axis abnormalities, specifically hypercortisolaemia, with increased urinary free cortisol levels or dexamethasone non-suppression, also occur in primary affective disorder. The corticotrophin-releasing factor infusion (CRF) test in patients with Cushing's syndrome reveals an augmented adrenocorticotrophic hormone (ACTH) response, while patients with primary depression have a blunted response. In doubtful cases, treatment of depression should be instituted; the resolution of HPA axis abnormalities suggesting a primary affective disorder.

The majority of cases of Cushing's syndrome are considered to be due to pituitary overproduction of ACTH, related to primary disturbance of the pituitary or the hypothalamus (Cushing's disease), and resulting in secondary hyperplasia of the adrenal cortex. Longer duration of this syndrome may place patients at increased risk of affective psychopathology (Dorn *et al.* 1995). The 'organic', endocrine origin of psychiatric syndromes in these patients is supported by data showing the improvement or resolution of psychiatric symptoms with successful treatment of the endocrine disorder (Kelly *et al.* 1996; Pérez-Echeverría 1985). It is also supported by correlations found in most studies between severity of depression or other psychopathological dimensions and levels of cortisol (Starkman *et al.* 1986) or ACTH (Lobo *et al.* 1988; Pérez-Echeverría 1985).

Since such correlations have not been found in some reports, a family history of affective disorder, or a substance other than cortisol produced by the adrenal under excessive pituitary and/or hypothalamic stimulation have been implicated in the aetiology of depressive symptoms (Cohen 1980). Hypersecretion of corticotrophin-releasing factor has been hypothesized as contributing to HPA axis hyperactivity and perhaps to certain signs and symptoms of primary, major depression (Nemeroff 1989). However, this hypothesis of production of affective disturbances in Cushing's disease is weak, since CRF may presumably be suppressed (Gold *et al.* 1986). A hypothesis of glucocorticoid-associated brain damage has also been formulated (Martignoni *et al.* 1992), and the cognitive disturbance found in Cushing's patients has been related to structural deficits, including reduced hippocampal volume, correlated with high cortisol levels (Starkman *et al.* 1992).

Resolution of depression and/or psychiatric syndromes usually follows medical and/or surgical treatment of the endocrine disorder (Kelly *et al.* 1996), unless there is history of previous psychiatric disorder. However, the response is often delayed (1–3 months), and treatment of severe depression should be instituted while awaiting the response of both physical and psychiatric disturbances. Vigorous antidepressive medication and/or electroconvulsive therapy (ECT) may be necessary, but antidepressants should usually be discontinued when the hypercortisolaemia has been controlled for several months.

Inhibitors of corticosteroid production (e.g. ketoconazole, metyrapone, aminoglutethimide), rather than antidepressant drugs, have also been recommended in treating depressive and other disabling symptoms (Sonino & Fava 2001), but response may be delayed for months (Cohen 1980). The possibility that cognitive dysfunction caused by glucocorticoids can be pharmacologically managed has been suggested (Belanoff *et al.* 2001).

Addison's disease

The output of adrenal steroids is low in Addison's disease, resulting in most cases from destruction of the adrenal cortices, mainly due to autoimmune mechanisms. In a small proportion of cases, hypothalamic or pituitary pathology or the administration of exogenous steroids may produce the disturbance. Few studies have examined associated psychiatric symptoms in a standardized manner.

Typical addisonian symptoms are a gradual and progressive apathy, lethargy and fatigue. Similarly, loss of drive and initiative are common manifestations. Clinical psychiatric studies have reported psychopathological syndromes in up to 80% of cases and depression in half (Cleghorn 1965). Fluctuations in mood are common, and severity of symptoms tends to oscillate in relation to the severity of the endocrinopathy. Psychotic symptoms such as delusions are very rare, but florid delirium with hallucinations and paranoid ideas has been described in severe cases. Changes in perceptual threshold have also been reported (Reus 1987). Memory difficulties and other cognitive disturbances observed in patients with Addison's disease might be influenced by apathy. Addisonian crisis may be preceded by psychopathological manifestations. Stress or abrupt suppression of treatment with adrenal steroids may produce a severe crisis with signs of acute circulatory shock.

Early dementia, primary depression, neurotic illness, anorexia nervosa and chronic fatigue syndrome (CFS) should be considered in the differential diagnosis. However, the possibility that CFS might be a form of Addison's disease (Baschetti 2000) or the result of low hypothalamic-pituitary-adrenal activity has also been considered. Definitive diagnosis is usually accomplished with laboratory investigations of endocrine function.

The insufficiency of steroids, in particular glucocorticoids, is considered to be fundamental in the production of psychiatric symptoms (Reus 1987). Increased axonal conductivity, and elevated CRF or ACTH have all been suggested as important metabolic factors (Johnstone *et al.* 1990).

Replacement therapy is usually quite satisfactory in resolving both the physical and psychopathological manifestations of Addison's disease. Glucocorticoids are suggested by some to be more effective than mineralocorticoids in alleviating the psychiatric symptoms (Lishman 1998). The education of patients to adjust dosages of medication according to circumstances is considered to be important. A patient's identification card may help in case of an emergency. Patients should also be alerted to their sensitivity to drugs with central nervous system depressant potential, and patients treated with lithium may need higher doses of mineralocorticoids.

Phaeochromocytoma

Tumours typified by an excess of catecholamine production are mostly found in the chromaffin cells of the adrenal medulla. Their output may be paroxysmal or continuous and therefore symptoms are subject to great variation. Classical descriptions of the acute episodes include frequent and marked mental symptoms, which may closely mimic panic attacks and include fear and feelings of impending death; confusion may be seen afterwards. Some cases may present less abruptly, the anxiety being less severe, but accompanied by feelings of faintness and palpitations. Anxiety syndromes are predictable in view of the well-established effects of catecholamines on stress responses. It has also been suggested that attacks may be precipitated by emotional factors (Lishman 1998).

Some reports suggest that psychopathological syndromes may be less frequent or typical as initially suggested. Starkman *et al.* (1985) documented in a sample of 17 patients that none of them described the severe apprehension or fear characteristic of panic attacks and only one patient received a diagnosis of possible panic disorder; two met criteria for generalized anxiety disorder, and two for major depressive episode. The illness behaviour during episodes of illness may also suggest hysteria or agitated depression, and these entities should be considered in the differential diagnosis (Guerrieri *et al.* 2002).

A careful medical history is essential to establish the diagnosis, and hyperthyroidism should be considered in the differential diagnosis. In cases of phaeochromocytoma examination reveals marked hypertension during the attacks and also usually in between attacks, and the essential investigation is the demonstration of greatly increased levels of catecholamines in the plasma or urine, or of their metabolites in 24-hour samples of urine. Psychiatric symptoms in these patients, including anxiety syndromes, tend to resolve with the removal of the tumour.

Acromegaly

Acromegaly, the disease due to overproduction of pituitary growth hormone, has been associated with psychiatric manifestations, but the existing documentation is limited and recent studies suggest lower rates of psychiatric morbidity than previously described. Case reports have described alterations of personality, the patients showing lack of spontaneity and initiative and lack of consideration for others, as well as changes of mood and brief periods of impulsive behaviour (Lishman 1998). Some later reports tend to support these initial findings, and the case series of Richert et al. (1987) describes 'uniform psychopathological symptoms' including loss of drive, affective disorders such as dejection and irritability and 'strikingly uniform personality traits' of conscientiousness, reliability and industriousness.

However, this study found that the psychopathological symptoms were not dependent on the level of the increased growth hormone, and more recent reports could not confirm the thesis of a uniform psychopathology in these patients. Furthermore, Abed et al. (1987) studied 51 acromegalic patients with standardized instruments, including a psychiatric interview, and concluded that there was no increase in psychiatric morbidity in general, nor an increased incidence of depression, in comparison with general population and patient samples. If psychiatric symptoms are observed in individual cases consideration needs to be given to the emotional impact of the illness, particularly due to altered appearance from skeletal overgrowth, as well as to the effects of hormonal changes on mental state.

REFERENCES

Abed, R. T., Clark, J., Elbadawy, M. H., et al. (1987). Psychiatric morbidity in acromegaly. *Acta Psychiatrica Scandinavica*, **75**, 635–9.

Baschetti, R. (2000). Chronic fatigue syndrome: a form of Addison's disease. *Journal of Internal Medicine*, **247**, 737–9.

Bauer, M. S. and Whybrow, P. C. (1990). Rapid cycling bipolar affective disorder. II. Treatment of refractory rapid cycling with high-dose levothyroxine: a preliminary study. *Archives of General Psychiatry*, **47**, 435–40.

Baumgartner, A. (1993). Thyroid hormones and depressive disorders – critical overview and perspectives. Part 1: Clinical aspects. *Nervenarzt*, **64**, 1–10.

Belanoff, J. K., Gross, K., Yager, A., *et al.* (2001). Corticosteroids and cognition. *Journal of Psychiatric Research*, **35**, 127–45.

Bresler, S. A., Logan, W. S. and Washington, D. (2000). Hyperparathyroidism and psychosis: possible prelude to murder. *Journal of Forensic Science*, **45**, 728–30.

Brown, G. G., Preisman, R. C. and Kleerekoper, M. (1987). Neurobehavioral symptoms in mild primary hyperparathyroidism: related to hypercalcemia but not improved by parathyroidectomy. *Henry Ford Hospital Medical Journal*, **35**, 211–15.

Buckman, M. T. and Kellner, R. (1985). Reduction of distress in hyperprolactinemia with bromocriptine. *American Journal of Psychiatry*, **142**, 242–4.

Carroll, B. J., Feinberg, M., Greden, J. F., *et al.* (1981). A specific laboratory test for the diagnosis of melancholia. Standardization, validation, and clinical utility. *Archives of General Psychiatry*, **38**, 15–22.

Cleghorn, R. A. (1965). Surgery and the psyche. *Journal of International College of Surgeons*, **44**, 561–6.

Cohen, S. I. (1980). Cushing's syndrome: a psychiatric study of 29 patients. *British Journal of Psychiatry*, **136**, 120–4.

Correa, N., Opler, L. A., Kay, S. R., *et al.* (1987). Amantadine in the treatment of neuroendocrine side effects of neuroleptics. *Journal of Clinical Psychopharmacology*, **7**, 91–5.

Deary, I. J. and Frier, B. M. (1996). Severe hypoglycaemia and cognitive impairment in diabetes. *British Medical Journal*, **313**, 767–8.

Dorn, L. D., Burgess, E. S., Dubbert, B., *et al.* (1995). Psychopathology in patients with endogenous Cushing's syndrome: 'atypical' or melancholic features. *Clinical Endocrinology (Oxford)*, **43**, 433–42.

Eiber, R., Berlin, I., Grimaldi, A., *et al.* (1997). Insulin-dependent diabetes and psychiatric pathology: general clinical and epidemiologic review. *Encephale*, **23**, 351–7.

Engum, A., Bjoro, T., Mykletun, A., *et al.* (2002). An association between depression, anxiety and thyroid function – a clinical fact or an artefact? *Acta Psychiatrica Scandinavica*, **106**, 27–34.

Fava, M., Fava, G. A., Kellner, R., *et al.* (1982). Depression and hostility in hyperprolactinemia. *Progress in Neuropsychopharmacology and Biological Psychiatry*, **6**, 479–82.

Fourman, P., Rawnsley, K., Davis, R. H., *et al.* (1967). Effect of calcium on mental symptoms in partial parathyroid insufficiency. *Lancet*, **2**, 914–15.

Gold, P. W., Loriaux, D. L., Roy, A., *et al.* (1986). Responses to corticotropin-releasing hormone in the hypercortisolism of depression and Cushing's disease. Pathophysiologic and diagnostic implications. *New England Journal of Medicine*, **314**, 1329–35.

Guerrieri, M., Filipponi, S., Arnaldi, G., *et al.* (2002). Unusual clinical manifestation of pheochromocytoma in a MEN2A patient. *Journal of Endocrinological Investigation*, **25**, 53–7.

Hudson, J. I., Hudson, M. S., Griffing, G. T., *et al.* (1987). Phenomenology and family history of affective disorder in Cushing's disease. *American Journal of Psychiatry*, **144**, 951–3.

Jalenques, I., Tauveron, I., Albuisson, E., et al. (1993). Prevalence of anxiety and depressive symptoms in patients with type 1 and 2 diabetes. *Revue médicale de la Suisse romande*, **113**, 639–46.

Joborn, C., Hetta, J., Palmer, M., et al. (1986). Psychiatric symptomatology in patients with primary hyperparathyroidism. *Uppsala Journal of Medical Sciences*, **91**, 77–87.

Joborn, C., Hetta, J., Rastad, J., et al. (1988). Psychiatric symptoms and cerebrospinal fluid monoamine metabolites in primary hyperparathyroidism. *Biological Psychiatry*, **23**, 149–58.

Johnstone, P. A., Rundell, J. R. and Esposito, M. (1990). Mental status changes of Addison's disease. *Psychosomatics*, **31**, 103–7.

Kalmijn, S., Mehta, K. M., Pols, H. A., et al. (2000). Subclinical hyperthyroidism and the risk of dementia. The Rotterdam study. *Clinical Endocrinology (Oxford)*, **53**, 733–7.

Kathol, R. G. (2002). Endocrine disorders. In *The American Psychiatric Publishing Textbook of Consultation-liaison Psychiatry: Psychiatry in the Medically Ill*, 2nd edn., ed. M. G. Wise and J. R. Rundell. Washington, DC: American Psychiatric Publisher, pp. 563–7.

Kathol, R. G. and Delahunt, J. W. (1986). The relationship of anxiety and depression to symptoms of hyperthyroidism using operational criteria. *General Hospital Psychiatry*, **8**, 23–8.

Kathol, R. G., Turner, R. and Delahunt, J. (1986). Depression and anxiety associated with hyperthyroidism: response to antithyroid therapy. *Psychosomatics*, **27**, 501–5.

Kelly, W. F., Kelly, M. J. and Faragher, B. (1996). A prospective study of psychiatric and psychological aspects of Cushing's syndrome. *Clinical Endocrinology (Oxford)*, **45**, 715–20.

Kupka, R. W., Nolen, W. A., Post, R. M., et al. (2002). High rate of autoimmune thyroiditis in bipolar disorder: lack of association with lithium exposure. *Biological Psychiatry*, **51**, 305–11.

Linder, J., Brimar, K., Granberg, P. O., et al. (1988). Characteristic changes in psychiatric symptoms, cortisol and melatonin but not prolactin in primary hyperparathyroidism. *Acta Psychiatrica Scandinavica*, **78**, 32–40.

Lishman, W. A. (1998). Endocrine diseases and metabolic disorders. In *Organic Psychiatry: the Psychological Consequences of Cerebral Disorder*, 3rd edn. Oxford: Blackwell Science, pp. 507–69.

Lloyd, C. E., Dyer, P. H. and Barnett, A. H. (2000). Prevalence of symptoms of depression and anxiety in a diabetes clinic population. *Diabetic Medicine*, **17**, 198–202.

Lobo, A., Pérez-Echeverría, M. J., Jimenez-Aznarez, A., et al. (1988). Emotional disturbances in endocrine patients. Validity of the scaled version of the General Health Questionnaire (GHQ-28). *British Journal of Psychiatry*, **152**, 807–12.

Lobo, A., Huyse, F., Herzog, T., et al. (1992). *Profiles of Psychiatric and Physical Co-morbidity*. Paper read before the E. C. L. W. Health Service Study Conference: Amsterdam.

Maguire, G. A. (2002). Prolactin elevation with antipsychotic medications: mechanisms of action and clinical consequences. *Journal of Clinical Psychiatry*, **63**(Suppl. 4), 56–62.

Martignoni, E., Costa, A., Sinforiani, E., et al. (1992). The brain as a target for adrenocortical steroids: cognitive implications. *Psychoneuroendocrinology*, **17**, 343–54.

Mauri, M., Sinforiani, E., Bono, G., et al. (1993). Memory impairment in Cushing's disease. *Acta Neurologica Scandinavica*, **87**, 52–5.

Mayou, R., Peveler, R., Davies, B., *et al.* (1991). Psychiatric morbidity in young adults with insulin-dependent diabetes mellitus. *Psychological Medicine*, **21**, 639–45.

Nemeroff, C. B. (1989). Clinical significance of psychoneuroendocrinology in psychiatry: focus on the thyroid and adrenal. *Journal of Clinical Psychiatry*, **50**(Suppl.), 13–20.

Oliveira, M. C., Pizarro, C. B., Golbert, L., *et al.* (2000). Hyperprolactinemia and psychological disturbance. *Arquives de Neuropsiquiatria*, **58**, 671–6.

Oomen, H. A., Schipperijn, A. J. and Drexhage, H. A. (1996). The prevalence of affective disorder and in particular of a rapid cycling of bipolar disorder in patients with abnormal thyroid function tests. *Clinical Endocrinology (Oxford)*, **45**, 215–23.

Pérez-Echeverría, M. J. (1985). Correlaciones entre trastornos endocrinológicos, niveles hormonales en sangre, variables de personalidad y alteraciones psicopatológicas. Unpublished Ph.D. Thesis, Universidad de Zaragoza.

Petersen, P. (1968). Psychiatric disorders in primary hyperparathyroidism. *Journal of Clinical Endocrinology and Metabolism*, **28**, 1491–5.

Pieri-Balandraud, N., Hugueny, P., Henry, J. F., *et al.* (2001). Hyperparathyroidism induced by lithium. A new case. *Review Medicine Interne*, **22**, 460–4.

Pratty, J. S., Ananth, J. and O'Brien, J. E. (1986). Relationship between dystonia and serum calcium levels. *Journal of Clinical Psychiatry*, **47**, 418–19.

Reus, I. V. (1987). Disorders of the adrenal cortex and gonads. In *Handbook of Clinical Psychoneuroendocrinology*, ed. C. B. Nemeroff and P. T. Loosen. New York: Guilford Press, pp. 71–84.

Richert, S., Strauss, A., Fahlbusch, R., *et al.* (1987). Psychopathologic symptoms and personality traits in patients with florid acromegaly. *Schweizer Archfür Neurologic und Psychiatrie*, **138**, 61–86.

Simon, N. M., Blacker, D., Korbly, N. B., *et al.* (2002). Hypothyroidism and hyperthyroidism in anxiety disorders revisited: new data and literature review. *Journal of Affective Disorders*, **69**, 209–17.

Sonino, N. and Fava, G. A. (2001). Psychiatric disorders associated with Cushing's syndrome. Epidemiology, pathophysiology and treatment. *CNS Drugs*, **15**, 361–73.

Starkman, M. N., Schteingart, D. E. and Schork, M. A. (1981). Depressed mood and other psychiatric manifestations of Cushing's syndrome: relationship to hormone levels. *Psychosomatic Medicine*, **43**, 3–18.

Starkman, M. N., Zelnik, T. C., Nesse, R. M., *et al.* (1985). Anxiety in patients with pheochromocytomas. *Archives of Internal Medicine*, **145**, 248–52.

Starkman, M. N., Schteingart, D. E. and Schork, M. A. (1986). Cushing's syndrome after treatment: changes in cortisol and ACTH levels, and amelioration of the depressive syndrome. *Psychiatry Research*, **19**, 177–88.

Starkman, M. N., Gebarski, S. S., Berent, S., *et al.* (1992). Hippocampal formation volume, memory dysfunction, and cortisol levels in patients with Cushing's syndrome. *Biological Psychiatry*, **32**, 756–65.

Stern, R. A., Robinson, B., Thorner, A. R., *et al.* (1996). A survey study of neuropsychiatric complaints in patients with Graves' disease. *Journal of Neuropsychiatry and Clinical Neuroscience*, **8**, 181–5.

Trzepacz, P. T., McCue, M., Klein, I., *et al.* (1988). A psychiatric and neuropsychological study of patients with untreated Graves' disease. *General Hospital Psychiatry*, **10**, 49–55.

White, R. E., Pickering, A. and Spathis, G. S. (1996). Mood disorder and chronic hypercalcemia. *Journal Psychosomatic Research*, **41**, 343–7.

Wilkinson, G., Borsey, D. Q., Leslie, P., *et al.* (1998). Psychiatric morbidity and social problems in patients with insulin-dependent diabetes mellitus. *British Journal of Psychiatry*, **153**, 38–43.

World Health Organization. (1992). *The ICD-10 Classification of Mental and Behavioural Disorders. Clinical Descriptions and Diagnostic Guidelines*: Geneva: World Health Organization.

19

Diabetes

Khalida Ismail and Robert Peveler

Introduction

Diabetes mellitus is one of the most common chronic diseases worldwide and is characterized by chronic hyperglycaemia. The prevalence of detected diabetes is around 3–4% in the general population and increasing largely due to the epidemic of obesity and to improved survival rates (Amos *et al.* 1997). Diabetes mellitus presents specific challenges to the liaison psychiatrist additional to those common to chronic disease conditions as the management and prognosis is largely based on the patient taking responsibility for multiple self-care tasks such as diet, exercise, weight reduction, self-monitoring of glucose, foot care and injection sites and adhering to oral medication and insulin injections.

Despite the high prevalence of diabetes in the general medical setting and good evidence that mental health problems are common and reduce life expectancy, the development of diabetes-specific liaison mental health services is sporadic and piecemeal. We begin by giving an outline of the clinical features of diabetes. This is followed by a review of the psychiatric and psychological factors associated with diabetes. Finally a summary of the evidence of the effectiveness of pharmacological and psychological interventions is examined.

Clincial features of diabetes mellitus

An increasing understanding of the aetiology of diabetes and advances in treatment recently led to a new classification comprising four types of diabetes based on pathology of the underlying condition rather than on the nature of

Handbook of Liaison Psychiatry, ed. Geoffrey Lloyd and Elspeth Guthrie. Published by Cambridge University Press. © Cambridge University Press 2007.

treatment (Alberti & Zimmett 1998; Expert Committee on the Diagnosis and Classification of Diabetes Mellitus 1997).

Type 1 diabetes represents around 10% of all cases of diabetes and includes immune-mediated and idiopathic forms which lead to absolute insulin deficiency. It used to be called insulin-dependent or juvenile onset diabetes. It has a rapid onset of a few months to weeks characterized by fatigue, weight loss, polyuria and polydypsia. Its peak ages of onset are around 5 years and 18 years. There is often a 'honeymoon' phase during the first year in which the physiological need for exogenous insulin is transiently less and glycaemic control is deceptively good.

Type 2 diabetes represents around 85% of all cases of diabetes and it may originate from insulin resistance and relative insulin deficiency or from a secretory defect. It is a disease of adult onset with a mean age of onset at around 60 years. Factors associated with an increased risk for type 2 diabetes are obesity, being of African and Indian subcontinent ethnicity, material deprivation and having genetic predisposition and physical inactivity.

Type 3 diabetes covers a wide range of specific types of diabetes including pancreatic failure secondary to alcohol-induced pancreatitis. Type 4 diabetes is gestational diabetes.

The aim of diabetes management is to maintain glycaemic levels within, or as close as possible to, the normal range. Chronic hyperglycaemia increases the risk of serious diabetic microvascular complications such as nephropathy, retinopathy and neuropathy and macrovascular conditions such as coronary heart disease and cerebrovascular disease which herald a deterioration in functioning and reduced life expectancy. In type 4 diabetes, persistent hyperglycaemia is associated with an increased risk of adverse maternal and birth outcomes. Two large scale multicentre randomized controlled trials have demonstrated that intensive medical management can improve glycaemic control and reduce rate of complications in type 1 (DCCT Research Group 1993) and type 2 diabetes (UK Prospective Diabetes Study (UKPDS) Group 1998). At the end of the Diabetes Control and Complications Trial in type 1 diabetes the improvements were not sustained in the intervention arm and it has been argued that the increased psychological support may have biased the observed benefits (Lorenz *et al.* 1996). In the UK Prospective Diabetes Study for type 2 diabetes, the authors suggested that adherence difficulties for patients may have accounted for the observed progressive increase in glycated haemoglobin even in the intensively managed group (UK Prospective Diabetes Study (UKPDS) Group 1998).

Psychiatric disorders in diabetes mellitus

Depression

Depression is the most common psychiatric disorder observed in diabetes mellitus. There is evidence supporting an association with depressive disorders at each stage of the natural history of diabetes.

Depressive disorders prior to onset of diabetes

The notion that diabetes is psychogenic in its origins has been suggested for many centuries. Thomas Willis in 1679 speculated that prolonged sorrow was linked to the onset of diabetes. In the 19th and early 20th century, there was a theory that anxiety or stressful lives could cause emotional glycosuria (Meninger 1935).

There is putative evidence that depression may be a risk factor for the onset of type 2 diabetes (Knol *et al.* 2006). In the Epidemiological Catchment Area Study in 1981 major depressive disorder measured by the Diagnostic Interview Schedule was prospectively associated with more than a twofold increase in the incidence of cases of self-report type 2 diabetes 13 years later (Eaton *et al.* 1996). In a prospective study of Japanese men, depressive symptoms were associated with a similar over twofold increased risk for a clinical diagnosis of type 2 diabetes over a four-year period (Kawakami *et al.* 1999).

Concurrence of depression and diabetes

Population-based cross-sectional studies that have used diagnostic research interviews and where cases of diabetes and the controls have been derived from the same population have reported that the prevalence of depressive disorders is around two to three times higher in patients with diabetes than in healthy controls (Wells *et al.* 1989; Weyerer *et al.* 1989; Zhang *et al.* 1991). This increase is not specific to diabetes as similar or higher rates are found in other chronic medical conditions (Wells *et al.* 1989; Weyerer *et al.* 1989). Studies that have used depression rating scales have not consistently found an association between depressive symptoms and self-report of diabetes (Murrell *et al.* 1983; Palinkas *et al.* 1991). Smaller highly selected hospital samples (Popkin *et al.* 1988; Robinson *et al.* 1988) have found a greater increase in depressive symptoms and disorders compared to healthy controls.

In a systematic review conducted in 1993, the mean weighted prevalence of current depression in people with diabetes was estimated to be around 15% with a range from 8% to 20% (Gavard *et al.* 1993).

Incidence of depression in diabetes

One US prospective cohort of around 100 youths with newly diagnosed type 1 diabetes found that the incidence of depression was 28% during a 10-year follow-up period, the majority of which occurred within the first year following diagnosis (Kovacs *et al.* 1997). This is in contrast to a smaller US cohort study of 57 youths which did not show an increase of psychiatric symptoms compared to a healthy matched control group over a 10-year follow-up period (Jacobson *et al.* 1997a). A small highly select cohort study of depressed patients with diabetes showed a poorer outcome with recurrent or chronic depression than those who were not depressed at baseline (Lustman *et al.* 1988).

Depression and glycaemic control

There is good cross-sectional evidence that depressive symptoms and disorders are associated with poorer glycaemic control (Eaton *et al.* 1992; Lustman *et al.* 1988; Lustman *et al.* 1997a) although not all agree (Robinson *et al.* 1988).

A recent thorough meta-analytic review of the literature reported that there was a small but significant association between depression and glycaemic control as measured by the glycated haemoglobin with a pooled effect size of 0.17 (Lustman *et al.* 2000a). The meta-analysis did not find a difference by type of diabetes, although individual studies suggest that the association between depressive symptoms and glycaemic control may be stronger in type 1 compared to type 2 diabetes (de Groot *et al.* 1999; Van Tilburg *et al.* 2001). Nearly all the studies had one or more methodological limitations with small sample sizes, lack of control group, self-report measures of depression or depressive symptoms or mixed type 1 and 2 diabetes samples (Lustman *et al.* 2000). No causal inference could be made and prospective studies are needed to examine whether depression increases the risk of poor glycaemic control and/or whether poor self-care of diabetes and poor glycaemic control can lead to depressive mood states.

Depression and complications

Recent meta-analyses of cross-sectional studies have demonstrated a significant association of depression and diabetes complications (de Groot *et al.* 2001). Most studies are marred by the same methodological limitations as with studies that have examined the association between depression and glycaemic control described above.

There is a general lack of longitudinal data to indicate whether depression increases the risk for developing complications. The US cohort study of 66 youths with type 1 diabetes found that depression was an independent risk factor for diabetic retinopathy 10 years later (Kovacs *et al.* 1995). On the other hand stressful life events (risk factors for depression) were not associated with increased mortality or onset of macrovascular disease in a random sample of 160 people with diabetes (Lloyd *et al.* 1991). Recent work in a cross-sectional study of 184 patients with type 2 diabetes found that anxiety, depression and negative beliefs about illness influence physical and mental functioning, but not metabolic control (Paschalides *et al.* 2004).

Despite the methodological limitations of many studies there is overall consistent evidence that depression is common in diabetes, may be a potential risk factor for diabetes and is associated with suboptimal glycaemic control and complications and mortality (Katon *et al.* 2005; Zhang *et al.* 2005). It is mostly undetected and untreated (Lustman & Harper 1987) and has a doubly disabling effect (Jacobson *et al.* 1997b).

Eating disorders

The particular clinical problems that occur when patients have both diabetes mellitus and an eating disorder have been highlighted in case reports since the 1970s. Anorexia nervosa (AN), bulimia nervosa (BN) and the milder forms of eating disorder have all been described; in the main the clinical features seen in such patients resemble closely those of non-diabetic patients, with one important exception. This difference is that patients with diabetes have available to them an additional means of weight control: the under-use or omission of insulin to promote glycosuria. Dieting, binge-eating, vomiting and other means of weight control all tend to worsen glycaemic control, and are probably therefore associated with an increased risk of early microvascular complications (Rydall 1997). Such features are often found in those patients with self destructive behaviours who are admitted with recurrent episodes of ketoacidosis.

There has been considerable interest in the question of whether or not people with diabetes are at increased risk of developing an eating disorder. Most of the existing studies of this question are inconclusive by reason of methodological limitations. Early studies tended to rely on self-report measures of eating disorder features; many have also been based upon clinic populations that are unlikely to be representative of the overall population of people with diabetes, and have not included appropriate control groups. Furthermore most lack adequate power to be sure of their conclusions. Perhaps the best recent study of prevalence is that of Jones *et al.* which found no excess of cases of anorexia nervosa or bulimia nervosa but a suggestion that there was some excess of milder forms of eating problem (Jones *et al.* 2000). Even if the overall prevalence is not raised, some form of disturbance of eating habits and attitudes may affect up to 10−15% of adolescent and young adult females. Such disturbance is strongly associated with poor self-care and the increased risk of microvascular complications has now been demonstrated (Bryden *et al.* 1999, 2003).

The first step in successful management of such disorders is detection, but this can be difficult as many patients may be secretive or ashamed of their behaviour and unwilling to divulge details in the clinic setting. Poor glycaemic control, repeated episodes of ketoacidosis or hypoglycaemia or fluctuation in body weight are all important clues. Sensitive but direct enquiries about attitudes to body shape and weight and methods of weight management should be made. Screening questionnaires such as the Eating Attitudes Test may help but are not diagnostic. Specific forms of treatment such as cognitive-behavioural therapy are likely to be of benefit, but practitioners providing such treatments need to have a good understanding of the management of diabetes if they are to be effective.

Substance misuse

Alcohol is hypothesized to be diabetogenic. Suggested mechanisms include weight gain, pancreatitis and long-term effects on insulin secretion and insulin resistance. The evidence for an association between alcohol consumption and diabetes is inconsistent. Some well-designed large population-based prospective cohort studies in men have shown an inverse association between amount of alcohol consumption and incident cases of diabetes (Ajani *et al.* 2000; Rimm *et al.* 1995) although other similarly well-designed studies have found a positive association (Kao *et al.* 2001). An inverse association between alcohol consumption and incident cases of diabetes in women has also been reported (Hu *et al.* 2001), but again this is controversial (Kao *et al.* 2001). One of the reasons for these discrepancies may relate to the more general observation that there is a U-shaped association between alcohol intake and mortality. It has been suggested that individuals who are not currently drinking or drinking less are 'sick quitters' in that their reduction is in response to ill health (Shaper *et al.* 1988). Most of the studies have used lifetime self-report measures of alcohol which are likely to underestimate alcohol consumption, especially in women where the stigma is the greatest.

The prevalence of problem drinking does not appear to be raised in diabetes population patients but even so alcohol consumption is associated with reduced diabetes self-care behaviours (Johnson *et al.* 2000; Spangler *et al.* 1993) and worse glycaemic control (Peveler *et al.* 1993) and it may be an independent risk factor for developing diabetes complications (Adler *et al.* 1997; Kohner *et al.* 1998).

Anxiety disorders

Anxiety disorders often coexist with depression (Kovacs *et al.* 1997). Needle phobia is one of the most common anxiety disorders referred to liaison mental health. Needle phobia is classified in the Diagnostic and Statistical Manual-IV (DSM-IV) as 'blood-injection-injury phobia' and in the International Classification of Diseases-10 (ICD-10) as 'blood injury phobia'. There is intense fear associated with seeing blood or receiving an injection. Unlike other specific phobias, the autonomic response is typically although not universally vaso-vagal (an initial increase in heart rate followed by a decrease in heart rate and a drop in blood pressure). The lifetime prevalence of blood-injection-injury phobia has been estimated at around 3.5% in the general population (Bienvenu & Eaton 1998) with a 50–70% preponderance in females and in persons with less education. Whether the prevalence of DSM-IV or ICD-10 needle phobia is higher in patients with diabetes than in the general population is not known. Despite this, phobic symptoms and anxieties related to self-injection of insulin and self-monitoring of blood glucose are common and associated with difficulties in adhering to diabetes self-care and consequently increased glycaemic levels (Berlin *et al.* 1997; Bienvenu & Eaton 1998; Mollema *et al.* 2001).

Psychotic disorders

A possible association between schizophrenia and diabetes has long been suggested, and seems to predate the availability of effective drug treatments (Braceland *et al.* 1945; Freeman 1946). A number of recent well-conducted prevalence studies have underlined this association (e.g. Sernyak *et al.* 2002), although as most patients now receive medication it is more difficult to disentangle the effects of the illness and its treatments. The prevalence of diabetes in schizophrenia is approximately 10% (Koro *et al.* 2002) but rises with age, and up to 20–25% of patients may have clinically important glucose dysregulation over the age of 60 years.

Attempts to identify different causal factors have included analysis of case reports; population prevalence studies, pharmaco-epidemiological studies, including post-marketing surveillance and prescription event monitoring; and *post hoc* analysis of data from randomized trials. Concern has been raised about the use of some atypical antipsychotic drugs and the risks of developing diabetes (Lindenmayer *et al.* 2003). In a population-based sample of patients with schizophrenia nested in the UK General Practice Research Database, an age- and sex-matched case control study showed that prior use of olanzapine was significantly associated with a sixfold increase in incident cases of diabetes (as defined by use of insulin and/or oral antidiabetic agents) compared to randomly selected controls not taking any antipsychotic medication and a fourfold increase compared to controls taking conventional antipsychotic medication (Dixon *et al.* 2000; Koro *et al.* 2002). There was a smaller and non-significant association between prior use of risperidone and cases of diabetes.

The causal mechanisms are complex and at present poorly understood. One of the main side-effects of atypical antipsychotics is weight gain which is of course diabetogenic. People with schizophrenia are prone to unhealthy lifestyles, and social factors such as inadequate rehabilitation once psychosis has settled may lead to a sedentary existence, both of which are associated with obesity. There is some evidence that olanzapine has a direct effect on glucose metabolism as suggested by case reports of ketoacidosis. Given the serious implications for morbidity and mortality attributable to diabetes and adherence difficulties in people with schizophrenia, general psychiatrists do need to be aware of the diabetogenic risk of atypical antipsychotics. If evidence mounts of this risk major ethical issues such as informed consent and risk—benefit analysis may adversely impact on the use of atypical antipsychotics.

In October 2003 an international group of diabetologists and psychiatrists met to review the literature relating to the association, and to create pragmatic guidelines for the management of diabetic risk in patients with severe mental illness (Holt *et al.* 2005). The group concluded that the reasons why individuals with schizophrenia are more prone to developing diabetes than the general population are poorly defined, but likely to be multifactorial. The role of antipsychotic medications in the development of diabetes and other prediabetic states remains controversial, but they concluded that the attributable risk is low. Traditional risk factors most probably account for much of the diabetes seen in schizophrenia populations, suggesting that routine screening and aggressive risk-factor management are especially important in this patient group.

Personality disorders

The notion of the diabetic personality is rooted in 19th century medicine when psychogenic factors were considered in the onset of diabetes (Meninger 1935) but it is now generally discredited (Dunn & Turtle 1981). No personality trait has been consistently identified to be associated with the onset of, or co-exist with, diabetes. There has been no cohort study examining whether personality traits predict the onset of diabetes. One cross-sectional study using the Cloninger Tridimensional Personality Questionnaire on 139 people with diabetes found that opportunistic, alienated and explosive temperaments were most often associated with poor glycaemic control (Lustman *et al.* 1991). A follow-up study of 105 patients with type 2 diabetes participating in a randomized controlled trial showed that in the Revised NEO Personality Inventory the neuroticism domain was associated with better glycaemic control at baseline but associations with different personality domains and glycaemic control were inconsistent at 6- and 12-month follow-up. (Lane *et al.* 2000). Most studies have been flawed by methodological limitations such as study design, selection bias and small samples. Research in this area as in other chronic diseases is hampered by the more complex question of reverse causality, that is to what extent does the life experience of diabetes affect personality development.

Psychological problems

There are a number of psychological problems specific to diabetes which, whilst they do not fall into any psychiatric classification, can present with marked morbidity and distress and are of clinical significance to the liaison psychiatrist. Various authors present these problems in different ways but the same diabetes-specific themes recur such as fear of hypoglycaemia, fear of complications, self-destructive behaviours, family functioning and adjustment reactions.

Fear of hypoglycaemia

Hypoglycaemia is much more common in type 1 than type 2 diabetes. The consequences of hypoglycaemia can be distressing and disabling. Physical sequelae vary, from dizziness and impaired concentration, emotional and behavioural changes, physical injury and seizures to life-threatening coma. Some patients develop hypoglycaemia unawareness which is loss of the early physiological signs of falling blood sugars. Others find it difficult to distinguish symptoms of anxiety from those of hypoglycaemia. Psychological sequelae of hypoglycaemia include shame, guilt and embarrassment if it occurs in public or the workplace and helplessness if it occurs when the individual is alone. Some patients develop such a disabling fear of future hypoglycaemia attacks that they avoid them by maintaining higher blood sugar levels than medically advised. Others will find themselves in the clinical phenomenon of 'chasing blood sugars' where they are in a distressing cycle of excessively checking and responding to their blood sugars in order to avoid high and low sugar levels.

Adjustment problems

Adjusting to diabetes is a complex process that involves a reappraisal of, and adaptation of one's lifestyle, relationships and occupation. For people with type 1 diabetes, the initial relief of a diagnosis and immediate benefit from insulin therapy is often replaced by a bereavement phase which if prolonged or excessive can lead to delayed acceptance. Children can appear to adjust to living with diabetes but they often enter a rebellious phase during adolescence that can continue into early adult life. This is compounded by physiological changes which place new demands on the diabetes regime. In type 2 diabetes, patients are often presented with the diagnosis on routine screening or during investigations for other health problems. They may not perceive an urgency to change lifelong unhealthy lifestyles. Poorer psychological adjustment to diabetes does appear to be associated with poorer glycaemic control (Bryden *et al.* 2001; Polonsky *et al.* 1995; Welch *et al.* 1994) but the evidence base for factors associated with poor adjustment is barely understood. Clinically, themes relating to stigma, peer pressure, anger and resentment, fear of diabetes complications and non-diabetes related social stressors may predominate (Rubin & Peyrot 2001).

Self-destructive behaviours

This term is used to described a group of patients with type 1 diabetes who have serious difficulties in self-management manifested by severe fluctuations in glucose levels, frequent admissions for recurrent diabetic ketoacidosis and recurrent severe hypoglycaemia in the context of severe chronic poor glycaemic control (Gill 2001). It replaces the subgroup of patients who were labelled as having 'brittle diabetes', usually young females. The complications and mortality rates in this subgroup are high. Brittle diabetes was believed to have an underlying physiological explanation but this has not been substantiated and it is probably also related to psychological problems, including eating disorder psychopathology (see above). The evidence for one or more distinct psychological risk factors is still in its infancy. Social problems are associated with psychiatric morbidity and with admissions for poor control (Mayou *et al.* 1991; Wilkinson *et al.* 1988; Wrigley & Mayou 1991). Many diabetes services will search for evidence for manipulative, deceitful, factitious behaviours such as hiding insulin or adding glucose to the urine. Slowly but thankfully the emphasis is moving away from one of blame or malingering to paying closer attention to identifying past or current child abuse and neglect, family conflicts or other social stressors such as domestic violence which may be perpetuating the diabetes self-neglect.

Health beliefs

As with any illness, unhelpful illness beliefs can be barriers to self-care. Unhelpful diabetes-specific beliefs and behaviours such as fear of hypoglycaemia, fear of self-injecting, barriers to initiating and optimizing insulin therapy (Hampson *et al.* 1990, 1995; Wilson *et al.* 1986) and reduced self-efficacy (Bailey 1996) have been found to be associated with poorer glycaemic control. Although these studies are cross-sectional they support a cognitive-behavioural model for understanding adherence in diabetes.

Family factors

A number of small prospective cohort studies of children and adolescents with type 1 diabetes have shown that family functioning, in particular maternal attitudes (Jacobson *et al.* 1994) and maternal psychiatric status (Kovacs *et al.* 1997), are associated with glycaemic control. In a naturalistic 10-year cohort study of around 100 youths with newly diagnosed type 1 diabetes, maternal psychopathology, in particular maternal depression, was associated with depressive disorders in children and young adults with type 1 diabetes (Kovacs *et al.* 1997). The first year following diagnosis was the peak period for the onset of psychiatric disorders.

Interventions

The two main aims for offering psychiatric treatments to people with diabetes are to improve their diabetes control and to reduce psychological distress. Therapeutic interventions generic to psychiatry are in general applicable to people with diabetes.

Pharmacological interventions

Tricyclic antidepressants for depression in diabetes have been associated with hypoglycaemia. It has been suggested that this may be due to a direct effect of the antidepressant on blood glucose but the evidence for this is poor. The alternative explanation is that improvement in depression improves diabetes self-care related cognitions and behaviours. In a double-blind placebo-controlled study nortriptyline was compared with placebo in patients with diabetes stratified by their depression status. Nortriptyline did reduce depressive symptoms compared to placebo in the depressed group. However it appeared to have a direct effect on worsening glycaemic control regardless of depression status (Lustman *et al.* 1997b). The selective serotonin reuptake inhibitor, fluoxetine, improved both mood and glycaemic control, although there is no evidence to distinguish whether this is a direct effect on insulin action or an indirect effect on improving self-care (Lustman *et al.* 2000b). A recent study has suggested that a new antidepressant duloxetine may be beneficial for the reduction of pain in patients with diabetic neuropathy (Goldstein *et al.* 2005), as may sodium valproate (Kochar *et al.* 2004). Both these findings require further substantiation.

Psychotherapy

There have been many studies examining the effectiveness of non-pharmacological approaches in improving diabetes control and/or psychiatric morbidity, but one of the main difficulties is that educational and psychological approaches have often been combined in such a way as to be unable to distinguish between them. Diabetes is unique in that patient education has been one of the cornerstones of diabetes care. With the discovery of insulin and improvements in prognosis it was apparent that knowledge about diabetes, diet and insulin therapy was necessary if patients were to lead independent lives. Patient education theory uses two general methods, 'didactic' and 'enhanced' (sometimes also termed collaborative, therapeutic or behavioural). Didactic education involves instruction, giving information and advice and teaching skills. Enhanced education also includes behavioural instruction, teaching skills such as how to do self-monitoring, setting goals in dietary, exercise and blood glucose, problem solving such as negotiating diets at social functions, sporting activities or on holidays. In enhanced education, social learning theory was developed by Bandura, in which the view that peer support may enhance knowledge acquisition was introduced (Bandura 1986). This was followed by piecemeal inclusion of behavioural or cognitive psychological techniques, such as relaxation therapy and biofeedback, or coping strategies resulting in the theoretical foundation of many interventions being so blurred or combined that a distinction cannot always be made. The importance of this is twofold: first it is difficult to distinguish which methods are actually effective, and second, educational and psychotherapeutic skills are different, requiring different training needs and expertise and even clinical application to different patient populations.

Several recent systematic reviews have examined educational and psychological approaches in diabetes (Hampson *et al.* 2001; Norris *et al.* 2001). Some very thorough reviews were reluctant to pool the data in a meta-analysis because of the obvious heterogeneity of the interventions (Griffin *et al.* 1998; Norris *et al.* 2001; Snoek & Skinner 2002). One review did pool data from a combination of educational and psychosocial interventions in adolescents with type 1 diabetes and found that there was a mild-to-moderate effect of these interventions in improving glycaemic control (effect size 0.3 which is equivalent to 0.66% reduction in glycated haemoglobin) and in reducing psychological distress (Hampson *et al.* 2001).

Psychotherapy for type 1 diabetes

Individual randomized controlled trials of more conventional forms of psychotherapy in type 1 diabetes suggest that psychological treatments may be more effective in improving glycaemic control compared to education or usual care controls albeit only with a small effect. These include family therapy (Satin *et al.* 1989; Sundelin *et al.* 1996; Wysocki *et al.* 2000) for children and adolescents, techniques from cognitive-behaviour therapy such as problem solving (Halford *et al.* 1997), relaxation therapy (Feinglos *et al.* 1987), and stress management (Boardway *et al.* 1993), and techniques based on psychoanalytic theory such as cognitive analytic theory (Fosbury *et al.* 1997). None of these studies were based on representative samples, all were inadequately powered, and none described or used clinical trial methodology to current standards.

Psychotherapy for type 2 diabetes

The majority of randomized controlled trials in type 2 diabetes have used one or more practical strategies grounded in cognitive-behaviour therapy (CBT). The interventions placed emphasis on behavioural techniques for weight reduction, as this is one of the most important outcomes for improving glycaemic control in type 2 diabetes. Techniques have included relaxation therapy (Aikens *et al.* 1997; Jablon *et al.* 1997; Lane *et al.* 1993), problem solving (White *et al.* 1986), contract setting (Boehm *et al.* 1993; Wing *et al.* 1985). Only a handful of studies made use of the wider range of cognitive-behaviour techniques (Henry *et al.* 1997; Kenardy *et al.* 2002; Lustman *et al.* 1998; Ridgeway *et al.* 1999; Wing *et al.* 1991). Some of the more recent studies tended to apply the CBT principles to specific problem areas in diabetes such as depression (Lustman *et al.* 1998) and binge eating (Kenardy *et al.* 2002) for which specific manuals were developed. Two studies added counselling (D'Eramo-Melkus *et al.* 1992) and motivational interviewing (Smith *et al.* 1997) to the behavioural modification or education. The majority of these studies suggest a mild to modest improvement in glycaemic control and reduction in weight, but methodological problems similar to those in randomized controlled trials in type 1 diabetes prevail except for the occasional study (Lustman *et al.* 1998).

A systematic review and meta-analysis of the effectiveness of psychological therapies in improving glycaemic control in type 2 diabetes has been published recently (Ismail *et al.* 2004). The main outcome was long-term glycaemic control measured by percentage of glycated haemoglobin. Twenty-five trials were eligible for the review. In 12 trials, the mean percentage glycated haemoglobin was lower in people assigned a psychological intervention than in the control group (usual care, education, waiting list, or attention control); the pooled mean difference was −0.32 equivalent to an absolute difference of −0.76%. There were non-significant differences in blood glucose concentration and weight gain. Psychological distress was significantly lower in the intervention groups. The authors concluded that in type 2 diabetes, there are improvements in long-term glycaemic control and psychological distress but not in weight control or blood glucose concentration in people who receive psychological therapies.

Other interventions which have shown benefits in non-randomized evaluations and require further investigation include rehabilitation and empowerment (Keers *et al.* 2006) and motivational interviewing for teenagers with diabetes (Channon *et al.* 2005)

Summary

Psychiatric disorders are common in diabetes and are associated with poor diabetes control, complications and increased mortality. They are disabling, poorly detected and inadequately treated. Diabetes is also an important complication of major psychiatric illnesses such as schizophrenia. There have been recent developments to identify specific psychological problems in diabetes such as depression, diabetes-specific fears and binge eating. The emphasis on diabetes education as a solution for impaired adherence is giving way to a more psychological understanding of the person living with diabetes as a chronic disease, but the availability of diabetes-specific liaison mental input is extremely limited. Future research should include a focus on better psychological models of diabetes-specific problems such as adherence in type 2 diabetes and self-destructive behaviour in type 1 diabetes, which should inform future psychological interventions.

REFERENCES

Adler, A., Boyko, E., Ahroni, J., *et al.* (1997). Risk factors for diabetic peripheral sensory neuropathy. Results of the Seattle Prospective Diabetic Foot Study. *Diabetes Care*, **20**, 1162–7.

Aikens, J., Kiolbasa, T. and Sobel, R. (1997). Psychological predictors of glycemic change with relaxation training in non-insulin-dependent diabetes mellitus. *Psychotherapy and Psychosomatics*, **66**, 302–6.

Ajani, U., Hennekens, C., Spelsberg, A., *et al.* (2000). Alcohol consumption and risk of type 2 diabetes mellitus among US male physicians. *Archives of Internal Medicine*, **160**, 1025–30.

Alberti, K. and Zimmett, P. (1998). for the WHO consultation. Definition, diagnosis, and classification of diabetes mellitus and its complications. Part 1. Diagnosis and classification of diabetes mellitus. Provisional report of a WHO consultation. *Diabetic Medicine*, **15**, 539–53.

Amos, A., McCarty, D. and Zimmet, P. (1997). The rising global burden of diabetes and its complications: estimates and projections to the year 2010. *Diabetic Medicine*, **14**, S7–85.

Bailey, B. (1996). Mediators of depression in adults with diabetes. *Clinical Nursing Research*, **5**, 28–42.

Bandura, A. (1986). *Social Foundations of Thought and Action: a Social Cognitive Theory.* Englewood Cliffs, NJ: Prentice Hall.

Berlin, I., Bisserbe, J., Eiber, R., *et al.* (1997). Phobic symptoms, particularly the fear of blood and injury, are associated with poor glycemic control in type 1 diabetes mellitus. *Diabetes Care*, **20**, 176–8.

Bienvenu, O. and Eaton, W. (1998). The epidemiology of blood-injection-injury phobia. *Psychological Medicine*, **28**, 1129–36.

Boardway, R., Delamater, A., Tomakowsky, J., *et al.* (1993). Stress management training for adolescents with diabetes. *Journal of Pediatric Psychology*, **18**, 29–45.

Boehm, S., Schlenk, E., Raleigh, E., *et al.* (1993). Behavioral analysis and behavioral strategies to improve self-management of Type II diabetes. *Clinical Nursing Research*, **2**, 327–44.

Braceland, F., Meduna, L. and Viachulis, J. (1945). Delayed action of insulin in schizophrenia. *American Journal of Psychiatry*, **102**, 108–10.

Bryden, K. S., Neil, A., Mayou, R. A., *et al.* (1999). Eating habits, body weight, and insulin misuse. *Diabetes Care*, **22**, 1956–60.

Bryden, K., Peveler, R., Stein, A., *et al.* (2001). Clinical and psychological course of diabetes from adolescence to young adulthood. *Diabetes Care*, **24**, 1536–40.

Bryden, K. S., Dunger, D. B., Mayou, R. A., *et al.* (2003). Poor prognosis of young adults with type 1 diabetes: a longitudinal study. *Diabetes Care*, **26**(4), 1052–7.

Channon, S., Huws-Thomas, M. V., Gregory, J. W., *et al.* (2005). Motivational Interviewing with Teenagers with Diabetes. *Clinical Child Psychology and Psychiatry*, **10**(1), 43–51.

DCCT Research Group. (1993). The effect of intensive treatment of diabetes on the development and progression of longterm complications in insulin-dependent diabetes mellitus. *New England Journal of Medicine*, **329**, 977–86.

de Groot, M., Jacobson, A., Samson, J., *et al.* (1999). Glycemic control and major depression in patients with type 1 and type 2 diabetes mellitus. *Journal of Psychosomatic Research*, **46**, 425–35.

de Groot, M., Anderson, R., Freedland, K., *et al.* (2001). Association of depression and diabetes complications: a meta-analysis. *Psychosomatic Medicine*, **63**, 619–30.

D'Eramo-Melkus, G., Wylie-Rosett, J. and Hagan, J. (1992). Metabolic impact of education in NIDDM. *Diabetes Care*, **15**, 864–9.

Dixon, L., Weiden, P., Delahant, J., *et al.* (2000). Prevalence and correlates of diabetes in national schizophrenia samples. *Schizophrenia Bulletin*, **26**, 903–12.

Dunn, S. and Turtle, J. (1981). The myth of the diabetic personality. *Diabetes Care*, **4**, 640–6.

Eaton, W., Mengel, M., Mengel, L., *et al.* (1992). Psychosocial and psychopathologic influences on management and control of insulin-dependent diabetes. *International Journal of Psychiatry and Medicine*, **22**, 105–17.

Eaton, W., Armenian, H., Gallo, J., *et al.* (1996). Depression and risk for onset of type II diabetes. A prospective population-based study. *Diabetes Care*, **19**, 1097–102.

Expert Committee on the Diagnosis and Classification of Diabetes Mellitus. (1997). Report of the expert committee on the diagnosis and classification of diabetes mellitus. *Diabetes Care*, **20**, 1183–97.

Feinglos, M., Hastedt, P. and Surwit, R. (1987). Effects of relaxation therapy on patients with Type 1 diabetes mellitus. *Diabetes Care*, **10**, 72–5.

Fosbury, J., Bosley, C. M., Ryle, A., *et al.* (1997). A trial of cognitive-analytical therapy in poorly controlled Type 1 patients. *Diabetes Care*, **20**, 959–64.

Freeman, H. (1946). Resistance to insulin in mentally disturbed soldiers. *Archives of Neurology and Psychiatry*, **56**, 74–8.

Gavard, J., Lustman, P. and Clouse, R. (1993). Prevalence of depression in adults with diabetes. An epidemiological evaluation. *Diabetes Care*, **16**, 1167–78.

Gill, G. (2001). Does brittle diabetes exist? In *Difficult Diabetes*, ed. G. Gill, J. Pickup and G. Williams. Oxford: Blackwell Science, pp. 151–67.

Goldstein, D. J., Lu, Y., Detke, M. J., *et al.* (2005). Duloxetine vs. placebo in patients with painful diabetic neuropathy. *Pain*, **116**(1–2), 109–18.

Griffin, S., Kinmouth, A. L., Skinner, C., *et al.* (1998). Educational and psychosocial interventions for adults with diabetes. *Report to the British Diabetic Association*. London: British Diabetic Association.

Halford, W., Goodall, T. and Nicholson, J. (1997). Diet and diabetes (II): a controlled trial of problem solving to improve dietary self-management in patients with insulin dependent diabetes. *Psychology and Health*, **12**, 231–8.

Hampson, S., Glasgow, R. and Toobert, D. (1990). Personal models of diabetes and their relations to self-care activities. *Health Psychology*, **9**, 632–46.

Hampson, S., Glasgow, R. and Foster, L. (1995). Personal models of diabetes among older adults: relation to self-management and other variables. *The Diabetes Educator*, **21**, 300–7.

Hampson, S., Skinner, T., Hart, J., *et al.* (2001). Effects of educational and psychosocial interventions for adolescents with diabetes mellitus: a systematic review. *Health Technology Assessment*, **5**(10), 1–79.

Henry, J., Wilson, P., Bruce, D., *et al.* (1997). Cognitive-behavioural stress management for patients with non-insulin dependent diabetes mellitus. *Psychology, Health and Medicine*, **2**, 109–18.

Holt, R. I. G., Peveler, R. C. and Byrne, C. D. (2004). Schizophrenia, the metabolic syndrome and diabetes. *Diabetic Medicine*, **21**(6), 515–23.

Hu, F., Manson, J., Stampfer, M., *et al.* (2001). Diet, lifestyle, and the risk of Type 2 diabetes mellitus in women. *New England Journal of Medicine*, **345**, 790–7.

Ismail, K., Winkley, K. and Rabe-Hesketh, S. (2004). Systematic review and meta-analysis of randomised controlled trials of psychological interventions to improve glycaemic control in patients with type 2 diabetes. *Lancet*, **363**(9421), 1589–97.

Jablon, S., Naliboff, B., Gilmore, S., *et al.* (1997). Effects of relaxation training on glucose tolerance and diabetic control in Type II diabetes. *Applied Psychophysiology and Biofeedback*, **22**, 155–69.

Jacobson, A., Hauser, S., Willett, J., *et al.* (1997a). Psychological adjustment to IDDM: a 10 year follow-up of an onset cohort of child and adolescent patients. *Diabetes Care*, **20**, 811–18.

Jacobson, A., de Groot, M. and Samson, J. (1997b). The effects of psychiatric disorders and symptoms on quality of life in patients with Type 1 and Type 2 diabetes mellitus. *Quality of Life Research*, **6**, 11–20.

Jacobson, A. M., Hauser, S. T., Lavori, P., *et al.* (1994). Family environment and glycaemic control: a four year prospective study of children and adolescents with insulin dependent diabetes mellitus. *Psychosomatic Medicine*, **56**, 401–9.

Johnson, K., Bazargan, M. and Bing, E. (2000). Alcohol consumption and compliance among inner-city minority patients. *Archives of Family Medicine*, **9**, 964–70.

Jones, J., Lawson, M., Daneman, D., *et al.* (2000). Eating disorders in adolescent females with and without type 1 diabetes: cross sectional study. *British Medical Journal*, **320**, 1563–6.

Kao, W., Puddey, I., Boland, L., *et al.* (2001). Alcohol consumption and the risk of type 2 diabetes mellitus. *American Journal of Epidemiology*, **154**, 748–57.

Katon, W., Rutter, C., Simon, G., *et al.* (2005). The association of comorbid depression with mortality in patients with type 2 diabetes. *Diabetes Care*, **28**(11), 2668–72.

Kawakami, N., Shimizu, H., Takatsuka, N., *et al.* (1999). Depressive symptoms and occurrence of type 2 diabetes among Japanese men. *Diabetes Care*, **22**, 1071–6.

Keers, J. C., Bouma, J., Links, T. P., *et al.* (2006). One-year follow-up effects of diabetes rehabilitation for patients with prolonged self-management difficulties. *Patient Education and Counseling*, **60**(1), 16−23.

Kenardy, J., Mensch, M., Bowen, K., *et al.* (2002). Group therapy for binge eating in Type 2 diabetes: a randomized trial. *Diabetic Medicine*, **19**, 234−9.

Knol, M., Twisk, J., Beekman, A., *et al.* (2006). Depression as a risk factor for the onset of type 2 diabetes mellitus. A meta-analysis. *Diabetalogia*, **49**, 837−45.

Kochar, D. K., Rawat, N., Agrawal, R. P., *et al.* (2004). Sodium valproate for painful diabetic neuropathy: a randomized double-blind placebo-controlled study. *QJM: An International Journal of Medicine*, **97**(1), 33−8.

Kohner, E., Aldington, S., Stratton, I., *et al.* (1998). United Kingdom Prospective Diabetes Study, 30: diabetic retinopathy at diagnosis of non-insulin-dependent diabetes mellitus and associated risk factors. *Archives of Ophthalmology*, **116**, 297−303.

Koro, C., Fedder, D., L'Italien, G., *et al.* (2002). Assessment of independent effect of olanzapine and risperidone on risk of diabetes among patients with schizophrenia: population based nested case-control study. *British Medical Journal*, **325**, 243.

Kovacs, M., Mukerji, P., Drash, A., *et al.* (1995). Biomedical and psychiatric risk factors for retinopathy among children with IDDM. *Diabetes Care*, **18**, 1592−9.

Kovacs, M., Goldston, D., Obrosky, D., *et al.* (1997). Psychiatric disorders in youths with IDDM: rates and risk factors. *Diabetes Care*, **20**, 36−44.

Lane, J., McCaskill, C., Ross, S.L., Feinglos, M. and Surwit, R. (1993). Relaxation training for NIDDM. *Diabetes Care*, **16**, 1087−94.

Lane, J., McCaskill, C., Willians, P., *et al.* (2000). Personality correlates of glycemic control in type 2 diabetes. *Diabetes Care*, **23**, 1321−5.

Lindenmayer, J.-P., Czabor, P., Volavka, J., *et al.* (2003). Changes in glucose and cholesterol levels in patients with schizophrenia treated with typical or atypical antipsychotics. *American Journal of Psychiatry*, **160**, 290−6.

Lloyd, C., Robinson, N., Stevens, L., *et al.* (1991). The relationship between stress and the development of diabetic complications. *Diabetic Medicine*, **8**, 146−50.

Lorenz, R., Bubb, J., Davis, D., *et al.* (1996). Changing behavior: practical lessons from the Diabetes Control and Complications Trial. *Diabetes Care*, **19**, 649−52.

Lustman, P. and Harper, G. (1987). Nonpsychiatric physicians' identification and treatment of depression in patients with diabetes. *Comprehensive Psychiatry*, **28**, 22−7.

Lustman, P., Griffith, L. and Clouse, R. (1988). Depression in adults with diabetes. Results of 5-yr follow-up study. *Diabetes Care*, **11**, 605−12.

Lustman, P., Frank, B.L. and McGill, J.B. (1991). Relationship of personality characteristics to glucose regulation in adults with diabetes. *Psychosomatic Medicine*, **53**, 305−12.

Lustman, P., Griffith, L., Freedland, K., *et al.* (1997a). The course of major depression in diabetes. *General Hospital Psychiatry*, **19**, 138−43.

Lustman, P., Griffith, L., Clouse, R., *et al.* (1997b). Effects of nortriptyline on depression and glycaemic control in diabetes: results of a double-blind, placebo-controlled trial. *Psychosomatic Medicine*, **59**, 241−50.

Lustman, P., Griffith, L., Freedland, K., *et al.* (1998). Cognitive behavior therapy for depression in type 2 diabetes mellitus. A randomized, controlled trial. *Annals of Internal Medicine*, **129**, 613–21.

Lustman, P., Anderson, R., Freedland, K., *et al.* (2000a). Depression and poor glycaemic control. A meta-analytic review of the literature. *Diabetes Care*, **23**, 934–42.

Lustman, P., Freedland, K., Griffith, L., *et al.* (2000b). Fluoxetine for depression in diabetes: a randomized double-blind placebo-controlled trial. *Diabetes Care*, **23**, 618–23.

Mayou, C., Peveler, R., Davies, B., *et al.* (1991). Psychiatric morbidity in young adults with insulin-dependent diabetes mellitus. *Psychological Medicine*, **21**, 639–45.

Meninger, W. (1935). Psychological factors in the etiology of diabetes. *Journal of Nervous and Mental Disease*, **81**, 1–13.

Mollema, E., Snoek, F., Ader, H., *et al.* (2001). Insulin-treated diabetes patients with fear of self-injecting or fear of self testing. Psychological comorbidity and general well-being. *Journal of Psychosomatic Medicine*, **51**, 665–72.

Murrell, S., Himmelfarb, S. and Wright, K. (1983). Prevalence of depression and its correlates in older adults. *American Journal of Epidemiology*, **117**, 173–85.

Norris, S., Engelgau, M. and Venkat Naryan, K. (2001). Effectiveness of self-management training in type 2 diabetes. *Diabetes Care*, **24**, 561–87.

Palinkas, L., Barrett-Connor, E. and Wingard, D. (1991). Type 2 diabetes and depressive symptoms in older adults: a population-based study. *Diabetic Medicine*, **8**, 532–9.

Paschalides, C., Wearden, A. J., Dunkerley, R., *et al.* (2004). The associations of anxiety, depression and personal illness representations with glycaemic control and health-related quality of life in patients with type 2 diabetes mellitus. *Journal of Psychosomatic Research*, **57**, 557–64.

Peveler, R., Davies, B., Mayou, R., *et al.* (1993). Self-care behaviour and blood glucose control in young adults with type 1 diabetes mellitus. *Diabetic Medicine*, **10**, 74–80.

Polonsky, W., Anderson, B., Lohrer, P., *et al.* (1995). Assessment of diabetes-related distress. *Diabetes Care*, **18**, 754–60.

Popkin, M., Callies, A., Lentz, R., *et al.* (1988). Prevalence of major depression, simple phobia, and other psychiatric disorders in patients with longstanding Type 1 diabetes mellitus. *Archives of General Psychiatry*, **45**, 64–8.

Ridgeway, N., Harvill, D., Harvill, L., *et al.* (1999). Improved control of Type 2 diabetes mellitus: a practical education/behavior modification program in a primary care clinic. *Southern Medical Journal*, **92**, 667–72.

Rimm, E., Chan, J., Stampfer, M., *et al.* (1995). Prospective study of cigarette smoking, alcohol use and the risk of diabetes in men. *British Medical Journal*, **310**, 555–9.

Robinson, N., Fuller, J. and Edmeades, S. (1988). Depression and diabetes. *Diabetic Medicine*, **5**, 268–74.

Rubin, R. and Peyrot, M. (2001). Psychological issues and treatments for people with diabetes. *Journal of Clinical Psychology*, **57**, 457–78.

Rydall, A. C., Rodin, G. M., Olmstead, M. P., *et al.* (1997). Disordered eating behavior and microvascular complications in young women with insulin dependent diabetes mellitus. *New England Journal of Medicine*, **336**, 1849–54.

Satin, W., La Greca, A., Zigo, M., *et al.* (1989). Diabetes in adolescence: effects of multifamily group intervention and parent simulation of diabetes. *Journal of Pediatric Psychology*, **14**, 259–75.

Sernyak, M., Douglas, L., Alarcon, R., *et al.* (2002). Association of diabetes mellitus with use of atypical neuroleptics in the treatment of schizophrenia. *American Journal of Psychiatry*, **159**, 561–6.

Shaper, A., Wannamethee, G. and Walker, M. (1988). Alcohol and mortality in British men: explaining the U-shaped curve. *Lancet*, **2**, 1267–73.

Smith, D., Heckemeyer, C., Kratt, P., *et al.* (1997). Motivational interviewing to improve adherence to a behavioural weight-control program for older obese women with NIDDM. *Diabetes Care*, **20**, 52–4.

Snoek, F. and Skinner, T. (2002). Psychological counselling in problematic diabetes: does it help? *Diabetic Medicine*, **19**, 265–73.

Spangler, J., Konen, J. and McGann, K. (1993). Prevalence and predictors of problem drinking among primary care diabetic patients. *Journal of Family Practice*, **37**, 370–5.

Sundelin, J., Forsander, G. and Mattson, S.-E. (1996). Family-oriented support at the onset of diabetes mellitus: a comparison of two group conditions during 2 years following diagnosis. *Acta Paediatrica*, **85**, 49–55.

UK Prospective Diabetes Study (UKPDS) Group. (1998). Intensive blood-glucose control with sulphonylureas or insulin compared with conventional treatment and risk of complications in patients with type 2 diabetes (UKPDS). *Lancet*, **352**, 837–53.

Van Tilburg, M., McCaskill, C., Lane, J., *et al.* (2001). Depressed mood is a factor in glycaemic control in Type 1 diabetes. *Psychosomatic Medicine*, **63**, 551–5.

Welch, G., Dunn, S. and Beeney, L. (1994). A measure of psychological adjustment to diabetes. In *Handbook of Psychology and Diabetes: A Guide to Psychological Measurement in Diabetes Research and Practice*, ed. C. Bradley. Amsterdam: Harwood Academic Publishers.

Wells, K., Golding, J. and Burnam, M. (1989). Affective, substance use, and anxiety disorders in persons with arthritis, diabetes, heart disease, high blood pressure, or chronic lung conditions. *General Hospital Psychiatry*, **11**, 320–7.

Weyerer, S., Hewer, W., Pfeifer-Kurda, M., *et al.* (1989). Psychiatric disorders and diabetes – results from a community study. *Journal of Psychosomatic Research*, **33**, 633–40.

White, N., Carnahan, J., Nugent, C., *et al.* (1986). Management of obese patients with diabetes mellitus: comparison of advice education with group management. *Diabetes Care*, **9**, 490–6.

Wilkinson, G., Borsey, D., Newton, L., *et al.* (1988). Psychiatric morbidity and social problems in patients with insulin-dependent diabetes mellitus. *British Journal of Psychiatry*, **153**, 38–43.

Wilson, W., Ary, D., Biglan, A., *et al.* (1986). Psychosocial predictors of self care behaviors (compliance) and glycaemic control in non-insulin-dependent diabetes mellitus. *Diabetes Care*, **9**, 614–22.

Wing, R., Epstein, L., Nowalk, M., *et al.* (1985). Behavior change, weight loss, and physiological improvements in Type II diabetic patients. *Journal of Consulting and Clinical Psychology*, **53**, 111–22.

Wing, R., Marcus, M., Epstein, L., *et al.* (1991). A 'family-based' approach to the treatment of obese Type II diabetic patients. *Journal of Consulting and Clinical Psychology*, **59**, 156–62.

Wrigley, M. and Mayou, R. (1991). Psychosocial factors and admission for poor glycaemic control: a study of psychological and social factors in poorly controlled insulin dependent diabetic patients. *Journal of Psychosomatic Research*, **35**, 335–43.

Wysocki, T., Harris, M., Greco, P., *et al.* (2000). Randomized controlled trial of behavior therapy for families of adolescents with IDDM. *Journal of Pediatric Psychology*, **25**, 22–33.

Zhang, J., Markides, K. and Lee, D. (1991). Health status of diabetic Mexican-Americans: results from the Hispanic HANES. *Ethnic Diseases*, **1**, 273–9.

Zhang, X., Norris, S., Gregg, E., *et al.* (2005). Depressive symptons and mortality among persons with and without diabetes. *American Journal of Epidemiology*, **161**(7), 652–60.

20

HIV and AIDS

Russell Foster and Ian Everall

Introductory topics

Introduction

The psychiatric care of individuals infected with HIV encompasses a wide range of issues which, as for other chronic and life-threatening illnesses, include biological, social and psychological factors (Table 20.1). Due to the diversity of these issues, deliverance of mental health care for those with HIV infection or disease is best carried out in a multidisciplinary team setting involving co-ordination and co-operation between HIV physicians, social services, community mental health teams, child and adolescent mental health services and voluntary sector organizations as appropriate. HIV liaison psychiatry attempts to integrate the medical, psychological and social aspects of HIV and can make a unique contribution to the care and management of affected individuals (Clark & Everall 1997). In this chapter, the main aspects of HIV in the adult population and its effects on mental state are considered in terms of epidemiology, clinical manifestations and management. In addition, the impact of HIV on the mental health of two special populations – children and older adults – is considered briefly.

Epidemiology of psychiatric morbidity in those infected with HIV

Routes of transmission of HIV include sexual transmission, transmission in blood/blood products, and vertical transmission, from mother to child. In the UK the groups with the highest prevalence are homosexual men, sub-Saharan African populations (primarily due to heterosexual transmission), and intravenous drug users. Recent figures suggest that the prevalence of HIV infection in

Handbook of Liaison Psychiatry, ed. Geoffrey Lloyd and Elspeth Guthrie. Published by Cambridge University Press. © Cambridge University Press 2007.

Table 20.1. Biological, social and psychological aspects of HIV infection.

Biological	Organic illnesses
	Pre-existing medical/psychiatric conditions
	Effects of substance use
	Effects of medications
Social	HIV testing issues
	Culture-specific issues
	Community support
	Housing/environment
	Relationships
	Stigma/discrimination
	Social support/isolation issues
	Financial security/work-related problems
	Independence and wellbeing
	Control
Psychological	Loss and bereavement issues
	Sexual expression
	Self-respect
	Death/dying
	Chronic illness issues
	Personality issues
	Deliberate self-harm and suicide
	Identity/body image
	Spiritual issues

the UK is 0.11% as compared to 0.35% in Western Europe (WHO fact sheet 2000). Of these, homosexual men account for a large proportion of cases, although other at-risk groups, such as heterosexual sub-Saharan African populations, are showing increasing rates of infection (McHenry *et al.* 2002). A study has noted that those with pre-existing mental health problems are at an elevated risk of acquiring HIV infection (Stoskopf *et al.* 2001).

Current figures pertaining to the prevalence of psychiatric morbidity in target populations suggest that 61.4% of an adult population in the United States receiving care for HIV have used mental health or drug and alcohol services (Burnam *et al.* 2001) and approximately 27% of HIV-infected patients in another study were receiving psychotropic medication (Vitiello *et al.* 2003). Antidepressants were the most widely prescribed (21%), followed by anxiolytics (17%), antipsychotics (5%) and psychostimulants (3%). A study reported by Ellis *et al.* (1994) in London revealed that the most common psychiatric presentations to adult liaison services were organic, affective and adjustment disorders and

Table 20.2. Possible landmark events in HIV disease.

Initial diagnosis of HIV infection
Initiation of anti-HIV or opportunistic infection therapy
Development of HIV disease
Complicating illnesses
Discontinuation of therapy
Peer-group illness and death
Death and dying

personality problems, with high rates of substance abuse (44% as compared to 30% in a matched control group). A later, American, study reported that almost half (48%) of a HIV-infected population had a diagnosable psychiatric disorder, with major depression (36%) the most common condition (Bing *et al.* 2001). This was followed by dysthymia (27%), generalized anxiety disorder (16%) and panic attacks (11%).

Clinical presentations of psychiatric illness in HIV-affected individuals

The range of psychiatric illnesses that can develop in those infected with HIV is diverse and will vary depending on the stage of the infection. A number of specific psychiatric disorders will be considered later, whereas here we highlight particular recognized 'life events' in HIV disease, as summarized in Table 20.2 (Welsby & Richardson 1995). Typically these include the time at HIV testing when notified of a positive result, during asymptomatic stages of infection, during symptomatic stages of infection and in the final stages of disease. These will be considered briefly in turn.

Period of post-positive HIV test notification

Receiving a positive HIV test result is an understandably stressful experience. In some an acute stress reaction, or a more prolonged adjustment disorder, can develop. Some individuals presenting for a HIV test can also have a pre-existing mental health problem and are at greater risk of developing mental health problems following diagnosis (Catalan *et al.* 1992). In some cases there may be a causal relation between pre-existing psychiatric illness and the acquisition of HIV, for example poor self-esteem may be associated with inability to have safer sex. Interestingly, it has been noted that individuals who voluntarily seek HIV testing may have raised rates of psychopathology (Perry *et al.* 1990). In rare instances, an individual may claim to be infected with HIV and later found to be malingering (Huang *et al.* 2001) or even be suffering from Munchausen syndrome

(Oyewole 1996). Other recognized mental disorders include the 'worried well' (Forstein 1984), mania, or psychosis (El-Mallakh 1991).

Pre-test counselling is usually undertaken by specially trained counsellors. The counselling normally includes asking the person what they understand about the test, why they want a test (there may be lesser emphasis on this if the test is being performed as part of a series of investigations) and their views and concerns on how they would react to a positive test result (Catalan 1999). Potential social and financial implications should also be discussed. Post-test counselling, regardless of the outcome of the test, should review the person's knowledge of how HIV is transmitted, including safer sex. A positive test result will require a variable period of time in which suitable pastoral support is provided. When appropriate, the consequences of HIV infection, the detrimental effect it has on the immune system and the need for regular medical follow-up to monitor this should be discussed. Information about how immune damage can be prevented by taking antiretroviral drugs and how this decision will be made should involve a collaborative effort with the HIV physician. As this requires the patient understanding a large amount of complicated information such counselling often occurs over more than one session.

Although the efficacy of specific post-test counselling strategies is unclear and remains the subject of debate (Meursing & Sibindi 2000; Rotheram-Borus *et al.* 2000), a recent study has shown that post-test counselling by trained counsellors has been effective in encouraging HIV-infected individuals to seek and adhere to medical treatment (Eichler *et al.* 2002).

Development of opportunistic infections and HIV-related illnesses

Development of opportunistic infections and HIV-related illnesses are significant 'life events' for individuals infected with HIV. For some patients these illnesses may be viewed as a sign of their immunocompromised state, possible failure of antiretroviral therapy or even the 'beginning of the end'. These cognitions may either precipitate an adjustment/depressive disorder or exacerbate a premorbid mood disorder. Given the possible increased risk of suicide in individuals affected by AIDS (Marzuk *et al.* 1988) the clinician should be aware of these possible effects on both the patient and his or her family and friends, and consider appropriate interventions.

Initiation of anti-HIV or opportunistic infection therapy

Initiation of antiretroviral treatment or medications to prevent opportunistic infections is recognized as a potentially stressful time in a patient's HIV history. For patients it can signify that the virus has already caused significant damage to their immune system leaving them vulnerable to opportunistic infection, which may be accompanied by worries about episodes of illness, suffering and possibly death. Recognition and treatment of mental health problems at this point are very important as they have a significant negative impact upon patients' adherence with antiretroviral treatment (Murphy *et al.* 2000; Singh *et al.* 1996; Tuldra *et al.* 2000).

Poor adherence can result in antiretroviral treatment failure, markedly increased morbidity and subsequently mortality. First, patients on failing antiretroviral regimes may have to be switched to different drug combinations. These second- or third-line regimes may be more complicated than first line treatments and may be even more difficult to adhere to. Second, as treatment options fail the prognosis of the poorly adherent individual becomes less favourable as the immune system damage continues and the likelihood of becoming seriously ill or even dying increases. Hence recognition and treatment of depression or other mental health problems are essential to maximize the success of antiretroviral and other therapy.

Non-adherence to highly active antiretroviral therapy (HAART) medication can be a major problem (Mehta *et al.* 1997). Poor compliance has been shown to correlate with poorer outcomes including treatment failure (Ickovics *et al.* 2002). Adherence of taking less than 95% of medication correctly should be addressed using a number of different approaches, such as simplifying treatment regimes (where possible), consideration of temporary treatment interruption, attempting to minimize treatment side-effects and instituting appropriate educational strategies (Stone 2002). Factors noted to be specifically associated with non-adherence to treatment include unpleasant symptoms, adverse drug effects such as lipodystrophy, psychological distress, lack of social or family support, complexity of treatment regime, low patient self-esteem/coping ability and 'inconvenience' of treatment (Ammassari *et al.* 2002). The British HIV Association (BHIVA) has published helpful guidelines for adherence to medica-tion (www.aidsmap.org/about/bhiva/bhiva_adherence.asp).

Adherence rates in people with HIV and comorbid serious mental illness have been reported to range from 90% adherence in 40% of the subjects investigated, down to 31% displaying less than 50% adherence (Wagner *et al.* 2003). While these findings suggest that HIV infection in those with serious mental illness need not be a barrier to good medication adherence, this may have a substantial impact in selected individuals. To improve adherence, a number of strategies has been suggested, including support of community mental health nurses as part of the Care Plan Approach, collaboration between community mental health teams and HIV clinics, simplification of regimes, adjustment of the treatment schedule to fit the patient's lifestyle, and anticipation of side-effects to allow the patient to self-manage these (Trotta *et al.* 2002).

Dying and death

Death of partners, family or friends, can lead to a considerable amount of psychiatric morbidity, not all of which is recognized by clinicians. A number of issues may arise due to bereavement, and various psychotherapeutic approaches may be used to deal with these (Demmer 2001; Sikkema *et al.* 2000). On occasion, use of an appropriate antidepressant may be required as an adjunct to psychological intervention.

The terminal stages of AIDS result in a wide spectrum of concerns, such as the possible development of organic brain syndromes, as well as psychiatric syndromes, including changes in behaviour, depression and psychosis (Catalan *et al.* 1995). A number of HIV-infected individuals may experience the 'Lazarus syndrome' (Brashers *et al.* 1999; Scott & Constantine 1999). This refers to the 'new lease of life' afforded to some sufferers thanks to the efficacy of new combination therapies. Although the benefits of this may be positive, as yet there is no complete cure for AIDS and there may also be negative repercussions, with the resulting ambiguity and uncertainty resulting in further psychiatric morbidity. In addition, the 'fatigue' of longer-term survival may place an additional burden.

HIV and child psychiatry

Although HIV infection is rare in children in the UK, psychiatric manifestations such as HIV encephalopathy are relatively more common and hence affected children may present to psychiatric services in various ways. A number of factors will influence presentation, including parental and cultural views of HIV, presence of infection in parents, age of the child and reproduction issues. A child with HIV must be considered in relation to family, culture and community. Adequate psychosocial input must accompany any medical interventions, and input strategies should aim to alleviate distress and treat any accompanying psychiatric morbidity.

Children may acquire HIV by vertical transmission, through blood or blood products, and other routes, such as heterosexual transmission (Yeung & Gibb 2001). Regardless of the mode of infection, the multiple care issues remain complex and will require expert input from multidisciplinary services.

Children with HIV may have a number of central nervous system complications, which may manifest in diverse ways (Belman 1992), including developmental delay, speech/and language problems, cognitive problems, behavioural problems and emotional problems. Prognosis is variable, but survival has increased greatly since introduction of highly effective antiretroviral therapies so that most affected children are surviving into adult life (Hermoine Lyall 2002).

HIV and older adult psychiatry

The advances in treatment of HIV infection and its consequences has implications for the mental health of older adults, a group little considered as being at risk of HIV-related psychiatric morbidity (Hinkin *et al.* 2001). The known routes of transmission (sexual transmission, intravenous drug abuse and transfusion of blood and blood products) are also recognized in older adults (Hilton 1988) and should not be underestimated. The recognized spectrum of psychiatric morbidity is also seen in older individuals infected with HIV, although age has been noted as a protective factor from psychiatric illness in general (Regier *et al.* 1993). Older patients appear to have a greater rate of progression to AIDS following HIV infection (McArthur *et al.* 1993), with older adults reported to have higher rates of neurocognitive deficits in association with HIV infection (Janssen *et al.* 1992). Treatment of the older adult with HIV will be similar to that of younger adult groups, although special attention should be paid to the other needs of these populations. Additional complications such as the increased risks associated with cardiovascular disease or metabolic effects of HAART should also be taken into account.

Specific disorders

Introduction

Patients with HIV can experience the full gamut of recognized psychiatric disorders at any stage of infection, and the most important syndromes are summarized below. For a summary of the key features of each disorder see Table 20.3.

Organic and neuropsychiatric disorders in HIV

Organic and neuropsychiatric disorders in HIV are common, and may result from direct effects of HIV, opportunistic infections, effects of neoplasms, metabolic abnormalities, iatrogenic interventions and others (Everall 1995).

The prevalence of HIV dementia is somewhere in the region of 13% (Kilbourne *et al.* 2001), although exact figures are difficult to calculate. Since the introduction of HAART regimes, however, the incidence of HIV dementia has declined by up to 50% (Sacktor 2002).

Cognitive changes may be due directly to the effects of the HIV itself, secondary to opportunistic infection, following treatment or due to pre-existing psychological morbidity. These changes may be classified into early and late, and key features of HIV-related cognitive changes are summarized in Table 20.4. Treatment should be aimed at both the underlying cause of the presentation

Table 20.3. Summary of major psychiatric disorders in HIV.

HIV-associated dementia

Epidemiology: 11% (Kilbourne *et al.* 2001).

Clinical features: see Table 20.4.

Diagnosis: see Table 20.5.

Treatment: directed at cause, zidovudine reported to be particularly effective.
Social/behavioural and psychological approaches also useful.

Outcome: variable, poor prognostic factors include older age, lower IQ and somatic
symptoms of depression (Farinpour *et al.* 2003).

HIV and mania

Epidemiology: prevalence 1.2% (HIV-positive); 4.3% (AIDS; Ellen *et al.* 1999);
4% (HIV-positive; Kilbourne *et al.* 2001).

Treatment: valproate (first-line); lithium and carbamazepine (use with caution);
some evidence for risperidone, olanzapine and benzodiazepines (short-term).

Outcome: variable, probably similar to that for bipolar disorder.

HIV and psychosis

Epidemiology: schizophrenia: 0.2–15% (Sewell 1996).

Treatment: atypical antipsychotics (first-line); avoid depot preparations where possible.

Outcome: variable, related to treatment compliance, some cases reversible
(e.g. antiretroviral-induced psychosis – Foster *et al.* 2003).

HIV and affective disorders

Epidemiology: lifetime prevalence of depression 22–45% (Penzak *et al.* 2000).

Treatment: SSRI (first-line, especially fluoxetine and sertraline); TCA (use with caution).

Outcome: good, in one study 85% somewhat improved, 51% very much improved
(Treisman *et al.* 1994).

HIV and anxiety disorders

Epidemiology: 32% (Kilbourne *et al.* 2001).

Treatment: SSRI (for chronic anxiety); buspirone; benzodiazepines (short-term use only).

Outcome: variable, one study found no change at 2-year follow-up (Sewell *et al.* 2000).

HIV and personality disorders

Epidemiology: 36% (Turrina *et al.* 2001).

Treatment: no specific pharmacological treatment; psychological/supportive measures.

Outcome: variable.

HIV and suicide

Epidemiology: 9% of victims in one study HIV positive (Marzuk *et al.* 1997);
44.3% of HIV substance-dependent patients attempted suicide in recent study (Roy 2003).

Risk factors: female, younger age, family history of suicide, more childhood trauma,
higher neuroticism scores, more comorbidity with depression, more received
antidepressant medication (Roy 2003).

Outcome: no significant difference from general population (Dannenberg *et al.* 1996).

Table 20.4. Symptoms and signs of HIV dementia.

Early	Late
Forgetfulness	Disorientation
Poor concentration	Confusion
Balance problems	Peripheral neuropathies
Apathy	Slowed verbal responses
Withdrawal	Indifference to illness
Dysphoric mood	Organic psychosis
Behavioural changes	Incontinence
Dyspraxia	Carphologia (picking)

Possible laboratory and radiological findings

Early
CSF may show increased protein or lymphocytes with normal or low glucose.
    Head MRI/CT may show cortical atrophy and ventricular enlargement.

Late
Head CT/MRI may show cortical atrophy and white matter change.

(e.g. by using an appropriate antiretroviral agent or combination of agents for opportunistic infections) as well as controlling the presenting symptoms via the use of anxiolytics or neuroleptics as appropriate.

Before the development of combination antiretroviral therapy HIV dementia had an extremely poor prognosis, estimated at roughly six months post-onset (McArthur *et al.* 1993). With the new generation of antiretrovirals and combination therapy, however, this figure is no longer accurate, and the incidence of HIV dementia has declined considerably (Sacktor 2002).

A study by McArthur *et al.* in 1993 suggested that significant predictors of HIV-dementia included low haemoglobin and a low body mass index 1–6 months before development of AIDS, constitutional symptoms 7–12 months before onset of AIDS, and older age. Other identified risk factors include increasing age, intravenous drug use and a lower IQ (Farinour *et al.* 2003; Wang *et al.* 1995).

A number of clinical features define HIV-associated dementia, and Price and Brew (1988) have devised a rating scale with gradations ranging from stage 0 (no dementia) up to stage 4, end-stage dementia in which the affected individual may be mute, lacking in social and intellectual comprehension, paralytic and doubly incontinent. Although this classification has its limitations (Everall 1995), it formed the basis for later, ICD-10 and DSM-IV definitions. Table 20.5 summarizes the criteria for HIV-associated minor cognitive disorder, a variant of HIV-dementia. There may be a wide number of presenting symptoms which

Table 20.5. Criteria for HIV-associated mild neurocognitive disorder.

---

1. Acquired impairment in cognitive functioning, involving at least two ability domains, documented by performance of at least 1.0 standard deviation below the mean for age-appropriate norms on standardized neuropsychological tests. The neuropsychological assessment must survey at least the following abilities: verbal/language; attention/speeded processing; abstraction/executive; memory (learning, recall); complex perceptual-motor performance. Motor skills.

2. The cognitive impairment produces at least mild interference in daily functioning (at least one of the following): a. self-report of reduced mental acuity, inefficiency in work, home-making or social functioning; b. observation by knowledgeable others that the individual has undergone at least mild decline in mental acuity, with resultant inefficiency in work, home-making or social functioning.

3. The cognitive impairment has been present for at least one month.

4. The cognitive impairment does not meet criteria for delirium or dementia.

5. There is no evidence of another pre-existing cause of the mild neurocognitive disorder.

Source: Grant & Atkinson (1995).

require thorough investigation, including appropriate blood tests and imaging. It is important to rule out reversible infectious or metabolic causes, which may respond to appropriate treatment. A specific screening test may be of particular benefit (Power *et al.* 1995). Management is directed, where possible, at the precise cause of the disorder, and specific antiretroviral treatments (especially zidovudine) may be particularly effective (Gray *et al.* 1991; Portegies *et al.* 1989).

Although a number of adjunct agents have also been assessed for their efficacy in the treatment of HIV dementia, including nimodipine (Navia *et al.* 1998), tumour necrosis factor antagonists (Clifford *et al.* 2002) and gp120 analogues (Heseltine *et al.* 1998), none has yet to be fully clinically validated. Lithium may have utility in the treatment of HIV dementia (see review by Harvey *et al.* 2002) and animal studies suggest that lithium protects against HIV gp-120-mediated neurotoxicity (Everall *et al.* 2002). At present these adjunct agents remain to be fully evaluated and are not currently recommended first-line treatments.

Apart from pharmacological approaches to treatment, both psychological and social approaches should be utilized, and can help in the treatment of miscellaneous symptoms such as fatigue, pain, weight loss and sexual dysfunction.

HIV and psychosis

Psychotic disorders may occur in HIV-infected individuals as part of an existing illness or may arise secondary to HIV-associated consequences including antiretroviral therapy itself. A wide range of first-onset presentations has been described, including mania (El-Mallakh 1991) and psychosis (Foster *et al.* 2003;

Stevens *et al.* 2000). Psychotic symptomatology need not necessarily reflect a schizophreniform process, and the episode may resolve upon investigation and appropriate treatment of causative factors. For those individuals with pre-existing psychotic illnesses, careful management with neuroleptics and appropriate psychosocial interventions may be effective. Special precaution must be taken with clozapine due to increased risk of bone marrow toxicity (Dettling *et al.* 1988). A wide range of medications and illicit drugs may be contributory in some cases, and cessation or alteration of putative offending agents may ameliorate the psychotic presentation.

Affective disorders in HIV

Depression has been reported as occurring in at least 15–20% (Rabkin *et al.* 1997) and up to 84% (Anonymous 2002) of HIV-positive patients. Much of this depression is either not recognized or is insufficiently managed (Katz *et al.* 1996). It is therefore extremely important to assess and monitor depressive symptomatology in infected populations and to manage symptoms with appropriate medical, pharmacological, psychological and social input.

Treatment-resistant depression in HIV-infected individuals can pose a number of problems, and a hierarchical approach has been suggested (Franco-Bronson 1996) in which first-line agents include one of a serotonin-specific reuptake inhibitor (SSRI), buspirone or a psychostimulant, with a tricyclic antidepressant (TCA) as a second-line agent and electroconvulsive therapy (ECT) as third-line. It should be noted that the use of psychostimulants in HIV is comparatively rare, although there is some evidence that this approach may be useful (Breitbart *et al.* 2001). Additionally, anticholinergic side-effects with TCAs may be more severe in HIV-affected populations, thus limiting their utility.

Mania is a recognized presentation (El-Mallakh 1991) and may be an exacerbation of pre-existing bipolar disorder or may be secondary to organic disorders or medication. Although the exact prevalence of mania in HIV-infected individuals is unclear, one study suggests that the prevalence of 'secondary' mania (i.e. mania in the absence of a history of mood disorder in either the patient or the patient's family) is low, around 1.2% for HIV-infected individuals and 4.3% for those patients with AIDS (Ellen *et al.* 1999). Treatment using mood stabilizers requires caution, due to the possibility of increased side-effect profiles in HIV-affected individuals. Neuroleptics are extremely useful in this group, and may also be useful in AIDS mania.

Anxiety and related disorders

Not surprisingly, anxiety and related disorders are very common in HIV-infected persons, with a recent study revealing that of 101 patients infected with

HIV, 72.3% exhibited high levels of distress, 70.3% had high levels of anxiety, 45.5% were felt to be depressed and 53.5% were found to be experiencing 'significant' distress (Cohen *et al.* 2002). This study further noted that patients with high viral loads were more likely to be depressed and anxious, while those with higher CD4 counts (above 500 mm^3) were less likely to be depressed.

Medication may be warranted for treatment of chronic anxiety states, with an SSRI as the first choice to treat conditions such as generalized anxiety disorder, panic disorder, social phobia, post-traumatic stress disorder and obsessive-compulsive disorder, in association with appropriate psychosocial strategies. Other agents which may also be of use include buspirone, antihistamines (not terfenadine), and benzodiazepines, especially lorazepam and clonazepam.

Personality and lifestyle issues

Individuals infected with HIV who have comorbid personality disorders can present particular therapeutic challenges. Reports suggest a prevalence of personality problems (of any sort) ranging between 19% (Johnson *et al.* 1995) and 33% (Perkins *et al.* 1993). It has been noted that antisocial personality disorder is associated with increased risk of exposure to HIV, especially in the context of drug-taking (Compton *et al.* 1995). Borderline personality disorder may be associated with impulsive sexual behaviour (Hull *et al.* 1993), and it has been noted in hospital inpatients that HIV-infected patients had higher rates of borderline personality disorder than control patients (Ellis *et al.* 1994). It is thus important for the clinician to be aware of possible personality disorder in patients and to consider how these individuals deal with the multiple issues associated with HIV infection.

Management of HIV-positive individuals with personality disorders is complex; although medication is generally not appropriate as a primary treatment of personality problems, it may be useful for treating associated features such as depression or anxiety. There is anecdotal evidence that lamotrigine may be effective. Management will generally involve psychological approaches, ranging from general, consistent support to directed therapies, to deal with pre-existing concerns as well as post-diagnosis issues such as treatment adherence, changes in relationships, survival issues and others.

Drug and alcohol misuse

Dual diagnosis is common in HIV, with drug and alcohol problems associated with HIV infection at all stages of the natural history of the disorder. Prior to diagnosis there may be addiction/dependence issues, which may contribute directly or indirectly to HIV infection. Intravenous drug-users are a high-risk population for infection, and the care of these individuals is complex (see Cohn 2002, for review).

Despite the difficulties in managing these groups of patients, it has been shown that psychiatric treatment combined with concurrent treatment for substance abuse can result in decreased substance utilization and better clinical outcomes (Lyketsos *et al.* 1997).

Drug and alcohol misuse may interact adversely with prescribed medications (Antoniou & Tseng 2002; Kresina *et al.* 2002), leading to higher rates of cognitive impairment (Egan *et al.* 1990) and possibly to engagement in high-risk behaviours (Dausey & Desai 2003). In addition, adherence to treatment and attendance at clinics may be influenced by substance-related lifestyle factors (Coleman *et al.* 1988).

Treatment of substance abuse in HIV-infected individuals should aim to treat both the substance disorder as well as accompanying psychiatric problems. A number of options have been suggested, including the use of targeted treatment programmes such as methadone maintenance or the use of pharmacological modalities for specific addictions. Joint care approaches are also useful.

Suicide

Although it is unclear whether HIV infection itself is a trigger for suicide, the fact remains that suicide and HIV infection are interrelated, although the exact nature of this relationship remains controversial (Komiti *et al.* 2001). Suicidal behaviour may be influenced by a number of variables, such as HIV seropositivity (Cochand & Bovet 1998), drug abuse and previous psychiatric history, notably depression (Beckett & Shenson 1993). Assessment of suicidality should be a mandatory part of all psychiatric assessments, and a thorough risk assessment completed. In some cases hospitalization may be required, with medical or psychiatric liaison input as appropriate.

Assessment and treatment

Assessment of the HIV liaison patient

Assessment of the HIV liaison patient includes the usual evaluation of medical, social and psychological functioning, together with additional information concerning the history of the individual HIV patient's disease progression, complications, treatments and CD4/viral loads. The psychiatrist needs to liaise closely with the HIV physicians and be aware of the activity of the HIV infection and of any complications that have arisen. Further investigations should be arranged in conjunction with the medical team. Regular monitoring of viral load and CD4 count is important to determine appropriate treatment interventions, to assess progression and to help determine prognosis. Regular review of drug

Table 20.6. Professionals and others who may be involved in the psychiatric/social care of individuals with HIV and AIDS.

Statutory	Non-statutory
Psychiatrist	Voluntary organizations (e.g. Terrence Higgins Trust)
HIV physician	Patient groups
Psychologist	Religious organizations
Psychiatric nurses	Cultural organizations
General practitioner	
Other medical and nursing staff	
Social worker	
Occupational therapist	
Physical therapist	
Dietitian	

histories (prescribed and illicit) in the context of altered physical or psychological parameters is also recommended.

General management of psychiatric morbidity

The psychiatric management of individuals with HIV and AIDS may be complicated by biological manifestations of infections which may contribute to altered behaviour. The clinician should therefore liaise with others in the multidisciplinary management team. Table 20.6 lists those who may be involved in care. Social and supportive contributions of non-statutory organizations can be extremely useful adjuncts to clinical treatment. The location of treatment is also a factor, with most patients managed as outpatients, and inpatient admissions reserved for severe medical and/or psychiatric complications.

Physical treatments

Electroconvulsive therapy has been used infrequently in the treatment of HIV-infected individuals with psychiatric morbidity and full evaluation of its efficacy remains to be confirmed. However it has been shown to be useful in the treatment of major depression (Schaerf et al. 1989) as well as in the treatment of the rare HIV-associated stupor (Kessing et al. 1994).

Pharmacotherapy

Where possible, directed interventions should aim to treat the cause of psychiatric disorder in HIV-infected patients. When considering introduction of a psychotropic medication, a number of issues need to be considered, including medical, drug, psychiatric and social factors.

The mainstay of treatment of HIV/AIDS is with antiviral agents of three broad classes, nucleoside reverse transcriptase inhibitors, non-nucleoside reverse transcriptase inhibitors and protease inhibitors. A number of other antiviral agents may be used for specific infections (e.g. herpes simplex, cytomegalovirus) in addition to other anti-infectious agents. Certain of these agents can induce mood disturbances or even frank psychosis (Table 20.7; Foster *et al.* 2003, 2004), and thus careful and expert monitoring is required.

In general, treatment of psychiatric disorders in individuals infected with HIV is similar to that in non-infected persons. Although most psychopharmacological agents in current use may be used safely HIV-infected persons may be more vulnerable to adverse effects, higher medication doses, side-effects and interactions (Ayuso 1994). In addition, interaction with illicit drugs may further complicate the psychiatric presentation and its management.

Specific classes of agents

Tricyclic antidepressants

Although imipramine has been shown to be effective in treating depressed HIV-positive patients (Manning *et al.* 1990; Rabkin & Harrison 1990; Rabkin *et al.* 1994a), its side-effect profile may cause severe adversity which could limit adherence and hence the utility of this agent. It has been suggested that TCAs may be of most utility in depressed HIV patients who are otherwise generally well (Ochitill 1992).

Monoamine oxidase inhibitors

These agents have not been widely used in the treatment of depression in HIV-infected individuals, and the literature contains few reports about their use. They may interact dangerously with zidovudine and sulphonamides, and their use is not recommended.

SSRIs

These are the first-line choice for treatment of depression in HIV-infected individuals. A number of SSRIs have been shown to be of use in affected populations, including fluoxetine (Rabkin *et al.* 1999), sertraline (Rabkin *et al.* 1994b) and paroxetine (Elliott *et al.* 1998). Fluoxetine together with supportive group therapy has been reported to be superior to placebo (Zisook *et al.* 1998). Although the SSRIs have favourable side-effect profiles, they can have significant interactions with other psychotropic medications which may limit their utility in

Table 20.7. Reported psychiatric side-effects of antiretroviral medications used in the treatment of HIV/AIDS.

Antivirals used to treat herpes simplex and varicella zoster

Aciclovir	Depression, psychosis (Sirota *et al.* 1988)
Famciclovir	None reported
Valaciclovir	None reported
Idoxuridine	None reported
Inosine pranobex	None reported

Nucleoside reverse transcriptase inhibitors

Abacavir	Psychosis, mood changes, depression (Colebunders *et al.* 2002; Foster *et al.* 2003, 2004)
Didanosine	Mania (Brouillette *et al.* 1994)
Lamivudine	Mood disorders (Turjanski & Lloyd 2005)
Stavudine	None reported
Tenofovir	None reported
Zalcitabine	None reported
Zidovudine	Mania (Anonymous 1988; Maxwell *et al.* 1988; O'Dowd & McKegney 1988; Wright *et al.* 1989)

Protease inhibitors

Amprenavir	None reported
Delaviridine	None reported
Indinavir	Mood disturbance (Jewett & Hecht 1993)
Lopinavir	None reported
Nelfinavir	None reported
Ritonavir	None reported
Saquinavir	None reported

Non-nucleoside reverse transcriptase inhibitors

Efavirenz	Depression (Hoyt 2004; Lang *et al.* 2001; Lederer 2004; Puzantian 2002), mania (Blanch *et al.* 2001; Shah & Balderson 2003), psychosis (De La Garza *et al.* 2001; Hasse *et al.* 2005; Peyriere *et al.* 2001; Poulsen & Lublin 2003; Sabato *et al.* 2002) post-traumatic stress disorder (Moreno *et al.* 2003); miscellaneous symptoms (Allin *et al.* 2003; Peyriere *et al.* 2001)
Nevirapine	Depression, psychosis (Wise *et al.* 2002); vivid dreams (Morlese *et al.* 2002)

Agents active against cytomegalovirus

Foscarnet sodium	None reported
Valganciclovir	None reported

certain individuals. Their side-effect profile (including interference with sexual function) may decrease their efficacy and affect compliance.

Miscellaneous agents

A number of other agents have been suggested to be useful in the treatment of HIV-related depression, including nefazodone (Elliott *et al.* 1999), mirtazapine (Elliott & Roy-Byrne 2000), venlafaxine (Fernandez & Levy 1997), psychostimulants (Breitbart *et al.* 2001; Wagner *et al.* 2000) and testosterone (Rabkin *et al.* 1999, 2000a). Testosterone precursors such as DHEA (Rabkin *et al.* 2000b) and L-acetylcarnitine, a naturally occurring acetylcholine-like substance (De Simone *et al.* 1988) have also been investigated. In addition, it has been reported that smoking cannabis may be of benefit to those who are HIV-positive (Ogborne *et al.* 2000), although this remains controversial. Bupropion has been investigated but has not been found to be an effective treatment (Fichtner & Braun 1992; Haney 2002; Trachman 1992).

Alternative, herbal and other medications

Several alternative medications have been utilized in the treatment of various aspects of HIV, but there is insufficient evidence for their general use (Power *et al.* 2002; Vermani & Garg 2002) and they should only be considered with great care. St John's Wort has not been found to be an effective treatment of HIV-related depression (James 2000; Williams *et al.* 2001), and has been reported to interact dangerously with ritonavir (Hennessy *et al.* 2002; Hesse *et al.* 2001), efavirenz and nelfinavir (Hesse *et al.* 2001) as well as indinavir (Miller 2000; Piscitelli *et al.* 2000) and nevirapine (De Maat *et al.* 2001). Its use is therefore not recommended in HIV-infected populations.

Antipsychotics

Antipsychotics of all types are used for the treatment of psychotic illness in HIV-infected individuals. They are also useful in the management of diverse conditions such as nausea and delirium. There is an increased risk of extrapyramidal side-effects and neuroleptic malignant syndrome in psychotic patients with HIV encephalopathy as compared to non-AIDS psychotics (Burch & Montoya 1989; Horwath & Cournos 1999; Hriso *et al.* 1991; Shedlack *et al.* 1994). The use of clozapine in HIV-infected individuals remains controversial (Dettling *et al.* 1988; Lera & Zirulnik 1999) and is not currently recommended in this population.

Atypical antipsychotics are recommended as first-line treatment, and there is evidence that agents such as risperidone (Meyer *et al.* 1998; Singh *et al.* 1997; Zilikis *et al.* 1998) and haloperidol (Breitbart *et al.* 1996; Mauri *et al.* 1997;

Sewell *et al.* 1994) are useful agents. Olanzapine may also be useful (Meyer *et al.* 1998); however, there is currently insufficient evidence for its use to be universally recommended.

Mood stabilizers and anticonvulsants

It has been reported that these agents are poorly tolerated in HIV-infected patients who are immunosuppressed (Halman *et al.* 1993) and so anti-convulsants and mood stabilizers must be used cautiously (Romanelli *et al.* 2000). In addition, these agents may interact in complex ways with other prescribed agents. Lithium has been found to have multiple benefits in HIV and AIDS, and may have additional neuroprotective functions in addition to its mood-stabilizing effects (Everall *et al.* 2002; Harvey *et al.* 2002). Lithium has, however, been reported to cause toxicity at therapeutic levels in an AIDS patient (Tanquary 1993).

Anxiolytics

Benzodiazepines and hypnotics are widely used in psychiatry and may be useful in HIV-infected people with anxiety or insomnia. The long-term use of these agents is not recommended, and attention should be paid to treating the cause of the anxiety with non-pharmacological methods or where indicated, an antidepressant or antihistamines. Excessive sedation may result when benzodiazepines or zopiclone are administered with ritonavir (Dresser *et al.* 2000).

Adverse effects of antiretrovirals

Medications used in treatment regimes for HIV have a wide variety of side-effects which may limit their efficacy. Indeed, specific agents may have direct psychiatric effects which may initiate or exacerbate psychiatric morbidity. These are summarized in Tables 20.8 and 20.9.

Interactions between antiretroviral agents and psychotropics

A number of antiretroviral agents can interact with antipsychotics, antidepressants and other psychotropic medications. A review by Robinson and Qaqish (2002) implicates ritonavir and efavirenz as having the greatest number of interactions across all classes of psychopharmacologically active agents, with delavirdine and nevirapine having less broad-ranging interactions. In addition, zidovudine is reported to interact with sodium valproate and cause increased bone marrow toxicity. Levin *et al.* (2001) have reported that co-administration of venlafaxine and indinavir can lead to decreased plasma concentrations of indinavir. The use of this particular combination is thus not recommended.

Table 20.8. Reported interactions of antiretroviral agents with psychotropic drugs.

Class/agent	Antiretroviral	Effect on psychotropic
Antidepressants		
TCA	Ritonavir	Increase in serum concentration
SSRI	Ritonavir	Increase in serum concentration
Bupropion	Ritonavir	Increase in serum concentration, leading to seizures
Anxiolytics		
Buspirone	Delavirdine ?Efavirenz	Increase in serum concentration
Midazolam	Delavirdine	Increase in serum levels leading to excessive sedation/respiratory
Triazolam	?Efavirenz	Depression – contraindicated
Alprazolam	Delavirdine	Increase in serum levels
Clonazepam	?Efavirenz	
Lorazepam		Not reported
Temazepam		Not reported
Lorazepam	Ritonavir Nelfinavir	Decrease in serum concentration, leading to withdrawal
Mood stabilizers		
Carbamazepine	Amprenavir	Increased serum levels
	Ritonavir	Increased serum levels
Neuroleptics		
Chlorpromazine	Ritonavir	Increase in serum concentration
Clozapine	Ritonavir	
Haloperidol		Not reported
Perphenazine		Not reported
Thioridazine		Not reported
Pimozide	Delavirdine ?Efavirenz	Increase serum concentration, risk of cardiotoxicity – contraindicated
Quetiapine	Delavirdine ?Efavirenz	Increase serum concentration

Source: Adapted from Robinson & Qaqish (2002).

Psychological treatments

A number of psychological approaches have been used, both as primary therapeutic interventions and as adjuncts to psychopharmacological treatments. These include a variety of counselling, supportive and psychoeducational approaches, as well as psychotherapy (psychodynamic and interpersonal) and cognitive-behavioural therapy (CBT). Although the literature contains

Table 20.9. Reported interactions of psychotropic drugs with antiretroviral agents.

Antiretroviral	Psychotropic	Effect on antiretroviral
Amprenavir	Carbamazepine	↓Amprenavir effect
	Phenobarbital	↓Amprenavir effect
	Primidone	↓Amprenavir effect
	St John's Wort	↓Amprenavir effect
Delavirdine	Carbamazepine	↓Delavirdine effect
	Fluoxetine	↑Delavirdine effect
	Phenobarbital	↓Delavirdine effect
	Primidone	↓Delavirdine effect
Efavirenz	Carbamazepine	↓Efavirenz effect
	Phenobarbital	↓Efavirenz effect
	Primidone	↓Efavirenz effect
	St John's Wort	↓Efavirenz effect
Indinavir	Carbamazepine	↓Indinavir effect
	Phenobarbital	↓Indinavir effect
	Primidone	↓Indinavir effect
	St John's Wort	↓Indinavir effect
	Venlafaxine	↓Indinavir levels
Lopinavir/ritonavir	Carbamazepine	↓Lopinavir/ritonavir effect
	Phenobarbital	↓Lopinavir/ritonavir effect
	Primidone	↓Lopinavir/ritonavir effect
	St John's Wort	↓Lopinavir/ritonavir effect
Nelfinavir	Carbamazepine	↓ Nelfinavir effect
	Phenobarbital	↓ Nelfinavir effect
	Primidone	↓ Nelfinavir effect
	St John's Wort	↓ Nelfinavir effect
Ritonavir	Carbamazepine	↓ Ritonavir effect
	Primidone	↓ Ritonavir effect
	St John's Wort	↓ Ritonavir effect
Saquinavir	Carbamazepine	↓ Saquinavir effect
	Phenobarbital	↓ Saquinavir effect
	Primidone	↓ Saquinavir effect
	St John's Wort	↓ Saquinavir effect
Zidovudine	Valproate	↑ Zidovudine levels

Source: Adapted from Foster (2005).

comparatively few HIV-specific reports, the efficacy of these interventions in other situations suggests that they may be of benefit in the HIV/AIDS setting.

Counselling

Counselling has been shown to be an important and useful intervention in various stages of HIV disease progression, including pre-test (Adcock & Stewart-Moore 1996; Perry *et al.* 1990) and post-test (Perry *et al.* 1991). Psychoeducational strategies aimed at health maintenance (Jewett & Hecht 1993) and compliance with medication (Mehta *et al.* 1997) may also be effective.

Psychotherapy

Both psychodynamic and interpersonal therapies have been shown to be helpful. For example, individual and group psychodynamic therapy has been shown to be effective in gay men with HIV (Blechner 1997; Cadwell *et al.* 1994; Weiss 1997), and existential therapy has also been used with this group (Milton 1994).

Interpersonal therapy (IT) is a brief (12–16 weeks) weekly treatment, which focuses on improving interpersonal functioning (Klerman *et al.* 1984). In HIV-infected individuals it has been shown to be effective in association with antidepressants as well as by itself (Weissman 1997), and a randomized controlled trial comparing four different psychotherapeutic interventions in depressed HIV-positive patients (IT, CBT, supportive therapy (ST) and ST with imipramine) suggested that interpersonal therapy resulted in significantly greater improvements in depression measures than CBT or ST alone (Markowitz *et al.* 1995). This study also showed that ST with imipramine was of equal efficacy to IT.

Cognitive-behavioural therapy

Cognitive-behavioural therapy has been shown to be useful in the treatment of anxiety and mood symptoms (Blanch *et al.* 2002; Lutgendorf *et al.* 1997, 1998) and has also been shown to be a useful adjunct to antidepressant therapy (Lee *et al.* 1999). In addition, approaches based on CBT may be useful in reducing HIV-risk behaviours (Tallis 1995).

Social interventions

HIV and AIDS affect individuals, families, friends and the wider community in general. Hence the inclusion of social supports is an essential adjunct to successful treatment of any HIV-associated psychiatric mortality. Interventions which may be helpful include appropriate education strategies (either professional or lay), attention to finances, housing, social support and general needs issues.

Loss of independence may cause great distress and should be addressed early. The input of social workers, housing officials and others should be sought when required. A number of HIV-infected individuals may experience social isolation and stigmatization which may be helped by various HIV/AIDS support organizations.

Models of care

Although the impact of HIV in mental health is complex and wide-ranging, current systems of care that rely on a multidisciplinary approach appear to be effective, and interventions aimed at increasing quality (as well as quantity) of life should be implicated (Douaihy & Singh 2001).

Outcomes of intervention and prognosis

It is clear that improved treatment modalities have resulted in sustained survival generally in HIV-infected individuals, with prevention, early detection, intervention and multifaceted treatment strategies contributing to this overall decline in morbidity (Sacktor 2002). However, the appearance of resistance to antiretroviral medications may eventually result in increases in the prevalence of HIV and AIDS (Pillay 2001). New strategies such as measurement of HIV replication capacity may be useful in future patient management protocols (Maldarelli 2003).

REFERENCES

Adcock, J. and Stewart-Moore, J. (1996). Pre-test counselling for HIV. *British Journal of Midwifery*, **4**, 196–8.

Allin, M., Reeves, I., Tennant-Flowers, M., *et al.* (2003). Frequency of serious psychiatric adverse events with efavirenz. 5th International Workshop on Adverse Drug Reactions and Lipodystrophy, Paris, France. *Antiviral Therapy*, **8**, L85.

Ammassari, A., Trotta, M. P., Murri, R., *et al.* (2002). Correlates and predictors of adherence to highly active antiretroviral therapy: overview of published literature. *Journal of Acquired Immune Deficiency Syndrome*, **31**(Suppl. 3), S123–7.

Anonymous. (1988). Manic syndrome associated with zidovudine. *Journal of the American Medical Association*, **260**, 3587–8.

Anonymous. (2002). Depression is common among AIDS patients. Psych consult often is necessary. *Aids Alert*, **17**, 153–4.

Antoniou, T. and Tseng, A. (2002). Interactions between recreational drugs and antiretroviral agents. *Annals of Pharmacotherapy*, **36**, 1598–613.

Ayuso, J. L. (1994). Use of psychotropic drugs in patients with HIV infection. *Drugs*, **47**, 599–610.

Beckett, A. and Shenson, D. (1993). Suicide risk in patients with human immunodeficiency virus infection and acquired immunodeficiency syndrome. *Harvard Review of Psychiatry*, **1**, 27–35.

Belman, A. (1992). AIDS and the child's CNS. *Pediatric Clinics of North America*, **39**, 691–714.

Bing, E. G., Burnam, M. A., Longshore, D., *et al.* (2001). Psychiatric disorders and drug use among human immunodeficiency virus-infected adults in the United States. *Archives of General Psychiatry*, **58**, 721–8.

Blanch, J., Corbella, B., Garcia, F., *et al.* (2001). Manic syndrome associated with efavirenz overdose. *Clinical Infectious Diseases*, **33**, 270–1.

Blanch, J., Rousaud, A., Hautzinger, M., *et al.* (2002). Assessment of the efficacy of a cognitive-behavioural group psychotherapy programme for HIV-infected patients referred to a consultation-liaison psychiatry department. *Psychotherapy and Psychosomatics*, **71**, 77–84.

Blechner, M. J. (ed). (1997). *Hope and Mortality: Psychodynamic approaches to AIDS and HIV*. Hillsdale, NJ: The Analytic Press.

Brashers, D. E., Neidig, J. L., Cardillo, L. W., *et al.* (1999). 'In an important way, I did die': uncertainty and revival in persons living with HIV or AIDS. *AIDS Care*, **11**, 201–19.

Breitbart, W., Marotta, R., Platt, M., *et al.* (1996). A double-blind trial of haloperidol, chlorpromazine and lorazepam in the treatment of delirium in hospitalised AIDS patients. *American Journal of Psychology*, **153**, 231–7.

Breitbart, W., Rosenfeld, B., Kaim, M., *et al.* (2001). A randomized, double-blind, placebo-controlled trial of psychostimulants for the treatment of fatigue in ambulatory patients with human immunodeficiency virus disease. *Archives of Internal Medicine*, **161**, 411–20.

Brouillette, M., Chouinard, G. and Lalonde, R. (1994). Didanosine-induced mania in HIV infection. *American Journal of Psychiatry*, **151**, 1839–40.

Burch, E. and Montoya, J. (1989). NMS in an AIDS patient. *Journal of Clinical Psychopharmacology*, **9**, 228–9.

Burnam, M. A., Bing, E. G., Morton, S. C., *et al.* (2001). Use of mental health and substance abuse services among adults with HIV in the United States. *Archives of General Psychiatry*, **58**, 729–36.

Cadwell, S. A., Burnham, R. A. and Forstein, M. (eds). (1994). *Therapists on the Front Line: Psychotherapy with Gay Men in the Age of Aids*. Washington, DC: American Psychiatric Press, Inc.

Catalan, J. (1999). Psychological problems in people with HIV infection. In *Mental Health and HIV Infection*, ed. J. Catalan. London: UCL Press, pp. 21–46.

Catalan, J., Klimes, I., Day, A., *et al.* (1992). The psychosocial impact of HIV infection in gay men: a controlled investigation and factors associated with psychiatric morbidity. *British Journal of Psychiatry*, **161**, 774–8.

Catalan, J., Burgess, A. and Klimes, I. (1995). *Psychological Medicine of HIV Infection*. Oxford: Oxford University Press.

Clark, B. and Everall, I. P. (1997). What is the role of the HIV liaison psychiatrist? *Genitourinary Medicine*, **73**, 568–70.

Clifford, D. B., McArthur, J. C., Schifitto, G., *et al.* (2002). A randomized clinical trial of CPI-1189 for HIV-associated cognitive-motor impairment. *Neurology*, **59**, 1568–73.

Cochand, P. and Bovet, P. (1998). HIV infection and suicide risk: an epidemiological inquiry among male homosexuals in Switzerland. *Social Psychiatry and Psychiatric Epidemiology*, **3**, 230–4.

Cohen, M., Hoffman, R. G., Cromwell, C., *et al.* (2002). The prevalence of distress in persons with human immunodeficiency virus infection. *Psychosomatics*, **43**, 10–15.

Cohn, J. A. (2002). HIV-1 infection in injection drug users. *Infectious Disease Clinics of North America*, **16**, 745–70.

Colebunders, R., Hilbrands, R., De Roo, A., *et al.* (2002). Neuropsychiatric reaction induced by abacavir. *American Journal of Medicine*, **113**, 616.

Coleman, R. M., Curtis, D. and Feinmann, C. (1988). Perception of risk of HIV infection by injecting drug users and effects on medical clinic attendance. *British Journal of Addiction*, **83**, 1325–9.

Compton, W. M., Cottler, L. B., Shillington, A. M., *et al.* (1995). Is antisocial personality disorder associated with increased HIV risk behaviors in cocaine users? *Drug & Alcohol Dependence*, **37**, 37–43.

Dannenberg, A. L., McNeil, J. G., Brundage, J. F., *et al.* (1996). Suicide and HIV infection. Mortality follow-up of 4147 HIV-seropositive military service applicants. *Journal of the American Medical Association*, **276**, 1743–6.

Dausey, D. J. and Desai, R. A. (2003). Psychiatric comorbidity and the prevalence of HIV infection in a sample of patients in treatment for substance abuse. *Journal of Nervous and Mental Disease*, **191**, 10–17.

De la Garza, C. L., Paoletti-Duarte, S., Garcia-Martin, C., *et al.* (2001). Efavirenz-induced psychosis. *AIDS*, **15**, 1911–12.

De Maat, M. M., Hoetelmans, R. M., Math, R. A., *et al.* (2001). Drug interaction between St John's wort and nevirapine. *AIDS*, **15**, 420–1.

Demmer, C. (2001). Dealing with AIDS-related loss and grief in a time of treatment advances. *American Journal of Hospice and Palliative Care*, **18**, 35–41.

De Simone, C., Catania, S., Trinchieri, V., *et al.* (1988). Amelioration of the depression in HIV-infected subjects with L-acetyl carntine therapy. *Journal of Drug Development*, **3**, 163–6.

Dettling, M., Muller-Oerlinghausen, B. and Britsch, P. (1988). Clozapine treatment of HIV-associated psychosis – too much bone marrow toxicity? *Pharmacopsychiatry*, **31**, 156–7.

Douaihy, A. and Singh, N. (2001). Factors affecting quality of life in patients with HIV infection. *AIDS Reader*, **11**, 450–4, 460–1, 475.

Dresser, G. K., Spence, J. D. and Bailey, D. G. (2000). Pharmacokinetic-pharmacodynamic consequences and clinical relevance of cytochrome P450 3A4 inhibition. *Clinical Pharmacokinetics*, **38**, 41–57.

Egan, V., Crawford, J. R., Brettle, R. P., *et al.* (1990). The Edinburgh cohort of HIV positive drug users: current intellectual function is impaired, but not due to early AIDS dementia complex. *AIDS*, **4**, 651–6.

Eichler, M. R., Ray, S. M. and del Rio, C. (2002). The effectiveness of HIV post-test counselling in determining healthcare-seeking behavior. *AIDS*, **16**, 943–5.

Ellen, S. R., Judd, F. K., Mijch, Am., *et al.* (1999). Secondary mania in patients with HIV infection. *Australian and New Zealand Journal of Psychiatry*, **33**, 353–60.

Elliott, A. J. and Roy-Byrne, P. P. (2000). Mirtazapine for depression in patients with human immunodeficiency virus (letter). *Journal of Clinical Psychopharmacology*, **20**, 265–7.

Elliott, A. J., Uldall, K. K., Bergam, K., *et al.* (1998). Randomized, placebo-controlled trial of paroxetine versus imipramine in depressed HIV-positive outpatients. *American Journal of Psychiatry*, **155**, 367–72.

Elliott, A. J., Russo, J., Bergam, K., *et al.* (1999). Antidepressant efficacy in HIV-seropositive outpatients with major depressive disorder: an open trial of nefazodone. *Journal of Clinical Psychiatry*, **60**, 226–31.

Ellis, D., Collis, I. and King, M. (1994). A controlled comparison of HIV and general medical referrals to a liaison psychiatry service. *AIDS Care*, **6**, 69–76.

El-Mallakh, R. S. (1991). Mania in AIDS: clinical significance and theoretical considerations. *International Journal of Psychiatry in Medicine*, **21**, 383–91.

Everall, I. P. (1995). Neuropsychiatric aspects of HIV infection. *Journal of Neurology, Neurosurgery and Psychiatry*, **58**, 399–402.

Everall, I. P., Bell, C., Mallory, M., *et al.* (2002). Lithium ameliorates HIV-gp120-mediated neurotoxicity. *Molecular and Cellular Neuroscience*, **21**, 493–501.

Farinpour, R., Miller, E., Satz, P., *et al.* (2003). Psychosocial risk factors of HIV morbidity and mortality: findings from the Multicenter AIDS Cohort Study (MACS). *Journal of Clinical Experimental Neuropsychology*, **25**, 654–70.

Fernandez, F. and Levy, J. (1997). Efficacy of venlafaxine in HIV-depressive disorders. *Psychosomatics*, **38**, 173–4.

Fichtner, C. G. and Braun, B. G. (1992). Bupropion-associated mania in a patient with HIV infection. *Journal of Clinical Psychopharmacology*, **12**, 366–7.

Forstein, M. (1984). AIDS anxiety in the worried well. In *Psychiatric Implications of AIDS*, ed. S. Nichols and D. Ostrow. Washington, DC: American Psychiatric Press, pp. 50–60.

Foster, R. (2005). General principles of precribing in HIV. In *Maudsley Prescribing Guidelines 2005*, 8th edn., ed. D. Taylor, C. Paton and R. Kerwin. London: Martin Dunitz.

Foster, R., Olajide, D. and Everall, I. P. (2003). Antiretroviral-therapy induced psychosis: case report and brief review of the literature. *HIV Medicine*, **4**, 139–44.

Foster, R., Taylor, C. and Everall, I. P. (2004). More on abacavir-induced neuropsychiatric reactions. *AIDS*, **18**, 2449.

Franco-Bronson, K. (1996). The management of treatment-resistant depression. *Psychiatric Clinincs of North America*, **19**, 329–50.

Grant, I. and Atkinson, J. H. (1995). Psychiatric aspects of acquired immune deficiency syndrome. In *Comprehensive Textbook of Psychiatry, Volume VI*. ed. H. I. Kaplan and B. J. Sadock. Baltimore: Williams and Wilkins, pp. 1644–69.

Gray, F., Geny, C., Dournon, E., *et al.* (1991). Neuropathological evidence that zidovudine reduces incidence of HIV infection of the brain. *Lancet*, **337**, 852–3.

Halman, M., Worth, J. L., Sanders, K., *et al.* (1993). Anticonvulsant use in the treatment of manic syndromes in patients with HIV1 infection. *Journal of Neuropsychiatry*, **54**, 30–4.

Haney, M. (2002). Effects of smoked marijuana in healthy and HIV + marijuana smokers. *Journal of Clinical Pharmacology*, **42**, 34S–40S.

Harvey, B. H., Meyer, C. L., Gallichio, V. S., *et al.* (2002). Lithium salts in AIDS and AIDS-related dementia. *Psychopharmacological Bulletin*, **36**, 5–26.

Hasse, B., Gunthard, H. F., Bleiber, G., *et al.* (2005). Efavirenz intoxication due to slow hepatic metabolism. *Clinical Infectious Diseases*, **40**(3), 22–3.

Hennessy, M., Kelleher, D., Spiers, J. P., *et al.* (2002). St Johns wort increases expression of P-glycoprotein: implications for drug interactions. *British Journal of Clinical Pharmacology*, **53**, 75–82.

Hermoine Lyall, E. G. (2002). Paediatric HIV in 2002 – a treatable and preventable infection. *Journal of Clinical Virology*, **25**, 107–19.

Heseltine, P. N., Goodkin, K., Atkinson, J. H., *et al.* (1998). Randomized double-blind placebo-controlled trial of peptide T for HIV-associated cognitive impairment. *Archives of Neurology*, **55**, 41–51.

Hesse, L. M., von Molke, L. L., Shader, R. I., *et al.* (2001). Ritonavir, efavirenz, and nelfinavir inhibit CYP2B6 activity in vitro: potential drug interactions with bupropion. *Drug Metabolism and Disposition*, **29**, 100–2.

Hilton, C. (1998). General paralysis of the insane and AIDS in old age psychiatry: epidemiology, clinical diagnosis, serology and ethics – the way forward. *International Journal of Geriatric Psychiatry*, **13**, 875–85.

Hinkin, C. H., Castellon, S. A., Atkinson, J. H., *et al.* (2001). Neuropsychiatric aspects of HIV infection among older adults. *Journal of Clinical Epidemiology*, **54**, S44–52.

Horwath, E. and Cournos, F. (1999). NMS and HIV. *Psychiatric Services*, **50**, 564.

Hoyt, G. (2004). Life after Sustiva. *Survivors News* (Atlanta Ga) **15**(3), 8.

Hriso, E., Kuhn, T. and Maslev, J. (1991). Extrapyramidal symptoms due to dopamine blocking agents in patients with AIDS encephalopathy. *American Journal of Psychiatry*, **148**, 1558–61.

Huang, D. B., Salinas, P. and Dougherty, D. (2001). Feigned HIV in a malingering patient. *Psychosomatics*, **42**, 438–9.

Hull, J. W., Clarkin, J. F. and Yeomans, F. (1993). Borderline personality disorder and impulsive sexual behavior. *Hospital and Community Psychiatry*, **44**, 1000–2.

Ickovics, J. R., Cameron, A., Zackin, R., *et al.* (2002). Consequences and determinants of adherence to antiretroviral medication: results from Adult AIDS Clinical Trials Group protocol 370. *Antiviral Therapies*, **7**, 185–93.

James, J. S. (2000). St John's wort warning: do not combine with protease inhibitors, NNTRIs. *AIDS Treatment News*, **337**, 3–5.

Janssen, R. S., Nwanyanwu, O. C., Selik, R. M., *et al.* (1992). Epidemiology of human immunodeficiency virus encephalopathy in the United States. *Neurology*, **42**, 1472–6.

Jewett, J. F. and Hecht, F. M. (1993). Preventive health care, for adults with HIV infection. *Journal of the American Medical Association*, **269**, 1144–53.

Johnson, J. G., Williams, J. B., Rabkin, J. G., *et al.* (1995). Axis I psychiatric symptoms associated with HIV infection and personality disorder. *American Journal of Psychiatry*, **152**, 551–4.

Katz, M. H., Douglas, J. M. Jr, Bolan, G. A., *et al.* (1996). Depression and use of mental health services among HIV-infected men. *AIDS Care*, **8**, 433–42.

Kessing, L., LaBianca, J. H. and Bolwig, T. G. (1994). HIV-stupor treated with ECT. *Convulsive Therapy*, **10**, 232–5.

Kilbourne, A. M., Justice, A. C., Rabeneck, L., *et al.*, VACS 3 Project Team. (2001). General medical and psychiatric comorbidity among HIV-infected veterans in the post-HAART era. *Journal of Clinical Epidemiology*, **54**, S22–8.

Klerman, G. L., Weissman, M. M., Rounsaville, B. J., *et al.* (1984). *Interpersonal Psychotherapy of Depression*. New York: Basic Books.

Komiti, A., Judd, F., Grech, P., *et al.* (2001). Suicidal behaviour in people with HIV/AIDS: a review. *Australian and New Zealand Journal of Psychiatry*, **35**, 747–57.

Kresina, T. F., Flexner, C. W., Sinclair, J., *et al.* (2002). Alcohol use and HIV pharmacotherapy. *AIDS Research and Human Retroviruses*, **18**, 757–70.

Lang, J. P., Halleguen, O., Picard, A., *et al.* (2001). Apropos of atypical melancholia with Sustiva (efavirenz) (article in French). *Encephale*, **27**, 290–3.

Lederer, B. (2004). *The Great Depression.* www.poz.com.

Lee, M. R., Cohen, L., Hadley, S. W., *et al.* (1999). Cognitive-behavioural group therapy with medication for depressed gay men with AIDS or symptomatic HIV infection. *Psychiatric Services*, **50**, 948–52.

Lera, G. and Zirulnik, J. (1999). Pilot study with clozapine in patients with HIV-associated psychosis and drug-induced parkinsonism. *Movement Disorders*, **14**, 128–31.

Levin, G. M., Nelson, L. A., DeVane, C. L., *et al.* (2001). A pharmacokinetic drug-drug interaction study of venlafaxine and indinavir. *Psychopharmacology Bulletin*, **35**, 62–71.

Lutgendorf, S. K., Antonni, M. H., Ironson, G., *et al.* (1997). Cognitive-behavioural stress management decreases dysphoric mood and herpes simplex virus-type 2 antibody titres in symptomatic HIV-seropositive gay men. *Journal of Consulting and Clinical Psychology*, **65**, 31–43.

Lutgendorf, S. K., Antonni, M. H., Ironson, G., *et al.* (1998). Changes in cognitive coping skills and social support during cognitive behavioural stress management intervention and distress outcomes in symptomatic immunodeficiency virus (HIV)-seropositive gay men. *Psychosomatic Medicine*, **60**, 204–14.

Lyketsos, C., Fishman, M., Hotton, H., *et al.* (1997). The effectiveness of psychiatric treatment for HIV-infected individuals. *Psychosomatics*, **38**, 423–32.

Maldarelli, F. (2003). HIV-1 fitness and replication capacity: what are they and can they help in patient management? *Current Infectious Disease Reports*, **5**, 77–84.

Manning, D., Jacobsberg, L., Erhart, S., *et al.* (1990). The efficacy of imipramine in the treatment of HIV-related depression. *International Conference on Aids* (Abstract Number Th.B. 32), 20–23 June, 1990.

Markowitz, J. C., Klerman, G. L., Clougherty, K. F., *et al.* (1995). Individual psychotherapies for depressed HIV-positive patients. *American Journal of Psychiatry*, **152**, 1504–9.

Marzuk, P. M., Tierney, H., Tardiff, K., *et al.* (1988). Increased risk of suicide in persons with AIDS. *Journal of the American Medical Association*, **259**, 1333–7.

Marzuk, P. M., Tardiff, K., Leon, A. C., *et al.* (1997). HIV seroprevalence among suicide victims in New York City, 1991–1993. *American Journal of Psychiatry*, **154**, 1720–5.

Mauri, M. C., Fabiano, L., Bravin, S., *et al.* (1997). Schizophrenic patients before and after HIV infection: a case-control study. *Encephale*, **23**, 437–41.

Maxwell, S., Scheftner, W. A., Kessler, H. A., *et al.* (1988). Manic syndrome associated with zidovudine treatment. *Journal of the American Medical Association*, **259**, 3406–7.

McArthur, J. C., Hoover, D. R., Bacellar, M., *et al.* (1993). Dementia in AIDS patients: incidence and risk factors. Multicenter AIDS Cohort Study. *Neurology*, **43**, 2245–52.

McHenry, A., Evans, B. G., Sinka, K., *et al.* (2002). Numbers of adults with diagnosed HIV infection 1996–2005 – adjusted totals and extrapolations for England, Wales and Northern Ireland. *Communicable Diseases and Public Health*, **5**(2), 97–100.

Mehta, S., Moore, R. and Graham, N. (1997). Potential factors affecting adherence with HIV therapy. *AIDS*, **11**, 1655–70.

Meursing, K. and Sibindi, F. (2000). HIV counselling – a luxury or necessity? *Health Policy and Planning*, **15**(1), 17–23.

Meyer, J. M., Marsh, J. and Simpson, G. (1998). Differential sensitivities to risperidone and olanzapine in a human immunodeficiency virus patient. *Biological Psychology*, **44**, 791–4.

Miller, J. L. (2000). Interaction between indinavir and St. John's wort reported. *American Journal of Health-System Pharmacy*, **57**(7), 625–6.

Milton, M. (1994). The case for existential therapy in HIV-related psychotherapy. *Counselling Psychology Quarterly*, **7**, 367–74.

Moreno, A., Labelle, C. and Samet, J. H. (2003). Recurrence of post-traumatic stress disorder symptoms after initiation of antiretrovirals including efavirenz: a report of two cases. *HIV Medicine*, **4**, 302–4.

Morlese, J. F., Qazi, N. A., Gazzard, B. G., *et al.* (2002). Nevirapine-induced neuropsychiatric complications, a class effect of non-nucleoside AIDS 16 1840#reverse transcriptase inhibitors? *AIDS*, **16**(13), 1840–1.

Murphy, D. A., Roberts, K. J., Martin, D. J., *et al.* (2000). Barriers to antiretroviral adherence among HIV-infected adults. *AIDS Patient Care and STDs*, **14**(1), 47–58.

Navia, B. A., Dafni, U., Simpson, D., *et al.* (1998). A phase I/II trial of nimodipine for HIV-related neurological complications. *Neurology*, **51**(1), 221–8.

Ochitill, H. (1992). Prescribing antipsychotic drugs for patients with AIDS. *Drug Therapy*, **22**, 37–41.

O'Dowd, M. A., McKegney, F. P. (1988). Manic syndrome associated with zidovudine (letter). *Journal of the American Medical Association*, **260**, 3587.

Ogborne, A. C., Smart, R. G., Weber, T., *et al.* (2000). Who is using cannabis as a medicine and why: an exploratory study. *Journal of Psychoactive Drugs*, **32**(4), 435–43.

Oyewole, D. (1996). Munchausen's syndrome and HIV infection: a trap for the unwary. *British Journal of Clinical Practice*, **50**(3), 176.

Penzak, S. R., Reddy, Y. S. and Grimsley, S. R. (2000). Depression in patients with HIV infection. *American Journal of Health-System Pharmacy*, **57**(4), 376–86.

Perkins, D. O., Davidson, E. J., Leserman, J., *et al.* (1993). Personality disorder in patients infected with HIV: a controlled study with implications for clinical care. *American Journal of Psychiatry*, **150**(2), 309–15.

Perry, S. W., Jacobsberg, L., Fishman, B., *et al.* (1990). Psychiatric diagnosis before serological testing for HIV. *American Journal of Psychiatry*, **147**, 89–93.

Perry, S. W., Fishman, B., Jacobsberg, L., *et al.* (1991). Effectiveness of psychoeducational intervention in reducing emotional distress after HIV antibody testing. *Archives of General Psychiatry*, **48**, 143–7.

Peyriere, H., Mauboussin, J. M., Rouanet, I., *et al.* (2001). Management of sudden psychiatric disorders related to efavirenz. *AIDS*, **15**(10), 1323–4.

Pillay, D. (2001). The emergence and epidemiology of resistance in the nucleoside-experienced HIV-infected population. *Antiviral Therapy*, **6**(Suppl. 3), 15–24.

Piscitelli, S. C., Burstein, Ah., Chiatt, D., *et al.* (2000). Indinavir concentrations and St John's wort. *Lancet*, **355**(9203), 547–8.

Portegies, P., Gans, J., Lange, L. M., *et al.* (1989). Declining incidence of Aids dementia complex after introduction of zidovudine treatment. *British Medical Journal*, **299**, 819–21.

Poulsen, H. D. and Lublin, H. K. (2003). Efavirenz-induced psychosis leading to involuntary detention. *AIDS*, **17**(3), 451–3.

Power, C., Selnes, O. A., Grim, J. A., *et al.* (1995). The HIV dementia scale: a rapid screening test. *Journal of Aids*, **8**, 273–6.

Power, R., Gore-Felton, C., Vosvick, M., *et al.* (2002). HIV: effectiveness of complementary and alternative medicine. *Primary Care*, **29**(2), 361–78.

Price, R. W. and Brew, B. J. (1988). The AIDS dementia complex. *Journal of Infectious Disease*, **158**, 1079–83.

Puzantian, T. (2002). Central nervous system adverse effects with efavirenz: case report and review. *Pharmacotherapy*, **22**(7), 930–3.

Rabkin, J. G. and Harrison, W. M. (1990). Effect of imipramine on depression and immune status in a sample of men with HIV infection. *American Journal of Psychology*, **47**, 495–7.

Rabkin, J. G., Rabkin, R., Harrison, W., *et al.* (1994a). Imipramine effects on mood in depressed patients with HIV illness. *American Journal of Psychology*, **151**, 516–23.

Rabkin, R. G., Wagner, G. and Rabkin, R. (1994b). Effects of sertraline on mood and immune status in patients with major depression and HIV illness: an open trial. *Journal of Clinical Psychology*, **55**(1), 433–9.

Rabkin, J. G., Ferrando, S. J., Jacobsberg, L. B., *et al.* (1997). Prevalence of Axis I disorders in an AIDS cohort: a cross-sectional, controlled study. *Journal of Comparative Psychology*, **38**(3), 146–54.

Rabkin, J. G., Wagner, G. J. and Rabkin, R. (1999). Fluoxetine treatment for depression in patients with HIV and AIDS: a randomized, placebo-controlled trial. *American Journal of Psychology*, **156**, 101–7.

Rabkin, J. G., Wagner, G. J. and Rabkin, R. (2000a). A double-blind, placebo-controlled trial of testosterone therapy for HIV-positive men with hypogonadal symptoms. *Archives of General Psychiatry*, **57**, 141–7.

Rabkin, J. G., Ferrando, S. J., Wagner, G., *et al.* (2000b). DHEA treatment of men and women with HIV infection. *Psychoneuroendocrinology*, **25**, 53–68.

Regier, D., Farmer, M. E., Rae, D. S., *et al.* (1993). One-month prevalence of mental disorders in the United States and sociodemographic characteristics: the Epidemiologic Catchment Area Study. *Acta Psychiatrica Scandinavica*, **88**, 35–47.

Robinson, M. J. and Qaqish, R. B. (2002). Practical psychopharmacology in HIV-1 and Acquired Immunodeficiency Syndrome. *Psychiatric Clinics of North America*, **25**(1), 149–75.

Romanelli, F., Jennings, H. R., Nath, A., *et al.* (2000). Therapeutic dilemma: the use of anticonvulsants in HIV-positive individuals. *Neurology*, **54**(7), 1404–7.

Rotheram-Borus, M. J., Cantwell, S. and Newman, P. A. (2000). HIV prevention programs with heterosexuals. *AIDS*, **14**(Suppl. 2), S59–67.

Roy, A. (2003). Characteristics of HIV patients who attempt suicide. *Acta Psychiatrica Scandinavica*, **107**, 41–4.

Sabato, S., Wesselingh, S., Fuller, A., *et al.* (2002). Efavirenz-induced catatonia. *AIDS*, **16**(13), 1841–42.

Sacktor, N. (2002). The epidemiology of human immunodeficiency virus-associated neurological disease in the era of highly active antiretroviral therapy. *Journal of Neurovirology*, **8**(Suppl. 2), 115–21.

Schaerf, F. W., Miller, R. R., Lipsey, J. R., *et al.* (1989). ECT for major depression in four patients infected with human immunodeficiency virus. *American Journal of Psychology*, **146**(6), 782–6.

Scott, S. and Constantine, L. M. (1999). The Lazarus syndrome: a second chance for life with HIV infection. *Journal of the American Pharmaceutical Association (Wash)*, **39**(4), 462–6.

Sewell, D. D. (1996). Schizophrenia and HIV. *Schizophrenia Bulletin*, **22**(3), 465–73.

Sewell, D. D., Jeste, D. V., McAdams, L. A., *et al.* (1994). Neuroleptic treatment of HIV-associated psychosis. HNRC Group. *Neuropsychopharmacology*, **10**, 223–9.

Sewell, M. C., Goggin, K. J., Rabkin, J. G., *et al.* (2000). Anxiety syndromes and symptoms among men with AIDS: a longitudinal controlled study. *Psychosomatics*, **41**(4), 294–300.

Shah, M. D. and Balderson, K. (2003). A manic episode associated with efavirenz therapy for HIV infection. *AIDS*, **17**(11), 1713–14.

Shedlack, K. J., Soldato-Couture, C. S. and Swanson, C. L. (1994). Rapidly progressive tardive dyskinesias in AIDS. *Biological Psychology*, **35**, 147–8.

Sikkema, K. J., Kalichman, S. C., Hoffmann, R., *et al.* (2000). Coping strategies and emotional wellbeing among HIV-infected men and women experiencing AIDS-related bereavement. *AIDS Care*, **12**(5), 613–24.

Singh, N., Squier, C., Sivek, C., *et al.* (1996). Determinants of compliance with antiretroviral therapy in patients with human immunodeficiency virus: prospective assessment with implications for enhancing compliance. *AIDS Care*, **8**(3), 261–9.

Singh, A. N., Golledge, H. and Catalan, J. (1997). Treatment of HIV-related psychotic disorders with risperidone: a series of 21 cases. *Journal of Psychosomatic Research*, **42**, 489–93.

Sirota, P., Stoler, M. and Meshulam, B. (1988). Major depression with psychotic features associated with acyclovir therapy. *Drug Intelligence and Clinical Pharmacy*, **22**(4), 306–8.

Stevens, V. M., Neel, J. L. and Baker, D. L. (2000). Psychosis and nonadherence in an HIV-seropositive patient. *AIDS Reader*, **10**(10), 596–601.

Stoskopf, C. H., Kin, Y. K. and Glover, S. H. (2001). Dual diagnosis: HIV and mental illness, a population-based study. *Community Mental Health Journal*, **37**, 469–79.

Stone, V. E. (2002). Enhancing adherence to antiretrovirals: strategies and regimens. *Medscape General Medicine*, **4**(3), 22.

Tallis, F. (1995). Cognitive behavioural strategies for HIV sexual risk reduction. *Clinical Psychology and Psychotherapy*, **1**, 267–77.

Tanquary, J. (1993). Lithium neurotoxicity at therapeutic levels in an AIDS patient. *Journal of Nervous and Mental Disease*, **181**(8), 518–19.

Trachman, S. B. (1992). Buspirone-induced psychosis in a human immunodeficiency virus infected man. *Psychosomatics*, **33**, 332–5.

Treisman, G., Fishman, M., Lyketsos, G., *et al.* (1994). Evaluation and treatment of psychiatric disorders associated with HIV infection. In *HIV, AIDS and the Brain*, ed. R. W. Price and W. Perry. New York: Raven Press, pp. 239–50.

Trotta, M. P., Ammassari, A., Melzi, S., *et al.* (2002). Treatment-related factors and highly active antiretroviral therapy adherence. *Journal of Acquired Immune Deficiency Syndromes*, **31**(Suppl. 3), S128–31.

Tuldra, A., Furnaz, C. R., Ferrer, M. J., *et al.* (2000). Prospective randomized two-arm controlled study to determine the efficacy of a specific intervention to improve long-term adherence to highly active antiretroviral therapy. *Journal of Acquired Immune Deficiency Syndromes*, **25**(3), 221–8.

Turjanski, N. and Lloyd, G. G. (2005). Psychiatric side effects of medication: recent developments. *Advances in Psychiatric Treatments*, **11**, 58–70.

Turrina, C., Fiorazzo, A., Turano, A., *et al.* (2001). Depressive disorders and personality variables in HIV positive and negative intravenous drug-users. *Journal of Affective Disorders*, **65**(1), 45–53.

Vermani, K. and Garg, S. (2002). Herbal medicines for sexually transmitted diseases and AIDS. *Journal of Ethnopharmacology*, **80**(1), 49–66.

Vitiello, B., Nurnam, M. A., Bing, E. G., *et al.* (2003). Use of psychotropic medications among HIV-infected patients in the United States. *American Journal of Psychology*, **160**, 547–54.

Wagner, G. J., Rabkin, J. G and Rabkin, R. (2000). Effects of dextroamphetamine on depression and fatigue in men with HIV: a double-blind, placebo-controlled trial. *Journal of Clinical Psychology*, **61**(6), 436–40.

Wagner, G. J., Kanouse, D. E., Koegel, P., *et al.* (2003). Adherence to HIV antiretrovirals among persons with serious mental illness. *Aids Patient Care and STDs*, **17**(4), 179–86.

Wang, F., So, Y., Vittinghoff, E., *et al.* (1995). Incidence proportion of and risk factors for AIDS patients diagnosed with HIV dementia, central nervous system toxoplasmosis, and cryptococcal meningitis. *Journal of Acquired Immune Deficiency Syndromes and Human Retroviruses*, **8**, 75–82.

Weiss, J. J. (1997). Psychotherapy with HIV-positive gay men: A psychodynamic perspective. *American Journal of Psychology*, **51**(3), 387–402.

Weissman, M. N. (1997). Interpersonal psychotherapy: current status. *Keio Journal of Medicine*, **46**(3), 105–10.

Welsby, P. D. and Richardson, A. M. (1995). Palliative aspects of adult acquired immune deficiency syndrome. In *Oxford Textbook of Palliative Medicine*, ed. D. Doyle, G. W. C. Hanks and N. MacDonald. Oxford: Oxford University Press, pp. 737–57.

Williams, A., George, K., Willard, S., *et al.* (2001). Is St John's wort safe in HIV? *Advance for Nurse Practitioners*, **9**(6), 31.

Wise, M. E., Mistry, K. and Reid, S. (2002). Drug points: neuropsychiatric complications of nevirapine treatment. *British Medical Journal*, **324**(7342), 879.

World Health Organization. (2000). *Epidemiological Fact Sheet on HIV/AIDS and Sexually Transmitted Infections*. Geneva: WHO.

Wright, J. M., Sachdev, P. S., Perkins, R. J., *et al.* (1989). Zidovudine related mania. *Medical Journal of Australia*, **150**, 339–41.

Yeung, S. M. and Gibb, D. M. (2001). Paediatric HIV infection – diagnostic and epidemiological aspects. *International Journal of STD & AIDS*, **12**(9), 549–54.

Zilikis, N., Nimatoudis, I., Klosses, V., *et al.* (1998). Treatment with risperidone of an acute psychotic episode in a patient with AIDS. *General Hospital Psychiatry*, **20**, 384–5.

Zisook, S., Peterkin, J., Goggin, K. J., *et al.* (1998). Treatment of major depression in HIV-seropositive men. *Journal of Clinical Psychology*, **59**, 217–24.

21

Renal disease

Janet Butler

Overview of renal medicine

Renal services tend to be specialist settings serving patients from a wide geographical area. The age range of patients within a service covers the entire lifespan (Phipps & Turkington 2001) and once involved with renal services, many patients will remain under care for the rest of their lives. Although this chapter concentrates on adult patients with renal disease, much will also apply to paediatric settings. Other reviews provide information relating specifically to children (Cochat *et al.* 2000; Collier & Watson 1994; Davis 1999; Fischbach *et al.* 2005). Renal disease presents at all ages and includes acute presentations, with a sudden onset of renal failure, and more gradual presentations, with renal function deteriorating slowly over time. Some patients make a full recovery from their initial renal problem but many retain a lifelong condition. Medical management in the form of medication to achieve good blood pressure control and correct various biochemical abnormalities, specific dietary advice and general lifestyle interventions can slow disease progression, but patients with chronic renal failure usually progress to end-stage renal disease. At this stage, kidney function has deteriorated such that the glomerular filtration rate is below 10 ml/min (Renal Association 2002) and the patient requires renal replacement therapy to stay alive. Such therapy is provided by renal dialysis or transplantation. Some patients in renal services have primary renal diseases (e.g. inherited polycystic kidney disease), others have a multisystem disease (e.g. autoimmune conditions like systemic lupus erythematosus) or renal problems resulting from a pre-existing condition, most commonly diabetes or hypertension. Once in end-stage renal disease, patients are at high risk of multiple comorbid medical problems, with cardiovascular disease

Handbook of Liaison Psychiatry, ed. Geoffrey Lloyd and Elspeth Guthrie. Published by Cambridge University Press. © Cambridge University Press 2007.

being a particularly major problem and the dominant cause of premature death (Phipps & Turkington 2001).

Renal replacement therapy: dialysis and transplantation

Patients receiving renal replacement therapy often form the bulk of referrals from renal medicine to a liaison psychiatry service. Such patients have to engage with complex, multifaceted medical management. There are two main forms of dialysis, haemodialysis and peritoneal dialysis. The significant demands placed upon dialysis recipients make the risk of psychiatric disorders well recognized. Patients on dialysis require multiple medications since dialysis does not correct the full range of biochemical abnormalities resulting from renal failure. They also have significant fluid and dietary restrictions to avoid fluid overload and the build up of metabolites between dialysis sessions. For a haemodialysis patient with no urine output, the daily fluid restriction is in the order of 500 ml. With peritoneal dialysis, patients can usually drink slightly more since they can remove some excess fluid each day.

Haemodialysis is an intermittent form of dialysis requiring circulation of the patient's blood through a dialysis machine. This allows diffusible exchange of metabolites and fluid and usually occurs three times a week for around four hours at a time. Patients can feel unwell during haemodialysis due to large fluid shifts in the body and they often complain of feeling very tired immediately after a dialysis session. Problems with haemodialysis arise when arterio-venous access becomes difficult, or when factors such as cardiovascular instability limit the amount of fluid that can be removed in one session.

Peritoneal dialysis is the initial form of dialysis for 30–40% patients in the UK (The Renal Association 2002). It is most commonly provided by continuous ambulatory peritoneal dialysis performed by the patient. A 2–2.5-l bag of dialysis fluid is drained in and out of the abdomen via a surgically implanted indwelling peritoneal catheter. Exchange of metabolites, electrolytes and fluid occurs across the peritoneum. Patients usually need to perform four exchanges a day, each taking around one hour. The main medical problems with peritoneal dialysis are the risk of peritonitis, due to bacteria gaining entry to the abdomen via the catheter, and eventual peritoneal failure. Patients may also be distressed by associated factors such as abdominal distension and, although they can dialyse at home, patients do not necessarily perceive their treatment to be less intrusive than those receiving haemodialysis (Schlebusch 1986; The Renal Association 2002).

Transplantation is regarded as the treatment of choice for end-stage renal disease (Royal College of Surgeons 1999) since it corrects more biochemical abnormalities and is more cost-effective than dialysis (Brickman & Yount 1996). Despite this, like those on dialysis, patients facing, or having received, a transplant remain vulnerable to psychiatric illness. They are exposed to a variety of psychological stresses including the uncertainty of a transplant waiting list, issues involved in the decision to undergo a transplant donated by a family member, fear of rejection, reduction in medical supervision compared to dialysis and the lifelong need for immunosuppressant medication and medical monitoring. Despite still requiring medical treatment, in the UK, many patients lose social security benefits following transplantation and this can be a significant financial stress if the patient is unable to work.

Renal transplants usually come from a cadaveric donor (cadaveric transplant) but may come from a living person who is currently usually a close blood relative of the recipient (live related transplant). Patients face a waiting list for transplantation since the supply of cadaveric donor organs falls far short of that required (Renal Association 2002). In the UK in 1998, the median waiting time was 500 days and 13.5% of patients waited more than five years (Royal College of Surgeons 1999), although the waiting time tends to be shorter for children (UK Transplant 2001). Furthermore, the waiting list is growing due to improved survival of patients and an ageing population with increasing acceptance of the elderly onto renal replacement programmes. This has led to recommendations to increase the rate of transplants from live donors (Renal Association 2002; Royal College of Surgeons 1999).

After transplantation, the recipient's immune system recognizes the transplant as 'foreign'. This leads to an immune response causing the graft to fail unless the response can be suppressed. To reduce the risk of rejection, immune markers on the donor organ are matched as closely as possible to those of the recipient and the recipient takes immunosuppressant medication. Contrary to much public opinion, transplants are not a cure; even with adequate immunosuppression transplants will eventually fail, although death of the patient from other reasons is becoming more common, especially in the elderly (British Transplantation Society 1998). One, five and ten years post-transplantation, 13%, 24% and at least 50% transplants respectively are likely to have failed (UK Transplant 2001). The failure rate is slightly less with transplants from live donors and is higher for third and subsequent transplants. When renal transplants were first undertaken, some psychiatric criteria were taken to be absolute contraindications to transplantation (Rodin & Abbey 1992). However, although some units still report the use of psychiatric grounds to exclude patients from the transplant waiting list (Levenson & Glocheski 1995), there are now few if any psychiatric illnesses that should preclude a patient from receiving a transplant (Freeman et al. 1992). Transplants have been reported to be successful even in those with severe psychoses and it can be argued that patients would cope better with transplantation than with the demands of dialysis (Rodin & Abbey 1992). However patients with a history of significant psychiatric illness will be more vulnerable to psychiatric side-effects of medication and they are recognized to be a high-risk group for future psychiatric problems, so they may benefit from increased psychosocial support at times of increased stress such as when dialysis commences, a transplant starts to fail or when other negative events occur in their lives.

Psychological issues facing patients with renal disease

In common with other patients suffering chronic medical conditions, patients with renal disease have to face the loss of their pre-existing health and they may also suffer other losses such as loss of their job, curtailment of leisure activities, relationship breakdown and loss of self-esteem. They also need to adapt to a lifelong relationship with health professionals and the need for lifelong complex self-care involving diet, medication and lifestyle changes. Patients with chronic renal failure and end-stage renal disease are also required to adapt to an uncertain future, awareness of their own mortality and personal experience of healthcare rationing and limitations of medical care. Given the demands of dialysis and the possibility of live-related transplants, families of patients with renal disease may become more closely involved in medical issues than the families of patients with other chronic diseases (Table 21.1).

Table 21.1. Psychological themes that can be a problem for patients due to their renal disease.

Type of psychological problem	Examples of events triggering the problem
Loss	Own health, employment, leisure, bereavement, transplant failure
Uncertainty	Timing of renal replacement therapy, waiting list for transplantation, length of transplant survival
Guilt	Hereditary disease, transplantation
Awareness of own mortality	Dependency on dialysis machine, death of other patients
Awareness of the limitations of medical care	Limited haemodialysis places, transplant waiting list
Problems accepting the medical regime	Poor adherence to diet or fluid restrictions, drug regimes or clinic and dialysis appointments
Relationship difficulties	Role changes produced by need for dialysis, live donor kidney donation

Experience of events involving loss

The multiple losses experienced by patients with end-stage renal disease (Kimmel 2001a), increase their vulnerability to grief-like adjustment reactions and depression. Denial is one defence mechanism that some patients use following such losses (Phipps & Turkington 2001). Extreme denial can cause problems for the patient's management if it leads to non-compliance with the medical regime. However denial has also been shown to relate to fewer symptoms of mood disturbance (Fricchione *et al.* 1992) and may thus be a way of allowing a gradual adjustment to illness to occur (Phipps & Turkington 2001). Non-medical aspects of life are important for patients' psychological wellbeing (Hooper 1994) so helping and encouraging patients retain activities and relationships that they had before their renal disease was diagnosed is likely to reduce their experience of loss induced by renal failure.

Employment is widely regarded as an important factor determining quality of life. However improving the number of renal patients holding a full-time or part-time job appears to be very difficult (Kaplan De-Nour 1994). Scheduling evening dialysis slots, liaison with employers and taking occupational factors into account when discussing medication, fluid and dietary regimes may all be ways to help patients with end-stage renal disease stay in employment.

Experience of uncertainty

Uncertainty, and consequent anxiety, commonly accompanies chronic physical illness, including renal disease (Maguire & Haddad 1996). Patients cannot be exactly sure of when their disease will progress such that they need renal replacement therapy; those on haemodialysis know that one day their access sites may be exhausted, those receiving peritoneal dialysis live with the risk of peritonitis; those waiting for a transplant do not know when a suitably matched organ will be found, and after transplantation patients have to stay alert to early signs of rejection and they know that one day their transplant will fail.

Awareness of own mortality

Patients receiving dialysis are uniquely dependent upon a machine or technology to stay alive (Christensen & Ehlers 2002; Schlebusch 1986) and renal disease markedly increases the mortality rate. These facts and the nature of most end-stage renal disease services involving a community of patients who frequently meet each other mean that many patients with renal disease become aware of their own mortality and will know acquaintances, friends or even family members who have a deteriorating medical course or who die prematurely as a result of their renal disease (House & Thompson 1988). This may be a particularly poignant psychological stress for transplant recipients who know the recipient of the other kidney from the same cadaveric donor, a person sometimes known as a 'transplant twin'.

Awareness of the limitations of healthcare

Patients facing dialysis may not have a completely free choice as to which modality they receive, for example in the UK the number of haemodialysis places falls short of that required to provide for all patients requiring renal replacement therapy and some units are unable to offer haemodialysis unless it is medically necessary. If this is the case, then patients are likely to have more trust in future treatment decisions if they are made aware of the limited haemodialysis places, with the resulting need for them to start peritoneal dialysis, and there is sensitive explanation of their lack of opportunity to have a free choice of treatment options. Patients awaiting transplantation have a different awareness of the limitations of medical care. They have to face the fact that although all agree that transplantation is the treatment of choice for them, they have to wait an uncertain period of time due to the shortage of donor organs. They also have to adjust to the knowledge that their treatment requires either the death of another person or the loss of a kidney from a living donor who is usually a close relative (House & Thompson 1988).

Involvement of the family in medical issues

Families of patients with renal disease can be affected by the stresses of the patient's illness and treatment (Hooper 1994; Kimmel 2001a; Salmons 1980). Stresses imposed upon relationships can affect the amount of social support available to patients. This is particularly important in the light of findings that poor social support increases the risk of psychiatric illness, especially when patients have high levels of physical morbidity (Christensen & Ehlers 2002).

With the current trends to increase live donor transplants, families may be intimately involved in the patient's treatment when transplantation is considered. The decision to donate is complex (Eggeling 1999; Rodin & Abbey 1992) and potential donors are likely to experience ambivalent feelings about donation (Eggeling 1999; Switzer *et al.* 2000). Many studies suggest that donors do not suffer significant psychological problems and often report increased feelings of wellbeing, and a closer relationship with the recipient, after donation (Rodin & Abbey 1992). However there are few long-term studies looking at the psychological impact of donation from live donors and there is evidence that, if transplant failure occurs, donors and recipients of live donor transplants are more vulnerable to significant feelings of guilt and anger. This is an area that requires further research but liaison psychiatrists should be aware of possible benefits of family assessment or interventions in relation to referrals of patients with a transplant from a relative.

Psychiatric disorders in patients with renal disease

Given the wide range of ages affected by renal disease, the multiple causes of renal disease and the multifaceted treatment options it is not surprising that the full range of psychiatric disorders are seen within renal medicine. There is some evidence that rates of psychiatric disorder are higher in patients with end-stage renal disease than in those with other chronic medical conditions (Kimmel *et al.* 1998). Depression accounts for most psychiatric referrals in a variety of countries (Hailey *et al.* 2001; House 1987; Rustomjee & Smith 1996) but adjustment disorders (Hailey *et al.* 2001; House 1989) and delirium (Fukunishi *et al.* 2001) are also common. Anxiety disorders, organic disorders, eating disorders and substance abuse also occur in relation to renal disease.

Depression

Frequency of depression

Estimates of the prevalence of depression in patients with renal disease vary widely according to the population studied (Levenson & Glocheski 1995) and the assessment tool used to identify depression, but studies tend to suggest that 12–40% patients with end-stage renal disease meet diagnostic criteria for a mood disorder (Christensen & Ehlers 2002). Instruments designed to screen for depression, or which include physical symptoms of depression, will be more likely to suggest a patient is depressed than standardized diagnostic interview or diagnostic instruments that rely more on the psychological features of depression. Depression has been reported to be less common as the duration of renal disease increases (House 1987), being more likely surrounding diagnosis of renal disease or when a patient reaches end-stage renal disease. However other studies suggest that psychiatric disorder may be a bigger problem later in the course of renal disease (Kimmel *et al.* 1998). Existing literature suggests that depression is more common in patients on dialysis compared to those with a functioning transplant (House 1987). However depression is still relatively frequent in those with a transplant. Depression has been reported to occur in 20% transplant recipients (Schlebusch *et al.* 1989) and, although there is little research on the experience of transplant failure (McCauley & Johnson 1994), patients with a failed transplant may have a particularly high risk of psychological problems (McCauley & Johnson 1994).

It is essential that depression is identified since effective treatments exist and it is an important factor relating to quality of life (Cagney *et al.* 2000). There are conflicting reports regarding the impact of depression on mortality in end-stage renal disease (Kimmel 2001b; Kimmel *et al.* 2000), but some have found that depression increases the risk of death by the same magnitude as medical risk factors (Kimmel *et al.* 2000). Furthermore, although the decision to withdraw dialysis is often agreed to be the best option by the patient, their family and staff (Phipps & Turkington 2001), in some cases depression has been suggested to influence patient decisions (Christensen & Ehlers 2002).

Causes and diagnosis of depression

There are many causes for depression in patients with renal disease (Table 21.2). A history of depressive illness predating renal disease is a key risk factor (Sensky 1997). An organic mood disorder can be the result of an underlying autoimmune disease or the secondary hyperparathyroidism that is commonly found in end-stage renal disease. Furthermore many drugs taken by patients, particularly corticosteroids, can cause depression. Adverse life events, particularly those involving loss, are well-established risk factors for depressive illness. Patients with renal disease experience multiple losses throughout the course of their illness. Transplant failure is one such loss and, although levels of psychiatric illness are reported to be lower in transplant populations than those on dialysis (Christensen *et al.* 1991a; House 1987; Petrie 1989), there is evidence that patients with a failed transplant have particularly high levels of depression. Depressive symptoms have also been found in patients who have an unrealistically high expectation of life post-transplantation (Dubovsky & Penn 1980). This is particularly important in the light of suggestions that the benefits of transplantation may, at times, be overstated when the option of transplantation is discussed with patients (McCauley & Johnson 1994). However losses do not inevitably produce depression and, as with other physical illnesses, depression is often more closely associated with patients' beliefs about their disease rather than an objective measure of disease severity (Sacks *et al.* 1990). Different styles of thinking and behaving in response to stresses, such as whether patients believe that they have a

Table 21.2. Causes and risk factors for depression in patients with renal disease.

Past history of depression
Medication
Organic mood disorder
Life events involving 'loss'

Table 21.3. Medical conditions to distinguish from depression in patients with renal disease.

Drug side-effects
Uraemia
Electrolyte imbalances
Systemic disease

lot of control over their illness, have been related to the risk of depression although such beliefs interact with the medical experience. For example, Christensen and colleagues (1991b) found that patients on haemodialysis who believed that they had control over their health were less likely to be depressed if they had not previously had a failed transplant but they were more likely to be depressed following transplant failure.

As with other medical conditions, the diagnosis of depression can be more difficult in patients with renal disease (Table 21.3; Christensen & Ehlers 2002). Uraemia and electrolyte imbalances resulting from renal impairment produce fatigue, loss of appetite, weight loss, poor concentration, reduced libido and sleep disturbance, and immunosuppressant drugs taken by transplant recipients are associated with fatigue. Thus, as with other medical conditions, diagnosis of depression in patients with renal disease should rely more heavily on the psychological features such as anhedonia, guilt, loss of self-esteem, hopelessness and suicidal ideation (Craven *et al.* 1987). However assessment tools that include physical symptoms as indicators of depression, such as the Beck Depression Inventory could be useful to indicate patients who may be suffering from a depressive illness (Craven *et al.* 1988).

Adjustment disorders

Patients with renal disease have to adjust to many psychological issues and life events, all of these can produce an adjustment disorder. Levy (1977) described a specific adjustment reaction commonly seen in patients commencing renal replacement therapy. The process starts with a 'honeymoon phase' and progresses through 'discouragement and disenchantment' to long-term adaptation. Although common, adjustment disorders should not be ignored and dismissed as understandable reactions since they can cause considerable distress, progress to a clear depressive illness or anxiety disorder, and have been shown to persist (House 1989). Although adjustment reactions may be expected after increased physical morbidity, they can also occur following successful transplantation (Rodin & Abbey 1992). When detected, adjustment disorders should prompt exploration of the patient's perception of current stresses. For example, following transplantation, patients may find it difficult to adjust to the lesser degree of medical involvement (Schlebusch *et al.* 1989), they may miss the previous social contacts they developed in the dialysis unit or they may become particularly distressed at the physical changes produced by immunosuppressants or by the ongoing experience of fatigue.

Organic disorders

There are many potential causes of cerebral dysfunction in renal disease. Delirium is the commonest organic disorder (Fukunishi *et al.* 2001) and, although due to medical causes, it may be mistaken for a primary psychiatric illness and lead to a request for an urgent psychiatric opinion if behavioural disturbance is prominent and organic causes have not been considered. The rapid onset of confusion, disorientation and behavioural change should suggest the possibility of delirium particularly if there is a fluctuating clinical course, cardiovascular instability, visual hallucinations, pyrexia or the patient has recently had surgery, has presented in acute renal failure or is prescribed medication commonly associated with delirium.

Many systemic diseases affecting the kidney also affect the brain and so may produce an organic psychiatric disorder. Systemic vascular disease is common in patients with end-stage renal disease and there is an increased risk of cerebrovascular disease. The anticoagulation required for dialysis places patients at risk of cerebral haemorrhage, particularly if they have abnormal cerebral vasculature such as with a vasculitis or with a cerebral aneurysm associated with polycystic kidney disease. Systemic inflammatory diseases can cause organic mood disorders and organic psychoses. Systemic lupus erythematosus is associated with both renal and cerebral vasculitis and may result in an organic psychosis or behavioural changes. Such patients are also usually immunosuppressed due to medication to treat their primary disorder and so they are vulnerable to infections that result in delirium. In such cases a common diagnostic dilemma, that may result in referral to liaison psychiatry services, is whether psychiatric symptoms are due to the systemic disease or secondary infection. This can be difficult to differentiate.

Many drugs prescribed for renal disease are known to cause organic disorders (House & Thompson 1988). Steroid-induced psychoses used to be particularly common post-transplantation but are now only seen infrequently due to the use of lower doses of steroids in conjunction with other immunosuppressant medications (Rodin & Abbey 1992). However mood disorders and less commonly psychosis due to steroids still present in transplant and other patients receiving steroids, and neuropsychiatric complications are a rare, but well-recognized, side-effect of cyclosporin (House & Thompson 1988). Although steroids are typically thought to be associated with euphoria, depressive reactions are more common. Past psychiatric history increases the risk of drug-induced mood changes and so patients with a history of depression should be carefully monitored after prescription of steroids. Such drugs should be used with caution in patients with a history of bipolar affective disorder.

Anxiety disorders

Cross-sectional studies do not suggest that anxiety disorders are particularly common in renal populations. However some patients may experience anxiety symptoms related to their renal disease. A few patients develop a phobic response to needles which causes problems on a dialysis unit (Salmons 1980). Other patients, particularly if their renal failure has come on acutely, may have intense anxiety and even panic attacks when confronted with the need to attend the dialysis unit (Salmons 1980). Given the fact that about 40% patients starting renal replacement therapy are referred as emergencies without time to be counselled about treatment or introduced to the dialysis unit (Renal Association 2002), anxiety disorders may be more common than currently reported. Generalized anxiety states may present somatically with headaches or nausea which, like the somatic symptoms of depression, can cause diagnostic difficulty. Anxiety about the risk of transplant failure is extremely common immediately post-transplantation (Schlebusch *et al.* 1989). This usually diminishes with time but studies show that many patients retain significant fear of rejection. Fear of transplant failure or immunosuppression leading to disabling anxiety requires intervention. For example, patients may be severely curtailing their social activities due to fear of catching an infection or directly damaging their transplant. Patients with end-stage renal disease face many procedures and medications that produce physical changes to their body, such as facial swelling and hirsutism due to prednisolone and ciclosporin. This can result in anxieties related to body image and lowering of self-esteem.

Treatments for psychiatric illness in patients with renal disease

General issues

As with many patients referred to psychological services from a medical setting, the first issue needs to be an active engagement of the patient who may well be reluctant to attend (Bass 2000). The referral may be easier for the patient to accept if the liaison psychiatrist is an established member of the renal team and sees patients in the renal unit. However, even if this is not possible, it is good practice to establish the patient's expectations and fears relating to the referral and to explain the role of liaison psychiatry. A discussion of problems relating to the physical illness and the impact of the illness on the patient's life is a recommended starting point for many assessments in medical settings (e.g. Bass 2000). Patients may require persuasion to accept treatment for a psychological condition (Wuerth *et al.* 2001).

Pharmacological therapy

As in other medical conditions, drug interactions and side-effects need particular consideration when considering drug therapy for psychiatric illness in patients with renal disease. However, unlike many other conditions, if there is renal impairment it is also essential to consider pharmacokinetics and electrolyte imbalances carefully. Expert pharmacological advice should be sought when prescribing in renal disease (Table 21.4), but general guidelines are published, for example, in the *Maudsley Hospital Prescribing Guidelines* (Taylor *et al.* 2001), which are updated regularly. The *British National Formulary*, updated biannually, includes an appendix related to prescribing to patients with renal impairment. Many hospital pharmacies run drug information services that could provide further advice and a specialist renal pharmacy drug information service exists in Bristol. However, although drugs need to be used with particular care in renal disease, psychotropic medication should not be withheld since patients will still respond to appropriately prescribed medication. There are few large controlled trials of psychotropic prescribing in renal disease. However there is evidence of clinical benefits from antidepressants in depressed patients receiving dialysis (Kennedy *et al.* 1989; Wuerth *et al.* 2001) and a systematic review of patients with a variety of physical illnesses concluded that antidepressants are an effective treatment for depression (Gill & Hatcher 2002).

Many drugs or their active metabolites are renally excreted and so their half-life will be prolonged by renal impairment and dangerously toxic levels may arise if dose adjustments are not made. In general drugs should be prescribed in reduced doses or at less frequent intervals and an increase in dose should be titrated against

Table 21.4. Sources of advice relating to prescribing psychotropics in renal disease.

Local hospital drug information service

Specialist renal drug information service in Bristol (tel: 0117 9282 867)

Specialist psychiatric drug information service in the Maudsley Hospital, London
(tel: 0207 919 2317)

Current *British National Formulary*

Current Maudsley Hospital Prescribing Guidelines

clinical effect and tolerability (Taylor *et al.* 2001). Prescribing drugs that have a short half-life will minimize the duration of adverse effects should they occur. Drugs that are primarily renally excreted should be avoided. Many psychotropics are lipid soluble and highly protein bound so would not be expected to be significantly cleared by dialysis. However some drugs are not plasma bound and therefore accumulate between dialysis sessions with rapid reduction in drug levels occurring after dialysis. Such drugs should be taken after dialysis sessions. Drug side-effects, particularly postural hypotension, sedation and confusion, are thought to be more common in patients with renal failure (Taylor *et al.* 2001) and are thus another reason to initiate drugs at low doses if renal impairment is present (Table 21.5).

Nephrotoxic drugs should be avoided if possible and, if required, their use requires close monitoring of renal function and plasma drug levels. Most renal patients receive antihypertensive medication and many have significant cardiac disease so drugs with cardiac side-effects should be prescribed with care. Many patients on dialysis suffer significant constipation so drugs with anticholinergic side-effects should be avoided. Renal transplant survival is highly dependent upon adequate immunosuppression and so all drugs prescribed to transplant recipients should be checked for possible interactions with the immunosuppressants prescribed for that patient.

Metabolites of tricyclic antidepressants are renally excreted and so accumulate in renal impairment (Taylor *et al.* 2001). Thus patients are more vulnerable to toxic levels and dose-related side-effects. Plasma levels may be useful if there are concerns about dose increments. There are variable reports concerning the effect of renal failure on levels of selective serotonin reuptake inhibitors (Taylor *et al.* 2001), but many manufacturers advise that the drug be commenced at a low dose. Amisulpride and sulpiride are excreted renally and chlorpromazine has pronounced sedative and anticholinergic properties and many active metabolites; these antipsychotics are probably best avoided if possible when the patient has significant renal impairment (Taylor *et al.* 2001). Clozapine is contraindicated

Table 21.5. General rules for prescribing in renal disease.

Seek expert advice if not familiar with prescribing for the renal condition
Check for interactions with the other drugs that the patient is prescribed
Avoid nephrotoxic drugs
Use drugs with a short half-life
Start with low or reduced doses
Monitor the patient closely for side-effects and signs of toxicity
Titrate the dose against efficacy and tolerability

in severe renal disease and low doses and slow dose titration are needed if the drug is prescribed to a patient with mild-to-moderate renal impairment (*British National Formulary* 2002). Lithium is nephrotoxic and renally excreted so is contraindicated by the manufacturer in renal insufficiency. However there are reports of its use in renal disease when it is carefully monitored and used in lower doses (Phipps & Turkington 2001). There is little data concerning carbamazepine and sodium valproate as mood stabilizers in patients with renal impairment but serum levels are easily monitored.

Immunosuppressive regimes following renal transplantation are constantly being developed and patients may be involved in drug trials of new immunosuppressive agents. The risk of dangerous drug interactions with existing and new immunosuppressants is high and advice about psychotropic prescribing to this population should always be sought. Clinicians should also question patients about their use of herbal and 'alternative' medicines following the well-publicised reports of transplant loss in heart transplant recipients due to reduction in immunosuppressant levels with the use of St John's Wort. Benzodiazepines should be used with caution in renal disease to avoid oversedation since many such drugs have significantly prolonged half-lives with renal impairment (Phipps & Turkington 2001).

Psychosocial interventions

In view of the problems associated with prescribing in renal disease, non-pharmacological approaches should always be considered for patients with real impairment. There are few studies of psychosocial interventions in renal populations but those that are published have shown treatment efficacy (Friend *et al.* 1986; Hener *et al.* 1996; Koudi *et al.* 1997) and there is no reason to believe that interventions benefiting other patients should not be effective in those with renal disease (Sensky 1997).

Cognitive behavioural therapy is well established as an effective treatment for mild to moderate depressive disorders, panic attacks and phobic disorders. Treatment techniques are well described in a variety of books (e.g. Hawton *et al.* 1989; Wells 1997) and should be no different to those used for patients without renal disease, but practicalities such as timing of dialysis session and physical problems such as fatigue or infections may need to be taken into account and it may be important to address beliefs that are specific to the renal disease (Horne & Weinman 1994). Patients attending hospital dialysis or with a recent transplant already spend a large proportion of their time travelling to, and waiting in, hospital so they may attend therapy more easily if this can be co-ordinated with other hospital appointments. Although not psychiatric illnesses, other problems, such as non-adherence and family disturbance seen in patients with renal disease have been shown to relate to belief patterns (Horne & Weinman 1994), and may therefore be amenable to cognitive-behavioural techniques targeted to the salient maladaptive beliefs. However efficacy of treatments for these problems has not yet been widely researched or demonstrated.

Phobic disorders should also respond to psychological treatments shown to be effective in patients without renal disease. A needle phobia should respond to behavioural approaches based on systematic desensitization. The need for the patient to undergo dialysis may require the liaison psychiatrist to facilitate the start of psychological treatment more rapidly than occurs in general psychiatric settings. Social anxiety related to medication-induced bodily and facial changes may respond to cognitive-behavioural approaches used to treat social anxiety. The bodily changes from medication, surgery and dialysis access sites may elicit psychological distress that is more akin to that seen in disfigurement from a variety of causes including skin conditions, burns and trauma. In these cases the focus of treatment may need to be related more to dealing with body shame (Gilbert 2002) than social anxiety, although cognitive-behavioural approaches are still suggested to be useful (Kent & Thompson 2002).

Other problems referred to liaison psychiatrists

Non-adherence

Patients receiving dialysis are asked to stick to strict dietary and fluid restrictions and attend regular dialysis sessions. Failure to do this puts the patient's life at risk. However poor adherence to these behavioural requirements of dialysis is common (Horne *et al.* 2001; Kutner *et al.* 2002). Non-adherence to medication is common in dialysis (Curtin *et al.* 1999; Horne *et al.* 2001) and transplant recipients (Butler *et al.* 2004) and non-adherence to immunosuppressants is a major cause of transplant failure (Butler *et al.* 2004). Patients needing emergency dialysis due to biochemical problems or fluid overload resulting from dietary non-adherence can result in significant frustration among dialysis unit staff. Patients who have lesser degrees of apparent non-adherence may also be difficult for staff to understand and, if they have drunk too much, they will suffer unpleasant symptoms such as extreme breathlessness. Transplant failure due to non-adherence is seen as an avoidable cause of transplant loss and thus has significant avoidable financial and psychological costs to the health service and patient as well as placing a strain on scarce donor organs. The problems resulting from non-adherence can lead patients suspected of being, or proven to be, non-adherent being referred to liaison psychiatrists.

Discussion of non-adherence is likely to be easier if a non-judgemental, collaborative approach can be demonstrated to the patient (De Geest *et al.* 1995). For some patients an underlying psychiatric illness, particularly depression, may contribute to non-adherence (Kiley *et al.* 1993). Clearly, if present, a depressive illness should be treated appropriately. However for many patients with problems adhering to treatment, no such illness will be detected. Concerns about actual (Pruna & Fornairon 2000) or potential (Horne *et al.* 2001) side-effects of medication are widely thought to contribute to non-adherence. Some concerns may be amenable to modification, for example phobic anxiety resulting from the commonly experienced distress due to facial changes induced by immunosuppressant medication. Other concerns, such as the increased risk of malignancy with immunosuppression, may be better addressed by helping the patient weigh up the pros and cons of treatment and consider a plan of action should their feared outcome occur. Patients most commonly cite forgetting as the main reason for non-adherence (Kory 1999) and in such cases, simple behavioural measures to aid memory, such as pairing medication taking with daily activities or leaving prominent reminders, are likely to be beneficial (Butler & Cairns 2000). However there is increasing evidence that specific beliefs held by the individual and related to the illness and its treatment underlie non-adherence for some patients (Horne & Weinman 1994). As experts in eliciting and modifying individual's thoughts and feelings, psychiatric staff are ideally placed to identify reasons for non-adherence. Much more research is needed to identify key beliefs and develop effective interventions, but beliefs about the need for medication and concerns with the medication appear particularly relevant (Horne *et al.* 2001; Greenstein & Siegal 2000; Siegal & Greenstein 1997)

Problems transferring adolescents to adult services

As with other chronic diseases occurring in childhood, many adolescents with renal disease find the transition to adult clinics stressful. Non-adherence is reported to be particularly common at this time as are concerns about physical side-effects of medication and impingement of treatment regimes on daily life (Griffin & Elkin 2001). Paediatric clinics generally have a higher staff-to-patient ratio and have often been involved with the child's family and school. To help adolescents transfer smoothly to adult services some renal units have set up a 'transition clinic' run by staff with a particular interest in this group of patients. However, whatever sort of clinic the adolescent is to be transferred to, it is generally thought helpful for the young person to have the opportunity to look around the new unit and to meet staff and sometimes patients in the new setting prior to a full transfer (Cochat *et al.* 2000). The age of transfer varies in different units and should be partly determined by the patient's maturity and wishes (Collier & Watson 1994).

REFERENCES

Bass, C. (2000). Liaison psychiatry in the pain clinic. In *Liaison Psychiatry: Planning Services For Specialist Settings*, ed. R. Peveler, E. Feldman and T. Friedman. London: The Royal College of Psychiatrists, pp. 92–109.

Brickman, A. L. and Yount, S. E. (1996). Non-compliance in end-stage renal disease: a threat to quality of care and cost containment. *Journal of Clinical Psychology in Medical Settings*, **3**, 399–412.

British National Formulary. (2002). *British National Formulary.* British Medical Association and Royal Pharmaceutical Society of Great Britain.

British Transplantation Society. (1998). *Towards Standards for Organ and Tissue Transplantation in the United Kingdom.* British Transplantation Society.

Butler, J. A. and Cairns, H. (2000). Non-adherence in renal transplant recipients. *British Journal of Renal Medicine*, Summer, 21–4.

Butler, J. A., Roderick, P., Mullee, M., *et al.* (2004). Frequency and impact of nonadherence to immunosuppressants after renal transplantation: a systematic review. *Transplantation*, **77**(5), 769–76.

Cagney, K. A., Wu, A. W., Fink, N. E., *et al.* (2000). Formal literature review of quality of life instruments used in end-stage renal disease. *American Journal of Kidney Diseases*, **36**, 327–36.

Christensen, A. J. and Ehlers, S. L. (2002). Psychological factors in end-stage renal disease: an emerging context for behavioural medicine research. *Journal of Consulting and Clinical Psychology*, **70**, 712–24.

Christensen, A. J., Holman, J. M., Turner, C. W., *et al.* (1991a). A prospective examination of quality of life in end-stage renal disease. *Clinical Transplantation*, **5**, 46–53.

Christensen, A. J., Turner, C. W., Smith, T. W., *et al.* (1991b). Health locus of control and depression in end-stage renal disease. *Journal of Consulting and Clinical Psychology*, **59**, 419–24.

Cochat, P., De Geest, S. and Ritz, E. (2000). Drug holiday: a challenging child-adult interface in kidney transplantation. *Nephrology Dialysis and Transplantation*, **15**, 1924–7.

Collier, J. and Watson, A. R. (1994). Renal failure in children: specific considerations in management. In *Quality of Life Following Renal Failure*, ed. H. McGee and C. Bradley. Amsterdam: Harwood Academic Publishers, pp. 225–45.

Craven, J. L., Rodin, G. M. and Johnson, L. (1987). The diagnosis of major depression in renal dialysis patients. *Psychosomatic Medicine*, **49**, 482–92.

Craven, J. L., Rodin, G. M. and Littlefield, C. H. (1988). The Beck Depression Inventory as a screening device for major depression in renal dialysis patients. *International Journal of Psychiatry in Medicine*, **18**, 373–82.

Curtin, R. B., Svarstad, B. L. and Keller, T. H. (1999). Hemodialysis patients' noncompliance with oral medications. *ANNA Journal*, **26**, 307–16.

Davis, I. D. (1999). Pediatric renal transplantation: back to school issues. *Transplantation Proceedings*, **31**, 61S–2.

De Geest, S., Borgermans, L., Gemoets, H., *et al.* (1995). Incidence, determinants, and consequences of subclinical noncompliance with immunosuppressive therapy in renal transplant recipients. *Transplantation*, **59**, 340–7.

Dubovsky, S. L. and Penn, I. (1980). Psychiatric considerations in renal transplant surgery. *Psychosomatics*, **21**, 481–91.

Eggeling, C. (1999). Psychosocial consequences of transplantation for the counsellor and the donor. *British Journal of Renal Medicine*, Summer, 21–4.

Fischbach, M., Edefonti, A., Schroder, C., *et al.* (2005). The European Pediatric Dialysis Working Group. Hemodialysis in children: general practical guidelines. *Pediatric Nephrology*, **20**, 1054–66.

Freeman, A., Davis, L., Libb, J. W., *et al.* (1992). Assessment of transplant candidates and prediction of outcome. In *Psychiatric Aspects of Organ Transplantation*, ed. J. Craven and G. Rodin. Oxford: Oxford University Press, pp. 9–21.

Fricchione, G., Howanitz, E., Jandorf, L., *et al.* (1992). Psychological adjustment to end-stage renal disease and the implications of denial. *Psychosomatics*, **33**, 85–91.

Friend, R., Singletary, Y., Mendell, N. R., *et al.* (1986). Group participation and survival among patients with end-stage renal disease. *American Journal of Public Health*, **76**, 670–2.

Fukunishi, I., Kitaoka, T., Shirai, T., *et al.* (2001). Psychiatric disorders among patients undergoing haemodialysis therapy. *Nephron*, **91**, 344–7.

Gilbert, P. (2002). Body shame: a biopsychosocial conceptualisation and overview, with treatment implications. In *Body Shame*, ed. P. Gilbert and J. Miles. Hove, East Sussex: Brunner-Routledge, pp. 3–54.

Gill, D. and Hatcher, S. (2002). Antidepressants for depression in medical illness (Cochrane Review). In *The Cochrane Library*. Oxford: Update Software.

Greenstein, S. and Siegal, B. (2000). Evaluation of a multivariate model predicting non-compliance with medication regimens among renal transplant patients. *Transplantation*, **69**, 2226–8.

Griffin, K. J. and Elkin, T. D. (2001). Non-adherence in paediatric transplantation: a review of the existing literature. *Pediatric Transplantation*, **5**, 246–9.

Hailey, B. J., Moss, S. B., Street, R., *et al.* (2001). Mental health services in an outpatient dialysis practice. *Dialysis and Transplantation*, **30**, 732–9.

Hawton, K., Salkovskis, P., Kirk, J., *et al.* (1989). *Cognitive Behaviour Therapy for Psychiatric Problems: a Practical Guide*. Oxford: Oxford University Press.

Hener, T., Weisenberg, M. and Har-Evan, D. (1996). Supportive versus cognitive-behavioural programs in achieving adjustment to home peritoneal kidney dialysis. *Journal of Consulting and Clinical Psychology*, **64**, 731–41.

Hooper, J. (1994). Psychological care of patients in the renal unit. In *Quality of Life Following Renal Failure*, ed. H. McGee and C. Bradley. Amsterdam: Harwood Academic Publishers, pp. 181–209.

Horne, R. and Weinman, J. (1994). Illness cognitions: implications for the treatment of renal disease. In *Quality of Life Following Renal Failure*, ed. H. McGee and C. Bradley. Amsterdam: Harwood Academic Publishers, pp. 113–32.

Horne, R., Sumner, S., Jubraj, B., *et al.* (2001). Haemodialysis patients' beliefs about treatment: implications for adherence to medication and fluid/diet restrictions. *International Journal of Pharmacy Practice*, **9**, 169–75.

House, A. (1987). Psychosocial problems of patients on the renal unit and their relation to treatment outcome. *Journal of Psychosomatic Research*, **31**, 441–52.

House, A. (1989). Psychiatric referrals from a renal unit: a study of clinical practice in a British hospital. *Journal of Psychosomatic Research*, **33**, 363–72.

House, R. M. and Thompson, T. L. (1988). Psychiatric aspects of organ transplantation. *Journal of the American Medical Association*, **260**, 535–9.

Kaplan De-Nour, A. (1994). Psychological, social and vocational impact of renal failure: a review. In *Quality of Life Following Renal Failure*, ed. H. McGee and C. Bradley. Amsterdam: Harwood Academic Publishers, pp. 33–42.

Kennedy, S. H., Craven, H. and Roin, G. M. (1989). Major depression in renal dialysis patients: an open trial of antidepressant therapy. *Journal of Clinical Psychiatry*, **50**, 60–3.

Kent, G. and Thompson, A. R. (2002). The development and maintenance of shame in disfigurement: implications for treatment. In *Body Shame*, ed. P. Gilbert and J. Miles. Hove, East Sussex: Brunner-Routledge, pp. 103–16.

Kiley, D. J., Lam, C. S. and Pollak, R. (1993). A study of treatment compliance following kidney transplantation. *Transplantation*, **55**, 51–6.

Kimmel, P. L. (2001a). Psychosocial factors in dialysis patients. *Kidney International*, **59**, 1599–613.

Kimmel, P. L. (2001b). Psychosocial factors in adult end-stage renal disease patients treated with haemodialysis: correlates and outcomes. *American Journal of Kidney Diseases*, **53**, S132–40.

Kimmel, P. L., Thamer, M., Richard, C. M., *et al.* (1998). Psychiatric illness in patients with end-stage renal disease. *American Journal of Medicine*, **105**, 214–21.

Kimmel, P. L., Peterson, R. A., Weihs, K. L., *et al.* (2000). Multiple measures of depression predict mortality in a longitudinal study of chronic haemodialysis outpatients. *Kidney International*, **57**, 2093–8.

Kory, L. (1999). Nonadherence to immunosuppressive medications: a pilot survey of members of the transplant recipients international organization. *Transplantation Proceedings*, **31**, S14–15.

Koudi, E., Iacovides, A., Iordanidis, P., *et al.* (1997). Exercise renal rehabilitation programme. *Nephron*, **77**, 152–8.

Kutner, N. G., Zhang, R., McClellan, W. M., *et al.* (2002). Psychosocial predictors of non-compliance in haemodialysis and peritoneal dialysis patients. *Nephrology Dialysis and Transplantation*, **17**, 93–9.

Levenson, J. L. and Glocheski, S. (1995). End-stage renal disease. In *Psychological Factors Affecting Medical Conditions*, ed. A. Stoudemire. American Psychiatric Publishing, pp. 159–72.

Levy, N. B. (1977). Psychological studies of the Downstate Medical Centre of patients on haemodialysis. *Medical Clinics of North America*, **61**, 759–69.

Maguire, P. and Haddad, P. (1996). Psychological reactions to physical illness. In *Seminars in Liaison Psychiatry*, ed. E. Guthrie and F. Creed. Londan: Royal College of Psychiatrists, pp. 157–91.

McCauley, C. and Johnson, J. P. (1994). Transplant failure: psychosocial consequences and their management. In *Quality of Life Following Renal Failure*. ed. H. McGee and C. Bradley. Amsterdam: Harwood Academic Publishers, pp. 211–24.

Petrie, K. (1989). Psychological well-being and psychiatric disturbance in dialysis and renal transplant patients. *British Journal of Medical Psychology*, **62**, 91–6.

Phipps, A. and Turkington, D. (2001). Psychiatry in the renal unit. *Advances in Psychiatric Treatment*, **7**, 426–32.

Pruna, A. and Fornairon, S. (2000). European multicenter survey on noncompliance after solid organ transplantation. *Transplantation Proceedings*, **32**, 393–5.

Rodin, G. M. and Abbey, S. (1992). Kidney transplantation. In *Psychiatric Aspects of Organ Transplantation*, ed. J. L. Craven and G. M. Rodin. Oxford: Oxford University Press, pp. 145–63.

Rustomjee, S. and Smith, G. (1996). Consultation-liaison psychiatry to renal medicine: work with an in-patient unit. *Australian and New Zealand Journal of Psychiatry*, **30**, 229–37.

Sacks, C. R., Peterson, R. A. and Kimmel, P. L. (1990). Perceptions of illness and depression in chronic renal disease. *American Journal of Kidney Disease*, **15**, 31–9.

Salmons, P. H. (1980). Psychosocial aspects of chronic renal failure. *British Journal of Hospital Medicine*, **23**, 617–21.

Schlebusch, L. (1986). Medical psychology and psychonephrology: contributions of clinical psychology. *South African Journal of Psychology*, **16**, 47–56.

Schlebusch, L., Pillay, B. J. and Louw, J. (1989). Depression and self-report disclosure after live related donor and cadaver renal transplants. *South African Medical Journal*, **75**, 490–3.

Sensky, T. (1997). Depression in renal failure and its treatment. In *Depression and Physical Illness*, ed. M. M. Robertson and C. L. E. Katona. Chichester: John Wiley & Sons, pp. 359–75.

Siegal, B. R. and Greenstein, S. M. (1997). Postrenal transplant compliance from the perspective of African-Americans, Hispanic-Americans, and Anglo-Americans. *Advances in Renal Replacement Therapy*, **4**, 46–54.

Switzer, G. E., Dew, M. A. and Twillman, R. K. (2000). Psychosocial issues in living organ donation. In *The Transplant Patient: Biological, Psychiatric and Ethical Issues in Organ Transplantation*, ed. P. T. Trzepacz and A. F. DiMartini. Cambridge: Cambridge University Press, pp. 42–66.

Taylor, D., McConnell, H., McConnell, D., *et al.* (2001). *The Maudsley Prescribing Guidelines*. London: Martin Dunitz Ltd.

The Renal Association. (2002). *Treatment of Adults and Children with Renal Failure: Standards and Audit Measures*. London: Royal College of Physicians.

The Royal College of Surgeons. (1999). *The Report of the Working Party to Review Organ Transplantation.* London: The Royal College of Surgeons of England.

UK Transplant. (2001). *Renal Transplant Audit 1990–1998.* Bristol: UK Transplant.

Wells, A. (1997). *Cognitive Therapy of Anxiety Disorders: a Practice Manual and Conceptual Guide.* Chichester: John Wiley & Sons.

Wuerth, D., Finkelstein, S. H., Ciarcia, J., *et al.* (2001). Identification and treatment of depression in a cohort of patients maintained on chronic peritoneal dialysis. *American Journal of Kidney Diseases,* **37**, 1011–17.

22

Musculo-skeletal disorders

Chris Dickens and Graham Ash

Introduction

The term musculo-skeletal disorders describes a broad range of problems, with varying aetiologies and different natural histories, that are seen and treated in diverse treatment settings. These disorders have in common symptoms (with or without signs) in the muscles, skeleton or connective tissues, with associated functional disability.

It is beyond the scope of this chapter to describe all of the individual musculo-skeletal disorders along with their accompanying psychological/psychiatric features. Instead we have selected the four conditions that best represent the conditions within this group: rheumatoid arthritis, fibromyalgia, osteoarthritis and back pain. By discussing the features of these disorders we have covered the most common, and the most widely studied of the musculo-skeletal disorders.

Rheumatoid arthritis

Rheumatoid arthritis (RA) is a chronic inflammatory disorder of unknown aetiology affecting approximately 0.8% of the population, with women being affected three times more often than men. The brunt of this disorder falls on articular and periarticular tissues, resulting in a peripheral symmetrical inflammatory arthropathy. Destruction of joint cartilage and bony erosions can occur, which eventually lead to destruction of the joint. Some degree of extra-articular involvement is found in most sufferers. These extra-articular manifestations vary widely between subjects but may include systemic symptoms (anorexia, weight loss, myalgia), more localized abnormalities such as rheumatoid nodules, or involvement of the cardiovascular system (vasculitis, pericarditis), respiratory

Handbook of Liaison Psychiatry, ed. Geoffrey Lloyd and Elspeth Guthrie. Published by Cambridge University Press. © Cambridge University Press 2007.

system (pleural effusions, pulmonary fibrosis), or central nervous system (spinal cord compression, peripheral neuropathy).

Onset, most commonly in the third and fourth decades, is insidious in the majority of cases. The course of the illness is typically prolonged and characterized by relapses and remissions. As the disease advances progressive joint destruction results in limitations to joint movements, joint instability and deformities which result in increasing pain and functional disability.

Prevalence of psychiatric disorders

Psychiatric disorders are common in sufferers of rheumatoid arthritis. Prevalence figures vary widely in the published literature, though more conservative prevalence figures, obtained using standardized research interviews, indicate that about one-fifth of sufferers of RA have a psychiatric disorder. Creed *et al.* interviewed a mixed group of inpatients and outpatients with definite or classical rheumatoid arthritis using the Present State Examination and found that 21% of subjects had a psychiatric disorder: 12.5% of the group were found to be depressed and the remainder were anxious (Creed *et al.* 1990). This study also revealed that a population of RA sufferers of approximately equal size (19%) had psychiatric symptoms but did not meet criteria for psychiatric caseness.

Interestingly the prevalence of depression does not appear to vary according to gender in rheumatoid arthritis, with men and women being equally at risk (Fifield *et al.* 1996). This similarity in prevalence of depression in men and women with rheumatoid arthritis contrasts with the excess of depression in women seen in other chronic illness populations or in the general population at large (Creed *et al.* 2002; Melter *et al.* 1995). Reasons for this difference between RA and other chronic illnesses are not clear and further research is required in this area.

Aetiological factors in the development of psychiatric disorders in RA

Pain and depression

Depression may arise, in part, as a reaction to the experience of chronic pain. Cross-sectional studies have shown that depression is worse in people experiencing most pain (Dickens *et al.* 2002), though it is unclear whether depression is a reaction to the pain (Romano & Turner 1985), or whether depression contributes to the pain experience (Blumer & Heilbronn 1982). The majority of studies in this area have been cross-sectional in design, allowing no causal inferences to be drawn.

Disability and depression

Depression may be due to increasing disability. Prospective studies have shown that depression occurs following deterioration in functional ability, particularly with regards to activities that an individual regards as being important, e.g. visiting the family, going away on holiday. A 10% reduction in ability to perform these valued activities is followed by a sevenfold increase in depression over the subsequent year (Katz & Yelin 1995).

The mechanisms by which pain and disability may lead to depression are unclear. Though pain and disability are potent stressors and may increase the likelihood of depression, there is evidence to indicate that the pain and disability of rheumatoid arthritis are not sufficient in themselves to cause depression, except in the most advanced disease (Mindham *et al.* 1981). Factors such as social stresses and social isolation may be required for depression to develop in less severe RA.

The role of social stress

Social stresses have been shown to be associated with depression in RA as they have in the general population (Creed 1990; Kraaimaat *et al.* 1995; Murphy *et al.* 1988). Particularly important in causing depression are those stresses in which the degree of threat to the individual is great (Brown & Harris 1978). Dickens *et al.* found that marked social difficulties were more important than RA disease activity in predicting depression in ambulant patients, with both RA-related social difficulties and those independent of RA (e.g. caring for a sick relative, financial problems not related to RA) being required to cause depression (Dickens *et al.* 2003).

The role of social support

A number of studies have demonstrated that social support benefits patients with RA (Goodenow *et al.* 1990). In patients with RA, social support, and its actual or perceived availability, has been shown to be associated with better coping (Manne & Zautra 1989), increased perceptions of control of RA (Spitzer *et al.* 1995), and less psychological distress (Evers *et al.* 1997; Revenson *et al.* 1991). Not all social contacts are supportive, however, and critical or punishing comments are associated with increased psychological distress (Kraaimaat *et al.* 1995; Revenson *et al.* 1991).

Neuroticism

The importance of neuroticism has been confirmed in patients with rheumatoid arthritis. In a prospective study, patients with RA completed daily reports on joint pain and mood for a period of 75 days. Patients scoring higher on neuroticism experienced more chronic distress, regardless of the intensity of their pain (Affleck *et al.* 1992).

Neuropsychiatric problems in RA can also arise as the result of direct central nervous system (CNS) involvement. This is rare, however, and when it does occur usually takes the form of acute and chronic brain syndromes resulting from ischaemia or infarction associated with cerebral vasculitis (Ando *et al.* 1995; Ohta *et al.* 1998).

Problems related to treatments in RA

Since a number of treatments can be associated with immune dysregulation or immunosuppression, they predispose individuals to CNS and systemic infections that can result in neuropsychiatric manifestations.

Corticosteroid-induced psychiatric syndromes

Corticosteroids have dose-related psychiatric adverse effects, including mania, depression, mixed states, psychosis, anxiety, insomnia, and delirium. A previous psychiatric reaction to corticosteroids does not necessarily predict recurrent reactions with subsequent steroid treatment. The onset of psychiatric symptoms usually occurs within the first two weeks of corticosteroid treatment. Mood disorders are the most common psychiatric reaction. The psychiatric symptoms induced by corticosteroids most often resemble those of bipolar disorder (Brown & Suppes 1998). Delirium and psychosis (without mood symptoms) are less common. The preferred treatment for corticosteroid-induced psychiatric reactions is reduction of corticosteroid dosage, if possible, which improve psychiatric disorders attributable to the corticosteroids in over 90% of cases. Adjunctive psychopharmacological treatment may be necessary.

Impact of psychiatric illness in RA

Depression and symptom perception/reporting

Depression may influence the way a patient experiences or reports the symptoms of RA. Depression has been shown to be associated with more graphic verbal descriptions of the type of pain (e.g. excruciating, punishing) though not with the reported frequency of pain (MacKinnon *et al.* 1994). Depression also predicts greater disability, more disability days and more RA-related hospitalizations (Katz & Yelin 1993). Reduction in disability has been shown to follow improvement in depression in medical patients, though such changes are yet to be shown in RA patients specifically (Von Korff *et al.* 1992).

Depression and illness cognitions

Cognitive factors may be important in mediating the influence of depression on physical symptoms and signs in RA. Depression is associated with increased worry about illness and conviction of severe disease (Pilowsky 1993). Depressed RA patients perceive their illness as being more serious and feel hopeless about a cure compared to non-depressed RA patients and these negative appraisals of health status are not simply the result of depressed people having more severe illness (Murphy *et al.* 1999). Depression is associated with impairment of general coping, especially at high levels of pain (Brown *et al.* 1989).

Depression and illness behaviour

Depression has been shown to impact on health-seeking behaviours and health-care utilization in patients with RA (Macfarlane *et al.* 1999; Manning *et al.* 1992). Depressed RA patients are more likely to report physical symptoms (Murphy *et al.* 1999), less likely to be reassured by a doctor (Pilowsky 1993), and less likely to comply with medications (DiMatteo *et al.* 2000).

Assessment and treatments of psychiatric disorders

Despite their high prevalence and significant impact on the patient's illness and overall quality of life, psychiatric disorders remain mostly unrecognized and under-treated in patients with RA. This is partly attributable to a tendency to focus on the physical aspects of disease coupled with limited resources in some health-care systems. Furthermore, diagnosing depression in patients with rheumatological disorders is complicated as there is an overlap in symptoms of depression and rheumatological disorders (e.g. fatigue, weight loss, insomnia, and lack of appetite) such that the depression frequently goes unrecognized (Rifkin 1992).

Use of standardized psychiatric questionnaires, such as the Minnesota Multiphasic Personality Inventory, the Beck Depression Inventory and the Center for Epidemiologic Studies Depression Scale, in patients with RA tends to overestimate the prevalence of depression since many include somatic symptoms which may be attributable to the rheumatological disorders (Callahan *et al.* 1991; Pincus *et al.* 1996). Scales which have little somatic content such as the Geriatric Depression Scale (Sheikh & Yesavage 1989), the Hospital Anxiety and Depression (HAD) scale (Zigmond & Snaith 1983) or disease-specific instruments (Smedstad *et al.* 1995) may aid accurate diagnosis of depression in such patients. These self-rated questionnaires may be used by rheumatologists or specialist nurses to identify probable cases of psychiatric disorder. With additional training in the use of follow-up questions to confirm caseness of depression, rheumatologists can initiate anti-depressant treatment where indicated, thus avoiding referrals to psychiatrists in uncomplicated cases.

Complex cases may require more detailed assessment by a consultation-liaison psychiatrist. In addition to assessing current mental state, such a psychiatrist should explore the development of psychiatric symptoms and how these relate to the recent disease state and changes in management, availability of social support, psychosocial stresses resulting from pain and disability, but also stresses independent of the illness. Identification of maladaptive coping strategies to physical symptoms (e.g. 'I just lie down and wait for my symptoms to ease', 'I simply avoid activities that cause me pain') can identify potential targets for psychological interventions. Assessing past psychiatric history and family history will help identify which patients are most vulnerable to developing depression and other psychiatric disorders. Finally, investigating the patients' personal beliefs about the illness, such as the perceived causes, possible outcomes and likelihood of controlling disease progression through treatment can identify psychological mechanisms by which psychiatric problems have arisen.

Treatment of psychiatric disorders in RA

Intervention studies have shown that psychological treatments, mostly cognitive and behavioural, are effective in reducing psychological distress, and improving coping in subjects with rheumatological disorders (Bradley *et al.* 1987). In addition such therapies may reduce pain and improve functioning, though it is unclear whether any of these effects are mediated by changes to the inflammatory state or improvements in coping (Bradley *et al.* 1987; Sharpe *et al.* 2001).

Psychological interventions should always be considered in patients with rheumatoid arthritis who have psychiatric problems. Lack of immediate availability of such treatments often means that psychological therapies are reserved for more complex cases. Cognitive behavioural principles however, can be employed by non-psychologists to optimize patients' care. Newly diagnosed patients should be educated about the disease and its likely course, which is likely to facilitate adherence.

There is a wide choice of antidepressants currently available to clinicians, yet the majority of these drugs have not undergone assessment of efficacy in patients suffering from physical illness. Current evidence from studies in psychiatric and other chronic pain populations indicates that the variety of antidepressants when given in appropriate psychotherapeutic doses have roughly equal efficacy in the treatment of depression (Anderson *et al.* 2000). They do differ in their analgesic efficacy, tolerability and profile of drug interactions, however. Tricyclic antidepressants (TCAs) with the least-specific receptor activity, such as amitriptyline, appear to have the greatest analgesic efficacy (Onghena & Van Houdenhove 1992), even at low doses (e.g. 25 mg of amitriptyline) and independent of whether depression is present or not (Bromm *et al.* 1986). In higher doses tolerability and safety are poor, particularly in the elderly.

Newer drugs have comparable antidepressant efficacy, though their analgesic efficacy is yet to be established and they are more expensive. In general, serotonin-specific reuptake inhibitors (SSRIs), such as fluoxetine or citalopram, in doses up to recommended maxima should be considered as first-line treatment for depression in RA (Anderson *et al.* 2000). Gradually introduced TCAs, such as amitriptyline or dosulepin (not available in the USA), should be used in low dose (25–75 mg) for pain relief (Onghena & Van Houdenhove 1992). Combined use of TCAs and SSRIs greatly increases the risk of adverse events and should be avoided unless under expert guidance. Drug interactions may occur though this is not a problem with first- and second-line treatments for RA.

Fibromyalgia

Many patients present with widespread and longstanding rheumatic pain in the absence of the cardinal clinical signs of rheumatic disease. The management of such patients presents a significant challenge to healthcare professionals in both primary and specialist care.

The diagnosis of fibromyalgia was initially proposed as a descriptive label for a clinical syndrome characterized by widespread pain and increased sensitivity to pressure at various anatomical locations known as tender points (Yunus *et al.* 1981). The criteria defining the fibromyalgia syndrome have since broadened to include non-musculoskeletal symptoms such as fatigue, sleep disturbance, headache and irritable bowel. Presentations of this nature were previously explained by earlier medically oriented concepts such as muscular rheumatism, fibrositis, and neurasthenia.

The central clinical feature of the fibromyalgia syndrome is chronic widespread pain (CWP), which is measurable in epidemiological studies without the need for clinical assessment. The American College of Rheumatology (ACR) introduced research criteria in 1990 to distinguish fibromyalgia from other rheumatic disorders. The ACR criteria require a history of widespread pain affecting both sides of the body, at sites both above and below the waist, for at least three months, together with clinical evidence of altered pain threshold as reflected by increased tenderness in at least 11 of 18 specified musculoskeletal trigger points.

Criticism of the lack of specificity of the ACR criteria has lead to the proposal of a revised definition for use in epidemiological research, the Manchester definition (Hunt *et al.* 1999; Quintner & Cohen 1999). The Manchester definition, CWP (M), requires that widespread pain has been present for at least three months and this must specifically be reported in at least two sections of two contralateral limbs, and in the axial skeleton.

Prevalence of fibromyalgia and chronic widespread pain

The prevalence of chronic widespread pain has been measured in large-scale community epidemiological studies (Hunt *et al.* 1999; McBeth *et al.* 2001a;

Schochat & Raspe 2003). Fibromyalgia as defined by the ACR has a prevalence of around 13% in the adult working population, as against 4.7% for the more restrictively defined CWP (M). The prevalence of cases of CWP (M) increased with age and single marital status. No gender difference in prevalence has been apparent in community surveys despite the apparent predominance of female sufferers in clinical practice.

Within community samples cases of chronic widespread pain may be found without tender points and vice versa. Chronic widespread pain appears to be associated differentially with symptoms such as fatigue, psychological distress, number of tender points and sleep disruption, whereas positive tender points show independent associations with low physical mobility, pain, and bodily complaints.

Course of fibromyalgia and relationship to other disorders

Fibromyalgia has a persistent course in clinic and population samples (Ledingham *et al.* 1993). This study found that symptomatic outcome had improved in 26% of clinic attenders on follow-up over four years but worsened in 60% and this was often associated with high levels of anxiety and depression and marked functional disability.

Ledingham's clinic-based study found no evidence that fibromyalgia predates the onset of other disease, rheumatological or otherwise. However, a larger long-term population-based follow-up found an apparent relationship between regional and widespread pain (defined by ACR criteria) and increased mortality (Macfarlane *et al.* 2001; McBeth *et al.* 2003). The excess mortality was primarily due to malignant disorders, even allowing for potential confounding factors including diagnostic error or delay, although there was also an excess of deaths due to suicide and non-accidental injury. Whilst the finding of excess cancer mortality requires repetition, this study indicates that periodic diagnostic review is prudent in the course of clinical patient management, particularly in the event of the presentation of new pain symptoms.

Aetiology of fibromyalgia

Fibromyalgia belongs to a group of chronic pain disorders that present without any antecedent physical injury or identifiable evidence of ongoing tissue damage and no definitive evidence has emerged to support the hypothesis of an underlying pathology of the muscles and soft tissues (Shipley 2002).

Abnormalities of sleep have been demonstrated, which might potentially be relevant to aetiology. These include early morning awakenings, awakening feeling tired or unrefreshed, insomnia, and primary sleep disorders including sleep apnoea (Harding 1998). Patients with fibromyalgia show abnormalities on polysomnographic recording including disrupted sleep architecture and 'alpha–delta' sleep anomaly, which is reproduced in normal controls during stage 4 sleep deprivation or by experimentally induced deep pain. The relationship between poor sleep quality and pain intensity nevertheless cannot be assumed to be aetiological, although relevant to treatment.

Current views on the aetiology of fibromyalgia focus on the interaction of central pain processing and hypothalamo-pituitary-adrenal (HPA) axis dysfunction (Ashburn & Staats 1999). Clinical mechanical allodynia has been postulated as an underlying pathophysiological mechanism (Quintner & Cohen 1999). It is unclear whether this phenomenon is secondary to altered nociception or altered central attention to pain, and the onset of fibromyalgia remains unexplained.

Impairments of activation of the hypothalamic-pituitary portion of the hypothalamic–pituitary-adrenal axis and sympathoadrenal system have been shown in fibromyalgia patients (Buskila 2000). These result in reduced cortico-trophin and epinephrine response to hypoglycaemia. Patients with fibromyalgia may have a vulnerability to HPA axis dysfunction representing the long-term psychological and neurophysiological consequences of early psychosocial trauma (Winfield 1999, 2000).

Psychological factors and psychiatric disorders per se do not appear to be directly implicated in the onset of fibromyalgia. However, somatization, the tendency to display emotional distress in terms of somatic symptoms as a response to life stress, has been proposed as the process initiating the onset and subsequent persistence of pain complaints in fibromyalgia (McBeth et al. 2001a). It is relevant that McBeth and colleagues' study demonstrated that the onset of CWP in the community is predicted by the presence of psychological and behavioural features of the process of somatization. Central pain processing might putatively be altered through an interactive effect with the somatization process mediated by stress-induced disturbances of HPA axis function. Somatization has also been shown to be predictive of the persistence of widespread pain (McBeth et al. 2001b).

Relationship of psychiatric disorders in fibromyalgia

The majority of patients with fibromyalgia do not meet diagnostic criteria for a current psychiatric disorder at the time of presentation and there is little evidence in support of a direct causal relationship between affective disorder and onset of fibromyalgic symptoms (Goldenberg 1989; Walker et al. 1997). A large population-based case-control study found that the prevalence of psychiatric disorder in subjects with chronic widespread pain was around 16.9% compared to 11.9% for those without (Benjamin et al. 2000). Virtually all diagnoses were anxiety or mood disorders with only a few cases of somatoform disorder, the odds of having a mental disorder for subjects with CWP versus those without being 3.18 (95% confidence interval 1.97—5.11).

In secondary care, depressive and functional somatic symptoms show similar prevalence in patients with fibromyalgia to those in patients with other chronic medical conditions (Walker *et al.* 1997). However, patients with fibromyalgia show a higher lifetime prevalence of anxiety and depressive disorders and more frequently have family history of depression than patients with other rheumatic diagnoses. In Walker's clinic—based study nearly all the patients with fibromyalgia had a prior psychiatric diagnosis compared with less than half of the patients with rheumatoid arthritis. The patients with fibromyalgia had equal or greater functional disability, reported more medically unexplained physical symptoms and appeared to be less well adapted to their illness, despite the lack of demonstrable organic pathology in fibromyalgia.

Clinical management

From a rheumatological perspective fibromyalgia is viewed primarily as a chronic pain disorder. Other clinical features, such as persistent fatigue and disordered sleep, are seen as secondary consequences so that the initial pharmacological approach to treating the disorder is the management of pain (Shipley 2002). Non-steroidal anti-inflammatory drugs and centrally acting agents such as opioids and anticonvulsants are helpful to some patients but may be problematic in relation to adverse reactions and misuse.

In secondary care fibromyalgia patients tend to develop a psychological illness model consistent with the belief that they are suffering from an arthritic disorder. This frequently leads to the adoption of dysfunctional health behaviours such as exercise avoidance, consistent with secondary health beliefs, for example, that physical activity is harmful to their joints. Such behaviours lead to secondary disabilities such as loss of physical fitness and loss of daily living function.

Patients often have difficulty in accepting the diagnosis of fibromyalgia and need support from professionals whilst traversing the emotional and cognitive processes leading to psychological readjustment to their physical diagnosis. Psychiatric referral at an early stage in the patient's illness career is thus often met by anger and feelings of abandonment by the treating doctor, leading to hostility towards the psychiatrists and difficulties in engagement. The facilitation of early psychological reorientation from a 'cure-seeking' to a 'self-coping' model of illness is nevertheless an important aim in psychiatric management. Adoption of the liaison model of working with colleagues in rheumatology and other health professions thus has potential advantage over practice based on referral-consultation.

A rationale exists for the use of antidepressants in fibromyalgia for pain control and amitriptyline and related tricyclic antidepressants appear to be more effective than SSRIs (Lawson 2002). The analgesic action of antidepressants putatively involves the modulation of central serotonin and noradrenaline transmission but other mechanisms, such as potassium channel modulation and NMDA receptor antagonism, may be relevant to the action of amitriptyline. Treatment should be initiated at low dosage (10–25 mg at night) as patients are often sensitive to the sedative and anticholinergic side-effects of amitriptyline, and gradually increased over three to four weeks to 75–150 mg daily in divided doses, according to response and tolerance.

Randomized controlled trials (RCTs) of non-pharmacological interventions including exercise, electromyogram (EMG) biofeedback training, electrotherapy and acupuncture, patient education and self-management programmes, multi-modal treatment approaches, and other interventions have been subjected to systematic review (Sim & Adams 1999, 2002). Their study found aerobic exercise to be moderately effective as a single intervention alone although conclusions could not be drawn on the effectiveness of any specific combinations of interventions due to methodological difficulties. Another systematic review of RCTs involving exercise training also found that supervised aerobic exercise training has beneficial effects on physical capacity and FMS symptoms (Busch *et al.* 2002).

Complementary and alternative medicine (CAM) has gained increasing popularity, and acupuncture, herbal and nutritional supplements containing magnesium or S-adenosylmethionine (SAMe), and massage therapy have the best evidence for effectiveness with fibromyalgia syndrome (Holdcraft *et al.* 2003).

In practice, outcomes are likely to be better when patients are offered several treatment modalities as a package as single treatments are rarely sufficient to treat chronic pain disorders (Ashburn & Staats 1999). Pharmacological and non-pharmacological treatments appear to produce different outcomes (Karjalainen *et al.* 2000; Rossy *et al.* 1999). Rossy *et al.*'s meta-analysis found that antidepressants and non-pharmacological treatments lead to improvements in physical status and self-reported symptoms whereas non-pharmacological treatments alone were associated with improvement in psychological status and daily living functioning. There may nevertheless be potential for improvement in the psychological outcome of antidepressant therapy in clinical practice through more consistent usage of dosage regimes within the range associated with antidepressant efficacy.

Karjalainen and colleagues' (2000) systematic review was unable to demonstrate the efficacy in clinical practice of current multidisciplinary rehabilitation approaches. Multimodal treatment is nevertheless likely to be superior to single treatment modalities (Ashburn & Staats 1999). The optimal treatment package for fibromyalgia would appear to include non-pharmacological treatments, specifically exercise and cognitive-behavioural therapy, in addition to appropriate medication management as needed for sleep and pain symptoms.

Treatments with reasonable evidence of efficacy include psychoeducational approaches, cognitive-behavioural therapy, graded exercise programmes, and antidepressants and hypnotic medications. The main role for the liaison psychiatric team lies in diagnosis and management of comorbid psychiatric disorder, advice on antidepressant treatment, and the management of complex cases. Where psychiatric treatment is indicated patients are more likely to engage if this is offered within the rheumatological/pain clinic setting. Treatment of comorbid anxiety and depressive disorders should be expected to produce similar benefits to those seen in patients with rheumatoid arthritis.

Overall, treatments may be more effective in clinical practice than in research settings as fibromyalgia patients show considerable heterogeneity so that matching of specific treatments to individual patient characteristics may improve outcomes (Turk & Okifuji 2000). Careful clinical assessment will facilitate individualized care planning and will potentially optimize outcomes. The role of the liaison psychiatrist in management will include use of psychotherapeutic skills in engagement and promoting adjustment to the diagnosis of fibromyalgia, assessment and treatment of comorbid psychiatric disorder and substance misuse, liaison with other health professionals in formulating a treatment package, and specific advice on antidepressant therapy.

In conclusion, psychiatric management of fibromyalgia has broad similarities with the treatment of other functional somatic disorders such as chronic fatigue syndrome or irritable bowel disorder.

Osteoarthritis

Osteoarthritis (OA) is the most common of all joint diseases. Its prevalence in the population changes with age: less than 2% of women aged <45 years are affected compared to 30% between ages of 45 and 64 years, and 68% over 65 years. In the majority of cases the disorder is idiopathic although secondary OA can occur as the result of trauma. The pattern of joint involvement varies considerably. Previous joint overload, particularly repetitive trauma, has a considerable influence on the distribution of joint involvement. Clinically affected joints are painful, particularly on movement, and stiff after a period of inactivity. As the condition advances movements become limited and joint instability may occur.

The majority of people with OA in the general population are not greatly troubled by the disorder. Consequently the prevalence of psychological disorders in such community samples of people with OA is similar to that seen in the general population (Dexter & Brandt 1994). In secondary care, patients with OA of the knee or hand have been found to have slightly lower scores on a standardized assessment of depression compared to subjects with other musculoskeletal disorders (Hawley & Wolfe 1993). These results taken together would indicate that OA is less closely associated with depression than other musculoskeletal disorders such as RA, though studies of patients with more advanced OA are required.

The risk factors for depression when it does occur in OA include younger age, less education, higher pain and greater self-reported impact of the OA (Dexter & Brandt 1994; van Baar *et al.* 1998; Zautra & Smith 2001). Anxiety and hopelessness are associated with functional disability (Creamer *et al.* 2000).

There have been some studies examining the efficacy of antidepressants or psychological therapies in OA. Both antidepressants and cognitive behavioral therapy have been shown to be efficacious in the treatment of depression in patients with OA. Furthermore, improvement in depression is associated with reduced pain experience and less disability (Calfas *et al.* 1992; Lin *et al.* 2003).

Back pain

Chronic low back pain (CLBP) and associated disability is a major health and socioeconomic problem. In the United States, annual costs of low back disability have been estimated to be approximately $50 billion, with the average cost of a single case of work-related back pain exceeding $8000 (Hazard *et al.* 1996). It has been estimated that 70–80% of the costs for work-related low back claims are accounted for by 7–10% of patients who develop CLBP (Spengler *et al.* 1986).

Most people with CLBP have no identifiable pathophysiologic cause for their pain, or the severity of their pain is disproportionate to any pathological changes in the spine on X-ray or computed tomography scan.

Depression and psychological distress in chronic low back pain

Patients with chronic low back pain have three times the prevalence of major depression compared with individuals in the general population (Sullivan *et al.* 1992). In prospective studies, the presence of a depressive disorder has been demonstrated to increase the risk of developing chronic musculoskeletal pain three years later (Leino & Magni 1993; Magni *et al.* 1993, 1994; Von Korff *et al.* 1993). Even after eight years, previously depressed patients remain twice as likely to develop chronic pain when compared with non-depressed patients (Leino & Magni 1993; Magni *et al.* 1993, 1994; Von Korff *et al.* 1993). Older adults with depression symptoms are at even higher risk for developing back and hip pain.

Depression is also associated with a nearly fourfold increase in the likelihood of seeking a consultation for back pain (lasting for a period greater than three months).

In the Baltimore Epidemiologic Catchment Area Study, which is one of the largest prospective studies of mental health ever to be undertaken, householders were assessed at baseline, then 1 year later, and then 13 years later. In cross-sectional analyses undertaken at baseline, lifetime occurrence of depressive disorder was significantly correlated with lifetime prevalence of back pain (OR = 1.6, $p = 0.01$; Larson *et al.* 2004). During the 13-year follow-up, across the three data collection points, there was an increase in the risk for incident back pain when depressive disorder was present at baseline (OR = 1.9, 95% CI 1.03, 3.4). However, during the short-term follow-up period of one year, between baseline and wave 2, depressive disorder at baseline was unrelated to first-ever reports of back pain. Depressive disorder both at baseline and one year later was associated with a more than three times greater risk for a first-ever report of back pain during the 12–13-year follow-up period, in comparison to those who did not have depressive disorder at either the first or second assessment (OR = 3.4, 95% CI 1.4, 7.8). However back pain at baseline was not significantly associated with an increased risk for depression in the longitudinal analysis (OR = 0.8, 95% CI 0.5, 1.4).

The findings of this study suggest that depression is an independent risk factor for incident back pain independent of other characteristics often associated with back pain. Back pain does not appear to be a short-term consequence of depressive disorder but emerges over periods longer than one year.

Treatment interventions

The biopsychosocial model of chronic pain has gained widespread acceptance as the appropriate model for understanding chronic pain and has lead to the development of treatments emphasizing multidisciplinary care (Gatchel *et al.* 1995) and functional restoration (Hazard *et al.* 1989).

Both cognitive-behavioural and physical therapy approaches have shown evidence of efficacy. In a recent study of patients with acute low back pain, either cognitive behavioural therapy or preventative physical therapy was more likely to prevent long-term disability and sick leave than a minimal intervention of reassurance and advice (Linton *et al.* 2005). Physical therapy and exercise alone are also helpful (Geisser *et al.* 2005). A systematic review of trials of intensive multidisciplinary biopsychosocial rehabilitation for chronic low back pain found that psychological treatments were contributory to improvements in pain and function, whereas less intensive interventions were ineffective (Guzman 2002). Given the current knowledge base in this area, it seems sensible to suggest that psychological interventions in chronic low back pain are likely to have most effect if combined with physical therapy and rehabilitation approaches.

Conclusions

Psychological symptoms are common in patients with musculoskeletal disorders, and either occur as result of pain and disability brought about by the condition, or in certain conditions (e.g. low back pain) can also be aetiological risk factors for the development of the condition. Psychological treatments are effective in reducing psychological distress, and improving coping in subjects with a wide range of musculo-skeletal disorders. There is also a role for antidepressant treatment in patients with overt depressive symptoms. Lack of immediate availability of such treatments often means that psychological therapies are reserved for more complex cases, where the presence of powerful maintaining factors have resulted in chronic and enduring difficulties.

REFERENCES

Affleck, G., Tennen, H., Urrows, S., *et al.* (1992). Neuroticism and the pain-mood relation in rheumatoid arthritis: insights from a prospective daily study. *Journal of Consulting & Clinical Psychology*, **60**, 119–26.

Anderson, I. M., Nutt, D. J. and Deakin, J. F. W. (2000). Evidence based guidelines for treating depressive disorders with antidepressants: a revision of the 1993 British Association for Psychopharmacology guidelines. *Journal of Psychopharmacology*, **14**(1), 2–30.

Ando, Y., Kai, S., Uyama, E., *et al.* (1995). Involvement of the central nervous system in rheumatoid arthritis: its clinical manifestations and analysis by magnetic resonance imaging. *Internal Medicine*, **34**, 188–91.

Ashburn, M. A. and Staats, P. S. (1999). Management of chronic pain. *Lancet*, **353**(9167), 1865–9.

Benjamin, S., Morris, S., McBeth, J., *et al.* (2000). The association between chronic widespread pain and mental disorder: a population-based study. *Arthritis and Rheumatism*, **43**(3), 561–7.

Blumer, D. and Heilbronn, M. (1982). Chronic pain as a variant of depressive disease: the pain-prone disorder. *Journal of Nervous and Mental Disease*, **170**, 381–94.

Bradley, L. A., Young, L. D., Anderson, K. O., *et al.* (1987). Effects of psychological therapy on pain behaviour of rheumatoid arthritis patients. *Arthritis and Rheumatism*, **30**, 1105–15.

Bromm, B., Meier, W. and Scharein, E. (1986). Imipramine reduces experimental pain. *Pain*, **25**, 245–57.

Brown, G. and Harris, T. (1978). *Social Origins of Depression: A Study of Psychiatric Disorder in Women*. London: Tavistock.

Brown, E. S. and Suppes, T. (1998). Mood symptoms during corticosteroid therapy: a review. *Harvard Review of Psychiatry*, **5**, 239–46.

Brown, G. K., Nicassio, P. M. and Wallston, K. A. (1989). Pain coping strategies and depression in rheumatoid arthritis. *Journal of Consulting and Clinical Psychology*, **57**, 652−7.

Busch, A., Schachter, C. L., Peloso, P. M., *et al.* (2002). Exercise for treating fibromyalgia syndrome. *Cochrane Database Systematic Review*, **3**, CD003786.

Buskila, D. (2000). Fibromyalgia, chronic fatigue syndrome, and myofascial pain syndrome. *Current Opinion in Rheumatology*, **12**(2), 113−23.

Calfas, K. J., Kaplan, R. M., Ingram, R. E. (1992). One year evaluation of cognitive behavioral intervention in osteoarthritis. *Arthritis Care and Research*, **5**, 202−9.

Callahan, L. F., Kaplan, M. R. and Pincus, T. (1991). The Beck Depression Inventory, Center for Epidemiological Studies Depression Scale (CES-D), and general Well-Being Schedule Depression Subscale in rheumatoid arthritis. *Arthritis Care Research*, **4**, 3−11.

Creamer, P., Lethbridge-Cejku, M., Hochberg, M. C. (2000). Factors associated with functional impairment in symptomatic knee osteoarthritis. *Rheumatology*, **39**, 490−6.

Creed, F. (1990). Psychological disorders in rheumatoid arthritis: a growing consensus. *Annals of the Rheumatic Diseases*, **49**, 808−12.

Creed, F., Murphy, S. and Jayson, M. (1990). Measurement of psychiatric disorders in rheumatoid arthritis. *Journal of Psychosomatic Research*, **34**, 79−87.

Creed, F., Morgan, R., Fiddler, M., *et al.* (2002). Depression and anxiety impair health-related quality of life and are associated with increased costs in general medical inpatients. *Psychosomatics*, **43**, 302−9.

Dexter, P. and Brandt, K. (1994). Distribution and predictors of depressive symptoms in osteoarthritis. *Journal of Rheumatology*, **21**, 279−86.

Dickens, C. M., McGowan, L., Clark-Carter, D., *et al.* (2002). Depression in rheumatoid arthritis: a systematic review of the literature with meta-analysis. *Psychosomatic Medicine*, **64**, 52−60.

Dickens, C. M., Jackson, J., Tomenson, B., *et al.* (2003). Association of depression and rheumatoid arthritis. *Psychosomatics*, **44**, 209−15.

DiMatteo, M. R., Lepper, H. S. and Croghan, T. W. (2000). Depression is a risk factor for non-compliance with medical treatment: meta-analysis of the effects of the anxiety and depression on patient adherence. *Archives of Internal Medicine*, **160**(14), 2101−7.

Evers, A. W., Kraaimaat, F. W., Geenen, R., *et al.* (1997). Determinants of psychological distress and its course in the first year after diagnosis in rheumatoid arthritis patients. *Journal of Behavioral Medicine*, **20**, 504.

Fifield, J., Reisine, S., Sheehan, T. J., *et al.* (1996). Gender, paid work, and symptoms of emotional distress in rheumatoid arthritis patients. *Arthritis & Rheumatism*, **39**, 427−35.

Gatchel, R. J., Polatin, P. B. and Mayer, T. G. (1995). The dominant role of psychosocial risk factors in the development of chronic low back pain disability. *Spine*, **20**, 2702−9.

Geisser, M. E., Wiggert, E. A., Haig, A. J., *et al.* (2005). A randomized, controlled trial of manual therapy and specific adjuvant exercise for chronic low back pain. *Clinical Journal of Pain*, **21**, 463−70.

Goldenberg, D. L. (1989). Psychological symptoms and psychiatric diagnosis in patients with fibromyalgia. *Journal of Rheumatology Supplement*, **19**, 127−30.

Goodenow, C., Reisine, S. T. and Grady, K. E. (1990). Quality of social support and associated social and psychological functioning in women with rheumatoid arthritis. *Health Psychology*, **9**, 266–84.

Guzman, J., Esmail, R., Karjalainen, K., *et al.* (2002). Multidisciplinary biopsychosocial rehabilitation for chronic low back pain. *Cochrane Database Systematic Review*, **1**(1), CD000963.

Harding, S. M. (1998). Sleep in fibromyalgia patients: subjective and objective findings. *American Journal of the Medical Sciences*, **315**(6), 367–76.

Hawley, D. J. and Wolfe, F. (1993). Depression is not more common in RA: a 10 year longitudinal study of 6,153 patients with rheumatic disease. *Journal of Rheumatology*, **20**, 2025–31.

Hazard, R. G., Fenwick, J. W., Kalish, S. M., *et al.* (1989). Functional restoration with behavioral support: a one year prospective study of patients with chronic low back pain. *Spine*, **14**, 157–61.

Hazard, R. G., Haugh, L. D., Reid, S., *et al.* (1996). Early prediction of chronic disability after occupational low back injury. *Spine*, **21**, 945–51.

Holdcraft, L. C., Assefi, N. and Buchwald, D. (2003). Complementary and alternative medicine in fibromyalgia and related syndromes. *Best Practice Research Clinical Rheumatology*, **4**, 667–83.

Hunt, I. M., Silman, A. J., Benjamin, S., *et al.* (1999). The prevalence of chronic widespread pain in the community using the 'Manchester' definition of chronic widespread pain. *Rheumatology*, **38**, 275–9.

Karjalainen, K., Malmivaara, A., van Tulder, M., *et al.* (2000). Multidisciplinary rehabilitation for fibromyalgia and musculoskeletal pain in working age adults. *Cochrane Database Systematic Reviews*, **2**, CD001984.

Katz, P. P. and Yelin, E. H. (1993). Prevalence and correlates of depressive symptoms among persons with rheumatoid arthritis. *Journal of Rheumatology*, **20**, 790–6.

Katz, P. P. and Yelin, E. H. (1995). The development of depressive symptoms among women with rheumatoid arthritis. *Arthritis and Rheumatism*, **38**, 49–56.

Kraaimaat, F. W., Dam-Baggen, R. M. J. and Bijlsma, J. W. J. (1995). Association of social support and the spouse's reaction with psychological distress in male and female patients with rheumatoid arthritis. *Journal of Rheumatology*, **22**, 644–8.

Larson, S. L., Clark, M. R. and Eaton, W. W. (2004). Depressive disorder as a long-term antecedent risk factor for incident back pain: a 13-year follow-up study from the Baltimore Epidemiological Catchment Area Sample. *Psychological Medicine*, **34**, 211–19.

Lawson, K. (2002). Tricyclic antidepressants and fibromyalgia: what is the mechanism of action? *Expert Opinion on Investigative Drugs*, **11**(10), 1437–45.

Ledingham, J., Doherty, S. and Doherty, M. (1993). Primary fibromyalgia syndrome – an outcome study. *British Journal of Rheumatology*, **32**(2), 139–42.

Leino, P. I. and Magni, G. (1993). Depressive and distress symptoms as predictors of low back pain, neck shoulder pain and other musculoskeletal morbidity: a 10-year follow-up of metal industry employees. *Pain*, **52**, 89–94.

Lin, E., Katon, W., Von Korff, M., *et al.* (2003). Effects of improving depression care on pain and functional outcomes among older adults with arthritis. *Journal of the American Medical Association*, **290**, 2428–34.

Linton, S. J., Boersma, K., Jansson, M., *et al.* (2005). The effects of cognitive-behavioral and physical therapy preventive interventions on pain-related sick leave; a randomized controlled trial. *Clinical Journal of Pain*, **21**, 109–19.

Macfarlane, G. J., Morris, S., Hunt, I. M., *et al.* (1999). Chronic widespread pain in the community: the influence of psychological symptoms and mental disorder on healthcare seeking behaviour. *Journal of Rheumatology*, **26**(2), 413–19.

Macfarlane, G. J., McBeth, J. and Silman, A. J. (2001). Widespread body pain and mortality: prospective population based study. *British Medical Journal*, **323**(7314), 662–5.

MacKinnon, J. R., Avison, W. R. and McCain, G. A. (1994). Pain and functional limitations in individuals with rheumatoid arthritis. *International Journal of Rehabilitation Research*, **17**, 49–59.

Magni, G., Marchetti, M., Moreschi, C., *et al.* (1993). Chronic musculoskeletal pain and depressive symptoms in the National Health and Nutrition Examination. I. Epidemiologic follow-up study. *Pain*, **53**, 163–8.

Magni, G., Moreschi, C., Rigatti-Luchini, S., *et al.* (1994). Prospective study on the relationship between depressive symptoms and chronic musculoskeletal pain. *Pain*, **56**, 289–97.

Manne, S. L. and Zautra, A. J. (1989). Spouse criticism and support: their association with coping and psychological adjustment among women with rheumatoid arthritis. *Journal of Personality Social Psychology*, **56**, 608–17.

Manning, W. and Wells, K. B. (1992). The effects of psychological distress and psychological well-being on use of medical services. *Medical Care*, **30**, 541–53.

McBeth, J., Macfarlane, G. J., Hunt, I. M., *et al.* (2001a). Risk factors for persistent chronic widespread pain: a community-based study. *Rheumatology (Oxford)*, **40**(1), 95–101.

McBeth, J., Macfarlane, G. J., Benjamin, S., *et al.* (2001b). Features of somatization predict the onset of chronic widespread pain: results of a large population-based study. *Arthritis and Rheumatism*, **44**(4), 940–6.

McBeth, J., Silman, A. J. and Macfarlane, G. J. (2003). Association of widespread body pain with an increased risk of cancer and reduced cancer survival: a prospective, population-based study. *Arthritis and Rheumatism*, **48**(6), 1686–92.

Melter, H., Gill, B., Petticrew, M., *et al.* (1995). *The Prevalence of Psychiatric Morbidity Among Adults Living in Private Households*. London: HMSO.

Mindham, R. H. S., Bagshaw, A., James, S. A., *et al.* (1981). Factors associated with the appearance of psychiatric symptoms in rheumatoid arthritis. *Journal of Psychosomatic Research*, **25**, 429–35.

Murphy, S., Creed, F. H. and Jayson, M. I. V. (1988). Psychiatric disorders and illness behaviour in rheumatoid arthritis. *British Journal of Rheumatology*, **27**, 357–63.

Murphy, H., Dickens, C. M., Creed, F. H., *et al.* (1999). Depression, illness perception and coping in rheumatoid arthritis. *Journal of Psychosomatic Research*, **46**, 155–64.

Ohta, K., Tanaka, M., Funaki, M., *et al.* (1998). Multiple cerebral infarction associated with cerebral vasculitis in rheumatoid arthritis. *Rinsho Shinkeigaku – Clinical Neurology*, **38**, 423–9.

Onghena, P. and Van Houdenhove, B. (1992). Antidepressant-induced analgesia in chronic non-malignant pain: a meta-analysis of 39 placebo controlled studies. *Pain*, **49**, 205–19.

Pilowsky, I. (1993). Dimensions of illness behaviour as measured by the Illness Behaviour Questionnaire. *Journal of Psychosomatic Research*, **37**, 53–62.

Pincus, T., Callahan, L. F., Bradley, L., *et al.* (1996). Elevated MMPI scores for hypochondriasis, depression and hysteria in patients with rheumatoid arthritis reflect disease rather than psychosocial status. *Arthritis and Rheumatism*, **29**, 1466.

Quintner, J. L. and Cohen, M. L. (1999). Fibromyalgia falls foul of a fallacy. *Lancet*, **353**, 1092–4.

Revenson, T. A., Schiaffino, K. M., Majerovitz, S. D., *et al.* (1991). Social support as a double-edged sword: the relation of positive and problematic support to depression among rheumatoid arthritis patients. *Social Science & Medicine*, **33**, 807–13.

Rifkin, A. (1992). Depression in physically ill patients. *Postgraduate Medicine*, **92**, 147–54.

Romano, J. M. and Turner, J. A. (1985). Chronic pain and depression: does the evidence support a relationship? *Psychological Bulletin*, **97**, 18–34.

Rossy, L. A., Buckelew, S. P., Dorr, N., *et al.* (1999). A meta-analysis of fibromyalgia treatment interventions. *Annals of Behavioral Medicine*, **21**(2), 180–91.

Schochat, T. and Raspe, H. (2003). Elements of fibromyalgia in an open population. *Rheumatology*, **42**, 829–35.

Sharpe, L., Sensky, T., Timberlake, N., *et al.* (2001). A blind, randomized, controlled trial of cognitive-behavioural intervention for patients with recent onset rheumatoid arthritis: preventing psychological and physical morbidity. *Pain*, **89**, 275–83.

Sheikh, J. I. and Yesavage, J. (1989). Geriatric Depression Scale (GDS): recent evidence and development of a shorter version. *Clinical Gerontology*, **9**, 37–43.

Shipley, M. (2002). Fibromyalgia. *Medicine*, **30**(9), 81–4.

Sim, J. and Adams, N. (1999). Physical and other non-pharmacological interventions for fibromyalgia. *Baillière's Best Practice and Research. Clinical Rheumatology*, **13**(3), 507–23.

Sim, J. and Adams, N. (2002). Systematic review of randomized controlled trials of nonpharmacological interventions. *Clinical Journal of Pain*, **18**(5), 324–36.

Smedstad, L., Vaglum, P., Kvien, T., *et al.* (1995). The relationship between self-reported pain and sociodemographic variables, anxiety, and depressive symptoms in rheumatoid arthritis. *Journal of Rheumatology*, **22**, 514–20.

Spengler, D. M., Bigos, S. J., Martin, N. A., *et al.* (1986). Back injuries in industry: a retrospective study: I. Overview and cost analysis. *Spine*, **11**, 241–5.

Spitzer, A., Bar-Tal, Y. and Golander, H. (1995). Social support: how does it really work? *Journal of Advanced Nursing*, **22**, 850–4.

Sullivan, M. J., Reesor, K., Mikail, S., *et al.* (1992). The treatment of depression in chronic low back pain: review and recommendations. *Pain*, **50**, 5–13.

Turk, D. C. and Okifuji, A. (2000). Pain in patients with fibromyalgia syndrome. *Current Rheumatology Reports*, **2**(2), 109–15.

van Baar, M. E., Dekker, J., Lemmens, J. A., *et al.* (1998). Pain and disability in patients with osteoarthritis of the hip or knee: the relationship with articular, kinesiological and psychological characteristics. *Journal of Rheumatology*, **25**, 125–33.

Von Korff, M., Ormel, J., Katon, W., *et al.* (1992). Disability and depression among high utilizers of health care. A longitudinal analysis. *Archives of General Psychiatry*, **49**, 91–100.

Von Korff, M., LeResche, L. and Dworkin, S. F. (1993). First onset of common pain symptoms: a prospective study of depression as a risk factor. *Pain*, **55**, 251–8.

Walker, E. A., Keegan, D., Gardner, G., *et al.* (1997). Psychosocial factors in fibromyalgia compared with rheumatoid arthritis: I. Psychiatric diagnoses and functional disability. *Psychosomatic Medicine*, **59**, S65–7.

Winfield, J. B. (1999). Pain in fibromyalgia. *Rheumatic Disease Clinics of North America*, **25**, 55–79.

Winfield, J. B. (2000). Psychological determinants of fibromyalgia and related syndromes. *Current Review of Pain*, **4**, 276–86.

Yunus, M., Masi, A. T., Calabro, J. J., *et al.* (1981). Primary fibromyalgia (fibrositis): clinical study of 50 patients with matched normal controls. *Seminars in Arthritis Research*, **11**, 151–71.

Zautra, A. J. and Smith, B. W. (2001). Depression and reactivity to stress in older women with rheumatoid arthritis and osteoarthritis. *Psychosomatic Medicine*, **63**, 687–96.

Zigmond, A. S. and Snaith, R. P. (1983). The Hospital Anxiety and Depression Scale. *Acta Psychiatrica Scandinavica*, **67**, 361–70.

23

Oncology

Geoffrey Lloyd

Despite considerable advances in medical treatment cancer is still one of the most frightening diagnoses a doctor can convey to a patient. In the minds of most people malignancy is associated with severe pain, disfigurement, impaired quality of life and drastically reduced life expectancy. Surgical treatment is feared because it may result in altered appearance and body image. Chemotherapy and radiotherapy are also viewed apprehensively. Chemotherapy, in particular, is feared because of its association with nausea, vomiting, fatigue and hair loss.

Not surprisingly the prevalence of psychiatric disorders is high. Many studies have reported on the prevalence of psychiatric disorders in different groups of patients. Variations in reported rates are due to differences in sampling methods and the methods of assessment used. They do not necessarily reflect differences in the actual prevalence of psychiatric disorders in different types of malignancy. However some cancers are associated with particular problems involving anatomical loss, sexual difficulties and reduced fertility. Reviews of the literature have indicated that up to half of patients have a clinical disorder at any time (Cull 1990; McDaniel *et al.* 1995). Affective disorders are particularly common. Fallowfield *et al.* (1990) observed that a quarter of women developed an affective disorder following surgical treatment for breast cancer. Parle *et al.* (1996) conducted a prospective study of 600 cancer patients over a two-year period and found that 20% had an affective disorder. An American study, using the Brief Symptom Inventory, assessed a random sample of patients attending 12 oncology centres and found that 35% obtained scores consistent with a psychiatric disorder (Zabora *et al.* 1997). Sharpe *et al.* (2004a) found that 8% of patients attending a regional cancer centre had a major depressive disorder, most of whom were receiving no potentially effective therapy. These patients were assessed with a two-stage procedure; they first completed the Hospital Anxiety and Depression (HAD)

Handbook of Liaison Psychiatry, ed. Geoffrey Lloyd and Elspeth Guthrie. Published by Cambridge University Press. © Cambridge University Press 2007.

scale and those with elevated scores were then interviewed by telephone using the Structured Clinical Interview for DSM-IV (SCID).

Factors predisposing to psychiatric disorders

Although some other illnesses are associated with similar rates of psychiatric disorder there are several factors, more commonly associated with malignancy, which the clinician needs to consider when trying to understand the development of psychological symptoms.

Nature of the illness

Cancer remains a stigmatized type of illness. It is not a diagnosis which people feel comfortable discussing with their acquaintances or even with close friends and family. The anticipation of a reduced life expectancy is particularly difficult for patients with young families. Even after treatment that has apparently been successful, most patients live with the anxiety of a recurrence of the tumour and a fear that they will not live long enough to see their children grow up. Recurrent disease is often associated with intractable pain and many cancer patients fear the time when curative or even palliative treatment is no longer possible.

Several cancers are linked aetiologically to lifestyle factors. Smoking is the most clearly identified of these and has a well established predisposition to cancer of the lung, oropharynx and gastrointestinal tract among others. Heavy alcohol consumption over many years is known to predispose to oropharyngeal cancer, colorectal cancer and liver tumours. Sexual habits have also been invoked in the aetiology of some cancers particularly cancer of the cervix, which has been linked to a sexually promiscuous lifestyle. Indeed, the most important risk factor for cervical cancer is the number of sexual partners a woman has had. Infection with one of the human papilloma viruses provides the causal link and suggests that cervical cancer has an infective basis in many cases. Sexual habits play a part in those tumours that develop following AIDS. Kaposi's sarcoma and non-Hodgkin's lymphoma have an increased risk of over 300 and 100 times respectively (Boshoff & Weiss 2002). Other tumours with an increased prevalence in AIDS patients include angiosarcoma, Hodgkin's disease, some leukaemias, multiple myeloma and brain tumours.

Patients developing these cancers often harbour considerable feelings of guilt concerning their own contribution to their illness. There is a sense of remorse for a pattern of behaviour which they believe to have brought on their illness, a remorse which is often reinforced by public attitudes which are critical of smokers, heavy drinkers, drug addicts and the sexually promiscuous. The guilt is worsened by a realization that even if the lifestyle is modified it may be too late to alter the outcome of the illness. Even when there are no clearly defined lifestyle factors, some patients still blame themselves for the onset of their illness. They attribute it to a personal flaw or an inability to handle stress. Conversely some patients blame others for their illness. In the case of occupationally linked cancers there may be good reason for this. Several cancers, including cancer of the lung, bladder and scrotum, are associated with occupational processes and with specific chemicals used in an occupational setting. Employers may be held responsible if it is thought that inadequate precautions have been taken to protect employees from these toxic substances. The effects of passive smoking have become increasingly recognized and employers are taking steps to ban smoking from the workplace as otherwise there will be a large number of claims for compensation for an illness induced by avoidable factors at work.

Effects of treatment

Treatment for malignancy is often extremely unpleasant. Surgical intervention is required for many cancers at some stage. Breast cancer was previously treated with radical mastectomy, a procedure dreaded by most women who underwent it. The mutilating effects of the surgery and the sense of a loss of femininity have been described in numerous reports. Women fear a decline in their sexual attractiveness and rejection by their partners. They also complain of being lopsided. A further complication is the painful and visually embarrassing development of lympho-edema in the arm on the affected side. The morbidity of mastectomy has led to a more conservative surgical approach. Simple mastectomy or localized removal of the tumour ('lumpectomy') are now practised more often and if mastectomy is undertaken many women can be offered the choice of immediate breast reconstruction with an implant. For those who need to undergo a course of radiotherapy, reconstruction can be offered at a later date.

Men commonly develop sexual complication following surgery for prostatic cancer. Prostatectomy may also be followed by urinary incontinence which greatly restricts the patient's social life.

Colostomy also has a major psychological impact. The altered body appearance is difficult to accept. Patients may feel that they have become unclean and that their stoma bag may leak or give off offensive smells. Fears such as these tend to reduce self-confidence and restrict social life. A stoma is particularly difficult for those who are sexually active. Rejection by the sexual partner is a common anxiety, made worse if the surgical treatment has impaired sexual potency by damaging nerve supply to the pelvis. Other surgical procedures with profound psychological consequences include laryngectomy, glossectomy and limb amputation. Specific issues related to head and neck cancer are reviewed in Chapter 24.

Chemotherapy has many adverse effects which induce psychological symptoms. In addition to the effects on fertility, which are described below, chemotherapy can cause intense anxiety as a result of the nausea and vomiting which are so commonly experienced, even though antiemetic drugs have reduced their frequency. Nausea and vomiting may be so severe during the first one or two treatments that a conditioned reflex is established. The patient becomes anxious and nauseated at the prospect of returning for further treatment and may then refuse to attend even though it is realized that treatment is necessary to improve prognosis. A conditioned phobic anxiety response is thus established and in severe cases anxiety may be experienced even when driving past the hospital or when the hospital or its staff are mentioned by name. Loss of hair is often a source of distress, especially for women. Although the hair loss is usually reversible some patients become so affected that the provision of a wig is required to prevent social withdrawal and depression. Chemotherapeutic drugs, such as vincristine and L-asparaginase, can have a direct effect on cerebral function causing depression and delirium. Steroids, which are used in conjunction with chemotherapy, also have a well-recognized risk of inducing depression, mania or delirium.

Radiotherapy is better tolerated than chemotherapy. Nevertheless it can cause severe fatigue which can lead to depression. Irradiation to the brain appears to cause more profound fatigue than does irradiation to other areas. Cerebral atrophy is a recognized complication of brain irradiation and if sufficiently pronounced the patient shows clinical evidence of dementia.

Bone marrow transplantation is used in the treatment of leukaemias, lymphomas and solid tumours. It is usually given following chemotherapy and radiotherapy designed to destroy malignant cells. It involves the intravenous injection of bone marrow cells which locate to the recipient's marrow and then produce red and white blood cells and platelets. Allogenic transplantation uses healthy marrow or stem cells from a suitable donor. Autologous transplantation uses the patient's own marrow which has been harvested and frozen prior to chemotherapy and radiotherapy. Being considered for bone marrow transplantation is in itself a stressful experience (Baker *et al.* 1997) because the procedure carries a considerable morbidity and mortality. Once the transplantation has been completed the patient has to be treated in isolation but remains at high risk of several potentially fatal opportunistic infections including herpes simplex, cytomegalovirus, *Pneumocystis carinii* and various fungal infections. There is also the possibility of graft versus host disease in those who have undergone allogenic grafting. Patients have to wait anxiously for evidence that their haematological system is recovering and many monitor their blood counts closely. For those who survive, the outcome is generally good with improved quality of life due to changes in functional limitations and somatic symptoms (Broers *et al.* 2000).

Reduced fertility

Radiotherapy and chemotherapy both have harmful effects on gonadal function and the consequences for sexual function and fertility can cause profound emotional distress, contributing to the development of a depressive disorder in the patient, partner or both. Not surprisingly marital discord is not unusual.

The testis is particularly susceptible. The effects of radiotherapy and chemotherapy are mainly on the germinal epithelium, resulting in reduced spermatogenesis. There may also be evidence of hypogonadism. In some malignant conditions there is evidence of reduced spermatogenesis even before treatment starts. During radiotherapy all necessary precautions are taken to shield the testes from exposure to radiation. If chemotherapy is planned the least toxic regime is chosen without reducing efficacy. The effects of treatment on fertility need to be discussed fully with the patient when treatment is being planned. Recovery of testicular function is possible but if it does not recover, storing frozen sperm, cryopreservation, is now widely available for men who indicate they wish to consider fathering children once treatment has been completed. Advanced in-vitro fertilization techniques can improve the chances of fertility if the semen is of poor quality.

Ovarian function is also suppressed following treatment and because there is an absolute number of oocytes the chances of recovery are slight, particularly if the woman is in her late twenties or older at the time of treatment. Women need to be well informed of the likelihood of reduced fertility and of the various options which are available to improve the chances of conception and a successful pregnancy. Counselling should be available to enable the woman to discuss the options at length and to come to a considered and unhurried decision. Amenorrhoea is common and is accompanied by reduced libido and other manifestations of a premature, artificial menopause. Hormone replacement therapy should be considered unless it is contraindicated for other medical reasons. Oocytes can be harvested under ultrasound guidance after artificial ovarian stimulation. Following cryopreservation, in-vitro fertilization can then be attempted. There have also been encouraging reports of pregnancy occurring after cryopreservation of ovarian tissue which is subsequently reimplanted on the ovarian pedicle.

Other organic factors

Cerebral tumours, both primary and secondary, are well known to predispose to psychiatric symptoms in a proportion of cases. These may develop before focal neurological signs, epilepsy or evidence of raised intracranial pressure become manifest and the patient may then initially present to a psychiatrist. Psychiatric symptoms more commonly develop during the course of the illness, once the tumour has been diagnosed. Cognitive changes are well recognized. Disturbance of the level of consciousness is probably the commonest sign and may be accompanied by the entire range of symptoms to fulfil a diagnosis of delirium. Cognitive changes can occur without impairment of consciousness. If the changes affect global intellectual capacity the patient appears to have a dementing process. On the other hand there may be focal deficits such as dysphasia, dyspraxia or an amnesic syndrome. Personality change, without other evidence of dementia, can be a presenting feature of a tumour of the frontal lobe, particularly when this is slowly growing and has not yet caused overt neurological signs. Frontal lobe tumours can also present with classical symptoms of a depressive illness. The onset of psychiatric symptoms for the first time in middle age or later, without any obvious psychological predisposing factors, should raise the suspicion that there is an underlying physical cause and underline the need for thorough medical assessment.

The remote effects of cancer can also lead to the development of neuropsychiatric disorders. In some cases these result from metabolic complications such as hypercalcaemia or hyponatraemia. In other cases the aetiology is thought to be immunologically mediated due to the production by the tumour of antibodies with antineuronal activity. These clinical effects are known as the paraneoplastic syndromes. Encephalomyelitis is one of the complications and typically presents with a clinical picture of delirium. Sometimes the pathology is limited to the limbic system and the resulting limbic encephalomyelitis presents with a rapid onset of memory loss which may be accompanied by anxiety and depression.

Previous stress and psychiatric disorder

Psychiatric disorders following cancer have close links with a patient's mental state prior to diagnosis. There have been suggestions that stressful life events predispose to cancer (Ramirez et al. 1989). The authors of this study found that severely threatening life events were significantly more often experienced by women who developed a first recurrence of breast cancer compared with women whose cancer remained in remission. However the evidence for these claims is conflicting and a subsequent study from the same unit did not replicate the observation (Graham et al. 2002). Stressful life events have a better-established relationship with depressive illness so any patient who has had to deal with a separate major adversity when cancer becomes manifest is more likely to develop depression.

Likewise if a patient has already been depressed prior to diagnosis the depression is likely to recur or to become exacerbated. There is evidence that people who suffer from psychiatric illness are more likely to develop cancer. In an extensive review of the literature Harris and Barraclough (1998) found that the mortality rate from natural causes was twice that expected among a total population of over

50 000 in all psychiatric treatment settings. The death rate from cancer was significantly raised but when analysed by gender this observation applied only to women. The reasons for these observations are not understood but are probably linked to lifestyle habits. The implications for clinical practice are that women who develop cancer are more likely to have been psychiatrically ill prior to diagnosis. The onset of cancer will almost certainly make matters worse for many of them.

Communication with staff

The importance of effective communication has already been discussed in Chapter 4. Nowhere is this more important than in an oncology setting. Providing information to a patient with cancer often involves imparting bad news, both when cancer is initially diagnosed and when clinical examination or special investigations indicate that it has recurred after treatment. Breaking bad news is a task with which many doctors feel uncomfortable. However the manner in which it is handled has an important influence on the level of psychological distress which the patient experiences.

The responsibility for imparting bad news to a patient usually falls to a doctor, either the primary care doctor or a senior hospital specialist. It is appropriate that this is the usual practice but many doctors feel ill-equipped to handle this type of clinical consultation. They find it difficult for several reasons:

- lack of formal training
- uncertainty of patient's reaction
- fear of increasing patient's distress
- damage to doctor–patient relationship
- uncertainty about responding to the patient's questions.

When the medical information about an illness conveys a gloomy prognosis this should not be withheld from the patient. Any notion of protecting patients from bad news is regarded as patronizing and outmoded. However the doctor should consider whether it might be preferable to give this type of information in the presence of a relative. This possibility should be explored with the patient. It is often appropriate to break the news gradually, during more than one consultation, particularly if the patient has a poor understanding of the illness at first. Several logical steps in the process have been recommended (Lloyd & Bor 2004). These are summarized here:

1. *Personal preparation.* Take sufficient time. Consider the patient's existing knowledge of the illness and the patient's personal resources. Prepare for questions the patient may ask. Prepare for dealing with the emotional response.

2. *Physical setting.* Use a room that provides privacy. Whenever possible do not give bad news in an open ward or corridor or over the telephone. The doctor should be seated at a similar level to the patient. This should convey that the doctor is not in a hurry and is going to stay to respond to any questions the patient wishes to ask.

3. *Talking to the patient and responding to concerns.* Proceed slowly and express empathy. Find out what the patient already knows and understands and what he/she wishes to know. Give information incrementally and summarize what the information means. Discuss how the patient has coped with personal difficulties previously. Instil realistic hope.

4. *Arrange follow-up.* A further consultation should be arranged to provide support, to contain the patient's anxiety and to clarify any points which have not been understood at the first interview.

5. *Feedback to colleagues.* Other members of the multidisciplinary team should be informed as soon as possible about the meeting with the patient and know what the patient and relatives have been told.

Screening for cancer

Screening for disease has become a routine practice for several cancers. Regular mammography has been shown to reduce the mortality of breast cancer in older women through earlier detection. It also allows more conservative treatment to be carried out. Cytological examination of cervical smears has long been a standard procedure for detecting precancerous lesions of the cervix and colonoscopy is used to detect cancer at an early stage in those who are predisposed to cancer of the colon, for example those with a family history of polyposis coli. Predictive DNA testing, which provides people with an estimate of the likelihood of their developing a particular disease, is being carried out with increasing frequency but can create some difficult therapeutic decisions for those with positive results. Women who are found to have one of the genes for breast cancer, BRCA1 and 2, are faced with the choice of having regular screening with mammography or undergoing prophylactic bilateral mastectomies. The benefits of screening have to be weighed up against the possible disadvantages, including inducing psychological distress before testing and exacerbating this in those with positive or equivocal results. Fortunately the evidence suggests that screening does not induce psychological symptoms for most who participate in it. A review by Marteau and Croyle (1998) noted that uptake for genetic testing is much higher when effective treatments or preventive strategies are available. Those who undergo screening usually expect negative results while those who believe themselves to be at high risk because of their family history are more prepared for positive results. People receiving positive results are more likely to be distressed but this distress is not usually very severe. Much depends on the quality of counselling which is available before and after testing. Although much research is still required into the most appropriate forms of counselling it is probably important to arrange counselling prior to testing so that the limitations of the test can be discussed together with the implications of a positive or negative result. Further counselling must be arranged once the result is known. A study of the emotional impact of predictive genetic testing found that adults who were low in optimism or self-esteem were more likely to become clinically anxious and it was recommended that counselling should be targeted at those low in psychological resources (Michie *et al.* 2001).

Do psychological factors influence the prognosis?

Many clinicians believe that the way people cope with cancer influences the outcome of the illness. It is implied that those who become significantly anxious or depressed do less well in terms of survival than those who respond with more positive attitudes. There have been a number of studies which have attempted to find support for this hypothesis. Greer *et al.* (1979) identified four different coping styles in a prospective study of women with breast cancer. These were termed fighting spirit, denial, stoic acceptance and helplessness/hopelessness. The coping styles were significantly associated with outcome, recurrence-free survival at five years being positively associated with fighting spirit or denial. Conversely those who coped with stoic acceptance or helplessness/hopelessness had a worse prognosis. These observations were confirmed when outcome was assessed again after eight years.

An important factor which reduces survival is delayed presentation. It seems logical to suspect that psychological factors may have a bearing on this but studies which have attempted to provide support for this belief have failed to do so (Burgess *et al.* 2000; Ramirez *et al.* 1999).

A well-known controlled study reported by Spiegel *et al.* (1989) found that survival time in patients with advanced breast cancer was increased for those who attended weekly group meetings which provided practical and educational support. A similar finding was reported by Fawzy *et al.* (1993) for patients with malignant melanoma who attended what were described as psychoeducational groups. These observations are intriguing but attempts to replicate them have not provided similar conclusions (Goodwin *et al.* 2001). A review by Gwikel *et al.* (1997) concluded that for early malignancy there was inconsistent evidence that psychological factors influenced disease progression, while for advanced malignancy biological factors were paramount, and psychological factors less important, in determining outcome.

Psychiatric disorders and their management

Any of the clinical syndromes described in Chapter 4 may be seen in patients being treated for cancer. Adjustment disorders are probably the commonest. In a survey of patients attending three oncology centres in the United States Derogatis *et al.* (1983) found a 47% prevalence of psychiatric disorder according to operational criteria. A clinical syndrome was diagnosed in 43% while 3% were considered to have a personality disorder. Adjustment disorders accounted for two-thirds of all psychiatric diagnoses. These reactions tend to develop early during the course of the illness, when the patient has to take in the implications of the illness and anticipate the need for treatment. Later on they may develop when follow-up consultations with a doctor are anticipated or when investigations such as blood tests and magnetic resonance imaging (MRI) scans are arranged.

The incidence of delirium in cancer patients is not known but clinical observation suggests that it is common. It is difficult to assess in a standardized manner because it is so evanescent, hence few research studies have been conducted. However it can be a major source of distress because of the frightening hallucinatory experiences and secondary delusions that are so characteristic of the condition. Accurate detection is important so that symptomatic treatment can be given and the underlying causes corrected.

Anxiety may become more prolonged than is compatible with a diagnosis of an adjustment disorder. It tends to be pervasive and unremitting. Specific phobic anxiety can develop in response to treatment, particularly chemotherapy. Watson *et al.* (1992) found that 23% of patients undergoing chemotherapy experienced anticipatory nausea. This can be so severe that patients develop a phobic response and refuse to complete their treatment. Phobic anxiety can also be triggered by being exposed to unfamiliar medical technology such as radiotherapy machines. If this problem is not treated the patient may drop out of treatment and the chances of cure or remission are lost.

Screening questionnaires have been used in several research studies to identify those likely to have developed a psychiatric disorder. The Hospital Anxiety and Depression Scale (HADS; Zigmond & Snaith 1983) is one of the most commonly used instruments. Pinder *et al.* (1993) assessed a series of women with advanced breast cancer and found that 25% obtained scores that indicated that they were probable cases of anxiety and/or depression and were therefore likely to benefit from psychosocial intervention. Clinical anxiety was not related to any sociodemographic or disease factors. Clinical depression was more prevalent among patients in lower socioeconomic classes and among those with poor performance status. A lower prevalence was found by Sharpe *et al.* (2004a) in the study referred to previously in this chapter. These authors have developed a nurse-delivered multicomponent intervention for major depression and preliminary results suggest the intervention is effective in reducing the severity of depression (Sharpe *et al.* 2004b). Fallowfield *et al.* (2001) had previously observed that doctors find it difficult to diagnose psychiatric illness in cancer patients. Much of the morbidity goes unrecognized and untreated and it was recommended that clinicians need training in communication skills to help them elicit psychological problems during consultations.

Suicide is a risk that has to be assessed in any patient who is depressed and cancer patients who are depressed are known to be at increased risk. Harris and Barraclough (1994) conducted a literature search of reports of 63 medical disorders said to have an increased suicide risk. Malignant neoplasms as a group and head and neck cancers in particular were among the disorders associated with an increased risk of suicide. The risk was highest immediately following diagnosis, one study indicating that 40% of the suicides occurred within the first year. There was a suggestion that the risk was highest in those with advanced or rapidly progressive disease. There was also a link with tumour site. The highest rates were reported for tumours of the lung, upper airways, gastrointestinal tract, central nervous system, pancreas and kidney. Lower risk was associated with tumours of the breast and female genital tract, probably reflecting the lower risk of suicide among women in general.

Sexual dysfunction is common among cancer patients. Loss of desire, impotence and anorgasmia are the most frequent complaints. During chemotherapy many patients experience a profound loss of libido due to the debilitating effects of the treatment but sexual interest is usually regained when treatment is completed. Sexual problems following surgery such as mastectomy or colectomy with colostomy usually result from a perceived loss of attractiveness on the part of the patient and partner. Referral to a therapist trained in psychosexual medicine often helps these patients. Psychosexual therapists can also help patients with hormone-dependent tumours who have undergone medical or surgical hormone removal.

Emotional support

Much distress can be averted if the cancer doctor can provide emotional support throughout the course of the patient's illness. Patients generally welcome an open relationship and develop trust if they believe the doctor is being frank with them about the nature of the illness, the treatment and the prognosis. Many studies have confirmed that patients wish to be as fully informed as possible. Medical concerns that disclosing the truth about cancer would be psychologically detrimental have not been borne out. Once the diagnosis has been established and discussed with the patient it is important to allow distress to be expressed and acknowledged and to enable further questions to be asked. This is a process which will need to be conducted over a number of consultations. Patients often feel inhibited from mentioning their emotional concerns, believing that nothing can be done for them or that doctors and nurses are too busy or not sufficiently interested to respond to their problems. For their part, professional staff often distance themselves from emotional problems, partly as a means of self-protection and partly because they fear that they will not be able to manage the patient's emotional response. There is also a widely held belief that depression is inevitable at some stage in the treatment of cancer and that it is largely untreatable.

To overcome these barriers doctors need to ask open-ended but directive questions about patients' understanding of their illness, their emotional response and their worries about the effects on their family and social network. It is important to demonstrate an empathic approach and to pick up on any cues the patient may give about emotional problems. If the doctor or nurse reflects these back the patient will realize that the psychological as well as the physical dimension of the illness is being taken into account.

Counselling

Many cancer centres have established specific counselling services to help manage the emotional problems associated with cancer. This development has been made easier by the practice of concentrating cancer treatment in large regional centres so that there is a sufficient demand for professionals to help manage the increasing numbers of patients who are receiving treatment. Counsellors are trained in communication skills and in the principles of counselling within a cancer service. They usually have a background in nursing, psychology or psychotherapy. They may already have an extensive knowledge of cancer and cancer services but if not they need to acquire this knowledge during their training because counselling incorporates an educational role which is important for correcting any misunderstanding about the diagnosis, treatment and prognosis. Counsellors must not be used as an excuse for doctors to avoid imparting information and exploring psychological issues, but in the context of a busy service a counsellor is likely to be able to spend more time in face-to-face contact with the patient. Counsellors are well placed to detect any serious disorder of mood, anxiety or psychotic symptoms which require assessment and treatment by a psychiatrist. It is therefore important for a counsellor to have ready access to a psychiatrist and a psychologist who themselves have experience of working in an oncology service. This access is facilitated if there are regular meetings where cases are discussed and supervision is provided.

Providing information

Given that lack of information is a common complaint among cancer patients it is not surprising that there has been a proliferation of services established to help fill the information gap. Cody and Slevin (2002) have listed some of the better known services in the UK, Europe, the United States and Australia. One of the first to be established in the UK was the British Association for Cancer United Patients, founded by a physician, Vicky Clement-Jones, who herself had developed cancer and who was struck by the lack of information available to patients. Now known as CancerBACUP this is a national service which provides information and support by telephone and letter and on-line. It is staffed by trained oncology nurses who have access to up-to-date information across the range of malignant disorders. They are supported by a medical advisory board whom they can consult for advice on more obscure problems. The organization publishes leaflets and booklets which advise on symptom control, sexuality, diet, complementary therapies and living with cancer. Other organizations provide advice and support for patients and families coping with specific problems such as colostomy, laryngectomy, breast cancer and leukaemia.

Psychological therapies

Specific psychological treatment is needed for some problems. Behaviour therapy based on relaxation and desensitization successfully treats those who develop phobic anxiety towards certain aspects of their care. These phobias include having blood taken, receiving chemotherapy and undergoing radiotherapy. Clinicians need to be able to refer rapidly to a clinical psychologist or a nurse who has trained in behaviour therapy.

Spiegel et al. (1981) evaluated the effect of group support for women with breast cancer and found that, compared with the control group, those who participated in the treatment groups had lower levels of mood disturbance, fewer maladaptive coping responses and fewer phobic symptoms. The groups were designed to be supportive and to foster a high degree of cohesion. There was relatively little confrontation. Treatment focused on improving relationship with family, friends and physicians and living as fully as possible in the face of a terminal illness. When the survival of patients was subsequently examined it was found that those in the treatment groups also had longer survival times (Spiegel et al. 1989). Fawzy et al. (1993) have shown similar effects for psychological treatment among patients with malignant melanoma. Patients were treated in a group setting, the intervention consisting of enhancement of problem-solving skills, stress management, and psychological support. The patients in the treatment group showed significantly lower depression, fatigue and total mood disturbance and also had longer survivals. However in the study reported by Goodwin *et al.* (2001) group therapy did not prolong survival time but it did improve patients' mood and reduce perception of pain.

A cognitive behavioural treatment has been developed specifically for cancer patients (Moorey & Greer 1989). Referred to as adjuvant psychological therapy this focuses on the individual meaning of cancer and on the patient's coping strategies, namely what the patient thinks and does to reduce the threat posed by cancer. Several techniques are employed during the sessions which are conducted with individual patients and, where appropriate, with a partner. Treatment aims at identifying personal strengths and fostering these to raise self-esteem. Overcoming helplessness and promoting a fighting spirit are also facilitated and the patient is taught to identify and challenge negative automatic thoughts underlying the anxiety and depression. Activities are encouraged that provide a sense both of achievement and pleasure, enabling some control over the patient's life to be regained. Expression of feelings and open communication with a partner are encouraged and patients are also taught techniques of progressive muscular relaxation.

Applying these techniques, in a controlled study, to patients with a wide range of cancers Greer *et al.* (1992) showed that patients undergoing therapy had lower levels of anxiety, psychological symptoms and psychological distress after four months than did the control group who received no treatment. These effects were maintained on longer follow-up. However Moynihan *et al.* (1998) did not find positive results when they applied a similar therapeutic approach to men with testicular cancer. Cognitive behaviour therapy is not widely available for cancer patients but it is being used in some large cancer centres to help patients cope with the psychological distress of their illness. More evaluation is required to determine which patients are likely to respond to this approach.

Physical treatments for depression

Few controlled trials of antidepressant drugs have been conducted with cancer patients but there is some evidence to support their efficacy (Costa *et al.* 1985; Evans *et al.* 1988). They are used widely in clinical practice and the selective serotonin reuptake inhibitors (SSRIs) have replaced the older tricyclic group as the drugs of first choice. Given that many cancer patients are already taking a number of other drugs, it is important to minimize drug interactions and citalopram and sertraline are the safest in this respect. However SSRIs may not be the best antidepressants to use in women taking tamoxifen for breast cancer because there is evidence that they reduce blood levels of tamoxifen metabolites (Jin *et al.* 2005).

For resistant, severe depression electroconvulsive treatment (ECT) can be used safely, even for those with cerebral tumours, but no controlled trials of ECT have been conducted in patients with cancer.

Complementary therapies

Complementary therapies have acquired a great following among the general public, in contrast to the scepticism they meet from the medical profession. Patients with cancer may be particularly attracted to non-conventional treatments if they believe that orthodox medicine has little to offer them. Faith healing, homeopathy, aromatherapy and reflexology are among the treatments to which patients resort. To date no type of complementary therapy has been found to be effective in a controlled trial but many patients report beneficial effects and are willing to spend substantial sums of money if they think they are deriving benefit. Research is urgently required to establish whether any of the currently available therapies have more than a placebo effect.

REFERENCES

Baker, F., Marcellus, D., Zabora, J., et al. (1997). Psychological distress among adult patients being evaluated for bone marrow transplantation. *Psychosomatics*, **38**, 10–19.

Boshoff, C. and Weiis, R. (2002). AIDS-related malignancies. *National Review of Cancer*, **2**, 373–82.

Broers, S., Kaptein, A. A., Le Cessie, S., et al. (2000). Psychological functioning and quality of life following bone marrow transplantation: a 3-year follow-up study. *Journal of Psychosomatic Research*, **48**, 11–21.

Burgess, C. C., Ramirez, A. J., Smith, P., et al. (2000). Do adverse life events and mood disorders influence delayed presentation of breast cancer? *Journal of Psychosomatic Research*, **48**, 171–5.

Cody, M. and Slevin, M. (2002). Support services for cancer patients. In *Oxford Textbook of Oncology*, 2nd edn., ed. R. L. Souhami, I. Tannock, P. Hohenberger, et al. Oxford: Oxford University Press, pp. 1079–87.

Costa, E., Mogos, I. and Toma, T. (1985). Efficacy and safety of mianserin in the treatment of depression in women with breast cancer. *Acta Psychiatrica Scandinavica*, **72**, 85–92.

Cull, A. (1990). Psychological aspects of cancer and chemotherapy. *Journal of Psychosomatic Research*, **34**, 129–40.

Derogatis, L. R., Morrow, G. R., Fetting, J., et al. (1983). The prevalence of psychiatric disorders among cancer patients. *Journal of the American Medical Association*, **249**, 751–7.

Evans, D. L., McCartney, C. F. and Haggery, J. J. (1988). Treatment of depression in cancer patients is associated with better life adaptation: a pilot study. *Psychosomatic Medicine*, **50**, 72–6.

Fallowfield, L., Hall, A., Maguire, G. P., *et al.* (1990). Psychological outcomes in women with early breast cancer. *British Medical Journal*, **301**, 1394.

Fallowfield, L., Ratcliffe, D., Jenkins, V., *et al.* (2001). Psychiatric morbidity and its recognition by doctors in patients with cancer. *British Journal of Cancer*, **84**, 1011–15.

Fawzy, I. F., Fawzy, N. W., Hyun, C. S., *et al.* (1993). Effects of an early structured psychiatric intervention, coping and affective state on recurrence and survival 6 years later. *Archives of General Psychiatry*, **50**, 681–9.

Goodwin, P. J., Leszcz, M., Ennis, M., *et al.* (2001). The effect of group psychosocial support on survival in metastatic breast cancer. *New England Journal of Medicine*, **345**, 1719–26.

Graham, J., Ramirez, A., Love, S., *et al.* (2002). Stressful life experiences and risk of relapse of breast cancer: observational cohort study. *British Medical Journal*, **324**, 1420.

Greer, S., Morris, T. and Pettingale, K. W. (1979). Psychological response to breast cancer: effect on outcome. *Lancet*, **ii**, 785–7.

Greer, S., Moorey, S., Baruch, J. D. R., *et al.* (1992). Adjuvant psychological therapy for patients with cancer: a prospective randomised trial. *British Medical Journal*, **304**, 675–80.

Gwikel, J. G., Behar, L. C. and Zabora, J. R. (1997). Psychosocial factors that affect the survival of cancer patients: a review of research. *Journal of Psychosocial Oncology*, **15**, 1–34.

Harris, E. C. and Barraclough, B. M. (1994). Suicide as an outcome for medical disorders. *Medicine (Baltimore)*, **73**, 297–8.

Harris, E. C. and Barraclough, B. (1998). Excess mortality of mental disorder. *British Journal of Psychiatry*, **173**, 11–53.

Jin, Y., Desta, Z., Stearns, V., *et al.* (2005). CYP2D6 genotype, antidepressant use and tamoxifen metabolism during adjuvant breast cancer treatment. *Journal of the National Cancer Institute*, **97**, 30–9.

Lloyd, M. and Bor, R. (2004). *Communication Skills for Medicine*, 2nd edn. Edinburgh: Churchill Livingstone.

Marteau, T. M. and Croyle, R. T. (1998). Psychological responses to genetic testing. *British Medical Journal*, **316**, 693–6.

McDaniel, J. S., Musselman, D. L., Porter, M. R., *et al.* (1995). Depression in patients with cancer: diagnosis, biology and treatment. *Archives of General Psychiatry*, **52**, 89–99.

Michie, S., Bobrow, M. and Marteau, T. M. (2001). Predictive genetic testing in children and adults: a study of emotional impact. *Journal of Medical Genetics*, **38**, 519–26.

Moorey, S. and Greer, S. (1989). *Psychological Therapy for Patients with Cancer: a New Approach*. Oxford: Heinemann Medical.

Moynihan, C., Bliss, J. M., Davidson, J., *et al.* (1998). Evaluation of adjuvant psychological therapy in patients with testicular cancer: randomised controlled trial. *British Medical Journal*, **316**, 429–35.

Parle, M., Jones, B. and Maguire, P. (1996). Maladaptive coping and affective disorders in cancer patients. *Psychological Medicine*, **26**, 735–44.

Pinder, K. L., Ramirez, A. J., Black, M. E., *et al.* (1993). Psychiatric disorders in patients with advanced breast cancer: prevalence and associated factors. *European Journal of Cancer*, **29A**, 524–7.

Ramirez, A. J., Craig, T. K., Watson, J. P., *et al.* (1989). Stress and relapse of breast cancer. *British Medical Journal*, **298**, 291–3.

Ramirez, A. J., Westcombe, A. M., Burgess, C. C., *et al.* (1999). Factors predicting delayed presentation of symptomatic breast cancer: a systematic review. *Lancet*, **353**, 1127–31.

Sharpe, M., Strong, V., Allen, K., *et al.* (2004a). Major depression in patients attending a regional cancer centre: screening and unmet treatment needs. *British Journal of Cancer*, **90**, 314–20.

Sharpe, M., Strong, V., Allen, K., *et al.* (2004b). Management of major depression in outpatients attending a cancer centre: a preliminary evaluation of a multicomponent cancer nurse-delivered intervention. *British Journal of Cancer*, **90**, 310–13.

Spiegel, D., Bloom, J. R. and Yalom, I. (1981). Group therapy for patients with metastatic cancer. *Archives of General Psychiatry*, **38**, 527–33.

Spiegel, D., Bloom, J. R., Kraemer, H. C., *et al.* (1989). Effect of psychosocial intervention on survival of patients with metastatic cancer. *Lancet*, **2**(8668), 888–91.

Watson, M., McCarron, J. and Law, M. (1992). Anticipatory nausea and emesis, and psychological morbidity: assessment of prevalence among outpatients on mild to moderate chemotherapy regimens. *British Journal of Cancer*, **66**, 862–6.

Zabora, J. R., Blanchard, C. G., Smith, E. D., *et al.* (1997). Prevalence of psychological distress among cancer patients across the disease continuum. *Journal of Psychosocial Oncology*, **15**, 73–87.

Zigmond, A. S. and Snaith, R. P. (1983). The Hospital Anxiety and Depression Scale. *Acta Psychatrica Scandinavica*, **67**, 361–70.

24

Head and neck cancer

Gerry Humphris

Introduction

Head and neck cancer is the sixth most common cancer worldwide and within the developed world ranks third (Boyle *et al.* 1992; Parkin *et al.* 1999). Ninety per cent of these cancers are squamous cell carcinomas, and comprise 4% of all cancers in the USA and 5% in the UK. Internationally there has been an increase in central and eastern Europe (Macfarlane *et al.* 1994). An incidence of 10.2 lip, mouth and pharyngeal cancers per 100 000 population in the UK in 1996 was reported (2940 new cases) (Quin 2001). Men are more likely than women to succumb to the disease by a ratio of 3:1 although this disparity between the sexes is becoming less pronounced in the UK.

Mortality rates are high at 54% overall (Johnson 2002). A cohort of 200 oral cancer patients from the north-west of England showed an overall two-year survival probability of 72% falling to 64% at five years (Woolgar *et al.* 1999). Prognosis of small oral cancer lesions is better than large lesions. For instance, the median survival time of a patient with a lesion greater than 4 cm in diameter is four years less than a patient of similar age with a smaller lesion (Platz *et al.* 1986). The overall health of head and neck cancer patients tends to be worse than their age-matched counterparts in the general public (Funk *et al.* 1997).

Recurrence rates for head and neck cancer are comparatively high. In the series of 200 patients reported by Woolgar *et al.* (1999) the local recurrence rate resulting in death was 18%. In total 38% had relapse with further malignancy (comprising local and regional disease, metachronous primary tumours or systemic metastases) following initial treatment.

Handbook of Liaison Psychiatry, ed. Geoffrey Lloyd and Elspeth Guthrie. Published by Cambridge University Press. © Cambridge University Press 2007.

Investigation

Primary care doctors detect most tumours on complaint of soreness in the mouth by their patients, and although general medical practitioners (GMPs) were enthusiastic about their role in detecting mouth cancer they were adamant that this task should be the major remit of the dentist (Ogden 2003). Referral guidelines are available for health professionals (British Dental Association 2000; Department of Health 2000). Although screening has been investigated as a possible intervention to reduce mortality due to this disease, many practical difficulties have been reported (Jullien *et al.* 1995; Rodrigues *et al.* 1998; Speight *et al.* 1993) unless conducted opportunistically (Lim *et al.* 2003).

Treatment

Survival rates for head and neck cancer have remained virtually static over the past 30 years (La Vecchia *et al.* 1997; Swango 1996). Having said this, survival is dependent on severity, with tumours that are diagnosed early eminently curable (Sanderson & Ironside 2002). Treatment consists of three modalities including surgery, radiotherapy and chemotherapy, either singly or in combination. Many head and neck cancer patients are treated with high-dose radiotherapy, which as a consequence also irradiates associated sensitive tissues such as mucous membranes, nerves and circulatory structures (Specht 2002). Increasing intensity of treatment has produced significant improvements to outcome but has raised the incidence of side-effects (Specht 2002). Delay (greater than six weeks) in starting radiotherapy following surgery has been shown to be detrimental to five-year local recurrence rate in head and neck cancer patients (Huang *et al.* 2003).

Public health issues

There is a lack of knowledge of oral cancer among the wider public (Bhatti *et al.* 1995; Canto *et al.* 1998; Horowitz *et al.* 1998; Humphris *et al.* 1999; Warnakulasuriya *et al.* 1999). Some attempts have been made recently to improve public awareness, especially for signs and symptoms (Cruz *et al.* 2002; Humphris *et al.* 2001a, b). Some mass-media approaches have been planned to encourage recognition of the disease, highlight risk factors and encourage earlier seeking for advice and assessment of suspicious lesions (Conway *et al.* 2002). Positive messages can be presented as early identification improves survival markedly (Hollows *et al.* 2000). There is some evidence that these health education programmes have stronger effects with people at higher risk, for example smokers (Boundouki *et al.* 2004; Humphris & Field 2004). Calls have been made for educational programmes to be focused on health professionals to alert them to the early identification of the disease and encouraging their patients to reduce high-risk behaviours such as smoking tobacco and excess alcohol intake (Horowitz *et al.* 2000).

Prevention

The prevention of head and neck cancer has relied principally on early identification, a careful review programme for patients with precancerous signs and exhortations to quit smoking and moderate excessive alcohol consumption. A further example is the recommendation to those originating from the Indian subcontinent to refrain from chewing 'paan' which is a known carcinogen and responsible for elevated levels of oral cancer in this ethnic group (Pearson *et al.* 2001).

Chemoprevention

The role of chemoprevention has been investigated with some encouraging possibilities signalled in current research trials (Ogden & Macluskey 2000). However, the benefits of these procedures are dependent on high compliance and also reducing high-risk behaviours such as tobacco smoking.

Risk factors

Tobacco

Approximately 30–40% of treated patients continue to smoke following initial treatment (Allison 2001). Patients who continue to smoke after diagnosis of head and neck cancer show a fourfold increase in recurrence rate compared to a control group (Stevens *et al.* 1983) and treatment is compromised (Browman *et al.* 1993).

Alcohol

Alcoholism prior to diagnosis is correlated with increased mortality five years post-diagnosis (Deleyiannis *et al.* 1996). Patients who drink heavily and smoke suffer an increased risk as 'tobacco synergizes with alcohol' (Johnson 2001). This risk is 'super-multiplicative' for the mouth. According to Johnson the rise in oral cancer in the West is a result of increased alcohol consumption.

Diet

There is mounting evidence that diet plays a small but independent role in the risk profile of oral and oropharyngeal cancers. Some studies are arguing that a high intake of vegetables and fruits confers a beneficial effect on the risk of developing these cancers (Sanchez *et al.* 2003).

Oral hygiene

Little evidence has been reported for a link between poor oral hygiene and oral cancer (Zakrzewska 1999), although a report from Poland suggests an independent effect of low frequency of toothbrushing and dental visits (Lissowska *et al.* 2003).

Sexual practices

The association between the human papilloma virus and oral cancer risk has been reported (Giovannelli *et al.* 2002; Herrero *et al.* 2003). This virus, implicated already in cervical cancer, may be a causative agent in oral cancer. Hence a number of studies have attempted to associate sexual practices with oral cancer risk. Some international studies report mixed findings (Herrero *et al.* 2003). In India for example, men who engage in oral sex were at greater risk (OR 3.14) whereas women with more than one sexual partner during life were at increased risk (OR 9.93) (Rajkumar *et al.* 2003). The Polish study quoted above found no effect of sexual practices on risk estimates (Lissowska *et al.* 2003). The difficulties of gaining information through interviews and relying on factual memories make this investigation difficult.

Psychological morbidity associated with diagnosis and treatment

An article in the *British Journal of Cancer* reported that oncologists are poor at recognizing distress in cancer patients (Sollner *et al.* 2001). The study was conducted in Austria with patients ($n=239$) diagnosed with various sites of disease. Interestingly, this limitation was greatest in patients with lung, and head and neck cancer. Although recognition of anxiety and depression by health professionals is poor, many studies have catalogued the incidence and prevalence of psychological distress in patients suffering with cancer (Sellnick & Crooks 1999). (See Chapter 23.)

An important threat to the overall wellbeing of patients with head and neck cancer is increased psychological distress (Frampton 2001; Hassanein *et al.* 2001). Considerable effort has been expended to estimate the level of psychological morbidity in patients recently diagnosed with cancer and at longer-term follow-up (Rogers *et al.* 1999, 2002). Head and neck cancer patients ($n=107$) who have serious disease (odds ratio, 5.77) or who live alone (odds ratio, 4.83) were found to be more likely to suffer psychological distress (Kugaya *et al.* 2000). The patients were assessed by structured psychiatric interview and by the Hospital Anxiety and Depression Scale (HAD) screening instrument (Zigmond & Snaith 1983). What is less clear is how both anxiety and depression develop over time following initial diagnosis of cancer (Nordin 2001). Although distress (30% 'cases') has been found in long-term survivors (> six years; Bjordal & Kaasa 1995), the immediate impact of diagnosis and treatment is an important phase for detailed study (Hammerlid *et al.* 1999a). This uncertainty explains a general issue that arises in psycho-oncolgy, as there is little consensus for when interventions are best placed to assist patients with cancer (Fawzy 1999).

One of the most extensive studies of anxiety and depression in this group has shown a high incidence of anxiety (35%) soon after diagnosis, and peak levels of depression (30%) about three months following initial treatment (Hammerlid *et al.* 1999a). Rates of anxiety and depression were estimated from using a cut-off score of seven on each subscale of the HAD to indicate a 'possible' case. Examining the profiles of these two assessments of psychological distress over the course of 12 months reveals some interesting findings. First, anxiety rises soon after diagnosis, whereas depression takes 3 months to reach a peak. Secondly, the rates of both constructs return almost to pretreatment

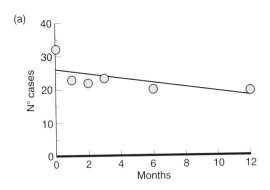

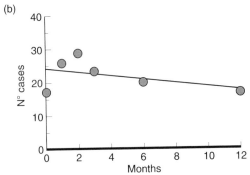

Figure 24.1. Possible cases (scores ≥8) of (a) anxiety and (b) depression on the Hospital Anxiety and Depression subscales on cohort of patients with head and neck cancer (Hammerlid *et al.* 1999a).

level by 12 months (see Figure 24.1). Local work in the north-west of England by Humphris and Rogers using the same measures had shown comparable rates at 3 months following treatment (anxiety: 37%, depression: 28%, $n = 87$; Humphris 2001).

Moderators of psychological distress

A number of factors are associated with the extent of distress experienced from diagnosis and treatment of this disease (see Table 24.1). As previously mentioned disease characteristics and course of treatment can have some influence on the patients' responses; however, psychosocial variables have been clearly implicated in the development of anxiety and depression in this group.

Quality-of-life studies

In the head and neck and oral cancer field there has been a rapid increase in the number of studies investigating patients' quality of life (Ringash & Bezjak 2001). In the period from 1980 to 1998 there have been 108 articles on oral and oropharyngeal cancers. Of these, 14 were published in the 1980s whereas 94 were in the 1990s with 21 studies reported in 2000 alone (Rogers 2002). A variety of instruments have been developed (see Table 24.2) and eight of these measures have been critically reviewed (Ringash & Bezjak 2001). For a description of the studies from 1980 up to 1998 see Rogers *et al.* (1999), and for an update Rogers (2002).

Cross-sectional and longitudinal studies have been conducted (Bjordal *et al.* 1998; Graeff 2000; Hassan & Weymuller 1993; Rogers *et al.* 1999, 2002; Weymuller *et al.* 2000). All measures have the capability to produce numerical

Table 24.1. Moderators of psychological distress in head and neck cancer patients.

Quality of life
Information
Fears of recurrence
Illness representations
Self-care behaviour
Intrusive thoughts
Appearance
Social support

Table 24.2. Selected quality-of-life instruments used in head and neck cancer studies.

	Abbreviation	Developer
General cancer-related measures		
European Organization of Research and Treatment of Cancer Quality of Life Core Questionnaire	EORTC-QoL C33[a]	Aaronson *et al.* (1993)
Specific disease-related measures		
European Organization of Research and Treatment of Cancer Quality of Life Head and Neck Questionnaire	EORTC-QoL H&N35	Bjordal & Kaasa (1992); Bjordal *et al.* (1994)
University of Washington Quality of Life Questionnaire	UoW-QoLv4[b]	Hassan & Weymuller (1993)
Functional Assessment of Cancer Therapy H&N	FACT-HN	List *et al.* (1996)
Performance Status Scale for Head and Neck Cancer	PSS-HN	List *et al.* (1990)

Notes: [a]Recommended version; [b]latest published version (Rogers *et al.* 2002).

scores that enable comparative analysis across patient groups. The scale scores derived have been used as additional outcome measures for evaluating new treatment procedures (Kuntz & Weymuller 1999). One set of investigators has conducted an in-depth analysis of the free written comments of patients supplied on the final sheet of the instrument form (Millsopp *et al.* 2003). Free-text comments were made on 40% of questionnaires and their frequency was independent of clinico-demographic characteristics. The majority of comments referred to head and neck (39%), medical (35%) and psychological (20%) issues, although other issues were also noted including social (11%) and administrative (16%). The free-text statements were negative in 55% of cases. Twenty-four per cent of the comments were not part of a validated health-related quality of life (HRQoL) head and neck measure and therefore gave information about additional concerns. Free-text is not widely used in research because of the inherent problems with analysis, however for the clinician and the team in a cancer unit greater insight can be gained with this approach.

One important longitudinal study was conducted in Sweden of 232 head and neck cancer patients over a three-year period from diagnosis. Quality of life was studied using the EORTC QLQ-C30, which assesses core aspects, and the EORTC QLQ H&N35, a specific module for head and neck cancer (Hammerlid *et al.* 2001). In addition anxiety and depression were assessed adopting the

HAD scale. After three years two-thirds (66%) of the patients were still alive. The health-related quality of life reduced to its lowest point immediately after treatment. However, virtually all of the subscales returned to pretreatment levels after 12 months. Dry mouth, sexual responsiveness and dentition were significant problems which tended not to improve with time. There were very few changes occurring between the one- and three-year assessments. Mental distress made the strongest improvement after three years, whereas global quality of life increased as the next most significant change. Depression and physical functioning predicted independently global quality of life at three years. Patients with advanced disease (stages III and IV) scored poorly on virtually all HRQoL domains which exacerbated over time. Other longitudinal studies tracking HRQoL adopting standardized instruments have reported a rise of quality of life on virtually all domains to pretreatment levels after one year post-treatment (Rogers *et al.* 1998). A smaller study using the FACT-H&N and the HAD scale with 58 outpatients with head and neck cancer from first week of treatment to one month post-treatment found physical and functional well-being improving, but depression showed no significant change (Rose & Yates 2001).

The extensive work of de Graeff and de Leeuw with longitudinal assessment of quality of life and depression in head and neck cancer patients at the University Medical Centre of Utrecht has shed light on the prediction of HRQoL. Raised depressive symptoms at pretreatment predicted similar difficulties at 6 and 12 months later including physical functioning (de Graeff *et al.* 2000a). Prediction of depressed status (Centre of Epidemiological Studies Depression scale) was 81% and 67% at the two time periods, 6 and 12 months respectively. These percentages increased to 89% and 82% if the patients' physical symptoms at the time of assessment were entered into the explanatory model. The authors recommend that the routine screening of psychosocial variables and physical symptoms before treatment may help to identify patients who may be susceptible to depression on recovery from surgery and/or radiotherapy for head and neck cancer (de Leeuw *et al.* 2000a). This group have reported similar analyses for a cohort of 107 patients and found a gradual improvement in depressive symptomatology over the course of three years (de Graeff *et al.* 2000b). They also report that prediction using eight pretreatment variables (tumour stage, sex, depressive symptoms, openness to discuss cancer in the family, available appraisal support, received emotional support, tumour-related symptoms and size of informal social network) determined which patients were depressed at six months to three years after treatment (de Leeuw *et al.* 2001).

The field of quality-of-life assessment has been the focus of debate recently to determine the clinical usefulness apart from the research benefits in assessing newly developed treatments (Rampling *et al.* 2003). Opinions vary although some consensus has been agreed on the minimum data required to assess the value of the therapeutic input of a particular treatment centre or intervention (Rogers & Radford 2002). However key questions still remain in the interpretation of the scores derived from these measures. These are recognized as problems for oncology in general and not just the head and neck speciality, and can be summarized as when to use proxy respondents, the phenomena of 'response shift' and interpreting QoL results from a meaningful clinical perspective (Sprangers 2002).

An interesting finding in a six-year longitudinal study with 133 patients with head and neck cancer was that the intensity of psychosocial complaints, that is feeling angry, irritable, tense, and anxious, was significantly associated with remaining recurrence-free ($p = 0.007$; de Boer *et al.* 1998). The only other variable (out of 16 variables entered simultaneously) that had a greater predictive power was extent of nodal metastases ($p = 0.003$). A lack of physical self-efficacy, that is physical ability and confidence, was also related to recurrence ($p = 0.018$).

Information

Patients vary considerably in the extent of the information that they wish to receive from healthcare providers. Some evidence suggests that the adequacy of information received by patients with head and neck cancer has implications for positive recovery some two to six years later (de Boer *et al.* 1999). Although patients may not appear to exhibit detailed knowledge of the options available for treatment, or the recommended practices for rehabilitation and aftercare following initial treatment, they will have their own beliefs and expectations. These will be based upon their own experiences of family members and/or friends who may have received treatment for cancer already. Of course it is likely that these contacts will have suffered other cancers and the range and types of treatments may differ significantly from those recommended for oral and oropharyngeal cancer. This issue of illness and treatment representations is discussed later in this chapter. Patients suffer undue anxiety because they do not understand the treatment they receive which is partially a function of the supply of limited information in a comprehensible form (Krupat *et al.* 2000). A number of authorities and voluntary groups have produced materials to satisfy the need for information reported by a sizeable proportion of patients. These organizations produce electronically accessible versions of leaflets and booklets aimed at patients at all stages of the diagnostic and treatment process. Little research has yet been reported on the frequency of access of this material and it is possible that the

Table 24.3. Sources of information for patients, carers and healthcare personnel.

Organization	Website
Restorative Dentistry Oncology	www.rdoc.org.uk
Faculty of Dental Surgery, Royal College of Surgeons of England. *Clinical Guidelines: the Management of Oncology Patients*	www.rcseng.ac.uk/fds/clinical_guidelines
Cancer Research UK	www.cancer.org.uk
International Psycho-Oncology Society	www.ipos-society.org
Cancer BACUP	www.cancerbacup.org.uk
National Cancer Institute	www.cancer.gov/cancer_information
Patient-centred cancer information	www.ican4u.com
Oral Cancer Foundation	www.oralcancerfoundation.org

typical patient with head and neck cancer will not have easy access or the computer skills to utilize this resource. Notable examples of websites that feature topic areas of relevance to patients, carers and health personnel are listed in Table 24.3.

Some authors have attempted to assess the level of information that patients require. For example, a systematic approach has been reported which tests a new measure of information needs for cancer patients (Mesters *et al.* 2001). This presents results in a study of 133 head and neck cancer patients which confirms that the new scale assesses two aspects: information on help and support that may be available, and on disease and treatment. Increased information needs were apparent in those who were more anxious and depressed. There were significant changes over time post-treatment (6, 13 and 52 weeks) in the amount of information required on disease and treatment.

In a different study with 49 patients questioned about their hospital experience following treatment for oral cancer it was found that those who were dissatisfied with the level of information were not reassured by family support, suggesting that the hospital service has a unique role in helping to explain uncertainties following treatment (Broomfield *et al.* 1997).

Fears of recurrence

Once treatment has been completed, some relief may be expressed due to fewer demands being placed upon the individual and immediate carers. However, this eagerly awaited step is often tinged with increased anxiety and distress

(Maher 1982). The stage has been referred to as the 'neutral time' when recurrence fears or the Damocles syndrome surfaces (Hurt *et al.* 1994). Although there are few studies that assess fears of recurrence, some evidence suggests that it is a major concern. For example, in a sample of 362 Canadians treated for a malignancy not less than six months previously 42% reported that fear of recurrence was their greatest concern (Charles *et al.* 1996).

The work of Maguire and colleagues has shown that health-related concerns have the potential to cause depression (Harrison & Maguire 1994). What appears to have the potential to precipitate an episode of depression is when these health concerns are not allowed expression during contact with the healthcare services. One concern not specifically addressed by the Maguire team was fear of recurrence. However, in a reanalysis of the verbatim reports originally coded as concerns about illness, treatment and the future collected at the CR-UK (formerly CRC) Unit of Psychological Medicine at the Christies Hospital, University of Manchester, the most frequently quoted comment was fear of recurrence (Winter 2002). A survey by Broomfield and Humphris showed that fear of recurrence was indeed the most frequently ranked concern of the 13 concerns listed in a questionnaire developed by Maguire *et al.* (Broomfield 1998).

One study has reported the relationship of concerns with psychological disorder in 50 consecutive head and neck cancer patients in India (Chaturvedi *et al.* 1996). These patients showed a significant relationship between the number of concerns and 'caseness'. However, these investigators did not focus on recurrence fears specifically. From a series of interviews ($n = 10$) with oral facial cancer patients (squamous cell carcinomas, all treated by surgery alone or adjunct radiotherapy) at the Regional Maxillofacial Unit at Aintree, Liverpool, uncertainty about the future and whether the disease would return was a common theme of discussion.

A cognitive formulation has been proposed to explain how patients' fears of recurrence are raised (Lee-Jones *et al.* 1997). Strikingly, the patients described their experience of recovery as one of frequent false alarms predicated by unusual sensations, such as tingling, pins and needles, rapid swelling and sensitivity to hot and cold. These sensations were interpreted as triggers to indicate the return, or the development of new, symptoms. This pattern of experiences fits the Common Sense Model of Illness developed by Leventhal (Leventhal *et al.* 1980, 1984, 1992). This and other work prompted the development of the AFTER (Adjustment to Fears, Threat or Expectation to Recurrence) intervention described later. Psychological distress and fears of recurrence were noted at three and seven months following initial treatment. The association between fears of recurrence and psychological distress are illustrated in Table 24.4 showing

Table 24.4. Prospective study: association of fears of recurrence with anxiety and depression as assessed by the HAD scale subscales.

	3 months			7 months		
	n	(%)	Base	n	(%)	Base
Anxiety possible caseness						
Fear of recurrence						
No concern	1	(3.1)	15^a	2	(8.7)	23^c
Concern	31	(43.1)	72	24	(40.0)	60
Depression possible caseness						
Fear of recurrence						
No concern	0	(0)	15^b	5	(21.7)	23^d
Concern	24	(33.3)	72	14	(23.3)	60

Notes: $^a p = 0.008$; $^b p = 0.009$; $^c p = 0.006$; $^d p = 0.88$.

a relationship at both time-points, especially at three months, for both anxiety and depression. The levels of concern of recurrence were high at both occasions (see Figure 24.2; Humphris *et al.* 2003).

The original pilot study for the AFTER intervention surveyed cross-sectionally 100 patients with orofacial cancer and found a high incidence of recurrence fears that were unrelated to the extent of the disease or when the diagnosis was made (Humphris *et al.* 2003). In a follow-up study where 50 patients were revisited successfully two years later these fears were found to be relatively stable (rs = 0.67; Lee-Jones 1998). The point prevalence of concerns about the cancer returning was 65% in both the baseline and two-year follow-up samples (see Figure 24.2). This is consistent with other reports of long-term survivors of head and neck cancer (Campbell *et al.* 2000).

Although the risk of recurrence is an important issue for patients, this concern is not always immediately obvious to the clinician (de Swann 1990). There are several explanations for this. Patients may prefer to keep recurrence concerns to themselves or deny the possibility of a recurrence. Also staff tend to avoid the topic of recurrence and attend to the specifics of providing medical treatment.

Self-care behaviour

An important study of self-care behaviour immediately after surgery was conducted by virtue of a reliable direct observation scale of basic hygiene, such

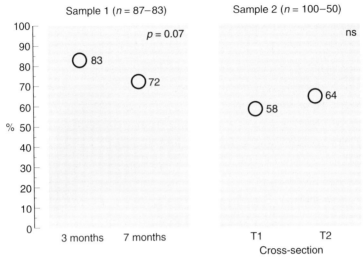

Figure 24.2. Recurrence concerns (slight or greater) in two consecutive samples of oropharangeal patients in Liverpool, UK. Sample 1 consisted of new patients assessed at three and seven months following initial treament. Sample 2 comprised initially 100 attenders at outpatient review clinic followed-up (*n* = 50) two years later. McNemar tests performed between two time-points for both samples. ns: not significant. (Humphris *et al.* 2003.)

as grooming and re-socialization, such as interaction with staff and friends (Dropkin 2001). The study was unique in using objectively defined observations at regular scheduled times during waking hours of the day on the ward. Clear associations were found to support the interpretation that in a matter of days, those patients who started looking after themselves made speedier recoveries. Patients who tried to cope and re-socialize needed to view themselves close up (in a mirror), touch their own facial defects, and expose them to others.

High-risk behaviour: smoking

An association between smoking behaviour and various indices of psychological distress and a specific health concern (fear of recurrence) has been found (Humphris & Rogers 2004). Two sets of results converged to demonstrate a clear relationship between tobacco consumption and raised levels of anxiety and depression. First, the comparison between consistent smokers and non-smokers established raised levels of mental distress in those that smoked at all points of assessment following treatment, with the exception at baseline. Separate analyses of subgroups of patients provided a second source of support. Early tobacco consumption following treatment was predictive of psychological distress at final follow-up a year later. This effect was observable even when initial levels of distress were held constant. Contrary to considered opinion that smoking is based upon patients self-medicating to minimize distress (e.g. Lerman *et al.* 1996) this result would tend to fit the view that smoking itself may be responsible in part for increasing levels of anxiety and depression (Pomerleau *et al.* 2000).

Non-smokers were also investigated in detail. The 30 patients, who claimed to be ex-smokers, were asked to estimate the duration of their smoking habit (in months). This smoking history estimate predicted distress at follow-up assessment. Such a finding if replicated would support the work of Watkins *et al.* and others who have shown that prolonged nicotine abstinence can cause or contribute to a negative affective state (Pomerleau *et al.* 2000; Watkins *et al.* 2000). Loewenstein puts forward the view that smoking is integrally bound up with neurochemical changes in the reward and motivation centres of the brain (referred to as the visceral account of addiction; Loewenstein 1996, 2001). Continued craving and averting this uncomfortable state is regarded as a mechanism which drives smoking behaviour including the inability to maintain long-term abstinence (Swan *et al.* 1996). A possible explanation is that longer-term use of tobacco is not necessarily a response to reduce outside aversive experiences but as a response to reduce craving. This effect may eventually undermine mental health status.

Fears of recurrence may be a trigger to patients to quit smoking (Spitz *et al.* 1990). A cross-sectional study of patients with head and neck cancer ($n = 55$) showed that some patients who stopped smoking after treatment had a tendency to blame themselves for their cancer (Christensen *et al.* 1999). However, such a belief was only associated with reduced smoking when they also possessed the clear additional opinion that a recurrence would be a direct result of their smoking. Therefore further studies should concentrate on the issue of the contingency between patients, beliefs and concerns about recurrence, smoking behaviour and self-blame.

Patient reaction to recurrence

There are few research studies investigating the psychological reactions to recurrent cancer, and virtually none specific to head and neck cancer. An early report concludes that patients with a recurrence respond according to their reaction to their initial cancer diagnosis (Schmale 1976). For many patients their experience of a recurrence is a renewed sense of uncertainty for the future, grief and feelings of injustice (Chekryn 1984). Some authors have viewed a recurrence as a traumatic event (Cella *et al.* 1990). Suzanne Mahon has published two interesting reports of patient reactions to a recurrence (Mahon *et al.* 1990), one qualitative and the other quantitative. The latter study reported on how patients ($n = 40$, mixed cancer tumours) view the recurrence and to what degree they regard a recurrence differently from their original diagnosis of cancer. In addition they collected patient views of the worst psychological aspects associated with a recurrence. Patients who had been alerted to the fact that the disease might return (30%) believed that they never were clear of the disease, even after treatment. Half the sample believed that there was always a possibility, whereas 20% were surprised, especially as they had been expecting a long disease-free period and had trusted their physician implicitly. The majority of patients (78%) reported that the recurrence was more distressing than the initial diagnosis. They believed that the threat of death was 'more real', treatments would be more severe with greater side-effects, and treatment decisions more difficult. Fear of uncontrollable pain and feeling more fatigued was also a common experience. Nearly half (45%) believed that the recurrence was due to some misdemeanour on their part. On the Psychological Adjustment to Illness Scale (PAIS) the recurrent cancer patients scored one to two standard deviations above a comparison group of patients with cancer. Similarly, two-thirds (67%) of patients scored above the cut-off point of 20 on either the thought intrusiveness or the avoidance scales.

The second study reported by Mahon was qualitative, focusing on the transcripts of 20 patients with mixed cancers and single or multiple recurrences (Mahon & Casperson 1997). A wide range of reactions to recurrence were found that were qualitatively different from their initial response to diagnosis. Patients reported that they felt they could not be prepared for the recurrence. A more extensive study would be required to confirm this finding, however there are important implications for healthcare which they must be aware of.

One of the triggers that some patients relate in interviews is the feature of disfigurement. For example the patients who view themselves in the mirror following initial surgery and focus on the scar on their face or neck will very often find that thoughts of recurrence surface. For some these thoughts may become difficult to dismiss (Brewin *et al.* 1998).

Appearance

There is considerable variation in the concerns that patients express about appearance changes. An early study of 152 head and neck cancer patients showed that 82% had adapted to their disfigurement (West 1977). This finding would tend to suggest that patients rate appearance concerns as less important than those associated with treatment for example. West proposed that the time spent on the ward with others of similar status prepares the patient for discharge into the social world on leaving the hospital. Other investigators have alerted clinicians to unspoken distress at scarring and disfigurement resulting directly from surgery or radiotherapy. A study conducted in Liverpool has followed a cohort of 278 patients over 18 months during the period of 1995 to 1999. Extensive disease involving neck dissection to remove involved lymph nodes had a strong negative effect on appearance ratings. Tumour size was less strongly associated with appearance, but those with larger tumours tended to rate themselves less positively than those with small tumours (Millsopp *et al.* 2006). This work within the UK is consistent with a Canadian study where 82 head and neck cancer patients were found to show a strong association between the level of disfigurement and depression (Katz *et al.* 2003). In addition the value of social support was shown to act as a buffer to women of their disfigurement.

In a cross-sectional survey of patients ($n = 211$) from various outpatient groups (burns, head and neck cancer, dermatology, general plastics, etc.) it was shown that ratings of, first, how the disfigurement had affected lifestyle, and, second, how noticeable was the condition, highest in the head and neck cancer group ($n = 14$). This set of findings was supported by the additional result that the level of distress suffered from the disfigurement was not predicted by clinician ratings of severity (Rumsey *et al.* 2003).

Some understanding of the variation of self-reports of appearance can be inferred from the results of a longitudinal study of 67 oral and oral-pharyngeal cancer patients conducted in the north-west of England. Ratings of appearance on a simple five-point rating scale at three and six months following treatment were predicted significantly by the patients' self-reported depression level as assessed by the HAD depression subscale at pretreatment (Humphris *et al.* 2000). As previously mentioned head and neck cancer patients express a variety of concerns, which include recurrence fears and appearance. Many of these concerns are unresolved and coping strategies that tend to be employed include, avoidance, distraction and the use of alcohol (Chaturvedi *et al.* 1996; Winter 2002). According to Chaturvedi a number of patients cope by drawing on support from family and friends, a feature that has started to attract interest among services and research teams in this field of head and neck cancer.

Social support

Immediate carers suffer considerable distress at their relative's diagnosis and course of treatment. General reports across oncology samples of patients and carers show rates of probable cases of psychiatric morbidity at 20 and 30%, whereas patients with advanced disease are found at 30–50% level of probable caseness (Pitceathly & Maguire 2003). Unfortunately the point prevalence of distress amongst carers during the course of treatment and recovery has not been reported with any confidence. A study comparing 51 patients with head and neck cancer and 44 partners on a number of mental status and QoL scales showed that partners were more distressed (Vickery *et al.* 2003). Somewhat surprisingly, no research in the head and neck field at the time of writing has shown that carers' adjustment actually influences patients. It is interesting that one study of breast cancer patients has shown that husbands who are distressed impact negatively on their spouses (Northouse *et al.* 1995).

The ability to sustain a recovery from treatment is crucially dependent on the level of support that the patient enjoys (Stam *et al.* 1991). Both surgery and radiotherapy to the face and neck influence important structures responsible for self-image. In addition, the ability to enter socially into the world can be markedly undermined. This particular cancer, more than most, challenges many aspects of the survivor to communicate with those immediately involved and those more distant. An important distinction is the difference between available and received support. Available support is considered as a relatively stable construct that may have associations with longer-term adjustment whereas received support is a function of the frequency and quality of the social contacts and appears to act as a buffer for the individual. Patients treated for head and neck cancer are more likely to receive little in the way of social support other than the link with the specialist unit. A statistically sophisticated study by the Utrecht group contributes some valuable findings in an under researched area within the head and neck cancer speciality (de Leeuw *et al.* 2000b). They studied 197 patients pretreatment and followed them six months later. Two competing models were tested, namely social support influenced depression or vice versa. Results were clear, as they showed that available support led to less depressive symptomology. This relationship was at its strongest in patients with few physical complaints. Received support was unrelated to depression and the authors believed that this form of support may be detrimental in those with few physical complaints, reinforcing the view that providing support needs to be targeted appropriately.

Psychological interventions

A number of key features of psychological interventions can be identified: decrease psychological sequelae (e.g. pain, depression, panic, anxiety), enhance adjustment, acceptance and QoL (Cassileth 1995). Guidelines have been suggested for the psychological assessment and treatment of patients with cancer and these are appropriate for head and neck cancer patients (Sellnick & Crooks 1999). For example the consensus statement included the following:

1. Basic psychological support should be available for all people with cancer.
2. All health providers should be able to provide psychosocial support.
3. Psychotherapeutic interventions should be encouraged:
   - for patients with adjustment problems
   - patients who request psychotherapy
   - carers of cancer patients who are in need.

Screening for depression is recommended (Berard *et al.* 1998). The Hospital Anxiety and Depression scale has been used extensively for cancer patients. Support for specific assessment of these two psychological constructs has remained firm (Johnston *et al.* 2000; Kugaya *et al.* 2000). Others advocate the Centre for Epidemiologic Studies Depression scale for screening depression (de Graeff *et al.* 2000a; de Leeuw *et al.* 2000a).

There have been a number of calls for introducing greater emotional support for head and neck cancer patients (Chaturvedi *et al.* 1996; Frampton 2001; Hutton & Williams 2001; Rose & Yates 2001). Pilot work describing the design and implementation of two types of intervention have been reported with some encouraging preliminary results (Hammerlid *et al.* 1999b). Despite having small patient numbers the value of psychological intervention was supported. The first study tested the effect of long-term group psychotherapy with newly diagnosed patients. Of the eight patients who completed the therapy and assessments some improvement in quality of life was found. The greatest improvement (i.e. from diagnosis to one-year follow-up) was emotional functioning in the intervention group compared to the controls. The second study observed 14 patients taking part in a one-week psychoeducational programme delivered one year following surgery. Positive changes (15% reduction in the proportion of patients scoring >7 on either scale of the HAD) were reported.

A psychosocial support programme was evaluated with head and neck cancer patients ($n = 144$) using a longitudinal, prospective, case-control study (Petruson *et al.* 2003). The support programme consisted of visits from the cancer team, including a weekly visit during treatment and then once a month for the first six months following treatment, and then again one and three years after diagnosis. Of the 81 patients offered the support, 15 did not want to participate, 11 did not attend the first visit and 3 died, leaving 52 patients in the study group. The control group consisted of 232 patients of whom 92 were matched to the study group on tumour location, stage, gender and age. At one year follow-up the control group had a clinically and statistically better global quality-of-life score but this difference was not sustained at three years. One possible explanation for the lack of improvement in QoL was explained by the authors as a design problem.

The study assigned patients to the study group who lived within 30 minutes of the cancer centre. Those who lived outside this limit were designated controls. It was found on *post hoc* analysis that the study group was more likely to live alone. It was found that depression levels were higher in the study (57%) compared to the control (35%) group. The trend was apparent from three months although none of these comparisons of the depression data were statistically significant. The authors stressed the need for improved training for hospital personnel to recognize patients with affective disorders. Another explanation offered was that patients in the study group became dependent on the visits as satisfaction levels with the intervention were high at one year whereas HRQoL did not improve.

An intervention programme for a mixed group of patients with cancer found little effect of the active arm of the study. In this well-powered study ($n = 450$) making information of the patients' needs, QoL and psychosocial scores available to the healthcare team was not helpful at follow-up assessment of QoL or psychological adjustment. However, a closer inspection of those who were moderately or severely depressed at baseline did show a significant reduction in depression at follow-up (McLachlan *et al.* 2001).

The AFTER intervention was designed to identify and reduce patients' fears of recurrence following primary treatment for orofacial cancer (Humphris 2001). The intervention consisted of six structured sessions to be delivered by a specialist nurse and featured the encouragement of the patient to express their concerns over future disease and what prompted them (e.g. symptoms) to seek reassurance from self-checking or professional review. The randomized controlled trial to test the intervention demonstrated a short-term effect that reduced worries about cancer, anxious preoccupation and increased global quality of life. Some patients who participated in the AFTER intervention stated that they would have preferred to have the intervention sooner following their initial treatment (surgery or surgery and radiotherapy).

A case-based approach to intervening psychologically has been outlined (White 2001), which identifies four areas of common difficulty featured by cancer patients in general and pertinent to many patients with head and neck cancer. These include tackling avoidance, facilitating control, promoting social support and handling uncertainty. Many of these problems can be assisted with the sensitive application of cognitive behavioural therapy, although for advanced cancers these issues may become subsumed by existential issues (Kissane *et al.* 1997).

Conclusion

The psychological care of the patient with head and neck cancer is a neglected area and moreover is traditionally a less developed service compared to more common cancers. However, clear features of the disease and its treatment indicate the need to study and intervene with this patient group. Due to the natural progression of the disease and the likelihood of recurrence healthcare personnel are encouraged to identify the key concerns expressed by patients and their carers. The literature demonstrates an interest in understanding the psychological processes that interfere with improving self-care practices of patients and preventing good recovery from initial treatment. A clear impetus is required to improve general awareness of this cancer to allow programmes targeted to prevent the risk factors so far identified expressing themselves in the form of new disease.

REFERENCES

Aaronson, N. K., Ahmedzai, S., Berman, B., *et al.* (1993). The European Organization for Research and Treatment of CancerQLQ-C30: A Quality-of-Life Instrument for Use in International Clinical Trials in Oncology. *Journal of the National Cancer Institute*, **85**(5), 365–76.

Allison, P. (2001). Factors associated with smoking and alcohol consumption following treatment for head and neck cancer. *Oral Oncology*, **37**(6), 513–20.

Berard, R., Boermeester, F. and Viljoen, G. (1998). Depressive disorders in an outpatient oncology setting: prevalence, assessment, and management. *Psychooncology*, **7**(2), 112–20.

Bhatti, N., Downer, M. and Bulman, J. (1995). Public knowledge and attitudes on oral cancer: a pilot investigation. *Journal of International Health Education*, **32**, 112–17.

Bjordal, K. and Kaasa, S. (1992). Psychometric validation of the EORTC Core Quality of Life Questionnaire, 30-item version and a diagnosis-specific module for head and neck cancer patients. *Acta Oncologica*, **31**, 311–21.

Bjordal, K. and Kaasa, S. (1995). Psychological distress in head and neck cancer patients 7–11 years after curative treatment. *British Journal of Cancer*, **71**, 592–7.

Bjordal, K., Ahlner-Elmqvist, M., Tollesson, E., *et al.* (1994). Development of a European Organisation for Research and Treatment of Cancer (EORTC) questionnaire module to be used in quality of life assessments in head and neck cancer patients. *Acta Oncologica*, **33**, 879–85.

Bjordal, K., Hammerlid, E., Ahlner-Elmqvist, M., *et al.* (1998). Quality of life in head and neck cancer patients: validation of the European Organisation for Research and Treatment of Cancer Quality of Life Questionnaire-H&N35. *Journal of Clinical Oncology*, **17**, 1008–19.

Boundouki, G., Humphris, G. and Field, E. (2004). Knowledge of oral cancer, anxiety and screening intentions: longer term effects of a patient information leaflet. *Patient Education and Counseling*, **53**, 71–7.

Boyle, P., Macfarlane, G. J., Zheng, T., *et al.* (1992). Recent advances in the epidemiology of head and neck cancer. *Current Opinion in Oncology*, **4**, 471–7.

Brewin, C., Watson, M., McCarthy, S., *et al.* (1998). Intrusive memories and depression in cancer patients. *Behaviour Research and Therapy*, **36**(12), 1131−42.

British Dental Association. (2000). *Opportunistic Oral Cancer Screening: a Management Strategy for Dental Practice* (Occasional Paper No. 6). London: British Dental Association.

Broomfield, D. (1998). A Study to Determine Information Needs of General Practice Staff in the Care of Cancer Patients. Unpublished PhD thesis, University of Liverpool, Liverpool.

Broomfield, D., Humphris, G., Fisher, S., *et al.* (1997). The orofacial cancer patient's support from the general practitioner, hospital teams, family, and friends. *Journal of Cancer Education*, **12**(4), 229−32.

Browman, G., Wong, G., Hodson, I., *et al.* (1993). Influence of cigarette smoking on the efficacy of radiation therapy in head and neck cancer. *New England Journal of Medicine*, **328**(3), 159−63.

Campbell, B., Marbella, A. and Layde, P. (2000). Quality of life and recurrence concern in survivors of head and neck cancer. *Laryngoscope*, **110**(6), 895−906.

Canto, M., Horowitz, A., Goodman, H., *et al.* (1998). Maryland veterans' knowledge of risk factors for and signs of oral cancers and their use of dental services. *Gerodontology*, **15**(2), 79−86.

Cassileth, B. (1995). The aim of psychotherapeutic intervention in cancer patients. *Support Care Cancer*, **3**, 267−9.

Cella, D., Mahon, S. and Donovan, M. (1990). Cancer recurrence as a traumatic event. *Behavioral Medicine*, **16**, 15−22.

Charles, K., Sellick, S., Montesanto, B., *et al.* (1996). Priorities of cancer survivors regarding psychosocial needs. *Journal of Psychosocial Oncology*, **14**(2), 57−72.

Chaturvedi, S., Shenoy, A., Prasad, K., *et al.* (1996). Concerns, coping and quality of life in head and neck cancer patients. *Support Cancer Care*, **4**, 186−90.

Chekryn, J. (1984). Cancer recurrence: personal meaning, communication, and marital adjustment. *Cancer Nursing*, **7**, 491−8.

Christensen, A., Moran, P., Ehlers, S., *et al.* (1999). Smoking and drinking behaviour in patients with head and neck cancer: effects of behavioural self-blame and perceived control. *Journal of Behavioural Medicine*, **22**(5), 407−18.

Conway, D., Macpherson, L., Gibson, J., *et al.* (2002). Oral cancer: prevention and detection in primary dental healthcare. *Primary Dental Care*, **9**(4), 119−23.

Cruz, G., Le Geros, R., Ostroff, J., *et al.* (2002). Oral cancer knowledge, risk factors and characteristics of subjects in a large oral cancer screening program. *Journal of the American Dental Association*, **133**(8), 1064−71.

de Boer, M., van den Bourne, B., Pruyn, J., *et al.* (1998). Physical and psychological correlates of survival and recurrence in patients with head and cancer: results of a 6-year longitudinal study. *Cancer*, **83**, 2567−79.

de Boer, M., McCormick, L., Pruyn, J., *et al.* (1999). Physical and psychological correlates of head and neck cancer: a review of the literature. *Otolaryngology − Head & Neck Surgery*, **120**(3), 427−36.

de Graeff, A., de Leeuw, J., Ros, W., *et al.* (2000a). Pretreatment factors predicting quality of life after treatment for head and neck cancer. *Head and Neck*, **22**(4), 398−407.

de Graeff, A., de Leeuw, J., Ros, W., *et al.* (2000b). Long-term quality of life of patients with head and neck cancer. *Laryngoscope*, **110**(1), 98–106.

de Leeuw, J., de Graeff, A., Ros, W., *et al.* (2000a). Prediction of depressive symptomatology after treatment of head and neck cancer: the influence of pre-treatment physical and depressive symptoms, coping, and social support. *Head and Neck*, **22**(8), 799–807.

de Leeuw, J., de Graeff, A., Ros, W., *et al.* (2000b). Negative and positive influences of social support on depression in patients with head and neck cancer: a prospective study. *Psychooncology*, **9**, 20–8.

de Leeuw, J., de Graeff, A., Ros, W., *et al.* (2001). Prediction of depression 6 months to 3 years after treatment of head and neck cancer. *Head and Neck*, **23**(10), 892–8.

de Swann, A. (1990). Affect management in a cancer ward. In *The Management of Normality: Critical Essays in Health and Welfare*. London: Routledge, pp. 31–56.

Deleyiannis, F. W.-B., Thomas, D., Vaughan, T., *et al.* (1996). Alcoholism: independent predictor of survival in patients with head and neck cancer. *Journal of National Cancer Institute*, **88**(8), 542–9.

Department of Health. (2000). *Referral Guidelines for Suspected Cancer*. www.dh.gov.uk/publicationsandstatistics/lettersandcirculars (accessed September 2006).

Dropkin, M. (2001). Anxiety, coping strategies, and coping behaviors in patients undergoing head and neck cancer surgery. *Cancer Nursing*, **24**(2), 143–8.

Fawzy, F. (1999). Psychological interventions for patients with cancer: what works and what doesn't. *European Journal of Cancer*, **35**(11), 1559–64.

Frampton, M. (2001). Psychological distress in patients with head and neck cancer: review. *British Journal of Oral Maxillofacial Surgery*, **39**(1), 67–70.

Funk, G., Karnell, L., Dawson, C., *et al.* (1997). Baseline and post-treatment assessment of the general health status of head and neck cancer patients compared with United States population norms. *Head and Neck*, **19**(8), 675–83.

Giovannelli, L., Campisi, G., Lama, A., *et al.* (2002). Human papillomavirus DNA in oral mucosal lesions. *Journal of Infectious Diseases*, **185**(6), 833–6.

Graeff, D. (2000). Long-term quality of life of patients with head and neck cancer. *Laryngoscope*, **110**, 96–106.

Hammerlid, E., Ahlner-Elmqvist, M., Bjordal, K., *et al.* (1999a). A prospective multicentre study in Sweden and Norway of mental distress and psychiatric morbidity in head and neck cancer patients. *British Journal of Cancer*, **80**(5–6), 766–74.

Hammerlid, E., Persson, L.-O., Sullivan, M., *et al.* (1999b). Quality-of-life effects of psychosocial intervention in patients with head and neck cancer. *Otolaryngology – Head and Neck Surgery*, **120**, 507–16.

Hammerlid, E., Silander, E., Hornestam, L., *et al.* (2001). Health-related quality of life three years after diagnosis of head and neck cancer – a longitudinal study. *Head and Neck*, **23**(2), 113–25.

Harrison, J. and Maguire, P. (1994). Predictors of psychiatric morbidity in cancer patients. *British Journal of Psychiatry*, **165**, 593–8.

Hassan, S. and Weymuller, E. (1993). Assessment of quality of life in head and neck cancer patients. *Head and Neck*, **15**, 485–96.

Hassanein, K., Musgrove, B. and Bradbury, E. (2001). Functional status of patients with oral cancer and its relation to style of coping, social support and psychological status. *British Journal of Oral Maxillofacial Surgery*, **39**(5), 340–5.

Herrero, R., Castellsague, X., Pawlita, M., *et al*. (2003). Human papillomavirus and oral cancer: the International Agency for Research on Cancer multicenter study. *Journal of National Cancer Institute*, **95**(23), 1772–83.

Hollows, P., McAndrew, P. and Perini, M. (2000). Delays in the referral and treatment of oral squamous cell carcinoma. *British Dental Journal*, **11**(7), 262–5.

Horowitz, A., Moon, H., Goodman, H., *et al*. (1998). Maryland adults' knowledge of oral cancer and having oral cancer examinations. *Journal of Public Health Dentistry*, **58**(4), 281–7.

Horowitz, A., Drury, T., Goodman, H., *et al*. (2000). Oral pharyngeal cancer prevention and early detection. Dentists' opinions and practices. *Journal of American Dental Association*, **131**(4), 453–62.

Huang, J., Barbara, L., Brouwers, M., *et al*. (2003). Does delay in starting treatment affect the outcomes of radiotherapy? A systematic review. *Journal of Clinical Oncology*, **21**(3), 555–63.

Humphris, G. (2001). *Fear of Recurrence in Orofacial Cancer Patients: the Development and Testing of a Psychological Intervention* (No. CP1031/0102). London: Cancer Research Campaign.

Humphris, G. and Field, E. (2004). Oral cancer information leaflet has benefit for smokers in primary care: results from two randomised control trials. *Community Dentistry and Oral Epidemiology*, **32**, 143–9.

Humphris, G. and Rogers, S. (2004). The association of cigarette smoking and anxiety, depression and fears of recurrence in patients following treatment of oral and oropharyngeal malignancy. *European Journal of Cancer Care*, **13**, 328–35.

Humphris, G., Duncalf, M., Holt, D., *et al*. (1999). The experimental evaluation of an oral cancer information leaflet. *Oral Oncology*, **35**, 575–82.

Humphris, G., McNally, D. and Rogers, S. (2000). Mood, Facial Appearance and Self-Decrepancy in Oral Facial Cancer Patients. Paper presented at the British Division of the International Association of Dental Research, 48th Annual Meeting, 12–15 April 2000, Liverpool, UK.

Humphris, G., Ireland, R. and Field, E. (2001a). Immediate knowledge increase from an oral cancer information leaflet in primary care health service attenders: a randomized controlled trial. *Oral Oncology*, **37**(1), 99–102.

Humphris, G., Ireland, R. and Field, E. (2001b). Randomized trial of the psychological effect of information about oral cancer in primary care settings. *Oral Oncology*, **37**(7), 548–52.

Humphris, G., Rogers, S., McNally, D., *et al*. (2003). Fear of recurrence and possible cases of anxiety and depression in orofacial cancer patients. *International Journal of Oral and Maxillofacial Surgery*, **32**, 486–91.

Hurt, G., McQuellon, R. and Barrett, R. (1994). After treatment ends: neutral time. *Cancer Practice*, **2**(6), 417–20.

Hutton, J. and Williams, M. (2001). An investigation of psychological distress in patients who have been treated for head and neck cancer. *British Journal of Oral Maxillofacial Surgery,* **39**(5), 333–9.

Johnson, N. (2001). Tobacco use and oral cancer: a global perspective. *Journal of Dental Education,* **65**(4), 328–39.

Johnson, N. (2002). Epidemiology of premalignant and malignant lesions. In *Oxford Textbook of Oncology,* volumes 1 & 2, ed. R. Souhami, I. Tannock, P. Hohenberger, *et al.* Oxford: Oxford University Press, pp. 1247–92.

Johnston, M., Pollard, B. and Hennessey, P. (2000). Construct validation of the hospital anxiety and depression scale with clinical populations. *Journal of Psychosomatic Research,* **48**(6), 579–84.

Jullien, J., Zakrzewska, J., Downer, M., *et al.* (1995). Attendance and compliance at an oral cancer screening programme in a general medical practice. *European Journal of Cancer B Oral Oncology,* **31**B(3), 202–6.

Katz, M., Irish, J., Devins, G., *et al.* (2003). Psychosocial adjustment in head and neck cancer: the impact of disfigurement, gender and social support. *Head and Neck,* **25**(2), 103–12.

Kissane, D., Bloch, S., Miach, P., *et al.* (1997). Cognitive-existential group therapy for patients with primary breast cancer-techniques and themes. *Psychooncology,* **6**, 25–33.

Krupat, E., Fancey, M. and Cleary, P. (2000). Information and its impact on satisfaction among surgical patients. *Social Science and Medicine,* **51**, 1817–25.

Kugaya, A., Akechi, T., Okuyama, T., *et al.* (2000). Prevalence, predictive factors, and screening for psychologic distress in patients with newly diagnosed head and neck cancer. *Cancer,* **88**(12), 2817–23.

Kuntz, A. and Weymuller, E. (1999). Impact of neck dissection on quality of life. *Laryngoscope,* **109**, 1334–8.

La Vecchia, C., Tavani, A., Franceschi, S., *et al.* (1997). Epidemiology and prevention of oral cancer. *Oral Oncology,* **33**(5), 302–12.

Lee-Jones, C. (1998). A Two Year Follow-up Study Investigating Fear of Recurrence in Orofacial Cancer Patients. Unpublished Doctorate, University of Wales, Bangor.

Lee-Jones, C., Humphris, G., Dixon, R., *et al.* (1997). Fear of cancer recurrence: a literature review and formulation to explain exacerbation of recurrence fears. *Psycho-Oncology,* **6**, 95–105.

Lerman, C., Audrain, J., Orleans, C., *et al.* (1996). Investigation of mechanisms linking depressed mood to nicotine dependence. *Addiction and Behaviour,* **21**(1), 9–19.

Leventhal, H., Meyer, D. and Nerenz, D. (1980). The common sense representation of illness danger. In *Contributions to Medical Psychology,* ed. S. Rachman. Oxford: Pergamon Press, pp. 7–30.

Leventhal, H., Nerenz, D. and Steele, D. (1984). Illness representations and coping with health threats. In *Handbook of Psychology and Health, Volume IV: Social Psychological Aspects of Health,* ed. A. Baum, S. Taylor and J. Singer. Hillsdale, NJ: Erlbaum, pp. 219–52.

Leventhal, H., Diefenbach, M. and Leventhal, E. A. (1992). Illness cognition: using common sense to understand treatment adherence and affect cognition interactions. *Cognitive Therapy and Research,* **16**(2), 143–63.

Lim, K., Moles, D., Downer, M., *et al.* (2003). Opportunistic screening for oral cancer and precancer in general dental practice: results of a demonstration study. *British Dental Journal*, **194**, 497–502.

Lissowska, J., Pilarska, A., Pilarski, P., *et al.* (2003). Smoking, alcohol, diet, dentition and sexual practices in the epidemiology of oral cancer in Poland. *European Journal of Cancer Prevention*, **12**(1), 25–33.

List, M., Ritter-Sterr, C. and Lansky, S. (1990). A performance status scale for head and neck cancer patients. *Cancer*, **66**, 564–9.

List, M., D'Antonio, L., Cell, D., *et al.* (1996). A performance status scale for head and neck cancer patients and the functional assessment of cancer therapy – head and neck. A study of utility and validity. *Cancer*, **77**, 2294–301.

Loewenstein, G. (1996). Out of control: visceral influences on behaviour. *Organisational Behaviour and Human Decision Processes*, **65**, 272–92.

Loewenstein, G. (2001). A visceral account of addiction. In *Smoking*, ed. P. Slovic. London: Sage Publications, pp. 188–215.

Macfarlane, G. J., Boyle, P., Evstifeeva, T., *et al.* (1994). Rising trends of oral cancer mortality among males worldwide: the return of an old public health problem. *Cancer Causes and Control*, **5**, 259–65.

Maher, E. L. (1982). Anomic aspects of recovery from cancer. *Social Science and Medicine*, **16**, 907–12.

Mahon, S. and Casperson, D. (1997). Exploring the psychosocial meaning of recurrent cancer: a descriptive study. *Cancer Nursing*, **20**(3), 178–86.

Mahon, S. M., Cella, D. F. and Donovan, M. I. (1990). Psychosocial Adjustment to Recurrent Cancer. *Oncology Nursing Forum*, **17**(3, Suppl.), 47–52.

McLachlan, S.-A., Allenby, A., Matthews, J., *et al.* (2001). Randomized trial of coordinated psychosocial interventions based on patient self-assessments versus standard care to improve the psychosocial functioning of patients with cancer. *Journal of Clinical Oncology*, **19**(21), 4117–25.

Mesters, I., Van den Bourne, B., de Boer, M., *et al.* (2001). Measuring information needs among cancer patients. *Patient Education and Counseling*, **43**(3), 253–62.

Millsopp, L., Humphris, G., Lowe, D., *et al.* (2003). Free text UoW QoL paper. *Head and Neck*, **25**(12), 1042–50.

Millsopp, L., Brandon, L., Humphris, G., *et al.* (2006). Facial appearance after operations for oral and oropharangeal cancer: a comparison of casenotes and patient-completed questionnaire. *Head and Neck*, **44**, 358–63.

Northouse, L., Laten, D. and Reddy, P. (1995). Adjustment of women and their husbands to recurrent breast cancer. *Research Nursing and Health*, **18**, 515–24.

Ogden, G. (2003). Oral cancer prevention and detection in primary healthcare. *British Dental Journal*, **195**(5), 263.

Ogden, G. and Macluskey, M. (2000). An overview of the prevention of oral cancer and diagnostic markers of malignant change: 1. Prevention. *Dental Update*, **27**(2), 95–9.

Parkin, D., Pisani, P. and Ferlay, J. (1999). Estimates of the worldwide incidence of twenty-five major cancers in 1990. *International Journal of Cancer*, **80**, 827–41.

Pearson, N., Croucher, R., Marcenes, W., *et al.* (2001). Prevalence of oral lesions among a sample of Bangladeshi medical users aged 40 years and over living in Tower Hamlets, UK. *International Dental Journal*, **51**(1), 30–4.

Petruson, K., Silander, E. and Hammerlid, E. (2003). Effects of psychological intervention on quality of life in patients with head and neck cancer. *Head and Neck*, **25**, 576–84.

Pitceathly, C. and Maguire, P. (2003). The psychological impact of cancer on patients, partners and other key relatives: a review. *European Journal of Cancer*, **39**, 1517–24.

Platz, H., Fries, R. and Hudec, M. (1986). *Prognoses of Oral Cavity Carcinomas: Results of a Multicentre Retrospective Observational Study*. Munich: Carl Hanser Verlag.

Pomerleau, C., Marks, J. and Pomerleau, O. (2000). Who gets what symptom? Effects of psychiatric cofactors and nicotine dependence on patterns of smoking withdrawal symptomatology. *Nicotine & Tobacco Research*, **2**(3), 275–80.

Quin, M. (2001). *Cancer Trends in England and Wales 1950–1999*. (Studies on medical and population subjects No. 66.) London: Stationery Office.

Rajkumar, T., Sridhar, H., Balaram, P., *et al.* (2003). Oral cancer in Southern India: the influence of body size, diet, infections and sexual practices. *European Journal of Cancer Prevention*, **12**(2), 135–43.

Rampling, T., King, H., Mais, K., *et al.* (2003). Quality of life measurement in the head and neck cancer radiotherapy clinic: is it feasible and worthwhile? *Clinical Oncology (Royal College of Radiologists)*, **15**(4), 205–10.

Ringash, J. and Bezjak, A. (2001). A structured review of quality of life instruments for head and neck cancer patients. *Head and Neck*, **23**(3), 201–13.

Rodrigues, V., Moss, S. and Tuomainen, H. (1998). Oral cancer in the UK: to screen or not to screen. *Oral Oncology*, **34**, 454–65.

Rogers, S. (2002). *Quality of Life and Functional Outcomes After Oral and Oropharyngeal Cancer*. Cheshire: Astraglobe.

Rogers, S. and Radford, K. (2002). Quality of life issues – beyond primary treatment. In *Effective Head and Neck Cancer Management: Third Consensus Document*. London: British Association of Otorhinology Head and Neck Surgery.

Rogers, S., Humphris, G., Lowe, D., *et al.* (1998). The impact of surgery for oral cancer on quality of life as measured by the Medical Outcomes Short Form 36. *European Journal of Cancer: Oral Oncology*, **34**, 171–9.

Rogers, S., Fisher, S. and Woolgar, J. (1999). A review of quality of life assessment in oral cancer. *International Journal of Maxillofacial Surgery*, **28**, 99–117.

Rogers, S., Gwanne, S., Lowe, D., *et al.* (2002). The addition of mood and anxiety domains to the University of Washington quality of life scale. *Head and Neck*, **24**, 521–9.

Rose, P. and Yates, P. (2001). Quality of life experienced by patients receiving radiation treatment for cancers of the head and neck. *Cancer Nursing*, **24**(4), 255–63.

Rumsey, N., Clarke, A. and White, P. (2003). Exploring the psychological concerns of outpatients with disfiguring conditions. *Journal of Wound Care*, **12**(7), 247–52.

Sanchez, M., Martinez, C., Nieto, A., *et al.* (2003). Oral and oropharyngeal cancer in Spain: influence of dietary patterns. *European Journal of Cancer Prevention*, **12**(1), 49–56.

Sanderson, R. and Ironside, J. (2002). Squamous cell carcinoma of the head and neck. *British Medical Journal*, **325**, 822–7.

Schmale, A. (1976). Psychological reactions to recurrences, metastases or disseminated cancer. *International Journal of Radiation Oncology and Biological Physics*, **1**, 515–20.

Sellnick, S. and Crooks, D. (1999). Depression and cancer: an appraisal of the literature for prevalence, detection, and practice guideline development for psychological interventions. *Psycho-oncology*, **8**, 315–33.

Sollner, W., DeVries, A., Steixner, E., *et al.* (2001). How successful are oncologists in identifying patient distress, perceived social support, and need for psychosocial counselling? *British Journal of Cancer*, **84**(2), 179–85.

Specht, L. (2002). Oral complications in the head and neck radiation patient. Introduction and scope of the problem. *Support Care Cancer*, **10**(1), 36–9.

Speight, P., Downer, M. and Zakrzewska, J. E. (1993). Screening for oral cancer and precancer. A report of the UK Working Group on Screening for Oral Cancer and Precancer. *Community Dental Health*, **10**(Suppl. 1), 1–89.

Spitz, M., Fueger, J., Chamberlain, R. (1990). Cigarette smoking patterns in patients after treatment of upper aerodigestive tract cancers. *Journal of Cancer Education*, **5**(2), 109–13.

Sprangers, M. (2002). Quality of life assessment in oncology. Achievements and challenges. *Acta Oncologica*, **41**(3), 229–37.

Stam, H., Koopmans, J. and Mathieson, C. (1991). The psychological impact of a laryngectomy: a comprehensive assessment. *Journal of Psychosocial Oncology*, **9**, 37–58.

Stevens, M., Gardner, J., Parkin, J., *et al.* (1983). Head and neck cancer survival. *Archives of Otolaryngology*, **109**(11), 746–9.

Swan, G., Ward, M. and Jack, L. (1996). Abstinence effects as predictors of 28-day relapse in smokers. *Addiction and Behaviour*, **21**(4), 481–90.

Swango, P. (1996). Cancers of the oral cavity and pharanx in the United States: an epidemiologic overview. *Journal of Public Health Dentistry*, **56**, 309–18.

Vickery, L., Latchford, G., Hewison, J., *et al.* (2003). The impact of head and neck cancer and facial disfigurement on the quality of life and their partners. *Head and Neck*, **25**(4), 289–96.

Warnakulasuriya, K., Harris, C., Scarrott, D., *et al.* (1999). An alarming lack of public awareness towards oral cancer. *British Dental Journal*, **187**, 319–22.

Watkins, S., Koob, G. and Markou, A. (2000). Neural mechanisms underlying addiction: acute positive reinforcement and withdrawal. *Nicotine and Tobacco Research*, **2**(1), 19–37.

West, D. (1977). Social adaptation patterns among cancer patients with facial disfigurements resulting from surgery. *Archives of Physical and Medical Rehabilitation*, **58**(11), 473–9.

Weymuller, E., Yueh, B., Deleyiannis, F., *et al.* (2000). Quality of life in head and neck cancer. *Laryngoscope*, **110**(Suppl. 94), 4–7.

White, C. (2001). Cancer. In *Cognitve Behaviour Therapy for Chronic Medical Problems* Chichester: Wiley, pp. 95–122.

Winter, E. (2002). An Exploration of Whether Certain Coping Strategies are Optimal for Use with Certain Cancer-Related Concerns. Unpublished MPhil, University of Manchester, Manchester.

Woolgar, J., Rogers, S., West, C., *et al.* (1999). Survival and patterns of recurrence in 200 oral cancer patients treated by radical surgery and neck dissection. *Oral Oncology*, **35**(3), 257–65.

Zakrzewska, J. (1999). Oral cancer: clinical review. *British Medical Journal*, **318**, 1051–4.

Zigmond, A. S. and Snaith, R. P. (1983). The hospital anxiety and depression scale. *Acta Psychiatrica Scandinavica*, **67**, 361–70.

25

Palliative care

Matthew Hotopf and Max Henderson

Context

Palliative care arose as a discipline in the 1960s with the birth of the modern hospice movement. From its earliest origins palliative care championed what has come to be known as a 'patient-centred' approach to delivering care. In patients with advanced cancer (who remain the core patient group served by most palliative care services) the focus of care was to improve the quality, rather than the duration, of life. Symptom control — especially pain control — was key to this, but also a new approach to patient care in which the need for open and honest communication of diagnosis and prognosis was emphasized. The naïve view that by failing to inform the dying patient of his predicament, the doctor was somehow protecting him from unbearable distress was challenged. Palliative care also emphasizes the familial, social, cultural and spiritual context in which care is provided, and death and its aftermath are managed. Underpinning this is a multidisciplinary approach to the provision of care, with many hospices employing social workers, chaplains, other spiritual advisers, as well as bereavement counsellors, psychiatrists and psychologists.

Hospices are the most obvious means by which palliative care has been developed; however palliative care is not confined to them. The role of hospices is to provide more than terminal care; admissions may take place months or even years before death, in order to bring troublesome symptoms under control. Many hospices provide home-care, where clinical nurse specialists, with the back-up of medical and other staff, provide ongoing support to patients at home. In general hospitals palliative care services have been established which frequently act in a similar way to liaison psychiatry teams — advising the clinical team responsible for the patient's care on pain and other symptom management, and being a channel for referral to other agencies such as hospices or home-care teams.

Handbook of Liaison Psychiatry, ed. Geoffrey Lloyd and Elspeth Guthrie. Published by Cambridge University Press. © Cambridge University Press 2007.

In most hospice-based services the emphasis of palliative care remains patients with advanced cancer. Many provide care for patients with terminal neurological diseases such as motor neurone disease. There have been calls for the same sorts of services to be provided for patients with advanced heart failure, severe stroke, end-stage respiratory disease and other terminal illnesses, and palliative care is gradually influencing the development of services around these groups (Addington Hall & Higginson 2001). Palliative care teams in hospital settings generally have a wider diagnostic case-mix.

Psychiatry perhaps shares more with palliative care than many other medical disciplines (Ferrando 2000). Hospices often accept admissions for psychosocial indications. Both specialities are especially concerned with improving symptoms and function. Both emphasize the importance of the biopsychosocial approach, and the wider context of the patient's family and culture. Both have moved from providing care in specific inpatient facilities, to providing care at home, and in general hospital settings. Psychiatrists have also played a prominent role in the development of palliative care. The writings of John Hinton, Colin Murray Parkes and Elizabeth Kübler Ross were powerful and influential calls for improving communication and recognizing the distress associated with dying and bereavement.

The liaison psychiatrist's job in palliative care shares much with other settings. The most obvious role is in assessing and helping to manage individual patients. However it is not enough solely to provide a narrow clinical role, as this risks reducing the skill of clinical teams in managing distressed patients. Another vital role is education of staff. Psychiatrists also have a role in developing policies and advising on service developments. In this chapter the clinical assessment of patients with advanced disease is discussed, followed by a description of a number of common clinical problems that may be referred to psychiatrists working in palliative care. First models of coping in advanced disease are discussed.

Models of coping in advanced disease

It would be wrong to assume that when patients are referred to palliative care they have crossed an imaginary line at which point all concerned are aware that the disease will be fatal. Not only do palliative care teams sometimes care for individuals whose condition becomes stable or is cured; but also information about the disease and prognosis is usually not available at a single point in time. Patients usually live with a period of uncertainty, which is not simply due to inadequate communication with doctors. Frequently patients go back and forth to hospital having complicated diagnostic procedures and treatments which, if not curative, slow the progress of disease. In the midst of all this, the patient is confronted by good and bad news — sometimes at the same time. Thus coping with advanced disease is more complicated than 'coming to terms' with a static fact that death will come in, say, three months' time.

In 1969 Elizabeth Kübler-Ross published *On Death and Dying* (Kübler-Ross 1969), an account of her experience running a seminar with assistance of hospital chaplains, in which patients with advanced and incurable disease were interviewed. The book is a wise and sharply observed description of the suffering of patients with advanced disease. Kübler-Ross' study was essentially a qualitative one, in which she described five 'stages' in the process of dying. These are denial and isolation, anger, bargaining, depression and acceptance. At each stage different emotions or defence mechanisms dominate. It is certainly possible to find evidence to back up each of these stages. For example, Hinton observed denial in his classic study of dying patients in a general hospital (Hinton 1963) 'not infrequently patients would speak seriously of death and then apparently dismiss it from their minds, talking in rather vague terms of future plans'.

Kübler-Ross' model has been widely criticized on both methodological and theoretical grounds. The methodological problems are obvious — her account makes no attempt to describe the sample from which the often vivid case descriptions are drawn. For example, some have commented that her sample may have been predominantly young cancer patients. The experience of dying in older people may be greatly different, when there is a sense that life has run its full course. The theoretical criticisms are more damning. It is obvious that patients go backwards and forwards between 'stages' and often experience several different emotional responses simultaneously. However, the aspect of the model which has drawn the fiercest opprobrium has been the implication that in order to reach acceptance (and therefore a 'good' death) the individual has to go through the previous stages. Kübler-Ross was therefore accused of having described a 'correct' way to die, and the model has been viewed by many as prescriptive.

As Kübler-Ross' model fell out of fashion, new 'task-based' models were proposed (Corr 1992, 1999; Doka 1995). These models are influenced by work on coping, and see the dying individual as an active participant who has certain tasks to accomplish. Such tasks are summarized by Doka as:

- responding to the physical fact of the disease
- taking steps to cope with the reality of the disease
- preserving self-concept and relationships with others in the face of disease
- dealing with affective, existential, and spiritual issues created or reactivated by disease.

Each of these tasks may differ according to the stage of disease. Immediately after the diagnosis is made, the task of responding to the physical fact of the disease equates to understanding the illness. Different individuals may approach this task in very different ways — some may actively seek out as much information as possible, others are more passive. In the chronic stage of the disease, the task of preserving self-concept and relationships may involve a reappraisal of key relationships — friends who had seemed close at earlier stages of life may have withdrawn, and new relationships may become more important. These models emphasize the active participation of the patient. They are also very broad, taking in physical, psychological, social and spiritual dimensions and are therefore 'holistic'. They also attempt to be non-judgemental and emphasize the autonomy of the individual.

Noble though many of the aspirations of task-based approach are, the breadth and flexibility of these models weakens their explanatory power. They do not generate testable hypotheses, nor do they allow one to explain patients' behaviour in a clinical setting. They are perhaps better understood as a framework on which to describe the process of dying. Finally the proponents of such models appear too eager to be non-judgemental. It is not the case, as (Doka 1995) states, that 'no way of coping is inherently more desirable'. Some coping mechanisms are manifestly less helpful than others.

Leventhal's self-regulatory model (Leventhal & Cameron 1987) has been influential in health psychology as a means of predicting health behaviour. The model includes three processes — representation of the health threat (which might include symptom perceptions and the patient's understanding of the symptom's potential causes or consequences); a coping strategy (which might include active approaches such as seeking medical attention or passive strategies such as avoidance and denial); and appraisal, in which the individual judges the effectiveness of his or her coping strategy. Individual differences in health behaviour are therefore predicted by the perception of symptoms; the coping style and appraisal. Greer and Watson (1987) have described five coping styles in patients with cancer: fighting spirit, helplessness—hopelessness, anxious preoccupation, fatalism and positive avoidance. Individual coping styles are predictive of mood. For example, individuals with fighting spirit, who have optimism about the prognosis, a belief that the disease and life are controllable and a determination to cope with the situation, have less anxiety and depression than those with the helpless—hopeless coping styles (Watson *et al.* 1991). Attractive though such models may be, they have developed from work on early cancer, and it is not clear whether they have similar explanatory power in advanced disease — it may be, for example, that individuals with fighting spirit find the realization that they will succumb to their disease most difficult to manage.

The practice of liaison psychiatry in palliative care settings

Referrals

As in any other setting, patients and their families may be anxious about, or hostile to, referral to a psychiatrist. In our experience, such attitudes are less prominent in patients with advanced disease (where distress is perhaps recognized to be understandable, and therefore less stigmatizing) than in patients with medically unexplained symptoms. It is helpful to make time available to discuss potential referrals with clinical teams. Sometimes a simple management plan can be devised without the need for an assessment, and this can build the confidence of the referring team in managing patients with psychiatric disorders. Those who refer to the service should be aware of what is likely to be offered, and should be open about the referral with the patient.

The assessment

Patients with advanced disease may be unable to withstand a prolonged assessment. If this seems likely, it is important to focus the interview on specific topics, rather than attempt a comprehensive psychiatric evaluation. In our experience it is surprisingly rare for patients not to be able to give a full history in one sitting, however we always make it clear at the start that the patient can take a break at any point if required.

History

It is logical to start with a history of the disease. Apart from demonstrating that the psychiatrist can listen empathically and understand the patient's physical illness, this also allows an assessment of the patient's psychological response. Was there prolonged delay in presenting with a breast lump, which might indicate an avoidant coping style or denial of disease? Did the patient believe that the GP or surgeon mis-handled his or her care, and now feels aggrieved that the disease was not diagnosed earlier? How was he or she told about the diagnosis? Did the patient feel revulsion at her mastectomy scar? Did the patient believe that the cancer had been cured after chemotherapy? How surprised was he or she when liver metastases were discovered? How ill does the patient feel now? What does he or she think is the likely prognosis? The answers to these questions are often surprising. Patients may have a logical understanding of the function of a hospice ('it's where you come to die'), but hold out a strong belief that they will be cured. They may continue to avoid the use of words like 'cancer' and prefer euphemisms like 'growth'. During the assessment the psychiatrist needs to strike a balance between colluding with the patient who may be denying illness or its implications, and being overly challenging and thereby threaten the patient's engagement with the assessment. Having gained an understanding of the psychological response to the disease, and the disease's progress itself, the main psychiatric complaint may be explored in the usual way.

The personal history should take the usual format, but is often a particularly helpful process which patients find useful in putting their current experiences into perspective. The family history should include experiences of bereavements and family history of the disease the patient is suffering from. The patient's previous experience of death, for example how the patient's parents died, is highly relevant to his or her current predicament. Patients who have greatest difficulty adapting to their diagnoses, or bereavement, often have disturbed early experiences with abuse or inadequate parenting. A history of stable relationships is almost certainly protective against depression and anxiety. Occupational history is also important – in patients of working age, it is very common that work stopped at around the time of diagnosis, and current psychiatric problems are a result in the change in role the disease has brought about – sometimes unnecessarily. The history should also include a detailed description of current social networks, the current 'typical day' and a clear account of level of dependency and functional impairments. The mental state is described in more detail for each of the common presentations.

Common presentations in palliative care

In our practice, the reasons commonly given for requesting an assessment are:
- depression
- anxiety
- disturbed behaviour (delirium, dementia and psychosis)
- mental incapacity
- requests for euthanasia or physician-assisted suicide.

Depression

As in any other groups of patients with established physical disease, comorbid depression is a familiar problem. In palliative care depression may have dramatic consequences. Clinicians in palliative care are frequently presented with patients who appear to have 'given up' or 'turned their face to the wall'. Such patients may stop eating and drinking, and through cachexia and immobility die earlier than would have been expected given the severity of their disease under these circumstances. Requests for euthanasia or physician-assisted suicide are also common problems.

Diagnosis

Current definitions of depressive disorders are problematic in patients with advanced disease. First, some mood change under these circumstances is understandable. Second, some of the biological and cognitive symptoms of depression may be a direct consequence of physical disease. Various alternatives have been raised to deal with this problem. Endicott (1984) proposed the use of a series of criteria whereby biological symptoms of depression are replaced with more mood-based symptoms (see Table 25.1). Chochinov studied this approach in a case series of hospice patients, and found that the prevalence of depression did not change when the substitution criteria were applied, and that the same patients were diagnosed with depression whichever approach was used (Chochinov *et al.* 1994). This study also assessed the use of alternative diagnostic thresholds – setting case definitions at higher than usual levels. As might be expected, this led to a reduction in the prevalence. Depression is a syndrome and depressive symptoms which make up the syndrome all lie on a continuum, making any definition essentially arbitrary (House 1988). Therefore it may be more helpful to consider what the level of severity and chronicity of depression should be present before specific treatments are used.

This theoretical debate does little to help the clinician. In the setting of advanced disease, it is possible that medicalizing 'normal' distress is as harmful as failing to diagnose 'pathological' depression. Patients who are in a state of emotional turmoil, but not depressed, need support and assistance in maximizing their self-efficacy, and giving a diagnosis of depression may push them into yet another sick role, which may be unhelpful. Our approach is to keep an open mind, but to diagnose depression according to features which we believe distinguish it from distress. These features are:

1. Lack of reactivity of affect: patients with depression maintain a low affect throughout the interview, whereas those with more transient distress show greater fluctuation in mood – they may often appear miserable and tearful at the start of the interview, but after 30 minutes the mood lifts.

2. Anhedonia: even in advanced disease, many patients are able to enjoy visits from grandchildren, but the ability to experience pleasure is typically missing in depression.

Table 25.1. Endicott substitution criteria.

---

1. Change in appetite/weight → tearfulness, depressed appearance
2. Sleep disturbance → social withdrawal, decreased talkativeness
3. Fatigue/loss of energy → brooding self-pity, pessimism
4. Diminished ability to think or concentrate/indecision → lack of reactivity

---

3. Cognitive features of depression such as prominent guilt and worthlessness are uncommon under other circumstances.

Recognition of depression and screening for cases

It is probable that depression is underdiagnosed and treated in palliative care settings, as indeed it is in primary care and general hospitals (Lloyd-Williams et al. 1999). Case-finding questionnaires such as the Hospital Anxiety and Depression scale (Zigmond & Snaith 1983) and the Beck Depression Inventory (Beck et al. 1961) have been used, with satisfactory sensitivity and specificity (for a review see Hotopf et al. 2001). Many patients who are very frail will not be able to complete such questionnaires, leading (Chochinov et al. 1997) to the provocative idea that a single-item question 'have you been depressed most of the time in the last two weeks?' would perform as well as established screening questionnaires. The results of this study were striking, as the single question had perfect sensitivity and specificity. More recent work has failed to replicate this result (Lloyd-Williams et al. 2003), presumably because the original paper had not used the screening question independently of the gold-standard interview. Using screening questionnaires is not an alternative to clinical awareness, and recognition of depression (especially in withdrawn patients) is a key educational goal for palliative care staff.

Differential diagnosis of depression

In palliative care settings the need to detect physical illnesses which can present with depressed mood is less vital than in other liaison psychiatry settings. It is certainly theoretically possible that a patient may have hypothyroidism as well as advanced cancer, but it is rare. More important is recognizing aspects of the known disease and current treatment which may have affected mood. Steroid therapy, hypercalcaemia, cerebral metastases and chemotherapies may all cause lowering of mood. Temporal associations between such factors and mood changes should be sought in the history.

Prevalence of depression in advanced disease

Hinton's cross-sectional study of patients dying of cancer in King's College Hospital found high rates of depression (with only one-third having a 'normally cheerful' mood) which was stable before death. Our systematic review of depression in palliative care has since confirmed very high rates of depression (Hotopf et al. 2001). Studies that simply ask about depression as a symptom find as many as 40% of patients endorsing the symptom, with 93% judged to have some degree of psychological distress (Edmonds et al. 1998). Other studies which have used questionnaires such as the Hospital Anxiety and Depression Scale (Zigmond & Snaith 1983) find rates of patients scoring above threshold of between 16 and 50%

(Faull *et al.* 1994; Fulton 1997). Studies that use more robust psychiatric interviews to make operationally defined diagnoses of depression have found up to one-third of patients with advanced disease suffer from depression (Chochinov *et al.* 1995; Hopwood *et al.* 1991a; Power *et al.* 1993).

Who becomes depressed? Younger age is probably a risk factor, with older patients having reduced prevalence (Hinton 1963). Whilst this is in keeping with population-based surveys, which show prevalence to fall with age, it is probably more marked than would be expected on this alone. Female gender is a far less pronounced risk factor compared with surveys in the general population (Plumb & Holland 1981). Spirituality is probably a protective factor, as is social support. The relationship with pain is weaker than one might anticipate with some studies failing to detect an association (Melvin *et al.* 1995; Sze *et al.* 2000), but others showing a strong association (Hopwood *et al.* 1991b). Certain types of cancer (e.g. head and neck disease which may interfere with speech and have dramatic cosmetic consequences) or treatments (e.g. mutilating surgery) may also heighten risk. There is also growing interest in the relationship between depression and release of illness-behaviour cytokines such as interleukin-6 (McDaniel *et al.* 1995; Musselman *et al.* 2001).

Impact and prognosis of depression

Few studies have assessed the prognosis of depression in patients with advanced disease. Edmonds *et al.* (1998) found it to be an especially persistent symptom. Depression is likely to have a number of important consequences in advanced disease. Many studies have shown that depression is a risk factor for mortality in earlier stages of physical disease. It seems probable that even in advanced cancer, individuals with depression succumb more quickly due to immobility and inadequate nutrition. It is also likely that depression increases perception of pain and other physical symptoms, as it does in healthy populations. Depression is likely also to impact on service use and costs. Finally depression may have an adverse effect on carers (Given *et al.* 1993; Kurtz *et al.* 1995) and ultimately bereavement outcome, if the family perceives the patient to have died in a state of anguish and misery.

Treatment of depression

There are a few specific considerations to take account of in the management of depression in advanced disease. First, time may be short. If antidepressants take two weeks to start working their use is limited in dying individuals. The implication of this is clear — early recognition and treatment of depression is particularly crucial in this setting. Second, it is often difficult to monitor treatment effects when so much else is changing. Patients may experience dramatic fluctuations in physical symptoms and it is sometimes difficult to know whether an improvement in depression is due to, for example, pain having been effectively managed, or a new antidepressant having been prescribed. When patients are highly symptomatic, it is also difficult to assess side-effects of antidepressants. Third, some of the medications commonly used in palliative care, most obviously steroids, can have a direct impact on mood. Finally, whilst there are a handful of randomized controlled trials for the treatment of depression in physical disease, very few of these are in palliative care samples, presumably due to the difficulties of researching this group.

There are probably only three randomized controlled trials to have assessed treatments of depression in samples of patients with advanced disease (Ly *et al.* 2002). Of these, one used thioridazine which is now withdrawn from the UK market (Johnston 1972). A placebo-controlled trial of mianserin indicated that the antidepressant was effective (Costa *et al.* 1985). A comparative study of fluoxetine and desipramine indicated no convincing advantages of either treatment (Holland *et al.* 1998). There are no randomized controlled trials on psychotherapy. Treatment therefore has to be based on what is known about treating depression in physically ill populations, with a few observations from palliative care.

Choice of psychotropic medication

Since all antidepressants have approximately the same efficacy, the choice is based on matching the side-effect profile against the patient's symptoms. Given that many patients are elderly and frail, tricyclic antidepressants are not a first-line treatment. The one exception is when a patient has been started on a tricyclic in low dose for neuropathic pain, where the dose is cautiously increased, rather than switching to an alternative class. Selective serotonin reuptake inhibitors are widely used as first-line treatments. They lack some of the more severe side-effects of tricyclics such as postural hypotension, but are not necessarily better tolerated. Patients who are cachectic and have suffered severe nausea from chemotherapy may be understandably reluctant to be prescribed yet another drug which causes nausea. Newer antidepressants with actions on both serotonin and noradrenaline may have some advantages in this group. Mirtazapine for example has the useful side-effect of causing increased appetite and weight gain, which patients find an attractive feature.

The psychostimulants (methylphenidate, dexamfetamine and pemoline) have been used in the management of depression and fatigue in advanced disease, especially in North America. Their advantages are said to be their rapid action and effectiveness against severe psychomotor slowing and fatigue. There is some evidence that they are effective in the short-term management of fatigue in HIV patients (Breitbart *et al.* 2001), but no randomized controlled trials into their efficacy in depression. In our view the treatment (which causes sleep disturbance, nervousness, motor tics, dyskinesias and possible psychotic symptoms) is still experimental and should not be given outside the context of randomized controlled trials.

Choice of psychotherapy

The time restraints on treating depression in palliative care are such that it is rarely possible to provide formal psychotherapy in this setting. Instead, certain important elements of the main psychotherapeutic modalities should be extracted and used where appropriate. We use elements of supportive, couple and cognitive behavioural therapies in working with patients, as well as making use of psychodynamic formulations where appropriate.

Supportive psychotherapy techniques include allowing the patient to ventilate emotions, and responding to these in a non-judgemental manner. Cognitive behavioural approaches to depression in advanced disease may involve diary keeping, problem solving, activity scheduling, monitoring, questioning and challenging automatic thoughts. Couple or family approaches include using a family member as a cotherapist. Communication problems are extremely common within couples, and seeing couples together often allows strong emotions to be ventilated in a safe environment. Couples can also be helped to avoid 'mind reading', where one member of the dyad makes assumptions about how his or her partner is feeling without checking.

Anxiety

Compared to depression, anxiety has received much less attention in the literature (Chochinov 2000; Chochinov & Breitbart 2000). In those studies reporting prevalence, the rates vary from 1.1% (Minagawa *et al.* 1996) to over 70% (Breitbart *et al.* 1995). Such disparity relates strongly to the methodological heterogeneity of the studies but to some degree reflects the confusion that exists clinically — distinguishing between distress and pathology is as difficult as with depression.

Patients are frequently reluctant to complain of psychological symptoms, and many doctors and nurses will avoid discussion of these sensitive areas (Barraclough 1997). Anxiety, like depression, is often felt to be universal, understandable and resistant to intervention (Massie 1989). These difficulties are compounded by the overlap between physical symptoms of anxiety and common symptoms of advanced disease (and its treatment), most obviously breathlessness but also sweating, dry mouth and tremor. Such symptoms will often be managed 'physically' with psychological considerations less attended to.

Whilst psychiatric diagnoses are often a cause of anxiety symptoms, the prevalence of pure anxiety disorders in palliative care is not known. Anecdotally, anxiety symptoms are more commonly part of an adjustment disorder or a mixed anxiety and depressive disorder. Such an overlap is particularly relevant to palliative care. Anxiety has been suggested to arise from 'threat' life events and depression from 'loss' life events (Barraclough 1997). Patients with advanced disease are commonly in a position of being exposed to both. The threat is of further, perhaps increasingly distressing, symptoms and an awareness that they are dying. The loss can come in a number of forms, including loss of independence, loss of social and occupational roles and, in time, loss of function.

Whilst anxiety symptoms are in themselves distressing, their impact can be greater than just the immediate discomfort. Avoidance of situations believed to be associated with anxiety can occur — for example agoraphobic features can have a disabling effect on the patient's life. These can in turn impact on the patient's family or carer who may have to accompany the patient or take on tasks normally performed by the patient. The 'physical' nature of many anxiety symptoms can increase patients' vigilance for bodily symptoms and can be interpreted as sinister developments in the underlying disease.

Management of anxiety

The management of anxiety symptoms in palliative care must start with a careful assessment. This will include a clear description of the symptoms with information about triggers, both physical and emotional. The assessment must go on to examine the impact these symptoms are having on the patient's life and the strategies the patient is currently using to deal with them. Of course possible physical differential diagnoses must be considered but equally the patient's broader mental state should be examined, in particular for an underlying depressive disorder.

Simple anxiety symptoms can arise from concerns about the illness or its treatment. The role of information, education and reassurance should not be underestimated. Patients are at times just relieved that this aspect of their distress has been acknowledged and taken seriously. Whilst there should be a reluctance to medicalize distress, drugs do have a significant role to play in the management of anxiety. Benzodiazepines are used frequently within palliative care, especially for the short-term management of severe and overwhelming anxiety. They are well tolerated, act swiftly and palliative care doctors and nurses are comfortable and familiar with their use. Such familiarity can lead to situations where the threshold for benzodiazepine use is lowered; use increases and alternative methods are not considered. The impact of such prescribing habits on patients' and doctors willingness to discuss emotional matters further, and side-effects such as confusion and unwanted drowsiness have not been assessed in this setting.

Antidepressant drugs can treat the mixed anxiety and depression states which appear commonly but are also of use in the treatment of panic disorder and generalized anxiety disorder (Kasper & Resinger 2001). The choice of antidepressant in this situation again depends on which particular side-effects the patient may be able to best tolerate — evidence exists that serotonin-specific reuptake inhibitors can be as effective as tricyclic antidepressants.

There has been almost no research on psychotherapies such as cognitive behavioural therapy in the management of anxiety in palliative care, although studies are under way. These treatments have been helpful in early cancer (Moorey et al. 2003). Such approaches are limited both by the availability of therapists and for some patients by the timescale involved. However for a significant proportion of patients the use of cognitive techniques, including the exploration of underlying beliefs about symptoms and identification of maladaptive coping styles, could be beneficial.

Disturbed behaviour

There are a large number of reasons why patients with advanced disease, particularly those in hospices, might present with confusion or disturbed behaviour. These include delirium, comorbid cognitive impairment and longstanding psychotic illnesses. In addition, a significant number of hospice patients will experience terminal delirium in the days before death (Lawlor et al. 2000a,b).

Delirium

Patients with advanced disease have many risk factors for developing an acute confusional state (Casarett & Inouye 2001). These include increasing age, physical illnesses, which can directly increase the risk, or make patients more susceptible to intercurrent infections, and exposure to drugs that impair cognitive function. Estimates of the prevalence of delirium range between 28% (Caraceni et al. 2000) and 85% (Massie, et al. 1983), making it a very common problem. Unfortunately delirium is often missed amongst the plethora of other symptoms (Inouye et al. 2003; Roth-Roemer et al. 1997). A number of assessment tools are available to assist identification of these patients — Confusion Assessment Method (Inouye et al. 1990), Memorial Delirium Assessment Scale (Breitbart et al. 1997), Bedside Confusion Scale (Sarhill et al. 2001) and the Delirium Rating Scale (Mattis 1988) have all been used in published studies. They may be particularly helpful in picking up patients with the hypoactive form of delirium.

The presence of delirium can have a number of unwelcome consequences. Disturbed behaviour can interfere with the appropriate provision of palliative care to the patient, for example the accurate assessment and optimal management of pain (Bruera *et al.* 1992). The interference with communication can impact adversely on the relationship the patient has with his family, increasing their distress (Boyle *et al.* 1998; Breitbart *et al.* 2000; Gordon *et al.* 1997; Lawlor *et al.* 2000b). One study has shown that delirium is a marker for poor outcome, as delirious patients had a significantly shorter life expectancy than non-delirious patients (Caraceni *et al.* 2000).

Delirium should not be thought of as inevitable or untreatable. An elegant study by Inouye confirmed that appropriate management of the patient and their environment can be effective (Inouye *et al.* 1999). Amelioration of sleep deprivation, immobility, visual and hearing impairments and dehydration can reduce the incidence of delirium (see Chapter 12).

Management of delirium

The American Psychiatric Association's guidelines on delirium are applicable to the management of patients with advanced disease (American Psychiatric Association 1999). These suggest that haloperidol is the treatment of choice, starting with low doses (0.5–1 mg four times daily) and titrated upwards, monitoring closely for adverse reactions. Patients with cerebral disease may be sensitive to extrapyramidal side-effects. Other possible treatments include atypical antipsychotics (such as risperidone, olanzapine and quetiapine) or novel drugs like ondansetron or rivastigmine. Several studies within palliative care have shown that symptoms can be effectively treated in up to 69% of patients (Cobb *et al.* 2000; Gagnon *et al.* 2000; Lawlor *et al.* 2000b). Patients in whom medication or dehydration are identified as potential causal factors seem to respond particularly well (Lawlor *et al.* 2000b). The presence of advanced disease does not preclude the possibility of delirium tremens secondary to alcohol withdrawal, and this should always be considered (see Chapter 8).

Dementia

Patients in the palliative care system will include, if only on the basis of age, a significant number of patients with common dementing illnesses such as Alzheimer's-type dementia, Lewy body disease, and cerebrovascular disease. Some patients have an established diagnosis of dementia, but in many the chronic cognitive impairment may have gone undetected. The prevalence in this patient group is not known. The presence of cognitive impairment can have an impact on the way palliative care is received and given (Nowels *et al.* 2002). Cognitively impaired patients may be less able to accurately communicate their needs, or to follow instructions about medication. Capacity may be impaired. Existing cognitive impairment is a risk factor for a superimposed delirium (Boyle *et al.* 1998), and may make assessments about the effectiveness of its management difficult.

With dementia, the focus is less on treatment than on recognition, both that the patient has a degree of cognitive impairment, and what particular difficulties this causes the patient and his or her carer. The Mini Mental State Examination (Folstein *et al.* 1975), although perhaps a little unwieldy for routine practice, is widely used, as is the shorter Abbreviated Mental Test Score (Hodkinson 1972). A recent attempt to use a single screening question alone was unsuccessful (Kibiger *et al.* 2003), though alternatives are being assessed. The liaison psychiatrist has a role both in assisting other staff in assessing cognitive function and in educating staff, patients and families about the implications of impaired cognitive function. It is important to remember that depression rates are elevated in both cognitively impaired patients (Lyketsos & Olin 2002) and their carers (Pinquart & Sorensen 2003).

It has been argued that conditions such as the Alzheimer's-type dementia are terminal diseases, meriting palliative care in their own right (Shuster 2000). The limited numbers of patients who receive palliative care for Alzheimer's disease, together with the communication difficulties alluded to, have led to the suggestion that cognitively impaired patients represent an excluded group (Henderson 2004). There is an ongoing discussion within palliative care as to how the challenge of providing appropriate palliative care for this growing group of patients should be met.

Established psychotic illness

Patients with longstanding mental health problems frequently require medical and nursing care for advanced disease. Most of these cause no difficulties at all, but an exacerbation of an underlying psychotic illness should be considered in a patient presenting with disturbed behaviour. Most of these patients will be engaged with mental health services or will be well known to the general practitioners. The liaison psychiatrist may have a role in communicating with the community mental health teams, and planning for discharge from the hospice.

Assessment of mental capacity

As discussed above, cognitive impairments and depression are both common in the palliative care setting, and psychiatrists are sometimes asked to assess mental capacity. Mental capacity is a legal concept and its exact definition differs in different legislatures. In England and Wales, the Mental Capacity Act (2005) states that a person may be incapacitated if, because of an impairment of brain or mind:

1. he/she is unable to understand the information relevant to the decision;
2. he/she is unable to retain the information relevant to the decision;
3. he/she is unable to use or weigh the information relevant to the decision as part of the process of making the decision; or
4. he/she is unable to communicate the decision (whether by talking, using sign language or any other means).

Patients are assumed to have mental capacity unless there is good evidence to doubt it. Mental capacity is situation specific – so a patient may lack capacity to make a choice about treatment, but may have capacity to give a relative enduring power of attorney or make a will (see also Chapter 3).

Our research on general hospital inpatients finds that mental incapacity related to making a treatment decision is very common, with as many as 40% of patients during some point of their hospital admission being unable to understand, retain or communicate decisions regarding treatment preferences (Raymont *et al.* 2004). In most instances such difficulties are caused by cognitive impairment in this frail, elderly and acutely-ill sample. Mental incapacity is infrequently detected by clinicians, probably because in most instances the patients acquiesced to treatment and accepted their doctor's advice.

Occasionally patients refuse treatments, or insist on living in circumstances which are dangerous. Very occasionally there is grave concern that a relative is attempting to extort money from a vulnerable patient by coercing him or her into writing a new will or signing enduring power of attorney. Under such circumstances a careful assessment of capacity is indicated. When patients refuse to accept medical advice, this is commonly due to a break-down in communication with the clinical team, and may be a form of protest by the patient. The psychiatrist's task under these circumstances is to try to improve understanding on both sides.

If a decision is made that the patient lacks capacity, the next step is to assess the patient's best interests. If the patient has made an advanced directive over his or her care, this should be respected unless current circumstances have not been foreseen. In assessing best interests, the relatives should be consulted, as should other healthcare professionals such as the patient's general practitioner. It is important to take into account any previously expressed views the patient may have had.

Suicide and deliberate self-harm

As a group, palliative care patients have two important risk factors for completed suicide – they are an elderly population and by definition they have physical illness. This and the high rates of depression and pain associated with advanced disease are probably responsible for the high rates of suicide in palliative care patients reported in the few studies which have measured it (Ripamonti *et al.* 1999). However, suicide rates are probably higher still in patients with early cancer (Crocetti *et al.* 1998).

Clinically, deliberate self-harm and suicide are not uncommon. Deliberate self-harm is covered in Chapter 11; however there are a few considerations which are especially germane to palliative care. First, patients with advanced disease may have access to lethal methods in the form of opiate medication. If there are genuine concerns about suicide risk it is important to ensure that supplies are small and a responsible family member is aware of this possibility. Second, the assessment when self-harm has taken place should be no different from that used in any other setting. The aim is to gather information on the attempt, in order to judge the degree of intent, diagnose underlying psychiatric disorders, and come to a judgement of the risk of repetition. The case history in Box 25.1 demonstrates how confused some doctors can be when confronting suicidal behaviour in this setting. Third, if admission following deliberate self-harm is indicated, where should this be? Ideally joint medical/psychiatric wards would be available to care for frail medically ill patients requiring psychiatric admission. If the risk of repetition is not considered to be imminent, the patient is very

---

Box 25.1 Deliberate self-harm in palliative-care patients.

A 63-year-old woman with metastatic breast cancer was admitted to a hospice after taking an overdose of paracetamol. She had disclosed the overdose to her husband 30 minutes after taking the overdose. He persuaded her to go to the local Accident and Emergency department. A junior doctor had assessed her, but because she had not wanted treatment had written. 'Patient refuses treatment. In view of her advanced cancer, her wishes are to be respected'. The doctor had then arranged transfer to the hospice. When admitted, a psychiatrist saw her and persuaded her to take acetylcysteine. The patient was stabilized, and quickly admitted to regretting the overdose. Psychiatric assessment revealed a moderately severe depressive illness which was treated with antidepressants and supportive psychotherapy. She made a good recovery from her depression, continued to express amazement that she had attempted to end her life, and died comfortably of natural causes six months later.

The case demonstrates that:
- The presence of advanced disease can sometimes lead to inappropriate management by doctors. The desire to 'respect the wishes' of the patient would presumably have been absent under other circumstances.
- Desire for death, even in the context of a suicide attempt, fluctuates.
- Depression in this context is treatable.

frail, and the clinical team feels confident in managing the patient, transfer to a hospice may be greatly preferable than to a psychiatric ward. Finally, there are circumstances where the resuscitation of patients who have attempted suicide, and have advanced disease, may be inappropriate. The fact that the patient has chosen to kill himself should not lead to over-zealous attempts at resuscitation, if under other circumstances, a deterioration would have been treated in a non-invasive manner.

When patients commit suicide, it is sensible to review the case with the clinical team, in an unthreatening way. Following a suicide of a patient under the care of the hospice, we routinely hold a team meeting (and invite the general practitioner) to establish the facts of the case. Whilst the psychiatrist should have a supportive role in the aftermath of suicide, it is probably not helpful to provide emotional debriefing, although hospices might expect this. The psychiatrist also has a role in advising the hospice on the development of guidelines for the management of suicidal behaviour.

Euthanasia and physician-assisted suicide

In the UK, euthanasia and physician-assisted suicide (PAS) are illegal, whilst the act of suicide itself is legal. In the Netherlands, Switzerland, and the state of Oregon in the USA, voluntary euthanasia or physician-assisted suicide have been decriminalized, if not legalized. Recent 'right-to-die' cases have given the topic renewed publicity in the UK, and in clinical settings it is not uncommon to be asked to see a patient because he or she has requested euthanasia.

Why might individuals with advanced disease request euthanasia? A Canadian qualitative study of HIV patients (Lavery *et al.* 2001) suggested there were two main factors — disintegration and loss of community. Disintegration referred to fears of uncontrolled physical symptoms, loss of independence and becoming a burden on carers. Loss of community referred to loss of occupational roles, inability to form new relationships, and stigmatization by others. Both disintegration and loss of community ultimately led to a loss of self. Similar broad themes have been identified in qualitative work in terminally-ill cancer patients (Kelly *et al.* 2002).

Will-to-live changes over time. In an elegant descriptive study (Chochinov *et al.* 1999) Chochinov and colleagues were able to demonstrate substantial fluctuations in will-to-live among palliative care patients even over the course of a day. Desire for death was predicted by symptoms (anxiety, depression, shortness of breath), but the importance of each symptom changed as death approached — psychological distress becoming less prominent in the terminal stages. Emanuel *et al.* (2000) also demonstrated considerable fluctuation in terms of interest in use of euthanasia. Ganzini *et al.* (1998), in a survey of 100 patients with motor neurone disease, demonstrated that whilst many (56%) expressed an interest in physician-assisted suicide, only one individual actually wanted to receive it at the time of the interview. Approximately one-third expressed a desire to have medication available for future use.

It will come as no surprise to psychiatrists that depression is a powerful risk factor for wishes to hasten death. For example, Chochinov *et al.* (1995) found that occasional wishes to die were common (44.5%). Of the smaller proportion (8.5%) who had a serious and pervasive desire to die, 58.5% suffered from depression, compared to 7.7% in the remaining sample. Brown *et al.* (1986) found similar results. Further work in HIV patients (at a time when the diagnosis had considerably higher mortality) found a high proportion supporting physician-assisted suicide and wanting this as a possible option in the future (Breitbart *et al.* 1996). Those who expressed an interest were more likely to be depressed, isolated, or to fear being a burden on others. Finally a major study of 988 terminally-ill patients with mixed diagnoses found that the 10% who would seriously consider using euthanasia if available were younger, had greater pain and more depressive symptoms than those who would not (Emanuel *et al.* 2000).

Spirituality is another important concept in desire for death. Spirituality is a complex dimension which is distinguished from participation in organized religious practice. It has been defined as 'the way in which people understand their lives in view of their ultimate meaning and value' — as such it is unsurprising that spirituality is a protective factor against depression. However, there is some evidence that individuals with high spirituality who become depressed are less likely to desire a hastened death (McClain *et al.* 2003).

What do these findings suggest in clinical practice in an environment where euthanasia is not available? How should a clinician respond to expressions that a patient wants euthanasia? First, a high proportion of respondents to surveys on this topic have a broadly sympathetic view of euthanasia. Expression of a desire for euthanasia at some point in the future is not uncommon, and such expressions are best explored in an open-minded way. They should not automatically be a trigger for referral to a psychiatrist, but the clinicians should be encouraged to explore fears that the illness will lead to a loss of dignity, uncontrolled pain or of the patient becoming a burden. Such fears are then best addressed in their own right, with appropriate explanations and reassurances.

Second, many individuals who express a desire for euthanasia in the future may use this as a means of maintaining a degree of control over their destiny. In jurisdictions where euthanasia is outlawed, such control may appear illusory, but it is important to recognize the underlying sentiment. Clinicians in palliative care may need support from psychiatrists to plan this. Third, a high proportion of patients who request a wish to end their lives will have depression, and this should be treated energetically.

Psychiatry has an important role in the wider debate on euthanasia, for two main reasons – first, because of the importance of psychiatric disorders, and in particular depression, on desire for death, and the fact that such disorders are potentially treatable. Second, because of the role of psychiatrists in assessing mental capacity in patients with medical illness. The legislatures that have decriminalized euthanasia and/or PAS, limit the procedures to individuals who are competent to give their consent. However, the cognitive processes which underpin capacity are complex and dimensional. When assessments of capacity are applied to an individual clinical decision, this complexity has to be synthesized into a single 'yes/no' answer. It is a sound principle that in judging mental capacity, the threshold should be proportionate to the importance of the decision. Ending a life requires a higher level of capacity compared with lesser procedures. Thus the assessment of mental capacity under such circumstances should be especially rigorous and detailed. As well as ensuring that patients have capacity, the act of euthanasia must be truly voluntary. There is substantial evidence that this is not the case in the Netherlands (Hendin 1997) where patients may in subtle ways be coerced by family members and medical enthusiasts into pursuing euthanasia. We do not believe that current 'safeguards' in the Netherlands and elsewhere are sufficient to guarantee that euthanasia is truly voluntary.

REFERENCES

Addington Hall, J. and Higginson, I. (2001). *Palliative Care for Non-cancer Patients.* Oxford: Oxford University Press.

American Psychiatric Association. (1999). *Practice Guidelines for the Treatment of Patients with Delirium.*

Barraclough, J. (1997). ABC of palliative care. Depression, anxiety, and confusion. *British Medical Journal*, **315**(7119), 1365–8.

Beck, A. T., Ward, C. H. and Mendelson, M. (1961). An inventory for measuring depression. *Archives of General Psychiatry*, **4**, 561–71.

Boyle, D. M., Abernathy, G., Baker, L., *et al.* (1998). End of life confusion in patients with cancer. *Oncology Nurses Forum*, **25**, 1335–43.

Breitbart, W., Bruera, E., Chochinov, H., *et al.* (1995). Neuropsychiatric syndromes and psychological symptoms in patients with advanced cancer. *Journal of Pain and Symptom Management*, **10**(2), 131–41.

Breitbart, W., Rosenfeld, B. D. and Passik, S. D. (1996). Interest in physician-assisted suicide among ambulatory HIV-infected patients (see comments). *American Journal of Psychiatry*, **153**(2), 238–42.

Breitbart, W., Rosenfeld, B., Roth, A., *et al.* (1997). The Memorial Delirium Assessment Scale. *Journal of Pain and Symptom Management*, **13**(3), 128–37.

Breitbart, W., Rosenfeld, B., Pessin, H., *et al.* (2000). Depression, hopelessness, and desire for hastened death in terminally ill patients with cancer. *Journal of the American Medical Association*, **284**, 2907–11.

Breitbart, W., Rosenfeld, B., Kaim, M., *et al.* (2001). A randomized, double-blind, placebo-controlled trial of psychostimulants for the treatment of fatigue in ambulatory patients with human immunodeficiency virus disease. *Archives of Internal Medicine*, **161**(3), 411–20.

Brown, J. H., Henteleff, P., Barakat, S., *et al.* (1986). Is it normal for terminally ill patients to desire death? *American Journal of Psychiatry*, **143**(2), 208–11.

Bruera, E., Miller, L., McCallion, J., *et al.* (1992). Cognitive failure in patients with terminal cancer: a prospective study. *Journal of Pain and Symptom Management*, **7**(4), 192–5.

Caraceni, A., Nanni, O., Maltoni, M., *et al.* (2000). Impact of delirium on the short term prognosis of advanced cancer patients. Italian Multicenter Study Group on Palliative Care. *Cancer*, **89**(5), 1145–9.

Casarett, D. J. and Inouye, S. K. (2001). Diagnosis and management of delirium near the end of life. *Annals of Internal Medicine*, **135**(1), 32–40.

Chochinov, H. M. (2000). Psychiatry and terminal illness. *Canadian Journal of Psychiatry*, **45**(2), 143–50.

Chochinov, H. M. and Breitbart, W. (2000). *Handbook of Psychiatry in Palliative Medicine*, 1st edn. Oxford: Oxford University Press.

Chochinov, H. M., Wilson, K. G., Enns, M., *et al.* (1994). Prevalence of depression in the terminally ill: effects of diagnostic criteria and symptom threshold judgements. *American Journal of Psychiatry*, **151**(4), 537–40.

Chochinov, H. M., Wilson, K. G., Enns, M., *et al.* (1995). Desire for death in the terminally ill. *American Journal of Psychiatry*, **152**(8), 1185–91.

Chochinov, H. M., Wilson, K. G., Enns, M., *et al.* (1997). Are you depressed? Screening for depression in the terminally ill. *American Journal of Psychiatry*, **154**(5), 674–6.

Chochinov, H. M., Tataryn, D., Clinch, J. J., *et al.* (1999). Will to live in the terminally ill. Comment. *Lancet*, **354**(9181), 816–19.

Cobb, J. L., Glanyz, M. J., Nicholas, P. K., *et al.* (2000). Delirium in patients with cancer at the end of life. *Cancer Practice*, **8**, 172–7.

Corr, C. A. (1992). A task-based approach to coping with dying. *Omega – Journal of Death and Dying*, **24**(2), 82–94.

Corr, C. A. (1999). Dying and its interpreters: a review of selected literature and some comments on the state of the field. *Omega – Journal of Death and Dying*, **39**(4), 239–59.

Costa, D., Mogos, I. and Toma, T. (1985). Efficacy and safety of mianserin in the treatment of depression of women with cancer. *Acta Psychiatrica Scandinavica*, **72**(Suppl. 320), 85–92.

Crocetti, E., Arniani, S., Acciai, S., *et al.* (1998). High suicide mortality soon after diagnosis among cancer patients in central Italy. *British Journal of Cancer*, **77**(7), 1194–6.

Doka, K. J. (1995). Coping with life-threatening illness: a task model. *Omega – Journal of Death and Dying*, **32**, 111–22.

Edmonds, P. M., Stuttaford, J. M., Peny, J., *et al.* (1998). Do hospital palliative care teams improve symptom control? Use of a modified STAS as an evaluation tool. *Palliative Medicine*, **12**(5), 345–51.

Emanuel, E. J., Fairclough, D. L. and Emanuel, L. L. (2000). Attitudes and desires related to euthanasia and physician-assisted suicide among terminally ill patients and their caregivers. Comment. *Journal of the American Medical Association*, **284**(19), 2460–8.

Endicott, J. (1984). Measurement of depression in patients with cancer. *Cancer*, **53**(Suppl.), 2243–8.

Faull, C. M., Johnson, I. S. and Butler, T. J. (1994). The hospital anxiety and depression (HAD) scale: its validity in patients with terminal malignant disease. *Palliative Medicine*, **8**(1), 69.

Ferrando, S. J. (2000). Commentary: integrating consultation-liaison psychiatry and palliative care. *Journal of Pain and Symptom Management*, **20**(3), 235–6.

Folstein, M. F., Folstein, S. E. and McHugh, P. R. (1975). Mini-mental state. A practical method for grading the cognitive state of patients for the clinician. *Journal of Psychiatric Research*, **12**(3), 189–98.

Fulton, C. L. (1997). The physical and psychological symptoms experienced by patients with metastatic breast cancer before death. *European Journal of Cancer Care*, **6**(4), 262–6.

Gagnon, B., Allard, P., Masse, B., *et al.* (2000). Delirium in terminal cancer: a prospective study using daily screening, early diagnosis and continuous monitoring. *Journal of Pain and Symptom Management*, **19**, 412–26.

Ganzini, L., Johnston, W. S., McFarland, B. H., *et al.* (1998). Attitudes of patients with amyotrophic lateral sclerosis and their care givers toward assisted suicide. Comment. *New England Journal of Medicine*, **339**(14), 967–73.

Given, C. W., Stommel, M., Given, J., *et al.* (1993). The influence of cancer patients' symptoms and functional states on patients' depression and family caregivers reaction and depression. *Health Psychology*, **12**(4), 277–85.

Gordon, D. S., Carter, H. and Scott, S. (1997). Profiling the care needs of the population with dementia: a survey in central Scotland. *International Journal of Geriatric Psychiatry*, **12**(7), 753–9.

Greer, S. and Watson, M. (1987). Mental adjustment to cancer: its measurement and prognostic importance. *Cancer Surveys*, **6**, 439–53.

Henderson, M. (2004). Mental health needs. In *Death, Dying and Social Differences*, ed. B. Monroe and D. Oliviere. Oxford: Oxford University Press.

Hendin, H. (1997). *Seduced By Death: Doctors, Patients, and the Dutch Cure*. New York: Norton.

Hinton, J. M. (1963). The physical and mental distress of the dying. *Quarterly Journal of Medicine*, **32**, 1–21.

Hodkinson, H. M. (1972). Evaluation of a mental test score for assessment of mental impairment in the elderly. *Age and Ageing*, **1**(4), 233–8.

Holland, J. C., Romano, S. J., Heilgenstein, J. H., *et al.* (1998). A controlled trial of fluoxetine and desipramine in depressed women with advanced cancer. *Psycho-oncology*, **7**, 291–300.

Hopwood, P., Howell, A. and Maguire, P. (1991a). Screening for psychiatric morbidity in patients with advanced breast cancer: validation of two self-report questionnaires. *British Journal of Cancer*, **64**, 353–6.

Hopwood, P., Howell, A. and Maguire, P. (1991b). Psychiatric morbidity in patients with advanced cancer of the breast: prevalence measured by two self-rating questionnaires. *British Journal of Cancer*, **64**, 349–52.

Hotopf, M., Ly, K. L., Chidey, J., *et al.* (2001). Depression in advanced disease – a systematic review: 1. Prevalence and case finding. *Palliative Medicine*, **16**, 81–97.

House, A. (1988). Mood disorders in the physically ill – problems of definition and measurement. *Journal of Psychosomatic Research*, **32**, 345–53.

Inouye, S. K., van Dyck, C. H., Alessi, C. A., *et al.* (1990). Clarifying confusion: the confusion assessment method. A new method for detection of delirium. *Annals of Internal Medicine*, **113**(12), 941–8.

Inouye, S. K., Bogardus, S. T., Jr, Charpentier, P. A., *et al.* (1999). A multicomponent intervention to prevent delirium in hospitalized older patients. *New England Journal of Medicine*, **340**(9), 669–76.

Inouye, S. K., Foreman, M. D., Mion, L. C., *et al.* (2003). Nurses recognition of delirium and its symptoms: comparison of nurse and researcher ratings. *Archives of Internal Medicine*, **161**, 2467–73.

Johnston, B. (1972). Relief of mixed anxiety – depression in terminal cancer patients: effect of thioridazine. *New York State Journal of Medicine*, **72**(18), 2315–17.

Kasper, S. and Resinger, E. (2001). Panic disorder: the place of benzodiazepines and selective serotonin reuptake inhibitors. *European Neuropsychopharmacology*, **11**(4), 307–21.

Kelly, B., Burnett, P., Pelusi, D., *et al.* (2002). Terminally ill cancer patients' wish to hasten death. *Palliative Medicine*, **16**, 339–45.

Kibiger, G., Kirsh, K. L., Wall, J. R., *et al.* (2003). My mind is as clear as it used to be: a pilot study illustrating the difficulties of employing a single-item subjective screen to detect cognitive impairment in outpatients with cancer. *Journal of Pain and Symptom Management*, **26**(2), 705–15.

Kübler-Ross, E. (1969). *On Death and Dying*, 1st edn. New York: Macmillan.

Kurtz, M. E., Kurtz, J. C., Given, C. W., *et al.* (1995). Relationship of caregiver reactions and depression to cancer patients' symptoms, functional states and depression: a longitudinal study. *Social Science and Medicine*, **40**, 837–46.

Lavery, J. V., Boyle, J., Dickens, B. M., *et al.* (2001). Origins of the desire for euthanasia and assisted suicide in people with HIV-1 or AIDS: a qualitative study. Comment. *Lancet*, **358**(9279), 362–7.

Lawlor, P. G., Fainsinger, R. L. and Bruera, E. D. (2000a). Delirium at the end of life: critical issues in clinical practice and research. *Journal of the American Medical Association*, **284**(19), 2427–9.

Lawlor, P. G., Gagnon, B., Mancini, I. L., *et al.* (2000b). Occurrence, causes, and outcome of delirium in patients with advanced cancer: a prospective study. *Archives of Internal Medicine*, **160**(6), 786–94.

Leventhal, H. and Cameron, L. (1987). Behavioural theories and the problem of compliance. *Patient Education and Counselling*, **10**, 117–38.

Lloyd-Williams, M., Friedman, T. and Rudd, N. (1999). A survey of antidepressant prescribing in the terminally ill. *Palliative Medicine*, **13**, 243–8.

Lloyd-Williams, M., Dennis, M., Taylor, F., *et al.* (2003). Is asking patients in palliative care, Are you depressed? appropriate? Prospective study. *British Medical Journal*, **327**(7411), 372–3.

Ly, K. L., Chidey, J., Addington Hall, J., *et al.* (2002). Depression in palliative care – a systematic review: 2. Treatment. *Palliative Medicine*, **16**, 279–84.

Lyketsos, C. G. and Olin, J. (2002). Depression in Alzheimer's disease: overview and treatment. *Biological Psychiatry*, **52**(3), 243–52.

Massie, M. J. (1989). Depression. In *Handbook of Psychooncology*, ed. J. Holland and J. Rowland. New York: Oxford University Press.

Massie, M. J., Holland, J. and Glass, E. (1983). Delirium in terminally ill cancer patients. *American Journal of Psychiatry*, **140**(8), 1048–50.

Mattis, S. (1988). *Dementia Rating Scale Professional Manual*. Odessa, FL: Pychological Assessment Resources Inc.

McClain, C. S., Rosenfeld, B. and Breitbart, W. (2003). Effect of spiritual well-being on end-of-life despair in terminally-ill cancer patients. Comment. *Lancet*, **361**(9369), 1603–7.

McDaniel, J. S., Musselman, D. L., Porter, M. R., *et al.* (1995). Depression in patients with cancer. Diagnosis, biology, and treatment. *Archives of General Psychiatry*, **52**, 89–99.

Melvin, T. A., Ozbek, I. N. and Eberle, D. E. (1995). Recognition of depression. *Hospice Journal*, **10**(3), 39–46.

Minagawa, H., Uchitomi, Y., Yamawaki, S., *et al.* (1996). Psychiatric morbidity in terminally ill cancer patients. A prospective study. *Cancer*, **78**(5), 1131–7.

Moorey, S., Frampton, M. and Greer, S. (2003). The Cancer Coping Questionnaire: a self-rating scale for measuring the impact of adjuvant psychological therapy on coping behaviour. *Psycho-oncology*, **12**, 331–44.

Musselman, D. L., Miller, A. H., Porter, M. R., *et al.* (2001). Higher than normal plasma interleukin-6 concentrations in cancer patients with depression: preliminary findings. *American Journal of Psychiatry*, **158**, 1252–7.

Nowels, D. E., Bublitz, C., Kassner, C. T., *et al.* (2002). Estimation of confusion prevalence in hospice patients. *Journal of Palliative Medicine*, **5**(5), 687–95.

Pinquart, M. and Sorensen, S. (2003). Differences between caregivers and noncaregivers in psychological health and physical health: a meta-analysis. *Psychology and Aging*, **18**(2), 250–67.

Plumb, M. and Holland, J. (1981). Comparative studies of psychological function in patients with advanced cancer. II. Interviewer-rated current and past psychological symptoms. *Psychosomatic Medicine*, **43**, 243–54.

Power, D., Kelly, S., Gilsenan, J., *et al.* (1993). Suitable screening tests for cognitive impairment and depression in the terminally ill – a prospective prevalence study. *Palliative Medicine*, **7**(3), 213–18.

Raymont, V., Bingley, W., Buchanan, A., *et al.* (2004). The prevalence and predictors of mental incapacity in medical in-patients. *Lancet*, **364**, 1421–7.

Ripamonti, C., Filiberti, A., Totis, A., *et al.* (1999). Suicide among patients with cancer cared for at home by palliative-care teams. *Lancet*, **354**(9193), 1877–8.

Roth-Roemer, S., Fann, J. and Syrjala, K. (1997). The importance of recognizing and measuring delirium. *Journal of Pain and Symptom Management*, **13**(3), 125–7.

Sarhill, N., Walsh, D., Nelson, K. A., *et al.* (2001). Assessment of delirium in advanced cancer: the use of the bedside confusion scale. *American Journal of Hospice and Palliative Care*, **18**(5), 335–41.

Shuster, J. L., Jr. (2000). Palliative care for advanced dementia. *Clinics in Geriatric Medicine*, **16**(2), 373–86.

Sze, F. K., Wong, E., Lo, R., *et al.* (2000). Do pain and disability differ in depressed cancer patients? *Palliative Medicine*, **14**, 11–17.

Watson, M., Greer, S., Rowden, L., *et al.* (1991). Relationships between emotional control, adjustment to cancer and depression and anxiety in breast cancer patients. *Psychological Medicine*, **21**, 51–7.

Zigmond, A. S. and Snaith, R. P. (1983). The Hospital Anxiety and Depression Scale. *Acta Psychiatrica Scandinavica*, **67**, 361–70.

26

Cosmetic procedures

David Veale

Introduction

Whatever the reader thinks of aesthetic cosmetic surgery, it is a popular lifestyle choice and attractiveness is a valued attribute in all societies. More than 50% of women and slightly fewer than 50% of men report dissatisfaction with their appearance (Garner 1997). Not surprisingly, many such individuals turn to cosmetic procedures to enhance their appearance. In the USA, 6.6 million procedures were performed in 2002 (American Society for Aesthetic Plastic Surgery 2003). This represents an increase of 1600% over the past decade. Many new procedures have been introduced which are non-surgical and, in the USA, the top six procedures in order of popularity are botox injections, chemical peel, microdermabrasion, laser hair removal, sclerotherapy and collagen injections. The most popular surgical procedures are rhinoplasty, mammaplasty augmentation or lift, liposuction, blepharoplasty, rhytidectomy (face-lift), and mammaplasty reduction. No such figures are available in the UK but, so far as one can tell, the profile is similar to the USA. It is estimated by market analysts that approximately £200 million per annum is spent on cosmetic procedures in the UK in the private sector and that 25% of all bank loans are given for cosmetic surgery.

The availability of cosmetic surgery in the National Health Service (NHS) is patchy. It is viewed by purchasers as a low priority, and there is a clear stigma against psychological distress and handicap caused by minor disfigurement or anomalies. In conditions of disfigurement, there is no relationship between the degree of disfigurement and distress flowing from it; on the contrary, minor physical disfigurement may be associated with great distress and handicap and vice versa (Robinson 1997). This is a difficult concept for health purchasers to understand and a liaison psychiatrist may be given the invidious task of helping to

Handbook of Liaison Psychiatry, ed. Geoffrey Lloyd and Elspeth Guthrie. Published by Cambridge University Press. © Cambridge University Press, 2007.

set priorities to determine which patients should be funded by the NHS. Cook *et al.* (2003) have examined the clinical guidelines from 32 health authorities. Guidelines mostly concerned arbitrary sets of cosmetic procedures and lacked any evidence base. Most guidelines permit surgery 'exceptionally' for psychological reasons. They found that the guidelines did not appreciably alter surgeons' decisions which were made on a number of criteria:

1. The cost of the procedure (for example moles were routinely operated upon as it was easier for the surgeon to operate than to explain why surgery could not be offered).
2. Whether the patient sought restoration or improvement of appearance (an ugly scar might be operated upon because it was restoration to normality).
3. The degree of abnormality.
4. The degree to which the patient was seen to deserve the treatment (for example a woman who has made the effort to lose a considerable amount of weight but is left with an overhanging apron might be granted a tummy tuck while one who is seen to be requesting a quick fix would not).
5. The impact on the future quality of life (for example a young girl unable to form a relationship might be operated on while an older woman in a stable relationship was refused).

Some surgeons described feeling pressured to offer surgery by some patients' emotional and insistent presentations and believed that some patients contrived their presentation in the attempt to elicit the desired surgical decision. Cosmetic procedures to be performed within the NHS would appear to be a suitable topic for guidelines from the National Institute for Health and Clinical Excellence (NICE).

Liaison psychiatrists are sometimes asked to assess the suitability of patients prior to cosmetic surgery. Indeed, in some NHS hospitals, a psychologist or liaison psychiatrist may be asked to evaluate routinely all patients prior to cosmetic surgery but there is no evidence base to justify this practice. In the private sector, the National Care Standards Commission has set down a standard that 'referral to appropriate psychological counselling is available if clinically indicated prior to surgery' (Department of Health 2000:73). In the UK private sector, it is uncommon for a psychiatrist or a psychologist to be asked by a surgeon to assess patients prior to surgery and there is no operational criterion in the national care standards to clarify when 'appropriate psychological counselling' is clinically indicated. Alternatively, psychiatrists are sometimes consulted by a patient's parent or partner, the assessment being requested from concern that the surgery is not necessary, especially when the relatives are being asked to pay. In such situations, the patient believes that surgery is the only solution to perceived problems. This chapter will attempt to guide the reader through the minefield of cosmetic surgery and especially its role in psychosis, body dysmorphic disorder, amputee identity disorder and eating disorders. The decision about whether to proceed with cosmetic surgery lies with the surgeon and the patient. The role of a psychiatrist or psychologist is to advise the surgeon and patient on the patient's psychiatric status and whether the expectations are realistic. Surgeons want clear advice on whether to operate or not. The first problem is that patients are aware of this and may be economical with the truth about some of their symptoms and expectations. The second problem is the lack of prospective data.

Psychosocial effects of cosmetic surgery

Sarwer *et al.* (1998a,b) and Castle *et al.* (2002) have reviewed the literature on psychosocial outcomes after cosmetic surgery and identified only 36 longitudinal studies of varying design and quality. Most were investigations of patients undergoing a specific procedure (e.g. rhinoplasty) and the follow-up period ranged from post-operative to 10 years after the procedure (in one study). Only 11 studies included a control group. Overall, most patients were satisfied with the results of the surgery and felt more self-confident after it. However many of the studies had methodological problems, such as the absence of blind raters or valid assessment measures. However, surgeons' headaches and claims for negligence arise from the minority of patients who are dissatisfied with their outcomes. There are no good, large, prospective studies on predictors of dissatisfaction and poor psychosocial outcome. Putative factors associated with poor outcome include being male, young, suffering from depression or anxiety and having a personality disorder (Castle *et al.* 2002). Other authors have suggested that the nature and degree of surgical change ('type-change' procedures, e.g. rhinoplasty, are more difficult to adjust to than 'restorative' procedures, e.g. rhytidectomy; Sarwer *et al.* 1998b). The extent of changes in sensation following the procedure (a feeling of skin-tightening after a rhytidectomy or loss of nipple sensation after breast augmentation) may also influence outcome, with greater sensory disturbances making worse adjustment likely (Pruzinsky & Edgerton 1990). Lastly, the patient's expectation of outcome appears to be important: a distinction may be drawn between expectations regarding the self (e.g. improve body image and improve self-confidence) and expectations relating to external factors (e.g. the patient's wish to please their partner). The latter is associated with lower levels of satisfaction. However it should be emphasized that these putative factors have not been properly evaluated in any prospective studies.

Cosmetic surgery is usually contraindicated in three groups of patients. The first group is patients with psychosis, mania or severe depression, whose judgement about the need for surgery may be impaired or who may have systematized delusions or command hallucinations about cosmetic surgery or the surgeon.

The second group in whom cosmetic surgery might be contraindicated are those with eating disorders, who might be attracted to procedures such as liposuction or abdominoplasty. However there is no data to guide the clinician. Screening for a history of bulimia would be important if only because of the possibility of electrolyte imbalance and cardiac arrhythmias during surgery. There are no prevalence studies of eating disorders presenting in a cosmetic surgery clinic or prospective outcome studies in patients with eating disorders. There is likely to be a publishing bias of negative case reports. McIntosh *et al.* (1994) describes two women who had breast augmentation. After cognitive behaviour therapy, they regretted having surgery and became more concerned about the possible health risks of the implants. Yates *et al.* (1998) report two cases of eating disorders, both women. In the first, breast augmentation provided a decrease in symptoms of bulimia for about three months. The second woman had a chin and nose reconstruction. She experienced a remission of her eating disorder for about a month. Both appeared pleased with the results of their surgery but disappointed with the recurrence of their eating disorder. Lastly Losee *et al.* (1987) report improvements in several, but not all, patients with symptoms of eating disorder with breast reduction.

It may be difficult to distinguish between a diagnosis of an eating disorder and body dysmorphic disorder (BDD). The diagnostic criteria for BDD in the Diagnostic and Statistical Manual (DSM-IV) state that the preoccupation must not be better accounted for by the dissatisfaction that occurs in an eating disorder. No such exclusion is made in the International Classification of Diseases (ICD-10). This is a grey area as there are a significant number of individuals with disordered eating who do not fulfil the criteria for anorexia or bulimia nervosa but might have Eating Disorder Not Otherwise Specified (EDNOS). The boundaries between BDD and an eating disorder are not clear. For example Rosen *et al.* (1995) described a sample of BDD patients who were different to those reported from other centres. They were all female, 38% were preoccupied with their weight and shape alone, and they were generally less handicapped and less socially avoidant than BDD patients described in most other centres. Such patients often had periods of disordered eating or excessive exercise.

The third group in whom cosmetic surgery is usually contraindicated is those with a diagnosis of BDD. The psychopathology and characteristics of BDD will be described briefly before discussing cosmetic surgery. Body dysmorphic disorder is characterized by a preoccupation with an 'imagined' defect in one's appearance or, in the case of a slight physical anomaly, the person's concern is markedly excessive

(American Psychiatric Association 1994). Table 26.1 includes screening questions for the diagnosis of BDD. The term 'dysmorphophobia' is now falling into disuse probably because ICD-10 has discarded it and subsumed it under that of hypochondriacal disorder.

There is frequent comorbidity in BDD, especially for depression, social phobia and obsessive-compulsive disorder (OCD; Neziroglu *et al.* 1996; Phillips & Diaz 1997; Veale *et al.* 1996a). There is also heterogeneity in the presentation of BDD from individuals with comorbid borderline personality disorder to others with muscle dysmorphia (Pope *et al.* 1997), or those who are severely depressed. The most common preoccupations concern the skin, hair, nose, eyes, eyelids, mouth, lips, jaw and chin. However any part of the body may be involved and the preoccupation is frequently focused on several body parts simultaneously (Phillips *et al.* 1993). Complaints typically involve perceived or slight flaws on the face, asymmetrical or disproportionate body features, thinning hair, acne, wrinkles, scars, vascular markings, and pallor or ruddiness of complexion. Sometimes the complaint is extremely vague and amounts to no more than a general perception of ugliness. BDD is characterized by time-consuming behaviours such as mirror gazing, comparing particular features to those of others, excessive camouflage, skin-picking, and reassurance seeking. There is usually avoidance of social situations and of intimacy. Alternatively such situations are endured with the use of alcohol or illegal substances as can occur with social phobia.

Table 26.1. Screening questions for the diagnosis of body dysmorphic disorder.

---

1. Do you currently think a lot about your appearance? What features are you unhappy with? Do you feel your feature(s) are ugly or unattractive?
2. How noticeable do you think your feature(s) is to other people?
3. On an average day, how many hours do you spend thinking about your feature(s)? Please add up all the time that your feature is on your mind and make the best estimate.
4. Does your feature(s) currently cause you a lot of distress?
5. How many times a day do you usually check your feature(s)? (For example looking in a mirror or other reflective surfaces like a shop window or feeling the affected part with your fingers.)
6. How often do you feel anxious about your feature(s) in social situations? Does it lead you to avoid social situations?
7. Has your feature(s) had an effect on dating or on an existing relationship?
8. Has your feature(s) interfered with your ability to work or study, or your role as a homemaker?

The prevalence of BDD in the community is reported as 0.7% in two studies (Faravelli *et al.* 1997; Otto *et al.* 2001), with a higher prevalence of milder cases in adolescents and young adults (Bohne *et al.* 2002). Surveys of BDD patients attending a psychiatric clinic tend to show an equal sex ratio. They are usually single or separated (Neziroglu & Yaryura-Tobias 1993; Phillips & Diaz 1997; Phillips *et al.* 1993; Veale *et al.* 1996a). Although the age of onset of BDD is during adolescence, patients are usually diagnosed 10–15 years later (Phillips 1991; Phillips & Diaz 1997; Veale *et al.* 1996a). Patients may be secretive because they think they will be viewed as vain or narcissistic. They are therefore more likely to present to mental health practitioners with symptoms of depression or social anxiety unless they are specifically questioned about symptoms of BDD (Grant *et al.* 2001). BDD patients are the most distressed and handicapped of all the body image disorders with a high rate of depression and suicide. Phillips *et al.* (2000) used a quality-of-life measure and found a degree of distress that is worse than that of depression, diabetes or bipolar disorder. The best evidence-based treatments demonstrate modest efficacy for cognitive behaviour therapy in two randomized controlled trials (RCTs) (Rosen *et al.* 1995; Veale *et al.* 1996b) and for serotonin-specific reuptake inhibitor antidepressants in two RCTs (Hollander *et al.* 1999; Phillips *et al.* 2002). These form the basis of recommending either cognitive-behaviour therapy or a serotonin-specific reuptake inhibitor in the National Institute for Health and Clinical Excellence (NICE) guidelines on OCD and BDD (www.nice.org.uk/page.aspx?0=cg31).

Body dysmorphic disorder in psychiatric clinics

In a series of 50 BDD patients in the UK, 26% had managed to obtain one or more cosmetic operations but no outcome data were collected (Veale *et al.* 1996b). There are two retrospective surveys that reported on the outcome of cosmetic surgery in BDD patients seen in a psychiatric clinic. Phillips *et al.* (2001) reported on the outcome of 58 patients seeking cosmetic surgery. The large majority (82.6%) reported that symptoms of BDD were the same or worse after cosmetic surgery. The most common outcome following surgery was no change in overall BDD severity (58%) and no change in the concern with the treated body part (48.3%). More patients worsened in overall BDD severity (24.3%) than improved (17.4%). However, in terms of the treated body part, more patients reported a decrease (34.5%) than an increase (17.2%) in concern. No data is provided on satisfaction for the procedures.

Veale (2000) reported on 25 BDD patients in the UK who had had a total of 46 procedures. Ten patients had had one procedure, ten patients had had two procedures, four patients had had three procedures, and one patient had had four procedures. Three patients claimed that they were not preoccupied by their appearance prior to the surgery and that their symptoms of BDD developed only after surgery, which they believed had been done badly. The numbers for several procedures are small but the satisfaction ratings tended to be higher for mammaplasty, rhytidectomy and pinnaplasty. Mammaplasty and pinnaplasty (but not rhytidectomy) tended to lead to an overall decrease in preoccupation and handicap. Repeated surgery tended to lead to increasing dissatisfaction. Some operations, such as rhinoplasty, appear to be associated with higher degrees of dissatisfaction. Mammaplasty and pinnaplasty tended to have relatively higher satisfaction ratings. These operations tend to be unambiguous in that patients can usually describe the problem that concerns them and their desired outcome and the cosmetic surgeon can understand their expectations.

The satisfaction rating was relatively low for rhinoplasty, which was the most common procedure. The nose is also the most usual location for complaint by BDD patients (Veale *et al.* 1996a). Rhinoplasty tended to be associated with an increase in preoccupation and handicap. Most of the patients in the study had multiple concerns about their appearance. After half of the procedures the preoccupation transferred to another area of their body. When patients were dissatisfied with their operation, they often felt guilty or angry with themselves or the surgeon at having made their appearance worse, thus further fuelling their depression and exacerbating their feeling of failure to achieve their ideal. This in turn tended to increase further mirror gazing and craving for more surgery.

The main weaknesses of studies in psychiatric clinics are that the data are retrospective and there is a selection bias of patients in favour of treatment failures. Mental health practitioners are unlikely to be consulted by people who are satisfied with their cosmetic surgery and whose symptoms of BDD improve.

Body dysmorphic disorder in cosmetic surgery clinics

Body dysmorphic disorder is not uncommon in cosmetic surgery clinics and there have been five prospective surveys. In the first, Ishigooka *et al.* (1998) reported that in a Japanese cosmetic surgery clinic, 15% of the patients had BDD. No outcome data reported on their cosmetic surgery. In a second study, Sarwer *et al.* (1998c) assessed 132 women of whom 100 completed a screening questionnaire for BDD. They found that 5% had BDD. Of these, three were requesting a rhytidectomy, one a rhinoplasty and one an abdominoplasty. There were two further women (one requesting breast reduction, one laser resurfacing) whose defects were not regarded as 'imagined or slight'. They were however similar to BDD sufferers in that they were significantly preoccupied and significantly distressed or handicapped by their defects. None of the seven patients were operated on at the clinic in question.

Vindigni *et al.* (2002) reported that a staggering 53% of patients seeking cosmetic surgery were diagnosed with BDD. Of these, the majority (82%) were classified as mild, 10% were moderate and 8% were severe. The mild cases had cosmetic surgery but no outcome data were available. The study raises a number of questions about their interpretation of the diagnostic threshold and the outcome of cosmetic surgery in their 'mild' cases.

Aouizerate *et al.* (2003) report on a study in 132 subjects (8 males, 124 females) who consulted one cosmetic surgeon over a six-month period at a University hospital in France. The plastic surgeon independently rated a physical defect scale and all patients were later interviewed with the BDD Diagnostic Module. They found the prevalence of BDD to be 9.1% in subjects seeking cosmetic surgery, the prevalence being higher in men. Among subjects with no or minimal defect, the rate was 40%. No follow-up data on outcome after surgery were provided.

Lastly, Veale *et al.* (2003) recruited patients seeking cosmetic rhinoplasty in the UK using a screening questionnaire, the BDDQ (Phillips *et al.* 1995). Six out of 29 patients were identified preoperatively as having possible BDD but in this pilot study it was not possible to validate the self-report screening questionnaire with an interview. The BDDQ may have been over-sensitive in this population since all the patients were satisfied with their rhinoplasty. The interpretation was that a group of patients with subclinical or mild BDD had been identified who were satisfied by cosmetic rhinoplasty. This study and the one by Vindigni *et al.* (2002) suggest that mild BDD may be relatively common in cosmetic surgery clinics and the diagnostic criteria for BDD may need tightening if the net is not to be cast too wide. Some operations such as rhinoplasty may attract BDD patients more than other procedures. Alternatively the diagnosis of BDD by itself may not be a contraindication to surgery and that additional factors such as an unrealistic psychosocial outcome may be more important.

There may be difficulties in making a diagnosis of BDD in a cosmetic clinic and deciding when the patient has a minor physical anomaly or when it becomes a more significant 'anomaly' and when the concern becomes 'markedly excessive'. It is worth remembering that aesthetic cosmetic surgery is about enhancing a normal appearance and therefore most patients will look perfectly 'normal' to the examining doctor. Alternatively a surgeon may describe the appearance in medical jargon, when it is still part of a normal variation. However patients will latch onto it like a medical diagnosis to prove that they have an abnormal appearance. The major unanswered question is what predicts satisfaction with cosmetic surgery and when do symptoms of BDD improve? There are no prospective data but one study has examined the differences between 23 individuals without BDD in a cosmetic surgery clinic who were satisfied with their rhinoplasty against 16 patients in a psychiatric clinic diagnosed with BDD (Veale *et al.* 2003). The BDD patients were selected if they craved rhinoplasty but for various reasons had not obtained it, for example they could not afford it or had a fear of the operation failing.

The BDD group was significantly younger than the rhinoplasty patients but there was no significant difference between the sexes. As expected, BDD patients had greater psychological morbidity compared to rhinoplasty patients. They had higher scores on the Yale Brown Obsessive Compulsive Scale (YBOCS) modified for BDD (Phillips *et al.* 1997), and anxiety and depression on the Hospital Anxiety and Depression scale (HAD; Zigmond & Snaith 1983). The mean scores of the BDD patients were all in the clinical range while the rhinoplasty patients were not. BDD patients were more distressed and reported much greater interference in their social and occupational functioning and in intimate relationships because of their nose. They were more socially anxious and more likely to avoid situations because of their nose. They were more likely to check their nose in mirrors or to feel it with their fingers. BDD patients were more likely to believe that cosmetic surgery would significantly alter their life (for example, obtain a new partner or job). BDD patients were significantly more likely to be dissatisfied with other areas of their body. They were likely to have attempted 'DIY' surgery in the past. (Examples of 'DIY' surgery included using a pair of pliers in an attempt to make their nose thinner; applying tape to flatten the nose or placing tissue up one side of their nose to try to make it look more curved.) In summary, BDD patients who desire cosmetic rhinoplasty are a quite different population from those patients who obtain routine cosmetic rhinoplasty. There are a number of clues from this study to assist in the development of a short screening questionnaire or structured interview to assist cosmetic surgeons to identify individuals with BDD who are unsuitable for cosmetic surgery. Table 26.2 summarizes some of the key issues to explore with patients who are being assessed for cosmetic surgery. However good the interview, patients may be economical with the truth and even when a surgeon identifies possible symptoms of BDD, they may not agree to a referral to a mental health practitioner and merely take themselves to another surgeon. More prospective research is required to enable practitioners to identify BDD patients and to explain when cosmetic surgery can be recommended for them.

In the USA, a patient made an unsuccessful claim against her surgeon on the grounds that he should have refrained from operating on her in view of her BDD (Kaplan 2001). Such cases may well increase and it is very important for a psychiatrist to document recommendations to the patient and surgeon and ensure they both receive written communications. In a few cases cosmetic surgery may lead to satisfaction with the surgery especially when the desired outcome is unambiguous (e.g. mammaplasty). Where there are multiple concerns, then the

Table 26.2. Issues to explore in assessment for cosmetic surgery.

1. How noticeable do you think your feature(s) is to other people?
2. Have most of your family or friends discouraged you from having a cosmetic procedure?
3. When you describe what it is that you dislike about your feature(s) to others (family, friends), do you feel they understand exactly what you mean?
4. What would be your main motivation for altering your feature?
5. To what degree do you believe that having a cosmetic procedure will improve your social life?
6. To what degree do you believe that having a cosmetic procedure will improve dating or an existing intimate relationship?
7. To what degree do you believe that having a cosmetic procedure will improve your ability to work or study?
8. To what extent are you also worried with other areas of your body?
9. Have you ever tried to alter the appearance of your feature(s) by yourself?

preoccupation is likely to transfer to a different area of the body. At worst cosmetic surgery leads to dissatisfaction and symptoms of BDD may intensify. Rarely, dissatisfied patients with BDD may resort to harassment and violence against a surgeon (Lucas 2002). At this stage it is very difficult to predict which patients may be satisfied, other than where the symptoms are mild and when patients do not expect any significant change in their symptoms of BDD and psychosocial situation.

'DIY' cosmetic surgery

Body dysmorphic disorder patients have been described who, either in desperation at being turned down for cosmetic surgery, or because they could not afford it, have performed their own 'DIY' cosmetic surgery in which they attempted by their own hand to alter their appearance dramatically (Veale 2000). Examples of procedures include a young man who was preoccupied by his skin which he believed was too 'loose'. He had consulted a cosmetic surgeon who had turned down his request for a face-lift. In desperation, he used a staple gun on both sides of his face to try to keep his skin taut. The staples fell out after 10 minutes and he narrowly missed damaging his facial nerve. Another example is a woman, preoccupied by her skin and the shape of her face, who filed down her teeth in order to alter the appearance of her jaw-line. She stopped when a relative agreed to pay for her to receive cosmetic dental surgery. Lastly, a man preoccupied by his facial skin said he had used sandpaper as a form of dermabrasion to remove scars and to lighten his skin. All cases were dissatisfied with the results of their attempts at surgery, and there was an increase in their preoccupation and symptoms of BDD.

The motivation for DIY surgery is complex but it appears to be primarily an attempt either to camouflage a perceived defect or to try to achieve an unrealistic ideal. It does not fit the existing classification of self-harm by Favazza and Rosenthal (1993). It has a similar poor psychological outcome in so far as nearly all the patients were dissatisfied with their handiwork and found their symptoms of BDD exacerbated. It reflects the extreme measures that some patients take and is mirrored in the high rate of attempted suicide in this population (Veale *et al.* 1996b).

Implications for cognitive-behaviour therapy

If cosmetic surgery is an issue for a BDD patient, then it is recommended that the patient is asked for a commitment not to have any surgery, dermatological or beauty treatments whilst they are receiving psychological therapy. Fortunately many patients do not have the financial resources to pursue these expensive options and just dream of winning the lottery. If they do decide to have an operation, therapy can be suspended until the patient returns. A common presentation is patients who are dissatisfied with previous surgery and blame the surgeon for not doing what they requested or making their appearance worse. They may therefore desire a surgical revision and subsequent surgeons may reinforce this desire. Some surgeons may covertly blame previous surgeons for poor workmanship and give hope of improvement. This in turn increases the frustration and anger of the patient. It is usually impossible for a mental health practitioner to make a judgement on such matters!

When patients are preoccupied by cosmetic surgery or dermatological treatment as a solution, they may be helped by a cost-benefit analysis. This consists of asking the patient to complete a list of advantages or benefits of cosmetic surgery and the disadvantages or costs and to repeat the exercise on costs and benefits of the cognitive behaviour therapy being offered. If they have not already done so, then you can raise disadvantages such as the cost, the possibility of the surgery going wrong, or the symptoms of BDD becoming worse. It can be highlighted that cosmetic surgery is an industry and there are always surgeons willing to operate. Make it clear that you are not opposed to cosmetic surgery per se and would encourage each patient to speak to other dissatisfied BDD patients (such as through the charity OCD Action which has many members with BDD). Another option is to ask the patient to delay surgery until psychological treatment has been completed. In other cases, it is impossible to engage patients in therapy until they have had surgery. In such cases, it is often helpful to contact patients a few months after surgery to enquire about their progress.

Even when patients agree to stop seeking cosmetic surgery, the next goal is attitudinal change and modifying the dream of changing their appearance. This is often seen in mirror gazing and 'mental cosmetic surgery' when patients alter their appearance in their mind. Although this is lot cheaper and less risky than 'real' cosmetic surgery, it is a major obstacle in therapy for overcoming BDD. It is a sign of a difficulty in testing out alternative hypotheses and engaging in therapy.

Amputee identity disorder

Amputee identity disorder (AID) is often confused with BDD. It is a term used to describe individuals who desire one or more digits or limbs to be amputated and in whom current psychiatric treatment is unsuccessful (Furth *et al*. 2000; Smith & Fisher 2003). In the face of opposition from surgeons, some patients may hasten amputation (e.g. chainsaw wound) or carry out self-amputation (for example on a railway line). Although such individuals are preoccupied with becoming disabled, they do not believe (as in BDD) that their limbs are defective or ugly or wish to alter their limb cosmetically. They feel that one or more limbs are not part of their 'self' (a form of reverse 'phantom limb') and that amputation will lead to becoming more able-bodied. Follow-up of patients who have had amputation is generally successful compared to the results in BDD (Fisher & Smith 2000). Prior to amputation, individuals with AID may live as if they had a disability when they are known as 'pretenders'. For example, if the patient believes that he or she should be paraplegic, he or she may live with a wheelchair, crutches or leg braces. This condition is more akin to a gender identity disorder in which an individual feels that his or her genitalia do not belong to them and that he or she is trapped in the wrong body. AID is not a sexual fetish and should not be confused with individuals (known as apotemnophilia 'devotees') who have a special interest in or sexual desire for people who are disabled. AID used to be known as apotemnophilia but this term is more suitable for patients in whom there is a sexual fetish (Money *et al*. 1977). It is certainly one of the most bizarre psychiatric disorders described but it is fortunately rare. Such patients have usually been assessed by specialists in gender identity disorder in the UK.

Body sculpting

There is another group of individuals who either sculpt their body as a form of art or seek to transform their body to become an animal. An example is 'Tigerman' (http://xx-blue-streak-xx.tripod.com) (2003). No cosmetic surgeon will assist him and so all his surgery is done without anaesthetic by a friend. As far as I am aware he has not been psychiatrically evaluated. There is no particular indication of psychiatric disorder, however, though he may be regarded as a highly eccentric individual with beliefs akin to over-valued ideas.

REFERENCES

American Psychiatric Association. (1994). *Diagnostic & Statistical Manual of Mental Disorders –* 4th edition. Washington DC: American Psychiatric Association.

American Society for Aesthetic Plastic Surgery. (2003). *Cosmetic Surgery National Data Bank – 2002 Statistics.* New York: American Society for Aesthetic Plastic Surgery.

Aouizerate, B., Pujol, H., Grabot, D., *et al.* (2003). Body dysmorphic disorder in a sample of cosmetic surgery applicants. *European Psychiatry,* **18,** 365–8.

Bohne, A., Wilhelm, S., Keuthen, N. J., *et al.* (2002). Prevalence of body dysmorphic disorder in a German college student sample. *Psychiatry Research,* **109,** 101–4.

Castle, D. J., Honigman, R. J. and Phillips, K. A. (2002). Does cosmetic surgery improve psychosocial wellbeing? *Medical Journal of Australia,* **176,** 601–4.

Cook, S. A., Rosser, R., Meah, S., *et al.* (2003). Clinical decision guidelines for NHS cosmetic surgery: analysis of current limitations and recommendations for future development. *British Journal of Plastic Surgery,* **56,** 429–36.

Department of Health. (2000). *National Minimum Standards and Regulations for Independent Health Care.* London: TSO.

Faravelli, C., Salvatori, S., Galassi, F., *et al.* (1997). Epidemiology of somatoform disorders: a community survey in Florence. *Social Psychiatry & Psychiatric Epidemiology,* **32(1),** 24–9.

Favazza, A. R. and Rosenthal, R. J. (1993). Diagnostic issues in self-mutilation. *Hospital and Community Psychiatry,* **44,** 134–40.

Fisher, K. and Smith, R. (2000). More work is needed to explain why patients ask for amputation of healthy limbs. *British Medical Journal,* **320,** 1147.

Furth, G. M., Smith, R. and Kubler-Ross, E. (2000). *Amputee Identity Disorder: Information, Questions, Answers and Recommendations About Self-demand Amputation.* Bloomington, 1st Books Library.

Garner, D. M. (1997). The 1997 body image survey results. *Psychology Today,* **31,** 30–94.

Grant, J. E., Won Kim, S. and Crow, S. J. (2001). Prevalence of clinical features of body dysmorphic disorder in adolescent and adult psychiatric inpatients. *Journal of Clinical Psychiatry,* **62,** 517–22.

Hollander, E., Allen, A., Kwon, J., *et al.* (1999). Clomipramine vs desipramine crossover trial in body dysmorphic disorder: selective efficacy of a serotonin reuptake inhibitor in imagined ugliness. *Archives of General Psychiatry,* **56,** 1033–42.

Ishigooka, J., Mitsuhiro, I., Makihiko, S., *et al.* (1998). Demographic features of patients seeking cosmetic surgery. *Psychiatry and Clinical Neuroscience,* **52,** 283–7.

Kaplan, R. (2001). What should plastic surgeons do when crazy patients demand work? *New York Observer*, 23 February.

Losee, J. E., Serletti, J. M., Kreipe, R. E., *et al.* (1987). Reduction in mammaplasty in patients with bulimia nervosa. *Annals of Plastic Surgery*, **39**, 443−6.

Lucas, P. (2002). Body dysmorphic disorder and violence: case report and literature review. *Journal of Forensic Psychiatry*, **13**, 145−56.

McIntosh, V. V., Britt, E. and Bulik, C. N. (1994). Cosmetic breast augmentation and eating disorders. *New Zealand Medical Journal*, **107**, 151−2.

Money, J., Jobaris, R. and Furth, G. (1977). Apotemnophilia. *Journal of Sexual Research*, **13**, 125.

Neziroglu, F. and Yaryura-Tobias, J. A. (1993). Body dysmorphic disorder: phenomenology and case descriptions. *Behavioural Psychotherapy*, **21**, 27−36.

Neziroglu, F., McKay, D., Todaro, J., *et al.* (1996). Effects of cognitive behavior therapy on persons with body dysmorphic disorder and comorbid Axis II diagnoses. *Behavior Therapy*, **27**, 67−77.

Otto, M. W., Wilhelm, S., Cohen, L. S., *et al.* (2001). Prevalence of body dysmorphic disorder in a community sample of women. *American Journal of Psychiatry*, **158**, 2061−3.

Phillips, K. A. (1991). Body dysmorphic disorder: the distress of imagined ugliness. *American Journal of Psychiatry*, **148**, 1138−49.

Phillips, K. A. (2000). Quality of life for patients with body dysmorphic disorder. *Journal of Nervous & Mental Disease*, **188**, 170−5.

Phillips, K. A. and Diaz, S. F. (1997). Gender differences in body dysmorphic disorder. *Journal of Nervous & Mental Disease*, **185**, 570−7.

Phillips, K. A., McElroy, S. L., Keck, P. E., Jr, *et al.* (1993). Body dysmorphic disorder: 30 cases of imagined ugliness. *American Journal of Psychiatry*, **150**, 302−8.

Phillips, K. A., Atala, K. D. and Pope, H. G. (1995). *Diagnostic Instruments for Body Dysmorphic Disorder. New Research Programs and Abstracts*. Miami, FL: American Psychiatric Association, p. 57.

Phillips, K. A., Hollander, E., Rasmussen, S. A., *et al.* (1997). A severity rating scale for body dysmorphic disorder: development, reliability, and validity of a modified version of the Yale-Brown Obsessive Compulsive Scale. *Psychopharmacology Bulletin*, **33**, 17−22.

Phillips, K. A., Grant, J., Siniscalchi, J., *et al.* (2001). Surgical and non psychiatric medical treatment of patients with body dysmorphic disorder. *Psychosomatics*, **42**, 504−10.

Phillips, K. A., Albertini, R. S. and Rasmussen, S. A. (2002). A randomized placebo-controlled trial of fluoxetine in body dysmorphic disorder. *Archives of General Psychiatry*, **59**, 381−8.

Pope, H. G., Jr, Gruber, A. J., Choi, P., *et al.* (1997). Muscle dysmorphia. An underrecognized form of body dysmorphic disorder. *Psychosomatics*, **38**, 548−57.

Pruzinsky, T. and Edgerton, M. T. (1990). Body-image change in cosmetic plastic surgery. In *Body-images: Development, Deviance, and Change*, ed. T. F. Cash and T. Pruzinsky. New York: Guilford Press, pp. 217−36.

Robinson, E. (1997). Psychological research on visible differences in adults. In *Visibly Different. Coping With Disfigurement*, ed. R. Lansdown, N. Rumsey, E. Bradbury, *et al.* Oxford: Butterworth-Heinemann, pp. 102−11.

Rosen, J. C., Reiter, J. and Orosan, P. (1995). Cognitive-behavioral body image therapy for body dysmorphic disorder. *Journal of Consulting & Clinical Psychology*, **63**, 263–9.

Sarwer, D. B., Pertschuk, M. J., Wadden, T. A., *et al.* (1998a). Psychological investigations of cosmetic surgery patients: a look back and a look ahead. *Plastic & Reconstructive Surgery*, **101**, 1136–42.

Sarwer, D. B., Wadden, T. A., Pertschuk, M. J., *et al.* (1998b). The psychology of cosmetic surgery: a review and reconceptualization. *Clinical Psychology Review*, **18**, 1–22.

Sarwer, D. B., Wadden, T. A., Pertschuk, M. J., *et al.* (1998c). Body image dissatisfaction and body dysmorphic disorder in 100 cosmetic surgery patients. *Plastic & Reconstructive Surgery*, **101**, 1644–9.

Smith, R. and Fisher, K. (2003). Healthy limb amputation: ethical and legal aspects. *Clinical Medicine*, **3**, 188.

Veale, D. (2000). Outcome of cosmetic surgery and 'DIY' surgery in patients with body dysmorphic disorder. *Psychiatric Bulletin*, **24**, 218–21.

Veale, D., Boocock, A., Gournay, K., *et al.* (1996a). Body dysmorphic disorder. A survey of fifty cases. *British Journal of Psychiatry*, **169**, 196–201.

Veale, D., Gournay, K., Dryden, W., *et al.* (1996b). Body dysmorphic disorder: a cognitive behavioural model and pilot randomised controlled trial. *Behaviour Research and Therapy*, **34**, 717–29.

Veale, D., De Haro, L. and Lambrou, C. (2003). Cosmetic rhinoplasty in body dysmorphic disorder. *British Journal of Plastic Surgery*, **56**, 546–51.

Vindigni, V., Pavan, C., Semenzin, M., *et al.* (2002). The importance of recognizing body dysmorphic disorder in cosmetic surgery patients: do our patients need a preoperative psychiatric evaluation? *European Plastic Surgery*, **25**, 305–8.

Yates, A., Shisslak, C. M., Allender, J. R., *et al.* (1998). Plastic surgery and the bulimic patient. *International Journal of Eating Disorders*, **7**, 557–60.

Zigmond, A. and Snaith, R. P. (1983). The hospital depression and anxiety scale. *Acta Psychiatrica Scandinavica*, **67**, 361–70.

27

Perinatal and gynaecological disorders

Kathryn M. Abel

Introduction

The interface between obstetrics, gynaecology and psychiatry is complex. All women require access to obstetric or gynaecological services via primary care or hospital specialists at some point in their lives. It is likely that the only medical care many women have received is associated with aspects of their reproductive health. Their experience is not of illness and the need for medical intervention, but of a necessary contact in the setting of their general wellbeing. However, women are repeatedly subject to intimate and often painful examination in the context of wellness. Added to this, matters of sexual health, sexual behaviour, fertility and childbirth are sensitive, open to inappropriate judgement and fraught with difficult choices, whilst being inextricably set within a culture that may be different for each woman. Reproductive choices have been profoundly influenced by recent technologies and interventions. These increase the choices (and the risks) for women and provide a complex interplay between the social and the personal.

More than ever, clinicians in obstetric/gynaecological (OB/GYN) settings need to be aware of the potential psychological implications of normal reproductive events across a woman's life. They are also increasingly called upon to work together with psychiatrists in the care of women with existing mental health problems. These women do not necessarily experience different outcomes of reproductive health. For some mentally ill women, their reproductive lives may represent an opportunity to take part in community life in a way that features of their illness may otherwise prevent.

The challenge for clinicians is to develop a range of effective and sensitive interfaces which recognize the overlap between reproductive experiences and psychological wellbeing (Stewart *et al.* 2001). This chapter seeks to emphasize the place of women's mental health requirements in the context of normal

Handbook of Liaison Psychiatry, ed. Geoffrey Lloyd and Elspeth Guthrie. Published by Cambridge University Press. © Cambridge University Press 2007.

reproductive events. It is divided into two parts: the first part focuses on ways in which menstruation, pregnancy, childbirth and menopause are specifically related to women's mental health and covers practical aspects of treatment in each case. Although it covers some of the risks of mental health problems associated with childbirth itself, its remit is not to cover motherhood and mental illnesses in detail; several good texts are available which deal with these issues in greater detail. The second part addresses ways in which gynaecological contact may interact with psychological wellbeing. This chapter does not cover sexually transmitted diseases or gynaecological cancers.

Psychological aspects of the reproductive life cycle

Menstruation

The concept of a systematic change in physiological and psychological function across the menstrual phase is not new (Frank 1931). Whether in some women this represents a medical syndrome remains controversial. Some view premenstrual syndrome (PMS) as a culture-bound syndrome that constitutes a negotiated reality between those who treat it and those who suffer (Morokoff 1991). Although it is true to say that premenstrual symptoms encourage a negative view of women as weak, emotional and unable (or unfit) to work, if women are asked, most experience mild changes in energy levels, appetite, breast tenderness, abdominal swelling and reduced self-esteem in a reliable pattern across their menstrual phase which they manage with lifestyle adjustments (*Drugs and Therapeutics Bulletin* 1992a; O'Brien 1987). Morgan *et al.* (1996) reported that women have increased feelings of inadequacy in the absence of demonstrable changes in cognitive function. Changes in cognitive abilities have been demonstrated with menstrual phase and hormone levels (Hamspon 1990; Kimura 1996; Sommer 1982) consistent with women's perception of altered function particularly in the context of more severe menstrually-associated disorder.

Reporting of perimenstrual mood disturbance is extremely common, particularly in young women under 25 (Wittchen *et al.* 2002) and 30–50% of women experience premenstrual symptoms severe enough to lead them to seek medical help at some stage in their life. Several psychoneuroendocrine studies have found that healthy ovulating women experience more stress, lower mood, more negative cognitions and poor self-appraisal and higher stress responses in the premenstrual and early menstrual phases of their cycle, which may be due to diminishing levels of oestrogen (see Collins *et al.* 1985; Kirschbaum *et al.* 1992, 1999). Women approaching menopause may have more severe mood changes in the luteal phase of their cycles as oestrogen levels are further diminished in this group.

Between 2 and 12% of women are debilitated by severe disturbances of mood and behaviour, recurring consistently and solely before a menstrual period and which severely disrupt all aspects of life (Angst *et al.* 2001; Kendler *et al.* 1992; Wittchen *et al.* 2002). This is known as premenstrual dysphoric disorder (PMDD; American Psychiatric Association 1994). The symptoms of PMDD are shown in Table 27.1 and diagnostic criteria in Table 27.2. Diagnosis should be confirmed prospectively by means of daily diary ratings of symptoms over two consecutive cycles. These should show symptom deterioration in the luteal phase, with at least one week free from symptoms in the follicular phase. Hypothalamic-pitutary-adrenal axis (HPA) activity alters systematically across the menstrual phase (see Kudielka *et al.* 2000), but there are few consistent pathophysiological findings in women with menstrual mood disturbance or PMDD, and no evidence of differences in gonadal steroid levels. It is likely that dysregulation of HPA and other key neurotransmitter systems (β-endorphin, cholinergic, serotonergic, adrenergic), possibly from genetic susceptibility, make some women particularly vulnerable to physiological fluctuations of gonadal steroids.

Table 27.1. Symptoms of PMDD.

- Depressed mood, tension and anxiety, emotional lability
- Irritability and anger, poor concentration, loss of interest in usual activities
- Altered eating and sleeping patterns and functional impairment
- Breast tenderness, 'bloating', tiredness and headaches

Table 27.2. PMDD diagnostic criteria.

- A constellation of severe symptoms starting after ovulation (luteal phase)
- Symptoms occur during last week of luteal phase
- Symptoms must disappear completely at onset of menses (days 2–3)
- At least one week free from symptoms in the follicular phase
- 11 core symptoms described: must have at least five of these and one of these five must be depressed mood, marked anxiety or tension, marked affective lability, or persistent marked anger or irritability
- 30% worsening of at least five symptoms between week of luteal phase and menses
- Symptoms for most months of the previous year
- Symptoms over at least two consecutive cycles
- Symptoms lead to real impairment in woman's functioning in work, school, social activities or relationships
- Diagnosis must be made by prospective daily diarizing of symptoms
- Women >45 years should have menopausal status evaluated

Major depressive disorder, panic disorder and substance abuse commonly coexist with PMDD (Breaux *et al.* 2000; Endicott *et al.* 1999; Pearlstein *et al.* 1990; Wittchen *et al.* 2002) and require treatment before any residual premenstrual symptoms can be assessed. Approximately 35% of PMDD women suffer major depression in their lifetimes and are also more likely to experience postpartum depression (see Yonkers 1997a). Premenstrual exacerbation of depression is well recognized and thought to relate to increased rates of admission and attempted suicide at this time (Baca *et al.* 1998; Chaturvedi *et al.* 1995; Wittchen *et al.* 2002). Panic disorder and anxiety symptoms commonly worsen premenstrually, especially in women with PMDD (Yonkers 1997b). Bingeing behaviour in bulimia may be exacerbated premenstrually, although the evidence for this is limited (Price *et al.* 1987). Menstrual patterns of symptom exacerbation have also been reported in post-traumatic stress disorder and dissociative disorders associated with a past history of abuse (Jensvold *et al.* 1989).

Treatment issues

Treatment of PMDD is summarized in Table 27.3. Managing women with PMDD begins with validating their experiences; screening out other psychiatric and medical disorders and assessing nutritional intake are also important preliminary steps. High levels of caffeine, salt and alcohol may all worsen PMDD. Some types of contraception may also worsen symptoms. Simple behavioural measures such as adequate sleep, relaxation, regular exercise and a healthy diet may also be important. Blake *et al.* (1998) reported evidence for cognitive-behavioural therapy (CBT) in PMDD and some reports suggest that light therapy may also be effective

Table 27.3. Treatments for PMDD.

Drug treatments for psychological symptoms	Drug treatments for physical symptoms	Nutritional treatments	Psychobehavioural treatments
First-line: SSRIs (sertraline, fluoxetine, paroxetine, citalopram) TCAs (clomipramine)	Diuretics NSAIDs Simple analgesia	*Reduce:* alcohol caffeine sugar carbohydrates salt	Cognitive and behavioural therapy Relaxation therapy Exercise Coping skills training
Second-line: Anxiolytics as treatment with anxiety symptoms (buspirone, alprazolam)		*Supplement diet:* calcium carbonate vitamin B_6	

although the placebo response is high (20–40%) in this group (Dimmock *et al.* 2000). Evidence of benefit with the selective serotonin reuptake inhibitors (SSRIs) is strongest for fluoxetine (the only SSRI licensed for PMDD in the UK) and sertraline and apply to highly selected patients without coexisting psychological or medical disorder (*Drugs and Therapeutics Bulletin* 2002). Up to 70% of such women with proven PMDD may have a worthwhile response to treatment with an SSRI. Relapse of the symptoms is usual when treatment is stopped, and there are few reliable data on long-term treatment beyond six months but women tend to relapse within two months of stopping treatment. A recent meta-analysis found no significant difference in symptom reduction whether an SSRI was given continuously or only in the luteal phase (Dimmock *et al.* 2000). However, no randomized double-blind trial has adequately compared these approaches directly. Empirical use of SSRIs for 'premenstrual syndrome' is not justified (*Drugs and Therapeutics Bulletin* 2002). Treatment with an SSRI should not be started without an adequate prospective assessment of symptoms and careful clinical evaluation to exclude other disorders that might require a different approach to treatment. The commonest side-effect of long-term treatment is sexual dysfunction.

Few studies have compared SSRIs with other relevant treatments for PMDD. Hormonal treatments for PMDD have encompassed both oestrogen and progesterone. In two studies, transdermal oestradiol was more effective than placebo for symptoms of PMS/PMDD, but a further (small) study of conjugated oestrogens was negative (see Yonkers *et al.* 2000). Only 1 of 10 double-blind studies of over 400 women found progesterone to be effective in PMS/PMDD (for review see Yonkers *et al.* 2000). Other pharmacological treatments without controlled trial evidence include the use of diuretics during symptomatic days; prostaglandin inhibitors (e.g. ibuprofen, naproxen sodium) during symptomatic days; and vitamin E and magnesium throughout the cycle.

Calcium carbonate has been shown to decrease symptom scores by 48% compared with 30% placebo; vitamin B_6 is twice as effective as placebo in PMS. Evening primrose oil may be of benefit in reducing physical and some psychological symptoms (*Drugs and Therapeutics Bulletin* 1992b).

Fertility treatments

Up to 15% of couples suffer with infertility (Speroff *et al.* 1994). Postponed childbearing and decreasing sperm quality are likely to increase these rates and the demand for treatments. The capacity to access treatment is determined by age, and wealth, as most health authorities do not offer treatments within the National Health Service. Menning (1980) described a sequence akin to shock with surprise, denial, anger, isolation, guilt and grief followed by resolution if the acceptance of infertility were to be successfully worked through by a couple. Marital relationships are invariably strained by involuntary childlessness: a sense of failure in the infertile party, guilt about past behaviour even if it is unrelated to fertility, anger from the 'healthy' partner; enforced sexual intercourse regimes; repeated and long-lasting unsuccessful interventions. Wright *et al.* (1991) reported that women were much more likely than men to report psychiatric symptoms in association with a couple's infertility including distress, anger, anxiety, low self-esteem and depression, and as many as 25% of women compared to 12% of men have been reported to suffer mild depression following repeated failed treatments (Newton *et al.* 1990).

Other pressures on couples include the financial burden with costs per cycle of treatment in the thousands. Even if some health authorities offer one free cycle, couples are likely to need more than one treatment (15% success from one-cycle in-vitro fertilization (IVF); 25% from gamete intra-fallopian transfer (GIFT)). Successful pregnancy may also be fraught with anxiety after a prolonged wait and few attempts have been made to assess the impact of anonymous donor egg or sperm on the family (Kovacs *et al.* 1993). Couples undergoing fertility treatment need ongoing support from formal and informal sources. Some centres have a framework of counselling for couples and self-help groups. The psychological impact of hormonal manipulation is considered below.

Pregnancy

Pregnancy should always be considered by clinicians when prescribing medical interventions to any woman of reproductive age. It is a common mistake to assume that women with mental illness are not sexually active. These women should be offered regular reproductive health assessments and preconception education or counselling by familiar (preferably female) members of the psychiatric team. Methods of current contraception must be explored, as well as the risks and benefits of continuing medication should a woman become pregnant during treatment. The significance of mental illness during pregnancy and the post-partum period is manifold (see NICE 2007).

The most recent Confidential Enquiry into maternal deaths during the perinatal period in England and Wales (1996–1998) revealed that suicide was at least as important as death due to hypertensive disorders, with 20 suicides reported during this triennium (Department of Health 1999). Although up to half the pregnancies in England and Wales are unplanned, women with mental illness are especially likely to have an unplanned pregnancy. The risks to the foetus of untreated mental illness in a mother are unquantified, and the risks of exposure to psychotropic medication poorly understood (see Briggs *et al.* 1999). What is known is that the offspring of mentally ill women have lower birth weights, poorer neonatal condition, and more birth complications than healthy controls (Barkla & McGrath 2000; McNeil *et al.* 1983, 1984). Low-birth-weight infants have higher perinatal mortality in general (Wilcox & Russell 1983), whilst mothers of low-birth-weight children are more likely to have depressive and anxiety symptoms (Langkamp *et al.* 2001; Wadhwa *et al.* 1993). The offspring of mentally ill parents are also more likely than those of healthy women to be stillborn or to die in the perinatal period, and these increased risks of mortality are sustained to adulthood (Webb *et al.* 2005). In the next few years further data will emerge describing in greater detail the mortality, morbidity, social and forensic outcomes of these vulnerable children.

Mood disorders in pregnancy

Whilst symptoms of anxiety are common during pregnancy, especially in the first trimester of the first pregnancy, and around the time of now routine testing for foetal abnormality, the prevalence of anxiety disorders in pregnancy is unclear (Steiner & Born 2002). New-onset panic disorder is thought to be relatively rare during pregnancy; existing panic and phobic anxiety disorder is thought to abate (Hertzberg & Wahlbeck 1999; Wisner *et al.* 1996). About a quarter of women report worsening of symptoms during pregnancy (Cohen *et al.* 1994). The puerperium however sees more than a third of women worsen (Hertzberg & Wahlbeck 1999). Little is known about obsessive-compulsive disorder in pregnancy. Studies of postnatal depression report high levels of obsessive and ruminative thoughts in mothers (Jennings *et al.* 1999) and parents (Abramowitz *et al.* 2003) about either self-harm or harm to the infant, although these are rarely enacted. The long-term effects of maternal depression on offspring are yet to be quantified, but some evidence suggests these children are more likely to present with behavioural problems at school and may be at greater risk of cognitive difficulties (Alpern & Lyons-Ruth 1993; Cooper & Murray 1995, 1997; Essex *et al.* 2001).

During pregnancy many women report depressive symptoms which may be important in themselves as predictors of subsequent depressive disorder. Symptoms seem to fluctuate through pregnancy with peaks coinciding with most physical discomfort in the first and third trimesters and the anxiety in anticipation of childbirth (Evans *et al.* 2001; Kumar & Robson 1984; Steiner & Yonkers 1998); anxiety is an important feature of perinatal depression (Stuart *et al.* 1998). Depressive symptoms often 'overlap' with those of pregnancy (e.g. loss of energy, fatigue and sleep disturbance; Altshuler *et al.* 1998) and may be difficult to diagnose. Although only 10–16% actually suffer a depressive episode (Gotlib *et al.* 1989; Llewellyn *et al.* 1997), for those with a long history of depression, the risk of depressive relapse during pregnancy is especially high (Altshuler *et al.* 1998).

Risk factors associated with the development of a depressive episode during pregnancy are similar to those conferring risk at other times and include a personal or family history of depression or mood disorder, the lack of a supportive relationship, marital distress, dysfunctional attributional style and higher age at pregnancy, although adolescent mothers are most likely to suffer depressive episodes (Kitamura *et al.* 1993).

The risk of depression in particular groups such as asylum seekers is as yet unquantified despite its increasing relevance in clinical practice. These women have often suffered traumatic experiences and live in grossly impoverished circumstances with little or no support. They may be difficult to detect because of isolation, language barriers and a lack of culturally sensitive services. Particular effort should be made to engage interpreters for antenatal appointments; psychiatric assessment may also be made at this time.

Treatment issues

Treatment of perinatal depression is summarized in Table 27.4. Wisner *et al.* (2000) present a useful overview of the dilemmas facing women and clinicians alike in the treatment of women with depression during pregnancy. Ideally, depressive symptoms in at-risk women should be monitored regularly by staff with mental health training. The use of recognized rating scales has the advantage of being quick, easily applied by non-psychiatric staff and can form an objective assessment of symptoms when a woman is seen by a number of doctors and different healthcare workers over time.

The management of women who attend antenatal booking clinics and are already on maintenance antidepressant (AD) therapy is summarized in Table 27.4. Women who are well, but at high risk of depressive illness (previous episodes, strong family history) may benefit from education, counselling and enhanced social support prior to childbirth (Dennis 2004; Gordon & Gordon 1960). These kinds of interventions should be considered from the first trimester onwards. If women are well when maintained on an antidepressant, they may still wish to consider stopping treatment prior to conception; this option should be discussed with a local psychiatric team. Women who continue to experience significant residual depressive symptoms who wish to become pregnant may still be offered a trial of discontinuation of medication, and may benefit from non-medical interventions such as psychological support or CBT, depending on local resources. These alternatives should also be considered in women keen to remain on treatment where the clinical indication is not as strong. In both cases prophylaxis against a post-partum relapse may be achieved through the reintroduction of AD medication late in the third trimester or even early puerperium (Wisner *et al.* 1994).

Table 27.4. Perinatal management of depression.

	Women well on maintenance treatment	Women currently depressed on/off maintenance therapy	Well women at high risk of depression (untreated)
Pre-conception Assess for high risk: Recurrent Severe Poor function when ill	• Discuss and document contraception • Education • Counsel (genetic) • Review risk • Review prescription: If past mild symptoms or single moderate/severe: (i) non-drug therapies (ii) withdraw over 4–6 weeks If past single severe symptoms or recurrent severe past illness: (i) continue (ii) change to safer AD (iii) lower dose (iv) psychotherapies • Consider checking plasma level for baseline therapeutic level • Engage MDT	• Discuss and document contraception • Education • Counsel (genetic) • Review prescription: If mild symptoms: (i) non-drug therapies (ii) withdraw over 4–6 weeks If moderate/severe: (i) continue (ii) change to safer AD[a] (iii) lower dose (iv) psychotherapies • Consider checking plasma level for baseline therapeutic level • Engage MDT[b]	• Psychiatric review • Education • Counsel (genetic)
First trimester	• Education • Review prescription: (i) withdraw (ii) continue (iii) change to safer AD (iv) lower dose (v) psychotherapies • Consider/add non-pharmacological prescription • Consider checking plasma level	*Mild/moderate symptoms* MDT review and care • Psychiatric review • Monitor mood • Education Supportive therapies (consider CBT[c], IPT[d]) • AD (especially if past history or high risk) *Severe symptoms* Discuss with patient and family Consider: • psychiatric admission • AD +/− high potency classical APD • ECT[e]	MDT review • Psychiatric review • Education • Support • Monitor mood

Table 27.4. (*cont.*)

	Women well on maintenance treatment	Women currently depressed on/off maintenance therapy	Well women at high risk of depression (untreated)
Second trimester	• If remaining on ADs, consider increasing dose • Psychotherapeutic and educational supports	(as above) • Psychotherapeutic and educational supports	(as above) • Psychotherapeutic and educational supports
Third trimester	• If remaining on ADs, monitor symptoms and inform medical teams • Psychotherapeutic and educational supports	(as above) • Psychotherapeutic and educational supports	(Consider prophylactic AD) • Psychotherapeutic and educational supports
Post-partum	• Monitor neonate for signs of toxicity • Consider reducing dose of AD if increased in second trimester • Psychotherapeutic and parenting supports • Counsel regarding breastfeeding	*Mild/moderate: (as above)* • psychotherapeutic and parenting supports *Severe:* • admission to MBU[g] • AD +/− high potency classical APD[h] • ECT • Counsel regarding breastfeeding • Parenting support	• Consider prophylactic AD SSRI[f] • Counsel regarding breastfeeding • Psychotherapeutic and parenting supports

Notes: [a]AD: antidepressant;   [b]MDT: multidisciplinary team;   [c]CBT: cognitive behavioural therapy;
[d]IPT: interpersonal therapy;   [e]ECT: electroconvulsive therapy;
[f]SSRI: specific serotonin reuptake inhibitor;   [g]MBU: mother and baby unit;   [h]APD: antipsychotic drug.

Women who are at high risk of relapse and who wish to conceive should be given the option to have their AD dose reduced, with regular monitoring by psychiatric team and/or may switch to a 'safer' AD. Although no data exist to support the idea, there is a theoretical argument for checking AD plasma concentrations preconception in women on maintenance therapy. This preconception level may help clinicians to use the lowest effective dose and minimize total dose. As dosing requirements of ADs increase to an average of 1.6 times the prepregnancy dose (range 1.3−2.0) during the second trimester (Wisner *et al.* 1993), some clinicians routinely increase the dose of AD. If a plasma level has been measured preconception, or early in the first trimester, it can be used to titrate the dose in the latter half of pregnancy as discussed above.

The only population-based study of effects of antenatal AD exposure found that antidepressant use reported at the first prenatal visit was associated with premature delivery (Ericsson *et al.* 1999). Although there is no evidence that foetal exposure to tricyclics or SSRIs increases the risk of intrauterine growth retardation, foetal death or congenital abnormalities (Simon *et al.* 2002; Wisner *et al.* 2000), only one group has addressed the more pernicious possibility of behavioural teratogenicity (Nulman *et al.* 1997, 2002) and reported no adverse effects on IQ or language development following tricyclic or fluoxetine exposure.

A post-partum 'withdrawal syndrome' involving neonatal irritability, constant crying, restlessness, shivering, hypothermia, increased tonus, eating and sleeping difficulties and convulsions, has been described following use of ADs near term (Dahl *et al.* 1997; Nordeng *et al.* 2001; Nulman *et al.* 1997). These symptoms occur within a few days of birth and can last up to one month and may require treatment. The syndrome has been described with use of both tricyclics and SSRIs. Some suggest stopping ADs three to four weeks before the estimated date of delivery (EDD; Cohen *et al.* 1989a). However, description of this syndrome is based on anecdotal reports. Discontinuation of medication at this time when the risk of depressive illness is at its highest is not advised. Monitoring maternal AD drug concentration, especially close to term, and careful observation of the neonate for signs of toxicity are suggested alternative strategies (McElhatton *et al.* 1996).

Bipolar disorder and pregnancy

In a large American study, 45% of women with known bipolar affective disorder (BPAD) reported high levels of emotional disturbance during pregnancy and within the first month post-partum (Blehar *et al.* 1998). All women with a history of BPAD should be rigorously encouraged to plan both contraception and pregnancy. It is uncommon for women to have either a relapse or first episode of mania during pregnancy (Cott & Wisner 2003), but in such an event, she will usually require hospital admission. The outcomes of pregnancy in women with BPAD and affective psychosis are consistently worse than healthy women, with increased rates of prematurity, congenital malformation, stillbirth, neonatal death and low birth weight (Jablensky *et al.* 2005).

Treatment issues

All women with BPAD who become pregnant should be managed by the joint obstetric and mental health teams. Families and supportive others should be encouraged to take an active role. There is evidence to suggest that folic acid (0.4 mg per day) may prevent neural tube defects in all women, if given during the early stages of embryogenesis (Medical Research Council 1991). Both carbamazepine and sodium valproate are folic acid antagonists, so a higher dose (4 mg per day) of folic acid is recommended for women taking these mood stabilizers preconception. Discontinuation of mood stabilizers in non-gravid women with

BPAD is associated with a significant risk of relapse. This risk is greater following rapid discontinuation of medication (Faedda *et al.* 1993) and these risks remain in pregnancy (Viguera *et al.* 2002). Therefore, stopping treatment should be done with close liaison between the multiprofessional team and the patient and preferably planned for early pregnancy to provide prophylaxis for the longest period while at the same time minimizing foetal exposure (Cohen & Rosenbaum 1998). Treatment is summarized in Table 27.5.

If a woman does choose to stop medication she should be made aware that a relapse may put herself and her foetus at risk and may expose her to higher doses of medication and multiple drugs. If medication is withdrawn prior to conception, the option of recommencing medication towards term or in the first 48 hours post-partum should also be discussed. For women remaining on maintenance, monotherapy is recommended, and plasma levels should be kept at the lower limit of the therapeutic range to minimize the risk of teratogenesis. Patients should be switched to slow-release compounds or have doses divided to reduce plasma peaks of medication. Lithium levels should be taken monthly, along with urea and electrolyte (U/Es) and thyroid functions tests (TFTs). This should increase to fortnightly in the second trimester due to the rapid changes in drug metabolism and distribution. The dose of lithium usually needs to be increased as the pregnancy progresses, and by the third trimester, weekly lithium level tests are required to monitor the fall in plasma levels and/or alterations in renal or thyroid function.

Protocols for the measurement of anticonvulsant mood stabilizers (lamotrigine, valproate, carbamazepine) are less clear, but plasma levels should probably be checked equally frequently and the dose of medication adjusted accordingly. All women on a mood stabilizer require a detailed ultrasound scan during the second trimester to screen for anomalies, such as neural tube or cardiac defects; those receiving lithium should also be considered for a foetal echocardiogram.

Clear plans for delivery should be discussed in the third trimester. Given the high rate of relapse in women with BPAD (see below), some advocate a planned delivery via caesarean section. This approach allows careful management of mental state and lithium levels between the obstetric and psychiatric teams. Alternatively, if vaginal delivery is planned, it is generally advised that lithium plasma concentration is reduced prior to delivery, because of the volume changes and possible dehydration that may occur at delivery. Some advocate reducing the lithium dose by 25–30% on the day before the EDD. Since the majority of women do not deliver on their EDD, a more practical solution is to reduce the dose by 50% (or to the pre-pregnancy dose) at the onset of labour (Calabrese & Gulledge 1985).

Even when maintenance medication has been stopped successfully antenatally, the greatest risk of relapse remains the post-partum period. Prophylaxis may be

Table 27.5. Perinatal management of bipolar affective disorder.

	Women well on maintenance treatment	Women currently ill	Women at high risk of a manic episode

Preconception Assess high risk: recurrent illness severe illness suicidality poor function when ill Encourage rigorous planning of conception	• Discuss and document contraception
	• Education
	• Counsel (genetic)
	• Review risk
	  (i) withdraw medication slowly
	or
	(ii) continue medication:
	  • monotherapy
	  • lowest therapeutic dose (lithium best data)
	  • reduce plasma peaks (divided dose/slow release)
	  • baseline plasma levels
	  • CBZ^a/VP^b: folic acid 4 mg
	  • Support
		• Multiprofessional care (usually in hospital)
		• Discuss and document contraception
		• Educate
		• Counsel
		• Support
			• Psychiatric review
			• Educate
			• Counsel (genetic)
			• Support

First trimester	As above Lithium monthly plasma level U/E^d + TFT^e CBZ/VP: plasma level	• Psychiatric admission • ADP^c high potency +/– BZs^f if demanded (lorazepam, clonazepam) +/– Mood stabilizer +/– ECT^g	As above
Second trimester	As above Lithium fortnightly plasma level U/E + TFT Detailed US^h +/– Echocardiogram of foetus CBZ/VP: detailed US Plasma level	As above	As above
Third trimester	As above Lithium weekly plasma level U/E + TFT 50% dose reduction or	As above	As above (consider mood stabilizer)

Table 27.5. (cont.)

	Women well on maintenance treatment	Women currently ill	Women at high risk of a manic episode
	preconception dose at labour CBZ: vitamin K (10 mg per day) From 36 to 40 weeks: • discuss mode of delivery • inform anaesthetic team		
Post-partum	• Maintain hydration • Monitor neonate for signs of toxicity Lithium check plasma level CBZ: vitamin K 1 mg (im) to neonate Discuss protected sleep Discuss breastfeeding	• Admission to MBU[i] if available • ADP high potency +/− BZs if demanded + Mood stabilizer +/− ECT Support for partner Discuss protected sleep Discuss breastfeeding	• Consider mood stabilizer (within 48 hours) Discuss protected sleep

Notes: [a]CBZ: carbamazepine; [b]VP: sodium valproate; [c]ADP: antipsychotic; [d]U/E: urea and electrolytes; [e]TFT: thyroid function tests; [f]BZs: benzodiazepines; [g]ECT: electroconvulsive therapy; [h]US: ultrasound scan (of foetus); [i]MBU: mother and baby unit.

achieved by administering medication close to term. Evidence supporting this approach is limited to a few studies involving lithium administration (Cohen *et al.* 1995). Data for the prophylactic potential of other mood stabilizers are lacking and further research is urgently required in this area. There is increasing use of atypical antipsychotic drugs in the maintenance treatment of BPAD, but few data are available for their use in pregnancy or lactation (Llewellyn & Stowe 1998).

Despite these measures, there have been reports of neonatal toxicity in babies exposed to lithium at the time of delivery (Ananth 1978; Briggs 2002). Thus, some suggest withdrawal of medication in the month prior to delivery or towards the end of the third trimester, depending on individual needs. These toxic effects are, however, both rare and apparently self-limiting. They are usually absent by 14 days, corresponding with the delayed renal elimination of the drug in the neonate. Carbamazepine is an enzyme-inducing agent that leads to a reduction in vitamin-K-dependent clotting factors in the foetus. To prevent neonatal haemorrhage oral vitamin K (10 mg per day) should be administered to the mother from 36 weeks gestation and intramuscularly (1 mg) to the neonate post-partum.

Schizophrenia and pregnancy

Early literature reported that women with schizophrenia had reduced fertility, although many confounders such as ill health, poor nutrition, reduced capacity to make relationships and, latterly, the possible side-effects of neuroleptic medication are likely explanations. Now, however, conception rates may be increasing due to a combination of deinstitutionalization and antipsychotic agents that are less disruptive to the hypothalamic-gonadal axis (Miller 1997). Women with schizophrenia may still have fewer children than healthy women (Haukka *et al.* 2003; Howard *et al.* 2002), but most still become mothers (McGrath *et al.* 1999), and in UK samples, those who do, have more than one child (Howard *et al.* 2001, 2002).

Women with schizophrenia are less likely to plan their pregnancy than healthy women (McNeil *et al.* 1983; Miller 1997) and are more likely to have an unwanted pregnancy, to become pregnant through rape and to harbour negative feelings about their pregnancy (Miller & Finnerty 1996). Pregnancy *may* be a time of increased wellbeing and an opportunity for women with schizophrenia to be accepted in society; but in general, schizophrenic symptoms do not improve and often worsen during pregnancy (Davies *et al.* 1995a; McNeil *et al.* 1984). Subtle cognitive deficits may affect a woman's capacity to monitor herself in pregnancy and to comply with antenatal care; psychosis may also prevent the recognition of the onset of labour (Spielvogel & Wile 1992). Bennedsen (1998) reported that women with schizophrenia attended fewer antenatal care visits and were at increased risk of interventions such as caesarean section, vaginal assisted delivery, amniotomy, and pharmacological stimulation of labour. Children of women with schizophrenia suffer more stillbirths, congenital malformations and infant death than offspring of healthy women (Bennedsen 1998; Bennedsen *et al.* 2001; Coverdale *et al.* 1997; Jablensky *et al.* 2005; Nilsson *et al.* 2002), but do not have a greater risk than women with other psychiatric disorder (King-Hele *et al.* 2007 in press). There is a need to give women with schizophrenia specific and careful education about, and preparation for, childbirth and delivery, to prevent potentially harmful outcomes.

Whilst for some, motherhood has a very positive impact on health and results in reduced social stigma, a more meaningful work role and improved social networks (Schwab *et al.* 1991), the extra stressors involved in childrearing become particularly potent in this vulnerable population and only about half the women with schizophrenia who become mothers manage to continue caring for their infants long term (Hearle & Mcrath 2000). Fears about losing custody of their infants may trigger deterioration in mental state (Apfel & Handel 1993). The need to optimize conditions for mothers with schizophrenia is clear (e.g. Howard *et al.* 2001), yet these mothers are often the most materially and socially deprived.

Treatment issues

Some would advise avoiding haloperidol and other conventional antipsychotic drugs (APDs) in women with schizophrenia who wish to conceive because most women develop secondary hyperprolactinaema which suppresses ovarian function (see Smith *et al.* 2002; Wieck & Haddad 2003). Indeed, even women who report no menstrual disturbance have ovarian suppression with conventional agents (Smith *et al.* 2002). Haloperidol also may cause troublesome anticholinergic side-effects and exacerbate postural hypotension of pregnancy. Most women with schizophrenia will not present to a clinician until 6–8 weeks gestation when organogenesis is nearly complete. As behavioural teratogenicity (Coyle *et al.* 1976) may occur on a different timescale, review of medication after this time is equally important. It is most likely that women with schizophrenia will remain on treatment throughout pregnancy and ideally this should consist of monotherapy. An unresolved dilemma for clinicians and women alike is the increasing use of atypical APDs which are generally better tolerated than conventional agents. Most data for their use in pregnancy are available for clozapine and olanzapine from the manufacturer's database. Although it is still recommended that women be changed to a high potency, classical agent such as trifluoperazine or haloperidol, this decision has to be made individually for each woman. Classical APDs carry an increased risk of extrapyramidal movement disorder (which is dose related) and clinicians also need to be aware of the risk of relapse when changing drug. In addition some drugs have a particular risk of hyperprolactinaemia. Conventional agents, such as haloperidol and sulpiride, and atypical APDs, such as risperidone and amisulpiride, are especially likely to raise prolactin in women. This may affect capacity to conceive as discussed above, but its effect on pregnancy and lactation is unknown.

As pregnancy progresses, gut absorption of APDs reduces, plasma volume increases, the entry of these compounds into the brain may reduce and renal clearance increases. All these factors may reduce the efficacy of APDs. Close monitoring of women by the multidisciplinary team is vital, so that drug dose can be titrated against symptom control. If a woman becomes floridly psychotic during pregnancy, hospital admission (preferably to a specialist mother-and-baby facility) is necessary to determine the need for medication, if not already known. Following delivery, the newborn should be monitored for a number of well-described side-effects of exposure to APDs in utero. These include jaundice, hypo- and hyperactivity, intestinal obstruction, and less specific effects such as poor feeding, reduced movement and vasomotor instability. Although many women with schizophrenia improve symptomatically after childbirth, those with unstable illness or high risk factors (poor compliance, prominent negative symptoms, severe illness, isolation, previous children in care), prophylactic admission to a specialist mother-and-baby unit should be considered in the early postnatal period. It is good practice to encourage the mother to visit the unit before labour if this is planned.

Anxiety disorders and pregnancy

Pregnancy is associated with a significant increase in general symptoms of anxiety in all women and has a variable effect on the anxiety disorders ranging from resolution to worsening of symptoms (Altshuler *et al.* 1998; Cohen *et al.* 1989b; Klein *et al.* 1995). The association between high levels of anxiety in a mother and foetal outcome are variable. Whilst some data show an association between high maternal stress and shorter gestation and low birth weight (Copper *et al.* 1996) others have not (Perkin *et al.* 1993). Teixera *et al.* (1999) suggested that maternal anxiety in the third trimester is associated with increased uterine artery resistance as a causal factor in the association of low birth weight and anxiety in mothers. However, these findings are very preliminary in small numbers and the authors were unable to make causal associations between their cross-sectional measures of blood flow and maternal mental state. Many studies with low-quality evidence have suggested that maternal exposure to stress is associated with poor obstetric and foetal outcome. A more recent epidemiological paper finds preterm delivery associated with maternal stress (Dole *et al.* 2003). Emerging high-quality evidence from the Danish population databases seems to be confirming at least that maternal exposure to extreme stress in the form of the death of a first-degree relative periconceptionally, or early in pregnancy (i.e. first trimester) can adversely affect pregnancy outcome (A. Khashan, personal communication, 2006) and possible longer-term risk of psychiatric disorder in childhood and early adulthood.

Treatment issues

Women taking anxiolytic medication who wish to conceive should consider reduction and cessation of drug therapy. Liaison with psychiatric colleagues is important, as these patients often have chronic, hard-to-treat symptoms that may interfere with obstetric management. Reduction of anxiolytics should be combined with alternative non-pharmacological interventions such as supportive and cognitive-behavioural therapy. Anxiolytics should be avoided during pregnancy (see Altshuler *et al.* 1996). If considered essential, prescription should be on a short-term basis at the minimum effective dose. Women on maintenance therapy should be managed as described above. In women who develop anxiety disorder during the first trimester, most can be managed non-pharmacologically with education, supportive care, and reassurance. Pharmacological therapy should be reserved for the most severe cases. Anxiety symptoms tend to abate in the second trimester as women have relief from some of the physical symptoms and reassurance from ultrasound data about the health of the foetus. Few women require anxiolytic maintenance therapy during pregnancy, but those remaining on medication throughout the second trimester should have a detailed ultrasound scan during this period. Anaesthetists and paediatricians should be warned about concurrent use of sedatives prior to delivery.

Teenage pregnancy

The UK has the highest rates of teenage pregnancy in the European Union (Office of National Statistics 2001). Teenage pregnancy is thought to be associated with deprivation and low social class and a positive attitude to childbearing, rather than a negative attitude to contraception (Stevens-Simon *et al.* 1996; Zabin & Hayward 1993). Some young women choose motherhood as a positive role in an impoverished environment with few life options (Drake 1996). Others seek pregnancy as a confirmation of fertility following previous sexual abuse (Rainey *et al.* 1995). Younger mothers are more likely to abort pregnancies, deny and conceal pregnancy, and have worse obstetric outcome (e.g. more low-birth-weight babies), poverty, lack of support and social isolation. In addition their physical health is worse during pregnancy than that of older mothers, with increased rates of hypertension, anaemia and preterm labour and delivery (Scholl *et al.* 1994). Young women may also be more likely to abuse substances, tobacco and alcohol during pregnancy and this is partly associated with higher psychosocial stress and a previous experience of sexual or physical abuse (Scafidi *et al.* 1997). It is perhaps unsurprising then that much evidence has suggested that increased levels of depression occur in teenage mothers compared with older mothers up to five years after their child's birth (Moffitt *et al.* 2002; Williams *et al.* 1997). Most of these studies have used small samples of mothers and often relied on interviews to obtain evidence of mental illness (Hudson *et al.* 2000). Suicide in pregnant teenagers is higher in the first year after birth than in older pregnant women (Appleby 1991). The only large population-based study of mental health in teenage mothers found a greater long-term likelihood of different types of death, and particularly suicide, in teenage mothers (Olausson *et al.* 2004).

Teenage mothers have poor socioeconomic backgrounds (Gigante *et al.* 2004) and teenage motherhood is associated with subsequent low socioeconomic status (Hayes 1987). Depressive symptoms and other family background factors are in themselves associated with subsequent teenage pregnancy (Quinlivan *et al.* 2004), but long-term depression has been examined on very small data sets, often using questionnaires to determine the extent of the depression. One population-based study reported that marital status, rather than the age of the mother at birth, is the important factor in determining subsequent risk of depressive symptoms (Kalil & Kunz 2002).

Violence and pregnancy

Violence against women is endemic worldwide (World Health Organization 1997). Perhaps surprisingly, women are at greatest risk of violence, usually from their partner, during pregnancy (Richardson *et al.* 2002). Almost 30% of women who have experienced domestic violence at some point in their lifetime, report that the first incidence occurred during pregnancy (Helton *et al.* 1987). A woman who is assaulted during pregnancy is more likely to respond to the abuse with self-destructive behaviour that is detrimental to both mother and/or foetus; she is also more likely to abuse alcohol and drugs, both prescribed and illegal (Bhatt 1998). The problem for health workers is to enable women to disclose violence. On average women have experienced 35 episodes of violence before they make it known to others. Disclosure of domestic violence requires confidentiality, privacy, sensitive questioning and a non-judgemental attitude. For example, women must be given the opportunity to be seen alone and to be treated with confidentiality. Often women are terrified of the consequences of disclosure, but questioning is essential and unless asked directly, women are unlikely to disclose violence. Women have often cited not being asked as a reason for non-disclosure of domestic violence. In fact women are very willing to be asked about their experiences by health professionals, providing it is dealt with sensitively and effectively, and by trained health professionals (Mezey *et al.* 2002). For pregnant women, finding a place of safety needs careful multi-disciplinary planning with the mother and can provide a challenge even to experienced clinicians.

Abortion and miscarriage

Little data are available on the psychological effects of pregnancy termination or loss (Boyce *et al.* 2002). Shame, secrecy, and thought suppression are all associated with greater post-abortion depression, anxiety and hostility. A recent large US study reported that married women were at significantly higher risk of a depressive episode following termination, compared to single women. This was thought to reflect the release of burden for single women of not rearing a child on their own (Reardon & Cougle 2002). Others have reported that most women who abort an unintended pregnancy in the first trimester do not suffer any adverse outcomes at two years, unless there is a past history of depression (Major *et al.* 2000). For most women, negative emotional effects are transient (Butler 1996).

The prenatal loss of an infant was until recently considered a 'normal' event. The impact on parents is now recognized (Frost & Condon 1996; Klier *et al.* 2002). One prospective follow-up of 144 women at 8 and 18 months after miscarriage reported that at 8 months, non-pregnant women were experiencing emotional distress and the use of psychotropic medication was three times that of the age-matched controls. By 18 months, the proportion still reporting emotional problems and having received health care for depressive disorders remained high in those who had not conceived. Successful conception after miscarriage was related to lack of previous infertility, desire for a child, and the woman's age. No associations between the psychological status of the women after the miscarriage and the experience and outcome of a subsequent pregnancy were clearly demonstrated.

Foetal anomaly

Foetal anomaly is increasingly diagnosed prenatally or predictable from genetic programming. However, testing for anomaly is a decision incumbent on the parents as is the decision to abort should anomaly be found. These decisions provide for enormous psychological stress and require experienced counselling to aid people through this difficult process. Common indications for prenatal testing include increasing maternal age (> 35), a known balanced translocation in one parent, previous children with chromosomal disorders (e.g. trisomy) or neural tube defect, a parent with a dominant disorder, a mother who is a known X-linked carrier so that foetal gender or molecular diagnosis may be determined, and parents who are both carriers of recessive disorders. Depending on the parents' perception of risk, the decision to undergo testing may be more or less fraught, in part because of the added fear of damaging the foetus in the process. Couples need support for these decisions, for planning subsequent pregnancy, and for their sexual and marital relationship which is frequently strained by such an ordeal.

'Routine' testing of maternal serum concentrations of e.g. alpha fetoprotein for neural tube defects, may also be problematic and associated with much anxiety. This is particularly the case should an initial seven-week result be abnormal and women are required to await further screening. It has also been shown that in multiple screening tests although 8% of women may have abnormal results, only 1% of those will have an abnormal foetus (Carroll 1994).

In psychiatric disorders where drug or alcohol abuse is present or likely, women and parents need to be counselled about increasing the risk of anomalies in their infant should they continue to abuse substances during pregnancy.

Malformed infants

Psychological responses to a malformed child are very varied, but often constitute components of grief reactions to the 'loss of the expected infant'. Parents may experience numbness and inability to accept abnormality, guilt, disgust, poor attachment or rejection of the infant. Depending on the degree to which the child requires physical support, some parents cope by becoming absorbed in practical care and over-involved in parenting to the exclusion of other activities or relationships.

Childbirth: postnatal mood disorders

See the National Institute for Health and Clinical Excellence (NICE) Guidelines (2007) for an overview. By far the most common mood disturbance occurring within days of delivery are the 'blues'. Up to 90% of women may experience this transient emotional lability. These have significance from a nosological perspective as, if severe, they are predictors of a depressive episode. Accurate community prevalence rates have been hard to estimate for a number of reasons. Women are often reluctant to come forward for fear of losing their infants, being seen as bad mothers or simply because of their depressed state and a belief that nothing can be offered to them. One meta-analysis of nearly 13 000 women reported 13% mean prevalence for non-psychotic post-partum depression assessed after at least two weeks post-partum (O'Hara & Swain 1996). But rates vary with timing and method of assessment; higher rates (14%) are recorded when self-report measures like the Edinburgh Postnatal Depression Scale (Cox et al. 1987) are used or misinterpreted as clinical assessment (rather than screening) tools. The number of weeks within which post-partum depression must emerge (as opposed to a depressive episode independent of childbirth) has not been agreed (Cooper & Murray 1995; Cooper et al. 1988). The fourth edition of the Diagnostic and Statistical Manual of Mental Disorders (DSM-IV; American Psychiatric Association 1994) states that symptoms must have onset within four weeks post-partum in order for the episode to qualify for the 'post-partum onset' specifier. In clinical and research practice, many use a time-frame of anything up to three months (Wisner et al. 2002). The long-term impact of maternal mood disorder on offspring development remains uncertain (Cooper & Murray 1997; Martins & Gaffan 2000; Murray 1992; Murray et al. 2001, 2003).

Although breastfeeding has been shown to have an active anxiolytic effect (Altemus et al. 1995) pre-existing anxiety disorders tend to worsen post-partum.

Between 1 and 2% of the population suffer with bipolar affective disorder (BPAD; Kessler et al. 1994), whilst puerperal psychosis, an episode of mania or psychosis precipitated by childbirth, follows approximately 1 in every 1000 births. Terp and Mortensen (1998) obtained a relative risk of 6.8 for first-episode bipolar manic-depressive psychosis 2–28 days following delivery. This figure was even higher when only the first two weeks post-partum were considered. The link between bipolar disorder and puerperal psychosis is striking. The symptoms of both are very similar: rapid-onset affective psychosis with poor sleep, irritability, restlessness, disorganized behaviour and often florid hallucinations and delusions. Women who have suffered a first episode of puerperal affective psychosis are at greater risk of subsequent bipolar affective disorder (Davidson & Robertson 1985); women with BPAD have a 20–30% chance of suffering puerperal psychosis (Kendell *et al.* 1987). Affective disorder is also found to cluster in the families of individuals who have had an episode of puerperal psychosis. Relatives of a sufferer have a 10–50% risk of suffering with an affective disorder (see Jones & Craddock 2001). Jones and Craddock (2001) have also demonstrated that in women with BPAD and a family history of puerperal psychosis, the rate of subsequent puerperal psychosis is in the order of 57%. The implication is that a shared factor, either genes or environment or both, is responsible for this puerperal trigger to affective disorder in these women. The same group of investigators have also reported that a particular variation in the serotonin transporter gene conveys an increased risk of puerperal bipolar disorder (Coyle *et al.* 2000), although this has yet to be confirmed.

Treatment issues

Efficacy of treatments for women postnatally are unlikely to differ from efficacy when non-pregnant. However if women are breastfeeding, specific guidance should be sought from local specialists (see NICE Guidelines 2007). In general, for pharmacological treatments, women should be treated with the lowest possible doses of high-potency agents. If they wish to continue breastfeeding, feeds should coincide with trough drug levels. A full overview of treatment recommendations in the postnatal period is given in the recent NICE guidelines (2007). Prevention of recurrence of depression in the postnatal period has been reported with some, but not all, antidepressants (Wisner *et al.* 2001, 2004).

Menopause

Large epidemiological surveys do not support the notion of a nosologically distinct 'involutional melancholia' (Avis *et al.* 1994; Kaufert *et al.* 1992; Woods & Mitchell 1996). In the Massachusetts Women's Health Study, a prospective, five-year observational trial, investigators sought to ascertain whether a change in menopausal status had an effect on depression in a cohort of 2565 women aged 45–55 at baseline (Avis *et al.* 1994). No link was found between the onset of natural menopause and an increased risk of depression. However, women experiencing a lengthy perimenopause did have a moderately increased rate of depressive symptoms, although the depression was transitory. Furthermore, the increased incidence of depression was largely secondary to menopause symptoms rather than to menopause itself.

Similar results were reported from the Seattle Midlife Women's Health Study (Woods & Mitchell 1996) and the Manitoba Project (Kaufert *et al.* 1992). In both studies, no consistent relationship was found between menopausal status and depression or depressed mood in population-based cohorts. Menopausal status did not differentiate women with patterns of depressed mood from those without depressed mood.

These studies also suggested that psychosocial and cultural factors accounted for more variation in depressed mood and depression among women at menopause than menopause itself. Patterns of depressed mood were multifactorial and related to stressful life context, past and/or present health status, and social factors at midlife; the variable which best predicted subsequent depression was a previous history of depression. Hunter (1990) reported that past depression, along with cognitive and social factors, accounted for 51% of the variance in depressed mood reported by menopausal women. Stressful life events, e.g. illness or death of parents, children leaving home, career changes, divorce, or financial problems, which may occur at midlife, also can affect mood.

The incidence of mood disturbances is higher in perimenopausal women than in post-menopausal women and appears to be greatest in those with a prolonged menopause (27 months). Schmidt *et al.* (1997) suggest that ovarian steroid withdrawal vasomotor symptoms, such as hot flashes and night sweats, which occur in the perimenopausal and early post-menopausal periods, are associated with mood symptoms. Vasomotor symptoms are associated with sleeplessness, irritability, depression, and loss of an overall sense of wellbeing.

Many women experience minor mood changes at menopause and a subgroup of women may be more likely to relapse or develop de-novo depression in association with severe menopausal symptoms. It may be that women with previous depression, PMDD or postnatal depression are more likely to develop depression at menopause.

Psychotic disorders are thought to occur more commonly in post-menopausal women and paraphrenia may represent a distinct disorder. Some have suggested that schizophrenia worsens post-menopausally and that women require higher doses of medication following menopause (e.g. Grigoriadis & Seeman 2002). The data are however confounded by the same factors as studies of depressed mood and have not been replicated in epidemiological samples. Age at onset data suggest a second peak of incidence of schizophreniform disorder in women at around 45 years (Castle *et al.* 1998), but this has not been associated with changes in ovarian hormone status. Rapid cycling bipolar disorder may also deteriorate at menopause, although again the data are inconsistent (see Liebenluft 1997).

The Harvard Study of Moods (Harlow *et al.* 2003) suggests that early menopause (<40 years)/ovarian failure may be more common in women who have a lifetime history of major depression.

Psychological aspects of gynaecological disorders

Menstrual disturbances

Disturbances of menstruation are common. The HPA and hypothalamic-gonadal (HPG) axes are closely linked. Activation of the HPA axis, whatever the cause, dampens the normal pattern of menstrual cycling. At some point in their lives, most women have 'missed a period' in association with life's stresses. Psychological disorders are commonly associated with loss of menstruation. Anorexia nervosa is in part defined by a loss of menstrual periods. Bulimia may also include loss of periods. Chronic substance abuse can cause loss of periods especially if weight loss is prominent. It is now recognized that menstrual disturbances occur (commonly) in depression, anxiety and psychotic disorder (Smith *et al.* 2002; Wieck & Haddad 2003). Chronic hypoestrogenaemia and loss of menstrual cycles are associated with accelerated bone loss, an increased risk of cardiovascular disease and possible premature menopause or ovarian failure (Davies *et al.* 1995b; Fabbri *et al.* 1991; Halbreich *et al.* 1995; Peterson 1998).

For most psychiatric disorders however, the extent of the menstrual disturbance has not yet been quantified. Psychotropic drugs are at least a part of the cause (Smith *et al.* 2002; Wieck & Haddad 2003). Women with chronic psychiatric disorder need to be asked regularly about their menstrual health, while mental health professionals and patients must be educated about normal menstrual function. Smith *et al.* (2002) suggest 'clinical practice should incorporate routine inquiries about menstrual status, and evaluation of prolactin and gonadal steroid blood levels' and that 'non-prolactin raising antipsychotics should be considered as first-line treatment in young women'.

Polycystic ovarian syndrome

Polycystic ovarian syndrome (PCOS) frequently presents during adolescence and is the commonest cause of menstrual irregularity and hirsutism (Franks 2002). Symptoms include hirsuites, acne, weight gain and infertility in a young woman. The characteristic endocrine abnormalities include hypersecretion of androgens and luteinizing hormone. Metabolic dysfunction is also a feature of many young women with PCOS. Hyperinsulinaemia and insulin resistance, which can be regarded as an exaggeration of the normal metabolic changes that occur during puberty, are further amplified by obesity.

The aetiology of PCOS is uncertain, but there is evidence for a primary abnormality of ovarian androgen production which is manifest at puberty but may have its origins in childhood or even during foetal development (Abbott *et al.* 2002). It affects up to 30% of women and is genetically and phenotypically polymorphic. It may or may not be associated with anovulation. PCOS patients with unexplained infertility tend to have higher midfollicular luteinizing hormone and testosterone compared with healthy controls.

The prevalence of PCOS is significantly higher in women with unexplained infertility where hyperandrogenaemia contributes to subfertility in women with regular menses (Kousta *et al.* 1999). Psychological disturbance has not been systematically investigated in this group although the polymorphic nature of the disease would allow distinction between physiological and psychosocial effects of the disorder.

Pelvic pain

Dysmenorrhoea is pelvic pain of menstrual origin (Dagwood 1995). Between 50 and 70% of adolescent girls experience dysmenorrhea (Westhoff & Davis 2001). For some women the pain is regularly disabling and poorly responsive to simple analgesics (Pedron *et al.* 1998). Treatment with the oral contraceptive pill (OCP) may be of some benefit in this group (Westhoff & Davis 2001). Primary dysmenorrhoea is thought to be associated with elevated uterine prostaglandin levels. Secondary dysmenorrhoea is associated with discrete uterine pathology such as fibroids and endometriosis. Intermenstrual, non-cyclic pelvic pain of a gynaecological origin is more likely to be secondary to pathology such as ovarian cystic disease or pelvic adhesions. Pelvic pain should be distinguished from dyspareunia, which is painful intercourse (Binik *et al.* 2002) and vulval pain (Bodden-Heidrich *et al.* 1999; see below).

Chronic pelvic pain is usually defined as cyclic or acyclic pain lasting more than six months and its cause is usually discernible through careful history taking, pelvic examination and diagnostic laparoscopy. Non-organic chronic pelvic pain or pelvic pain syndrome is characterized by impairment of function in daily activities and often associated with depressive symptoms (Peters *et al.* 1991). It is women in this group who require comprehensive psychological evaluation. They are likely to have a diminished role within their family and within their relationships. Unlike other chronic pain syndromes, women with chronic pelvic pain have a high incidence of sexual abuse including incest, rape and molestation (approx. 50%) and may be more likely to have a past psychiatric history (Reiter & Gambone 1990). Chronic pelvic pain may have similar features to other syndromes with medically unexplained symptoms (see Chapter 7). One of the confusing aspects of pelvic pain is that women with organic pathology may also have psychological difficulties which compound the pain and mean that the extent of the pathology is poorly related to the extent of the pain. These reasons may explain why a multidisciplinary approach to chronic pelvic pain is successful (Peters *et al.* 1991).

Vulvovaginitis and vulvodynia

Vulval inflammation or vulvovaginitis is commonly associated with acute infections such as yeast infection and *Trichomonas vaginalis*. Usually these are transient and readily treatable. However, recurrent infections do occur and may lead to a range of problems such as vaginismus and subsequent dyspareunia (see below) and psychological symptoms associated with any chronic painful syndrome (Ridley 1998). Vulval dystrophy in post-menopausal or oestrogen-deficient women may also cause vulvovaginitis. Vulval carcinoma may be difficult to diagnose. Vulval pain without evidence of pathology is an increasing problem. A recent large Harvard study of 16 000 women estimated that 16% of women suffered with vulvodynia over their lifetimes (Harlow & Stewart 2003). The aetiology is unclear (Gordon *et al.* 2003); it is akin to chronic pain syndromes and childhood trauma (including sexual abuse); psychiatric disorder (Jadresic *et al.* 1993) and the OCP have all been cited as risk factors (Davis & Hutchison 1999). Antidepressant drugs may be effective in some women with vulvodynia (Stolar & Stewart 2002).

Hormone replacement therapy

Hormone replacement (oestrogen +/− progesterone) has been popular for many women suffering oestrogen withdrawal symptoms over the menopause. More recently data are emerging which suggest that in women without hot flashes, oestrogen-replacement therapy (HRT) reduces symptoms of depression (Schmidt *et al.* 2000), although not all data are consistent (Stephens & Ross 2002). Early observational studies reported a reduction in cardiovascular disease risk and mortality in post-menopausal women on HRT. However, the longer term effects of HRT (more than five years) are associated with an increased risk of mortality from cardiovascular disease, stroke and breast cancer in those with a family history of breast cancer (Bushnell 2005; Douketis 2005; Greiser *et al.* 2005; Langer *et al.* 2005). Current Department of Health guidelines suggest that treatment with HRT should be limited to two years if there are no contraindications. These include:
- a history or family history of breast cancer
- a history of womb cancer
- unusual vaginal bleeding

- severe liver disease
- previous stroke or deep-vein thrombosis, or untreated high blood pressure
- may be pregnant (still the most common reason for periods to stop, and a possibility for up to two years after the start of the menopause).

The method of HRT delivery (e.g. patches rather than tablets) may be altered if a woman has insulin-dependent diabetes or irritable bowel syndrome.

Many women seek non-medical treatment options. Whilst no evidence exists for their efficacy, they are increasingly popular among women concerned about adverse side-effects of HRT. They include black cohosh, a herbal root (may reduce hot flushes and vaginal dryness); ginseng which contains essential fatty acids (may help hot flushes); and agnus castus (may help hot flushes). Some plants have small amounts of natural oestrogens called phyto-oestrogens. Phyto-oestrogens are similar to the oestrogen in women's bodies but may only have 2% of the potency of human oestrogens. Eating foods such as soy high in phyto-oestrogens products may help relieve symptoms, e.g. hot flushes. Isoflavenoids extracted from soya are now available in capsule form although biological effects of phyto-oestrogens are likely to be greater in post-menopausal women when oestrogen receptors may not be occupied. Some phyto-oestrogens have been found to have bone-sparing effects in experimental animals and in some human subjects.

The impact of the OCP on women's mood remains controversial (for overview, see Rubino-Watkins *et al.* 1999).

Testosterone (oral or implants) is increasingly sought by women perimeno-pausally to increase energy levels and libido (see below). Few data on long-term effects are available however, and each woman should be assessed individually before prescribing androgens.

Cervical smear and human papilloma virus

Routine cervical or PAP smears are provided for menstruating women every three years as a form of health screening for gynaecological cancers (carcinoma of the female reproductive tract). As such, women are usually asymptomatic when told they have an abnormal smear. Cervical cancer is essentially considered a sexually transmitted disease following infection with the human papilloma virus (HPV) and women are increasingly aware of this. As an asymptomatic (young) woman, therefore, being told that you have cancer and possibly an ineradicable sexually transmitted disease may present a particular psychological burden. The communication of abnormal smear results, either by letter or by telephone call, is typically the responsibility of a practice nurse, and communications vary widely in the amount of information given to women. Phillips *et al.* (2002) audited the practice of informing women of abnormal smear results and concluded that the method and content of communications imparting mild or borderline abnormal smear results were very variable, but that the way in which women are informed about borderline or mildly abnormal smears can have a significant psychological impact. Newsom et al. (1996) reported that self-blame was an important predictor of depressive symptoms and illness following a diagnosis of cancer. A woman may believe she could have prevented cervical cancer, as it is associated with a sexually transmitted disease. Treatments for cervical cancer may also affect a woman's fertility with attendant adverse psychological effects.

Vaginismus

Vaginismus is a relatively uncommon syndrome (2% prevalence) resulting from involuntary contraction of the perivaginal musculature. It may be the result of pelvic pathology or fear (conscious or otherwise) of sexual penetration. Some vaginismus occurs with any attempt at vaginal penetration, with a tampon by the woman herself or at medical vaginal examination. Some is restricted to attempts at sexual intercourse. A past history of trauma, sexual or otherwise (e.g. a traumatic delivery) may be associated with vaginismus.

Dyspareunia is pain in association with intercourse and is defined as either superficial or deep. Menstrual exacerbation is not uncommon. Vulval and vestibular inflammation may cause superficial dyspareunia, although it is commonly idiopathic. Deep dyspareunia is commonly thought to be associated with organic pathology. A careful history of variations in pain with different partners, past history of sexual abuse and trauma (e.g. childbirth-related injury) are helpful in determining both causes and planning management. If dyspareunia is considered psychological in origin, a multidisciplinary approach similar to that in chronic pelvic pain is recommended.

Sexual dysfunction

'Female sexual dysfunction' has only recently been described and remains controversial (Heiman 2002). Abnormalities of sexual desire or arousal (low libido and anorgasmia) are increasingly recognized for the important health concern they represent for sufferers. At the same time clinicians should be able to reassure a woman when a change in sexual desire is likely to be temporary and to be expected, e.g. during treatment for infertility, during pregnancy (especially third trimester), following childbirth or as a result of surgery or chemotherapy. Sexual desire may be reduced by social as much as medical factors: a change of circumstance, a new relationship, an old relationship and relationship difficulties (e.g. infidelity in a partner), illness, medications, fatigue, menopause, hysterectomy, depression, anxiety, stress (see O'Donohue & Geer 1993). A careful history of change in sexual desire and behaviour is essential for distinguishing situational disorder or more global problems secondary to, say, illness or medication, e.g. oral contraceptive, SSRIs, benzodiazepines and antipsychotic drugs. Anorgasmia and sexual dysfunction are commonly associated with the use of SSRIs, and conventional neuroleptic medication is well known to be associated with hyperprolactinaemia which can reduce libido. Acute changes in sexual desire may be easier to treat than chronic low sexual desire. The latter may be associated with endocrine abnormalities such as diabetes or PCOS or to pervasive psychological trauma such as sexual abuse. Some have reported benefit from exogenous androgens in premenopausal women and following ovariectomy (Alexander & Sherwin 1993; Koehler 1998).

Low sexual desire and anorgasmia are likely to be much more common in women with psychiatric illness and appear to be largely ignored by clinicians (see Smith *et al.* 2002). Women should be given the opportunity to discuss their sexual lives and to do so in a woman-only environment (Department of Health 2002). Clinicians should offer women this opportunity. Sexual functioning depends on so many aspects of life and available treatments reflect this complexity. An increasing number of specialist clinics are available for referral where sexual therapists tailor interventions to the couple or individual.

Drugs and women

Women show different handling and metabolism, and side-effect profiles for a number of drugs (Roe *et al.* 2002). Rarely are sex differences in pharmacokinetics taken into account in prescription (Gleiter & Gundert-Remy 1996). In addition, psychotropic drugs may affect sexual and reproductive function (Robinson 2002). For example, valproic acid may be associated with PCOS, and antidepressants may produce elevated serum prolactin concentrations, especially with long-term administration. However, the frequency of antidepressant-induced hyperprolactinaemia is much lower than that seen with antipsychotics, and serious adverse clinical effects are uncommon. Other psychotropic drugs such as lithium, valproic acid, buspirone, carbamazepine and benzodiazepines are either only rarely associated with symptomatic hyperprolactinaemia or do not produce clinically important changes in prolactin concentrations (Marken *et al.* 1992). Obesity and diabetes induced by newer atypical APDs may have effects on both sexual desire and menstrual function. Monitoring women's reproductive and sexual health should be a routine aspect of therapeutic monitoring.

REFERENCES

Abbott, D. H., Dumesic, D. A. and Franks, S. (2002). Developmental origin of polycystic ovary syndrome – a hypothesis. *Journal of Endocrinology*, **174**, 1–51.

Abramowitz, J. S., Schwartz, S. A. and Moore, K. M. (2003). Obsessional thoughts in postpartum females and their partners. Content, severity and relationship with depression. *Journal of Clinical Psychology in Medical Settings*, **10**, 157–64.

Alexander, G. M. and Sherwin, B. B. (1993). Sex steroids, sexual behavior, and selective attention for erotic stimuli in women using oral contraceptives. *Psychoneuroendocrinology*, **18**, 273–8.

Alpern, L. and Lyons-Ruth, K. (1993). Preschool children at social risk: chronicity and timing of maternal depressive symptoms and child behavior problems at school and at home. *Development and Psychopathology*, **5**, 371–87.

Altemus, M., Deutster, P. A., Galliven, E., *et al.* (1995). Suppression of hypothalamic-pituitary-adrenal axis responses to stress in lactating women. *Journal of Clinical Endocrinology and Metabolism*, **80**, 2954–9.

Altshuler, L. L., Cohen, L., Szuba, M. P., *et al.* (1996). Pharmacologic management of psychiatric illness during pregnancy: dilemmas and guidelines. *American Journal of Psychiatry*, **153**, 592–606.

Altshuler, L. L., Hendrick, V. and Cohen, L. S. (1998). Course of mood and anxiety disorders during pregnancy and the postpartum period. *Journal of Clinical Psychiatry*, **59**(Supp. 2), 29–33.

American Psychiatric Association. (1994). *Diagnostic and Statistical Manual of Mental Disorders*, 4th edn. (DSMIV). Washington, DC: American Psychiatric Association.

Ananth, J. (1978). Side effects in the neonate from psychotropic agents excreted through breastfeeding. *American Journal of Psychiatry*, **135**, 801–5.

Angst, J. R., Sellaro, R., Merikangas, K. R., *et al.* (2001). The epidemiology of perimenstrual psychological symptoms. *Acta Psychiatrica Scandinavica*, **104**, 110–16.

Apfel, R. and Handel, M. H. (1993). *Madness and the Loss of Motherhood: Sexuality, Reproduction and Long Term Mental Illness.* Washington, DC: American Psychiatric Association, APA Press.

Appleby, L. (1991). Suicide after pregnancy and the first postnatal year. *British Medical Journal*, **302**, 137–40.

Avis, N. E., Brambilla, D., McKinlay, S. M., *et al.* (1994). A longitudinal analysis of the association between menopause and depression: results from the Massachusetts Women's Health Study. *Annals of Epidemiology*, **4**, 214–20.

Baca, G., Sanchez, A., Gonzalez, P., *et al.* (1998). Menstrual cycle profiles of suicidal behaviour. *Acta Psychiatrica Scandinavica*, **97**, 32–5.

Barkla, J. and McGrath, J. (2000). Reproductive, preconceptual and antenatal needs of women with schizophrenia. In *Women and Schizophrenia*, ed. J. David Castle, J. McGrath and J. Kulkani. New York, NY: Cambridge University Press, pp. 67–78.

Bennedsen, B. E. (1998). Adverse pregnancy outcome in women with schizophrenia: occurrence and risk factors. *Schizophrenia Research*, **33**, 1–26.

Bennedsen, B. E., Mortensen, P. B., Olesen, A. V., *et al.* (2001). Congenital malformations, stillbirths and infant deaths among children of women with schizophrenia. *Archives of General Psychiatry*, **58**, 674–9.

Bhatt, R. V. (1998). Domestic violence and substance abuse. *International Journal of Gynecology and Obstetrics*, **63**, S25–31.

Binik, Y. M., Reissing, E., Pukhal, C., *et al.* (2002). The female sexual pain disorders: genital pain or sexual dysfunction? *Archives of Sexual Behavior*, **31**, 425–9.

Blake, F. P., Salkorskis, A., Gath, D., *et al.* (1998). Cognitive therapy for premenstrual syndrome. *Journal of Psychosomatic Research*, **45**, 307–18.

Blehar, M. C., DePaulo, J. R., Gershon, E. S., *et al.* (1998). Women with bipolar disorder: findings from the NIMH genetics initiative sample. *Psychopharmacological Bulletin*, **34**, 239–43.

Bodden-Heidrich, R., Kuppers, V., Beckmann, M. W., *et al.* (1999). Psychosomatic aspects of vulvodynia: comparison with the chronic pelvic pain syndrome. *Journal of Reproductive Medicine*, **44**, 411–16.

Boyce, P. M., Condon, J. T. and Ellwood, D. A. (2002). Pregnancy loss: a major life event affecting emotional health and well-being. *Medical Journal of Australia*, **176**, 250–1.

Breaux, C. S., Hartlage, S. and Gehlert, S. (2000). Relationships of premenstrual dysphoric disorder to major depression and anxiety disorders. *Journal of Psychosomatic and Obstetrics Gynaecology*, **21**, 17–24.

Briggs, G. G. (2002). *Drugs in Pregnancy and Lactation: a Reference Guide to Fetal and Neonatal Risk*, 6th edn. Baltimore, MD: Williams & Wilkins, pp. 6201–51.

Bushnell, C. D. (2005). Oestrogen and stroke in women: assessment of risk. *Lancet Neurology*, **4**, 743–51.

Butler, C. (1996). Late psychological sequelae of abortion. Questions from a primary care perspective. *Journal of Family Practice*, **43**(4), 396–401.

Calabrese, J. R. and Gulledge, A. D. (1985). Psychotropics during pregnancy and lactation: a review. *Psychosomatics*, **26**, 413–26.

Carroll, J. C. (1994). Maternal serum screening. *Canadian Family Physician*, **40**, 1756–64.

Castle, D., Sham, P., Murray, R. M., *et al.* (1998). Differences in distribution of ages of onset in males and females with schizophrenia. *Schizophrenia Research*, **33**, 179–83.

Chaturvedi, S. K., Chandra, P. S., Gururaj, G., *et al.* (1995). Suicidal ideas during premenstrual phase. *Journal of Affective Disorder*, **34**, 193–9.

Cohen, L. S. and Rosenbaum, J. F. (1998). Psychotropic drug use during pregnancy: weighing the risks. *Journal of Clinical Psychiatry*, **59**, 18–28.

Cohen, L. S., Heller, V. L. and Rosenbaum, J. F. (1989a). Treatment guidelines for psychotropic drug use in pregnancy. *Psychosomatics*, **30**, 25–33.

Cohen, L. S., Heller, V. L. and Kelley, K. L. (1989b). Course of panic disorder in 24 pregnant women. In *CMF Syllabus and Proceedings Summary*, 142nd Annual Meeting of the American Psychiatric Association. Washington, DC: American Psychiatric Association.

Cohen, L. S., Sichel, D. A., Dimmock, J. A., *et al.* (1994). Impact of pregnancy on panic disorder: a case series. *Journal of Clinical Psychiatry*, **55**, 284–8.

Cohen, L. S., Sichel, D. A., Robertson, L. M., *et al.* (1995). Postpartum prophylaxis for women with bipolar disorder. *American Journal of Psychiatry*, **152**, 1641–3.

Collins, A., Eneroth, P. and Landgren, B.-M. (1985). Psychoneuroendocrine stress responses and mood as related to the menstrual cycle. *Psychosomatic Medicine*, **47**, 512–27.

Cooper, P. J. and Murray, L. (1995). Course and recurrence of postnatal depression: evidence for the specificity of the diagnostic concept. *British Journal of Psychiatry*, **166**, 191–5.

Cooper, P. J. and Murray, L. (1997). The impact of psychological treatments of postpartum depression on maternal mood and infant development. In *Postpartum Depression and Child Development*, ed. L. Murray and P. J. Cooper. New York: Guilford, pp. 201–20.

Cooper, P., Cambpell, E., Day, A., *et al.* (1988). Non-psychotic psychiatric disorder after childbirth: a prospective study of prevalence, incidence, course and nature. *British Journal of Psychiatry*, **152**, 799–806.

Copper, R. L., Goldenberg, R. L., Das, A., *et al.* (1996). The preterm prediction study: maternal stress is associated with spontaneous preterm birth at less than 35 weeks gestation. *American Journal of Obstetrics and Gynecology*, **175**, 1286–92.

Cott, A. D. and Wisner, K. L. (2003). Psychiatric disorders during pregnancy. *International Review of Psychiatry*, **15**, 217–30.

Coverdale, J. H., Turbott, S. H. and Roberts, H. (1997). Family planning needs and STD risk behaviour of female psychiatric out-patients. *British Journal of Psychiatry*, **171**, 69–72.

Cox, J. L., Holden, J. M. and Sagovsky, R. (1987). Detection of postnatal depression – development of the 10-item Edinburgh Postnatal Depression Scale. *British Journal of Psychiatry*, **150**, 782–6.

Coyle, I., Wayner, M. J. and Singer, G. (1976). Behavioral teratogenesis: a critical evaluation. *Pharmacology, Biochemistry and Behavior*, **4**, 191–200.

Coyle, N., Jones, I., Robertson, E., *et al.* (2000). Variation at the serotonin transporter gene influences susceptibility to bipolar affective puerperal psychosis. *Lancet*, **356**, 1490–1.

Dagwood, M. Y. (1995). 'Dysmenorrhea'. *Journal of Reproductive Medicine*, **30**(3), 154–67.

Dahl, M. L., Olhager, E. and Ahiner, J. (1997). Paroxetine withdrawal in a neonate. *British Journal of Psychiatry*, **171**, 391–2.

Davidson, J. and Robertson, E. (1985). A follow-up study of postpartum illness, 1946–1978. *Acta Psychiatrica Scandinavica*, **71**, 451–7.

Davies, A., McIvor, R. J. and Kumar, R. C. (1995a). Impact of childbirth on a series of schizophrenic mothers: a comment on the possible influence of oestrogen on schizophrenia. *Schizophrenia Research*, **16**, 25–31.

Davies, M. C., Gulekli, B. and Jacobs, H. S. (1995b). Osteoporosis in Turner's Syndrome and other forms of primary amenorrhoea. *Clinical Endocrinology*, **43**, 7416.

Davis, G. D. and Hutchison, C. V. (1999). Clinical management of vulvodynia. *Clinical Obstetrics and Gynecology*, **42**(2), 221–33.

Dennis, C. (2004). Preventing postpartum depression. Part II: a critical review of non-biological interventions. *Canadian Journal of Psychiatry*, **49**, 526–38.

Department of Health. (1999). *Confidential Enquiries into Maternal Deaths in the United Kingdom 1999*. Department of Health, pp. 140–53.

Department of Health. (2002). *Women's Mental Health. Into the Mainstream: Strategic Development of Mental Health Care for Women*.

Dimmock, P. W., Wyatt, K. M., Jones, P. W., *et al.* (2000). Efficacy of selective serotonin-reuptake inhibitors in premenstrual syndrome: a systematic review. *Lancet*, **356**, 1131–6.

Dole, N., Saviz, D. A., Hertz-Picciotto, I., *et al.* (2003). Maternal stress and preterm birth. *American Journal of Epidemiology*, **157**(1), 14–24.

Douketis, J. (2005). Hormone replacement therapy and risk for venous thromboembolism: what's new and how do these findings influence clinical practice? *Current Opinion in Hematology*, **12**, 395–400.

Drake, P. (1996). Addressing developmental needs of pregnant adolescents. *Journal of Obstetric, Gynecologic and Neonatal Nursing*, **25**, 518–24.

Drugs and Therapeutics Bulletin. (1992a). Managing the premenstrual syndrome. *Drugs and Therapeutics Bulletin*, **30**, 69–72.

Drugs and Therapeutics Bulletin. (1992b). Evening primrose oil and premenstrual syndrome. *Drugs and Therapeutics Bulletin*, **30**, 1–3.

Drugs and Therapeutics Bulletin. (2002). SSRIs in the management of premenstrual disorders. *Drugs and Therapeutics Bulletin*, **40**, 72.

Endicott, J. J., Amsterdam, J., Eriksson, E., *et al.* (1999). Is premenstrual dysphoric disorder a distinct clinical entity? *Journal of Women's Health & Gender-Based Medicine*, **8**, 663–79.

Ericsson, A., Kallen, B. and Wiholm, B. (1999). Delivery outcome after the use of antidepressants in early pregnancy. *European Journal of Clinical Pharmacology*, **55**, 503–8.

Essex, M. J., Klein, M. H., Miech, R., *et al.* (2001). Timing of initial exposure to maternal major depression and children's mental health symptoms in kindergarten. *British Journal of Psychiatry*, **179**, 151–6.

Evans, J., Heron, J., Francomb, H., *et al.* (2001). Cohort study of depressed mood during pregnancy and after childbirth. *British Medical Journal*, **323**, 257–60.

Fabbri, G., Petraglia, F., Segre, A., *et al.* (1991). Reduced spinal bone density in young women with amenorrhoea. *European Journal of Obstetrics, Gynecology and Reproductive Biology*, **41**, 117–22.

Faedda, G. L., Tondo, L., Baldessarini, R. J., *et al.* (1993). Occurrence after rapid versus gradual discontinuation of lithium in bipolar disorders. *Archives of General Psychiatry*, **50**, 448.

Frank, R. (1931). The hormonal causes of premenstrual tension. *Archives of Neurology and Psychiatry*, **26**, 1053–7.

Franks, S. (2002). Adult polycystic ovary syndrome begins in childhood. *Best Practice & Research Clinical Endocrinology & Metabolism*, **16**, 263–72.

Frost, M. and Condon, J. T. (1996). The psychological sequelae of miscarriage: a critical review of the literature. *Australian and New Zealand Journal of Psychiatry*, **30**, 54–62.

Gigante, D. P., Victora, C. G., Goncalves, H., *et al.* (2004). Risk factors for childbearing during adolescence in a population-based birth cohort in southern Brazil. *Pan American Journal of Public Health*, **16**(1), 1–10.

Gleiter, C. H. and Gundert-Remy, U. (1996). Gender differences in pharmacokinetics. *European Journal of Drug Metabolism and Pharmacokinetics*, **21**, 123–8.

Gordon, R. and Gordon, K. (1960). Social factors in prevention of postpartum emotional problems. *Obstetrics and Gynecology*, **15**, 433–88.

Gordon, A. S., Panahian-Jand, M., McComb, F., *et al.* (2003). Characteristics of women with vulvar pain disorders: responses to a web-based survey. *Journal of Sex & Marital Therapy*, **29**(Suppl. 1), 45–58.

Gotlib, I. H., Whiffen, V. E., Mount, J. H., *et al.* (1989). Prevalence rates and demographic characteristics associated with depression in pregnancy and the postpartum. *Journal of Consulting and Clinical Psychology*, **57**, 269–74.

Greiser, C. M., Greiser, E. M. and Doren, M. (2005). Menopausal hormone therapy and risk of breast cancer: a meta-analysis of epidemiological studies and randomized controlled trials. *Human Reproduction Update*, **11**, 561–73.

Grigoriadis, S. and Seeman, M. V. (2002). The role of estrogen in schizophrenia: implications for schizophrenia practice guidelines for women. *Canadian Journal of Psychiatry*, **47**, 437–42.

Halbreich, U., Rojansky, N., Palter, S., *et al.* (1995). Decreased bone mineral density in medicated psychiatric patients. *Psychosomatic Medicine*, **57**, 485–91.

Hamspon, E. (1990). Variations in sex-related cognitive abilities across the menstrual cycle. *Brain & Cognition*, **14**, 26–43.

Harlow, B. L. and Stewart, E. G. (2003). A population-based assessment of chronic unexplained vulvar pain: have we underestimated the prevalence of vulvodynia? *Journal of American Medical Women's Association*, **58**, 82–8.

Harlow, B. L., Wise, L. A., Otto, M. W., *et al.* (2003). Depression and its influence on reproductive endocrine and menstrual cycle markers associated with perimenopause: The Harvard study of moods and cycles. *Archives of General Psychiatry*, **60**, 29–36.

Hauka, J., Suvisaari, J. and Lonnqvist, J. (2003). Fertility of patients with schizophrenia, their siblings, and the general population: a cohort study from 1950 to 1959. *American Journal of Psychiatry*, **160**, 460–3.

Hayes, C. D. (1987). *Risking the Future: Adolescent Sexuality, Pregnancy and Childbearing.* Washington, DC: National Academy Press.

Hearle, J. and McGrath, J. (2000). Motherhood and schizophrenia. In *Women and Schizophrenia*, ed. D. J. Castle, J. McGRath and J. Kulkarni. Cambridge: Cambridge University Press.

Heiman, J. R. (2002). Psychological treatments for female sexual dysfunction: are they effective and do we need them? *Archives of Sexual Behavior*, **31**, 445–50.

Hertzberg, T. and Wahlbeck, K. (1999). The impact of pregnancy and puerperium on panic disorder: a review. *Journal of Psychosomatic Obstetrics and Gynecology*, **20**(2), 59–64.

Howard, L. M., Kumar, R. and Thornicroft, G. (2001). Psychosocial characteristics and needs of mothers with psychotic disorders. *British Journal of Psychiatry*, **178**, 427–32.

Howard, L. M., Kumar, R., Leese, M., *et al.* (2002). The general fertility rate in women with psychotic disorders. *American Journal of Psychiatry*, **159**(6), 991–7.

Hudson, D. B., Elek, S. M. and Campbell-Grossman, C. (2000). Depression, self-esteem, loneliness, and social support among adolescent mothers participating in the new parents project. *Adolescence*, **35**(139), 445–53.

Hunter, M. S. (1990). Psychological and somatic experience of the menopause: a prospective study. *Psychosomatic Medicine*, **52**, 357–67.

Jablensky, A. V., Morgan, V., Zubrick, S. R., *et al.* (2005). Pregnancy, delivery, and neonatal complications in a population cohort of women with schizophrenia and major affective disorders. *American Journal of Psychiatry*, **162**(1), 79–91.

Jadresic, D., Barton, S., Neill, S., *et al.* (1993). Psychiatric morbidity in women attending a clinic for vulval problems: is there a higher rate in vulvodynia? *International Journal of STD & AIDS*, **4**, 237–9.

Jennings, K. D., Ross, K., Popper, S., *et al.* (1999). Thoughts of harming infants in depressed and non-depressed mothers. *Journal of Affective Disorders*, **54**(1–2), 21–8.

Jensvold, M. F., Muller, K., Putnam, F., *et al.* (1989). *Abuse and PTSD in PMS Patients and Controls.* International Society of Psychosomatic Obstetrics and Gynaecology Biannual Meeting, Amsterdam, Netherlands, May 1989.

Jones, I. and Craddock, N. (2001). Familiality of the puerperal trigger in bipolar disorder: results of a family study. *American Journal of Psychiatry*, **158**, 913–17.

Kalil, A. and Kunz, J. (2002). Teenage childbearing, marital status, and depressive symptoms in later life. *Child Development*, **73**(6), 1748–60.

Kaufert, P. A., Gilbert, P. and Tate, R. (1992). The Manitoba project: a re-examination of the link between menopause and depression. *Maturitas*, **14**, 143–55.

Kendell, R. E., Chalmers, J. C. and Platz, C. (1987). Epidemiology of puerperal psychosis. *British Journal of Psychiatry*, **150**, 662–73.

Kendler, K. S., Silberg, J. L., Neate, M. C., *et al.* (1992). Genetic and environmental factors in the aetiology of menstrual, premenstrual and neurotic symptoms: a population-based twin study. *Psychological Medicine*, **22**, 85–100.

Kessler, R. C., McGonagle, K. A., Zhao, S., *et al.* (1994). Lifetime and 12 month prevalence of DSMIIIR psychiatric disorders in the United States: results from the National Comorbidity Survey. *Archives of General Psychiatry*, **51**, 8–19.

Kimura, D. (1996). Sex, sexual orientation and sex hormones influence human cognitive function. *Current Opinion in Neurobiology*, **6**, 259–63.

King-Hele, S., Pickles, A., Webb, R. T., *et al.* (2007). Cause-specific stillbirth and infant death in the offspring of people with psychiatric illness (in press).

Kirschbaum, C., Wust, S. and Hellhammer, D. H. (1992). Consistent sex differences in cortisol responses to psychological stress. *Psychosomatic Medicine*, **54**, 648–57.

Kirschbaum, C., Kudielka, B. M., Gaab, J., *et al.* (1999). Impact of gender, menstrual cycle phase and oral contraceptives on the activity of the hypothalamus-pituitary-adrenal axis. *Psychosomatic Medicine*, **61**, 154–62.

Kitamura, T., Shima, S., Sugawara, M., *et al.* (1993). Psychological and social correlates of the onset of affective disorders among pregnant women. *Psychological Medicine*, **23**, 967–75.

Klein, D. F., Skrobala, A. M. and Garfinkel, R. S. (1995). Preliminary look at the effects of pregnancy on the course of panic disorder. *Anxiety*, **1**, 227–32.

Klier, C. M., Geller, P. A. and Ritscher, J. B. (2002). Affective disorders in the aftermath of miscarriage: a comprehensive review. *Archives of Womens Mental Health*, **5**, 129–49.

Koehler, J. D. (1998). Sexual dysfunction. In *Primary Care in Obstetrics and Gynecology*, ed. J. S. Sanfilippo and R. P. Smith. New York: Springer, pp. 485–524.

Kousta, E., White, D. M., Cela, E., *et al.* (1999). The prevalence of polycystic ovaries in women with infertility. *Human Reproduction*, **14**, 2720–3.

Kovacs, G. T., Mushin, D., Kane, H., *et al.* (1993). A controlled study of the psychosocial development of children conceived following insemination with donor semen. *Human Reproduction*, **8**, 788–90.

Kudielka, B. M., Hellhammer, D. H. and Kirschbaum, C. (2000). Sex differences in human stress responses. In *The Encyclopaedia of Stress*, ed. G. Fink. London: Academic Press, pp. 429–34.

Kumar, R. and Robson, M. K. (1984). A prospective study of emotional disorders in childbearing women. *British Journal of Psychiatry*, **144**, 35–47.

Langer, R. D., Pradhan, A. D., Lewis, C. E., *et al.* (2005). Baseline associations between postmenopausal hormone therapy and inflammatory, haemostatic, and lipid biomarkers of coronary heart disease. The Women's Health Initiative Observational Study. *Thrombosis & Haemostasis*, **93**, 1108–16.

Langkamp, D., *et al.* (2001). *Mothers of Low Birth Weight Children are at Increased Risk of Depression* (Abstract). American Pediatric Academic Societies Annual Meeting, Baltimore, Maryland, May 2001.

Liebenluft, E. (1997). Issues in the treatment of women with bipolar illness. *Journal of Clinical Psychiatry*, **58**(Suppl.), 5–11.

Llewellyn, A. M. and Stowe, Z. N. (1998). Psychotropic medications in lactation. *Journal of Clinical Psychiatry*, **59**, 41–52.

Llewellyn, A. M., Stowe, Z. N. and Nemeroff, C. B. (1997). Depression during pregnancy and the puerperium. *Journal of Clinical Psychiatry*, **58**, 26–32.

Major, M., Cozzarelli, C., Cooper, M. L., *et al.* (2000). Psychological responses of women to first-trimester abortion. *Archives of General Psychiatry*, **57**, 777–84.

Marken, P. A., Haykal, R. F. and Fisher, J. N. (1992). Management of psychotropic-induced hyperprolactinemia. *Clinical Pharmacology*, **11**, 851–6.

Martins, C. and Gaffan, E. A. (2000). Effects of early maternal depression on patterns of infant-mother attachment: a meta-analytic investigation. *Journal of Child Psychology and Psychiatry*, **6**, 737–46.

McElhatton, P., Garbis, H. M., Elefant, E., *et al.* (1996). The outcome of pregnancy in 689 women exposed to therapeutic doses of antidepressants. A collaborative study of the European Network of Teratology Information Services (ENTIS). *Reproductive Toxicology*, **10**(4), 285–94.

McGrath, J., Hearle, J., Jenner, L., *et al.* (1999). The fertility and fecundity of patients with psychoses. *Acta Psychiatrica Scandinavica*, **99**, 441–6.

McNeil, T. F., Kaij, L. and Malmquist-Larsson, A. (1983). Pregnant women with nonorganic psychosis: life situation and experience of pregnancy. *Acta Psychiatrica Scandinavica*, **68**, 445–57.

McNeil, T. F., Kaij, L. and Malmquist, L. A. (1984). Women with non-organic psychosis: pregnancy's effect on mental health during pregnancy. Obstetric complications in schizophrenic patients. *Acta Psychiatrica Scandinavica*, **70**, 140–8.

Medical Research Council (Vitamin Study Research Group). (1991). Prevention of neural-tube defects: results of the medical research council vitamin study. *Lancet*, **338**, 131–7.

Menning, B. E. (1980). The emotional needs of infertile couples. *Fertility and Sterility*, **34**, 313–19.

Mezey, G., Bacchus, L., Bewley, S., *et al.* (2002). *An Exploration of the Prevalence, Nature and Effects of Domestic Violence in Pregnancy.* Violence Research Programme (VRP) summary findings. http://www1.rhbnc.ac.uk/sociopolitical-science/VRP/Findings/rfmezey.pdf.

Miller, L. J. (1997). Sexuality, pregnancy and family planning in women with schizophrenia. *Schizophrenia Bulletin,* **23,** 623–35.

Miller, L. J. and Finnerty, M. (1996). Sexuality, pregnancy, and childrearing among women with schizophrenia spectrum disorders. *Psychiatric Services,* **47,** 502–6.

Moffitt, T. E., E-Risk Study Team. (2002). Teen-aged mothers in contemporary Britain. *Journal of Child Psychology & Psychiatry & Allied Disciplines,* **43**(6), 727–42.

Morgan, M., Rapkin, A., Delia, L., *et al.* (1996). Cognitive functioning in premenstrual syndrome. *Obstetrics and Gynecology,* **88,** 961–6.

Morokoff, P. (1991). *Premenstrual Syndrome: Representation of a Cultural Conflict.* Washington, DC: Society for Behavioural Medicine.

Murray, L. (1992). The impact of postnatal depression. *Journal of Child Psychology and Psychiatry,* **33,** 543–61.

Murray, L., Sinclair, D., Cooper, P., *et al.* (1999). The socio-emotional development of five year old children of postnatally depressed mothers. *Journal of Child Psychology and Psychiatry,* **40,** 1259–72.

Murray, L., Woolgar, M., Cooper, P. J., *et al.* (2001). Cognitive vulnerability in five year old children of depressed mothers. *Journal of Child Psychology and Psychiatry,* **42,** 891–9.

Murray, J., Cooper, P. J., Wilson, A., *et al.* (2003). Controlled trial of the short and longterm effect of psychological treatment of postpartum depression: impact on the mother-child relationship and child outcome. *British Journal of Psychiatry,* **182,** 420–7.

NICE. (2007). *Antenatal and Postnatal Health: Clinical Management and Service Guidance.* National Institute for Health and Clinical Excellence.

Newsom, J. T., Knapp J. E. and Schulz, R. (1996). Longitudinal analysis of specific domains of internal control and depressive symptoms in patients with recurrent cancer. *Health Psychology,* **15,** 323–31.

Newton, C. R., Hearn, M. T. and Yuzpe, A. A. (1990). Psychological assessment and follow-up after in vitro fertilization: assessing the impact of failure. *Fertility and Sterility,* **54,** 879–86.

Nilsson, E., Lichtenstein, P., Cnattingius, S., *et al.* (2002). Women with schizophrenia: pregnancy outcome and infant death among their offspring. *Schizophrenia Research,* **58,** 221–9.

Nordeng, H., Lindemann, R., Perminov, K. V., *et al.* (2001). Neonatal withdrawal syndrome after in utero exposure to selective serotonin reuptake inhibitors. *Acta Paediatrica,* **90,** 288–91.

Nulman, I., Rovet, J., Stewart, D. E., *et al.* (1997). Neurodevelopment of children exposed in utero to antidepressant drugs. *New England Journal of Medicine,* **336,** 258–62.

Nulman, I., Rovet, J., Stewart, D. E., *et al.* (2002). Child development following exposure to tricyclic antidepressants or fluoxetine throughout fetal life: a prospective, controlled study. *American Journal of Psychiatry,* **159,** 1889–95.

O'Brien, P. M. S. (1987). Prevalence and epidemiology. In *Premenstrual Syndrome*. Oxford: Blackwell.

O'Donohue, W. and Geer, J. H. (1993). *Handbook on the Assessment and Treatment of Sexual Dysfunction*. New York: Pergamon.

O'Hara, M. W. and Swain, A. M. (1996). Rates and risk of postpartum depression – a meta-analysis. *International Review of Psychiatry*, **8**, 37–54.

Office of National Statistics, Singleton, N., Bumpstead, R., O'Brien, M., *et al.* (2001). *Psychiatric Morbidity Among Adults living in Private Households 2000*. London: Office for National Statistics.

Olausson, P.O., Haglund, B., Ringback Weitoft, G., *et al.* (2004). Premature death among teenage mothers. *British Journal of Obstetrics & Gynaecology*, **111**(8), 793–9.

Pearlstein, T. B., Frank, E., Rivera-Tover, A., *et al.* (1990). Prevalence of axis I and II disorders in women with late luteal phase dysphoric disorder. *Journal of Affective Disorders*, **20**, 129–34.

Pedron-Nuevo, N., Gonzalez-Unzaga, L. N. M., Cellis-Carrillo, R., *et al.* (1998). Incidence of dysmenorrhoea and associated symptoms in women aged 15–24 years. *Ginecologia y Obstetricia de Mexica*, **66**, 492–4.

Perkin, M. R., Bland, J. M., Peacock, J. L., *et al.* (1993). The effect of anxiety and depression during pregnancy on obstetric complications. *British Journal of Obstetrics and Gynaecology*, **100**, 629–34.

Peters, A. A. W., van Dorst, E., Jellis, B., *et al.* (1991). A randomized clinical trial to compare two different approaches in women with chronic pelvic pain. *Obstetrics and Gynecology*, **77**, 740–4.

Peterson, L. R. (1998). Estrogen replacement therapy and coronary artery disease. *Current Opinion in Cardiology*, **13**, 223–31.

Philips, Z., Johnson, S., Avis, M., *et al.* (2002). Communicating mild and borderline abnormal cervical smear results: how and what are women told? *Cytopathology*, **13**, 355–63.

Price, W., Torem, M. and DiMarzio, L. (1987). Premenstrual exacerbation of bulimia. *Psychosomatics*, **28**, 378–80.

Quinlivan, J. A., Tan, L. H., Steele, A., *et al.* (2004). Impact of demographic factors, early family relationships and depressive symptomatology in teenage pregnancy. *Australian & New Zealand Journal of Psychiatry*, **38**(4), 197–203.

Rainey, D. Y., Stevens-Simon, C. and Kaplan, D. W. (1995). Are adolescents who report prior sexual abuse at higher risk for pregnancy? *Child Abuse and Neglect*, **19**, 1283–8.

Reardon, D. and Cougle, J. (2002). Depression and unintended pregnancy in the National Longitudinal Survey of Youth: a cohort study. *British Medical Journal*, **324**, 151–2.

Reiter, R. C. and Gambone, J. C. (1990). Demographic and historic variables in women with idiopathic chronic pelvic pain. *Obstetrics and Gynecology*, **75**, 428–32.

Richardson, J., Coid, J., Petruckevitch, A., *et al.* (2002). Identifying domestic violence: cross-sectional study in primary care. *British Medical Journal*, **324**, 271–7

Ridley, C. M. (1998). Vulvodynia: theory and management. *Dermatologic Clinics*, **16**, 775–8.

Robinson, G. E. (2002). Women and psychopharmacology. *Medscape: Women's Health eJournal*, **7**, 1–8.

Roe, C. M., McNamara, A. M. and Motheral, B. (2002). Gender- and age-related prescription drug use patterns. *Annals of Pharmacotherapy*, **36**, 30−5.

Rubino-Watkins, M., Doster, J., Franks, S., *et al.* (1999). Oral contraceptive use: implications for cognitive and emotional functioning. *Journal of Mental and Nervous Disease*, **187**, 275−80.

Scafidi, F. A., Field, T., Prodromidis, M., *et al.* (1997). Psychosocial stressors of drug-abusing disadvantaged adolescent mothers. *Adolescence*, **32**, 93−100.

Schmidt, P. J., Roca, C. A., Bloch, M., *et al.* (1997). The perimenopause and affective disorders. *Seminars in Reproductive Endocrinology*, **15**, 91−100.

Schmidt, P. J., Nierman, L., Danceau, M. A., *et al.* (2000). Estrogen-replacement in perimenopause-related depression: a preliminary report. *American Journal of Obstetrics and Gynecology*, **183**, 414−20.

Scholl, T. O., Hediger, M. L. and Belsky, D. H. (1994). Prenatal care and maternal health during adolescent pregnancy: a review and meta-analysis. *Journal of Adolescent Health*, **15**, 444−56.

Schwab, B., Clark, R. and Drake, R. (1991). An ethnographic note on clients as parents. *Psychosocial Rehabilitation Journal*, **15**, 95−9.

Simon, G. E., Cunningham, M. L. and Davis, R. L. (2002). Outcomes of prenatal antidepressant exposure. *American Journal of Psychiatry*, **159**, 2055−61.

Smith, S., O'Keane, V. O. and Murray, R. M. (2002). The effects of antipsychotic-induced hyperprolactinaemia on the hypothalamic-pituitary-gonadal axis. *Journal of Clinical Psychopharmacology*, **22**, 109−14.

Sommer, B. (1982). Cognitive behaviour and the menstrual cycle. In *Behaviour and the Menstrual Cycle*, ed. R. C. Friedman. New York: Marcel Dekker, pp. 101−72.

Speroff, L., Galss, R. H. and Kase, N. G. (1994). *Clinical and Gynaecologic Endocrinology and Infertility*. Baltimore, MD: Williams & Wilkins.

Spielvogel, A. and Wile, J. (1992). Treatment and outcomes of psychotic patients during pregnancy and childbirth. *Birth*, **19**, 131−7.

Steiner, M. and Born, L. (2002). Anxiety and panic disorders. In *Women's Health: Principles and Clinical Practice*, ed. J. P. Pregler and A. H. DeCherney. Toronto: BC Decker, pp. 661−74.

Steiner, M. and Yonkers, K. (1998). *Depression in Women*. London: Martin Dunitz Ltd.

Steven-Simon, C., Kelly, L., Singer, D., *et al.* (1996). Why pregnant adolescents say they did not use contraceptives prior to conception. *Journal of Adolescent Health*, **19**(1), 48−53.

Stephens, C. and Ross, N. (2002). The relationship between hormone replacement therapy use and psychological symptoms: no effects found in a New Zealand sample. *Health Care for Women International*, **23**, 408−14.

Stewart, D. E., Rondon, M., Damiani, G., *et al.* (2001). International psychosocial and systemic issues in women's mental health. *Archives of Women's Mental Health*, **4**, 13−17.

Stolar, A. G. and Stewart, J. T. (2002). Nortriptyline for depression and vulvodynia. *American Journal of Psychiatry*, **159**, 316−17.

Stuart, S., Couser, G., Schilder, K., *et al.* (1998). Postpartum anxiety and depression: onset and comorbidity in a community sample. *Journal of Nervous and Mental Disease*, **186**, 420−4.

Teixera, J. M. A., Fisk, N. M. and Glover, V. (1999). Association between maternal anxiety in pregnancy and increased uterine artery resistance index: cohort based study. *British Medical Journal*, **318**, 153–7.

Terp, I. M. and Mortensen, P. B. (1998). Post-partum psychoses: clinical diagnoses and relative risk of admission after parturition. *British Journal of Psychiatry*, **172**, 521–6.

Viguera, A. C., Cohen, L. S., Baldessarini, R. J., *et al.* (2002). Managing bipolar disorder during pregnancy: weighing the risks and benefits. *Canadian Journal of Psychiatry*, **47**, 426–36.

Wadhwa, P. D., Sandman, C. A., Porto, M., *et al.* (1993). The association between prenatal stress and infant birth weight and gestational age at birth: a prospective investigation. *American Journal of Obstetrics and Gynecology*, **175**, 1286–92.

Webb, R. T., Abel, K. M., Pickles, A., *et al.* (2005). Mortality in offspring of parents with psychotic disorders: a critical review and meta-analysis. *American Journal of Psychiatry*, **162**, 1045–56.

Westhoff, C. L. and Davis, A. R. (2001). Primary dysmenorrhea in adolescent girls and treatment with oral contraceptives. *Journal of Pediatric and Adolescent Gynecology*, **14**, 3–8.

Wieck, A. and Haddad, P. M. (2003). Antipsychotic-induced hyperprolactinaemia in women: pathophysiology, severity and consequences: selective literature review. *British Journal of Psychiatry*, **182**, 50–6.

Wilcox, A. J. and Russell, I. T. (1983). Birth weight and perinatal mortality: II. On weight-specific mortality. *International Journal of Epidemiology*, **12**, 319–25.

Williams, S., McGee, R., Olaman, S., *et al.* (1997). Level of education, age of bearing children and mental health of women. *Social Science & Medicine*, **45**(6), 827–36.

Wisner, K. L. and Wheeler, S. B. (1994). Prevention of recurrent postpartum major depression. *Hospital Community Psychiatry*, **45**, 1191–6.

Wisner, K. L., Perel, J. M. and Sheeler, S. B. (1993). Tricyclic dose requirements across pregnancy. *American Journal of Psychiatry*, **150**, 1541–2.

Wisner, K. I., Zarin, D. A., Holmboe, E. S., *et al.* (1994). Risk-benefit decision making for treatment of depression during pregnancy and the postpartum. *Hospital and Community Psychiatry*, **45**, 444–50.

Wisner, K. L., Peindl, K. S. and Hanusa, B. H. (1996). Effects of childbearing on the natural history of panic disorder with comorbid mood disorder. *Journal of Affective Disorders*, **41**, 173–80.

Wisner, K. L., Zarin, D. A., Holmboe, E. S., *et al.* (2000). Risk benefit decision making for treatment of depression during pregnancy. *American Journal of Psychiatry*, **157**, 1933–40.

Wisner, K. L., Perel, J. M., Peindl, K. S., *et al.* (2001). Prevention of recurrent postpartum depression: a randomized clinical trial. *Journal of Clinical Psychiatry*, **62**, 82–6.

Wisner, K. L., Parry, B. L. and Piontek, C. M. (2002). Clinical practice. Postpartum depression. *New England Journal of Medicine*, **347**(3), 194–9.

Wisner, K. L., Perel, J. M., Peindl, K. S., *et al.* (2004). Prevention of postpartum depression: a pilot randomized clinical trial. *American Journal of Psychiatry*, **161**(7), 1290–2.

Wittchen, H.-U., Becker, E., Lieb, R., *et al.* (2002). Prevalence, incidence and stability of premenstrual dysphoric disorder in the community. *Psychological Medicine*, **32**, 119–32.

World Health Organization. (1997). *Violence Against Women Information Pack: a Priority Health Issue*. Geneva: WHO.

Woods, N. F. and Mitchell, E. S. (1996). Patterns of depressed mood in midlife women: observations from the Seattle Midlife Women's Health Study. *Research in Nursing and Health*, **19**, 111–23.

Wright, J., Duchensne, C., Sabourin, S., *et al.* (1991). Psychosocial distress and infertility: men and women respond differently. *Fertility and Sterility*, **55**, 100–8.

Yonkers, K. (1997a). The association between premenstrual dysphoric disorder and other mood disorders. *Journal of Clinical Psychiatry*, **58**(Suppl.), 19–25.

Yonkers, K. (1997b). Anxiety symptoms and anxiety disorders: how they are related to premenstrual disorder. *Journal of Clinical Psychiatry*, **58**(Suppl.), 62–9.

Yonkers, K. A., Bradshaw, K. D. and Halbreich, U. (2000). Oestrogens, progestins and mood. In *Mood Disorders in Women*, ed. M. Steiner, K. A. Yonkers and E. Eriksson. London: Martin Dunitz, pp. 207–32.

Zabin, L. S. and Hayward, S. C. (1993). *Adolescent Sexual Behaviour and Childbearing*. Newbury Park, CA: Sage.

28

The intensive care unit

Simon Turner, Daniel Conway, Jane Eddleston and Elspeth Guthrie

Introduction

Intensive care medicine is a relatively new speciality made possible by technological advances in artificial life support. Intensive care unit (ICU) development took its first steps at Copenhagen in 1952, with treatment using positive pressure ventilation of poliomyelitis cases. This success was copied worldwide during similar epidemics and now intensive care units are integral parts of most major acute hospital services.

In the UK there are over 200 ICUs admitting around 80 000 patients per year. Intensive care medicine is able to offer support for those suffering acute multiple organ failure, including pulmonary, haematological, hepatic, cardiovascular and renal replacement therapy. Data derived from the Case Mix Programme of the Intensive Care National Audit and Research Centre (www.icnarc.org) suggest that ICU mortality is high, with only 70% of admissions surviving to hospital discharge. Technological advances have created unique ethical dilemmas for those involved in the ICU, particularly regarding the withdrawal of life-supporting therapy in patients often unable to speak for themselves.

From the 1960s, increasing interest has developed in the psychological impact of the ICU environment. Research and clinical input has been provided by several disciplines: nursing, psychology and psychiatry.

One of the first reviews of the issues from a psychiatric perspective was by Kornfeld in 1969. He categorized the problems into four areas:
• psychiatric reactions to the conditions that led to ICU admission
• psychiatric reactions provoked by the unusual environment of the ICU
• psychiatric reactions that develop post-discharge
• the psychological welfare of staff working on ICUs.

Handbook of Liaison Psychiatry, ed. Geoffrey Lloyd and Elspeth Guthrie. Published by Cambridge University Press © Cambridge University Press 2007.

In this chapter, the issues are categorized in the same way, but the impact on relatives and approaches to liaison with the ICU are also discussed.

Epidemiology

Depression

Although there are now several studies of the prevalence of depression in ICU and critically ill patients, there are relatively few in which semi-structured psychiatric assessments have been employed to measure psychiatric disorder according to strict diagnostic criteria. Most studies have used self-report instruments, which record psychological symptom severity, or health-related quality of life. Several of the most recent studies are shown in Table 28.1 and there is a recent good review of psychological sequelae of inpatients post ICU by Weinert (2005). Self-report

Table 28.1. Recent studies of the prevalence of depression in ICU and critically ill patients at follow-up.

Study	Patients studied	Sample size	Assessment method	Prevalence
Eddleston et al. (2000)	ICU patients	143 at 3 months	HAD[a]	10% depressed 12% anxious
Weinert et al. (2003)	Acute respiratory failure	105 at 2 months post-onset	SCID[b]	15% depressed 15% adjustment disorder
Jackson et al. (2003)	Ventilated patients	33 at 6 months	GDS[c]	25% depressed at 6 months
Kress et al. (2003)	Acute respiratory failure	32 at approximately 1 year	BDI[d]	34% depressed at 1 year
Hopkins et al. (2004)	Acute respiratory stress syndrome survivors	66 at 1 year, 62 at 2 years	BDI	16% depressed at 1 year 23% depressed at 2 years
Chelluri et al. (2004)	Ventilated patients	154 at 1 year	CES-D[e]	32% depressed at 1 year

Notes: [a]HAD: Hospital Anxiety and Depression Scale (Zigmond & Snaith 1983);
[b]SCID: Structured Clinical Interview for DSM-IV Axis I Disorders (First *et al.* 1998);
[c]GDS: The Geriatric Depression Scale (Lyness *et al.* 1997);
[d]BDI: Beck Depression Inventory (Beck *et al.* 1961);
[e]CES-D: a self-report depression scale for research in the general population (Radloff 1977).

measures are always going to be less accurate than semi-structured interview assessments, but they do provide an estimate of the degree of psychological distress in these patients.

Eddleston *et al.* (2000) examined psychological morbidity in patients using the Hospital Anxiety and Depression Scale (HAD), three months after discharge from an ICU. A consecutive series of patients were tracked. Out of 370 admissions to the ICU, 227 patients were alive at three months post-discharge, and 143 agreed to participate in the study. Seventeen patients (12%) scored above a recognized cut-off point on the HAD for anxiety and 14 patients (10%) scored above cut-off for depression. Of these, 10% required referral for psychological or psychiatric intervention. There was no significant difference between men and women in terms of psychological morbidity. Twenty-three female patients and 16 male patients reported experiencing distressing flashbacks of their ICU experience within three months of discharge.

Other researchers have focused upon specific populations of critically ill patients. Using standard cut-offs for moderate-to-severe depression on a self-report inventory (Beck Depression Inventory (BDI) Beck *et al.* 1961), Hopkins and colleagues (2004) found that 16% of survivors of acute respiratory distress syndrome were depressed six months later. They also found that psychiatric symptoms worsened between years 1 and 2 post-recovery, although no risk factors could be identified.

Kress and colleagues (2003) found rates of depression of 34% (BDI > 20) in patients with acute respiratory failure, and a similar rate of depression (32%) was found in a large population of patients who had required ventilation, six months post-treatment (Chelluri *et al.* 2004). Weinert and colleagues (2003) used semi-structured psychiatric assessments in patients who had recovered from acute respiratory failure and found a prevalence of major depressive disorder of 15%. A further 15% were diagnosed as suffering from an adjustment disorder. It is interesting that the figures for an actual diagnosis of depression in this study were much lower than some of the other studies in which self-report measures were employed, but the overall prevalence of some form of psychological reaction was similar to the prevalence figures obtained from studies using self-report measures.

It is reasonable to conclude that approximately one-third of ICU/critically ill patients will suffer from psychological distress in the months following recovery and approximately half of these patients will have a depressive disorder.

Post-traumatic stress disorder

Post-traumatic stress disorder (PTSD) has also been studied in populations of ICU and critically ill patients. Schelling and colleagues (1998) looked at 80 patients previously admitted to the ICU specifically for treatment of acute respiratory distress syndrome (ARDS). The median time between discharge and assessment was four years. They were assessed using the German version of the Post-Traumatic Stress Syndrome 10-Questions Inventory (PTSS-10). The occurrence rate of PTSD was 27.5% in the ARDS patients. They were also assessed using the Short-Form 36 (SF-36) and compared with an age- and gender-matched control group. They showed moderate but statistically significant impairments in all eight dimensions of the SF-36. The most severe limitations in quality of life were found within the group of patients with PTSD. The researchers found a positive correlation between the later development of PTSD symptoms and the number of distressing symptoms that patients had experienced during their ICU treatment.

A more recent study by Capuzzo and colleagues (2005) assessed 84 ICU patients, one week and three months post-discharge. At the first assessment 6% of patients had no memory of being on the ICU, and only four described intrusive memories of the experience. Two further patients developed PTSD-like symptoms within three months of discharge, but overall the prevalence of PTSD was low.

Quality of life

Quality of life has been assessed by several researchers. Eddleston and colleagues (2000) used the SF-36 and found that ICU patients reported much poorer function in all domains, in comparison with population norms, with the exception of mental health. There was also a difference between age groups in terms of quality of life. Younger males (below 65 years) reported significantly poorer functioning than older males in relation to social functioning, and physical and emotional role limitation (Figure 28.1). The picture was more mixed for women: younger women reported better physical function than those 65 years or over, but poorer mental health (Figure 28.2).

Wehler and colleagues (2003) also evaluated quality of life in ICU patients. They found that pre-ICU chronic illness was associated with a deterioration in mental health, and that multiple organ dysfunction during ICU stay was associated with a poorer outcome in physical but not mental health six months post-ICU discharge.

Psychiatric reactions to severe illness on the ICU

Delirium

The incidence of delirium on the ICU ranges from 7 to 57% (Fish 1991). Such differences may be due to different populations of patients or due to differing methods of recognition of this syndrome. Delirium occurs right across the age spectrum on the ICU. In contrast, on a standard medical ward, delirium is far

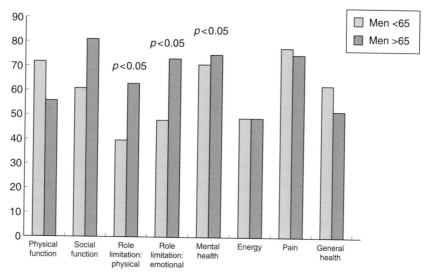

Figure 28.1. Mean scores on the short form (SF-36) for males below the age of 65 years versus those 65 years and older. (Eddleston *et al.* 2000.)

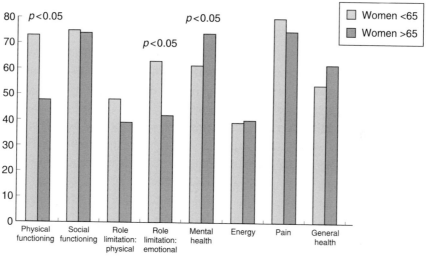

Figure 28.2. Mean scores on the short form (SF-36) for females below the age of 65 years versus those 65 years and older. (Eddleston *et al.* 2000.)

more prevalent in older patients. By its very nature, on the ICU, patients of all ages have severe or multiple medical problems sufficient to produce delirium.

Patients can become highly agitated and distressed when delirious. Some patients become highly distressed and misinterpret the events on the ICU ward. For example, patients can think that the unit is a concentration camp, that the uniformed nurses are guards and see nursing interventions with other patients as torture.

Treatment of delirium is required to reduce harmful behaviour to self and others, reduce distress and also to protect invasive treatments from being removed that are essential for the patient's survival. With all cases of delirium the most important focus for treatment is the underlying condition. But often this will not help fast enough and other interventions are needed.

When sedatives are given for delirium on the ICU they are usually delivered intravenously through established lines. This is useful in supplying the medications rapidly and in more reliable doses than through oral routes. Haloperidol is usually the treatment of choice for sedation of delirium on the ICU. In contrast, benzodiazepines and narcotics tend to worsen confusion rather than sedate effectively.

Haloperidol has a calming effect with less ability to provoke further confusion or worsen ongoing medical conditions, compared to other sedatives. It has this advantage due to its lack of antihistamine or anticholinergic properties. It has also been suggested that when given intravenously, haloperidol is less likely to cause extrapyramidal side-effects than when given orally (Menza *et al.* 1987).

It is important to review all the patient's medications. Many medications, particularly those with anticholinergic properties, have an ability to produce or worsen delirium. The usefulness of the medications should be reviewed and if possible, the regimen should be rationalized. Another issue relevant to medication review is that of drug withdrawal. Rapid drug withdrawal can precipitate delirium: particularly alcohol, benzodiazepine and narcotic withdrawal. This can occur when a patient has used drugs prior to admission and also when they have been used therapeutically at an early stage of treatment on the ICU. It may be appropriate to use benzodiazepines to reduce the symptoms of withdrawal and then wean the patient off at a slower rate.

There are also additional factors inherent in ICU treatments that are suspected to contribute to the production of delirium. Iatrogenic interventions, such as adding more than three new medications, the use of medications with sedating properties, sleep deprivation, catheterization and the use of immobilizing devices such as intravenous lines. The environment is also loud, unusual and confusing.

A liaison psychiatrist should manage delirium (see Chapter 12) in a similar fashion to that encountered on a general ward. A major role is to encourage staff to look beyond just medications and use environmental strategies, verbal reassurance and orientation. There are not the tensions present on general wards where there are sometimes pressures to move the patient on to a psychiatric ward. The severe medical needs of the patient make this option impossible.

Although some patients have no memory of their stay on the ICU, others can develop psychological distress in relation to abnormal perceptual experiences they suffer whilst acutely confused. These distressing images or ideas can haunt the patients for months after discharge, and can even sometimes lead to PTSD (MacKenzie & Popkin 1980). Patients and relatives can benefit from a clear explanation of the cause of any abnormal experiences, and reassurance that they are unlikely to recur if the individual remains physically well. Reassurance should be given that the patient is not suffering from 'madness', which is sometimes an unspoken fear.

Acute stress reactions and adjustment disorders

It is not too surprising that a common psychiatric reaction while on an ICU is acute stress disorder. Some patients can be completely unconscious during their stay on ICU. For others, however, the experience of being admitted to a strange and distressing environment will have a major impact. For some patients undergoing planned surgery there has been a degree of preparedness, but for most it is a major unexpected shock. In addition to the strange environment, patients will have difficulty communicating if they are intubated. Anxiety may be further amplified by discomfort and painful procedures. There can be a strong sense of loss of control. Rapid withdrawal of medications such as benzodiazepines can also lead to further feelings of anxiety.

The patient may express physical signs of distress such as motor agitation. This response if left untreated could potentially lead to physical deterioration and increased mortality rate. Objective observations for this kind of activity are not completely reliable in diagnosing anxiety, especially when patients are therapeutically paralysed. Some patients in apparent clinical comfort later recall they experienced significant fears and worry at the time (Wagner *et al.* 1997).

Benzodiazepines are frequently used for treatment of anxiety on the intensive care unit. Before this treatment is instigated it must be ensured that signs of agitation are not being produced by life-threatening illness such as hypoglycaemia. Delirium should also be considered as a cause as benzodiazepines can potentially worsen confusion. The adequacy of a patient's pain relief should also be reviewed. Benzodiazepines are given on ICUs in doses much higher than given for anxiety in general adult psychiatry or general practice populations (Table 28.2).

Benzodiazepine use, fortunately, does not appear to lead to significant problems with long-term dependence despite the higher doses used on the ICU. Conway *et al.* (2001) used information from the general practitioners of ICU survivors. Of 148 survivors 21 were discharged still on oral sedatives. At six months post-discharge only 10 continued to take these sedatives. There was no evidence of previous regular use of benzodiazepines in seven (5% of all ICU survivors) of these patients studied (Figure 28.3).

Medication is not the only answer, and it is important that staff are encouraged to talk to, reassure, and explain to patients what is going on. This is particularly important with patients who cannot respond verbally. Some staff are particularly uncomfortable about communicating with patients who are critically unwell and who cannot respond in the usual fashion. Nurses and doctors new to the unit may avoid talking to patients as they have not yet picked up the ability to lip read, or they may fear being asked direct questions about the likelihood of dying. For other

Table 28.2. Sedative use on ICU.

Name of drug	Bolus	Dose range infusion	Half-life	Active metabolites?
Midazolam	Up to 0.1 mg/kg	0.04–0.4 mg/kg per hour	3–11 hours	Yes: 1-hydroxy-midazolam
Diazepam	Up to 0.1 mg/kg	0.04–0.4 mg/kg per hour	20–120 hours	Yes: nordiazepam, temazepam and oxazepam
Lorazepam	0.02 mg/kg		8–15 hours	No
Propofol	Up to 0.1 mg/kg	0.005–0.1 mg/kg per hour	26–32 hours	No
Haloperidol	0.05–0.15 mg/kg	0.04–0.15 mg/kg per hour	18–54 hours	Yes

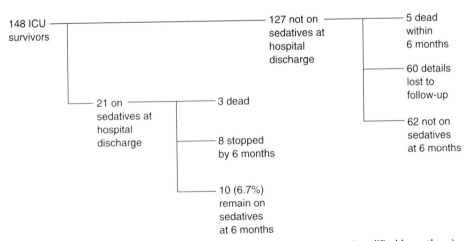

Figure 28.3. Flow diagram of long-term benzodiazepine use post-ICU (modified by authors).

far more experienced nursing staff, their own coping mechanisms in dealing with chronic distress may have led them to withdraw from patient contact and focus instead on the technical side of management (Hay & Oken 1972). Particular care must be taken with communication. Patients are able to recall whether they were spoken to rather than over. They can also recall overhearing conversations about other patients and assuming that nurses were discussing their own cases (Green 1996).

Overdoses and other suicide attempts

Patients who have made severe suicide attempts may spend a period of time on an intensive care unit. Many of these patients have had contact with psychiatric services in the past. A common cause of attempted suicide is depression. Other conditions, such as schizophrenia, substance dependence and personality disorder can also lead to severe life-threatening attempts. A liaison psychiatrist can have a useful role in co-ordinating future management of these patients. It is important to assess whether the patient remains suicidal and at high risk. In most cases, these patients do not present with an immediate high risk of reattempting self-harm as they feel too physically ill or weak while on the ICU.

Often the first input required is to review the medications while the patient is physically ill. In the short term it may be sensible to withdraw psychotropic medications if a patient is physically unwell. It is important to be alert to drug withdrawal effects as well as potential serotonergic syndrome symptoms. Serotonergic syndrome is a particular risk in overdoses of multiple types of antidepressants at the same time (Power *et al.* 1995), such as a selective serotonin reuptake inhibitor (SSRI) taken with a tricyclic antidepressant or a monoamine oxidase inhibitor (MAOI) (Kam & Chang 1997). Due to the relative safety of SSRIs in overdose in isolation, most patients who are admitted to ICU have either taken a combination of antidepressants, used large amounts of alcohol, or taken older antidepressants, such as the tricyclics. If tricyclic antidepressants have been taken it is important to review why they were given. They may have been prescribed by a general practitioner who was unaware of the patient's suicidal thoughts. In this case it would be appropriate to advise changing the medications to an SSRI. In other cases there may be legitimate reasons, such as a patient, being treated by a general psychiatrist, who has proved unresponsive to SSRIs and has responded in the past to tricyclics (Anderson *et al.* 2000).

Current studies of the outcome of patients admitted to ICU following overdose were drawn from periods before the widespread introduction of SSRIs. An Australian study showed mechanical ventilation was required in 79.5% of overdoses on the ICU and a short-term mortality rate of 2% (Henderson *et al.* 1993). A Scandinavian study found a mechanical ventilation rate of 100% and a mortality rate of 6.1% in overdose patients on an ICU (Strom *et al.* 1986). The highest mortalities were due to salicylate, propoxyphene and strong analgesics. Tricyclic antidepressants carried a mortality rate of 3%. In the following three years 18% of patients died, with a suicide rate of 10%.

It is important that all patients who are admitted to the ICU following an episode of self-harm receive a detailed psychosocial assessment before they are discharged. This should include a careful assessment of suicidal ideation and future risk of self-harm or suicide. Careful liaison with appropriate services (e.g. GP and psychiatry services) will be required. It is best that the assessment is carried out as soon as the patient is physically well enough to be interviewed, as there may be a risk of further self-harm whilst in hospital (see Chapter 11).

Psychiatric presentations unique to the ICU environment

'ICU psychosis' and 'ICU syndrome'

There are differing viewpoints about whether psychiatric conditions that are unique to, and produced by, the unusual environment of the ICU exist. The validity of the terms 'ICU psychosis' and 'ICU syndrome' has been questioned. It is helpful to take a historical approach to understand how these terms came about.

The initial interest in the impact of the medical environment came from studies of open-heart surgery recovery rooms in the 1960s. It was observed that delirium-like syndromes developed after lucid intervals of several days post-operatively. Physiology by this point was returning to normal and the condition appearing to stabilize after transfer from the recovery room. A theory was developed to explain this presentation which compared it to similar abnormal mental states that had been experimentally produced by sensory or sleep deprivation. It was proposed that the difficulties in sleep, the monotony of sound and vision from regularly hissing, flashing and bleeping equipment, in addition to the restriction of being bed-bound, could mimic these experiments and produce similar mental states (Kornfeld 1969). This theory was extended to psychotic states in the ICU environment and the term 'ICU psychosis' was coined.

Another similar term, 'ICU syndrome', came in to use. This condition was initially synonymous with ICU psychosis (McKegney 1966). Over the years this term was opened up to include more conditions. It continued to see the ICU as a significant provoking factor but now was defined as a syndrome of changed emotions which developed in a stressful environment (Kleck 1984).

Criticisms were directed at this terminology. It was said that ICU psychosis was a redundant, potentially harmful, term for what was essentially delirium in the setting of an intensive care unit (McGuire *et al.* 2000). Suggestions were also made that the supposedly lucid periods of a few days in the open-heart studies did not actually occur. It was proposed that the lucid interval was an artefact with heavy sedation and intubation masking psychological disturbances (Baxter 1974). If a lucid period does exist, there is disagreement over its duration. There have also been wide variations in the studies of rates of this presentation, varying from 7 to 72% (Granberg *et al.* 1996).

It is certainly important to be aware of the impact of the environment on patients whilst in the ICU, and also to be aware of the potential therapeutic benefits of environmental or supportive changes. In one study (Wilson 1972) 50 consecutive patients treated in an intensive care unit with no windows were compared with 50 patients treated on an intensive care unit with windows. Over twice as many patients developed delirium on the unit without windows. In contrast, age and type of surgical procedure had no effect on the incidence of delirium. Another much later paper showed a much more subtle environmental impact where ongoing media stories of a war appeared to affect the hallucinatory content of patients' experiences. Patients whose stays coincided with the Kosovo conflict were more likely to experience hallucinations with war or military themes (Skirrow *et al.* 2002).

It is hard to justify the use of the terms 'ICU psychosis' and 'ICU syndrome' as specific psychiatric diagnoses. The conditions do not have a unique set of symptoms, a different prognosis or particular treatment that would justify their use. They have been helpful, however, in highlighting important psychological changes that can occur in an ICU setting.

Difficulties with weaning patients off mechanical ventilation

A small number of patients can prove difficult to wean off mechanical ventilation following treatment for respiratory failure, even when they are physiologically fit for weaning. Psychological factors are thought to be relevant. Factors suggested are:

- fear of sudden death
- anger
- depression
- interpersonal conflict.

One small study of 10 psychiatric referrals for this problem reported background histories of previous psychiatric treatment and recent object loss through bereavement in the patients referred. These features were not, however, specific to those who proved difficult to wean. No non-physiologic differences were found between those who met the weaning criteria and those who did not (Mendel & Khan 1980).

Suggested practical approaches by the liaison psychiatrist to this problem are described in this paper. They include:

- making the weaning process slower and more gradual
- using a modified form of family therapy to explore interpersonal conflicts
- occasional use of psychotropic drugs.

The suggested medications are benzodiazepines, neuroleptics or antidepressants. All of these drugs should be used with caution in the context of respiratory difficulties.

Psychiatric presentations after discharge from ICU

Transfer to a general ward

The stress associated with a move from the intensive care unit to a ward has been termed either relocation or translocation stress (Cutler & Garner 1995). As with any stress, different people respond in different ways. Studies have shown that approximately 50% of patients view the move onto a general ward in positive terms. They see the move as one step closer to a return to home and independent living (Green 1996). For others the transition is more difficult. Anxiety levels may increase after the transfer (Kornfeld 1969). Patients can find it hard to adjust from the one-to-one relationship with a single nurse to being one patient amongst around 30 other patients managed by a limited number of nursing staff. Although being monitored by many machines can have negative consequences, such as alarms making patients anxious, for some the reduction in monitoring can be seen in negative terms. Close surveillance by technology can promote feelings of safety for patients and relatives (Russell 1999). The decrease in monitoring on a general ward can make a patient feel unsafe and vulnerable.

Psychotherapeutic insights about the patient–nurse relationship suggest that on the ICU a patient goes through a highly needy regressed state. The continuous presence and attention of a single nurse might be a dynamic re-enactment of the in-utero state of an infant being inseparable from its mother (Winship 1998). The severance of this powerful connection can be difficult for both parties. Other factors associated with relocation stress include lack of preparation for move, lack of predictability in the new environment and inconsistencies in care. Suggested strategies for reduction in stress have been described by Cutler and Garner (1995) and include:

- using an information booklet about impending changes in environment
- a visit from the new named nurse on ICU before the move
- gradual decrease in nursing attention and monitoring while not compromising patient care.

Discharge into the community

When ICUs were first developed the focus was exclusively on patients while they were on the unit with little follow-up. Over time it has been recognized that it is helpful to provide input after transfer onto the medical ward and also after discharge back into the community. Prior to this type of follow-up it was believed that there was little evidence of long-term adverse effects from the ICU experience (Baxter 1974). It is now clear after discharge that patients can present with depression, adjustment disorder or post-traumatic stress disorder requiring specialist input.

Specific psychiatric syndromes post-ICU discharge

Adjustment disorder

Adjustment disorders are prolonged gradual responses to severe stress. They are often a mixture of symptoms of anxiety and depression but can also involve behavioural problems. An admission to ICU can bring about significant lasting change to a patient's circumstances. They may no longer be fit enough to carry on their job or their interests. Their relationships and financial situation may be altered significantly for a prolonged period of time. Some patients will be less able to adjust to these changes than others. Patients may present with some mild depressive symptoms but not to the degree of warranting a diagnosis of depression. These patients may respond to supportive counselling and information about their condition. They may also need monitoring in case they go on to develop a major depressive illness.

Depression

Anxiety, rather than depression, appears to be the most common reaction of patients when they are on the ICU. Depression becomes more prominent after discharge to the general ward or to home. This is probably due to depression being produced by a slow mechanism of action, consistent with the neurotransmitter receptor hypothesis of affective disorders. At three months post-discharge, about 10% of patients have significant symptoms of depression (i.e. score above cut-off on the HAD; Eddleston et al. 2000). This is actually quite a low score and suggests that, given time, most people who are admitted to the ICU, and survive, manage to assimilate their experience, without the development of long-term psychiatric problems.

A study of referrals from an ICU follow-up clinic to a liaison psychiatrist (Turner et al. 2002) showed that those patients who go on to develop depression are highly likely to have a past history of depression; 78% of patients in the study who developed depression post-discharge from the ICU had a previous history of psychiatric illness. Some caution is required in generalizing the results of this study to other ICU populations, as the ICU in question was based in an inner city hospital, which served a population with high rates of social adversity.

The findings however suggest that all patients should be screened for a prior history of depression on admission to the ICU. This may involve checking GP's notes or making enquiries with relatives. Those identified should be closely monitored and certainly offered follow-up at three months post-discharge.

Treatment for depression can include supportive psychotherapy, social interventions or the use of medications. Care is required in selecting a safe treatment in the context of recent or ongoing poor physical health. The SSRIs are often chosen because of their relative safety compared to older antidepressants. Detection and treatment of depression is important in ICU and critically ill patients because of a variety of factors, including alleviating distress and improvement in quality of life and function. However, a recent study has suggested that depression is a significant risk factor for re-admission to ICU after discharge (Paratz *et al.* 2005). Other significant factors include age greater than 65 years, colonization, weakness, and comorbidities of either cardiac and/or respiratory disease.

Post-traumatic stress disorder

There are several factors associated with an intensive care admission that can potentially produce post-traumatic stress symptoms. Some patients may have experienced severe distress in the events leading up to admission, for instance, if the admission occurred following a road traffic accident, or a serious assault. For some patients the experience on the unit may be a traumatic experience, for instance undergoing mechanical ventilation, paralysis, painful procedures and being unable to communicate due to intubation can all cause distress. As mentioned earlier, periods of delirium with emotionally laden hallucinations and delusions can also lead to post-traumatic symptoms.

A postal questionnaire study (Scragg *et al.* 2001) looked at psychological trauma related to ICU treatment. Patients who suffered cerebral trauma, accidental and non-accidental injury were excluded from the study. This reduced the chances that any PTSD would be due to other causes apart from the ICU experience. Eighty patients returned completed questionnaires. Results indicated that 15% of these patients had a diagnosis of PTSD from scores on the Trauma Symptom Checklist 33 and the Impact of Events Scale.

Patients who are admitted to the unit with acute respiratory distress seem to be particularly prone to developing post-traumatic symptoms (Schelling *et al.* 1998). This study indicated that the patients most likely to experience problems in this group were those who had remembered multiple 'adverse events': episodes of extreme anxiety or physical discomfort during mechanical ventilation. These patients also showed significantly lower quality of life in the long term compared with survivors with no or only one adverse experience. The study also suggested that most of the adverse events occurred during the weaning process when the levels of sedation were required to be lower and consciousness was increased. A limitation of the Schelling study is that it relied on patients' memories of distress rather than objective measures at the time of admission. Studies of post-traumatic symptoms after myocardial infarction indicate that the patient's subjective interpretation of the incident is an important factor (Kutz *et al.* 1994). A similar process may be involved with ICU survivors.

It could be argued that the optimal approach to prevent psychological distress in patients would be to sedate them so heavily with medications so they retain no memories of intensive care. The benzodiazepines, such as lorazepam and midazolam, are seen as being ideal medications for this role as they have significant amnestic effects (Cheng 1996). In support of this argument, studies of patients recovering from road traffic accidents suggest that they do not develop post-traumatic symptoms if they were briefly unconscious and hence had no distressing memories of the accident (Mayou *et al.* 1993).

The real-life situation with sedation is more complex and research findings are often contradictory. From a practical perspective there would be phenomenal costs in keeping all patients at this high level of sedation. The general trend in ICU care is towards lower levels of sedation. There are also potentially negative psychological aspects of heavy sedation and marked amnesia. A total amnesia can lead to medically unrealistic expectations about recovery time to full health (Jones *et al.* 1994). This by itself can lead to psychological problems, and many patients appear to need a frame of reference, and an understanding of what has happened to them whilst they have been semi-conscious. This can be provided by encouraging recall and discussion of any half-formed memories and also by spending time with patients going through their notes and explaining in pragmatic terms what actually happened.

Benzodiazepines also do not always produce total amnesia. Their main effect is on long-term memory by impairing the acquisition and storage of new information. Painful and emotionally charged information appears more likely to be remembered, possibly because of the involvement of neuroendocrine stress responses (Wagner *et al.* 1997). It is possible that benzodiazepines could have a negative action by effectively screening out all neutral memories and just leaving a patient with affect-laden unpleasant memories.

A study of acute lung injury patients on the ICU (Nelson *et al.* 2000) found that patients who received a higher average dose of sedatives were actually more likely to experience symptoms of PTSD, but this was not of statistical significance. They postulated that the greater exposure to sedatives might be due to patients with anxious traits displaying more agitation and distress.

Another study (Jones *et al.* 2001) found that factual memories, however unpleasant, did not predict post-traumatic symptoms, and found instead that delusional memories without factual recall of the events on the ICU were much more predictive. It is hypothesized that the ICU experience of low external stimulation can cause an attentional shift. The attentional shift changes from external to internal stimuli; for example, visual hallucinations (Jones *et al.* 2000a).

To summarize, the general trend on ICUs is towards lighter sedation. The increased possibility for patients to remember more of their stay may be beneficial in the long run in providing patients with a realistic outlook towards their future speed of recovery. Staff on the ICU must understand that patients are often acutely aware of events and conversations on the ICU, even if they cannot respond or appear drowsy and confused. Care needs to be taken to ensure that patients are spoken to and reassured by staff to reduce the chances that they leave with unpleasant, potentially traumatizing, memories.

Follow-up clinics give the opportunity to pick up cases of post-traumatic stress disorder. The role of these clinics for 'debriefing' is unclear at this point as current opinion questions the effectiveness of this intervention and even suggests a possible detrimental effect (Van Emmerik *et al.* 2002). If post-traumatic stress disorder is identified in the follow-up clinic, this may require referral for specialist treatment.

Neurocognitive deficits

Critical illness can lead to significant impairments in neurocognitive function (Hopkins & Brett 2005). Hopkins and colleagues (1999) studied the neuropsychological sequelae of survivors of severe acute respiratory distress syndrome. One year post-discharge, 30% of patients showed evidence of generalized cognitive decline and over three-quarters (78%) were impaired in one or more neurocognitive domains (memory, attention, concentration or mental processing speed). The degree of hypoxaemia in these patients significantly correlated with neurocognitive impairment. After a further 12 months there had been some improvement, with 47% showing evidence of sustained neurocognitive deficits (Hopkins *et al.* 2005a).

Hopkins and Brett (2005) recently reviewed the findings of eight further cohort studies of neurocognitive function in critically ill patients. The prevalence of neurocognitive deficits ranged from 20% to 78%. Patients with acute respiratory distress syndrome had more profound difficulties than other critically ill patients, but even in patients without acute respiratory distress syndrome, significant problems were common. Two studies followed-up patients over a lengthy period (Rothenhausler *et al.* 2001; Suchyta *et al.* 2004) and showed that at least a quarter of patients have neurocognitive impairments six years post-discharge from ICU.

The kinds of neurocognitive problems experienced by ICU survivors include impaired executive function, slow psychomotor speed, impulsivity, generalized decline in intellectual ability, attention, memory and mental processing speed (Hopkins *et al.* 2005b). One study has suggested that the severity of cognitive impairment may be associated with depression (Jackson *et al.* 2003). Given the frequency of neurocognitive problems in patients post-ICU discharge, it is important that neurocognitive function is monitored during the recovery phase.

Psychiatric problems in ICU staff

The traumatic aspects of being on an ICU are not limited to patients. Significant problems can also be experienced by nurses and doctors. The environment is one of constant tension. The atmosphere has been compared to a tension-charged strategic war bunker (Hay & Oken 1972). Nurses have a high degree of responsibility for interpreting change where information is coming from many quarters. The nurses deal with patients all of whom are seriously ill. There is no respite through working with the less unwell or those who are significantly improved as they are transferred off the ward (Kornfeld 1969). The small size of the units enhances observation and accessibility, but this can lead to a lack of objectivity when a nurse is in such close proximity to pain and distress (Vreeland & Ellis 1969). The huge workload of monitoring and recording leads to repetitive routine. At the same the time nurses need to keep alert to subtle signs of an impending acute deterioration, 'like the mother who hears the faint cry of her baby over the commotion of a party' (Hay & Oken 1972). The high death rate can instil a sense of 'failure'. Continuing to nurse brain-dead patients before organ donation can be a particularly challenging experience for nurses (Pearson *et al.* 2001). The presence of many patients in a twilight state between life and death can directly challenge the sense of self and humanity (Hay & Oken 1972).

Nurses do have the advantage of working co-operatively in a group. Shared experiences, bonding and group social activities can be very helpful in coping with the stress. Younger nurses, in particular, benefit from belonging to the group. At later stages, when a nurse has other obligations such as family, tensions can occur and missing a social activity can be seen as disloyalty (Hay & Oken 1972). Not all nurses fit well into a group or there may be separate 'cliques'. This can lead at times of extreme stress on a unit to staff splitting along these lines or certain nurses being scape-goated by the group (Billig 1981).

Doctors tend to work in a more isolative manner; they have less opportunity to use group coping styles. They do have the advantage over ICU nurses of being able to leave the unit more easily due to obligations elsewhere, such as providing surgical anaesthesia. This can be used as a defence mechanism in difficult situations, but also can lead to tensions with nursing staff. For instance, nurses can feel abandoned, after unsuccessful resuscitations, not only with the 'mess' to clean up, but also with the sense of 'failure' and the job of passing of the bad news to relatives. Doctors also tend to isolate and deny feelings produced by the ICU experience. This coping mechanism can affect the relationships with patients, families and nurses. Some suggestions made to avoid these tensions are avoid perpetuating stereotypes, maximize continuity of physician care and maximize communication between and within professional groups (Youngner *et al.* 1979).

Distress in relatives

Intensive care admission should be viewed as a crisis for both patients and their families. Fear of death or permanent disability together with the inherent uncertainty that characterizes modern medicine can contribute to high levels of anxiety in relatives. Once the acute phase of illness is passed, other stressors present themselves as patients and families adjust to the long recovery process following critical illness. Relatives of the critically ill may experience powerful swings of emotion, from joy to despair in a day (Kleiber *et al.* 1994). A large prospective French study (Pochard *et al.* 2001) using the HAD score as a marker of psychological distress found a high prevalence of anxiety (HAD >10) in 69% of family members and a lower level of depression (34%) in families of patients within five days of ICU admission.

The behavioural response to stress amongst family members on ICU is known to include poor quality of sleep, reduction in nutrition and an increase in consumption of tobacco, alcohol and prescription medications (Halm *et al.* 1993). As the critically ill are often unconscious and sedated, their relatives are usually involved in clinical decision-making processes, particularly regarding the withholding and withdrawal of treatment. Around 7–12% of all ICU patients and 65–90% of those who die will have their relatives involved in these decisions, often when they are experiencing considerable distress themselves (Keenan *et al.* 1997). The burden of critical illness on relatives has been recognized by intensive caregivers and consequently research tools have been developed to assess and address relatives' needs. A descriptive study (Molter 1979) introduced the Critical Care Family Needs Inventory (CCFNI), a 45-item self-report questionnaire. Modified versions of the CCFNI have been validated, with different groups reporting consistent findings. The most important needs are 'to have questions answered honestly', 'to be assured that the best possible care was being given to the patient', 'to be called at home about changes in the condition of the patient', 'no perceived contradictions in information' and 'to know the expected outcome' (Azoulay *et al.* 2001; Bijttebier *et al.* 2001).

Even when needs are addressed and there is clinical improvement, further stresses may occur. Transfer anxiety or relocation stress has been reported in relatives, with up to 40% expressing negative or neutral feelings regarding transfer. Anxiety regarding unfamiliarity and reduced levels of care is common (Leith 1999). Unplanned or out-of-hours discharges can cause further distress and this is often associated with excess pressure on critical-care beds, emphasizing the finite resources within the healthcare system.

Physical and functional recovery from critical illness takes up to 12 months. Psychological morbidity following intensive-care discharge remains high for patients and relatives. Anxiety was detected in a third of relatives at six months (Jones *et al.* 2000b). Furthermore, signs of post-traumatic distress syndrome using the Impact of Events Score can be detected, particularly in those relatives with HADS > 13 at two weeks post-discharge. Recent work by the same group indicates that levels of anxiety (35%) and depression (15%) in relatives exceeded that in patients at three months post-ICU discharge, a pattern not seen in a control group of elective cardiac surgery patients (Young *et al.* 2005).

The psychosocial impact of critical illness on both patient and their relatives cannot be underestimated. Strategies to meet the needs of relatives and help them manage the emotional challenge of critical illness, sometimes long after their loved one has left the intensive care unit, need to be developed and thoroughly evaluated.

Different approaches to psychiatric liaison with ICU

One approach to the psychiatric problems presented on an ICU took a 'community-oriented' approach (Koumans 1965). There was less direct intervention with the patients involved and more indirect action via the care-giving social unit involved with the patients. The focus was on the nursing group. This was provided in the format of regular weekly discussions between the psychiatrist and the nursing staff. The issues regularly discussed were loss, the demands of distressed patients and relatives, reactions of staff and patients to stress and friction between team members. 'Difficult' patient problems were analysed, interpreted and approaches were suggested. Support for the medical staff was provided in a different format because of their greater fragmentation and regular turnover. This was provided by regular attendance at two ward rounds a week aiming to promote a shift in focus from a patient's distress or problematic behaviour to considering psychological and interpersonal issues.

Another approach reported (Billig 1981) used consultee-oriented, patient-centred and problem-oriented styles. This involved both a consultant and a resident in psychiatry being available. This involved regular attendance at morning ward rounds, involvement with monthly teaching sessions and availability to nursing staff for crises sessions when problems occurred. This was quite a labour-intensive approach but did have the benefit of the liaison psychiatrist becoming a valued member of the team, with sound trusting relationships.

Not many psychiatry services have the resources to devote such intensive input. An alternative approach described is to focus primarily on patients after discharge and to use the regular ICU follow-up clinic to assess referred patients (Turner *et al.* 2002). This sessional approach is more compatible with the constraints of normal day-to-day practice. While the liaison psychiatrist did not become a member of the ICU team it was still possible to build good working relationship with team members.

When patients who are still on the ICU need to be seen a normal psychiatric assessment is often not possible. Communication difficulties and sedation often limit standard history taking. The psychiatrist relies more on the medical notes and observations of staff and family (Gipson 1991). Non-verbal cues can be a useful source of information. If intubation is limiting communication closed questioning can be used, with the patient pointing to 'yes'/'no' written answers. Nurses in the ICU are often skilled lip readers. Joint assessments can therefore be useful in obtaining information from patients in a similar way to using a translator for a non-English speaking patient. Similar care must be taken to respect the patient's dignity in this situation.

Patients referred from the ICU can often present with highly complex problems. Examples of complex referrals made to the liaison service were five patients who had intentionally harmed themselves, all of whom had alcohol or drug misuse and multiple social adversities. Organic factors were felt to have a significant causal role in four referrals with problems such as systemic lupus erythematosus, diffuse brain injury and focal brain injury. This degree of complexity requires a mix of psychiatric, pharmacological and psychological skills particularly suited to a liaison psychiatrist (Turner *et al.* 2002).

REFERENCES

Anderson, I. M., Nutt, D. J. and Deakin, J. F. W. (2000). Evidence based guidelines for treating depressive disorders with antidepressants: a revision of the 1993 British Association for Psychopharmacology guidelines. *Journal of Psychopharmacology*, **14**, 3–20.

Azoulay, E., Pochard, F., Chevret, S., *et al.* (2001). French FAMIREA group meeting the needs of intensive care unit patient families: a multicenter study. *American Journal of Respiratory and Critical Care Medicine,* **163**, 135–9.

Baxter, S. (1974). Psychological problems of intensive care. *British Journal of Hospital Medicine,* **11**, 875–85.

Beck, A. T., Ward, C. H., Mendelson, M., *et al.* (1961). An inventory for measuring depression. *Archives of General Psychiatry,* **4**, 561–71.

Bijttebier, P., Vanoost, S., Delva, D., *et al.* (2001). Needs of relatives of critical care patients: perceptions of relatives, physicians and nurses. *Intensive Care Medicine,* **27**, 160–5.

Billig, N. (1981). Liaison psychiatry: a role on the medical intensive care unit. *The International Journal of Psychiatry in Medicine,* **11**, 379–86.

Capuzzo, M., Valpondi, V., Cingolani, E., *et al.* (2005). Post-traumatic stress disorder-related symptoms after intensive care. *Minerva Anesthesiologica,* **71**, 167–79.

Chelluri, L., Im, K., Belle, S., *et al.* (2004). Long-term mortality and quality of life after prolonged mechanical ventilation. *Critical Care Medicine,* **32**, 61–9.

Cheng, E. Y. (1996). Recall in the sedated ICU patient. *Journal of Clinical Anaesthesia,* **8**, 675–8.

Conway, D. H., Turner, S. J., Eddleston, J., *et al.* (2001). Sedation on intensive care: a pathway into dependence. *Care of the Critically Ill,* **17**, 170–1.

Cutler, L. and Garner, M. (1995). Reducing relocation stress after discharge from the intensive therapy unit. *Intensive and Critical Care Nursing,* **11**, 333–5.

Eddleston, J. M., White, P. and Guthrie, E. (2000). Survival, morbidity, and quality of life after discharge from intensive care. *Critical Care Medicine,* **28**, 2293–9.

First, M., Spitzer, R., Gibbon, M., *et al.* (1998). *Structured Clinical Interview for DSM-IV Axis I Disorders – non-patient edition (SCID-I/NP, Version 2.0).* Arlington VA: American Psychiatric Press.

Fish, D. N. (1991). Treatment of delirium in the critically ill patient. *Clinical Pharmacy,* **10**, 456–66.

Gipson, W. T. (1991). Fatigue and depression in the patient in the intensive care unit. *Primary Care,* **18**, 359–67.

Granberg, A., Engberg, I. B. and Lundberg, D. (1996). Intensive care syndrome: a literature review. *Intensive and Critical Care Nursing,* **12**, 173–82.

Green, A. (1996). An exploratory study of patients' memory recall of their stay in an adult intensive therapy unit. *Intensive and Critical Care Nursing,* **12**, 131–7.

Halm, M. A., Titler, M. G., Kleiber, C., *et al.* (1993). Behavioral responses of family members during critical illness. *Clinical Nursing Research,* **2**, 414–37.

Hay, D. and Oken, D. (1972). The psychological stresses of intensive care nursing. *Psychosomatic Medicine,* **34**, 109–18.

Henderson, A., Wright, M. and Pond, S. M. (1993). Experience with 732 acute overdose patients admitted to an intensive care unit over six years. *Medical Journal of Australia,* **158**, 28–30.

Hopkins, R. O. and Brett, S. (2005). Chronic neurocognitive effects of critical illness. *Current Opinion in Critical Care,* **11**, 369–75.

Hopkins, R. O., Weaver, L. K., Pope, D., *et al.* (1999). Neuropsychological sequelae and impaired health status in survivors of severe acute respiratory distress syndrome. *American Journal of Respiratory and Critical Care Medicine*, **160**, 50−65.

Hopkins, R. O., Weaver, L. K., Chan, K.J., *et al.* (2004). Quality of life, emotional, and cognitive function following acute respiratory distress syndrome. *Journal of the International Neuropsychological Society*, **10**, 1005−17.

Hopkins, R. O., Weaver, L. K., Collingridge, D., *et al.* (2005a). Two year neurocognitive, emotional and quality of life in acute respiratory distress syndrome. *American Journal of Respiratory and Critical Care Medicine*, **171**, 340−7.

Hopkins, R. O., Jackson, J. C. and Wallace, C. J. (2005b). Neurocognitive impairments in ICU patients with prolonged mechanical ventilation. *Program and Abstracts of the International Neuropsychology Society, 33rd Annual Meeting, 61.* 1−5 February, St Louis, Missouri, USA.

Jackson, J., Hart, R., Gordon, S., *et al.* (2003). Six-month neuropsychological outcomes of medical intensive care unit patients. *Critical Care Medicine*, **31**, 1226−34.

Jones, C., Griffiths, R. D., Macmillan, R., *et al.* (1994). Psychological problems occurring after intensive care. *British Journal of Intensive Care*, **4**, 46−53.

Jones, C., Griffiths, R. D. and Humpris, G. (2000a). Disturbed memory and amnesia related to intensive care. *Memory*, **8**, 79−94.

Jones, C., Skirrow, P., Griffiths, R. D., *et al.* (2000b). Predicting intensive care relatives at risk of post traumatic stress disorder. *British Journal of Anaesthesia*, **84**, 666−7.

Jones, C., Griffiths, R. D., Humphris, G., *et al.* (2001). Memory, delusions, and the development of acute posttraumatic stress disorder-related symptoms after intensive care. *Critical Care Medicine*, **29**, 687−8.

Kam, P. C. A. and Chang, G. W. M. (1997). Selective serotonin inhibitors: pharmacology and clinical implications in anaesthesia and critical care. *Anaesthesia*, **52**, 982−8.

Keenan, S. P., Busche, K. D., Chen, L. M., *et al.* (1997). A retrospective review of a large cohort of patients undergoing the process of withholding or withdrawal of life support. *Critical Care Medicine*, **25**, 1324−31.

Kleck, H. (1984). ICU syndrome: onset, manifestations, treatment, stressors and prevention. *Critical Care Quarterly*, **6**, 21−8.

Kleiber, C., Halm, M., Titler, M., *et al.* (1994). Emotional responses of family members during a critical care hospitalization. *American Journal of Critical Care*, **3**, 70−6.

Kornfeld, D. S. (1969). Psychiatric view of the intensive care unit. *British Medical Journal*, **1**, 108−10.

Koumans, A. J. R. (1965). Psychiatric consultation in an intensive care unit. *Journal of the American Medical Association*, **194**, 163−7.

Kress, J., Gehlbach, B., Lacy, M., *et al.* (2003). Long-term psychological effects of daily sedative interruption on critically ill patients. *American Journal of Respiratory and Critical Care Medicine*, **168**, 1457−61.

Kutz, I., Shabtai, H., Solomon, Z., *et al.* (1994). Post-traumatic stress disorder in myocardial infarction patients: prevalence study. *Israel Journal of Psychiatry and Related Sciences*, **31**, 48−56.

Leith, B. A. (1999). Patients' and family members' perceptions of transfer from intensive care. *Heart and Lung*, **28**, 210–18.

Lyness, J. M., Noel, T. K., Cox, C., *et al.* (1997). Screening for depression in elderly primary care patients. A comparison of the Center for Epidemiologic Studies-Depression Scale and the Geriatric Depression Scale. *Archives of Internal Medicine*, **157**, 449–54.

MacKenzie, T. B. and Popkin, M. K. (1980). Stress response syndrome occurring after delirium. *American Journal of Psychiatry*, **137**, 1433–5.

Mayou, R., Bryant, B. and Duthie, R. (1993). Psychiatric consequences of road traffic accidents. *British Medical Journal*, **307**, 647–51.

McGuire, B., Basten, C., Ryan, C., *et al.* (2000). Intensive care syndrome: a dangerous misnomer. *Archives of Internal Medicine*, **160**, 906–9.

McKegney, F. P. (1966). The intensive care syndrome: the definition, treatment and prevention of a new 'disease of medical progress'. *Connecticut Medicine*, **30**, 633–6.

Mendel, J. G. and Khan, F. A. (1980). Psychological aspects of weaning from mechanical ventilation. *Psychosomatics*, **21**, 465–71.

Menza, M. A., Murray, G. B., Holmes, V. F., *et al.* (1987). Decreased extrapyramidal symptoms with intravenous haloperidol. *Journal of Clinical Psychiatry*, **48**, 278–80.

Molter, N. C. (1979). Needs of relatives of critically ill patients. *Heart and Lung*, **8**, 332–9.

Nelson, B. J., Weinart, C. R., Bury, C. L., *et al.* (2000). Intensive care unit drug use and subsequent quality of life in acute lung injury patients. *Critical Care Medicine*, **28**, 3626–30.

Paratz, J., Thomas, P. and Adsett, J. (2005). Re-admission to intensive care: identification of risk factors. *Physiotherapy Research*, **10**, 154–63.

Pearson, A., Robertson-Malt, S., Walsh, K., *et al.* (2001). Intensive care nurses' experiences of caring for brain dead organ donor patients. *Journal of Clinical Nursing*, **10**, 132–9.

Pochard, F., Azoulay, E., Chevret, S., *et al.* The French FAMIREA group. (2001). Symptoms of anxiety and depression in family members of intensive care unit patients: ethical hypothesis regarding decision-making capacity. *Critical Care Medicine*, **29**, 1893–7.

Power, B. M., Pinder, M., Hackett, L. P., *et al.* (1995). Fatal serotonin syndrome following a combined overdose of moclobemide, clomipramine and fluoxetine. *Anaesthesia and Intensive Care*, **23**, 499–522.

Radloff, L. S. (1977). The CES-D scale: a self-report depression scale for research in the general population. *Applied Psychological Measurement*, **1**, 385–401.

Rothenhausler, H. B., Ehrentraut, S., Stoll, C., *et al.* (2001). The relationship between cognitive performance and employment and health status in long-term survivors of the acute respiratory distress syndrome: results of an exploratory study. *General Hospital Psychiatry*, **23**, 90–6.

Russell, S. (1999). An exploratory study of patients' perceptions, memories and experiences of an intensive care unit. *Journal of Advanced Nursing*, **29**, 783–91.

Schelling, G., Stoll, C., Haller, M., *et al.* (1998). Health-related quality of life and posttraumatic stress disorder in survivors of the acute respiratory distress syndrome. *Critical Care Medicine*, **26**, 651–9.

Scragg, P., Jones, A. and Fauvel, N. (2001). Psychological problems following ICU treatment. *Anaesthesia*, **56**, 9–14.

Skirrow, P., Jones, C., Griffiths, R. D., *et al.* (2002). The impact of current media events on hallucinatory content: the experience of the intensive care unit (ICU) patient. *British Journal of Clinical Psychology*, **41**, 87–91.

Strom, J., Thisted, B., Krantz, T., *et al.* (1986). Self-poisoning treated in an ICU: drug pattern, acute mortality and short-term survival. *Acta Anaesthesiologica Scandinavica*, **30**, 148–53.

Suchtya, M. R., Hopkins, R. O., White, J., *et al.* (2004). The incidence of cognitive dysfunction after ARDS. *American Journal of Respiratory Critical Care Medicine*, **169**, A18.

Turner, S. J., Ingleby, S. E., Eddleston, J. M., *et al.* (2002). Psychiatric perspectives on intensive care follow-up. *British Journal of Intensive Care*, **12**, 6–10.

Van Emmerik, A. A., Kamphuis, J. H., Hulsbosch, A. M., *et al.* (2002). Single session debriefing after psychological trauma: a meta-analysis. *The Lancet*, **360**, 766–71.

Vreeland, R. and Ellis, G. (1969). Stresses on the nurse in the intensive-care unit. *Journal of the American Medical Association*, **208**, 332–4.

Wagner, B. K. J., O'Hara, D. A. and Hammond, J. S. (1997). Drugs for amnesia in the ICU. *American Journal of Critical Care*, **6**, 192–201.

Wehler, M., Geise, A., Hadzionerovic, D., *et al.* (2003). Health-related quality of life of patients with multiple organ dysfunction: individual changes and comparison with normative population. *Critical Care Medicine*, **31**, 1094–101.

Weinert, C. (2005). Epidemiology and treatment of psychiatric conditions that develop after critical illness. *Current Opinion in Critical Care*, **11**(4), 376–80.

Weinert, C., Groom, J., Stibbe, C., *et al.* (2003). Depression and antidepressant therapy during recovery from acute respiratory failure. *American Journal of Respiratory Critical Care Medicine*, **167**, A437.

Wilson, L. M. (1972). Intensive care delirium: the effect of outside deprivation in a windowless unit. *Archives of Internal Medicine*, **130**, 225–6.

Winship, G. (1998). Intensive care psychiatric nursing – psychoanalytic perspectives. *Journal of Psychiatric and Mental Health Nursing*, **5**, 361–5.

Young, E., Eddleston, J., Ingleby, S., *et al.* (2005). Returning home after intensive care: a comparison of symptoms of anxiety and depression in ICU and elective cardiac surgery patients and their relatives. *Intensive Care Medicine*, **31**, 86–91.

Youngner, S., Jackson, D. L. and Allen, M. (1979). Staff attitudes towards the care of the critically ill in the medical intensive care unit. *Critical Care Medicine*, **7**, 35–40.

Zigmond, A. S. and Snaith, R. P. (1983). The Hospital Anxiety and Depression Scale. *Acta Psychiatrica Scandinavica*, **67**, 361–70.

29

The burns unit

Jonathan I. Bisson

Introduction

Burn trauma is a significant cause of mortality and morbidity. In 1999 192 males and 144 females died as a direct result of burn trauma in England and Wales (Office for National Statistics 2000). Frank *et al.* (1987) estimated that 731 000 emergency room visits and 60 900 hospital admissions occurred annually as a result of burn trauma in the USA. Wilkinson (1998) obtained data from six of the nine accident and emergency departments (AED) that served a UK population of 2.6 million. There were 3013 attendances as a result of burn trauma over a 1-year period representing 1% of the total AED workload.

It is no surprise that burn trauma can result in psychological distress. The burn trauma victim has many issues to contend with. Stressors often include the burn injury itself, pain, hospitalization, reduced functioning and permanent scarring. In addition the burn injury has often been sustained as a result of involvement in a frightening psychologically traumatic event. Individuals who sustain burn trauma also appear more likely to have pre-existing mental health difficulties than the general population (e.g. Patterson *et al.* 1993).

Nature and prevalence of psychiatric sequelae following burn trauma

Several authors and researchers have considered the psychological impact of burn trauma. The earliest studies were mainly descriptive in nature. Overall, the methodology employed has improved over time. The most recent studies have used well-validated measures to determine the presence of psychological sequelae although unfortunately, like the older studies, have relatively small sample sizes. Table 29.1 summarizes the data from studies with sample sizes over 100 that have

Handbook of Liaison Psychiatry, ed. Geoffrey Lloyd and Elspeth Guthrie. Published by Cambridge University Press. © Cambridge University Press 2007.

investigated the prevalence and predictors of psychological sequelae following burn trauma.

In a seminal paper Adler (1943) studied survivors of the Boston Coconut Grove nightclub fire in which 491 people died in November 1942. Twenty-five (54%) individuals were found to be suffering from psychiatric complications at three months. They were described as suffering from either 'general nervousness' ($n = 11$) with irritability, fatigue and insomnia or from 'anxiety neuroses' ($n = 14$) characterized by fears and anxiety that they were unable to control. After nine months 13 (28%) of the sample continued to display psychiatric complications. Nightmares that involved reliving scenes of the disaster in a more or less realistic manner were described in 15 (33%) individuals during their hospital stay and in 10 (22%) individuals after their discharge.

Bowden *et al.* (1980) interviewed 320 patients treated at the University of Michigan Burn Centre. The mean age was 29 years, the mean inpatient stay was 46 days and 24% of the sample were female. Of these, 13% were diagnosed as alcoholic before the burn. A specially developed questionnaire was completed during the interviews to determine level of self-esteem. Forty-seven (15%) individuals were classified as not having adequate self-esteem. Depression was not measured specifically in the study but 56 individuals indicated that they had wished themselves dead during treatment compared with 196 who had not. The 56 had significantly lower self-esteem. Unfortunately it was impossible to determine whether or not the low self-esteem detected preceded or was a consequence of the burn trauma.

White (1982) studied 142 consecutive patients with burn injuries admitted to Birmingham Accident Hospital. Ninety-three (65%) were male and 49 (35%) were female. All of the women sustained their burns in non-industrial accidents whereas only 34 (37%) of the men did. No information was given regarding age of the sample. Of the 76 individuals traced, interviewed and 'clinically rated' 24 (35%) were felt to have no sequelae, 17 (25%) mild sequelae, 13 (19%) moderate sequelae, 10 (15%) marked sequelae and 5 (7%) severe sequelae. The clinical presentations were of depression and anxiety states. Panic was described in 19 (25%), irritability in 22 (29%) and unhappiness or depression in 28 (37%).

Blank and Perry (1984) screened 189 adult burn trauma inpatients during two six-month periods. If delirium occurred then two weeks after a clear sensorium the Brief Psychiatric Rating Scale and the depression and anxiety subscales of the SCL-90 were administered. The impact of event scale was administered four weeks after the burn injury. Thirty-four (18%) (28 male and 6 female) fulfilled the DSM-III criteria for a diagnosis of delirium. Seven (28%) of the 25 survivors had severe psychological symptoms – either depression or post-traumatic stress disorder (PTSD).

Table 29.1. Studies containing data of the prevalence of psychological symptoms following burn trauma ($n > 10$).

Study	Setting	n	% Burn mean (SD)	Follow-up post-burn	Outcome measure	Completers n (%)	Mean (SD) outcomes	Prevalence psychological sequelae	Predictors of psychological sequelae
Adler[a] (1943)	USA	131	n.s.[b]	3 months 9 months	Psychological complications	46 (35%)	n.s.	26 (57%) 13 (28%)	Initial distress, nightmares, no loss of consciousness
Bowden et al. (1980)	USA	461	23 (n.s.)	up to 20 years	Low self-esteem	314 (68%)	n.s.	47 (15%)	Female sex, social support
White (1982)	UK	142	n.s.	1 year	Psychological sequelae	76 (54%)	n.s.	45 (65%)	% burn, initial distress, age 36–45, living alone, living with >2 children, time in hospital, initial anxiety or depression, personality disorder
Green et al. (1983)[c]	USA	500	n.s.	1 year 2 years	PEF[d] SCL-90[e] PEF SCL-90	147 (29%) 129 (26%)	2.1 (1.2) 0.7 (0.7) 1.7 (1.0) 0.6 (0.5)	36 (31%) n.s.	Presence at fire

Table 29.1. (*cont.*)

Study	Setting	n	% Burn mean (SD)	Follow-up post-burn	Outcome measure	Completers n (%)	Mean (SD) outcomes	Prevalence psychological sequelae	Predictors of psychological sequelae
Browne *et al.* (1985)		527		n.s., up to 12 years after					Unemployment, avoidance coping style, little recreational activity, loss of occupational status
Perry *et al.* (1987)	USA	134	20.7 (n.s.)	9 days	PTSD[f]	104	n.s.	43 (41%)	% burn, married, employed, younger age, pain, delirium, male sex, lack of responsibility
Ward *et al.* (1987)	USA	193	17.4 (17.6)	n.s., 108 (78%) > 2 years	BDI[g]	139 (72%)	n.s.	31 (22.3%)	Past psychiatric history, physical condition that contributed to burn trauma

Study	Country	N		Time	Measure				Findings
Sheffield et al. (1988)	USA	212	n.s., median 10	268 days	IES[h]	212 (100%) QOLI[i]	12.28 (n.s.) (n.s.) 9.34 (n.s.)	n.s.	Poor compliance with treatment
Perry et al. (1992)	USA	129	n.s.	2 months 6 months 1 year	PTSD PTSD PTSD	51 (40%) 40 (31%) 31 (24%)	n.s.	18 (35.3%) 16 (40%) 14 (45.2%)	Smaller burns, initial distress, less perceived social support, higher initial IES and POMS
Taal & Faber (1998)	Netherlands	1404	n.s.	1 to 2 years	IES	429 (31%)	19.8 (17.6)	33% >26	Burn-specific health problems (e.g. scarring), burn-related shame
Ehde et al. (1999)	USA	180	13.4 (9.8)	Within 24 hours	DSM-III-R PTSD symptoms	172 (96%)	n.s.	44 (24%) met symptom criteria	Poorer pre-burn mental health, larger burns

Notes: [a]Included patients with non-burn trauma injuries; [b]n.s: not significant; [c]patients who had suffered from delirium only; [d]PEF: Psychiatric Evaluation Form; [e]SCL-90 = Symptom Checklist; [f]PTSD: post-traumatic stress disorder; [g]BDI: Beck Depression Inventory; [h]IES: Impact of Event Scale; [i]QOLI: Quality of Life Index.

Perry *et al.* (1987) considered the records of adult burn trauma patients who had taken part in analgesic studies and were also interviewed using the Structured Clinical Interview for DSM-III to determine the presence or absence of PTSD. One hundred and four (78%) of the 134 who entered the analgesic studies had complete data and were therefore included. Forty-three (41%) of these patients satisfied PTSD symptom criteria at a mean of 9.4 days (SD = 3.1) post burn trauma. It was noted that their subjective rating of pain was greater than those without PTSD although the authors acknowledged that it was unknown whether the presence of PTSD increased pain perception or vice versa.

Ward *et al.* (1987) studied 193 of the 887 adult burn trauma victims treated at a burn unit in California between 1973 and 1979. They included all victims with total body surface area (TBSA) burns of 30% or more and a random sample of victims with smaller burns. One hundred and thirty-nine (72%) of the sample were located and interviewed. The mean age was 37.8 (SD 15.9) years and 27 (36%) were female. The mean time since burn trauma was not given but 31 (22%) were interviewed less than two years after the burn trauma, 65 (47%) between two and four years after and 43 (31%) more than four years after. On the Beck Depression Inventory 108 individuals (77.7%) scored below a cut-off of 10 and were considered not depressed, 13 (9.4%) scored between 10 and 14 and were considered to be mildly depressed and 18 (12.9%) scored over 14 and were considered to be moderately to severely depressed.

Sheffield *et al.* (1988) studied 212 patients admitted to a burn clinic in Minnesota, USA between 1977 and 1982. Mean inpatient stay was 22 days (range 0–193 days), the mean TBSA burn was not stated but the median was 10%, 91 sustained burns less than 10% and 121 greater than 10%. Outcome variables were administered at a mean of 246 days post-discharge from hospital (range 0–1980 days). The main psychological outcome variables were the impact of event scale and the quality-of-life index. Mean scores on these variables were 12.3 and 9.3 respectively (further details were not documented) which the authors considered to be within 'normal limits'. Twenty-one (10%) patients were referred for a psychiatric opinion and 14 (7%) received psychotherapy as a result, but no further details were given.

Difede *et al.* (1997) approached all new admissions to the New York Hospital Regional Burn Centre over a period of two years and interviewed 180 patients within two weeks of their burn injury. There were 133 (74%) males and 47 (26%) females, the mean age was 35.7 (SD 11.5), 74 (41%) were Black, 58 (32%) were White and 40 (22%) were Hispanic. Fifty-nine (33%) had a history of alcoholism recorded, 39 (22%) a history of drug abuse and 21 (12%) a history of psychiatric disorder. Mean TBSA burn was 14.9% (SD 11.4%), mean Impact of

Events Scale (IES) avoidance was 12.4 (SD 9.8), IES intrusion was 14.1 (SD 10.5) and Profile of Mood States (POMS) 5.29 (SD 5.34).

Taal and Faber (1998) identified all patients registered as hospitalized in the Netherlands in 1994 or 1995 with burn injury as the main discharge diagnosis (1523 individuals). Questionnaires were sent to those who could be located one to two years post-burn; 429 (31.4%) individuals responded. The mean age at time of discharge was 38.3 (SD 17.4), 64% were male, 44 (24%) met DSM-IIIR criteria for all three PTSD symptom clusters based on their self-report.

Bisson (2000) reviewed 24 studies (total $n = 2879$) and concluded that the research strongly suggested that a significant number of individuals would develop psychological difficulties following burn trauma. The main psychological sequelae reported were symptoms of anxiety, depression and PTSD. The quality of the research considered (including the studies described above) was variable and with some exceptions the quality overall was relatively poor. Common methodological problems included small numbers, problematic recruitment methods, large dropout rates with patients unaccounted for in the final analysis, the absence of systematic interviews and the absence of well-validated questionnaire measures. These factors along with the marked differences in the dimensions of the traumatic event, the percentage burn, outcome measures, thresholds for 'caseness' and assessment times make direct comparison of the different studies considered difficult.

Within the first three months of a burn trauma the 12 studies that considered the prevalence of psychological sequelae found rates between 7% and 54% with a mean of 29.8% (SD = 13.4%). The nine studies that considered the prevalence rate between three months and one year after the burn trauma found psychological sequelae rates between 19% and 65% with a mean of 34.4% (SD = 13.6%). The eight studies that considered the prevalence rate over one year after the burn trauma found psychological sequelae rates between 15% and 75% with a mean of 35.3% (SD = 20.3%). Of the nine studies that measured the prevalence of psychological sequelae at least two time points after the burn trauma, six found that there was a decrease in the prevalence over time, and three an increase over time. It can be concluded that psychological sequelae appear to be relatively common following burn trauma. The exact prevalence is difficult to estimate from the research currently available and although it is clear that psychological difficulties can continue for many years after the burn trauma there are contradictory findings in the literature regarding whether the natural course is for an increase or a decrease in prevalence over time.

In addition to depression and anxiety and post-traumatic-stress-like symptoms, the nature of psychological sequelae following burn trauma can be complex and include fear avoidance (Sgroi *et al.* 2005), effects on autobiographical memory

(Stokes *et al.* 2004) and a variety of psychosocial problems and difficulties (Weichmann & Patterson 2004).

Predictors of psychological reactions to burn trauma

There are many possible factors that could explain why some individuals appear to develop psychological sequelae following burn trauma and some individuals do not. It is perhaps commonly assumed that the greater TBSA burn an individual sustains the more likely that individual is to develop a distressing psychological reaction. An association between the severity of the traumatic event and adverse psychological outcome has been found following other traumatic events (e.g. Kessler *et al.* 1995). However, trauma research suggests that this is not a linear relationship and that many other factors may affect outcome. In addition to the TBSA burn other factors are likely to contribute to the severity of the trauma of an acute burn injury. For example, a 5% TBSA burn sustained as a result of an explosion in which many other people were involved is likely to be more traumatic than a 5% burn as a result of boiling water.

Most of the research into predictors of psychological reactions to burn trauma has been through the prevalence studies discussed above. This has been done by considering the presence of psychological sequelae in subgroups of individuals (e.g. males/females, higher percentage burn/lower percentage burn), by performing correlation co-efficients to consider relationships between a variety of variables or by performing more complex statistical tests such as regression analyses to explore the contribution of various factors to the main psychological outcome measure. Such analyses are exploratory and prone to error but they suggest factors that should be subjected to study in more detail in the future. It is therefore extremely important to interpret the research results with caution. One of the difficulties in critically appraising several of the available studies is that the full results and statistics are not presented, leaving the reader with no knowledge of the magnitude of any relationship or the degree of confidence that this relationship is true.

Table 29.1 includes a column that indicates the factors found to be predictive of poorer psychological outcome in the studies considered.

Bisson (2000) found that 23 of the studies he identified considered percentage TBSA burn. One found a relationship with a positive psychological outcome, 16 no association and six an association with increased psychological sequelae. Involvement of hands or face was considered in nine studies, with an association with negative outcome in four and no relationship in five. Past psychiatric history was considered in nine with no effect in five and an association with worse outcome in four. Sex was considered in 11 studies with no effect in nine, one found an association between negative outcome and male sex and one between negative outcome and female sex. Age had no association with outcome in nine studies and an increased risk with younger age in one study and age 36–45 in another. Initial psychological symptoms were associated with poorer outcome in nine studies and no effect in one. Other factors were looked at less frequently. Factors associated with worse outcome in at least two studies were length of hospitalization (three studies), pain (three studies), others being to blame for what happened (three), perceived disfigurement (two), compensation issues (two) and avoidance coping style (two). The only factors associated with fewer psychological sequelae in at least two studies were social support (two) and loss of consciousness (two).

There are clearly some conflicting results but overall there appears to be an association between severity of burn and psychological distress, although this association does not seem likely to be a very strong one. Several other factors may be associated but need researching more thoroughly. There seems little doubt that apparently healthy individuals with little in the way of apparent vulnerability to psychiatric disorder can develop psychological difficulties following relatively minor burn trauma. The apparent relationships of initial distress and increased TBSA burn with poorer psychological outcome and higher initial distress and poorer psychological outcome are in keeping with research following other traumatic events (e.g. Brewin *et al.* 2000; Kessler *et al.* 1995), but along with other potential predictors of outcome following burn trauma need researching in larger studies.

Self-inflicted burn trauma

One group of burn trauma victims of particular concern to the liaison psychiatrist are those who self-inflict burn trauma. In 1999 24 males and 7 females died as a direct result of self-inflicted burn trauma in England and Wales (Office for National Statistics 2000). Sonneborn and Vanstraelen (1992) reviewed the records of inpatients admitted to the Welsh Regional Burns Unit over a 12-year period. Of the 5758 patients, 91 were said to have self-inflicted their burns but on examination of the case notes only 51 had a true diagnosis of self-inflicted burns. Questionnaires were sent to the patients' general practitioners and psychiatrists, if involved, regarding their psychiatric histories. The 51 individuals had 64 admissions (one individual was admitted four times) over the 12-year period and represented 1.1% of the total admissions. Forty-two were believed to have made a suicide act, the other nine were considered self-mutilators. There were 26 males and 25 females in the series. One-third used highly flammable liquid to ignite themselves, one-third set fire to their clothes, others included gas explosions, setting fire to house, chemicals and electricity.

A direct burn with a match or lighter caused 50% of the self-mutilation and 31% was done with chemicals. Mean TBSA was 1.4% for self-mutilation and 22% for suicide attempt; the mean inpatient stays were 25 and 39 days respectively. No self-mutilators died; 12 (28%) of the suicide attempts died. All the self-mutilators except one, who was transferred to a psychiatric hospital, were discharged home. Of the suicide attempts, 13 were discharged home, 20 were transferred to a psychiatric hospital and 3 were returned to prison. A past psychiatric history was found in 74%; 55% of suicide attempts had previously attempted. In the attempted suicide group 11 (25%) were diagnosed as having schizophrenia, 16 (38%) an affective disorder, 7 (17%) personality disorder and 6 (14%) alcohol abuse or dependence. In the self-mutilators personality disorder was the commonest diagnosis with six (67%) being given this diagnosis. Of concern only 15 individuals appeared to be referred for psychiatric consultation during their inpatient stay although this figure is challenged by the number of individuals who were transferred to a psychiatric bed.

Relatives

There has been limited research into the psychological impact of burn trauma in the relatives of those burned. Bisson (2000) identified five studies including 149 individuals. The prevalence of significant psychological symptoms ranged between 36% and 61% at some point following their relative's burn trauma with up to seven years follow-up. The quality of the existing research is poor overall. Methodological shortcomings include small sample sizes, absence of comparison of symptoms with the burn trauma victim or an alternative control and the absence of the use of well-validated questionnaires or structured interviews. Most of the research to date has concerned parents of children who describe significant psychological sequelae. The studies that have considered relatives of adult burn trauma victims have also found significant psychological sequelae amongst them. Even if they have not witnessed the actual traumatic event they are likely to have endured other traumatic experiences. For example being informed that a close relative has sustained burn trauma and seeing the effects of the burn for the first time are likely to represent major traumatic experiences. The studies revealed significant symptoms of PTSD in this population and highlighted the potential psychological and emotional needs of burn trauma victims' relatives. Few studies have considered variables associated with the development of psychological sequelae. Those that have done have produced inconsistent results but possible associations have been found with measures of initial depression, intrusive thoughts, TBSA burn and guilt. It is apparent that this area is under-researched and that more studies are required to determine the true prevalence and predictors of psychological sequelae in relatives of acute burn trauma victims.

Management

Unfortunately there is little systematic research on the best way to deal with psychological sequelae following burn trauma. It is important to focus on ensuring that burns units provide an environment and package of care that openly acknowledges the importance of psychosocial factors, deals with them in a caring and sympathetic manner and identifies individuals with specific needs. Individuals with mental health difficulties should receive an accurate mental health assessment and management plan tailored to their individual needs using treatments that have been shown to be effective for similar difficulties in other populations.

Delirium

A common initial psychiatric presentation on the burns unit is delirium (see Chapter 12). The universal management principles for delirium must be applied, i.e. investigation for and treatment of the underlying organic cause, environmental considerations (nurse in cubicle, orientate with clock, TV, newspaper, etc., ensure adequate lighting, consistency of staff and familiar faces such as relatives) and psychological aspects (acknowledge distress, break down complicated tasks, ensure use of sensory aids). If medication is needed then an antipsychotic, orally when possible; e.g. quetiapine 25–50 mg or haloperidol 0.5–1 mg, may be helpful. When oral administration is difficult parenteral administration of medication may be necessary, for example with haloperidol, lorazepam or Diazemuls.

Early intervention

Attempts have been made to offer early intervention to victims of acute burn trauma to prevent the later development of psychological sequelae. Both psychological and pharmacological approaches have been used. Bisson *et al.* (1997a) studied 130 acute burn trauma victims admitted to a regional burns unit. They were randomly allocated to an individual psychological debriefing (PD) that lasted between 30 minutes and 2 hours or to no intervention. There were no significant differences between the groups at 3-month follow-up but at 13-month follow-up PD was associated with significantly worse outcome as judged by scores on the IES and Hospital Anxiety and Depression Scale (HAD). Interestingly 52% of the PD group described PD as 'definitely useful'. Caution should be exercised in interpreting the results as the severity of the burn was slightly more extreme in the PD group, and almost twice as many of the PD group described significant previous trauma although this did not appear to affect outcome. The results of systematic reviews of randomized controlled trials of one-off psychological interventions following other traumatic events suggests that such interventions are neutral overall and do not appear to warrant routine delivery following any traumatic event (Rose *et al.* 2001). There are more promising results for the use of multiple session cognitive behavioural interventions starting one month after the trauma for acute stress disorder sufferers (e.g. Bryant *et al.* 1998).

There have been a few trials of medication shortly after burn trauma although all are small and in need of replication with larger samples and better methodological designs. Stanovic *et al.* (2001) reported a case series of 10 burn trauma victims where risperidone 0.5–2 mg was administered as a result of clinically distressing acute stress symptoms. All reported a reduction of re-experiencing and hyper-arousal symptoms and improved sleep. Clearly it is difficult to determine the importance of this and a randomized controlled trial would be necessary to explore this further. Saxe *et al.* (2001) reported interesting results from a series of 24 children with acute burn trauma. Children who received higher doses of morphine had a greater reduction of PTSD symptoms over six months, leading to some interesting questions for further research. Imipramine has been compared with chloral hydrate in one small, randomized controlled trial of 25 child burn trauma victims aged between 2 and 19 (Robert *et al.* 1999). Children with acute stress disorder symptoms for at least two days and nights without a significant reduction in symptoms on the second night were included in the study. Those who received imipramine (1 mg/kg, maximum dose 100 mg) for seven days had a significantly greater reduction of their acute stress disorder symptoms than the chloral hydrate (25 mg/kg, maximum dose 250 mg) group.

Later intervention

There have been no randomized controlled trials of later psychological or pharmacological interventions for burn trauma victims. However, there is a strong evidence base for the use of psychopharmacological and psychological treatments for conditions such as depressive episodes, post-traumatic stress disorder and anxiety disorders. Given the current lack of information specifically regarding later intervention for burn trauma victims it can be strongly argued that current best practice would be to offer evidence-based interventions for these and other psychiatric conditions if present.

A key issue for many burn trauma victims is adjustment to the physical impact of their burn injuries. This can include reduced functioning, scarring, body image issues, relationship difficulties including sexual difficulties and issues around temperature regulation. Many of these difficulties are exacerbated if accompanied by psychological distress. It is important that clinicians and therapists dealing with burn trauma victims have a basic knowledge of physical issues. Facilitation of meetings with burn trauma specialists, access to information on prognosis and contact with individuals who have sustained burn trauma previously can all be helpful. Individuals often require support and time to undergo a process similar to a bereavement reaction as a result of their losses.

A cognitive-behavioural approach can be very useful in dealing with many of the issues faced by burn trauma victims. For example an individual with burn scars can often magnify the importance of these, feel unattractive and a failure as a result. This often leads to avoidance of social situations and a restricted lifestyle. It is important not to minimize the impact of the burn trauma but to work in partnership with the individual to reduce psychological distress and improve functioning. Challenging distorted cognitions and a graded exposure approach to help individuals confront situations they have started to avoid, interact with other people and develop strategies to deal with reactions of other people can be beneficial. It may also be helpful to liaise with other specialists involved in the rehabilitation process such as physiotherapists, occupational therapists and camouflage specialists.

Providing a liaison psychiatry service to the burns unit

It is apparent that individuals suffer a variety of psychiatric sequelae following burn trauma and that there is a need for liaison psychiatry input to burns units. Antebi (1993) described the first 12 months of a consultation-liaison psychiatry service to a burns unit in the UK. Burns unit staff requested regular meetings to explore staff concerns about particular patients and rapid access to psychiatric assessment and treatment of specific patients with involvement in discussion of management issues. Even when a formal psychiatric disorder was not present Antebi argued that a psychiatric assessment helped staff to make sense of an individual's presentation.

Mendelsohn (1983) wrote about his experiences at a burns centre in New York. He described four phases of recovery following severe burn trauma, all potentially requiring different types of input. The first phase is dominated by physical issues, pain often being a key issue. In the second phase the full impact of the trauma becomes apparent and treatment to restore functioning is often accompanied by feelings of depression. In the third, recuperative, phase the individual is planning to re-enter life and society, often with prominent identity issues. The fourth phase or social phase involves coping with disfigurement and dysfunction outside the protective environment of the burns unit. He advocated the need for regular team meetings and staff support describing the many difficult issues staff often have to deal with, such as dealing with severely ill individuals, some of whom die.

Individuals are often inpatients for a prolonged period of time, leading to strong bonds being formed. Staff have to view disfigurement and individual's reactions to this as well as the unavoidable infliction of pain on debridement. He argued that the most important thing for the burn trauma victim is warm human contact and that individuals need honest clear information about impairment, treatment and prognosis to promote a sense of control.

There is no evidence that to provide standard interventions to everyone is likely to help. It is apparent that the majority of burn trauma victims do not go on to develop major psychiatric sequelae. As with many liaison psychiatry services, it would therefore seem appropriate to advocate a stepped care approach. Ideally there should be a named person from the department of liaison psychiatry who liaises closely with the burns unit and is their first point of contact. An experienced liaison psychiatry nurse would likely be best placed to take on this role. There should be written information regarding the psychosocial impact of burn trauma and details of self-help organizations for further information such as the charity Changing Faces. Open expression of feelings, emotions and difficulties should be encouraged and considered normal. The staff on the unit should receive training regarding normal psychological reactions following burn trauma, psychiatric difficulties that may be encountered and how to manage them.

Ideally a system should be developed on the burns unit where general nursing and medical care includes psychosocial support and those with more significant difficulties are identified and further assessed by the liaison psychiatry service. There are several potential ways of screening. Standard questionnaires such as the Trauma Screening Questionnaire (Brewin *et al.* 2002) can be used. Individuals who scored above a cut-off would then be offered further assessment, although concerns have been expressed that the routine use of such instruments can be intrusive. Another approach is to ask the burns unit staff to identify individuals they have concerns about and request further assessment of them. It has been shown that the initial impression of staff with no formal mental health training can be a useful predictor of those who go on to develop psychiatric sequelae in facial assault victims (Bisson *et al.* 1997b). Finally, depending on the level of liaison psychiatry input funded, a mental health professional attached to the unit could briefly screen everyone personally or maintain a low threshold for further assessment.

The assessment/screening can often provide an opportunity for brief education regarding the normal trauma response and how to deal with it. Ideally this input would be provided by non-mental health professionals under supervision and be seen as part of routine care. When more significant mental health issues are suspected individuals should be offered a full assessment to determine the presence of psychiatric disorder or other issues and an appropriate management plan developed. As stated previously conditions such as depression and PTSD should be treated according to evidence-based guidelines. Ideally individuals would be able to choose between different pharmacological and psychological approaches. For example, individuals suffering from post-traumatic stress disorder can be offered treatment with antidepressant medication, cognitive-behavioural therapy and eye movement desensitization and reprocessing (Bisson 2002). The more complex the presentation the more complex the intervention that is likely to be required. It is common for individuals to require input from several members of a multidisciplinary liaison psychiatry team and a comprehensive mental health care plan following discharge from the burns unit.

If an individual has a self-inflicted burn trauma, particularly as a result of a suicide attempt, it is important that an urgent full mental health assessment is arranged. This should include a full risk assessment with particular vigilance being taken to accurately assess the risk of a further suicide attempt. This may result in appropriate precautions being required during their inpatient stay on the burns unit such as one-to-one nursing with a registered mental nurse.

Conclusion

Psychological difficulties following burn trauma are common. Departments of liaison psychiatry have a key role to play in the provision of a service that caters for burn trauma victims' psychosocial needs. The service is likely to include the education of staff, development of systems that provide basic education to all patients and their relatives, detects individuals who have more significant needs and co-ordinates and provides evidence-based management for these.

REFERENCES

Adler, A. (1943). Neuropsychiatric complications in victims of Boston's Coconut Grove disaster. *Journal of the American Medical Association*, **123**, 1098–101.

Antebi, D. (1993). The psychiatrist on the burns unit. *Burns*, **19**, 43–6.

Bisson, J. I. (2000). The Effectiveness of Psychological Debriefing for Victims of Acute Burn Trauma. DM Thesis, University of Southampton.

Bisson, J. I. (2002). Post-traumatic stress disorder. *Clinical Evidence*, **7**, 913–19.

Bisson, J., Jenkins, P., Alexander, J., *et al.* (1997a). A randomised controlled trial of psychological debriefing for victims of acute burn trauma. *British Journal of Psychiatry*, **171**, 78–81.

Bisson, J. I., Shepherd, J. P. and Dhutia, M. (1997b). Psychological sequelae of facial trauma. *Journal of Trauma, Injury, Infection and Critical Care*, **43**, 496–500.

Blank, K. and Perry, S. (1984). Relationship of psychological processes during delirium to outcome. *American Journal of Psychiatry*, **141**, 843–7.

Bowden, M. L., Feller, I., Tholen, D., *et al.* (1980). Self-esteem of severely burned patients. *Archives of Physical Medicine Rehabilitation*, **61**, 449–52.

Brewin, C. R., Andrews, B. and Valentine, J. D. (2000). Meta-analysis of risk factors for posttraumatic stress disorder in trauma-exposed adults. *Journal of Consulting and Clinical Psychology*, **68**, 748–66.

Brewin, C. R., Rose, S., Andrews, B., *et al.* (2002). Brief screening instrument for post-traumatic stress disorder. *British Journal of Psychiatry*, **181**, 158–62.

Browne, G., Byrne, C., Brown, B., *et al.* (1985). Psychosocial adjustment of burn survivors. *Burns*, **12**, 28–35.

Bryant, R. A., Harvey, A. G., Dang, S. T., *et al.* (1998). Treatment of acute stress disorder: a comparison of cognitive-behavioral therapy and supportive counselling. *Journal of Consulting and Clinical Psychology*, **66**, 862–6.

Difede, J., Jaffe, A. B., Musngi, G., *et al.* (1997). Determinants of pain expression in hospitalized burn patients. *Pain*, **72**, 245–51.

Ehde, D. M., Patterson, D. R., Wiechman, S. A., *et al.* (1999). Post-traumatic stress symptoms and distress following acute injury. *Burns*, **25**, 587–92.

Frank, H. A., Berry, C., Wachtel, T. L., *et al.* (1987). The impact of thermal injury. *Journal of Burn Care and Rehabilitation*, **8**, 260–2.

Green, B. L., Grace, M. C., Lindy, J. D., *et al.* (1983). Levels of functional impairment following a civilian disaster: the Beverly Hills supper club fire. *Journal of Consulting and Clinical Psychology*, **51**, 573–80.

Kessler, R. C., Sonnega, A., Bromet, E., *et al.* (1995). Post-traumatic stress disorder in the national comorbidity survey. *Archives of General Psychiatry*, **52**, 1048–60.

Mendelsohn, I. E. (1983). Liaison psychiatry and the burn center. *Psychosomatics*, **24**, 235–43.

Neal, L. A., Busuttil, W., Rollins, J., *et al.* (1994). Convergent validity of measures of post-traumatic stress disorder in a mixed civilian and military population. *Journal of Traumatic Stress*, **7**, 447–55.

Office for National Statistics. (2000). *1999 Mortality Statistics Cause England and Wales.* London: HMSO.

Patterson, D. R., Everett, J. J., Bombardier, C. H., *et al.* (1993). Psychological effects of severe burn injuries. *Psychological Bulletin*, **113**, 362–78.

Perry, S. W., Cella, D. F., Falkenberg, J., *et al.* (1987). Pain perception in burn patients with stress disorders. *Journal of Pain Symptom Management*, **2**, 29–33.

Perry, S., Difede, M. A., Musngi, R. N., *et al.* (1992). Predictors of post-traumatic stress disorder after burn injury. *American Journal of Psychiatry*, **149**, 931–5.

Robert, R., Blakeney, P. E., Villarreal, C., *et al.* (1999). Imipramine treatment in pediatric burn patients with symptoms of acute stress disorder: a pilot study. *Journal of the American Academy of Child and Adolescent Psychiatry*, **38**, 873–82.

Rose, S., Bisson, J. and Wessely, S. (2001). *A Systematic Review of Brief Psychological Interventions ('debriefing') for the Treatment of Immediate Trauma Related Symptoms and the Prevention of Post-traumatic Stress Disorder.* The Cochrane Library, Oxford: Update Software Inc.

Saxe, G., Stoddard, F., Courtney, D., *et al.* (2001). Relationship between acute morphine and the course of PTSD in children with burns. *Journal of the American Academy of Child and Adolescent Psychiatry*, **40**, 915–21.

Sgroi, M. I., Willebrand, M., Ekselius, L., *et al.* (2005). Gerhard. Fear-avoidance in recovered burn patients: association with psychological and somatic symptoms. *Journal of Health Psychology*, **10**, 491–502.

Sheffield, C. G., Irons, G. B., Mucha, P., *et al.* (1988). Physical and psychological outcome after burns. *Journal of Burn Care and Rehabilitation*, **9**, 172–7.

Sonneborn, C. K. and Vanstraelen, P. M. (1992). A retrospective study of self-inflicted burns. *General Hospital Psychiatry*, **14**, 404–7.

Stanovic, J. K., James, K. A. and Vandevere, C. A. (2001). The effectiveness of risperidone on acute stress symptoms in acute burn patients: a preliminary retrospective pilot study. *Journal of Burn Care and Rehabilitation*, **22**, 210–13.

Stokes, D. J., Dritschel, B. H. and Bekerian, D. A. (2004). The effect of burn injury on adolescents, autobiographical memory. *Behaviour Research and Therapy*, **42**, 1357–65.

Taal, S. A. and Faber, A. W. (1998). Posttraumatic stress and maladjustment among adult burn survivors 1–2 years postburn. *Burns*, **24**, 285–92.

Ward, H. W., Moss, R. L., Darko, D. F., *et al.* (1987). Prevalence of postburn depression following burn injury. *Journal of Burn Care and Rehabilitation*, **8**, 294–8.

Wiechman, S. A. and Patterson, D. R. (2004). ABC of burns: psychosocial aspects of burn injuries. *British Medical Journal*, **329**, 391–3.

Wilkinson, E. (1998). The epidemiology of burns in secondary care, in a population of 2.6 million people. *Burns*, **24**, 139–43.

White, A. C. (1982). Psychiatric study of patients with severe burn injuries. *British Medical Journal*, **284**, 465–7.

30

Psychocutaneous disorders

Nora Turjanski

Introduction

A relationship between dermatological conditions and psychological factors has long been observed. It has been estimated that approximately a third of the patients presenting with dermatological disorders have some psychological comorbidity (Rostenberg 1960). Several possible mechanisms explain this association. The dermis and brain share a common embryological origin. Also, because the skin is exposed to view, dermatological conditions that affect appearance may elicit reactions from other people that impact on the sufferer (Van Moffaert 1992).

The term psychocutaneous disorder describes several distinct psychiatric disorders in which the skin is affected. Koblenzer (1999) has proposed that these conditions can be loosely grouped into:

- psychiatric disorders in which the skin is the focus of symptoms
- dermatological disorders in which psychological distress contributes to the degree of severity
- psychiatric disorders secondary to chronic dermatological or disfiguring conditions.

Patients with psychocutaneous disorders usually attend dermatology clinics and may be reluctant to accept referral to a psychiatrist (Table 30.1).

Psychiatric disorders that have the skin as primary target

Psychogenic parasitosis

Psychogenic parasitosis includes conditions in which a person has a belief that he or she is suffering an infestation with living organisms despite a lack of evidence that such infestation exists.

Handbook of Liaison Psychiatry, ed. Geoffrey Lloyd and Elspeth Guthrie. Published by Cambridge University Press. © Cambridge University Press 2007.

Table 30.1. Psychocutaneous disorders.

Psychiatric disorders that have the skin as a primary target
- Psychogenic parasitosis
  Delusions of parasitosis
- Self-inflicted skin disorder syndromes
  Dermatitis artefacta
  Self-inflicted dermatosis: pruritus
  - prurigo nodularis
  - chronic lichen simplex
  - neurotic or psychogenic excoriations
  Trichotillomania
- Obsessional concerns: body dysmorphic disorder

Dermatological disorders influenced by psychological factors
- Pruritus and urticarias
- Acne vulgaris
- Psychogenic purpura syndromes
- Alopecia areata
- Chronic inflammatory skin disease
Psoriasis
Atopic dermatitis

Psychological reactions to chronic dermatological or disfiguring conditions

Note: Modified form Koblenzer (1999).

The differential diagnosis of psychogenic parasitosis includes a true parasitic infestation and medical disorders such as tuberculosis, lymphoma, syphilis, diabetes mellitus, renal and hepatic diseases, and vitamin B_{12} and folate deficiency. A variety of neurological conditions such as Parkinson's disease, Huntington's disease, cerebral infarct and brain tumours should also be excluded. Psychogenic parasitosis can result from use of toxics such as amphetamines, methylphenidate, cocaine or alcohol and medications like phenelzine (a monoamine-oxidase inhibitor) and corticosteroids (Arnold 2000; Koblenzer 1999).

From a psychiatric perspective beliefs of infestation may be sustained with a variable degree of conviction spanning from the non-delusional to the delusional. Therefore, a patient complaining of being infested with parasites may be suffering from obsessional thoughts or from a delusional disorder. Some patients may present with both obsessional and delusional thinking (Arnold 2000).

Delusions of parasitosis (Ekbom's disease)

Delusional parasitosis or delusions of infestation may be part of the spectrum of psychotic symptoms in schizophrenia or an affective psychosis. However, at times patients may have an isolated delusion of infestation without other associated psychotic symptoms. Monosymptomatic delusion of parasitosis (MDP) was initially described by Ekbom in 1938. Thereafter it has been generally mentioned in case reports or small series (Trabert 1995).

It has been suggested that MDP is an uncommon condition, although its true prevalence is unknown as sufferers present to dermatologists rather than to psychiatrists, but also to pest control agencies and entomologists (Lyell 1983). It appears to have an equal sex distribution in younger patients and a 3:1 female to male ratio in patients older than 50 years. Onset may be at any age with the highest incidence between the ages of 50 and 80 (Lyell 1983; Trabert 1995). MDP presents as a 'folie a deux' in up to 15% of cases, more commonly affecting spouses or mother—son, mother—daughter relationships (Bourgeois *et al.* 1992; Trabert 1999).

The presentation usually includes a history of potential or actual exposure to organisms which leads to delusional elaboration. Social isolation, visual or auditory impairment as well as recent psychosocial stressors may contribute to its development (Koblenzer 1999). Patients with this condition believe that they are infested with parasites. They report seeing and feeling parasites on the surface or under their skin and are dominated by anxiety and profound preoccupation with this delusional belief. Patients give a detailed history of the characteristics and life cycles of the parasites and of their skin lesions. They describe parasites located anywhere including their scalp or under their nails. Patients may complain that the parasites appear or disappear through natural body orifices or that they are invisible. Their stories may be very convincing. Patients take much effort in trying to rid themselves of the infestation. Usually they attempt treating it themselves washing the affected areas repeatedly, applying insecticides or introducing needles under their skin to pick out the alleged parasites. They may burn their clothes in an attempt to stop the 'infestation' (Koblenzer 1999). Patients may experience associated tactile hallucinations such as crawling, biting or stinging (Arnold 2000). These beliefs are held with unshakeable conviction and a psychological explanation is adamantly rejected.

Patients with MDP sometimes bring a box containing some 'evidence' of the presence of the offending agent. When examined microscopically the box tends to contain small parts of excoriated skin, blood, nails or dirt. Patients may present with intact skin or with excoriations, ulcers and linear scars on easily reached areas of the body. Lesions tend to be more profuse on the side of the body accessible to their dominant hand. There may be dermatitis secondary to the use of caustics and insecticides. The skin lesions tend to involve the face, especially ears, nose and eyes. Forearms, legs, and trunk may also be affected. Pathological findings are non-specific. On rare occasions there is an additional infection or underlying scabies (Koblenzer 1999).

Patients with MDP have a history of moving from doctor to doctor in search of somebody who will believe them. Although MDP is an encapsulated delusion it tends to have a severe impact on patients' lives. Social isolation and loss of employment often result from this disorder. There are occasional reports of severe mutilations (Wang & Lee 1997), of patients committing suicide (Monk & Rao 1994) and of violence against others (Bourgeois *et al.* 1992).

Related disorders are formication and bromosis. Formication is an unpleasant form of tactile hallucinations. Patients feel the movements of animals or insects crawling over the body or under their skin. It is especially associated with illicit drugs and toxic states. Delusions of bromosis describe patients who believe they emit a bad body odour that drives people away from them.

The treatment of psychogenic parasitosis and of the related disorders requires appropriate diagnosis, excluding any metabolic, toxic or neurological cause. Dermatological treatment is topical and symptomatic.

Psychiatric treatment depends on the underlying psychopathology. If possible patients should be referred to the psychiatric services. Obsessional patients may be more tolerant of this referral while patients with delusional beliefs usually reject it despite their intense suffering. If that is the case, a useful approach is an emphatic attitude from the dermatologist without colluding with the delusions. Frequent brief visits to the dermatologist help to maintain continuity and establish a rapport, which will then enable appropriate treatment (Koblenzer 1999; Koo & Pham 1992). When referral to the psychiatrist is not accepted the dermatologist should tactfully initiate treatment with an antipsychotic. Uncontrolled trials suggest that pimozide in doses of up to 12 mg a day is useful in this condition (Ait-Ameur *et al.* 2000; Koblenzer 1999; Koo & Pham 1992; Munro 1988). There are uncontrolled reports of efficacy with atypical antipsychotics such as risperidone, which have a safer profile of side-effects (Elmer *et al.* 2000; Koo & Lee 2001; Wenning *et al.* 2003). Antidepressants are useful in patients with depression or associated obsessive-compulsive symptoms. The role of psycho-therapy in the treatment of this condition is unclear (Ait-Ameur *et al.* 2000; Arnold 2000).

It has been suggested that approximately half of the patients with MDP will respond to treatment with antipsychotics although symptomatic improvement may require several months of treatment (Arnold 2000; Bhatia *et al.* 2000). Recovery is not usually associated with acquisition of insight. Relapses may occur and maintenance therapy is then required (Koblenzer 1999).

Self-inflicted skin disorders

The International Classification of Disease-10 (ICD-10) defines factitious disorders as those characterized by physical or psychological symptoms that are intentionally produced or feigned in order to assume the sick role. However, there is a confusing use of this terminology. Factitious syndrome is sometimes used in the literature to refer to all disorders that present with self-inflicted lesions including delusional parasitosis. In this chapter the ICD-10 definition of factitious disorder will be followed.

Koblenzer (1999) has suggested that self-inflicted lesions should be grouped as follows according to whether the patient acknowledges the self-inflicting nature of the lesions:

1. Dermatitis artefacta or factitious dermatitis: the patient denies responsibility for the lesions; the motivation may be conscious or unconscious. This disorder should be differentiated from malingering in which the lesions are produced consciously but deceitfully to obtain or preserve a secondary gain as opposed to the psychological gain that motivates patients with factitious disorder. This distinction can be difficult to make in practice.

2. Self-inflicted dermatosis and cutaneous compulsions: self-inflicted lesions and lesions that result from conscious and repetitive actions.

Dermatitis artefacta

Dermatitis artefacta comprises a variety of lesions that are induced by the patient to obtain a psychological gain. This condition is seen more commonly in females with female-to-male ratios ranging from 3:1 to 20:1 (Koblenzer 2000). Although it can occur at any age it is more frequent in adolescents and young adults. The patient usually inflicts lesions on her or himself but lesions can be produced in others, especially in children, in which case it is a form of Munchausen's syndrome by proxy. This particular form of dermatitis artefacta results from a dysfunctional mother—child relationship and reflects physical and emotional abuse. Most commonly adult sufferers have a personality disorder with borderline traits (Koblenzer 1987). Cutaneous injuring is often a tension-releasing habit (Van Moffaert 1992). In less severe cases, self-injurious behaviour may result from anxiety or an adjustment disorder. Psychosocial stressors are commonly present as well as a secondary gain, of which the patient is not consciously aware, which maintains the self-destructive behaviour. A large proportion of patients have worked in healthcare or have relatives who have worked in healthcare services.

Patients present to the physician with a variety of lesions. The morphology of the lesions depends on how these were inflicted, either by scratching, or by use of mechanical means, application of toxic or caustic materials, or heat. Lesions can be single or multiple, bilateral and symmetrical, small or extensive. They are often linear or have a geometric outline and are clearly demarcated from normal skin. They can be bizarre in outline with surface necrosis. The lesions can masquerade as numerous clinical conditions. The damage to the skin may be superficial or severe. It may leave scarring and on occasions may require amputation if blood supply has been occluded by ligatures. Skin lesions tend to be within easy reach of the dominant hand. Facial involvement, including lesions in the periocular areas, is relatively common (Ugurlu *et al.* 1999). Pathological findings are non-specific and depend on how the injuries were induced.

Lyell described the 'hollow history' provided by the patient with unobtainable descriptions about possible causes and evolution of the lesions (Lyell 1979). The patient remains undisturbed by the disfiguring effects and eventual pain caused by these lesions. He or she appears compliant with treatment but the condition has an unremitting course. Admission to hospital or occlusive bandaging transiently improves the lesions but occlusive dressings are later removed and the lesions perpetuated. The patient denies any responsibility for these lesions. The diagnosis is based in the morphology of the lesions, affect and personality of the patient as well as prior presence of unexplained medical illnesses and psychosocial stress (Koblenzer 1999).

Treatment requires the development of a therapeutic alliance between physician and patient. The patient's denial of psychic distress and the negative feelings evoked in the physician may make management difficult. The patient experiences confrontation as a threat and this will provoke further acting out or withdrawal from treatment. Therefore issues of aetiology should be avoided. An empathic approach may gradually allow recognition of the distress and enable the patient to accept a psychiatric referral. When psychiatric referral is refused by the patient the appropriate use of psychotropics by dermatologists may be useful. Underlying psychological conditions such as depression require appropriate drug treatment. High doses of serotonin-specific reuptake inhibitors (SSRIs) or low doses of atypical antipsychotic agents may be helpful (Garnis-Jones *et al.* 2000; Gupta & Gupta 2001; Koblenzer 2000). Less severe cases may be able to relinquish symptoms with support. Psychotherapy may be of help in more severe cases. The prognosis depends on the underlying psychological problem. In children a less severe and short-lasting illness may improve with parental education that allows the family to identify the stressors. More severe cases require involvement of a child psychiatrist or eventually child-care agencies. In adults the prognosis is poor except in mild transient cases, which developed in response to stress (Koblenzer 2000).

The condition has a fluctuating course with relapses depending on the circumstances of the patient's life. It has been suggested that a way to minimize lesions and costs is for the dermatologist to continue seeing the patients for supervision and support independently of the presence of lesions (Koblenzer 2000).

Self-inflicted dermatosis

Pruritus

Pruritus is common in dermatological disorders. Itching, a subjective sensation that leads to a desire to scratch, is the predominant symptom of inflammatory skin disease. Stress and pruritus have a complex association. Scratching may be a response to stress and in turn stress can reduce the itch threshold (Arnold 2000; Picardi & Abeni 2001).

Pruritus can be caused by a variety of metabolic conditions or be psychogenic in origin. Psychogenic pruritus could be localized or diffuse and lead to profuse excoriation. Pruritus may be associated with psychogenic parasitosis as already described (Greaves & Wall 1999). Common underlying psychological disturbances include depression and anxiety, which should be treated appropriately (Greaves & Wall 1999). SSRIs are potentially beneficial. Tricyclic antidepressants such as doxepin, amitriptyline and trimipramine are also useful in urticaria and pruritus due to their histamine H_1-blocking effects (Gupta & Gupta 2001). Behavioural interventions such as aversion therapy and token economy have also been advocated for this condition (Van Moffaert 1992; Daniels 1973).

Specific forms of chronic pruritus may result from habitual scratching and include:

1. Prurigo nodularis: this condition has an unclear aetiology. Some patients complain of intense itching, while others have habitual scratching. These patients present with hard irregular nodules in the skin of arms or legs. Treatment includes topical measures and adequate diagnosis and treatment of any underlying psychiatric condition including depression and anxiety (Habif 2004).

2. Chronic lichen simplex: this is an eczematous eruption caused by repeated habitual scratching. The person derives pleasure from intense scratching of the inflamed area. The role of stress remains controversial (Habif 2004; Picardi & Abeni 2001). Most frequently it affects the legs, genito-anal areas, wrists and ankles, eyelids, back and side of neck, ears, extensor forearms and scalp. The skin in the area is covered by a thick plaque with accentuation of skin lines. Appropriate treatment of this condition requires that the patient stops scratching. However this habit may occur during sleep and therefore the affected area has to be covered. Steroids may be helpful. Naltrexone may be helpful to reduce pruritic symptoms. Helpful techniques are habit-reversal training and cognitive-behavioural therapy (Habif 2004).

3. Neurotic or psychogenic excoriations: patients present with skin lesions caused by scratching or picking in response to an itch or to extract imaginary pieces of material that they feel are embedded or protruding from the skin

(Fruensgaard *et al.* 1979). Itching and digging become compulsive rituals. Patients are fully aware that they induce the lesions but are unable to resist the compulsion. It has an incidence of approximately 2% in dermatological clinics with a predominance of women (Arnold *et al.* 2001). It may occur at any age although it is frequently secondary to acne which begins in adolescence but can persist into adulthood (Van Moffaert 1992). There are lesions of similar size and shape. They are grouped in areas that can be easily reached such as arms, legs and upper back. Recurrent picking at crusts delays healing and may leave behind white scars surrounded by hyperpigmentation (Habif 2004; Koblenzer 1987).

Patients with chronic pruritus usually have perfectionist and compulsive traits. They may present with repressed aggression and self-destructive behaviour and report that attempting to resist excoriation is ego-dystonic. They may experience increased tension before the picking with transient relief afterwards (Stein & Hollander 1992). Skin-picking has been considered to fit within the spectrum of obsessive-compulsive and impulse-control disorders (Arnold *et al.* 1998, 2001; Stein & Hollander 1992; Wilhelm *et al.* 1999).

Patients sometimes describe a preoccupation with an irregularity of the skin or concerns about having smooth skin. On occasions, the degree of the preoccupation is severe enough to meet criteria for body dysmorphic disorder (BDD; Arnold *et al.* 1998; Phillips & Taub 1995). Patients may pick at their skin as a way to eradicate the 'defect'. In patients with skin picking resulting from BDD there is a higher psychosocial morbidity (Phillips & Taub 1995). Rarely, the severity of the skin picking has a delusional quality. The patient may induce deep wounds with resulting infections and severe morbidity (O'Sullivan *et al.* 1999).

The spectrum of severity ranges from an occasional symptom which only surfaces under stress to a severe compulsive behaviour that affects every aspect of the patient's life. This condition has also been associated with depression and with other body image problems such as eating disorders (Arnold *et al.* 2001). A significant psychosocial stressor has been found in up to 90% of patients. Dermatological treatment includes topical steroids and occlusion. Patients should be encouraged to substitute the ritual of applying lubricants to the affected skin instead of the ritual of digging (Habif 2004).

Psychiatric treatment will depend on symptom severity. Mild cases usually resolve with empathic support and dermatological measures. Longer-standing or more severe cases require additional measures. Psychiatric screening may identify an underlying disturbance. Depression should be appropriately treated. Because of its association with obsessive-compulsive behaviour SSRIs are the current drugs of choice for skin-picking disorder, but case reports include treatment with doxepin, clomipramine, naltrexone, pimozide and olanzapine

(Arnold *et al.* 2001; O'Sullivan *et al.* 1999; Phillips & Taub 1995). There are reports of successful treatment with behavioural interventions, especially with habit reversal techniques, but no controlled studies have been reported (Arnold *et al.* 2001). In certain cases insight oriented psychotherapy may be useful (Van Moffaert 1992).

Trichotillomania

The essential feature is recurrent pulling of the individual's own hair which results in hair loss. This may be associated with an increased sense of tension before the act or attempts to resist the urge to pull the hair. It may have a compulsive quality. There is a sense of gratification or relief when pulling the hair. In ICD-10 trichotillomania is classified as a habit and impulse disorder. Transient periods of hair pulling in childhood may be considered a 'habit' with a self-limiting course. Trichotillomania may be a manifestation of any psychiatric disorder but may also present as an isolated symptom.

The peak onset is in childhood. Females predominate after the age of two with a female-to-male ratio of 5:1. When the condition starts in adolescence it is more difficult to treat due to the accompanying shame and denial (Koblenzer 1999). It has been suggested that this condition reflects a dysfunctional family environment which results in poor impulse control. In early childhood hair pulling may reflect an anxiety disorder (Wright & Holmes 2003).

It usually affects the scalp hair, but other body hair may be pulled as well. Plucking may be confined to special times and places with a ritualized manipulation of the pulled hairs or ingestion which may lead to the formation of trichobezoars and thence to intestinal obstruction. The affected areas present with hairs at different stages of growth scattered around empty follicles. Treatment is similar to that of neurotic excoriations (Koblenzer 1999; Sticher *et al.* 1980).

Body dysmorphic disorder or dysmorphophobia

Patients with body dysmorphic disorder (BDD) have an intense preoccupation with an imagined defect of their body or skin or with a gross exaggeration of a minor defect in appearance. To fulfil Diagnostic and Statistical Manual-IV (DSM-IV) criteria of BDD the preoccupation must additionally cause significant distress or impairment in social, occupational or other areas of functioning. In ICD-10, BDD is classified under hypochondriacal disorder (see also Chapter 26).

The preoccupation in BDD may present with a variable degree of conviction ranging from an overvalued idea to a delusional belief. BDD appears to have some relationship to obsessive-compulsive and mood disorders, but a significant proportion of patients are psychotic (Phillips *et al.* 1994). Commonly, patients present with ideas or delusions of reference, believing that people around them notice their 'defect' and evaluate them accordingly (Veale 2004).

Body dysmorphic disorder usually begins during adolescence (Phillips *et al.* 1993). Although some series contain more females and others more males, large adult series have found that DBB affects the genders equally (Phillips & Diaz 1997; Veale 2004). The estimated prevalence in the population is 0.7% with a higher peak amongst adolescents and young adults (Bohne *et al.* 2002; Faravelli *et al.* 1997; Otto *et al.* 2001). The site of the body that becomes target of the preoccupations tends to differ between sexes and is culturally influenced (Phillips & Diaz 1997). Comorbidity varies according to gender, with bulimia nervosa being more common in women and alcohol abuse or dependence in men. Depression is equally prevalent in both genders (Koblenzer 1999; Phillips & Diaz 1997).

Patients usually present preoccupied with their 'defect'. Any part of the body may be affected although most commonly the preoccupations are centred on the skin, hair, nose or other facial features (Phillips *et al.* 1993). The complaint may be very specific or patients may have a vague sense of ugliness (Veale 2004). Patients with BDD repeatedly check their appearance in mirrors and other reflective surfaces. They have to reassure themselves about their appearance, even using a magnifying glass to check their 'defect'. Although checking is aimed to reduce the anxiety it has the opposite effect of intensifying the preoccupation. Thus some patients will subsequently avoid mirrors, covering them or removing them from their environment (Veale 2004).

Patients spend many hours engaged in excessive grooming. They may attempt to camouflage the perceived defect with make-up or clothes (Veale 2004). Skin picking is a frequent manifestation with consequent skin infection and scarring (O'Sullivan *et al.* 1999). Every aspect of the patient's life is affected. There is little insight. Shame, self-consciousness and therefore social withdrawal are common resulting in school refusal or social phobia. In adolescents a majority experience academic difficulties (Albertini & Phillips 1999). In adults there is a significant level of social interference (Phillips & Diaz 1997). Severe cases have a high rate of hospitalizations (Phillips & Diaz 1997). Numerous doctors are consulted with demands for treatment, especially surgery. Suicidal ideation and suicidal attempts are relatively common with similar rates in both genders (Koblenzer 1999; Phillips & Diaz 1997; Veale 2004).

Emerging data suggest that psychiatric treatment of BDD is effective. Because of its relationship with obsessive-compulsive disorders, SSRIs are the current first-line antidepressants. This recommendation also applies to BDD presenting in children and adolescents (Albertini & Phillips 1999; Phillips 1996). In adults, antidepressants should be used in high doses for at least 12 weeks (Veale 2004).

Delusional cases require additional antipsychotic treatment. Low doses of antipsychotic may be used as adjunct treatment in resistant cases that failed to respond to two or more SSRIs (Veale 2004). There is some evidence that cognitive behavioural therapy is effective (Phillips 1996; Veale 2004).

Body dysmorphic disorder patients commonly present to dermatologists or to cosmetic surgeons. Patients often request surgical interventions and other drastic cosmetic procedures although results are usually unsatisfactory. In a reported study of BDD patients 45% had received at least one dermatological treatment and 20% had undergone a surgical procedure (Phillips *et al.* 2001). The nose is one of the commonest preoccupations in BDD and therefore requests for surgical rhinoplasty were seen in almost half of these patients (Phillips *et al.* 2001). Retrospective surveys suggest a poor outcome of dermatological treatments and cosmetic surgery without marked changes in the severity of BDD symptoms. Patients tend to have repeated interventions, transfer the preoccupation to another area of the body and generally be dissatisfied with results. However, it has been observed that in a small proportion of patients with mild BDD (cases without multiple concerns about their body and without comorbidity) cosmetic surgery may be of benefit (Phillips *et al.* 2001; Veale *et al.* 2003).

Dermatological disorders influenced by psychological factors

The role of emotional stress on the course of various skin disorders is frequently accepted by both dermatologists and patients. However, dermatologists' perception of the patients' psychological wellbeing is influenced by their conceptual models of illness. There is some evidence that dermatologists tend to underestimate the degree of psychiatric morbidity in patients with skin disorders (Sampogna *et al.* 2003). Traditionally, it has been accepted that stress has an impact in psoriasis, alopecia areata, atopic dermatitis and urticaria. The role of stressful events has been less clear in vitiligo, acne, lichen planus and seborrhoeic dermatitis (Picardi & Abeni 2001). However, there are few properly controlled studies and hard evidence of a causative link between stress and these dermatological conditions remains scant (Picardi & Abeni 2001). Nevertheless, there is evidence of an association between certain dermatological conditions and increased psychopathology, although the directionality of the causation is unclear.

Pruritus and urticarias

Pruritus and urticarias of any origin can be affected by stress as previously described. It is unclear what percentage is purely psychogenic. Anxiety and depression may be contributory factors and if present should be treated.

Tricyclic antidepressants have potent antihistaminic effects and may relieve pruritus of many origins (Arnold 2000; Koblenzer 1999). Urticaria is characterized by circumscribed pruritic areas of oedema affecting the superficial dermis. It is a common condition with peak presentation between the ages of 20 and 40. It has an equal ratio of male to female in children but in adulthood is more common in women (Koblenzer 1987). It can be acute or chronic. Psychological factors have been implicated in some forms of urticarias (Picardi & Abeni 2001). In chronic urticaria there is a frequent association with depression and anxiety. Adrenergic urticaria develops acutely after an emotional stress and is associated with increased blood levels of adrenaline and noradrenaline. It resolves after treatment with β-adrenoreceptor blockers such as propranolol (Shelley & Shelley 1985).

Acne vulgaris

Acne vulgaris is a common disease of sebaceous glands presenting with a variety of skin lesions, some of which can become secondarily infected and develop scars. Usually this condition develops in adolescence when sebaceous gland activity increases and resolves spontaneously after several years although it may persist in some individuals. In adolescence it is more common in men. The aetiology is multifactorial (Strauss & Thiboutot 1999). There is an association between degree of severity of the acne and degree of anxiety, depression and poor self-image (Gupta & Gupta 1998). This association is bidirectional. Patients often report that acne is aggravated by stress, which in turn may interfere with patients' psychosocial functioning. Acne is frequently the cause of much emotional distress and social dysfunction. Reduction in severity of acne with dermatological treatment improves anxiety and depression but it has also been claimed that biofeedback assisted relaxation may improve acne (Arnold 2000).

Psychogenic purpura syndromes

This condition, also known as autoerythrocyte sensitization syndrome or Gardner–Diamond syndrome, is characterized by the spontaneous appearance of purpura with normal blood and coagulation tests. Generally this disorder is preceded by exposure to surgery or trauma (Archer-Dubon *et al.* 1998). Within hours, patients present with inflammatory skin changes including localized warmth, erythema, swelling and pruritus (Arnold 2000; Koblenzer 1999). Severe pain, malaise and chills, nausea and localized dysaesthesia, as well as bleeding through seemingly intact skin have been observed. Stress triggers relapses. The aetiology is unknown. Autoimmune mechanisms and increased cutaneous fibrinolytic activity have been implicated (Archer-Dubon *et al.* 1998). Patients tend to have pronounced underlying psychopathology. Psychopenic purpura has been described in dissociative (conversion) disorder and also in factitious disorders. The differentiation between the two often remains unclear as in many patients it is difficult to prove intentional self-injury. Interestingly, these lesions have been reported to be reproduced under suggestion and hypnosis (Koblenzer 1999). Patients with psychogenic purpura are vulnerable and require protection from excessive interventions. Antidepressants as well as psychotherapy have been claimed to be effective (Archer-Dubon *et al.* 1998; Koblenzer 1999).

Alopecia areata

Alopecia areata consists of patches of hair loss in well-demarcated areas of smooth skin. It usually involves the scalp but may affect other body hair such as eyelashes or eyebrows in patches. Some patients may present with total hair loss. There is an equal incidence in men and women and peak presentation is between the third and fifth decades of life. Patients may suffer several episodes of alopecia, with 30% never recovering hair growth after the first episode (Arnold 2000). The aetiology of alopecia remains uncertain, although mounting research points towards genetic and autoimmune mechanisms (Price 2003). The role of psychiatric factors remains controversial. Stressful events may trigger the condition in vulnerable individuals (Brajac *et al.* 2003; Picardi & Abeni 2001). Psychiatric referral is indicated in persistent cases. Some patients may benefit from treatment with antidepressants and psychotherapy.

Chronic inflammatory skin disease

Stress may trigger or exacerbate inflammatory disorders in predisposed patients (Picardi & Abeni 2001). The chronicity of these disorders as well as the characteristics of the lesions may in turn induce psychological disturbance.

Psoriasis

Psoriasis is a chronic relapsing disorder which presents with characteristic skin lesions involving the vasculature as well as the epidermis. The morphology of the skin lesions varies from pinpoint plaques to extensive lesions covered with silvery scales or pustular formations. Additionally, psoriasis may be associated with nail dystrophy and arthritis. It affects males and females equally with peak onset in the third decade of life. Early onset is associated with greater severity and a worse response to treatment. For most patients it is a life-long condition with unpredictable relapses (Christophers & Mrowietz 1999; Habif 2004).

The pathogenesis of psoriasis is incompletely understood. Genetic, immuno-logical and environmental factors affect its development and prognosis (Christophers & Mrowietz 1999; Habif 2004). Psoriasis can be induced by β-adrenergic blockers and lithium amongst other medications. Lithium-induced psoriasis resolves with its discontinuation (Krahn & Goldberg 1994).

There is conflicting literature regarding the role of psychosocial stressors in psoriasis. In some patients stress appears to play an important part in the clinical course of this condition. It has been suggested that upsetting life events precede the onset of psoriasis in up to 70% of cases and relapses in up to 90% (Picardi & Abeni 2001). However, the majority of the studies that have examined this association have been uncontrolled or have had methodological problems. Nevertheless, they provide anecdotal evidence of an association between stress and psoriasis (Picardi & Abeni 2001). Recent attention has also focused on the impact of psoriasis on the patient's psychosocial functioning. The chronic course and resulting impaired appearance may affect vulnerable individuals. Feelings of shame and stigmatization may affect all areas of patient's life. A variety of psychopathological disorders appears to be increased in patients with psoriasis (Fried *et al.* 1995; Gupta & Gupta 1998). Depression and obsessionality as well as alcoholism are common findings (Koblenzer 1999).

Adequate psychosocial interventions may improve the course of the disease (Arnold 2000). Patients' psychopathology should be treated according to the degree of severity. Mild cases may be helped by support groups, empathy and relaxation techniques. More severe psychopathology should be treated appropriately.

Atopic dermatitis

Atopic dermatitis is a chronic relapsing skin disorder characterized by pruritus and inflammation. It often begins as an eruption but repeated scratching leads to lichenification, excoriations and infections (Leung *et al.* 1999). It is a common condition with an estimated prevalence of 12% in urban communities (Rothe & Grant-Kels 1996). It can commence at any age but onset during the first five years of life is seen in the great majority of patients. Usually there is a family history of atopic dermatitis. Patients present with dry skin, papules, lichenification, eczematous inflammation and intense itching (Leung *et al.* 1999).

Atopic dermatitis is a multifactorial disorder. Its aetiology includes a genetic and immunological predisposition and environmental triggering factors. Suggestions of a specific personality profile have not been substantiated (Buske-Kirschbaum *et al.* 2001). Increased stress may precipitate or aggravate this condition although the evidence for this remains weak (Buske-Kirschbaum *et al.* 2001; Picardi & Abeni 2001). Stress-induced mechanisms include increased scratching with the consequent releasing of mediators of inflammation. This causes increased itching which in turn promotes scratching, thus perpetuating the cycle (Buske-Kirschbaum *et al.* 2001). It appears that there is a higher rate of anxiety and depression in patients with atopic dermatitis, although this may be a bidirectional association (Arnold 2000; Buske-Kirschbaum *et al.* 2001).

Addressing the psychosocial impact of the condition may be of help and some studies have suggested efficacy of behavioural approaches, relaxation and biofeedback.

Psychological reactions to chronic dermatological or disfiguring conditions

The psychological impact of skin disease has been under-researched, especially in dermatological conditions that result in impaired physical appearance (Papadopoulos et al. 1999). Depression and suicidal ideation are not uncommon in patients suffering disfiguring dermatological conditions. Adolescents and young adults may be more vulnerable to develop depression as a result of the cosmetic impact on their body image and self-esteem (Gupta & Gupta 1998). Completed suicide has been reported in patients suffering with acne or BDD with or without overt psychiatric comorbidity (Cotterill & Cunliffe 1997). Facial scarring as well as longstanding and debilitating inflammatory skin diseases have also been associated with completed suicide (Cotterill & Cunliffe 1997).

There are indications that other skin conditions that induce visible changes such as vitiligo also impact on the individual's self-esteem and psychosocial functioning (Agarwal 1998; Papadopoulos et al. 1999). There is some evidence that cognitive-behavioural therapy (CBT) may help reduce the feelings of stigmatization and improve the psychosocial adjustment of people with vitiligo. Researchers have made preliminary claims that this in turn may affect the progression of the vitiligo (Papadopoulos et al. 1999).

In recent decades there has been an increase in the rate of survival of patients with burn injuries. Studies of burn survivors report increased psychopathological symptoms with up to 40% presenting some form of psychological impairment 12 months after the event. The extent of the burns and facial disfigurement correlates with the prevalence of psychological disturbance (Madianos et al. 2001). A large number of survivors suffer from post-traumatic stress disorder (PTSD) and mood disorders. Pain, somatic complaints and motor impairment also contribute to the distress (Madianos et al. 2001). Those patients most at risk of disfiguring may benefit from early psychiatric and psychosocial intervention (Madianos et al. 2001). (See Chapter 29.)

Face transplantation is now a realistic treatment for people with severe facial disfigurement from burns, trauma or malignant disease. It involves complete removal of the facial soft tissue from a cadaver and transplanting this onto a suitable recipient with the aim of providing a more normal facial appearance than can be achieved by reconstruction alone. There are obvious ethical and psychological problems associated with this procedure, both for the recipient and the deceased donor's family. Careful selection of recipients will be required and appropriate psychological support should be available before the procedure is undertaken. Recipients will need close follow-up to ensure that any psychological problems which develop post-operatively are identified and treated.

REFERENCES

Agarwal, G. (1998). Vitiligo: an under-estimated problem. *Family Practice*, **15**(Suppl. 1), S19−23.

Ait-Ameur, A., Bern, P., Firoloni, M. P., *et al.* (2000). Delusional parasitosis or Ekbom's syndrome. *Revue de Medecine Interne*, **21**(2), 182−6.

Albertini, R. and Phillips, K. A. (1999). Thirty-three cases of body dysmorphic disorder in children and adolescents. *Journal of the American Academy of Child and Adolescent Psychiatry*, **38**(4), 453−9.

Archer-Dubon, C., Orozco-Topete, R. and Reyes-Gutierrez, E. (1998). Two cases of psychogenic purpura. *Revista de Investigacion Clinica*, **50**(2), 145−8.

Arnold, L. M. (2000). Dermatology. In *Psychiatric Care of the Medical Patient*, 2nd edn., ed. A. Stoudemiere, B. S. Fogel and D. B. Greenberg. New York: Oxford University Press, pp. 821−33.

Arnold, L. M., McElroy, S. L., Mutasim, D. F., *et al.* (1998). Characteristics of 34 adults with psychogenic excoriation. *Journal of Clinical Psychiatry*, **59**(10), 509−14.

Arnold, L. M., Auchenbach, M. B. and McElroy, S. L. (2001). Psychogenic excoriation. Clinical features, proposed diagnostic criteria, epidemiology and approaches to treatment. *CNS Drugs*, **15**(5), 351−9.

Bhatia, M. S., Jagawat, T. and Choudhary, S. (2000). Delusional parasitosis: a clinical profile. *International Journal of Psychiatry in Medicine*, **30**(1), 83−91.

Bohne, A., Keuthen, N. J., Wilhelm, S., *et al.* (2002). Prevalence of symptoms of body dysmorphic disorder and its correlates: A cross-cultural comparison. *Psychosomatics*, **43**, 486−90.

Bourgeois, M. L., Duhamel, P. and Verdoux, H. (1992). Delusional parasitosis: folie a deux and attempted murder of a family doctor. *British Journal of Psychiatry*, **161**, 709−11.

Brajac, I., Tkalcic, M., Dragojevic, D. M., *et al.* (2003). Roles of stress, stress perception and trait-anxiety in the onset and course of alopecia areata. *Journal of Dermatology*, **30**(12), 871−8.

Buske-Kirschbaum, A., Geiben, A. and Hellhammer, D. (2001). Psychobiological aspects of atopic dermatitis: an overview. *Psychotherapy and Psychosomatics*, **70**(1), 6−17.

Christophers, E. and Mrowietz, U. (1999). Psoriasis. In *Fitzpatrick's Dermatology in General Medicine*, 5th edn., ed. I. M. Freedberg, A. Z. Eisen, K. Wolff, *et al.* New York: McGraw-Hill, pp. 495−521.

Cotterill, J. A. and Cunliffe, W. J. (1997). Suicide in dermatological patients. *British Journal of Dermatology*, **137**, 246−50.

Daniels, L. K. (1973). Treatment of urticaria and severe headache by behaviour therapy. *Psychosomatics*, **14**, 347−51.

Elmer, K. B., George, R. M. and Peterson, K. (2000). Therapeutic update: use of risperidone for the treatment of monosymptomatic hypochondriacal psychosis. *Journal of the American Academy of Dermatology*, **43**(4), 683–6.

Faravelli, C., Salvatori, S., Galassi, F., *et al.* (1997). Epidemiology of somatoform disorders: a community survey in Florence. *Social Psychiatry & Psychiatric Epidemiology*, **32**, 24–9.

Fried, R. G., Friedman, S., Paradis, C., *et al.* (1995). Trivial or terrible? The psychosocial impact of psoriasis. *International Journal of Dermatology*, **34**(2), 101–5.

Fruensgaard, K., Hjortshoj, A. and Nielsen, H. (1979). Neurotic excoriations. *International Journal of Dermatology*, **17**, 761–7.

Garnis-Jones, S., Collins, S. and Rosenthal, D. (2000). Treatment of self-mutilation with olanzapine. *Journal of Cutaneous Medicine and Surgery*, **4**(3), 161–3.

Greaves, M. W. and Wall, P. D. (1999). Pathophysiology and clinical aspects of pruritus. In *Fitzpatrick's Dermatology in General Medicine*. 5th edn., ed. I. M. Freedberg, A. Z. Eisen, K. Wolff, *et al.* New York: McGraw-Hill, pp. 487–93.

Gupta, M. A and Gupta, A. K. (1998). Depression and suicidal ideation in dermatology patients with acne, alopecia areata, atopic dermatitis and psoriasis. *British Journal of Dermatology*, **139**, 846–50.

Gupta, M. A. and Gupta, A. K. (2001). The use of antidepressant drugs in dermatology. *Journal of the European Academy of Dermatology and Venereology*, **15**(6), 512–18.

Habif, T. P. (2004). *Clinical Dermatology. A Colour Guide to Diagnosis and Therapy*, 4th edn. Philadelphia: Mosby.

Krahn, L. E. & Goldberg, R. L. (1994). Psychotropic medications and the skin. In *Psychotropic Use in the Medically Ill*, vol. 21, ed. P. A. Silver. Basel: S Karger AG, pp. 90–106.

Koblenzer, C. S. (1987). *Psychocutaneous Disease*. Orlando: Grune & Stratton.

Koblenzer, C. S. (1999). Psychological aspects of skin disease. In *Fitzpatrick's Dermatology in General Medicine*, 5th edn., ed. I. M. Freedberg, A. Z. Eisen, K. Wolff, *et al.* New York: McGraw-Hill, pp. 475–86.

Koblenzer, C. S. (2000). Dermatitis artefacta. Clinical features and approaches to treatment. *American Journal of Clinical Dermatology*, **1**(1), 47–55.

Koo, J. and Lee, C. S. (2001). Delusions of parasitosis. A dermatologist's guide to diagnosis and treatment. *American Journal of Clinical Dermatology*, **2**(5), 285–90.

Koo, J. Y. M. and Pham, C. T. (1992). Psychodermatology. Practical guidelines on pharmacotherapy. *Archives of Dermatology*, **128**, 381–8.

Leung, D. Y. M., Tharp, M. & Boguniewicz, M. (1999). Atopic dermatitis (atopic eczema). In *Fitzpatrick's Dermatology in General Medicine*, 5th edn., ed. I. M. Freedberg, A. Z. Eisen, K. Wolff, *et al.* New York: McGraw-Hill, pp. 1464–80.

Lyell, A. (1979). Cutaneous artefactual disease: a review amplified by personal experience. *Journal of the American Academy of Dermatology*, **1**, 391–407.

Lyell, A. (1983). The Michelson lecture, delusions of parasitosis. *British Journal of Dermatology*, **108**, 485–99.

Madianos, M. G., Papaghelis, M., Ioannovich, J., *et al.* (2001). Psychiatric disorders in burn patients: a follow-up study. *Psychotherapy and Psychosomatics*, **70**, 30–8.

Monk, B. E. and Rao, J. (1994). Delusions of parasitosis with fatal outcome. *Clinical and Experimental Dermatology*, **19**, 341–2.

Munro, A. (1988). Monosymptomatic hypochondriacal psychosis. *British Journal of Psychiatry*, **153**(Suppl.), 37–40.

O'Sullivan, R., Phillips, K. A., Keuthen, N. J., *et al.* (1999). Near-fatal skin picking from delusional body dysmorphic disorder responsive to fluvoxamine. *Psychosomatics*, **40**, 79–82.

Otto, M. W., Wilhelm, S., Cohen, L. S., *et al.* (2001). Prevalence of body dysmorphic disorder in a community sample of women. *American Journal of Psychiatry*, **158**(12), 2061–3.

Papadopoulos, L., Bor, R. and Legg, C. (1999). Coping with the disfiguring effects of vitiligo: a preliminary investigation into the effects of cognitive behavioural therapy. *British Journal of Medical Psychology*, **72**, 385–96.

Phillips, K. A. (1996). Body dysmorphic disorder: diagnosis and treatment of imagined ugliness. *Journal of Clinical Psychiatry*, **57**(Suppl. 8), 61–4.

Phillips, K. A. and Diaz, S. F. (1997). Gender differences in body dysmorphic disorder. *The Journal of Nervous and Mental Disease*, **185**, 570–7.

Phillips, K. A. and Taub, S. L. (1995). Skin picking as a symptom of body dysmorphic disorder. *Psychopharmacology Bulletin*, **31**(2), 279–88.

Phillips, K. A., McElroy, S. L., Keck, P. E. Jr, *et al.* (1993). Body dysmorphic disorder: 30 cases of imagined ugliness. *American Journal of Psychiatry*, **150**(2), 302–8.

Phillips, K. A., McElroy, S. L., Keck, P. E. Jr., *et al.* (1994). A comparison of delusional and non-delusional body dysmorphic disorder in 100 cases. *Psychopharmacology Bulletin*, **30**(2), 179–86.

Phillips, K. A., Grant, J., Siniscalchi, J., *et al.* (2001). Surgical and non-psychiatric medical treatment of patients with body dysmorphic disorder. *Psychosomatics*, **42**(6), 504–10.

Picardi, A. and Abeni, D. (2001). Stressful life events and skin diseases: disentangling evidence from myth. *Psychotherapy and Psychosomatics*, **70**, 118–37.

Price, V. H. (2003). Therapy of alopecia areata: on the cusp and in the future. *Journal of Investigative Dermatology Symposium Proceedings*, **8**(2), 207–11.

Rostenberg, A. Jr. (1960). The role of psychogenic factors in skin disease. *Archives of Dermatology*, **81**, 81–3.

Rothe, M. J. and Grant-Kels, J. M. (1996). Atopic dermatitis: an update. *Journal of the American Academy of Dermatology*, **35**, 113.

Sampogna, F., Picardi, A., Melchi, C. F., *et al.* (2003). The impact of skin diseases on patients: comparing dermatologists' opinions with research data collected on their patients. *British Journal of Dermatology*, **148**, 989–95.

Shelley, W. B. and Shelley, E. D. (1985). Adrenergic urticaria: a new form of stress-induced hives. *Lancet*, **2**(8463), 1031–3.

Stein, D. J. and Hollander, E. (1992). Dermatology and conditions related to obsessive-compulsive disorder. *Journal of the American Academy of Dermatology*, **26**, 237–42.

Sticher, M., Abramovits, W. and Newcomer, V. D. (1980). Trichotillomania in adults. *Cutis*, **26**(1), 97–101.

Strauss, J. S. & Thiboutot, D. M. (1999). Diseases of the sebaceous glands. In *Fitzpatrick's Dermatology in General Medicine*, 5th edn., ed. I. M. Freedberg, A. Z. Eisen, K. Wolff, *et al.* New York: McGraw-Hill, pp. 769–84.

Trabert, W. (1995). 100 years of delusional parasitosis. Meta-analysis of 1223 case reports. *Psychopathology*, **28**(5), 238–46.

Trabert, W. (1999). Shared psychotic disorder in delusional parasitosis. *Psychopathology*, **32**(1), 30–4.

Ugurlu, S., Bartley, G. B., Otley, C. C., *et al.* (1999). Factitious disease of periocular and facial skin. *American Journal of Ophthalmology*, **127**, 196–201.

Van Moffaert, M. (1992). Psychodermatology: an overview. *Psychotherapy and Psychosomatics*, **58**, 125–36.

Veale, D. (2004). Body dysmorphic disorder. *Postgraduate Medical Journal*, **80**, 67–71.

Veale, D., De Haro, L. and Lambrou, C. (2003). Cosmetic rhinoplastia in body dysmorphic disorder. *British Journal of Plastic Surgeons*, **56**, 536–51.

Wang, C.-K. and Lee, J. Y.-Y. (1997). Monosymptomatic hypochondriacal psychosis complicated by self-inflicted skin ulceration, skull defect and brain abscess. *British Journal of Dermatology*, **137**, 299–302.

Wenning, M. T., Davy, L. E., Catalano, G., *et al.* (2003). Atypical antipsychotics in the treatment of delusional parasitosis. *Annals of Clinical Psychiatry*, **15**, 233–9.

Wilhelm, S., Keuthen, N. J., Deckerbasch, T., *et al.* (1999). Self-injurious skin-picking: clinical characteristics and co-morbidity. *Journal of Clinical Psychiatry*, **60**(7), 454–9.

Wright, H. H. and Holmes, G. R. (2003). Trichotillomania (hair pulling) in toddlers. *Psychological Reports*, **92**(1), 228–30.

31

Genitourinary disorders

David Osborn

Introduction

Genitourinary medicine attracted the attention of liaison psychiatrists decades before the emergence of HIV. Although many psychiatrists are accustomed to working in HIV departments, fewer contemporary practitioners have experience of general genitourinary medicine (GUM) clinics. Psychiatric sequelae of HIV are described separately in Chapter 20, allowing this chapter to focus specifically on other genitourinary diseases, which deserve both clinical and research emphasis within liaison psychiatry. The focus is on conditions such as genital herpes, gonorrhoea, genital warts, chlamydia and non-specific urethritis. The journey includes historical concepts such as 'syphilophobia', mutations of which retain relevance today. A wealth of studies in the 1970s and 1980s demonstrated disproportionate rates of common mental illness in genitourinary medicine outpatients and these rates persist into modern times. As in other fields of medicine, much of this morbidity goes unrecognized. The primary psychiatric diagnoses that may present in the GUM setting are discussed, before examining some of the causes, and the implications for treatment and service development.

The historical perspective and syphilophobia

As a sexually transmitted disease, syphilis held a uniquely prominent position in psychiatry during the nineteenth and twentieth centuries. Before penicillin (the treatment of choice for the condition) approximately 10% of new psychiatric inpatients were diagnosed with neurosyphilis (Hutto 2001). General paresis of the insane was a devastating condition appearing many years after the initial syphilitic infection. It rendered the patient demented and physically incapacitated, although the exact psychiatric presentation of the disease varied from case to case.

Handbook of Liaison Psychiatry, ed. Geoffrey Lloyd and Elspeth Guthrie. Published by Cambridge University Press. © Cambridge University Press 2007.

When the illness was first described, the typical presentation was manic in nature. However, this subtype quickly gave way to demented or depressed manifestations. The disease is now so uncommon that routine testing of psychiatric inpatients for syphilis is deemed unnecessary and cost-ineffective. Although the 1990s saw an upsurge in the incidence of syphilis in the USA this has now declined, and syphilis testing is reserved for high-risk groups (Hutto 2001). These include those demonstrating neurological or psychological symptoms of neurosyphilis, as well as psychiatric inpatients infected with HIV (Hutto & Adimora 2000). There have been recent small outbreaks of syphilis in UK cities (Doherty *et al.* 2002). This underscores the necessity of remaining mindful of syphilis when considering differential psychiatric diagnoses.

General awareness of the fatal effects of syphilis was accompanied by greater public anxiety about infection. In the 1940s and 1950s, there were several scientific reports of people attending GUM clinics with pathological concern about the possibility of being infected with a venereal disease such as syphilis. The anxiety symptoms would present regardless of actual risk of infection and constituted a considerable and increasing proportion of clinic attendees. MacAlpine (1957) used the term 'syphilophobia' to describe a case series of 24 patients referred by the GUM clinic at St Bartholomew's Hospital. This term had already been employed for a century to describe morbid fear of syphilis infection. Other authors employed a wider term 'venereophobia' (Kite & Grimble 1963; Oates & Gomez 1984). The latter authors discussed the exact form taken by venereophobia. They concluded that prevailing public disease concern, such as syphilis, herpes or HIV determines the exact focus of the health anxiety that presents within the GUM clinic. The common feature is an inappropriate or abnormal concern regarding the possibility of infection. Thus, as syphilis became treatable, less common and therefore less pertinent to the conscious mind, so non-specific urethritis, gonorrhoea, and latterly herpes and HIV would step in as the prevailing health concern.

A case vignette by Oates and Gomez (1984) illustrates the nature of syphilophobia. They describe a woman who 'haunted' (sic) the GUM clinic, convinced that she had contracted syphilis from her husband. Her rationale was rooted in his younger years as a sailor and possible engagement in risky sexual behaviour on his travels. As her concerns gained momentum, she blamed her imagined infection for a miscarriage in her distant past. She was consumed with fear and felt unable to discuss her problems in any detail, outside the GUM clinic. Her presentation was characterized by a preponderance of 'pseudoneurological symptoms' and her final diagnosis was a depressive episode. One of MacAlpine's (1957) case series was a medical student who developed a conviction of syphilitic infection while preparing for his final exams. Somatic symptoms such as headache, shin pains and eye strain were all misinterpreted as impending paralysis of the insane, optic atrophy and tabes dorsalis. Another man had spent years 'tramping the British Isles in quest of somebody who would agree ... he had hereditary syphilis'.

The key feature of venereophobia, whatever the nature of the feared disease, is preoccupation with ill health and a repetitive seeking of medical reassurance and investigation for disease. Previous commentators highlight the considerable suffering and potentially poor prognosis of such venereophobic presentations. Kite and Grimble (1963) noted two recent cases of suicide associated with the condition, reported in the *British Medical Journal*. No single psychiatric diagnosis satisfactorily explains all venereophobic presentations. The early descriptions of venereophobia noted a wide variety of associated psychiatric conditions, from anxiety presentations to depression and frank psychosis.

The prevalence of psychiatric morbidity in GUM clinics

The early case series of psychiatric morbidity in GUM settings galvanized efforts to quantify the extent of the problem. Although case series highlight the types of psychiatric illness that exist, they tell us little about how common a condition really is. Equipped with newly validated screening tools such as the General Health Questionnaire (GHQ), researchers in the 1970s and 1980s revealed a heavy burden of psychological suffering amongst GUM clinic attendees. Cross-sectional surveys suggested that between 20 and 40% of clinic attendees scored as psychiatric 'cases'. A summary of these results appears in Table 31.1. The largest studies include a GHQ survey by Ikkos *et al.* (1987), where 37.6% of 852 attendees scored above threshold, and an earlier survey by the same research team, where 42.8% of 381 attendees were GHQ 'cases' (Fitzpatrick *et al.* 1985). Importantly, psychological distress was not contingent on the presence or absence of genitourinary disorder. Statistically, psychological distress was equally as common in those with or without confirmed physical disease (Catalan *et al.* 1981; Mayou 1975). In other words, 'venereophobia' is not the sole psychiatric problem in GUM clinics. Those with confirmed sexually transmitted infections (STIs) are just as likely to be distressed. Fitzpatrick *et al.* (1985) made an attempt to quantify the actual prevalence of venereophobia. Only 4% of clinic attendees fulfilled the venereophobia criteria, with no detectable STI but an unwarranted degree of concern about STIs on an illness concern questionnaire. If venereophobia is strictly defined as abnormal concern in the absence of an STI, then it does not explain the majority of psychological morbidity detected in the GUM cross-sectional surveys.

Almost two decades on, a North London study including 774 GUM clinic attendees revealed that psychological symptoms have not abated over the years

Table 31.1. Prevalence of psychological problems in studies of STI clinic populations.

Authors	Year	n	Instrument	% scoring as cases	95% CI
Erbelding et al.[a]	2004	201	SCID[b]	45	38−52
Osborn et al.			HAD[c] A ≥ 8	50.3	46.8−53.8
	2002	774	HAD D ≥ 8	16.4	13.8−19.0
			A or D ≥ 8	51.9	48.3−55.4
Barczak et al.[a]			HAD A ≥ 8	40	30.4−49.6
	1988	100	HAD D ≥ 8	14	7.2−20.8
			A or D ≥ 8	N/D[d]	N/D
Ikkos et al.	1987	852	GHQ[e]	37.6	34.4−40.9
Fitzpatrick et al.	1985	381	GHQ	42.8	37.8−47.9
Catalan et al.	1981	140	GHQ	40	31.9−48.1
Mayou	1975	100	SSI[f]	20	10−28
Pedder & Goldberg	1970	219	GHQ	29.7	23.6−35.8

Notes: [a] Prevalence data not all reported in paper, but derived;
[b] SCID: Structured Clinical Interview for the Diagnostic and Statistical Manual, 4th Edition;
[c] HAD: Hospital Anxiety and Depression scale (A: anxiety subscale, D: depression subscale);
[d] N/D: not derivable;   [e] GHQ: General Health Questionnaire;
[f] SSI: semi-structured interview.

(Osborn *et al.* 2002). Sexual attitudes, practices and morality may have changed, but rates of psychological distress remain similar. Anxiety predominated with 50.3% of people scoring as possible cases on the Hospital Anxiety and Depression (HAD) scale with fewer positive cases of depression (16.1%). Critics have suggested that these results are eminently predictable and (more importantly) of little clinical significance for a number of reasons. First, psychiatric screening instruments do not generate formal psychiatric diagnoses, so perhaps this distress does not equate to actual psychiatric conditions. Second, the experience of attending the clinic should be considered. Genitourinary medicine involves intimate history taking, embarrassing examinations, genital swabs and the possibility of a stigmatized infection, surely enough to engender anxiety in even the most liberal individuals. Many people may then shed their anxiety within moments of leaving the clinic.

Although it may be tempting to dismiss the psychological symptoms of this population as transient or inevitable, there are compelling counter-arguments. First, the HAD scale has been validated in a GUM clinic, against the Structured Clinical Interview for Diagnostic and Statistical Manual (DSM)-III (SCID) (Barczak *et al.* 1988). In other words, the majority of HAD cases would attract formal DSM psychiatric diagnoses of anxiety or depressive disorders. Comparisons with recent studies in other medical settings give further context. The proportion of GUM attendees who are HAD cases is at least as high as for patients suffering with long-term cancer, for those with newly diagnosed head and neck tumours and even for those about to undergo neurosurgery for intracranial neoplasms (Osborn *et al.* 2002). This is confirmed by a recent GUM study which employed the fourth edition of the SCID in Baltimore, Maryland. In this survey 45% of 201 attendees attracted an Axis I diagnosis using DSM-IV (Erbelding *et al.* 2004). With this weight of evidence it seems unacceptable to dismiss the repeated findings of psychological distress as artefact.

While there is convincing evidence of unmet psychological needs within the general GUM setting, longitudinal data are lacking. The natural history of such distress is therefore unknown and we can only speculate. Mayou (1975) emphasized the need for information regarding the psychological progress and needs of the GUM clinic population, yet little has been forthcoming. This lack of cohort data is somewhat predictable given the barriers which hinder such research efforts. This is a sensitive research field where protection of an individual's data and the need for anonymity override scientific desire for accurate follow-up information through tracing of individuals. All that can be stated with confidence is that at the point of contact many GUM clinic attendances are associated with formal psychiatric diagnoses. The course of these conditions remains unclear.

Specific psychiatric conditions presenting in GUM clinics

The following sections describe specific illnesses found in GUM settings. Where applicable, the relevance of various International Classification of Disease (ICD)-10 diagnoses is discussed. Of course, almost any psychiatric condition may exist comorbidly in patients attending GUM clinics. The conditions described in the section are therefore clinical pictures where psychiatry and GUM overlap through more than a chance association.

Psychotic illnesses

With neurosyphilis almost banished to history, psychoses rarely present as direct complications of GUM disease or treatment. However, the hypochondriacal beliefs characteristic of venereophobia have often been observed to attain the delusional intensity indicative of a psychotic illness. Careful history taking and examination of the mental state will allow determination of the exact diagnosis for such psychoses. In the context of depressed mood and affect the hypochondriacal nature of the delusions is mood congruent and therefore diagnostic of a depressive psychosis (F32.3). In the absence of depressed mood, delusions of an infection such as syphilis, gonorrhoea or another STI are suggestive of either a mono-symptomatic persistent delusional disorder (F22) or even a schizophreniform illness (F20) should the delusions be accompanied by first-rank symptoms, formal thought disorder or a perplexed, blunted or incongruent affect.

A condition with a similar diagnostic spectrum, aetiology and prognosis is Ekbom's syndrome, a term usually reserved to describe delusions of para-sitic infestation often encountered in dermatology clinics (see Chapter 30). Interestingly, Ekbom's syndrome itself may present in the GUM clinic. The patient is convinced he/she is infested with pubic lice or scabies, but clinical evidence of the parasites is lacking. Although the mode of transmission of such parasites is not always sexual, the focus of symptoms in the genital region and the sexual connotations steer the patient towards the GUM department. In such cases, the characteristic pruritis and excoriation of Ekbom's syndrome focus on the groin area. Careful examination and investigation must exclude infection, before elucidating the psychiatric diagnosis. If a psychotic diagnosis is established, diagnosis and indeed treatment must follow the same principles as for other psychotic hypochondriacal venereophobias.

Management of GUM psychoses will depend on the precise diagnosis and symptom profile. Depressive episodes will require antidepressant therapy in adequate doses for six months to a year. Antipsychotic medication will also be required, and in severe or resistant cases inpatient treatment and electroconvulsive therapy may be considered. There is little evidence that one antidepressant or antipsychotic is likely to achieve better results over any other in these conditions. Adequate doses of atypical agents such as risperidone, olanzapine or quetiapine are now first-line treatments for new-onset psychosis. The efficacy of lower doses of older antipsychotics such as haloperidol make them first choice for previous responders or those who do not tolerate the side-effects of atypical antipsychotics, such as weight gain. Referral to psychiatric services is not always the appropriate course of action. The mention of a psychiatrist to a patient who is convinced of the physical basis of his/her current infection can disrupt any trust and introduce turbulence to any therapeutic relationship with the GUM practitioner. Sometimes pharmacological advice from a psychiatrist will be sufficient. However, the presence of any significant current risk, especially of self-harm, must take precedence and requires prompt psychiatric review.

If enough insight can be engendered to allow psychiatric referral, a number of treatment options may be considered alongside pharmacological intervention. In particular, individual cognitive therapy may be efficacious for psychotic symptoms including delusions, although results will vary between individuals (Turkington & McKenna 2003). Such therapy can certainly reap wide-ranging benefits for the dysphoria associated with these psychotic conditions. One core element of this therapy is a gradual challenge of the distorted logic which entrenches the hypochondriacal delusions, with a slow fostering of insight.

Affective illnesses

Although 'possible depression' was present in 16.1% of our London survey (Osborn *et al.* 2002), affective disorders are recognized far less frequently in busy GUM clinics. Since the core features of depression (F32–33) include low mood, decreased self-esteem and a depressive cognitive style, it is easy to see how the depressed patient may develop ruminations regarding STIs. Cognitively, these ruminations may be purely hypochondriacal, or they may be a secondary manifestation of a wider network of negative interpretations including guilt about past behaviours and an exaggeration of perceived risk of infection. The depressed state may encourage negative evaluations of past sexual behaviours leading the individual to seek reassurance and even to believe that s/he is infected with gonorrhoea or some other stigmatized condition. While some GUM attendances may be precipitated or perpetuated by depressive symptomatology, recent GUM diagnosis can also play a causal role in depressive disorders. Only careful history taking can determine the sequence.

When a depressive episode is detected, the diagnosis and risks must be established. A screen for subtle hypochondriacal delusions, indicative of a psychosis and direct questioning regarding suicidal ideation are essential. Any positive findings require a more urgent treatment strategy to optimize patient safety.

Hypomanic or manic disorders (F30–31) seem unlikely to be over-represented in the GUM clinic since the illnesses are characterized by inflated senses of self-worth and invincibility. Concerns about contracting sexual infections or guilt about sexual conquests are contrary to the classic manic mental state with unfounded positivity and confidence. It is worth emphasizing that elated mood states place a patient at marked risk of reckless sexual behaviour. Manic infallibility, increased libido and an excessive feeling of sexual attractiveness may induce sexual risk taking of a manner far removed from the individual's usual repertoire. Decreased perception of personal vulnerability obscures concerns about safe sexual activity and this carries the concomitant risks of contracting sexually transmitted diseases. The person with bipolar affective disorder is a candidate for more intensive education and screening in GUM settings, and by psychiatric teams managing such patients, particularly in the manic phase of the illness.

There is little to delineate the treatment of affective disorders in GUM settings from general treatment paradigms for these conditions. There are no major risks of specific drug toxicity or interactions with commonly prescribed GUM medications. In the rare cases where steroids are prescribed, their potential for inducing psychoses and depression should be remembered. The psychiatric sequelae of antiretroviral therapy are discussed in the section on HIV (see Chapter 20).

More severe cases of depression require antidepressant therapy. First-line agents include the serotonin specific reuptake inhibitors (SSRIs) or newer agents such as venlafaxine or mirtazapine. Side-effect profiles are a key consideration. In general, the GUM population is a sexually active one, and this may influence the prescription. The serotonergic agents confer a risk of gastrointestinal and sexual problems (including anorgasmia and delayed ejaculation). The older tricyclic antidepressants may generate anticholinergic symptoms and cardiac toxicity, an important consideration in the presence of any risk of overdose.

Psychological treatment is often equally effective as drug treatment for depressive illnesses, and may be the preferred choice of many patients (Parker *et al.* 2003). The appropriate form of therapy depends on both the cognitive and psychodynamic formulations. In general, when depression is accompanied by negative cognitions such as guilt about sex, a cognitive-behavioural approach may be more fruitful. When relationship difficulties (past or present) form a core of the condition, interpersonal therapy should be considered. In common with other areas of liaison psychiatry, the exact treatment plan must be tailored to each individual and hinges on careful psychiatric assessment and the local availability of expert psychological therapists.

Anxiety, somatoform and hypochondriacal disorders

The section on epidemiology highlighted the extraordinary prevalence of anxiety symptoms in GUM clinic attendees. The debilitating suffering caused by such anxiety symptoms may be neglected or marginalized, in both psychiatric and medical settings. This oversight is exaggerated in countries like the UK where general psychiatric health services divert attention to 'severe and enduring mental illnesses'. Such terms are usually equated with psychoses and aligned with concepts such as dangerousness rather than actual psychological suffering. This marginalizes the distress of anxiety disorders, however severe and enduring they may be. Anxiety disorders are therefore usually managed in the primary-care setting. It is essential that the exclusion of anxiety disorders from general adult psychiatric care is not mirrored in the GUM setting.

For anxiety disorders in GUM clinics the strict boundaries of ICD-10 can be difficult to apply. Teasing out a diagnosis of anxiety disorder rather than a somatoform disorder or hypochondriacal disorder is seldom straightforward. Considerable symptom overlap and comorbidity exist. Biological symptoms of anxiety including sweats, palpitations, dizziness and nausea often accompany the anxious cognitions. These include overt inappropriate ruminations about the infection with one STI or another. These in turn may precipitate somatic symptoms such as groin pain, itch or even discharge. As a framework, the relevant diagnostic categories are as follows. If somatic GUM symptoms are accompanied by multiple symptoms in other biological systems the diagnosis of undifferentiated somatoform disorder should be made (F45.1). However, when symptoms are chronic (years) and wide ranging, an ICD-10 diagnosis of somatization disorder (F45.0) is appropriate. If the somatic symptoms are restricted to the genito-urinary system, then the precise ICD diagnoses are persistent somatoform pain disorder (F45.4) or somatoform autonomic dysfunction of the genitourinary system (F45.3.34).

When the overriding feature is one of abnormally intense concern about the possibility of genitourinary infections, the primary diagnosis is hypochondriacal disorder (F45.2). The syndrome constitutes classic venereophobia and fits particularly neatly with a cognitive-behavioural formulation. The individual develops negative automatic thoughts regarding the possibility of an STI. Frequently such beliefs emerge from misinterpretation of innocuous bodily, and especially genital, sensations.

The management of anxiety disorders in the GUM setting is contingent on the core diagnosis and psychopathology. Pharmacological agents are often overlooked but the anxiolytic properties of many of the serotonergic antidepressants should be considered, especially those with licences for panic disorder (paroxetine and citalopram) and generalized anxiety disorder (venlafaxine), in the right diagnostic context. In the absence of risk of cardiac disease or self-poisoning the tricyclic antidepressants also warrant consideration.

Psychological management is usually the first-line therapeutic approach. When abnormal illness behaviour and somatic or hypochondriacal ruminations are core features, a cognitive approach is most commonly applied. The rationale is outlined by Miller *et al.* (1988), who base their theoretical framework of HIV hypochondriasis on previous descriptions of venereophobia. They describe illness preoccupation and seeking of medical reassurance as the core elements, making a cognitive behavioural approach the treatment of choice. The behavioural symptoms may include repetitive checking for symptoms of STIs. This can include scrutiny for penile discharge, for genital blemishes, and for lymphadeno-pathy. The zealous self-examination may itself induce the very somatic symptoms which are so feared. These self-inflicted signs are held as proof of infection and shame. The treatment of this behavioural pattern centres on careful education, challenging the cognitive distortions and breaking the cycle by reducing behavioural responses such as ruthless self-examination.

Personality disorders

Certain personality disorders (F60–61) predispose to impulsive behaviour and repetitive sexual risk behaviour, almost by definition. It is no surprise that people with such disorders are frequent attenders of GUM clinics. It would be misleading to generalize about their risk behaviours, presentation or treatment needs. Some will provide challenges to the therapeutic relationship, yet most people with personality disorders will traverse the clinic unrecognized. Recent evidence from North America suggests an excess of people with antisocial personality disorder in GUM attendees (Erbelding *et al.* 2004). This work, set in one geographical area with little ethnic diversity, has limitations in its generalizability, but raises interesting questions regarding the sexual risk-taking behaviour that results in GUM clinic attendance. An accompanying editorial (Aral 2004) championed the vital link between physical and mental disorder which underpins all liaison psychiatry. Whatever the reason, STIs, mental disorders and social adversity do cluster together. Possible explanations are wide ranging. They include factors such as substance misuse, personal and socioeconomic deprivation, as well as common genetic or intrauterine factors which determine life-course, experience and health. This model of common aetiology may be a key element in understanding the relationship between GUM and psychiatry. Examination of such complex, common pathways may therefore provide the foundation for future research.

Sexual dysfunction and assault

Direct clinical experience indicates that sexual dysfunction is common in many GUM patients. Catalan *et al.* (1981) attempted to quantify this problem in Oxford. Some form of sexual dysfunction was experienced by 25% of 70 male and 40% of 70 female attendees. The most common male problems were premature ejaculation (9%) and erectile impotence (6%) whilst coital orgasmic dysfunction (37%), loss of libido (13%) and dyspareunia (11%) were the most common female problems. While the women with sexual dysfunction were more likely to score as psychiatric cases on the GHQ, the men were not. In other words, sexual dysfunction is not simply a cause or a marker of other psychiatric disturbance in this population. The majority of these patients expressed a desire for help with their sexual difficulties. The authors recognized that this might be unrealistic since it would increase the workload of already busy GUM departments. Other GUM researchers had commented on the level of sexual dysfunction in GUM clinics, but Catalan *et al.* (1981) concluded that the prevalence of such problems may be no greater than in other clinics such as family planning and gynaecology. That is not to say that this sexual dysfunction should be ignored, rather that it does not differentiate GUM patients from others. A more important point relates to the predictors of sexual dysfunction. Although the clinic staff expected sexual problems in people who attended without confirmed evidence of STIs, dysfunction was in fact equally common irrespective of a positive STI diagnosis. This tendency to label attendees without STIs as psychologically or sexually disturbed is an inaccurate but repetitive finding, which is discussed in a subsequent section.

Genitourinary medicine clinics often provide a central role in assessing and supporting victims of sexual assault. Such patients need careful screening for potential STIs, and equally importantly require the offer of short- and long-term psychological support. The exact nature of this support will depend on the individual, their psychological presentation and the availability of specialist local services for rape victims.

Explanations and aetiology of psychological distress

Much speculation and research have focused on the aetiology of excess psychological morbidity detected in GUM settings. Why do people worry excessively about STIs rather than other clinical conditions? Why are rates of probable common mental illness so high when the GHQ or HAD scale are routinely used as screening instruments? The diseases are on the whole curable or manageable, they are not usually progressive or fatal and do not confer major physical disability, but something singles them out and produces increased levels of psychological suffering.

Sex, society and guilt

The mode of transmission of STIs is an obvious factor. Sex delineates these diseases from other illnesses. Sexual activity holds a different yet key place in both Western and non-Western society. Sex is imbued with a range of powerful attributes such as prowess, guilt, morality and embarrassment. Maybe the reason for anxiety in GUM clinics is that simple. People are ashamed to discuss their sexual activity, and ashamed of the stigma attached to STIs. Case series of psychiatric referrals from GUM clinics confirm this pattern. Kite and Grimble (1963) described high rates of guilt about extramarital sex and promiscuity. They outlined a variety of inner psychological conflicts including religious, altruistic, marital or sexual concerns. Guilt about sexual activity was their most prominent finding, but even at that time they were surprised by this, given the increasing sexual frankness. The source of the guilt will be evident in the individual history. It might involve sexual infidelity or personally unaccepted homosexual activity or desire which produces cognitive dissonance. If sexual guilt remains the key to psychological distress in modern days it seems remarkable, and at odds with liberalized attitudes to sexual activity. Oates and Gomez (1984) place the blame squarely on mixed social attitudes to sex.

Sex is inescapable throughout the modern multi-media. Millions of column inches are dedicated to the minutiae of people's sexual preferences and performance and satisfaction. Sex provides endless public fascination and yet is associated with mockery, judgement and even retribution. This provides the perfect substrate for excessive anxiety and concern about the consequences of sexual activity.

Illness behaviour

Abnormal illness behaviour refers to maladaptive or inappropriate forms of response to health, and encompasses an individual's perceptions and evaluations of symptoms. The relevance of the concept has been investigated as a model of psychological distress in the GUM setting. Early work derived from the small proportion of GUM patients who were referred to psychiatrists rather than from the majority of people suffering distress in the GUM clinic. However, Fitzpatrick *et al.* (1985) empirically assessed GHQ cases for a range of psychological disturbances as well as for distress which specifically related to their current condition and presentation. They concluded that illness concern with the current (GUM) situation was the prevalent stressor, and other measures of general psychological distress were actually lower than in other populations who score as cases on the GHQ. Ikkos *et al.* (1987) used a validated instrument to tease out specific aspects of illness behaviour in people who scored as GHQ cases, and compared results with findings from other settings. Such cases in the GUM clinic displayed levels of general hypochondriasis higher than any comparison group apart from psychiatric inpatients. This work lends epidemiological weight to the notion that general hypochondriasis is one of the key factors explaining high rates of distress in GUM clinics. The cognitive distortions which characterize this hypochondriasis have already been discussed. Negative automatic thoughts about infection may result from endless checking for symptoms, and from misinterpretation of normal bodily sensations.

Epidemiological associations

Limited insight has been provided by statistical investigation of psychiatric distress in this setting. In line with general population findings, the first studies suggested that women were more at risk. Otherwise psychological distress showed no consistent association with sexual orientation, with presence or absence of confirmed STIs or with a range of other factors. The availability of accessible multivariate analysis has shed a little further light. Our own work suggested that unemployment, current physical GUM symptoms and attending for an HIV test were the only factors independently associated with psychological distress (Osborn *et al.* 2002). The anxiety of HIV testing is a predictable finding (see Chapter 30). This presumably represented a group including the worried well (Miller *et al.* 1988) and those with genuine concern about possible exposure to HIV. Unemployment is a consistent predictor of psychiatric distress in psychiatric epidemiology. Overall, the evidence consistently highlights that physical GU symptoms induce distress in attendees which then results in excessive hypochondriacal concern.

Qualitative studies

In-depth interviews are often more powerful and rich in content than cross-sectional surveys. One such study involved 17 women with a diagnosis of chlamydia (Duncan *et al.* 2001). The women identified stigma as one of their chief sources of stress. They had pre-existing negative opinions about STIs which reflected stereotypical views about who is 'at risk'. After their own STI diagnosis, they feared rejection by others and especially by sexual partners. Clearly they felt others would hold the same negative views about people who have suffered STIs, and now they would be judged by those criteria. This study confirms the importance of sexual attitudes, stigma and guilt, but it also emphasized that other factors are important. Women also feared for their future fertility. This is an important emphasis for chlamydia screening. Programmes which overemphasize the risk of infertility may have a major psychosocial impact on women diagnosed with such conditions. We have recently embarked on a further qualitative study where GUM patients who score as a case on the HAD scale are interviewed regarding the causes of their distress. Preliminary findings confirm that a range of issues, including stigma and fear, as well as factors totally unrelated to the clinic contribute to the psychological suffering.

Sexual risk-taking behaviour

A further explanation for higher rates of psychological disturbance in the GUM setting relates to the sexual behaviours of people with mental illnesses. If individuals who are depressed or anxious are more likely to engage in unsafe sex, they will be more vulnerable to STIs and will need to consult more. These attendances may be precipitated by regret about the behaviour, or by the emergence of STI symptoms. A further contribution is alcohol and substance misuse, acting as both a cause and effect of common mental illnesses. Substance misuse is also a strong predictor of unsafe sexual activity and of STIs, so the pathway between mental illness and STI attendance is clearly plausible. The extent to which mental illness predicts STI transmission is as yet unclear. It has now been singled out as one of the most important issues for prevention strategies in a field where the incidence of STIs continues to alarm public health physicians (Adler 1997; Aral 2004). If mental health does indeed predict sexual health, this may necessitate specific strategies to foster safe sexual practice designed for both mental health and sexual health settings (Aral 2004).

Herpes genitalis

Although psychological distress is associated with sexually transmitted infections in general, no individual STIs consistently predict this distress. However one infection, genital herpes, attracted special attention, particularly before the discovery of HIV. In the early 1980s, herpes was conceptualized as a sexual epidemic, potentially ruining the sexual lives of millions of sufferers. Public campaigns resulted in widespread fear of the condition (Oates & Gomez 1984).

Psychological aspects of the disease drew attention when sufferers reported that stress seemed to precipitate recurrences of the condition. Studies often focused on those with frequent relapses of genital herpes, and suggested that stress, personality and sexual maturity might all influence the course of the infection. Drob et al. (1985) studied 42 sufferers of recurrent genital herpes. They concluded that psychological distress was very common and ensued from a number of sources. These included ethical issues such as confiding in sexual partners, the social meaning of genital herpes (including media sensationalization and jokes about herpes), and avoidance of sexual intimacy following diagnosis.

With the advent of HIV, public concern regarding herpes has diminished. Mindel (1996) has reviewed the psychological complications of genital herpes, including the role of stress in precipitating recurrences. There is an attractive theoretical biological model whereby acute stress may weaken the immunological system, perhaps through adrenaline release, or through hypothalamic function and neurotrophic factor release. Anecdotal reports of stress preceding recurrences have not been supported by more rigorous study. Daily accounts of stress and examination for recurrence only show stress levels increasing at the point of recurrence, rather than before. In other words, stress is a consequence rather than cause of recurrent herpes attacks. Those with frequent attacks represent a minority of cases, although this does not diminish their need for psychological support. Interestingly, long term antiviral therapy, which reduces the frequency of attacks, also benefits the psychological health of people with recurrent genital herpes (Carney et al. 1993).

In summary, the causes of psychological disturbance in GUM clinics are multifactorial and include established psychiatric risk factors such as gender and social deprivation. However, the specifics of GUM distress include exaggerated concern for GUM symptoms and result in a high prevalence of hypochondriacal type cognitions. The stigma attached to sex and GUM is a powerful contributor as are the perceived sequelae including female infertility. However, as in all psychiatric disciplines, individual factors unrelated to the clinic also play their part to warrant careful consideration of each person's own presentation and history.

Recognition of psychological distress and referral

The high levels of psychological disturbance in GUM clinics are not matched by high levels of referral to psychiatrists. Although any number from 20 to 50% of patients may score as distressed, fewer than 1% are referred to mental health services (Frost 1985; Osborn *et al.* 2002; Pedder & Goldberg 1970). When recognition, rather than referral, is explored GUM staff are generally inaccurate in their estimation of which patients are cases on instruments such as the GHQ. This is no different from other medical settings. It is a predictable sequel of very busy clinics providing brief infection-focused interviews. There is evidence that doctors are suspicious of hypochondriasis in the GUM setting. They are more likely to diagnose psychological problems in those without a confirmed STI diagnosis (Catalan *et al.* 1981; Osborn *et al.* 2002), perhaps because they are unable to attribute the clinical presentation to a more familiar STI diagnosis. All results are not consistent, for instance Fitzpatrick *et al.*'s (1985) results contradict this theory. This alerts us to the difficulty of drawing generalizable conclusions from the small numbers of doctors involved in local cross-sectional surveys. Each GUM study has involved only one individual clinic and therefore a handful of doctors. Further sampling bias may be present since these clinics are all ones where psychological research is taking place. Therefore one might expect detection rates to be even lower at sites without such a mental health focus.

The important clinical question is whether the detection of psychological distress is of benefit in this setting. Although half the clinic patients may score as cases, no one would suggest that half the clinic attendees need referring to a psychiatrist. Questions regarding the clinical course of GUM psychological distress are central to this decision. If much of it is transient in nature, simple reassurance may be adequate for many people. Since sexual guilt, stigma and illness concern are key elements in the distress, these are good candidates for brief education and support in the clinic process. There is evidence that patients want to discuss their distress. Catalan *et al.* (1981) revealed that the majority of their sample would have liked further help regarding their psychological problems.

There are sound medical reasons to emphasize the recognition of psychological symptoms in this population. Firstly, acknowledgement of the factors which contribute to psychological distress is likely to strengthen the doctor–patient relationship. This in turn will improve compliance with treatment regimens, with benefits for individual and public health by reducing further transmission of STIs. One specific aspect of treatment compliance in the GUM setting is attendance at a follow-up appointment to confirm treatment success. When GUM doctors recognize the distress of their patients, reattendance is significantly improved (Osborn *et al.* 2002). There is less evidence that psychological disturbance itself may affect reattendance, perhaps because there is such diversity within the clinic. Some may be anxious and more likely to attend, while others may be distressed or indifferent and less likely to comply. Women with higher scores on the psychoticism scale of the Eysenck Personality Questionnaire were observed to be less likely to attend their review appointments, as a result of decreased fear for their health (Hammond *et al.* 1989). Identification of these different subgroups requires more sophisticated research studies and analyses.

Clinical recommendations

The key observation in this field is the burden of psychological distress in people attending GUM clinics. Much of this is common mental illness, namely anxiety disorders and depression. Core components of these illnesses include somatization, illness concern and hypochondriasis. The strictly hypochondriacal and somatic forms of these illnesses, 'pure venereophobia' without the presence of depression or anxiety are important but less common. Despite changing attitudes to sex, the commonest causes for this morbidity continue to be stigma, sexual concern and guilt.

It is these findings that must continue to inform service development in the GUM setting. Efforts to destigmatize, educate and support GUM attendees may be potent methods of combating mental distress.

The prognosis of mental illness in this setting is uncertain, and anxiety may be transient for many attendees. Any referral to psychiatric services should be reserved for more complex or entrenched cases.

Clearly, management of psychological problems will vary from case to case. At the front line, sexual health counsellors have a wealth of experience in dealing with psychological reactions to STIs and sexual issues in general. They are well placed to assess the severity and nature of mental distress and refer to specialists as necessary.

Ideally all GUM settings would have on site access to the expertise of a liaison psychiatrist. Several authors have stressed the benefits of such in-house psychiatrists (Bhanji & Mahony 1978; Fitzpatrick *et al.* 1985; Oates & Gomez 1984). Realistically, coverage is patchy within and between countries. Clinics with higher involvement in HIV care may have more funding for psychiatric input, which could also be utilized for general GUM clinic patients.

Psychology input is invaluable in this setting. The approach will depend on the presentation. Although there are no trials of cognitive behavioural therapy specifically for 'venereophobia', it seems likely that the models for other forms of hypochondriasis are applicable (e.g. Warwick *et al.* 1996). Such work will challenge the negative automatic thoughts about infection, the misinterpretation of bodily sensations and the abnormal health-seeking behaviour. Those with excessive sexual guilt may also be candidates for a more psychodynamic approach or for interpersonal therapy. Careful assessment by a psychiatrist or psychologist will allow determination of the best treatment model.

REFERENCES

Adler, M. W. (1997). Sexual health – a health of the nation failure. *British Medical Journal,* **314,** 1743–7.

Aral, O. S. (2004). Mental health. A powerful predictor of sexual health? Sexually transmitted diseases. *Sexually Transmitted Diseases,* **31**(1), 13–14.

Barczak, P., Kane, N., Andrews, S., *et al.* (1988). Patterns of psychiatric morbidity in a genito-urinary medicine clinic. A validation of the Hospital Anxiety and Depression Scale (HAD). *British Journal of Psychiatry,* **152,** 698–700.

Bhanji, S. and Mahony, J. D. H. (1978). The value of a psychiatric service within the venereal disease clinic. *British Journal of Venereal Diseases,* **54,** 266–8.

Carney, O., Ross, E., Ikkos, G., *et al.* (1993). The effect of suppressive oral acylclovir on the psychological morbidity associated with recurrent genital herpes. *Genitourinary Medicine,* **69,** 457–9.

Catalan, J., Bradley, M., Gallwey, J., *et al.* (1981). Sexual dysfunction and psychiatric morbidity in patients attending a clinic for sexually transmitted disease. *British Journal of Psychiatry,* **138,** 292–6.

Doherty, L., Fenton, K. A., Jones, J., *et al.* (2002). Syphilis: old problem, new strategy. *British Medical Journal,* **325,** 153–6.

Drob, S., Loemer, M. and Lifshutz, H. (1985). Genital herpes: the psychological consequences. *British Journal of Medical Psychology,* **58,** 307–15.

Duncan, B., Hart, G., Scoular, A., *et al.* (2001). Qualitative analysis of psychosocial impact of Chlamydia trachomatis: implications for screening. *British Medical Journal,* **322,** 195–9.

Erbelding, E. J., Hutton, H. E., Zenilman, J. M., *et al.* (2004). The prevalence of psychiatric disorders in sexually transmitted disease clinic patients and their association with sexually transmitted disease risk. *Sexually Transmitted Diseases,* **31**(1), 8–12.

Fitzpatrick, R., Ikkos, G. and Frost, D. (1985). The recognition of psychological disturbance in a sexually transmitted diseases clinic. *International Journal of Social Psychiatry,* **31**(4), 306–14.

Frost, D. P. (1985). Recognition of hypochondriasis in a clinic for sexually transmitted disease. *Genitourinary Medicine,* **61,** 133–7.

Hammond, D., Maw, R. D. and Mulholland, M. (1998). Personality types of women attending an STD clinic: correlation with keeping first review appointments. *Genitourinary Medicine,* **65**(3), 163–5.

Hutto, B. (2001). Syphilis in clinical psychiatry. A review. *Psychosomatics*, **42**, 453−60.

Hutto, B. and Adimora, A. (2000). Syphilis in psychiatric inpatients. Prevalence, treatment, and implications. *General Hospital Psychiatry*, **24**(4), 291−3.

Ikkos, G., Fitzpatrick, R., Frost, D., *et al.* (1987). Psychological disturbance and illness behaviour in a clinic for sexually transmitted diseases. *British Journal of Medical Psychology*, **60**, 121−6.

Kite, E. C. and Grimble, A. (1963). Psychiatric aspects of venereal disease. *British Journal of Venereal Disease*, **39**, 173−80.

MacAlpine, I. (1957). Syphilophobia. *British Journal of Venereal Disease*, **33**, 92−9.

Mayou, R. (1975). Psychological morbidity in a clinic for sexually transmitted disease. *British Journal of Venereal Disease*, **51**, 57−60.

Miller, D., Acton, T. M. G. and Hedge, B. (1998). The worried well: their identification and management. *Journal of the Royal College of Physicians of London*, **22**, 158−65.

Mindel, A. (1996). Psychological and psychosexual implications of Herpes simplex virus infections. *Scandinavian Journal of Infectious Diseases*, **100**(Suppl.), 27−32.

Oates, J. K. and Gomez, J. (1984). Venereophobia. *British Journal of Hospital Medicine*, **31**, 435−6.

Osborn, D. P. J., King, M. B. and Weir, M. (2002). Psychiatric health in a sexually transmitted infections clinic: effect on re-attendance. *Journal of Psychosomatic Research*, **52**, 267−72.

Parker, G., Roy, K. and Eyers, K. (2003). Cognitive behavior therapy for depression? Choose horses for courses. *American Journal of Psychiatry*, **160**(5), 825−34.

Pedder, J. and Goldberg, D. P. (1970). Disturbances in patients attending a venereal disease clinic. *British Journal of Venereal Disease*, **46**, 58−61.

Turkington, D. and McKenna, P. (2003). Is cognitive−behavioural therapy a worthwhile treatment for psychosis? *British Journal of Psychiatry*, **182**, 477−9.

Warwick, H. M., Clark, D. M., Cobb, A. M., *et al.* (1996). A controlled trial of cognitive-behavioural treatment of hypochondriasis. *British Journal of Psychiatry*, **169**, 189−95.

32

The emergency department

Andrew Hodgkiss

Introduction

Assessing and managing patients with mental health problems or substance misuse problems in the emergency department (ED) is one of the most crucial and challenging aspects of psychiatric practice in general hospitals. However, it has long been an unpopular, neglected, risky and rather controversial task. It remains unpopular with patients, mental health professionals and ED staff alike, though each group has its own distinct issues. Patients complain of an unsuitable physical environment, lack of privacy, long delays before being seen and inappropriate decision-making. Consultant psychiatrists have understandably shied away from taking responsibility for numerous high-risk decisions made under pressure of time by a large number of different trainee psychiatrists at all hours of the day and night. Academic psychiatrists have, with a few notable exceptions, avoided the ED as a research area so there is not yet much evidence to guide practice. Emergency department staff may see patients with mental health and substance misuse problems as a numerically small, but potentially high-risk, group and quietly resent being the unacknowledged out-of-hours support to local community mental health services.

Before the situation can be improved nationally one question has to be settled. Is mental health work in the ED simply emergency community psychiatry being practised in the wrong setting because of a lack of planning and resources (Harrison & Bruce-Jones 2003), or is it an example of a specialist liaison psychiatry service to a single department of the general hospital (Cassar *et al.* 2002; Henderson *et al.* 2003)? Should there be improved out-of-hours crisis teams in the community or rapid development of 24-hour liaison psychiatry services in EDs? It will be argued here that patients attending the ED with mental health problems constitute a distinct group that have every reason to be assessed and managed

Handbook of Liaison Psychiatry, ed. Geoffrey Lloyd and Elspeth Guthrie. Published by Cambridge University Press. © Cambridge University Press 2007.

initially at the general hospital. The argument hinges on the little we know of the epidemiology of such ED attenders.

Epidemiology and mode of presentation of patients with mental health and substance misuse problems in the ED

Studies based on self-report questionnaires, such as the General Health Questionnaire (GHQ) or Hospital Anxiety and Depression (HAD) scale, report that approximately one-third of all ED attenders obtain scores indicating the probability that they have a current psychiatric disorder. This rate persists at one-month follow-up (Salkovskis *et al.* 1990a). The practical value of this finding is limited by the potential scale of unaddressed need in the ED (for example it suggests that at St Thomas' Hospital, London with 105 000 ED attendees per annum, over 38 000 have undiagnosed psychiatric disorder!) and by the lack of any well-established method of intervention for this huge number of people.

An alternative approach has been to count retrospectively ED attendees diagnosed with psychiatric disorder or referred to liaison psychiatry services (Crawford & Kohen 1997; Ellis & Lewis 1997; House & Hodgson 1994). Ellis and Lewis noted a preponderance of men and that these tended to present outside normal working hours. One-third of the patients lived outside the immediate psychiatric catchment area of the local mental health service. Sixty-six per cent were self-referrals to the ED. Forty per cent had deliberately self-harmed. Depression, schizophrenia, alcohol dependence and personality disorder were the top four psychiatric diagnoses made. Twenty-seven per cent of the self-harm patients and 19% of those presenting with psychotic symptoms left the ED without being assessed by either the ED doctor or psychiatrist. Rates of absconding were highest in those who presented out-of-hours and were attributed to long waiting times in the ED.

Cassar *et al.* (2002) undertook a prospective study of all patients with overt mental health or substance misuse problems attending an inner-city ED over a three-month period. Seventy per cent presented out-of-hours. The patients were young (mean age 33), predominantly male, single and unemployed. Seventeen per cent had no fixed abode. Presenting complaints included deliberate self-harm (31%), alcohol misuse (20%) and psychotic illness (17%). Only one-third were in contact with mental health services. The absconding rate was 4%. These results largely replicate the findings of Ellis and Lewis.

This small, but consistent, epidemiological literature indicates that inner city EDs serve a group of patients that is distinct from those served by community mental health services in a number of important respects. Emergency departments mostly work with young men who are unemployed and precariously housed, who present out-of-hours with deliberate self-harm and/or alcohol dependence syndrome, who abscond if kept waiting and who go on to repeat the self-harm. Community mental health teams in the inner city are increasingly dedicated to those with severe and enduring mental illnesses (i.e. psychoses) who have permanent residence in the catchment area. There is a strong case to be made for developing distinctive 24-hour liaison psychiatry services in the ED of hospitals which serve an inner-city population.

Clinical skills for practising psychiatry in the ED

Before describing the resources and managerial arrangements required for a liaison psychiatry service in the ED it is worth outlining some of the specific clinical skills required in that setting. It will be apparent that some of these are quite removed from the experience most psychiatry trainees gain working with psychotic patients on adult psychiatry wards or preparing for postgraduate examinations. These skills need to be taught specifically to trainees to equip them for work in the ED. Nurses making the move from general adult psychiatry settings to liaison nursing also need to learn these skills.

Patients in the ED are often too uncooperative, or too unwell, to provide a clear history. In many cases staff literally do not know with whom they are dealing. The availability of medical records, in the form of existing ED notes, Care Programme Approach documentation or discharge summaries from recent psychiatric admissions, can transform the assessment and immediate management. The advent of electronic patient records is greatly strengthening assessment of the one-third of ED attenders with mental health problems who are known to local mental health services. An informant history may also be crucial and should be documented under a separate heading to facilitate consideration for removal from the ED medical record should the patient request their notes in future. Gathering background information quickly and flexibly, perhaps before the patient is sober or 'medically fit', is one important skill. Such 'parallel assessment' with the ED medical team maintains goodwill.

Fluent assessment skills are important when faced with new patients who have self-harmed, are substance dependent, personality disordered, psychotic or suicidal.

The importance of exploring epidemiological risk factors for completed suicide as well as identifying high-risk methods, presentations and statements after an act of self-harm is emphasized.

In cases of substance misuse the features of a dependence syndrome should be sought in the history of the presenting complaint while the rest of the history is devoted to actively seeking the predictable medical, psychiatric and social complications of the substance misuse (e.g. hepatitis B and C status for intra-venous drug misusers, past history of jaundice, gastrointestinal bleeds and withdrawal fits for alcohol-dependent patients).

The philosopher Ludwig Wittgenstein once asked how doctors make judge-ments about the veracity of statements concerning the subjective experience of others. He concluded that it is a skill learned by experience and that more experi-enced clinicians could give trainees a few tips (Wittgenstein 1958). Such is the dilemma of the psychiatrist faced with the allegedly suicidal or hallucinating homeless patient in the small hours of the morning. A judgement about the veracity of the complaint has to be made, based on as full an understanding as possible of the context in which it is uttered. For example, the pseudohallucina-tions of the patient with borderline personality disorder who repeatedly self-harms may well involve the voice of his abuser. The documented lack of benefit derived from a series of short previous admissions to adult psychiatry wards may help clinch the diagnosis.

Mental health professionals working in the ED need to have specific training in the immediate assessment and management of risk and the fuller assessment of risk. Immediate assessment is required when patients have been triaged but wish to leave prior to any medical assessment. Effective intervention in this circumstance is only likely if the professionals have confidence in their ability to identify patients at unacceptably high risk and in their understanding of duty of care in common law. A recently published algorithm is helpful in this situation (Royal College of Physicians and Royal College of Psychiatrists 2003). Many trusts have developed standardized instruments to facilitate fuller risk assessments. These cover risk of suicide, homicide, risk to children, risk of exploitation and of self-neglect. The use of these in the ED is encouraged for medicolegal reasons despite scientific reservations about their specificity and sensitivity.

Another skill that is required in the ED is known as interim care planning. This specifies various aspects of the care of the patient during the few hours they will spend in the ED. It is almost universally neglected, or left undocumented, by psychiatrists. Should they be left alone or guarded? By whom? Are they free to leave? Can they smoke outside or go to the hospital cafe? Which cubicle in the ED would be most suitable? Under what circumstances should medication be offered? What physical observations are indicated over the next three hours? What exact transfer arrangements are advised: minicab or ambulance, with a healthcare assistant, a general nurse or a police escort?

Knowledge of evidence-based management of common presentations to the ED is essential. As a minimum an awareness is required of the literature on evidence-based brief intervention after deliberate self-harm (Guthrie *et al.* 2001; Hawton *et al.* 1998) and after life-threatening trauma (see Chapters 11 and 38;

Rose & Bisson 1998). It is also important for staff to be aware of brief intervention methods for hazardous drinkers (see Chapter 8; Wright *et al.* 1998).

The ED has a central place in the hospital's response to a major incident. Most acute hospitals have now developed a major incident plan to be effected in response to a local disaster and mental health professionals working there need to be aware of their specified role in the plan.

Finally, an extensive working knowledge of local mental health and substance misuse services (both in the state-run and voluntary sectors) and housing services (including options for the homeless) is required if alternatives to unnecessary hospital admission are to be generated, especially out-of-hours. Permanent staff are better placed than rotating trainees to acquire and share this material. Psychiatrists working in an ED function at an important interface between acute hospital services and community mental health and social services. The efficiency with which they work has a major influence on how appropriately resources are used in hospital and in the community.

These few paragraphs are not an exhaustive list but give some idea of the range of knowledge and skills required to function as a mental health professional in the ED. It should be apparent that a rota of largely unsupervised trainee psychiatrists is not likely to deliver this and so alternative service models are required.

Resourcing and managing the service

The starting point for this work will vary from place to place and from country to country. For the purposes of this chapter it is assumed that an ED is currently served round the clock by a rota of junior psychiatrists who are on-site at the general hospital but employed by a separate mental health trust. One local consultant general adult psychiatrist has a community mental health team and some psychiatric beds to manage but also has nominal responsibility for the ED (and specifically for patients who have deliberately self-harmed). This would not be an unusual scenario in many district general hospitals in the UK. How can a safer and more effective service be fashioned from this starting point?

The first step is to propose that a steering group of senior clinicians and managers from both trusts be established to look at service development in the ED for patients with mental health problems. The lead consultant for the ED, or the consultant psychiatrist with responsibility for the ED, is best placed to do this. The founders should devise terms of reference, reporting lines and propose formal representation on the steering group. These aspects should be approved by the chief executives of both trusts before the meetings begin. Meetings should be regular, short, infrequent and carefully minuted. One and a half hours every eight weeks has proven sufficient at our large ED over the past decade. Representation should include clinical directors or lead clinicians, senior nurse managers and service managers from both trusts.

An early task for the steering group is to arrange a baseline quantification of need in the ED. Information about deliberate self-harm, substance misuse and mental health presentations tends not to be captured well by standard computerized ED activity systems. A special effort to measure activity over a short period, say three months, will probably be required. The data should include age, sex, address, mode of referral, presenting complaint and time of presentation of the patient; response time of the psychiatrist, psychiatric and medical diagnoses and total time in ED. Outcomes of assessment include discharge, admission to medical/surgical bed or Clinical Decision Unit (observation ward), psychiatric admission (informal or under Mental Health Act) and referral on to various agencies dealing with substance misuse and psychosocial problems.

Once the scale of the task has been defined the work of developing a bid for resources can begin. Rather than setting up a service to fail, specified response times for mental health professionals and maximum waiting times for patients should be factored in early in the planning process. Another important issue at this stage is to decide whether the ED will serve as the designated place of safety for people arrested by police in a public place but who are thought to be suffering from a mental illness. In England and Wales they are brought to a place of safety, often a hospital, under the provisions of Section 136 of the Mental Health Act (1983) to be assessed by a psychiatrist and an approved social worker. Similar arrangements operate in other parts of the UK. This decision will require negotiation with the local police as well as with the mental health trust. A clear local policy is essential if the safety of patients and public alike is to be protected. It is particularly important to agree that police officers should remain with the patient until hospital staff are satisfied that they themselves can ensure the immediate safety of the patient and others. If the ED is to serve this function there needs to be a space where severely behaviourally disturbed patients can be managed for several hours without disrupting the whole department.

Resources include health professionals, space and equipment. Teams of psychiatric liaison nurses, supported by trainee psychiatrists and a consultant liaison psychiatrist, are increasingly favoured nationally. Such nurses usually have considerable experience and are able to practise autonomously. In order to provide 24-hour nursing cover 365 days per year to an ED seeing 105 000 presentations per annum a team of nine or ten nurses is required. A team leader from a nursing background may be better placed than a consultant psychiatrist to provide professional and managerial supervision to this group. The role of the consultant liaison psychiatrist is to provide senior psychiatric cover to the ED, to supervise and educate trainee psychiatrists working in the ED, to take medicolegal responsibility when there are problems, to lead clinical supervision of the permanent team and to take a leading role at the steering group. Four or five dedicated programmed activity sessions per week of consultant time are required to support a large ED. The responsibility for educating and supporting general-trained staff in the ED in their work with the mentally ill should be shared between all permanent members of the ED liaison psychiatry team.

Devising adequate clinical supervision of a large, rotating group of trainee doctors in psychiatry is a major challenge. Induction to the ED, in addition to the more general induction to the mental health trust, is important. Policies and protocols for working in the ED setting are brought to their attention (including personal safety policy and risk assessment tools) as well as precise information on how to contact senior support. New doctors are shown round the ED and the importance of communication with the general staff is stressed.

The postgraduate education of trainees is largely influenced by the need to prepare them for professional examinations, and the management of psychiatric emergencies in the ED is only a tiny part of that curriculum. In addition, we find duty psychiatrists reluctant to seek advice from consultant psychiatrists out-of-hours. For these reasons it is helpful to hold a weekly 'ED discussion group' for all trainees participating in on-call rotas at the general hospital. At this meeting, led by the consultant liaison psychiatrist, core assessment skills are taught and awareness of relevant local services raised. Clinical experiences in the ED are reflected upon and any conflicts with ED staff aired. Issues raised in this forum can be taken to the steering group for resolution when necessary.

Suitable space for assessing and managing patients with mental health and substance misuse problems is difficult to find in an ED. If the department accepts patients detained under Section 136 of the Mental Health Act (or its equivalent) a dedicated room with two exits, some windows to provide natural light and ventilation, closed circuit television, panic alarms, suitable furnishings, sound proofing and a carefully written operational policy are required. Facilities for severely intoxicated patients tend to be limited to a choice between the waiting room and the observation ward until sobriety is achieved. This is increasingly recognized as unsatisfactory. Emergency departments in Australia and the USA often have dedicated spaces where intoxicated patients can be nursed.

In assessing many patients a balance has to be achieved between providing privacy on the one hand and ensuring safety on the other. For example, as a result of high-profile cases where patients have absconded from the ED to complete suicide, we now advocate using a cubicle directly opposite the nursing station, with the curtain open and a security guard present, for assessing patients who are judged to be at highest risk of suicide after triage. It is useful to devise clear policies for where adolescents (aged 16–18) will be admitted after self-harm and where psychotic patients will be nursed during the several hours it takes to complete assessments for detention under the Mental Health Act. Many observation wards, now often referred to as Clinical Decision Units, specifically exclude the latter from their admission criteria, leaving the patient in the main ED for long periods.

The UK government's waiting time initiative has provoked a searching re-examination of resources and systems. The analysis of so-called 'breach data' (i.e. the events leading to patients remaining in an ED for longer than four hours) reveals what takes most time in the department. Preliminary analysis indicates that sobering up intoxicated patients, finding psychiatric beds (especially for adolescents) and accessing approved social workers for Mental Health Act assessments out of hours can all be very time-consuming. Moving patients who have poisoned themselves from the main department to a medical Clinical Decision Unit for further management of the overdose is an essential prerequisite for meeting the four-hour waiting time target.

Office space is required for the liaison psychiatry team in the ED. A single bleep for the nurses and another for the duty psychiatry senior house officer are needed. These should never be left unmanned. Other basic equipment includes phones, a fax machine, computer with activity database and access to any local electronic patient record for mental health as well as the main ED computer system. Policies and protocols should include guidance for triage staff, CDU admissions, deliberate self-harm, responsibility for finding psychiatric beds and arranging admission, staff safety, risk assessment, major incident policy, incident reporting policy and special observation policy.

An exhaustive and authoritative guide to best practice has recently been published by the Royal College of Psychiatrists in association with the British Association for Accident & Emergency Medicine (2004). This report makes numerous recommendations for best practice, including specified response times for mental health professionals to EDs. For example it recommends that in urban areas patients should be seen by a member of the mental health team within 30 minutes of referral and, if they require assessment for compulsory admission, they should be seen by suitably qualified professionals within 60 minutes of referral. Recommended times are slightly longer in rural areas. This policy, if implemented widely, should reduce the time patients with mental health problems have to wait in the ED but its success will depend on having a sufficiently well-staffed service so that members of the clinical team can respond promptly.

Outcomes

What does an adequately resourced liaison psychiatry service in the ED achieve? At present there is simply not enough published research data to answer this question comprehensively. One thing such a service will predictably not achieve is the complete elimination of risk or of serious incidents (i.e. suicides and homicides after leaving the ED). This needs to be understood by those commissioning the service.

An important recent study from Leeds indicates that 39% of the people committing suicide in that city had attended the ED there in the 12 months before dying (median 38 days before death). About 40% of these had attended with deliberate self-harm (Gairin *et al.* 2003). These figures suggest some scope for prevention but how to achieve such prevention is unclear. Leeds had some of the best developed liaison psychiatry services in the UK during the period of this study.

The first demonstrable outcome is an accessible mental health service that seems to suit the behaviour of a population of rather disadvantaged and otherwise socially excluded patients. The ED liaison psychiatry service is well placed to serve those with mixed physical and mental health problems; for example, self-harm, delirium, low mood and alcohol dependence. It provides an emergency psychiatry resource outside working hours and is an important interface between acute hospital and mental health services.

If evidence-based interventions, such as problem-solving, cognitive-behaviour therapy or brief psychodynamic psychotherapy for deliberate self-harm and brief intervention for hazardous drinkers, are offered there can be statistically significant reductions in repetition of self-harm (Guthrie *et al.* 2001; Hawton *et al.* 1998; Salkovskis *et al.* 1990b) and in hazardous drinking (Wright *et al.* 1998) after contact with the ED liaison psychiatry service.

We have local evidence to support the view that liaison psychiatry services reduce the waiting times in the ED for those with mental health problems. The expansion of the psychiatric liaison nursing team from two to nine between 1999 and 2004 led to a decrease in length of stay in the ED from an average of eight hours to under four hours for 90% of patients.

The liaison psychiatry team can significantly reduce the proportion of patients with mental health problems leaving the ED unassessed. While Ellis and Lewis (1997) reported absconding rates of 19–27%, the figure for St Thomas' ED, which has the benefit of a 24-hour liaison nursing presence, is now around 2%.

There is weak local evidence for a reduced number of psychiatric admissions via the ED with the expansion of the liaison psychiatry service. Between 1999 and 2004 the number of mental health assessments per annum in St Thomas' ED remained fairly static while the percentage admitted to psychiatric beds fell from 20% to 11%. This indicates a role in 'gatekeeping' scarce inpatient resources.

No studies have yet measured the effect of a well-resourced liaison psychiatry service on the patient environment for all in the ED, on retention of general-trained staff in the ED or on ED referrer satisfaction. We would predict positive findings on all these outcome measures.

REFERENCES

Cassar, S., Hodgkiss, A., Ramirez, A., *et al.* (2002). Mental health presentations to an inner city accident and emergency department. *Psychiatric Bulletin,* **26**, 134–6.

Crawford, M. and Kohen, D. (1997). Urgent psychiatric assessment in an inner city A&E department. *Psychiatric Bulletin,* **21**, 625–6.

Ellis, D. and Lewis, S. (1997). Psychiatric presentations to an A&E department. *Psychiatric Bulletin,* **21**, 627–30.

Gairin, I., House, A. and Owens, D. (2003). Attendance at the accident & emergency department in the year before suicide: retrospective study. *British Journal of Psychiatry,* **183**, 28–33.

Guthrie, E., Kapur, N., Mackway-Jones, K., *et al.* (2001). Randomised controlled trial of brief psychological intervention after deliberate self poisoning. *British Medical Journal,* **323**, 135–8.

Harrison, A. and Bruce-Jones, W. (2003). Reforming psychiatric care. *Psychiatric Bulletin,* **27**, 276.

Hawton, K., Arensman, E., Townsend, E., *et al.* (1998). Deliberate self harm: systematic review of efficacy of psychosocial and pharmacological treatments in preventing repetition. *British Medical Journal,* **317**, 441–7.

Henderson, M., Hicks, A. and Hotopf, M. (2003). Reforming emergency care: implications for psychiatry. *Psychiatric Bulletin,* **27**, 81–2.

House, A. and Hodgson, G. (1994). Estimating needs and meeting demands. In *Liaison Psychiatry: Defining Needs and Planning Services,* ed. S. Benjamin, A. House and P. Jenkins. London: Gaskell, pp. 3–15.

Rose, S. and Bisson, J. (1998). Brief early psychological interventions following trauma: a systematic review of the literature. *Journal of Traumatic Stress,* **11**, 697–710.

Royal College of Physicians and Royal College of Psychiatrists. (2003). *The Psychological Care of Medical Patients.* London: RCP, p. 70

Royal College of Psychiatrists and British Association for Accident & Emergency Medicine. (2004). *Psychiatric Services to Accident & Emergency Departments (Council Report CR118).* London: RCPsych.

Salkovskis, P., Storer, D., Atha, C., *et al.* (1990a). Psychiatric morbidity in an accident & emergency department. *British Journal of Psychiatry,* **156**, 483–7.

Salkovskis, P., Atha, C. and Storer, D. (1990b). Cognitive behavioural problem solving in the treatment of patients who repeatedly attempt suicide: a controlled trial. *British Journal of Psychiatry,* **157**, 871–6.

Wittgenstein, L. (1958). *Philosophical Investigations,* 2nd edn. Oxford: Basil Blackwell, p. 227.

Wright, S., Moran, L., Meyrick, M., *et al.* (1998). Intervention by an alcohol health worker in an accident & emergency department. *Alcohol & Alcoholism,* **33**, 651–6.

Part IV

Treatment

33

Psychopharmacological treatment in liaison psychiatry

Ulrik Fredrik Malt and Geoffrey Lloyd

Introduction

There is still limited systematic research on the effectiveness of psychotropic drugs used in liaison psychiatry settings. Evidence-based psychopharmacology of the medically ill still must rely on relevant information from traditional evidence-based data sources such as the Cochrane Library (www.thecochranelibrary.com), clinical evidence by the BMJ publishing group (www.clinicalevidence.com), American College of Physicians (ACP) Journal Club (www.acpjc.org), Evidence-Based Mental Health (http://ebmh.bmjjournals.com), the TRIP Database Plus (www.tripdatabase.com) and systematic reviews accessible through PubMed (www.pubmed.gov). This chapter is primarily based on those databases supplemented by reviews (e.g. Strain *et al.* 2004) and clinical experience in liaison and general psychiatry.

Principles for drug selection

All drugs available in clinical psychiatry for the treatment of psychiatric disorders can be used in liaison settings. However, before choosing a specific drug, liaison psychiatrists must address seven additional important issues beyond those related to the indication for a psychotropic drug (Table 33.1).

In order to answer these seven questions, the liaison psychiatrist needs some basic knowledge about pharmacodynamics (what the drug does to the body on a neurobiological level, e.g. drug receptor profile) and pharmacokinetics (what the body does to the drug, e.g. drug metabolism), in particular with reference to the special difficulties of treating patients with organ failure.

Handbook of Liaison Psychiatry, ed. Geoffrey Lloyd and Elspeth Guthrie. Published by Cambridge University Press. © Cambridge University Press 2007.

Table 33.1. The seven key questions before choosing a psychotropic drug in liaison psychiatry.

To what extent will a specific psychotropic drug influence positively the pathophysiology of the underlying
somatic disease? (e.g. 5HT receptor antagonists and reuptake inhibitors and positive effect on detrusor
instability incontinence)

To what extent will a specific psychotropic drug influence negatively the pathophysiology of the underlying
somatic disease? (e.g. platelet dysfunction with increased bleeding risk due to SSRIs; olanzapine worsening
diabetes mellitus; QTc prolongation due to thioridazine)

To what extent can the side-effect profile (i.e. the receptor profile) of the drug be used to achieve additional
symptomatic benefits? (e.g. antimanic effects of topiramate in overweight patients; antidepressants
with $5HT_3$ antagonism to counteract disease-related nausea)

To what extent can the side-effect profile of the drug be counterproductive in the specific disease in question?
(e.g. NA-reuptake blocking drugs in patients with Sjøgren's syndrome may worsen dry mouth; treatment of
social phobia related to diarrhoea with SSRIs in patients with inflammatory bowel disease; anticholinergic
side-effects of drugs may worsen cognition)

To what extent will a psychotropic drug interact with other drugs already taken by the patient? (e.g. SSRIs
and $5HT_{1a+c}$ active migraine drugs with increased risk for serotonergic syndrome; carbamazepine may
induce changes in the metabolism of other drugs)

Can the patient take oral medication or is it necessary to use drugs that can be administered intravenously?

Is liver and/or kidney function impaired to such extent that metabolism of the drug is likely to be reduced
thus requiring reduced dosage?

Pharmacodynamics

Three main types of receptors have been identified: inotropic (fast-acting
receptors); g-protein coupled ('slow'-acting receptors) and nuclear receptors.
Most psychotropic drugs used today are aimed at g-protein coupled receptors, e.g.
serotonergic (5HT), noradrenaline (NA), dopamine (DA), glutamate (GLU) and
acetylcholine (ACh) receptors. Currently only a few drugs act on enzymes
(e.g. moclobemide), but such drugs and drugs acting on hormone regulation are
currently being studied in pre-marketing clinical trials (e.g. CRH-antagonists).
Currently, drugs acting primarily on ionotropic or nuclear receptors are not
available for daily clinical use.

The most important clinical implication of a drug's effect on receptors is the
relationship between receptor profile effect (agonism=stimulation; antagonism=
blockade) and symptomatic response including side-effects. The receptor profile
of the drug can predict symptomatic response (e.g. NA-receptor stimulation
properties will predict activation) or side-effects (e.g. $5HT_3$ receptor antagonism
predicts reduced level of nausea). Thus if one knows the main receptor profile of a
drug, it is much easier to tailor a specific drug to a specific person, facilitating
wanted and avoiding unwanted effects.

Table 33.2. Symptoms of serotonergic syndrome.

Early symptoms
Impaired ability to concentrate
Involuntary muscle movements (myoclonus)
Hyperreflexia
Muscle rigidity
Orthostatic hypotension
Confusion
(Normal levels of creatinine-phosphokinase)

Life-threatening severity
Dysarthria
High fever
Nystagmus
Localized or general muscle cramps (e.g. oculogyric crisis; opisthotonus)
Babinsky's test positive
Disseminated intravascular coagulation (DIC)
Myoglobulinuria and kidney failure

Pharmacodynamic effects may also be of particular interest in liaison psychiatry when a psychotropic drug is given together with other drugs. If, for example, a serotonergic active drug (e.g. selective serotonin reuptake inhibitor (SSRI)) is given to a patient already taking another drug acting on serotonin (e.g. serotonergic-acting anti-migraine drugs), this may increase the risk of serotonergic syndrome (pharmacodynamic interaction), the symptoms of which are listed in Table 33.2.

Pharmacokinetics
Phase I metabolism and cytochromes

Following oral administration, a drug may be removed by gut and liver. About 50% of a drug is metabolized in phase I. This first phase of metabolism consists of oxidation, reduction and hydrolysis by cytochrome P450 (CYP) and other enzymes. There is considerable variation in the serum concentration between individuals after taking the same amount of a drug. In fact, in two different individuals the serum concentration after taking the same dose may vary up to 20 times! When a patient does not respond to a regular dose, or suffers from unusual strong side-effects, the possibility of under- or over-dosing respectively should be considered. If possible, serum concentration of the drug in question should be measured to help determine further action.

However, the metabolism of a drug can to some extent be predicted by knowledge of the enzymatic 'make-up' of the patient and by other factors such as alcohol consumption, smoking and diet. The enzymes of the P450-3A subfamily of cytochromes (CYP-3A) are the most abundant of the human hepatic cytochromes. CYP-3A isoforms mediate the biotransformation of many drugs, including a number of psychotropic, cardiac, analgesic, hormonal, immunosuppressant, antineoplastic, and antihistaminic agents. Other important specific oxidative metabolizing enzymes include CYP-1A2, CYP-2C9, CYP-2C19, CYP-2D6 and CYP-2E1

Genetic polymorphism

Activity of CYP-3A varies among individuals, but there is no evidence of genetic polymorphism. Significant amounts of CYP-3A are present in the gastrointestinal tract, and may contribute to presystemic extraction of drugs such as ciclosporin.

In contrast to CYP-3A, the amount of CYP-2C9, 2C19 and 2D6 may vary due to genetic polymorphism. If a person lacks CYP-2D6, even low doses of a psychotropic drug metabolized by this isoenzyme (e.g. paroxetine) may lead to very high serum concentrations and intolerable side-effects. Contrarily, too much of this enzyme may be associated with almost non-detectable amounts of drug in serum and no clinical response (or side-effects) despite good compliance. In some European countries, genetic determination of CYP-2C9, 2C19 and 2D6 polymorphism is available as part of the clinical routine assessment of patients seen in liaison services.

The issue is complicated by the fact that some drugs are substrate for the same isoenzyme. If the enzyme capacity is genetically or by other mechanisms reduced (e.g. competition through co-administration of other drug metabolized by the same isoenzyme), clinically significant interactions may occur.

Other drugs, or food items, may inhibit or induce the activity of one or more of the isoenzymes (2D6 is not inducible). Such mechanisms may also severely interfere with the metabolism of a given psychotropic drug. Side-effects, or more rarely — life-threatening adverse events, may be the result.

The azole antifungal agents ketoconazole and itraconazole are potent inhibitors of human CYP-3A isoforms. Selective serotonin reuptake inhibitor antidepressants are also CYP-3A inhibitors, but much less potent than ketoconazole or itraconazole.

It is almost impossible to remember all possible interactions. For that reason, an interaction list should always be consulted before mixing medication. A comprehensive update of the current knowledge about clinically significant substrates, inhibitors and inducers of some key cytochromes can be found by consulting http://medicine.iupui.edu/flockhart/clinlist.htm.

Phase II metabolism and glucuronide conjugation

Following phase I, phase II metabolism is characterized by glucuronide conjugation plus sulphate and mercapturic acid conjugates. The metabolites created by this process are water soluble and can be excreted in the urine. Glucuronide conjugation is induced by smoking and reduced by alcohol. Olanzapine, oxazepam and the anti-epileptics valproate and lamotrigine are all substrates for uridinephosphatase-glucuronide-transferase (UGT) activity. Presently N-acetyltransferase and glutathione transferase are being characterized and developed. These probes are now being applied in various settings where the characterization of the activities of metabolizing enzymes is required. However, the assessment of the activity of those enzymes is currently not available for regular clinical use.

There is still much research needed to understand the effect of disease, e.g. renal and hepatic diseases, on metabolizing activities. Also the influence of liver transplantation on metabolism of drugs is insufficiently understood as is the role of metabolizing activities as aetiological risk factors in disease development. Despite these shortcomings in our knowledge, clinical experience indicates that even the most severely ill medical patients can be treated with psychotropic drugs without severe complications if liaison psychiatrists pay appropriate attention to the basic pharmacokinetic mechanisms outlined above.

Pharmacogenomics

Pharmacogenomics is the study of how an individual's genetic inheritance affects the body's response to drugs. Pharmacogenomics holds the promise that the psychiatrist may choose a drug which is tailor-made for an individual and adapted to each patient's own genetic makeup. It is a rapidly developing research area and it is likely that in the near future genetic tests will be available to help the psychiatrist in tailoring treatment to the individual's genetic characteristics. More information on the very interesting development of pharmacogenetics may be found on the Human Genome Project website (www.ornl.gov/sci/techresources/Human_Genome/medicine/pharma.shtml).

Psychotropic drugs used in liaison psychiatry

The availability of psychotropic drugs varies to some extent between countries within the European Union. In this chapter the most frequently used drugs will be discussed. National Formularies for practical information are available in all European languages. The *British National Formulary* (www.bnf.org) is the UK-based formulary.

Antidepressants

These drugs have a broad range of effects and are used to treat other conditions as well as depression. The first generation of these drugs, the tricyclic antidepressants (TCA), have largely been superseded as first-line treatment by second-generation drugs, the SSRIs, because of less troublesome side-effects. These drugs are also used for non-affective disorders, for example panic disorder, generalized anxiety disorder, post-traumatic stress disorder, obsessive-compulsive disorder, eating disorders, impulsive disorders and several behavioural disturbances associated with brain injury.

The main mechanisms of actions of the drugs currently available are listed in Table 33.3.

Antidepressants are commonly given orally, but intravenous administration is possible for clomipramine, amitriptyline, citalopram and mirtazapine. Citalopram and mirtazapine cause fewer side-effects and interactions than TCAs and should be first choice when i.v. delivery is needed in liaison psychiatry. This is discussed in more detail below.

Table 33.3. Psychotropic drugs used to treat and prevent anxiety, depression and impulse disorders.

Mechanism of action		Specific type of action	Examples
1. Inhibition of presynaptic monoamine reuptake	1.1	Selective inhibition of serotonin (5HT) (selective serotonin reuptake inhibitor; SSRI)	citalopram, escitalopram, fluoxetine, fluvoxamine, paroxetine, sertraline
	1.2	Selective inhibition of noradrenaline (NA) (noradrenergic reuptake inhibitors; NARI)	atomoxetine, reboxetine
	1.3	Selective inhibition of 5HT and NA (SNRIs)	duloxetine, milnacipran, venlafaxine
	1.4	Selective inhibition of DA and NA	bupropion
	1.5	Unselective presynaptic inhibition of monoamines (tricyclic antidepressants; TCA)	amitriptyline, clomipramine, desimipramine, dosulepin,

Table 33.3. (*cont.*)

Mechanism of action		Specific type of action	Examples
			doxepine, imipramine, nortriptyline, trimipramine
2. Antagonism of $5HT_2$ receptors plus additional effects		Additional effects	
	2.1	Antagonism of pre-synaptic α_2-receptors and $5HT_3$ post-synaptic receptors	mianserin, mirtazapine
	2.2	Melatonin agonism	agomelatine
3. Inhibition of monoamine oxidase	3.1	Reversible and selective inhibition of monoamine oxidase A (RIMA)	moclobemide
	3.2	Reversible and selective inhibition of monoamine oxidase B	selegiline
	3.3	Unselective inhibition of monoamine oxidases (MAOI)	isocarboxazid, phenelzine, tranylcypromine
4. Mood stabilizers	4.1	Glutamate modulators with additional effects (see text)	lamotrigine
	4.2	Gamma-amino-buturic acid (GABA) agonists with additional effects (see text)	valproic acid, gabapentine, pregabaline, topiramate
	4.3	GABA-agonists and noradrenaline-reuptake inhibition	carbamazepine, oxcarbazepine
	4.4	Intracellular	lithium
5. Others	5.1	Combined partial postsynaptic agonists with complete agonists on serotonin autoreceptors	buspirone
	5.2	Serotonin reuptake accelerator (i.e. opposite to the SSRIs)	tianeptine
	5.3	$D_2 5HT_2$ receptor antagonist	amoxapine

Indications for SSRIs

Selective serotonin reuptake inhibitors (see Table 33.3; 1.1) are effective in the treatment of most non-psychotic disorders seen in liaison psychiatry but the indications approved for their use vary between different countries. They are well tolerated; most side-effects are immediate and of short duration. Regular doses can be used in liaison settings but for patients with severe medical illnesses the starting dose should be half the regular dose. Sertraline is the drug of choice for treating depression in patients with a recent myocardial infarction or unstable angina.

Pharmacokinetics and dosing of SSRIs

The clinical effects of the different generic versions of the SSRIs are similar. However, there are subtle differences which make a difference when considering potential side-effects and interactions. For example, citalopram, escitalopram and sertraline are least likely to cause problematic pharmacokinetic interactions with other drugs. Fluvoxamine has the highest risk of causing harmful interactions (mainly by inhibiting CYP-1A and CYP-3A3-4). For these reasons, fluvoxamine is not recommended as the first drug of choice for patients with comorbid somatic disorders.

Paroxetine and fluoxetine both inhibit CYP-2D6 to a larger extent than the other SSRIs and may cause increased serum concentrations of other drugs metabolized by this enzyme. Their use in liaison psychiatry thus requires attention to possible interactions with other drugs metabolized by 2D6.

The long half-life (14 days) of fluoxetine's active metabolite, nor-fluoxetine, may cause a major problem when there is a need to stop the drug at short notice. However, in bulimia, where occasionally vomiting and thus loss of recently ingested drugs may be a problem, the long half-life of fluoxetine may be an advantage. Citalopram is the only SSRI currently available as an infusion.

Selective noradrenaline reuptake inhibitors (NARIs or NRIs)

The NARIs are especially suitable for drive-deficient 'anergic' states where the capacity for sustained motivation is lacking. Some studies also suggest an effect in attention-deficit hyperactivity disorders. Their lack of effect on serotonin means that they will not have the same inhibitive effect on sexual drive as SSRIs.

Combined serotonin and noradrenaline reuptake inhibitors (SNARIs)

Three drugs are currently available with this mechanism of action (see Table 33.3; 1.3): duloxetine, milnacipran and venlafaxine. Unlike duloxetine and venlafaxine, milnacipran appears to select serotonin transporters in binding and norepinephrine transporters in uptake, suggesting that milnacipran's binding and uptake inhibition profile more closely resembles that of the tricyclic antidepressants. There are few direct comparisons between duloxetine, milnacipran and venlafaxine. Until more data are available, the clinical effects should be considered to be similar.

In higher doses, venlafaxine may have some dopamine-reuptake blockade effects. In low dosages, however (e.g. 37.5–150 mg), venlafaxine acts like the SSRIs.

It has been suggested that SNARIs and noradrenergic and specific serotonin antidepressants (NASSAs; see below) may show faster action of onset than other antidepressants. The studies claiming this result were not designed to address this issue, however.

The main indications for duloxetine, milnacipran and venlafaxine are severe depressive episodes, e.g. depressive phase of bipolar spectrum disorders, physical symptoms and pain related to such disorders and generalized anxiety. They should be used for patients who have not responded to an SSRI. SNARIs may also have advantages in the treatment of severe cases of obsessive-compulsive disorder (OCD). Duloxetine has been found to be effective for the treatment of stress urinary incontinence (Dmochowski *et al.* 2003).

Interactions are few. Duloxetine is a moderately potent inhibitor of CYP-2D6 and caution should be used when CYP-2D6 substrates and inhibitors are coadministered with duloxetine. SNARIs can be combined with mirtazapine in order to increase the response rate in severe cases of depression. Blood pressure measurement should be undertaken before SNARIs are started and blood pressure should be monitored regularly thereafter.

Selective inhibition of noradrenaline and dopamine

Bupropion's effect on both noradrenaline and dopamine makes it an activating drug. Accordingly, the main indication has been depressive disorders within the bipolar spectrum associated with hypersomnia, fatigue and cognitive impairment. Some data favour the use of bupropion to treat attention-deficit hyperactivity disorder (ADHD). The lack of serotonergic effects also makes bupropion an alternative to serotonin-active drugs among patients who are intolerant to serotonin-related side-effects (e.g. sexual dysfunction).

The stimulating effects on the dopamine system mimic to a certain extent the effects of nicotine and reduce the need for nicotine in nicotine-dependent patients. Bupropion has been used successfully in smoking cessation programmes. It reduces withdrawal symptoms as well as weight gain and is effective for smoking cessation for people with and without a history of depression or alcoholism (Richmond & Zwar 2003). In some countries, including the UK, bupropion is currently only licensed as an anti-smoking drug.

Unselective presynaptic inhibition of monoamine reuptake ('tricyclic antidepressants')

The efficacy of TCAs is at least as good as for the new more selective antidepressant drugs. Their drawback is mainly their complicated receptor profile with abundant associated risk of pharmacodynamic and pharmacokinetic interactions. Their anticholinergic effects may worsen cognitive function in the elderly and even provoke confusion. They are also very toxic in overdose. For those reasons, TCAs are no longer recommended as the first treatment option for depressive or anxiety disorders in the medically ill. They continue to be used by neurologists and pain treatment specialists in the management of patients with chronic pain, whether or not this is associated with depression.

If used in liaison settings, the potential interaction with other drugs must be checked prior to administration. Lower doses are required in patients with liver disease and those who are severely ill. If TCAs are given to patients with cardiovascular disease lofepramine is probably the safest choice. Amitriptyline may be given intravenously, but there is an increased risk for cardiovascular complications.

Antagonism of postsynaptic 5HT2 receptors

Several drugs have 5HT2-blocking effects. Such effects are associated with reduced anxiety, sedation and lack of sexual side-effects. However, the drugs within this class differ very much with regard to other pharmacodynamic effects.

Mianserin is a postsynaptic $5HT_{2\&3}$ receptor blocker with a strong presynaptic α_2 receptor blocking effect and additional potent $H_{1\&2}$ and postsynaptic α_1 blocker effect. Mirtazapine has an almost identical receptor profile except for a much weaker effect on postsynaptic α_1 receptors. It is suggested, but not proven in controlled studies, that this difference may favour mirtazapine with regard to somewhat better antidepressant effect (no blocking of the post-synaptic α_1 transferred serotonin-stimulating effect of noradrenaline in the raphe area). Thus mirtazapine is often called a dual-action antidepressant, i.e. a noradrenergic and specific serotonergic antidepressant (NASSA).

The advantage of mianserin and mirtazapine in liaison settings is a low potential for interaction with other drugs. Their appetite-inducing and fast sleep-improving effects may also be an advantage as are their blocking properties on the post-synaptic $5HT_{2\&3}$ receptors, which reduce risk of sexual side-effects to placebo levels and counteract nausea. However, $5HT_3$ receptor antagonists do not show a significant prophylactic effect on delayed emesis seen sometimes after chemotherapy for cancer. The α_2-antagonistic effect may counteract the antihypertensive effect of clonidine, however.

Mirtazapine (Remergil) is available for intravenous administration. The drug is mixed with 500 ml 5% glucose. The solution is given as an infusion over two hours.

In patients with a medical disorder 6 mg per day is recommended for the first two days, followed by 9 mg per day during days 3 and 4. From day 5 onwards, 15 mg per day is given. If available, a measurement of serum concentration of mirtazapine is recommended after a week on stable dose. When changing to oral administration, the oral dose should be double that of the i.v. dose (e.g. 15 mg i.v. = 30 mg orally). Mirtazapine is primarily eliminated via the urine (75%). Renal clearances are decreased in patients with liver and/or kidney dysfunction, and in elderly patients. The dose should be adjusted accordingly.

Trazodone also has serotonin-reuptake inhibiting properties, but it lacks noradrenaline properties. In contrast to agomelatine, trazodone has antihistamine properties. Thus in countries where trazodone is marketed, it is frequently used among patients with depression and sleep disorders. Due to its anxiolytic and sedative effects it has also been suggested to have a potential option in the treatment of alcohol post-withdrawal insomnia. The same indication has been suggested for other $5HT_2$ antagonists like mianserin and mirtazapine.

Reversible and selective inhibition of monoamine oxidase A (RIMA)

Moclobemide is the only marketed drug acting selectively on monoamine oxidase A (MAOA). MAOA is responsible for inactivating noradrenaline and serotonin. The net effect of moclobemide is thus to increase the amount of NA and 5HT available for transmission. From a clinical point of view, moclobemide is rather activating and insomnia and lightheadedness are frequently reported side-effects. The exact place of moclobemide in the treatment of depressive disorders remains to be settled. Clinical experience may suggest that the drug's main role is in moderately severe episodes of depression within the bipolar spectrum disorders, perhaps more so among younger subjects (Lingjærde et al. 1995).

Moclobemide is metabolized by CYP-2C19 (note genetic polymorphism!). It also inhibits CYP-2D6. Combination with serotonin reuptake inhibitors or lithium should be avoided due to the risk for serotonin syndrome.

Reversible and selective inhibition of monoamine oxidase B (MAOB)

Selegiline inhibits MAOB which inactivates dopamine. Selegiline has a neuroprotective role due to its ability to reduce the generation of free radicals. The main indication is Parkinson's disease and it is not used to treat depression due to a rather weak antidepressant effect. Selegiline should not be combined with MAOA. The net effect is an unselective MAO inhibitor with the risk of severe side-effects.

Unselective monoamine oxidase inhibitors (MAOIs)

The unselective MAOIs have a strong inactivating effect on NA, 5HT and DA and include phenelzine, tranylcypromine and isocarboxazid. MAOIs are seldom indicated in liaison psychiatry in view of their toxicity and interactions with other drugs. Common side-effects are orthostatic hypotension and insomnia. Patients on MAOIs must stick to a strict diet avoiding food items containing tyramine, which may cause lethal hypertensive crisis. Liver damage may also be due to MAO inhibition.

Other drugs used to treat anxiety and depressive disorders and impulsive-related disorders

This group includes a variety of drugs with different mechanisms of action (see Table 33.3).

Tianeptine binds with neither serotonin nor adrenergic receptors, but accelerates the uptake of serotonin, in contrast to the SSRIs which inhibit reuptake. Interestingly, in controlled trials, the antidepressant effect of tianeptine seems to be similar to that seen with SSRIs. However, so far the evidence of its effect is limited. Depression and anxiety disorders are the main indications for tianeptine. Tianeptine lacks sedative, anticholinergic and cardiovascular adverse effects. This may suggest that it is particularly suitable for use in the elderly and in patients following alcohol withdrawal. However, there is insufficient research to back this assumption.

Amoxapine is marketed as an antidepressant. However, its receptor occupancy, in vitro and in vivo, and its effects in preclinical models are very similar to atypical antipsychotics. It seems to have some antipsychotic properties. It may worsen motor function among patients with Parkinson's disease (Sa *et al.* 2001) and tardive dyskinesias have been reported. Neuroleptic syndrome has also been reported when using amoxapine. Considering the complex actions of amoxapine and its neuroleptic-like properties, it should not be a first-choice option in the treatment of depression in liaison psychiatry.

Hypericum perforatum (St John's wort) is a herbaceous perennial plant whose extract has acquired some popularity in the treatment of depression, but its efficacy is weak (Hammerness *et al.* 2003). Some patients seen in liaison psychiatry practice may already be taking the drug. It is therefore important to be aware of side-effects, which include nausea, rash, fatigue, restlessness, photosensitivity, acute neuropathy and episodes of mania. Interaction with other antidepressant drugs can cause the serotonergic syndrome (Rodriguez-Landa & Contreras 2003). St John's wort may interact with some cytostatic drugs reducing their effect. In transplant patients this effect may lead to rejection.

Risks and side-effects of antidepressants

There is no absolute contraindication to the use of antidepressants in the medically ill. Before treatment is started patients should be informed of the potential side-effects, particularly nausea, headache and sexual dysfunction, and of the risk of a discontinuation/withdrawal syndrome. They should also be informed of the delayed clinical effect and of the need to continue treatment for at least four to six months after remission. It is usual to start with low doses in patients with severe physical illness. Patients starting an SSRI may experience initial anxiety, tension or akathisia. This may be alleviated by reducing the dose or by taking a small dose of a benzodiazepine. Evidence that SSRIs may reduce tamoxifen activity (Jin *et al.* 2005) suggests they should not be used to treat depression in women taking the drug for breast cancer.

The possibility that drugs with strong serotonergic effects may trigger suicide attempts or cause suicide has been much debated. Current evidence indicates no clear relation between SSRIs and suicide (Cipriani *et al.* 2005) but there may be an increase in suicidal thoughts and suicide attempts during the early stages of treatment (Malt *et al.* 1999). In some patients, the activating properties of SSRIs and SNARIs may remove the psychomotor inhibition before the depression improves. Doctors should plan frequent monitoring after initiating treatment and continue this until there are signs of clinical improvement. Benzodiazepines should be prescribed if needed.

The major side-effects with mianserin and mirtazapine are weight gain and sedation. Sedation is not related to dose, e.g. if sedation is a clinical problem on 30 mg mirtazapine, it will most likely be so at 15 mg too.

The existence of several side-effects suggest that trazodone is not an optimal first-line antidepressant in liaison psychiatry. Trazodone may be arrhythmogenic in some patients with pre-existing heart disease. It may cause orthostatic hypotension and syncope. Caution is required if it is given to patients receiving antihypertensive drugs; an adjustment in the dose of the antihypertensive medication may be required. Trazodone has also been associated with the occurrence of priapism, which may require surgical intervention.

Patients with temporal lobe epilepsy often suffer from concomitant depressive disorders. Current data suggest that antidepressants can be used successfully (e.g. SSRIs, mirtazapine, reboxetine) without serious adverse events or an increase in the frequency or severity of seizures (Kuhn *et al.* 2003).

Antidepressants in pregnancy and the puerperium

The use of antidepressants during pregnancy, in the postnatal period and during breastfeeding requires special attention. Since the introduction of TCAs in the 1950s, several thousands of women have been exposed to them during pregnancy and systematic follow-up studies have not found any increased risk of malformations compared to the population base rate.

Among the SSRIs, the data are less robust, but nevertheless reassuring. Data from more than 1000 women exposed to fluoxetine during the first trimester do not indicate any increased risk of malformation. Similar trends are reported in studies looking at other SSRIs such as citalopram, sertraline and fluvoxamine, although there have been reports of birth defects and cardiovascular abnormalities in the babies of women who have taken paroxetine. Data from 150 women exposed to the SNARI venlafaxine do not suggest any increased rate of malformations. Currently there are no published data on escitalopram. Given the longer experience with tricyclics nortriptyline, amitriptyline and imipramine are often recommended as the antidepressants of choice. However, SSRIs are used more frequently during pregnancy. If an SSRI is required fluoxetine has been studied the most.

Transient neonatal symptoms may occur following prenatal psychotropic medication exposure. Symptoms include mild respiratory distress and, less commonly, hypotonia. Symptoms are self-limiting and not associated with other neonatal conditions. Follow-up studies do not suggest adverse developmental has been studied the most effects (Oberlander et al. 2004).

The amount of antidepressant drugs found in breast milk is minimal. However, the reduced metabolic capacity of the newborn must be taken into account. After six months their ability to metabolize drugs is comparable to that of adults (Spigset & Hägg 1998).

Except for doxepine, most TCAs can be used safely when the mother is nursing. However, more data are available for the newer drugs. Drug concentrations found in breast milk are highest for fluoxetine; somewhat less for citalopram; lower for paroxetine and lowest for sertraline and fluvoxamine. Until data regarding escitalopram is available, one should assume findings comparable to those seen when giving citalopram.

Considering the small amounts of drug found in breast milk and the physical and psychological importance of breast milk, SSRIs and related drugs can be prescribed to nursing women (Misri & Kostaras 2002) although to date there are few controlled trials.

Indications for antidepressants in liaison psychiatry

Depression and anxiety

Depressive disorders accompanying physical illness should be treated to improve quality of life and treatment adherence. There is evidence to suggest that when depression or anxiety disorders occur together with a somatic disease, mortality increases significantly (Cole & Bellavance 1997) so treatment may also increase survival after some illnesses.

In general terms, antidepressants are effective and better than placebo when given to patients with depression and concomitant medical diseases.

A Cochrane study reviewed 18 studies including 838 patients with a range of physical diseases: cancer, diabetes, head injury, heart disease, HIV, lung disease, multiple sclerosis, renal disease, stroke and mixed somatic diseases (Gill & Hatcher 2003). Those studies showed that patients treated with antidepressants were significantly more likely to improve than those given placebo. Antidepressants should be given to those with moderate to severe depression. Psychological treatments, particularly counselling and cognitive-behaviour therapy, should be available for patients with mild depression and for those who express a wish for them.

Functional symptoms

Antidepressants have an important role in the management of physical symptoms unexplained by physical pathology. These include chronic pain, headache, facial pain and functional bowel disturbances.

Depression resistant to medication

Using electroconvulsive treatment (ECT)

If depression fails to respond to treatment with adequate courses of antidepressant medication from at least two different groups of drugs it is necessary to review the psychiatric diagnosis and to consider the possibility of an undiagnosed underlying physical illness which may cause depression (see Chapter 4). If the diagnosis of a depressive disorder remains valid, electroconvulsive treatment (ECT) should be considered. In addition to its use in drug-resistant depression ECT is indicated in depression with psychotic features, when there is a high risk of a suicide attempt and a quick response is required and when depression is associated with stupor and inadequate food and fluid intake. However there have been no controlled trials of ECT in a liaison setting.

There are no absolute contraindications to the use of ECT in physically ill patients. Relative contraindications include a history of recent myocardial infarction or stroke, raised intracranial pressure, chest infection and unstable cervical spine. Before considering giving ECT to a physically ill patient the opinions of a physician and anaesthetist should be sought. (For further information on ECT see Scott 2005.)

Neuroleptics

All neuroleptics share a dopamine receptor antagonism. Of the many receptors identified, D_2 effects are most important. The role of other dopamine receptors in relation to the efficacy of neuroleptics is not clearly established.

The first generation of neuroleptics included the phenothiazines and butyrophenones but they had a range of unpleasant side-effects including sedation, anticholinergic effects and extrapyramidal symptoms. Drugs developed subsequently had relatively less affinity for dopamine receptors compared to other receptors (e.g. $5HT_2$). For that reason, those drugs were called atypical (e.g. clozapine, olanzapine, quetiapine, risperidone, sertindole, ziprasidone, zotepine). It was long thought that those drugs had somewhat better effect on negative symptoms of schizophrenia and fewer side-effects. However, some of the other newer drugs do not have effects on $5HT_2$ receptors (e.g. amisulpride, aripiprazole), but on dopamine receptors only. Nevertheless, they have similar beneficial effects on negative symptoms and a comparable low frequency of side-effects. Thus the whole concept about what constitutes an atypical neuroleptic is being questioned (Leucht *et al.* 2003). In the following text the newer or 'atypical' neuroleptics are referred to as 'second-generation neuroleptics'.

The antipsychotic effect is characterized by gradual resolution of delusional cognitions and hallucinations. There is no clear correlation between a drug's degree of specific sedative effect and its antipsychotic effect. The antipsychotic effect develops rather slowly (over days and even weeks). If the delusions or hallucinations resolve the patient often acquires insight into their psychotic nature.

Neuroleptics also have a modest psychostimulant effect. Symptoms like apathy, lack of spontaneity and cognitive dysfunction improve. The exact mechanism of this effect is not clear, but D_1 stimulation in the frontal cortex has been postulated.

The specific, but not the non-specific, sedative effects of the different neuroleptics are similar. The first-generation antipsychotics are just as effective as the second-generation neuroleptics (Table 33.4). Neuroleptics differ, however, on their effect on other receptors, explaining differences in unspecific sedation, side-effect profiles and tolerability. These differences are of clinical importance (Table 33.4).

Indications for neuroleptics in liaison psychiatry

The main indication of neuroleptics in liaison psychiatry is non-alcohol delirium and other psychotic reactions that cannot be controlled by behavioural measures alone. Neuroleptics are sometimes also used in relatively low doses to treat anxiety and behavioural dysfunction in patients with severe personality disorders or mental retardation.

Which neuroleptic should be chosen?

In general terms, the antipsychotic effects of the different neuroleptics are equal. It is important to avoid any side-effects that may worsen the somatic disorder

Table 33.4. Receptor activity of commonly used neuroleptics.

Name	5HT$_{2A}$ antagonism (cortisol reduction?)	Muscarine$_1$ antagonism (dry mouth; cognitive impairment?)	Histamine$_1$ antagonism (weight gain, sedation)	α_1 (noradrenaline) antagonism (risk of orthostatic hypotension)	α_2 (noradrenaline) antagonism (antianxiety/ depression)	Comments
Amisulpride	0	0	0	0	0	Affinity for D$_{2\&3}$ receptors. No effect on D$_1$ receptors: advantage in patients with mostly negative symptoms and cognitive impairment? May increase prolactin.
Aripiprazole	++	?	0	+	?	Reduce, rather than raise, prolactin levels; lower rates than haloperidol for akathisia, extrapyramidal signs (EPS) and somnolence.
Olanzapine	+++	++	+++	+	+(+)	Sedative. It should be avoided if diabetes, lipid disturbance and severe overweight. Neurotoxic in patients with brain disorder? See text. Some M$_1$ effects
Quetiapine	+(+)	+	++	++	+	Some M$_1$ effects.
Risperidone	++++	(+)	(+)	+++(+)	+++	Marked effect on prolactin. Neurotoxic in patients with brain disorders? See text
Sertindole	++++	+	(+)	+++(+)	+++	Should be avoided if risk factors for prolonged QT$_c$-interval
Ziprasidone	++++	+	(+)	++	+(+)	Should be avoided if prolonged QT-interval. Some effects on NA and 5HT. Avoid lithium and SSRI combinations?
Zotepine	++	?	?	?	?	Inhibits NA-reuptake.
Clozapine	+++	++(+)	+++	+++(+)	++	Risk of blood dyscrasia and cardiovascular complications. Should be avoided if prolonged QT-interval
Haloperidol	+	+	+	+	+	Avoid combination with lithium and strong serotonergic-acting drugs

or increase the risk of complications. The second generation of neuroleptics (see Table 33.5) have as a group fewer side-effects and are usually preferred. However, to what extent haloperidol is associated with more side-effects than second-generation antipsychotics listed in Table 33.5 is debated. Current evidence may favour the view that the overall prevalence of neurologic side-effects may be somewhat higher in patients treated with haloperidol compared to drugs like amisulpride, aripiprazole, olanzapine, risperidone, sertindole, quetiapine, ziprasidone and zotepine.

Administration and dosage

Oral administration is most commonly used. In elderly and infirm patients, half the usual starting dose should be given. Most neuroleptics are metabolized by the

Table 33.5. Side-effects of neuroleptics.

Neurologic side-effects
- Akinetic syndrome
- Parkinsonism
- Akathisia
- Acute dystonia
- Tardive dystonia
- Tardive dyskinesia

Mental

Vegetative and cardiovascular
- Anticholinergic syndrome
- Dry mouth
- Orthostatic hypotension
- Prolonged QTc interval

Endocrine and metabolic
- Weight increase
- Lipid changes
- Diabetes
- Menstrual irregularities
- Sexual side-effects

Skin

Blood dyscrasias

Liver

Neuroleptic malignant syndrome

Other

liver and excretion through the kidney is the rule. Accordingly, in patients with liver or kidney failure, starting doses must be reduced and increased slowly.

Interactions

Drugs inducing or reducing liver enzyme activity (e.g. carbamazepine) may influence the serum levels of neuroleptics. Newer-generation antipsychotics are metabolized predominantly by cytochrome P450 (CYP) isoenzymes, particularly CYP-1A2 (clozapine and olanzapine), CYP-3A4 (clozapine, quetiapine and ziprasidone) and CYP-2D6 (olanzapine and risperidone). Many antidepressants are metabolized by CYP-2D6 and some antibiotics inhibit CYP-3A4. The potential of interactions with other drugs should therefore always be checked prior to adding a neuroleptic drug.

Pharmacodynamic interactions may also occur. Case reports suggest that both clozapine and haloperidol may cause transient neurological adverse events if combined with lithium therapy or high doses of serotonergic drugs. This risk may be increased in patients with organic brain syndromes. To what extent this also is valid for neuroleptics other than clozapine and haloperidol is uncertain. In view of reports of increased rate of stroke in some elderly patients with behavioural dysfunction treated with olanzapine or risperidone, it is recommended that doses of neuroleptics given to the elderly with organic brain syndromes should be kept as low as possible and combinations with high serum levels of serotonergic drugs should be avoided.

Some neuroleptics may reduce the efficacy of adrenaline and other sympathomimetic drugs. If so, adrenergic drugs are not suitable for treating neuroleptic-induced hypotension.

Side-effects

The side-effects associated with neuroleptics are listed in Table 33.5. If the patient is unconscious or cannot communicate, clinical examination and observation are necessary to diagnose unwanted side-effects. Neurological side-effects may manifest by increased muscle rigidity (check elbow movement) or generalized or local tremor. Cardiovascular side-effects are identified by monitoring of vital signs.

Neurologic side-effects

Akinetic syndrome is due to an exaggerated specific sedative effect provoked by too-high doses. The hypokinetic, indifferent state of mind typical for neuroleptics becomes more marked. The patient demonstrates lassitude, distant behaviour and loss of interest. Some may appear depressed or dysphoric. Symptoms improve on reduction of the dose.

Akathisia consists of a subjective feeling of inner restlessness and the urge to move without feeling anxiety. Objectively there are signs of increased activity such as rocking while standing or sitting, lifting feet as if marching on the spot and crossing and uncrossing the legs while sitting. The exact pathophysiology of akathisia is still unknown. Akathisia usually develops hours to days after initiating neuroleptic treatment or increasing the dose. It is treated by reducing the dose, changing to another drug or adding a drug that reduces akathisia. Clonazepam 0.5–3 mg per day or propranolol (20–80 mg per day) or other lipophilic beta-blockers seem to be the most consistently effective treatment for acute akathisia.

Acute dystonia consists of abnormal positioning or muscle spasms within hours to a week of starting drug treatment or of a rapid increase in the dose of a drug. Tonic cramps in the muscles of the eye, face, tongue, neck, and back are most frequent. Dystonia involving the tongue or oesophagus may present with difficulties in speaking and swallowing. This state may be misdiagnosed as a conversion disorder. Acute dystonia is often painful and very frightening and may seriously disturb the relationship between the doctor and the patient. Prevalence is higher among younger patients, males and cocaine abusers. Low serum calcium is a risk factor and the calcium metabolism of patients developing acute dystonia should always be examined. Biperiden 5 mg should be administered intramuscularly (in severe cases slowly intravenously) to treat the condition. This treatment is nearly always effective within a few minutes (i.v.) or up to 20 minutes (i.m.). Alternative treatment is diazepam 10 mg i.v. Further drug-induced dystonia can be prevented by adding anticholinergic drugs to treatment with neuroleptic drugs for a week. Prophylaxis includes adding anticholinergic drugs during the first week of treatment or starting treatment with second-generation neuroleptics which have lower prevalence of acute dystonia.

Parkinsonism is usually dose-related. The characteristic features of cogwheel rigidity, tremor, akinesis and shuffling gait may be accompanied by dysphoria and apathy. Treatment involves dose reduction. If this is insufficient the next option is to use antiparkinsonian drugs (e.g. biperiden, orphenadrine, procyclidine or benzatropine).

Vegetative and cardiovascular side-effects

An anticholinergic syndrome is sometimes seen when prescribing the first-generation high-dose neuroleptics. The symptomatology is due to central and peripheral inhibition of acetylcholine receptors. Symptoms from the central nervous system include anxiety, restlessness, hyperactivity, confusion, impaired memory and orientation, hallucinations and myoclonus. Peripheral nervous systems symptoms include tachycardia, widening of the pupils, warm and dry skin, dry mouth, urine retention and constipation. In minor cases stopping the drug is sufficient to abort the syndrome. In severe cases slow intravenous infusion of 1–2 mg physostigmine is needed. In the general hospital, continuous infusion of 2 mg per hour may be needed in some cases to block the anticholinergic syndrome.

Hypotension due to α_1-antagonism (see Table 33.4) may be a problem. The risk is highest when prescribing risperidone, quetiapine and sertindole. The risk is lowest using neuroleptics with little (e.g. haloperidol, olanzapine) or no (amisulpride) α_1-antagonism. In cases of refractory hypotension during neuraxial anaesthesia, conventional treatment with ephedrine and i.v. fluids is the first option. If this does not work, large doses of phenylephrine may be indicated (Williams & Hepner 2004).

Some neuroleptics, notably clozapine and thioridazine, have been associated with QTc prolongation. In the worst case this effect may lead to ventricular fibrillation and acute death. This effect on heart conduction may be augmented by concomitant administration with metabolic inhibitors.

The risk of ventricular fibrillation due to prolongation of the QTc interval beyond 500 ms is very low. However, among patients with risk factors for prolongation of the QTc interval (e.g. prolonged interval at start of treatment, cardiac disease, low potassium or magnesium, cocaine abuse, family history of acute cardiac death), caution is required and drugs like clozapine, thioridazine, sertindole and ziprasidone should be avoided.

In severely ill patients with risk factors, an ECG should be done prior to treatment independent of the type of neuroleptic prescribed, since all neuroleptics are associated with measurable QTc prolongation at steady-state peak plasma concentrations (Harrigan *et al.* 2004).

Endocrine and metabolic side-effects

Olanzapine and most of the first-generation neuroleptics are associated with weight gain. Atypical neuroleptics are associated with increased prevalence of diabetes mellitus. The risk is highest for olanzapine, lower for quetiapine and least for amisulpride, risperidone and ziprasidone. The disturbance in glucose control is not related to weight gain. Death due to ketoacidosis is a rare outcome if the emerging diabetes is overlooked. Olanzapine has also been shown to cause hyperlipidaemia.

All neuroleptics and some antidepressants (e.g. trazodone) may increase serum levels of prolactin. Among the new-generation neuroleptics, most reports are related to amisulpride and risperidone. Although disturbances such as galactor-rhoea, amenorrhoea, gynaecomastia and impotence have been reported following neuroleptic-induced prolactin elevation, the clinical significance of elevated serum prolactin levels is unknown for most patients.

Neuroleptic malignant syndrome

Neuroleptic malignant syndrome (NMS) or malignant hyperthermia occurs in fewer than 1 in 1000 patients treated with neuroleptics. The key symptoms are listed in Table 33.6. The generalized rigidity, described as 'lead-pipe', is a core feature of NMS, and is usually associated with myonecrosis. Cogwheeling, myoclonus and even catatonia and coarse tremors are often described along with other extrapyramidal signs. Mental status changes include clouding of consciousness ranging from stupor to coma, delirium, and the development of catatonia. The classic NMS patient appears awake but dazed, stuporous and mute. In over 80% of cases, rigidity or mental-status changes herald the onset of the syndrome. Exhaustion, agitation, and dehydration may predispose patients to the development of NMS.

Elevations in serum creatine phosphokinase are not specific to NMS. However, determination of the enzyme concentration remains important as a measure of severity of rhabdomyolysis and the risk of myoglobinuric renal failure. Other frequently described laboratory abnormalities include metabolic acidosis, hypoxia, low serum iron, elevations in serum catecholamines, electrolyte abnormalities and coagulopathies.

Other causes of high fever are the main differential diagnoses. Withdrawal of levodopa, or other dopamine agonists, in patients with Parkinson's disease or other disorders, has resulted in hyperthermic syndromes indistinguishable from NMS, reflecting the same mechanisms of acute dopaminergic deficiency. Illegal stimulants and hallucinogens have been associated with hyperthermia, seizures, rigidity, rhabdomyolysis and death. Antiparkinsonian and other anticholinergic drugs can result in atropinic toxicity manifested by fever without rigidity.

Table 33.6. Symptoms suggesting neuroleptic malignant syndrome (malignant hyperthermia).

Hyperthermia
Muscle rigidity
Autonomic instability (tachypnoea, tachycardia, oscillations in blood pressure, profuse sweating, diaphoresis, sialorrhoea, incontinence)
Mental confusion
Neutrophile leucocytosis
Increased creatine phosphokinase (CPK)

Withdrawal states, such as delirium tremens, can also be difficult to distinguish from NMS, when neuroleptics have been administered.

Treatment includes stopping the neuroleptic drug, lowering the fever and stimulating the blocked post-synaptic dopamine receptors. Benzodiazepines (e.g. lorazepam 1–2 mg i.v. every eight hours) are useful in reversing catatonia, easy to administer, and could be tried initially in most cases. Trials of bromocriptine (2.5–10 mg every eight hours), amantadine (100 mg every eight hours), or other dopamine agonists may be a reasonable next step in patients with moderate symptoms of NMS. Dantrolene appears to be beneficial primarily in cases of NMS involving significant rigidity and hyperthermia. It has been beneficial in rapidly reducing an extremely high temperature.

These medications are effective during the first few days of treatment of NMS. Following discontinuation of oral neuroleptics, the mean recovery time has been estimated at 7 to 10 days. About two-thirds of cases recover within a week, and nearly all within 30 days.

Advanced stages of psychotic disorders associated with catatonia (lethal catatonia) can progress to exhaustion, stupor, hyperthermia and death. Lethal catatonia may be mistaken as NMS. Electroconvulsive treatment appears to be the treatment of choice in lethal catatonia. If idiopathic lethal catatonia cannot be excluded and if NMS symptoms are refractory to other measures, ECT is the logical treatment of choice. ECT may also be tried in NMS cases in patients with prominent catatonic features, and in patients who develop a residual catatonic state or remain psychotic after NMS has resolved.

Neuroleptics in pregnancy and the puerperium

Neuroleptics in early pregnancy may increase the risk of foetal malformations. The risk of using haloperidol seems low, however. Among high-dose first-generation neuroleptics the risk of malformation of the limbs or larger organs has been estimated to be 3–5%. Less is known about the risk related to second-generation neuroleptics. In general terms, obesity and hyperglycaemia are associated with increased risk for malformations (Temple *et al.* 2003).

There are suggestions that second-generation neuroleptics may increase the prevalence of premature birth and spontaneous abortion, but the evidence is weak. The rule should be to keep the exposure of neuroleptics as low as possible during pregnancy. Most evidence is available for chlorpromazine and trifluoperazine and if a neuroleptic is considered essential one of these should be selected. Peak serum concentrations should be avoided (i.e. multiple small doses should replace one-a-day dosing). If a mother wishes to breastfeed sulpiride is the neuroleptic of choice because the amount secreted into milk is very low.

Longer-term effects

Tardive dyskinesia and tardive dystonia may also occur after long term use. Benzodiazepines may have something to contribute to the care of people with neuroleptic induced tardive dyskinesia but the use of this group of compounds should be considered experimental. Anticholinergic drugs are not proven to be effective. Small trials indicate that vitamin E protects against deterioration of tardive dyskinesia but there is no evidence that vitamin E improves symptoms (Soares & McGrath 2003). Tardive dyskinesia or dystonia are seldom problems in a liaison psychiatry setting. The reader is referred to textbooks of psychiatry and psychopharmacology for further discussion of these topics.

Special issues related to liaison settings

For many years the first-generation neuroleptics (i.e. haloperidol) have been the treatment of choice in patients with non-alcohol delirium. Recent double-blind studies have found that olanzapine and risperidone have effects equal to that of haloperidol but with fewer extrapyramidal side-effects (Skrobik *et al.* 2004).

However, a recent epidemiological study found that the use of first-generation neuroleptics doubled the risk for sudden cardiac death. This finding has been followed by reports of a threefold increase in the risk for stroke in dementia patients with behavioural problems treated with olanzapine and risperidone. To which extent these findings can be extrapolated to other second-generation antipsychotics (e.g. amisulpride, aripiprazole, quetiapine, ziprasidone, zotepine) remains unsettled.

These observations cast doubt on the traditional psychopharmacological treatments of delirium in liaison psychiatry. Until further evidence is available, it is probably wise to avoid olanzapine and risperidone in the treatment of delirium, at least in elderly patients with organic brain damage. Haloperidol and amisulpride may be safer alternatives.

Intramuscular-administrated zuclopenthixol (acetate formulation) is often used in emergency situations to treat severe confusion and psychotic states. However, a recent review found no data directly related to tranquilization, but that it may produce earlier sedation than oral haloperidol (Fenton *et al.* 2003). If a neuroleptic is chosen to treat delirium, the dose should be kept as low as possible by combining it with benzodiazepines in order to increase sedation. Drugs with minor effects on the cardiovascular systems should be prescribed (e.g. amisulpride, haloperidol, aripiprazole, zotepine). Olanzapine and risperidone should probably be avoided in patients with cardiovascular risk factors.

Antipsychotic drugs may be appropriate for psychotic symptoms associated with Alzheimer-type dementia but it is important to identify and correct any treatable somatic causes before commencing neuroleptics. Nonpharmacologic treatments are often effective, such as improving sensory function via hearing aids or eyeglasses, providing stimulation and improving orientation.

Dementia with Lewy bodies (DLB) is an increasingly recognized cause of dementia. It is characterized by progressive cognitive decline and attention deficits which typically fluctuate over time. Patients with DLB often experience Parkinson-like spontaneous motor features as well as recurrent visual hallucinations. Another frequent finding in DLB is rapid eye movement (REM) sleep disorder. Ideally, each of the major symptom domains associated with DLB (behavioural, motor and cognitive) should be treated, but drug interactions in these patients are a serious concern. In addition, many patients with DLB are hypersensitive to neuroleptics, which can induce severe extrapyramidal and other symptoms — sometimes ending in death. Anticholinergic drugs are the first pharmacotherapeutic choice. Improving sleep by mianserin or mirtazapine may be an option.

Mood stabilizers

The mood stabilizers used in psychiatry are listed in Table 33.3. The main indications in liaison psychiatry settings are behavioural disorders caused by organic brain dysfunction including temporal lobe epilepsy, acute mania, pain disorders and prophylactic treatment of bipolar disorders. Some patients may already be taking a mood stabilizer for a previously diagnosed bipolar affective disorder.

Lithium

Lithium has a narrow therapeutic window (serum level 0.6–1.0 mmol/l), and good compliance is crucial for safe treatment. Toxic symptoms may occur when serum concentration levels exceed 1.5 mmol/l. They include tremor, diarrhoea and mental confusion similar to a serotonergic syndrome (see Table 33.1). There is also risk for serotonergic syndrome if lithium is given together with a serotonergic agent (e.g. SSRI).

Lithium can be used safely in most liaison settings but should be avoided among patients with high risk of cardiac arrhythmias. Drugs that may interfere with lithium excretion should be used with caution. Examples include angiotensin-converting enzyme (ACE) inhibitors, thiazide diuretics and metronidazole.

If the patient is to undergo a major operation, lithium should be stopped two to four days prior to the operation. Huyse et al. (2006) recommend ensuring blood level of less than 0.6 mmol/l before major surgery is undertaken otherwise there is risk of toxic levels in relation to changes in electrolyte balance and possible hazardous interactions with neuromuscular-blocking agents. Lithium should be reinstated when the patient is stable haemodynamically.

Valproate, oxcarbazepine or benzodiazepines may be used if the patient develops a manic episode when stopping lithium. In severe cases, a neuroleptic may be necessary (see delirium).

Lithium affects the kidney, causing a nephrogenic diabetes insipidus syndrome. In a few cases renal function may be significantly impaired with the development of chronic renal failure and the need for dialysis and transplantation. Renal function must be monitored regularly and the need for continuous lithium treatment reassessed in conjunction with a renal physician. Alternative mood stabilizers should be used if the risk of relapse of a bipolar affective disorder is considered to be high.

Impaired thyroid function occurs in 4–10% of lithium-treated patients. The symptoms may be confused with those of depression or chronic fatigue. The treatment is adding thyroxine (T4) or choosing another mood stabilizer. Among patients with thyroid-related impaired cognition (i.e. autoimmune thyroid disorders), adding T3 may sometimes be a better alternative than T4.

Lithium may worsen some dermatological diseases, in particular psoriasis. Lithium is found in breast milk. There is a wide interpatient variability in the lithium dose offered to the infant through breast milk (0–30% of maternal weight-adjusted dose; Moretti et al. 2003). That indicates that therapeutic drug monitoring of lithium in milk and/or in infant's blood, coupled with close monitoring of adverse effects, is a rational approach.

Antiepileptics

Several antiepileptic drugs have been shown to have mood-stabilizing properties.

Valproate is commonly used as a prophylactic agent in bipolar I disorders and can also be used to treat acute manic episodes. The main problems in liaison setting are side-effects such as drowsiness, nausea and tremor, and interaction with other drugs. In women with epilepsy who are treated with valproate, especially in those who have gained weight during treatment, polycystic ovaries, hyperandrogenism, and menstrual disorders appear to be common (Isojarvi 2003). Due to the androgenic effects of valproate, valproate should not be given to subjects with any signs of hirsutism (e.g. 21-hydroxylase impairment). Valproate increases the risk of malformations and should be avoided during pregnancy.

Carbamazepine is also used as a mood-stabilizing drug, either on its own or as an adjunct to other therapy. It has multiple side-effects and a wide range of drug interactions. Due to its liver enzyme enhancing effects, the serum levels of carbamazepine may drop over time despite steady dosage. Carbamazepine may also interfere with thyroid function, and hypothyroidism is a real risk if carbamazepine is combined with lithium. The most severe side-effects of carbamazepine are blood dyscrasias and Stevens-Johnson syndrome.

Gabapentin and its successor pregabalin are mostly used to treat chronic pain. Their antimanic and antidepressive properties are weak. However, anxiolytic effects have been reported. This suggests that gabapentin or pregabalin may be useful as additional medication for the treatment of bipolar disorders associated with significant anxiety. Gabapentin and pregabalin are well tolerated and shows few interactions with other drugs.

Topiramate has some antimanic, but not antidepressant properties. It may adversely influence cognitive function. Its weight reducing properties have been exploited to treat obesity related to other mood stabilizers but it is not recommended as a treatment for obesity because of reports of psychotic reactions.

Lamotrigine has antidepressant effects and is established as a prophylactic drug in bipolar disorder where recurrent depressive episodes are the main clinical problem. Its effect on depression is at least as good as that found for lithium. It is necessary to titrate lamotrigine slowly upwards due to a risk of rash if the dose is increased too rapidly. At least four to six weeks are needed to reach therapeutic levels (estimated to be 8–25 µmol/l 12–24 hours after last intake). For that reason, lamotrigine is not very useful as an acute treatment of depression in liaison settings.

Mood stabilizers are best avoided during pregnancy. Lithium may in a few cases cause cardiac defects if taken during the first trimester while carbamazepine and valproate may cause a variety of foetal abnormalities including spina bifida. If it is thought to be essential that they are taken during pregnancy folic acid should be prescribed for at least one month before conception

Benzodiazepines and related sedative drugs

Benzodiazepines are GABA-A agonists. GABA receptors are widely distributed in the central nervous system, and receptors exist on presynaptic neurones releasing serotonin and noradrenaline. All benzodiazepines have anxiolytic, sedating, muscle-relaxing and anticonvulsant properties. The main indications are treatment of anxiety disorders, including acute stress responses, and sleeping problems. They are helpful as short-term treatment for patients who are distressed by anxiety before medical procedures such as intravenous therapy or magnetic resonance imaging (MRI) scanning. They are also used to treat alcohol withdrawal symptoms and as a supplement in the treatment of manic episodes, psychotic disorders and agitated depression. Chlordiazepoxide is the drug of choice for treating alcohol withdrawal, the dose being titrated against the severity of the withdrawal symptoms. For moderate to severe symptoms a starting dose of 20 mg four times daily is appropriate. This should be gradually tailed off over a period of five days. However, in several European countries chlordiazepoxide is not available. Benzodiazepines may be an alternative.

Due to their relatively high potential for abuse, benzodiazepines should preferably be prescribed for a limited period of time. Patients with a history of drug abuse or extreme avoidant behaviour may be at particular risk of developing abuse or dependence.

The benzodiazepines are differentiated from each other by their rate of absorption and by their half-life. Drugs with a rapid absorption have a greater potential for abuse (see Table 33.7). Drugs with a very short half-life are suitable for treating insomnia. Drugs with a longer half-life are mostly used to treat clinical anxiety. The drawback of a relatively long half-life is increased risk of hangover if used during the evening.

The main clinical side-effects are excessive drowsiness and daytime sedation. Among patients with respiratory problems, the effect on muscles may cause respiratory problems and the drugs should be avoided; low doses must be used if the drug is essential. Another clinical problem is the interaction with other sedating drugs and alcohol. Among the elderly they may lead to unsteady gait, falls and an increased risk of accidents.

An important, but infrequent, side-effect is paradoxical agitation. Following the ingestion of a benzodiazepine, the patient may develop confusion, excitation or dysphoria. This side-effect is seen mostly among children and the elderly with organic brain syndromes. In some patients with antisocial personality disorders or impulsive aggressive personality traits, benzodiazepines may provoke loss of imp-ulse control and aggressive outbursts. Benzodiazepines should not be prescribed to such patients. If sedation is needed a small dose of a neuroleptic is a better choice.

Benzodiazepines are secreted into breast milk and should be avoided during breastfeeding. If the drug is prescribed, the dose should be low and oxazepam should be preferred. They should also be avoided during pregnancy. There have been reports of an increased incidence of cleft palate if the drugs are taken during the first trimester. If taken during the third trimester they can cause the 'floppy baby' syndrome.

Among patients who have used high doses of benzodiazepines over extended periods of time, abrupt tapering may cause withdrawal symptoms which include light and sound hypersensitivity, tachycardia, increased blood pressure, sweating and gastrointestinal pain. Some subjects may develop seizures. If tapering is needed, reduction by one therapeutic dose a week (e.g. 5 mg diazepam) is a safe regime.

Cognition-improving drugs

Cognition improving drugs include donepezil, galantamine and rivastigmine. They are all cholinesterase inhibitors. The main indication is mild to moderate dementia of the Alzheimer type (DAT).

Table 33.7. Benzodiazepines and related drugs.

	Oral absorption (+ slow ++++ very rapid)	Half-life (hours)	Metabolization	Active metabolite (half-life, hours)	Comments
Treatment of anxiety and agitation					
Alprazolam	+++	11–15	CYP-3A4	12–15	Only short-term use. Abstinence common when tapered after long-term use
Diazepam	++++	20–80	CYP-2C19 CYP-3A4 metabolite: CYP-2C19	Desmethyl diazepam (35–200)	Avoid in the elderly and patients with liver failure Diazepam may itself inhibit CYP-3A4
Clonazepam	++++	20–50	CYP-3A4	None	Sedation may be marked
Oxazepam	+	5–20	Glucoronidation	None	Slow increase in serum concentration after ingestion Low risk of abuse. Fever problems in patients with liver failure
Lorazepam	++	12	Glucoronidation	None	Fever problems in patients with liver failure
Treatment of insomnia					
Flunitrazepam	+++	20		Desmethyl flunitrazepam (31)	Great risk of abuse; should be avoided
Nitrazepam	+++	21–28		None	Relatively long half-life Risk of hangover and daytime sedation
Zaleplon	++++	1			Few interactions For initial insomnia only
Zolpidem	++++	1–4	CYP-3A4	None	Insomnia during night
Zopiclone	++++	4–6 (7 in the elderly)	CYP1A2 & 2D6	About 15% active metabolite	Risk of abuse. Should only be used for short periods of time

Rivastigmine has a non-linear kinetic profile (bioavailability increases with dose and food intake) and is not metabolized by cytochrome P450 enzymes in contrast to donepezil and galantamine. The latter may interact with ketoconazole and kinidine (donepezil) and paroxetine, ketoconazaole and erythromycin (galantamine). Cholinesterase inhibitors may act synergistically with beta blockers and increase the inhibition of cardiac conductance.

Side-effects are mainly explained by peripheral cholinergic stimulation (e.g. nausea, abdominal pain, dyspepsia, headache, fatigue and insomnia). Among patients with severe heart disease, cholinesterase inhibitors may cause sinoatrial or atrioventricular block. Signs of overdose include salivation, restlessness, cold sweating, muscle weakness (risk of respiratory depression), bradycardia, low blood pressure, hypothermia, seizures and vomiting.

Evidence suggests that a cholinergic deficit resulting from a loss of cholinergic neurones is the biological basis of some of the neuropsychiatric manifestations of Alzheimer disease (DAT) and related dementias. The basal forebrain nuclei, the primary source of cholinergic projections to the cortex, become atrophied in DAT. Cholinesterase inhibitors (ChEIs) enhance neuronal transmission by increasing the availability of acetylcholine at the receptors. This effect is beneficial in improving or stabilizing many behavioural symptoms of DAT, particularly apathy and hallucinations (Wynn & Cummings 2004).

Overstimulation of the N-methyl-D-aspartate (NMDA) receptor by glutamate is implicated in neurodegenerative disorders. Memantine is a non-competitive NMDA antagonist that has been approved as an alternative to cholinesterase-inhibiting drugs. In a USA study, memantine reduced clinical deterioration in moderate-to-severe Alzheimer's disease and was not associated with a significant frequency of adverse events (Reisberg *et al.* 2003). Comparison with lamotrigine, another drug modulating glutamate, has not been done.

REFERENCES

Cipriani, A., Barbui, C. and Geddes, J. R. (2005). Suicide, depression and antidepressants. *British Medical Journal*, **330**, 373—4.

Cole, M. G. and Bellavance, F. (1997). Depression in elderly medical inpatients: a metaanalysis of outcomes. *Canadian Medical Association Journal*, **157**, 1055—60.

Dmochowski, R. R., Miklos, J. R., Norton, P. A., *et al.*; Duloxetine Urinary Incontinence Study Group. (2003) Duloxetine versus placebo for the treatment of North American women with stress urinary incontinence. *Journal of Urology*, **170**, 1259—63.

Fenton, M., Coutinho, E. S. F. and Campbell, C. (2003). Zuclopenthixol acetate in the treatment of acute schizophrenia and similar serious mental illnesses (Cochrane Review). In: *The Cochrane Library*, Issue 4. Chichester: John Wiley & Sons.

Gill, D. and Hatcher, S. (2003). Antidepressants for depression in medical illness (Cochrane Review). In: *The Cochrane Library*, Issue 4. Chichester: John Wiley & Sons.

Hammerness, P., Basch, E., Ulbricht, C., *et al.* Natural Standard Research Collaboration. (2003). St John's wort: a systematic review of adverse effects and drug interactions for the consultation psychiatrist. *Psychosomatics*, **44**, 271–82.

Harrigan, E. P., Miceli, J. J., Anziano, R., *et al.* (2004). A randomized evaluation of the effects of six antipsychotic agents on QTc, in the absence and presence of metabolic inhibition. *Journal of Clinical Psychopharmacology*, **24**, 62–9.

Huyse, F. J., Touw, D. J., van Schijndel, R. S., *et al.* (2006). Psychotropic drugs and the perioperative period; a proposal for a guideline in elective surgery. *Psychosomatics*, **47**, 8–22.

Isojarvi, J. I. (2003). Reproductive dysfunction in women with epilepsy. *Neurology*, **61**(Suppl. 2), S27–34.

Jin, Y., Desta, Z., Stearns, V., *et al.* (2005). CYP2D6 genotype. Antidepressant use and tamoxifen metabolism during adjuvant breast cancer treatment. *Journal of the National Cancer Institute*, **97**, 30–9.

Kuhn, K. U., Quednow, B. B., Thiel, M., *et al.* (2003). Antidepressive treatment in patients with temporal lobe epilepsy and major depression: a prospective study with three different antidepressants. *Epilepsy Behaviour*, **4**, 674–9.

Leucht, S., Barnes, T. R., Kiesling, W., *et al.* (2003). Relapse prevention in schizophrenia with new generation antipsychotics: a systematic review and exploratory meta-analysis of randomized controlled trials. *American Journal of Psychiatry*, **160**, 1209–22.

Lingjærde, O., Jørgensen, J., Støren, R., *et al.* (1995). A double-blind comparison of moclobemide and doxepin in depressed general practice patients. *Acta Psychiatrica Scandinavica*, **92**, 125–31.

Malt, U. F., Robak, O. H., Madsbu, H.-P., *et al.* (1999). The Norwegian naturalistic treatment study of depression in general practice (NORDEP) – I: Randomised double-blind study. *British Medical Journal*, **318**, 1180–4.

Misri, S. and Kostaras, X. (2002). Benefits and risks to mother and infant of drug treatment for postnatal depression. *Drug Safety*, **25**, 903–11.

Moretti, M. E., Koren, G., Verjee, Z., *et al.* (2003). Monitoring lithium in breast milk: an individualized approach for breast-feeding mothers. *Therapeutic Drug Monitoring*, **25**, 364–6.

Oberlander, T. F., Misri, S., Fritzgerald, C. F., *et al.* (2004). Pharmacologic factors associated with transient neonatal symptoms following prenatal psychotropic medication exposure. *Journal of Clinical Psychiatry*, **65**, 230–7.

Reisberg, B., Doody, R., Stoffler, A., *et al.* (2003) and the memantine study group. Memantine in moderate-to-severe Alzheimer's disease. *New England Journal of Medicine*, **348**, 1333–41.

Richmond, R. and Zwar, N. (2003). Review of bupropion for smoking cessation. *Drug and Alcohol Review*, **22**, 203–20.

Rodriguez-Landa, J. F. and Contreras, C. M. (2003). A review of clinical and experimental observations about antidepressant actions and side effects produced by *Hypericum perforatum* extracts. *Phytomedicine*, **10**, 688–99.

Sa, D. S., Kapur, S. and Lang, A. E. (2001). Amoxapine shows an antipsychotic effect but worsens motor function in patients with Parkinson's disease and psychosis. *Clinical Neuropharmacology*, **24**, 242–4.

Scott, A. I. F. (2005). College guidelines on electroconvulsive therapy: an update for prescribers. *Advances in Psychiatric Treatment*, **11**, 150–6.

Skrobik, Y. K., Bergeron, N., Dumont, M., *et al.* (2004). Olanzapine vs haloperidol: treating delirium in a critical care setting. *Intensive Care Medicine*, **30**, 444–9.

Soares, K. V. S. and McGrath, J. J. (2003). Vitamin E for neuroleptic-induced tardive dyskinesia (Cochrane Review). In: *The Cochrane Library*, Issue 4, Chichester: John Wiley & Sons.

Spigset, O. and Hägg, S. (1998). Excretion of psychotropic drugs into breast milk. *CNS Drugs*, **9**, 111–34.

Strain, J. J., Chiu, N. M., Sultana, K., *et al.* (2004). Psychotropic drug versus psychotropic drug update. *General Hospital Psychiatry*, **26**, 87–105.

Temple, R., Aldridge, V., Greenwood, R., *et al.* (2003). Association between outcome of pregnancy and glycaemic control in early pregnancy in type 1 diabetes: population-based study. *British Medical Journal*, **325**, 1275–6.

Williams, J. H. and Hepner, D. L. (2004). Risperidone and exaggerated hypotension during a spinal anesthetic. *Anesthesia and Analgesia*, **98**, 240–1.

Wynn, Z. J. and Cummings, J. L. (2004). Cholinesterase inhibitor therapies and neuro-psychiatric manifestations of Alzheimer's disease. *Dementia and Geriatric Cognitive Disorders*, **17**, 100–8.

34

The role of psychological treatments

Elspeth Guthrie and Tom Sensky

Introduction

Physical illness is associated with worry and uncertainty. People react differently to illness, and their distress can seldom be adequately conceptualized in purely biomedical terms. Coping with illness is a dynamic process, which changes over time. People need to manage the initial emotional shock of diagnosis, assimilate information, construct an understanding of the illness, and the limitations or the demands it imposes upon them, and formulate ways to cope. Major illness often requires patients and their families to re-evaluate their lives and make substantial changes.

General principles

Why psychological interventions?

Everyone's response to illness is different and is shaped by their own unique experience of the world. People's reaction to illness depends much more on psychological factors than factors directly attributable to the disease (Sensky & Catalan 1992). This applies particularly to anxiety and depression. Both are common among people with physical illnesses, and are influenced more by the person's appraisal of his or her circumstances than by factors related to the disease, such as severity of symptoms or prognosis. The same is true of suffering. Suffering can be understood as a perceived threat to the person's self (Cassell 1982), and such threats are common in physical illness (for example, a threat to physical prowess caused by arthritis or obstructive airways disease, or a threat to body image resulting from cancer).

Handbook of Liaison Psychiatry, ed. Geoffrey Lloyd and Elspeth Guthrie. Published by Cambridge University Press. © Cambridge University Press 2007.

Factors common to all psychological approaches in physical illness

All psychotherapies consist of two elements; professional service and personal attachment. There is a formal contractual arrangement between therapist and client, with the delivery of specific psychological technology and expertise. This takes place in the context of personal relationship, in which a bond develops between the two (or more) individuals engaged in the process. When people are physically ill, they are more vulnerable and frightened than usual, particularly if the illness involves a severe threat. This vulnerability can lead to increased attachment or dependency on their healthcare providers, which will include the therapist.

Although there are many different types of therapies and diverse approaches to the relief of psychological suffering, all psychotherapies have key common, specific ingredients (Gallo *et al.* 2005). These are listed in Box 34.1. Of all these factors, therapeutic alliance has been found consistently to correlate positively with therapeutic outcome (Horvath & Luborsky 1993). In short-term therapy a strong early alliance has been found to be important (Horvath & Symonds 1991). The therapeutic alliance has been conceptualized in a variety of different ways and key aspects are listed in Box 34.2.

There are several other factors which are common to psychological interventions for people with physical illness. For example, fear and uncertainty are common experiences of physical illness, particularly when it is potentially serious and/or enduring. The tolerance of such fear and uncertainty, and its management

---

Box 34.1 Specific common therapeutic factors (SCTF; Gallo *et al.* 2005).

- Therapeutic alliance
- Communicative style
- Regulation of expectancies
- Setting-building
- Collecting personal history
- To keep the patient in mind

Box 34.2 Key aspects of the therapeutic alliance.

- The ability of the patient to work purposefully in therapy
- The capacity of the patient and therapist to form a strong affective bond between them
- The therapist's skill at providing empathic understanding
- An agreement between the client and therapist regarding goals and tasks
- The ability of the therapist to identify and repair ruptures to the alliance

within the therapy, is often an important element of the intervention. Similarly, people who have a physical illness may sometimes feel unable to express distress to their families, to the professionals involved in their care, or to friends. Having the opportunity to express such distress within the psychotherapeutic relationship can be extremely helpful in some instances. Also, being able to achieve a different (and hopefully more productive) understanding of the self and of the experience of illness can sometimes give a person a sense of empowerment, which is often reduced by the experience of physical illness.

The context of therapy

Despite these potential benefits of psychological interventions, as well as the research evidence supporting their effectiveness (see below), patients as well as the professionals looking after their physical illness may be sceptical. For example, many people believe that being referred for a psychological intervention indicates that the professional referring them has judged that their adjustment to the illness is substantially worse than that of others with the same illness. Similarly, patients may sometimes equate referral for psychological intervention with the judgement that their problems are 'all in the mind'. Unless such beliefs are elicited early on in the therapy, and at least acknowledged, if not discussed, the patient is unlikely to persist with the therapy. Equally, most therapeutic interventions begin with the patient's own story, and accept this as an appropriate starting point, rather than contesting it. These points highlight the crucial importance of the process of engagement in psychological interventions with people with physical illness.

Therapists commonly make ground rules for their patients, such as setting aside regular and predictable times for seeing individual patients. In interventions with the physically ill, modifications to such ground rules may be not only appropriate but also essential. For example, therapy sessions may have to be scheduled to fit in with other treatments, and the duration of the sessions may have to be varied, for example because of fatigue.

As noted below (Relational therapies), some psychological interventions have a particular focus on the patient's emotional status and relationships. However, more generally, whatever the intended focus of the therapy, it is often appropriate to devote some time to helping the patient understand his or her interactions with medical, nursing and other professional staff as well as with family and friends, particularly when these interactions contribute to distress and suffering.

There are many different types of psychotherapy, but for the purposes of this chapter we have focused on three main approaches: basic supportive techniques and problem solving, relational therapies and cognitive-behavioural therapies.

A relatively greater proportion of the chapter is devoted to cognitive-behavioural therapies, because of the large evidence base supporting this kind of therapy for a wide variety of different psychological and emotional problems.

Basic supportive techniques and problem solving

Prevention

Simple psychological skills can be employed by most healthcare professionals to help patients navigate their way through the illness process. It is important to help patients utilize their own resources to manage illness or a change in circumstances brought about by illness. Too active a role (e.g. using tranquillizers to alleviate distress) may hinder rather than help the process of adjustment.

Patients should be provided with information about their illness, to help them come to an informed choice. People are different, however, and some may want more autonomy, and a say in their treatment, than others, who may prefer to receive more guidance from healthcare providers. We know relatively little about what actually people want from doctors, and recent research suggests that for certain conditions (e.g. breast cancer), patients may want doctors to play a more active, authoritative role in decision making, than has previously been assumed (Wright *et al.* 2004).

These findings tell us how important it is to treat each person as an individual case, and to discuss with that person how much he/she wants to be involved in active decision making about his/her illness. Other important considerations include:

- Simple advice and problem solving. Specialist nurses (e.g. diabetic nurses, midwives, Macmillan nurses) may be particularly helpful in relation to certain conditions. Helping patients with practical problems (e.g. access to benefits) may enable them to cope better emotionally with their illness.
- Illness and disability affect whole families, not just individuals. Relatives and carers require support in their own right and, in many cases, will be closely involved in the day-to-day management of the patient's condition. Families should always, if possible, be included in discussions about management (provided of course the patient agrees). Sometimes families can unwittingly hinder improvement by being overprotective. Relatives may need permission or encouragement to withdraw and allow the patient more independence.
- In a medical model of care it is easy to forget spiritual and cultural dimensions of people's lives. Many religious organizations offer support and help for people at times of adversity, and other forms of cultural support may be available.

Patient narratives

Patients with physical illness rarely get an opportunity within the confines of medical treatment to talk and express their feelings about their illness; how it has affected their lives; how it makes them feel; how they feel about their medical treatment; how they feel about medical and nursing staff; their fears, frustration, anger, despair, etc. Most hospital clinics are conducted at a frenetic pace, and there is usually very little opportunity for patients or staff to talk about the emotional impact of the illness.

A large component of psychological treatment with the physically ill (no matter what the orientation) involves listening to the patient's story of his/her illness. Most people need to make sense of their experience, and the changes in their life produced by the illness. In the most extreme examples, they may have to confront their own death.

Writing about experience appears to have a beneficial and cathartic effect. Work by Pennebaker and Seagal (1999) has shown that writing about emotionally significant events, in comparison with innocuous topics, has psychological benefits in healthy people. Patients with chronic physical illness (either asthma or rheumatoid arthritis) also appear to benefit from being asked to write about an emotionally stressful experience in comparison with an emotionally neutral topic (Stone *et al.* 2000). This suggests that relatively simple interventions in patients with physical illness, which encourage expression of feelings, reflection and assimilation, may bring about therapeutic benefits, without recourse to formal psychotherapy. Further work is required to determine which patients may benefit from these kinds of approaches.

Counselling

A variety of different forms of counselling are used throughout medical services, both in primary and secondary care. Educational counselling services are widespread and are used in both primary and secondary prevention programmes (e.g. van Vilsteren *et al.* 2005). In these programmes, counselling skills are utilized to deliver information, help people understand and assimilate the information, and change behaviour.

Many medical services employ counsellors or specialist nurses to provide support and help to people with serious medical conditions. The aim of these services is usually not to treat specific problems of anxiety or depression, which may arise in the context of illness, but to help people adjust to their illness and to give them space to talk about the impact of illness on their lives. Such services are rarely evaluated empirically but are usually very popular with patients and staff. They perhaps fill an important gap which has been left by conventional psychiatry and psychology services, which focus on the treatment of specific mental disorders, and are tied increasingly to a disease model of psychological problems.

There are many different schools of counselling but probably the most common form practised in the UK is person-centred counselling. This is essentially a non-directive form of counselling in which emphasis is placed upon the provision of a supportive and non-critical environment in which the individual can talk openly about his or her problems. The person is encouraged to find his/her own solutions to problems by reflection and a better understanding of the difficulties within the context of therapy. The counsellor will employ a variety of skills including attentive listening and empathic understanding.

There are very few evaluations of counselling in relation to medical illness. However, there have been two recent systematic reviews of the effectiveness of counselling in primary care (not with patients with physical illness) which both showed modest but positive effects over the short term (Rowland *et al.* 2000, 2002). Counselling may also be cost neutral in that there is a reduction in other healthcare use by patients who use counselling services (Rowland *et al.* 2002). More recently, counselling has been shown to be as effective as cognitive therapy for the treatment of depression in a primary-care setting (Ward *et al.* 2000). It is becoming clearer that the treatment setting for a particular intervention may influence its efficacy and effectiveness, and there is a clear difference between the effects of some treatments when used with patients in a secondary-care setting in comparison with primary care (Raine *et al.* 2002).

Problem solving

Problem-solving therapy (PST) is a clinical intervention approach aimed at increasing an individual's ability to cope with stressful problems. It is based on the observation that emotional symptoms are generally induced by problems of living, and has its theoretical roots in cognitive approaches to depressive disorders (Nezu *et al.* 1989; see below (Cognitive-behaviour therapy)). Problem-solving treatment has been developed as a specific, collaborative treatment, with three main steps: first, patients' symptoms are linked with their problems; second, the problems are defined and clarified; and third, an attempt is made to solve the problems in a structured way. By starting to tackle problems patients can begin to reassert control over their lives, and it is proposed that it is this regaining of control that lifts mood. This process usually involves six sessions with a therapist, with a total contact time of less than four hours (Hawton & Kirk 1989). The skills needed to deliver PST can be easily and rapidly taught to a range of health professionals including general practitioners and nurses.

In a series of studies carried out by a group based in Oxford, UK, PST has been shown to be valuable in primary care for anxiety and minor emotional disorders

(Catalan *et al.* 1991), and as effective as antidepressant medication in the treatment of major depression, when provided either by experienced general practitioners (Mynors-Wallis *et al.* 1995) or by trained nurses (Mynors-Wallis *et al.* 2000). In the general hospital, PST has been mainly used for the treatment and management of patients following self-harm. Several studies have shown encouraging results (see Chapter 11). The techniques however are generalizable to a wide number of different problems, including patients with physical disease or physical symptoms.

As an example of this PST has been used to help patients with cancer (Nezu *et al.* 2003). The conceptual relevance of PST for persons with cancer is embedded in a general problem-solving model of stress, whereby the experience of cancer is conceptualized both as a major negative life event and as the cause of a series of stressful daily problems and hassles. Both such sources of stress are further hypothesized to increase the likelihood that a cancer patient will experience significant psychological distress, including feelings of depression.

The ability to problem-solve is conceptualized as an important moderator of these relationships, which should attenuate the probability of experiencing distress, even when patients are confronted by cancer-related stressful events. Under similarly high levels of cancer-related stress, patients who are ineffective problem solvers report higher levels of depression as compared with their cancer-patient counterparts who are effective problem solvers.

Re-attribution techniques

Re-attribution techniques are brief psychological skills which can be learnt by general practitioners and healthcare professionals during a brief training course which lasts two to three days. They have been designed specifically to help health professionals manage patients with medically unexplained physical symptoms. They are described in detail in Chapter 36.

Relational therapies

Relational therapies focus upon emotions or feeling states and their relationship to interpersonal functioning. The basic premise underlying all these different types of therapy is that human beings are social animals and are shaped by the relationships that they form, as infants, children and adults. The earliest relationship, that between mother and infant, or main carer and infant, is crucially important in shaping identity, cognitive function and the ability to regulate and control feelings. As adults, the bonds that we form with others, play a key role in helping us maintain our sense of 'self'. If the bonds break down or become noxious, this may precipitate anxiety and depression. Relational therapies are based upon the premise that feelings, thoughts and relationships are intimately tied up with each other. How we feel and think about others affects how we behave towards them and this in turn effects how we feel inside about ourselves.

Physical illness is a major stressor and usually has a major impact on not only the individual who is affected but also his/her family. The physically ill person can feel vulnerable and needy of support. However, if the ill person has always been a 'strong person' they may find it difficult to accept support if it is offered. They will also find it difficult to ask for help, if help is not forthcoming.

Physical illness demands that families or couples talk to each other, often about things that they may never have discussed before. It is difficult for some people to communicate and talk about serious or life-threatening issues. People who are not previously used to communicating deeply with each other, may find themselves having to talk about issues that are challenging and difficult.

Physical illness makes us scared, or sad, or angry. Illness is often experienced as a loss, whether this a real loss (e.g. loss of a limb) or a psychological loss (e.g. loss of role due to poor physical health). Feelings can be confused and messy. Those who we love most may be the very people we turn our anger and frustration upon, when we can no longer keep those feelings inside.

Physical illness can make us feel vulnerable and we may become physically dependent upon others. This can have an enormous psychological impact upon our sense of who we are and how we get along with other people. A history of childhood problems or unhappiness or abuse can deeply affect how we cope with illness, and the changes imposed upon us, as a consequence of being physically unwell. Indeed, there is a complex relationship between childhood experience, emotional regulation (defensive style), and physical and mental health (Vaillant 1994).

Recent work in diabetes has shown that individuals with insecure styles of attachment are more likely than those whose attachments are secure to have poorer diabetic control (Ciechanowski *et al.* 2004). This can have serious long-term physical consequences.

Psychodynamic therapy

There has been much less empirical research into psychodynamic therapy than cognitive therapy. However, objective evidence for its effectiveness and efficacy is slowly building. A recent meta-analysis of studies published in the last 30 years yielded effect sizes on target problems of 1.39, general psychiatric symptoms of 0.90, and social functioning of 0.80 (Leichsenring *et al.* 2004). These effect sizes were stable and tended to increase at follow-up (1.57, 0.95 and 1.19, respectively). The effect sizes of therapy significantly exceeded those of waiting-list controls and treatments as usual. No differences were found between brief therapy and other forms of psychotherapy.

Long-term psychoanalytic therapy has also been shown to be of benefit in a recent meta-analysis (Lamb 2005). There are insufficient studies of relational therapies in the field of liaison psychiatry to carry out specific meta-analyses on their efficacy and effectiveness in discrete physical conditions. The evidence base is therefore much less robust than that for cognitive-behavioural approaches. It is reasonable, however, to assume that the evidence base will develop over the next decade, and preliminary studies have shown encouraging results in certain areas.

Interpersonal therapy

Interpersonal therapy (IPT) was developed as a time-limited therapy for major depression although it has been adapted to treat a variety of different disorders. In IPT, there are three phases of development. During the first phase, depression is diagnosed within a medical model and explained to the patient. The major problem associated with the onset of the depression is identified and an explicit treatment contract to work on this problem area is made with the patient. Problem areas are classified into three groups; grief, interpersonal disputes and role transitions. In the second phase of the therapy, the therapist and patient work on the identified problem area, exploring ways of helping the patient deal with the problem. In the final phase of the therapy, the termination is discussed, progress is reviewed and the remaining work outlined.

A recent systematic review has concluded that it is an effective treatment for depression, superior to placebo, and equivalent to antidepressants (de Mello *et al.* 2005). Interpersonal therapy has been used to good effect to treat depression in HIV-positive patients (Markowitz *et al.* 1995), and the basic approach is outlined in Markowitz *et al.* (1993). It has also recently been adapted for the treatment of post-traumatic stress disorder (PTSD) for patients who refuse repeated exposure to past trauma (Cutler *et al.* 2004), and piloted in a recent study (Bleiberg & Markowitz 2005). If such new work is proven to be of help, it will be a useful alternative to traditional cognitive approaches for PTSD, which is a common condition in liaison psychiatry.

Interpersonal therapy has also been adapted for use in hypochondriasis (Stuart & Noyes 2005). The therapy focuses upon the interpersonal consequences of being preoccupied with fears of illness. The patient's real distress is understood, and maladaptive communications are explored and modified so that others are more able to meet the patient's attachment needs. With a focus on communication in a time-limited frame, fostered by a strong collaborative relationship, IPT may be an alternative method to cognitive therapy for reducing hypochondriacal behaviour.

Psychodynamic interpersonal therapy or conversational model therapy

This form of treatment has been developed by a psychiatrist called Hobson (1985). It has elements of psychodynamic therapy and interpersonal therapy. It places greater emphasis on the patient–therapist relationship as a tool for resolving interpersonal issues than IPT, and there is less emphasis on the interpretation of transference than psychodynamic therapies.

Key features of the model include

1. The assumption that the patient's problems arise from or are exacerbated by disturbances of significant personal relationships.
2. A tentative, encouraging, supportive approach from the therapist, who seeks to develop deeper understanding with the patient through negotiation, exploration of feelings and metaphor.
3. The linkage of the patient's distress to specific interpersonal problems.
4. The use of the therapeutic relationship to address problems, and test out solutions in the 'here and now'.

Emphasis is placed upon identifying repeated patterns of behaviour within relationships which result in conflict and emotional distress. Support and encouragement are provided to the patient to challenge difficult problem areas in relationships and to develop more adaptive ways of coping.

It has equivalence to cognitive therapy for the treatment of depression (Shapiro *et al.* 1994) and has been adapted for use in medically unexplained symptoms, and evaluated in several large randomized controlled trials (Creed *et al.* 2003; Guthrie *et al.* 1991; Hamilton *et al.* 2000). It is cost effective, with the costs of therapy being recouped by reductions in healthcare use in the months post-therapy (Creed *et al.* 2003; Guthrie *et al.* 1999). It has also been used following self-harm and results in a reduction in repetition in the subsequent six months following the index episode (Guthrie *et al.* 2001).

Cognitive-behaviour therapy

Introduction

The essence of cognitive-behaviour therapy (which will be referred to in this chapter as cognitive therapy) is that emotions, behaviour and cognitions (thoughts, beliefs, assumptions, mental images, etc.) are all interlinked. According to the cognitive model, when a person shows distressing emotions like anxiety or depression, there are particular beliefs or other cognitions associated with these emotions. Similarly, behaviours which are maladaptive (such as persistent and extreme denial of symptoms or illness, or poor adherence to essential treatments) are also associated with beliefs or attitudes that are maladaptive. The person is unlikely to be fully aware of these maladaptive cognitions, and this is one reason why they, and the associated emotions and behaviours, persist.

Cognitive therapy aims to help patients gain awareness and understanding of their maladaptive beliefs, to understand how these are associated with unhelpful behaviours and/or distressing emotions, and to help patients modify these behaviours or beliefs for better adaptation. Because emotions, beliefs and behaviours are interlinked, modifying one is expected to lead to changes in the others.

The initial step in therapy is usually to help the patient to use his or her own experiences to demonstrate the link between behaviours, beliefs and emotions. Thus for example, for someone who repeatedly seeks reassurance that his symptoms are not indicative of serious illness, that reassurance is characteristically short-lived, and the behaviour counter-productive, can be explored not only in the sessions with the therapist, but also by getting the patient to keep a diary between sessions, quantifying at various times the extent of his worry and/or reassurance on a 0–10 scale. Having identified the behaviour as maladaptive, patient and therapist collaborate to devise ways of managing the problem behaviours and beliefs more effectively. Commonly, this is done by devising behavioural and/or cognitive experiments aiming to produce more favourable outcomes. Thus in the above example, a behavioural experiment might be for the patient to delay seeking reassurance for progressively longer periods, to demonstrate that he/she is able to tolerate the anxiety involved. A cognitive task might be to prepare a statement (and perhaps even to write the statement down on a 'cue card') regarding the unhelpful outcomes of reassurance-seeking, that the patient can remind him- or herself about when he/she experiences the urge to seek reassurance. Each of these tasks might be rehearsed in the therapy session, so that the patient has some confidence that the possible benefits of carrying out the tasks between sessions outweigh the perceived risks.

Often, the problems which form the focus for cognitive therapy are problems in the 'here and now', as in the above example. The example also illustrates that specific problems are often indicative of more general underlying maladaptive beliefs (for example, 'Any new or unusual bodily sensation may be the start of a myocardial infarction'). This focus on current problems is often helpful as a way of engaging the patient in treatment. In some cases, the entire focus of treatment can remain on the present and the recent past. However, beliefs that are maladaptive commonly have their origins in the more distant past, particularly during childhood, and when this occurs, it is an appropriate focus in therapy to make links between the present and the past.

Research studies of applications of cognitive therapy commonly involve the use of a treatment manual, as one way of maintaining consistency and quality in the treatment. However, particularly in routine clinical practice, the treatment relies on an individual case-based formulation, agreed by patient and therapist. This formulation aims to explain the presenting problems in terms of the links that have been discovered during the assessment process between the patient's cognitions, emotions and behaviour. As therapy progresses, the formulation may be revisited and revised.

Adaptation of cognitive therapy to work with people with physical illnesses

Cognitive therapy was initially applied predominantly to the treatment of depression (Beck *et al.* 1979) and anxiety (Beck *et al.* 1985). Given that both are common in people with physical illnesses, many of the standard cognitive therapy techniques can be used, as with people who have no physical illness. Thus, for example, patients can be asked to complete a thought record, to facilitate the identification of maladaptive thoughts or beliefs. The patient is asked to record what is happening, how they feel, and what thoughts they are aware of. This is commonly done at regular intervals during the day, or the patient may be encouraged to complete the record when he or she feels particularly badly. During therapy, further work can be done to identify maladaptive thoughts, and then to help the patient recognize these more effectively, to review them, and if necessary generate alternatives, rather than taking them as axiomatic. Behavioural and cognitive experiments, as described above, are an integral part of therapy, whether or not the patient has a physical illness or somatic symptoms.

A key principle in cognitive therapy is that the patient, rather than the therapist, is the expert in understanding the patient's problems. Questioning the patient about the presenting problems and his or her model of the illness allows the emergence of inconsistent or even incorrect beliefs, sometimes associated with particular behaviours. Where such beliefs are identified, and acknowledged as inconsistent or incorrect, they can be revised during further work during therapy.

When cognitive therapy is used to treat anxiety or depression in the absence of physical illness, the therapist commonly has a comprehensive understanding, based on training and previous experience, of the patient's problems. However, one of the most important differences between these common applications of cognitive therapy and treating people with physical illness is that the therapist cannot expect in every instance to understand comprehensively the patient's experience, because the therapist usually has no experience in treating the patient's physical illness. Part of the expertise required to manage the patient's problems lies completely outside the cognitive therapy sessions — with physicians, surgeons, nurse specialists, physiotherapists, and others. This is crucial to remember, because it means that neither patient nor therapist necessarily have the full range of expertise to answer all the questions that may arise during the therapy. In physical illness, the patient is not necessarily an expert in understanding all his or her problems. For example, someone who suffers from rheumatoid arthritis may decide that limiting her activities and mobility is the best approach to reducing pain. Such a decision may seem entirely plausible to a therapist who is unfamiliar with the treatment of rheumatoid arthritis. However, the patient is likely to have been advised by her rheumatologist or physiotherapist that limiting activities too severely is likely to lead to increased stiffness which will result in further pain and disability.

The focus of cognitive therapy has been noted to be on maladaptive behaviours or beliefs (these are sometimes called dysfunctional). Although such beliefs can be erroneous, they are not necessarily so. For example, in someone who is terminally ill, the belief that he will soon die may be entirely accurate, but may also become maladaptive if ruminating about the imminence of death prevents the patient from doing what he wants to (such as spending time with the family, settling personal affairs, etc.).

Cognitive factors in assessment

A detailed and careful assessment is essential for understanding the nature of the patient's problems and the likelihood of a positive outcome in therapy. For a detailed description of assessment in the physically ill, see Sensky (2004). The key areas are listed in Box 34.3.

Box 34.3 Cognitive factors in assessment of the physically ill.

- Illness model: what is the patient's understanding of his/her illness, how does this contribute to distress or maladaptive behaviours or beliefs, how can the patient modify or elaborate his/her understanding?
- Personalized formulation of the patient's problem.
- Affective disturbance: identification of anxiety or depression.
- Motivation: Prochaska's stages of change model is a useful framework (Prochaska *et al.* 1994).
- Coping: identification of emotion-focused and problem-focused strategies and their appropriateness to the illness situation.
- Life transitions: how is individual managing the impact of illness on his/her life and what can be learned from the way he/she has managed previous life transitions.
- The influence of others: notably doctors and other professionals, also family and friends, and the way these relationships are influenced by the patient's beliefs about his/her illness.
- Resilience: vulnerability factors and ways of responding to stress.

Illness models

Patients' models of their illness can be diverse and idiosyncratic. Unusual illness representations can often lead to greater understanding of underlying fears or anxieties, and should always be explored. A useful model or framework for describing illness beliefs has been developed by Moss-Morris and colleagues (2002) from the work of Leventhal and colleagues (1997) in relation to illness perception. The Revised Illness Perception Questionnaire (IPQ-R; Moss-Morris *et al.* 2002) is a useful measure in the assessment of illness and its impact upon the person.

Affective disturbance

Depression and anxiety are common among the physically ill. Anxiety can be quantified with the Health Anxiety Inventory (Salkovskis *et al.* 2002). Continuing anxiety which does not resolve is often linked to underlying fears or beliefs about the illness. Recognition of depression in physical illness is also important and is described in Chapter 5. Treatment with antidepressants can be used in conjunction with psychological treatments and should be considered if the patient's symptoms are severe.

Motivation

The success of psychological treatment is dependent upon the patient's ability to work in a collaborative way with the therapist. There is no magical cure. Prochaska's theory of stages of change is a useful framework for assessing health behaviours (Prochaska *et al.* 1994). The theory suggests that in deciding to carry out some health-related behaviour people go through defined stages: precontemplation, contemplation, preparation, action and maintenance. These stages can be used to assess someone's readiness to change.

Coping

Coping strategies can be classified as emotion-focused, which refer to strategies or actions which help contain distress, or problem-focused, which involve strategies to manage events or difficulties. In coping with illness, people have to do both.

Resilience

The response to illness varies across individuals and some are more prone than others to develop depression or other kinds of psychological symptoms. Some people can face quite extreme adversity and maintain a positive attitude and coping style. This resilience to stressors has been referred to as salutogenesis (Antonovsky 1987). Individuals who show high salutogenesis are characterized by being able to regard stressors as predictable, as having confidence in themselves to overcome difficulties and to judge it worthwhile to rise to challenges they face. It's possible that these abilities may be linked to a more generalized capacity to find meaning and to use meaning-based coping.

Illness as a series of life transitions

Serious illness can be construed as an example of a life or role transition, which requires major re-evaluation of the self and one's role in life. A useful concept in relation to this is the idea of response shift (Schwartz & Sprangers 2000). This refers to the change in the meaning of some aspect of the person's self-evaluation which is brought about by one or more of three main mechanisms: recalibration, alteration of values and reconceptualization. It is often useful to explore how the individual has managed previous transitions, such as getting married or getting divorced or starting or leaving employment.

Evidence for the effectiveness of cognitive therapy

Cognitive therapy is an effective treatment for anxiety and depression (Gloaguen *et al.* 1998; Scott 2001), and there are many randomized controlled trials of the treatment of anxiety or depression in the physically ill, using cognitive therapy (Antoni *et al.* 2001; Greer *et al.* 1992; Kostis *et al.* 1994; Sharpe *et al.* 2001; Wilhelmsen *et al.* 1994).

Cognitive therapy also results in other benefits including changes in attitudes towards illness, adherence to medication, and reductions in the severity of pain (e.g. reduction in low back pain; Turner & Jensen 1993) and other physical symptoms (e.g. peptic ulceration; Wihelmsen *et al.* 1994).

For some illnesses there have been sufficient interventions to justify systematic reviews and meta-analyses. These are summarized in Table 34.1. Most of these studies, but not all, have focused upon cognitive therapy interventions, but some have included other therapeutic modalities in the analyses.

The overall evidence suggests that cognitive therapy can be an extremely valuable and useful treatment for a variety of psychological issues that arise in the context of physical illness. It can also impact upon physical symptoms and the ways in which patients manage and cope with illness.

Conclusion

Psychological therapies can be helpful for patients with emotional problems or difficulties arising from, or contributing to, physical symptoms. However, there are severe difficulties with resource provision for such help, both in the UK and

Table 34.1. Systematic reviews, critical reviews and meta-analyses of trials of cognitive therapy and psychological treatments in physical illness.

Authors	Condition	Therapy	Type of review	Outcome
Blanchard (2005)	Irritable bowel syndrome	Cognitive-behavioural therapies (CBT)	Critical review	Good evidence for efficacy of CBT interventions. Long-term outcome is rarely evaluated.
Van Dixhoorn & White (2005)	Ischaemic heart disease	Relaxation training	Systematic review and meta-analysis (27 studies)	Cardiac effects: positive effects on frequency of occurrence of angina pectoris; arrhythmia and exercise-induced ischaemia. Return to work was improved.
Patel et al. (2005)	Needle phobia	Cognitive-behavioural therapies	Systematic review (3 studies)	Methodology differed but all had optimistic outcomes. Overall quality of evidence for treatment effectiveness is poor and outcome measures need further development.
Lackner et al. (2004)	Irritable bowel syndrome	Psychological treatment	Systematic review (32 studies)	Meta-analysis of efficacy data of 17 trials gave an odds ratio of 12 (95% CI 5.6 to 26.0. Number needed to treat = 2).
Astin et al. (2002)	Rheumatoid arthritis	Psychological interventions	Meta-analysis (6 studies)	Significant pooled effect sizes were found for pain (0.22), disability (0.27), coping (0.46).
Fleming et al. (2004)	Asthma	Psychotherapeutic interventions	No meta-analysis performed because poor quality of studies (12 studies)	Unable to draw firm conclusions for the role of psychological interventions in asthma due to the absence of an adequate evidence base.
Bailey (2002)	Back pain	Psychological treatment	Meta-analysis (146 interventions)	Psychological interventions showed small effects. No treatment of choice emerged.

Table 34.1. (cont.)

Authors	Condition	Therapy	Type of review	Outcome
Sim & Adams (2002)	Fibromyalgia	Non-pharmacological treatment	Systematic review (25 studies)	Methodological quality of studies was fairly low. Variation in studies made it hard to form conclusions across studies. Strong evidence did not emerge in respect to any single intervention, though preliminary support of moderate strength existed for aerobic exercise.
Looper & Kirmayer (2002)	Chronic fatigue syndrome	CBT	Critical review (4 studies)	Positive outcome for most studies.
Holroyd (2002)	Headache	CBT	Critical review (4 studies)	Psychological treatment superior to usual care.
Looper & Kirmayer (2002)	Hypochondriasis	CBT	Critical review (4 studies)	Psychological treatment superior to usual care.
Blanchard & Scharff (2002)	Irritable bowel syndrome	Psychological treatment	Critical review (11 studies)	Psychological treatments more effective than controls in most studies.
Raine et al. (2002)	Back pain	CBT	Systematic review (16 studies)	Sustained improvements in pain, depression and disability.
Rose et al. (2002)	Anxiety in chronic obstructive pulmonary disease (COPD)	Psychologically based treatments	6 randomized controlled trials but variability prevented a meta-analysis	No study was adequately designed to provide an assessment of psychological intervention aimed at anxiety in COPD. Secondary outcomes included impacts on breathlessness, disability and quality of life.
Soo et al. (2004)	Nonulcer dyspepsia	Psychological treatment	Systematic review (4 studies)	All showed evidence of effectiveness, however, data could not be pooled for a meta-analysis.

Table 34.1. (*cont.*)

Authors	Condition	Therapy	Type of review	Outcome
Yucha *et al.* (2001)	Hypertension	Biofeedback	Meta-analysis	Biofeedback resulted in a reduction in systolic blood pressure (SBP) and diastolic blood pressure (DBP). Only biofeedback (with related cognitive therapy and relaxation training) showed a significantly greater reduction in both SBP and DBP when compared with inactive control treatments.
Boulware *et al.* (2001)	Hypertension	Patient-centred behavioural interventions	Meta-analysis (232 studies)	Results show that counselling improved both SBP and DBP beyond the benefit caused by medications alone. However, there was no significant effect on BP related to training courses or self-monitoring.

continental Europe. This means that appropriate psychological treatments are not available for many patients who may benefit from them. More resources are urgently required but psychological services also need to be more creative in the way that treatment is delivered. Not all patients need the same length of treatment, and some may benefit from being seen only once or twice. It is possible that some patients may derive a great deal of benefit from being given the opportunity to talk about their illness. At present, seeing a psychotherapist is really the only opportunity that patients get to do this. There may be other, relatively cheaper ways, of providing these kinds of opportunities, if they are proven to be of benefit.

It may be possible to train non-mental-health staff to use simple psychological techniques to help patients. This has been done with health visitors in relation to the treatment of post-natal depression and Macmillan nurses in the field of cancer. Other technologies (e.g. computer therapy) are being developed and these may also be of benefit in the liaison setting for certain groups of patients.

Psychotherapy is not effectively targeted at present. Referrals for psychotherapy treatment in patients with physical illness are fairly random processes.

Further work needs to be done to identify, at an early stage, those patients who are most vulnerable to psychological distress, so that treatment can be provided quickly and efficiently. In addition, more intensive treatments are required for patients with chronic and complex problems. There are very few chronic pain programmes available or other intensive day or inpatient facilities which provide psychological treatment and rehabilitation.

REFERENCES

Antoni, M. H., Lehman, J. M., Kilbourn, K. M., *et al.* (2001). Cognitive-behavioural stress management intervention decreases the prevalence of depression and enhances benefit finding among women under treatment for early stage breast cancer. *Health Psychology*, **20**, 20–32.

Antonovsky, A. (1987). *Unraveling the Mystery of Health: How People Manage Stress and Stay Well.* San Francisco, CA: Jossey-Bass.

Astin, J. A., Beckner, W., Soeken, K., *et al.* (2002). Psychological interventions for rheumatoid arthritis: a meta-analysis of randomized controlled trials. *Arthritis & Rheumatism: Arthritis Care & Research*, **47**(3), 291–302.

Bailey, G. W. (2002). The psychological treatment of back pain: a meta-analysis. *Dissertation Abstracts International: Section B: The Sciences and Engineering*, **63**(1–B), 515.

Beck, A. T., Rush, A. J., Shaw, B. F., *et al.* (1979). *Cognitive Therapy of Depression.* New York: Guilford.

Beck, A. T., Emery, G. and Greenberg, R. L. (1985). *Anxiety Disorders and Phobias: a Cognitive Perspective.* New York: Basic Books.

Blanchard, E. B. (2005). A critical review of cognitive, behavioral, and cognitive-behavioral therapies for irritable bowel syndrome. *Journal of Cognitive Psychotherapy*, **19**, 101–23.

Blanchard, E. B. and Scharff, L. (2002). Psychosocial aspects of assessment and treatment of irritable bowel syndrome in adults and recurrent abdominal pain in children. *Journal of Consulting & Clinical Psychology*, **70**(3), 725–38.

Bleiberg, K. L. and Markowitz, J. C. (2005). A pilot study of interpersonal psychotherapy for posttraumatic stress disorder. *American Journal of Psychiatry*, **162**(1), 181–3.

Boulware, L. E., Daumit, G. L., Frick, K. D., *et al.* (2001). An evidence-based review of patient-centered behavioral interventions for hypertension. *American Journal of Preventive Medicine*, **21**, 221–32.

Cassell, E. J. (1982). The nature of suffering and the goals of medicine. *New England Journal of Medicine*, **306**, 639–45.

Catalan, J., Gath, D., Anastasiades, P., *et al.* (1991). Evaluation of a brief psychological treatment for emotional disorders in primary care. *Psychological Medicine*, **21**, 1013–18.

Ciechanowski, P., Russo, J., Katon, W., *et al.* (2004). Influence of patient attachment style on self-care and outcomes in diabetes. *Psychosomatic Medicine*, **66**, 720–8.

Creed, F., Fernandes, L., Guthrie, E., *et al.* North of England IBS Research Group. (2003). The cost-effectiveness of psychotherapy and paroxetine for severe irritable bowel syndrome. *Gastroenterology*, **124**(2), 303–17.

Cutler, J. L., Goldyne, A., Markowitz, J. C., *et al.* (2004). Comparing cognitive behavior therapy, interpersonal psychotherapy, and psychodynamic psychotherapy. *American Journal of Psychiatry*, **161**, 1567–73.

de Mello, M. F., de Jesus Mari, J., Bacaltchuk, J., *et al.* (2005). A systematic review of research findings on the efficacy of interpersonal therapy for depressive disorders. *European Archives of Psychiatry and Clinical Neuroscience*, **255**, 75–82.

Fleming, S. L., Pagliari, C., Churchill, R., *et al.* (2004). Psychotherapeutic interventions for adults with asthma. *Cochrane Database of Systematic Reviews*, **1**, CD002982.

Gallo, E., Ceroni, G. B., Neri, C., *et al.* (2005). Specific common therapeutic factors in psychotherapies and in other treatments. *Rivista di Psichiatria*, **40**, 63–81.

Gloaguen, V., Cottraux, J., Cucherat, M., *et al.* (1998). A meta-analysis of the effects of cognitive therapy in depressed patients. *Journal of Affective Disorders*, **49**, 59–72.

Greer, S., Moorey, S., Baruch, J. D. R., *et al.* (1992). Adjuvant psychological therapy for patients with cancer: a prospective randomised trial. *British Medical Journal*, **304**, 675–80.

Guthrie, E., Creed, F., Dawson, D., *et al.* (1991). A controlled trial of psychological treatment for irritable bowel syndrome. *Gastroenterology*, **100**, 450–7.

Guthrie, E., Moorey, J., Margison, F., *et al.* (1999). Cost-effectiveness of brief psychodynamic-interpersonal therapy in high utilizers of psychiatric services. *Archives of General Psychiatry*, **56**(6), 519–26.

Guthrie, E., Kapur, N., Mackway-Jones, K., *et al.* (2001). Randomised controlled trial of brief psychological intervention after deliberate self poisoning. *British Medical Journal*, **323**, 135–8.

Hamilton, J., Guthrie, E., Creed, F., *et al.* (2000). Randomized controlled trial of psychotherapy in patients with chronic functional dyspepsia. *Gastroenterology*, **119**(3), 661–9.

Hawkins, J. R. (2004). The role of emotional repression in chronic back pain: a study of chronic back pain patients undergoing psychodynamically oriented group psychotherapy as treatment for their pain. *Dissertation Abstracts International: Section B: The Sciences and Engineering*, **64**, 4038.

Hawton, K. and Kirk, J. (1989). Problem-solving. In *Cognitive Behaviour Therapy For Psychiatric Problems: a Practical Guide*, ed. K. Hawton, P. Salkovskis, J. Kirk, *et al.* Oxford: Oxford Medical Publications, pp. 406–27.

Hobson, R. F. (1985). *Forms of Feeling*. London: Tavistock Publications.

Holroyd, K. A. (2002). Assessment and psychological management of recurrent headache disorders. *Journal of Consulting and Clinical Psychology*, **70**, 656–77.

Horvath, A. O. and Luborsky, L. (1993). The role of the therapeutic alliance in psychotherapy. *Journal of Consulting & Clinical Psychology*, **61**, 561–73.

Horvath, A. O. and Symonds, B. D. (1991). Relation between working alliance and outcome in psychotherapy: a meta-analysis. *Journal of Counseling Psychology*, **38**, 139–49.

Kostis, J. B., Rosen, R. C., Cosgrove, N. M., *et al.* (1994). Nonpharmacological therapy improves functional and emotional status in congestive heart failure. *Chest*, **106**, 996–1001.

Lackner, J. M., Mesmer, C., Morley, S., *et al.* (2004). Psychological treatments for irritable bowel syndrome: a systematic review and meta-analysis. *Journal of Consulting and Clinical Psychology*, **72**, 1100–13.

Lamb, W. K. (2005). A meta-analysis of outcome studies in long-term psychodynamic psychotherapy and psychoanalysis. *Dissertation Abstracts International: Section B: The Sciences and Engineering*, **66**(2–B), 1175.

Leichsenring, F., Rabung, S. and Leibing, E. (2004). The efficacy of short-term psychodynamic psychotherapy in specific psychiatric disorders: a meta-analysis. *Archives of General Psychiatry*, **61**, 1208–16.

Leventhal, H., Benyamini, Y. and Brownlee, S. (1997). Illness representations: theoretical foundations. In *Perceptions of Health and Illness: Current Research and Applications*, ed. K. J. Petrie and J. Weinman. Amsterdam: Harwood Academic Publishers, pp. 19–45.

Looper, K. J. and Kirmayer, L. J. (2002). Behavioural medicine approaches to somatoform disorders. *Journal of Consulting and Clinical Psychology*, **70**, 810–27.

Markowitz, J. C., Klerman, G. L. and Perry, S. W. (1993). An interpersonal psychotherapeutic approach to depressed HIV-seropositive patients. In *Clinical Challenges in Psychiatry*, ed. W. H. Sledge and A. Tasman. Addleston, VA: American Psychiatric Publishing, pp. 37–59.

Markowitz, J. C., Klerman, G. L., Clougherty, K. F., *et al.* (1995). Individual psychotherapies for depressed HIV-positive patients. *American Journal of Psychiatry*, **152**, 1504–9.

Moss-Morris, R., Weinman, J. and Petrie, K. J. (2002). The Revised Illness Perception Questionnaire (IPQ-R). *Psychological Health*, **17**, 1–16.

Mynors-Wallis, L., Gath, D., Lloyd-Thomas, A., *et al.* (1995). Randomised controlled trial comparing Problem Solving Treatment with amitriptyline and placebo for major depression in primary care. *British Medical Journal*, **310**, 441–5.

Mynors-Wallis, L., Gath, D., Day, A., *et al.* (2000). Randomised controlled trial of problem solving treatment, antidepressant medication, and combined treatment for major depression in primary care. *British Medical Journal*, **320**, 26–30.

Nezu, A., Nezu, C. and Perri, M. (1989). *Problem Solving Therapy for Depression. Theory, Research and Clinical Guidelines*. New York: John Wiley.

Nezu, A. M., Nezu, C. M., Felgoise, S. H., *et al.* (2003). Project Genesis: assessing the efficacy of problem-solving therapy for distressed adult cancer patients. *Journal of Consulting and Clinical Psychology*, **71**, 1036–48.

Patel, M. X., Baker, D. and Nosarti, C. (2005). Injection phobia: a systematic review of psychological treatments. *Behavioural and Cognitive Psychotherapy*, **33**, 343–9.

Pennebaker, J. W. and Seagal, J. D. (1999). Forming a story: the health benefits of narrative. *Journal of Clinical Psychology*, **55**, 1243–54.

Prochaska, J. O., Velicer, W. F., Rossi, J. S., *et al.* (1994). Stages of change and decisional balance for 12 problem behaviours. *Health Psychology*, **13**, 39–46.

Raine, R., Haines, A., Sensky, T., *et al.* (2002). Systematic review of mental health interventions for patients with common somatic symptoms: can research evidence from secondary care be extrapolated to primary care? *British Medical Journal*, **325**, 1082–5.

Rose, C., Wallace, L., Dickson, R., *et al.* (2002). The most effective psychologically-based treatments to reduce anxiety and panic in patients with chronic obstructive pulmonary disease (COPD): a systematic review. *Patient Education & Counseling*, **47**, 311–18.

Rowland, N., Godfrey, C., Bower, P., *et al.* (2000). Counselling in primary care: a systematic review of the research evidence. *British Journal of Guidance & Counselling*, **28**, 215–31.

Rowland, N., Bower, P., Mellor, C., *et al.* (2002). Effectiveness and cost effectiveness of counselling in primary care. *Cochrane Database of Systematic Reviews*, **1**, CD001025.

Salkovskis, P. M., Rimes, K. A., Warwick, H. M., *et al.* (2002). The Health Anxiety Inventory: development and validation of scales for the measurement of health anxiety and hypochondriasis. *Psychological Medicine*, **32**, 843–53.

Schwartz, S. P. and Sprangers, M. A. (2000). *Adaptation to Changing Health: Response Shift in Quality of Life Research*. Washington, DC: American Psychological Association.

Scott, J. (2001). Cognitive therapy for depression. *British Medical Bulletin*, **57**, 101–13.

Sensky, T. (2004). Cognitive therapy with medical patients. In *American Psychiatric Association Press Review of Psychiatry*, ed. J. Wright, Vol 23. Washington, DC: American Psychiatric Publishing, pp. 83–121.

Sensky, T. and Catalan, J. (1992). Asking patients about their treatment: why their answers should not always be taken at face value. *British Medical Journal*, **305**, 1109–10.

Shapiro, D. A., Barkham, M., Rees, A., *et al.* (1994). Effects of treatment duration and severity of depression on the effectiveness of cognitive-behavioral and psychodynamic-interpersonal psychotherapy. *Journal of Consulting and Clinical Psychology*, **62**, 522–34.

Sharpe, L., Sensky, T., Timberlake, N., *et al.* (2001). A blind, randomized, controlled trial of cognitive-behavioural intervention for patients with recent onset rheumatoid arthritis: preventing psychological and physical morbidity. *Pain*, **89**, 275–83.

Sim, J. and Adams, N. (2002). Systematic review of randomized controlled trials of non-pharmacological interventions for fibromyalgia. *Clinical Journal of Pain*, **18**(5), 324–36.

Soo, S., Moayyedi, P., Deeks, J., *et al.* (2004). Psychological interventions for non-ulcer dyspepsia. *Cochrane Database Systematic Review*, **3**, CD002301.

Stone, A. A., Smyth, J. M., Kaell, A., *et al.* (2000). Structured writing about stressful events: exploring potential psychological mediators of positive health events. *Health Psychology*, **19**, 619–24.

Stuart, S. and Noyes, R. Jr. (2005). Treating hypochondriasis with interpersonal psychotherapy. *Journal of Contemporary Psychotherapy*, **35**, 269–83.

Turner, J. A. and Jensen, M. P. (1993). Efficacy of cognitive therapy for chronic low back pain. *Pain*, **52**, 169–77.

van Dixhoorn, J. and White, A. (2005). Relaxation therapy for rehabilitation and prevention in ischaemic heart disease: a systematic review and meta-analysis. *European Journal of Cardiovascular Prevention & Rehabilitation*, **12**, 193–202.

van Vilsteren, M. C., de Greef, M. H. and Huisman, R. M. (2005). The effects of a low-to-moderate intensity pre-conditioning exercise programme linked with exercise counselling for sedentary haemodialysis patients in The Netherlands: results of a randomized clinical trial. *Nephrology Dialysis Transplantation*, **20**, 141–6.

Vaillant, G. E. (1994). 'Successful aging' and psychosocial well-being: evidence from a 45-year study. In *Older Men's Lives*, ed. E. H. Thompson Jr. Thousand Oaks, CA: Sage Publications, pp. 22–41.

Ward, E., King, M., Lloyd, M., *et al.* (2000). Randomised controlled trial of non-directive counselling, cognitive-behaviour therapy, and usual general practitioner care for patients with depression. I: clinical effectiveness. *British Medical Journal*, **321**(7273), 1383–8.

Wilhelmsen, I., Haug, T. T., Ursin, H., *et al.* (1994). Effect of short-term cognitive psychotherapy on recurrence of duodenal ulcer: a prospective randomised trial. *Psychosomatic Medicine*, **56**, 440–8.

Wright, E. B., Holcombe, C. and Salmon, P. (2004). Doctors' communication of trust, care, and respect in breast cancer: qualitative study. *British Medical Journal*, **328**, 864.

Yucha, C. B., Clark, L., Smith, M., *et al.* (2001). The effect of biofeedback in hypertension. *Applied Nursing Research*, **14**(1), 29–35.

35

Problem cases

Damien Longson and Sarah Burlinson

Introduction

Every referral to liaison psychiatry presents its own set of clinical dilemmas. Some cases are straightforward and can be assessed and managed easily. Others are complex and require a whole host of liaison skills and a large investment of time. The complexity of the clinical case is often not obvious from the referral. The assessing liaison psychiatrist therefore requires a flexible working style and an enthusiasm for the challenges of 'problem cases' in order to thrive in a liaison psychiatry setting.

This chapter is composed of a number of 'problem cases'. They are intended to replicate the process of referral, assessment and management by liaison psychiatry. Although not all types of liaison referral are covered the principles of the process are similar. The cases are described in instalments, with portions of information being added in stages. This mirrors the referral process with a small amount of information available in the referral letter, more from direct contact with the treating team, more again from past notes, the patient and informants. After each section of information a series of questions are posed. These reflect some of the questions considered during the assessment. They are designed to stimulate independent thought and debate. There may be different but valid approaches to managing cases and discussion should highlight this and encourage a flexibility of approach. Some of the answers to the questions highlighted will be found in the relevant chapters of this book, for others you may need to search more widely. This mirrors real life where the assessing psychiatrist may know much of the information needed to assess and manage a case, but still needs to look further to answer specific questions, e.g. regarding drug interactions etc. The diversity of clinical scenarios and physical comorbidity in liaison patients ensures a continual process of self-education.

Handbook of Liaison Psychiatry, ed. Geoffrey Lloyd and Elspeth Guthrie. Published by Cambridge University Press. © Cambridge University Press 2007.

Case 1: 'I can't catch my breath, doctor'

Referral information

The respiratory physicians referred a 45-year-old hairdresser. She had moderately severe chronic obstructive airways disease and had been admitted to hospital every month for the previous year and a half. Each admission lasted approximately two weeks. Anxiety was thought to be contributing to her breathlessness. She had been treated with dosulepin in the past and advised to seek psychological help but she had been reluctant to accept this.

Pause for thought

- What do you know about the prevalence and nature of psychological illness in respiratory disease?
- What other medical information would you be interested in?
- What effect could you have on the financial consequences of this patient's illness?

Pre-assessment

Medical notes: Her lifestyle was more restricted than lung function tests would predict. There were no signs of an infective exacerbation of her airways disease when admitted to hospital. Her oxygen saturation was always normal with a low pCO_2.

Nursing staff: She was extremely anxious, particularly when discharge was pending.

Pause for thought

- How would you engage the patient in the assessment interview?
- What do you think about the discrepancy between the physical symptoms and the clinical findings?
- How would you discuss this with her?

Initial assessment

The patient's physician persuaded her to be assessed whilst an inpatient. The initial interview focused on her physical symptoms of breathlessness, tremor, fatigue and paraesthesia. Breathlessness occurred during minor exertion. She was unable to walk more than 2 m, reliant on oxygen when at home and housebound. She also had episodes of acute breathlessness at rest. These were characterized by a fear of dying, parasthesia and culminated in urinary incontinence. She thought her airways collapsed while bending over and was fearful of movement. She felt that doctors doubted the severity of her symptoms.

Prior to her illness she had a good work record. She had been a keen hockey player, actively participating at the local club. Since the onset of her illness she had stopped working and given up outside interests. Her husband worked full-time and she was lonely, staying at home with little social contact. She had no children. Her mother had been a sickly woman, suffering from chronic bronchitis. Her family and personal history were otherwise unremarkable.

She complained of difficulty sleeping but was wary of questions about psychological symptoms. Assessment of this was deferred.

Her medication consisted of prednisolone, aminophylline, beta-blockers and diuretics. She took the last daily dose of aminophylline shortly before bedtime. On the ward she had experienced short-lived benefit from diazepam. She had been on 50 mg daily of dosulepin for four months.

On mental state examination she looked well and had a mild tremor. She was not breathless. She was mildly irritable and uncomfortable with the interview situation. Her thought content was difficult to access. There was no evidence of psychosis.

Pause for thought

- What effect may her medication be having on her mental state and physical symptoms?
- What effect may her illness beliefs be having on her symptoms?

Further information

Family: Her husband said that his wife was irritable and that her physical health was deteriorating rapidly. He was convinced that her breathlessness was solely due to respiratory disease.

Nursing staff: The senior respiratory nurse was frustrated by the patient's frequent readmissions. She had found it hard to involve the husband in treatment.

Primary care physician: The primary care physician said the family bypassed him, going directly to the hospital for treatment.

Pause for thought

- What is the differential diagnosis?
- What should your objectives be for the next interview?
- How could you intervene to reduce the patient's distress?

Management and progress

A working diagnosis was made of panic disorder with poor adjustment to illness. Depressive illness was thought a possibility but further information was needed to verify this. She was advised to take the aminophylline in the early evening. Levels were in the normal range. She agreed to a further appointment.

She was next assessed as an outpatient. She was acutely breathless and clutched an oxygen mask to her face. Her respiratory rate was highly variable. Episodes of coughing provoked severe breathlessness but when distracted she was able to talk with little difficulty. She expressed her hopelessness, low mood and fear and had stopped most of her medication. She was tearful and depressed. She agreed to restart the medication, with the exception of the beta-blockers, diuretics and diazepam, and to increase the dosulepin to 100 mg at night. This was discussed with the respiratory physician and she was seen jointly in order to reinforce the treatment strategy. The patient agreed to a cognitive-behavioural assessment.

She was treated with cognitive-behaviour therapy at home. The focus was on anxiety management, graded exercise and activity scheduling. A joint visit was conducted with the respiratory clinical nurse specialist and her husband was involved with treatment. He clearly undermined her ability to cope with symptoms and was frightened by the panic attacks. He would telephone for an ambulance at the slightest sign of respiratory problems. They were taught how to differentiate between breathlessness due to panic and breathlessness due to an exacerbation of chronic obstructive airways disease.

Involvement of the primary-care physician during the early phase of an exacerbation was encouraged. The patient's mood and sleep gradually improved. She attended a pulmonary rehabilitation class and began to exercise. The panic attacks decreased in frequency and she learnt to control breathlessness using breathing exercises. During the four months following referral she had had only one short admission, was driving to visit friends on a regular basis and enjoying two-mile walks. She continued to have mild anxiety symptoms and occasional insomnia.

Final thoughts

- Cognitive-behaviour therapy can be useful in a range of chronic medical illnesses. What factors in a patient's history would suggest that this approach might be effective?
- Joint working with staff from other specialities can be one of the highlights and challenges of liaison psychiatry. What are the benefits to patients, physicians and liaison psychiatrists? What are the potential difficulties?
- Many patients with chronic physical illness are on a variety of medications. What effects may this have on their symptoms and your treatment? How can you enlist the help of your general medical colleagues without challenging their professionalism?

- Patients' physical and psychological symptoms may be improved by alterations to their medication regimens. Aminophylline can have alerting effects and in this case avoiding nocturnal administration coincided with a subjective improvement in sleep.
- This case involved treatment by a cognitive-behaviour therapist and liaison psychiatrist. What other disciplines may you want in a liaison team?

Case 2: 'No-one believes my pain'

Referral information

A 40-year-old ex-librarian was referred to the liaison psychiatry service. She had been diagnosed with fibromyalgia by the rheumatologists but remained in pain and confined to a wheelchair despite physiotherapy and medication. In the past she had been dependent on morphine and had had a period of inpatient treatment to withdraw from this. There was a history of deliberate self-harm.

Pause for thought

- What do you know about fibromyalgia?
- What questions do you think the rheumatologists want you to answer? How important is it to clarify this?
- Do you think self-harm is typical of fibromyalgia? How might this complicate your assessment?

Pre-assessment

Medical notes: The fibromyalgia had been extensively investigated with normal results. All attempts at treatment had been unsuccessful. The assessing physicians were clearly frustrated. In addition there was a complex history of recurrent leg ulcers with no clear cause.

Pause for thought

- What might be the cause of the recurrent leg ulcers?
- What might you speculate about the relationship between the patient and physicians at this stage?
- Is this clinical scenario unravelling as expected?

Initial assessment

The patient was happy to see a psychiatrist: 'That's all I've really wanted, someone to listen'. Widespread pain started shortly after the death of her mother four years previously. At this time she was unhappy both at work and home. She lived with her father who was both critical of her illness and expected her to take over her mother's role. She initially lost the use of her left leg. Her primary-care physician and family told her it was 'all in her head' and she tried to struggle on. The symptoms worsened and she stopped working. She moved to her own flat. She said 'It's nice being away from them. If I hadn't been ill I don't know what I would have done'. Over the years she had gradually become more disabled needing a wheelchair when out and a stick whilst at home.

Her pain was continuous. She was unable to wear close-fitting underwear due to the sensitivity of her skin. Holding light items such as writing material or cutlery was almost impossible. She felt disbelieved and was disparaging about previous treatment. During the course of her illness she had taken escalating amounts of morphine with little benefit and had eventually required a period of detoxification. Physiotherapy exacerbated her symptoms.

She lived alone on high-rate invalidity benefit with daily visits from a home help. She cared for her three-year-old niece on a regular basis. She appeared awkward when explaining how she was able to do this despite her disability. She had no confiding relationships.

She was raised by her parents who paid little attention to her feelings and were dismissive when she was unwell. She had difficulty making friends and was a miserable child. She began cutting herself at the age of 16 to relieve stress. This behaviour became more frequent at times of unhappiness. At the time of assessment she was cutting herself on a monthly basis. She had taken one overdose six years previously. She had been on a variety of antidepressant medication in the past, prescribed by the primary-care physician, and was currently taking dosulepin 75 mg daily and temazepam 20 mg at night.

Mental state examination revealed a thin woman in a wheelchair. She was well made-up, smiled brightly, appeared at ease and seemed to enjoy the occasion. She made no attempt to manoeuvre the chair herself. When asked to walk she did so stooped over in an exaggerated fashion. There were no abnormalities of speech and mood. There were no suicidal plans, health anxieties or psychotic phenomena.

Pause for thought

- What factors may have predisposed her to her current illness?
- What may be maintaining her disability?
- What questions are raised by her history and mental state examination?

Further information

Patient: The leg ulcers occurred whilst her mother was ill with cancer. They had been slow to heal and the district nurses were suspicious that she had interfered with the dressings. When occlusive dressings were applied the ulcers healed quickly.

Primary-care physician: He described her mother as 'a total hypochondriac'.

Psychiatry notes: There was a history of bulimia as a teenager and psychiatric day hospital treatment for dysthymia.

Pause for thought

- What is the differential diagnosis?
- What would be your management plan?

Management and progress

The patient appeared to have features of persistent somatoform pain disorder and borderline personality traits. The possibility of factitious disorder was also considered. Her early childhood experiences of not being heard and rejection had been mirrored by her adult experiences of healthcare services.

The following management plan was devised with the aim of reducing the utilization of inappropriate healthcare and further iatrogenic damage. The psychiatrist agreed to see her on a regular basis to provide her with emotional support and contain her health-seeking behaviour. Further referrals and investigations were discouraged. She was amenable to this and did not seek further investigation or referral. The prognosis in terms of her functional disability was felt to be poor due to the longstanding nature of her problems and the considerable secondary gain she had been experiencing. She attended appointments reliably and stopped self-harming. Her reported level of mobility, pain and invalidism remained unchanged.

Final thoughts

- At times international classification systems can appear unsatisfactory when confronted with complex patients. What do you think of the diagnoses this patient was given? Do patients who present with so many difficulties in several modalities fall neatly into existing classification systems?
- What treatment strategies may be useful in factitious disorder? Should you confront patients who feign symptoms? Is there any evidence base to guide you?
- Do the diagnostic difficulties prevent you from deciding on a management plan?

Case 3: 'They keep saying it's in my head'

Referral information

A 19-year-old university student was admitted to hospital with a worsening of mobility, thought to be due to a flare-up of her multiple sclerosis. However, the results of neurological examination were not consistent with her walking difficulties. The treating physician wondered if she was depressed and requested an opinion. Her primary-care physician had prescribed sertraline.

Pause for thought

- What do you know about the psychological sequelae of multiple sclerosis? How do these correlate with disease activity?
- What information would you want from the medical notes?
- Who would you contact for further information?

Pre-assessment

Psychiatry notes: An earlier assessment by a junior psychiatrist documented psychosocial problems but no evidence of depressive disorder. No psychiatric intervention or follow-up was offered.

Physiotherapy: Assessment by a physiotherapist revealed a lack of consistency in her level of disability. Mobility increased when relaxation and distraction techniques were used during treatment sessions.

Nursing staff: Nursing staff were surprised by her cheerfulness in the face of major disability at an early age.

Medical notes: These confirmed the diagnosis of multiple sclerosis. This had been made three months earlier on the basis of the clinical history, physical examination and magnetic resonance imaging. Neurological symptoms and signs had improved during her previous hospital admission and she had been discharged with mildly reduced power in her arm. Recent magnetic resonance imaging was unchanged from the original.

Pause for thought

- How are you going to approach the discrepancy between her symptoms and the clinical findings?
- How will you broaden the agenda in order to explore psychosocial difficulties?
- How would you liaise with the nursing staff in order to improve the therapeutic environment?

Initial assessment

The patient did not seem to mind seeing another psychiatrist. She spontaneously described her social problems. One year previously she had started a degree in economics. During the second term she became pregnant with twins. The father was a married man with four children. She was advised to have an abortion by her parents. Initially she agreed but later changed her mind and continued with the pregnancy, returning to live with her parents and older sister. She secretly continued to see her boyfriend. Two months after the birth of twin girls she developed a hemiplegia and was diagnosed with multiple sclerosis. She spent five weeks as an inpatient and a further two months in a rehabilitation centre. During this time she had limited contact with her daughters who were cared for by her sister. On returning to the family home she found it difficult to care for and bond with them. Her mother and sister were very critical of these attempts and dismissive of her physical difficulties. She became deeply unhappy only gaining solace from phone calls to her boyfriend who promised he would leave his wife and make a home with her. She sent him money to aid this project. Three days prior to her second admission she discovered he had no intention of leaving his wife and had spent the money on his own family. She felt her life was in a terrible mess.

She had had a difficult childhood. Her mother developed rheumatoid arthritis when she was two years old. She felt unloved and neglected due to her mother's illness. She did well at school but developed unexplained physical symptoms during her examinations. These resolved with the prescription of antidepressant medication by her general practitioner.

She was a white woman with good self-care, who walked with great difficulty using a Zimmer frame. She developed leg tremor when discussing her home difficulties. She spoke clearly but with little emotional expression. Her mood was euthymic. There were no psychotic symptoms. Detailed cognitive testing was normal.

Pause for thought

- Where do you go from here?
- How might this scenario make you feel?

Further information

Family: A family interview highlighted the difficult family dynamics. Her mother was extremely critical of any of her attempts at rehabilitation and mothering. She appeared envious of the amount of attention her daughter was receiving and often commented on her own disability unfavourably comparing her daughter's ability to cope with her own.

Pause for thought

- What is your diagnosis?
- What sort of interventions may be of benefit?
- How would you co-ordinate your management plan?

Management and progress

A working diagnosis of conversion disorder superimposed on multiple sclerosis was made. A second neurological opinion confirmed the discrepancy between her physical symptoms and neurological signs. She was keen to pursue rehousing and was assigned a social worker. The physiotherapist continued to work with her in conjunction with a cognitive-behaviour therapist. She was taught anxiety-management techniques and her mobility slowly improved.

She was discharged to her parent's house to wait for her own accommodation. Her mobility rapidly deteriorated and she was only able to crawl around the house. There were frequent arguments between mother and daughter and several telephone calls to the department from her mother during which she insisted 'something be done'. On several occasions the family requested she be admitted to the mental health unit. The patient failed to engage with cognitive-behaviour therapy. She would agree to goals but not attempt to achieve them. She frustrated the community physiotherapist by her lack of commitment. After three weeks new accommodation was available and with social services support she moved in. Her mobility gradually improved in her new accommodation. Her relationship with her family continued to be turbulent and she left the care of her twins to her sister.

Final thoughts

- The physical symptoms associated with multiple sclerosis are numerous. What factors from the above history would suggest some of this patient's symptoms were exacerbated by psychosocial factors?
- Conversion disorder and multiple sclerosis may coexist. What do you know about the prevalence of other psychological disorders in multiple sclerosis? What treatment strategies may be useful?
- Multiple sclerosis may also cause cognitive deficits. How prevalent are these and how could they be assessed? How may cognitive impairment affect the patient's ability to cope with the consequences of their diagnosis?

Case 4: 'I won't let it get the better of me!'

Referral information

An urgent assessment was requested on a 71-year-old man, recently diagnosed with bone metastases from prostate cancer two years previously. He was reported as being agitated. The pain clinic, cancer nurses and primary-care physician requested referral.

Pause for thought

- The reason for referral was not clear. What challenge does this present? How would you deal with this?
- What particular information would you want from the medical notes?
- From whom would you want further information?
- What do you know about psychological disorders in palliative care?

Pre-assessment

Nursing staff: The cancer nurses described variability in the patient's pain control. He was often reluctant to take his analgesia. This included morphine and gabapentin. He was irritable and difficult to assess.

Medical notes: His prognosis was considered poor and he was due to receive palliative radiotherapy.

Pause for thought

- What are the physical and psychological side-effects of these medications?
- Why could his pain be so variable?
- What might be contributing to his irritability?

Initial assessment

The patient was a hesitant historian with a tendency to minimize his symptoms. He was sad about his diagnosis but not scared of death. As a deeply religious man he felt guilty that he was unable to bear his condition without recourse to psychological help. During his illness he had experienced considerable pain that had recently come under good control following an increase in his analgesic medication. He had constant fatigue and insomnia. His wife described behavioural changes since the secondary spread was diagnosed. Periods of extreme agitation and restlessness occurred on a daily basis. During these he became breathless and perspired. He was irritable with poor appetite and insomnia. At times he would appear confused and forgetful.

He had been fit and well prior to the diagnosis of prostate cancer. The only psychiatric history was an episode of depressive illness following a job promotion into a stressful position 30 years previously. He lived with his wife in a supportive relationship. His son lived nearby with four children. There was no history of substance misuse and his personal and family history were unremarkable.

On mental state examination he was extremely thin and looked unwell. He was tired and struggled to concentrate. His speech was normal and mood anxious. He was rather guarded. No psychotic symptoms were detected. He scored 28/30 on the mini-mental state examination. Blood tests were normal with the exception of mild anaemia.

Pause for thought

- What are the differential diagnoses?
- How would you differentiate between these?
- What would your management plan be?
- What effect might the anaemia have on his physical and psychological symptoms?

Further information

Primary care physician: The patient was described as a very stoic gentleman who rarely attended the practice.

Pause for thought

- What factors would influence your choice of medication?
- Who do you need to liaise with regarding his management?
- Would you want any further investigations at this stage?

Management and progress

A working diagnosis of a mixed anxiety/depressive disorder was made in addition to a possibility of an organic brain syndrome as a result of medication, metastases or electrolyte abnormality. A cerebral tomography scan requested by the oncologists was normal. He was commenced on a trial of mirtazapine and reviewed in clinic one month later. He reported much improved sleep, energy and appetite. He began walking to his son's house on a daily basis. He had visibly gained weight and his wife reported no further episodes of agitation. She was however concerned by episodes of confusion, worse in the evening. She was advised to record his total analgesic medication, which varied considerably, to see if the episodes of confusion coincided with days of high medication use. Routine bloods were again normal.

A month later he became delirious and was admitted to the local cancer unit. The treating physicians asked for a psychiatric assessment, suggesting his confusion might be a psychological reaction to his diagnosis. When assessed he clearly had an organic confusional state. The physicians were unable to find an explanation and he was discharged home to his wife's dismay. He was readmitted a week later with a chest infection and died several days later.

Final thoughts

- Depressive symptoms and depressive illness are common in patients with cancer. How often is depressive illness in this context missed? What do you know about the negative sequelae of not diagnosing depressive illness in this patient group?

- How could you help general hospital staff improve their ability to detect and treat psychological illness in their patients?
- Some antidepressants may improve the unpleasant effects of cancer and its treatment such as weight loss, anorexia and nausea. Which particular antidepressants may you want to consider?
- Fatigue, anorexia and insomnia are common in patients with cancer. It can be difficult to determine whether these are due to the disease or a psychological disorder. What questions could you ask to tease out the relative aetiological contributions? What pragmatic approaches could be tried if you are unable to clarify this?

Case 5: 'Why won't she just take the treatment?'

Referral information

The physicians referred a 43-year-old woman, who had been admitted to hospital with a history of indeterminate length, characterized by severe weight loss, malaise, weakness, fatigue, sweats and general debility. After admission, investigations revealed that she was infected with the HIV virus, and that she had acquired a secondary *Mycobacterium cellulare* infection. However, she refused to give the physicians any additional background information, and she refused to discuss her treatment options or her diagnoses. They noted that she wasn't eating, despite a body mass index of less than 18, that she was uncommunicative, and that she appeared depressed. They asked the liaison psychiatrist for further advice.

Pause for thought

- What goes through your mind as you approach the patient?
- Who will you need to speak to?
- What are the issues you may need to consider?

Pre-assessment

Nurses: Reported that she had been pulling out her naso-gastric tube, urinating in bed, refusing to come out of room, and hoarding medication. They were angry and frustrated. Although the nurses knew that she was physically ill, they believed that she ought to be 'somewhere psychiatric'. As a consequence, the nurses were avoiding her room, and interacting with her in a hostile manner.

Medical staff: Understood everything about the physical treatment plan, but seemed to know little about her behaviour, as they were only having minimal contact with her. They admitted that there was probably some connection between her mental state and physical states, probably interdependent.

Medical notes: These revealed investigations as above, ongoing abnormalities in haematological and biochemical markers, as well as a spiking temperature. There were several angry comments in the notes about non-compliance.

Pause for thought

- What issues have you picked up? Think of relative contributions of organic and non-organic factors.
- What are the causes of the attitudinal issues? Are they affecting care? How would you change that?
- What do you need to do now?

Initial assessment

This turned out to be a very difficult interview. She said she was 'devastated' to have HIV, and she said that she didn't want treatment, even though she knew that her illness would be fatal. She admitted to previous psychiatric contact at a nearby hospital, but she wouldn't provide further details. Furthermore, she refused permission to contact her family or friends. On mental state examination she avoided all eye contact. There was marked poverty of speech and thought, and her affect was flat and unreactive. Her mood was objectively and subjectively low, although she denied thoughts of self-harm and there were no psychotic symptoms. The transference was predominantly of anger.

Pause for thought

- Are you making progress?
- What are the questions or issues you have been asked to contribute to?
- What do you know about the psychiatric consequences of HIV?

Further information

Local psychiatric hospital: Sister at the day hospital confirmed that she had a long history of low mood, and that she had been attending there for years. She has always seemed extremely socially isolated, and reluctant to engage in treatments or activities. Episodically she had also had superimposed episodes of acute low mood. She said that the staff were divided between a diagnosis of personality disorder, or of dysthymia with acute episodes of depression.

Primary-care physician: Said that she had been suffering from chronic low mood for years, and that she had been on antidepressants for at least the past seven years, to no benefit. He was at a loss to advise how the current situation should be managed.

Further interview: She was reviewed three more times during the period of assessment. Although no rapport was established, she did say that she lived alone and that she had no friends, hobbies or leisure activities. She said that she did not enjoy watching television, listening to the radio or reading. She made some passing reference to having been employed at some time, and to some previous relationship with whom she now had no contact. Her mental state on each occasion was unchanged — she seemed predominantly angry as well as probably low in mood.

Pause for thought

- She appears to have long-term non-compliance with medication — this time with undoubted potentially fatal consequences. She knows this. How would you manage the situation, and what advice would you give?
- How do you think the ward staff responded to her anger?
- It's getting to the point of a management plan ... what are you going to do?

Management and progress

Following protracted negotiations, the mental health staff agreed to nurse her on the psychiatric unit, supported by daily visits from medical and nursing staff from the general hospital. To everyone's surprise, her behaviour rapidly improved. Within days, she was mixing with other patients, eating and drinking, and there were no further episodes of antisocial behaviour. Furthermore, she started to comply with all her medication, including that for the *Mycobacterium cellulare*. Multidisciplinary assessment on the psychiatric unit concluded that she did not have a depressive disorder.

One month later, she returned to the general hospital for further treatment of the HIV infection. There was a brief period where old patterns of behaviour appeared to return, but the nurses were supported to manage the situation. When her atypical infection was controlled and she had been established on the treatment for HIV, she was discharged.

Final thoughts

- *Diagnosis:* it was unclear whether she was depressed, and if so, whether this was arising as a direct consequence of the HIV infection, or as an emotional reaction to a serious diagnosis. There certainly appeared to be a predisposition to psychological illness, but did this fully account for her mood at the time of presentation. A trial of antidepressants seemed like a good idea, but total non-compliance was a problem.
- *Capacity:* was unresolved — to what degree was a depressive disorder affecting her ability to come to a balanced decision? In any case, management of HIV and the atypical infections would require long-term compliance with treatment,

whereas she had demonstrated an established pattern of poor compliance. Should her original choice to refuse treatment have been respected? A multidisciplinary meeting was held, which concluded that short-term coercive management was ethical, to see if her mental state could be improved to the point where she would consider the benefits of further treatment.

- *Ward environment:* from the outset, there were clear tensions in the relationship between the patient and the nurses, apparently resulting in some deliberate antisocial behaviour (e.g. soiling the bedclothes). Nevertheless, she clearly needed to remain in an acute environment because of the severity of her physical illness. Would there be time to work on staff attitudes? Some were willing to try, but none could see how they would be able to spend sufficient time with her.

- *Attitudes:* apart from the diagnostic complexities of this case, the principal challenges were attitudinal. Why was everybody so angry? What was different on the psychiatry ward? What implications does this case have for the work of a liaison psychiatrist?

Case 6: 'He's not the person he used to be'

Referral information

The endocrinologists referred a 45-year-old man who had had a craniopharyngioma excised four years previously. As a consequence, he had reduced pituitary function, diabetes insipidus and hypothyroidism. At the last clinic appointment, he had reported recurrent headaches and his wife said that he had been very aggressive in the mornings. She had also reported that he was overeating at times, and that his sleep was very disturbed.

Pause for thought

- What will be the challenges of this consultation? How will you deal with them?
- What might be the problem? Will it be organic, functional or both? Could this be an atypical depressive disorder?
- Do you need to know more about the illnesses, treatments and consequences mentioned in the referral?

Pre-assessment

Psychiatric notes: This man had been seen three years previously, at which time the letter to the physicians stated that: 'there was considerable difficulty assessing this man as he does not speak English. He has a sub-acute organic state secondary to an excised craniopharyngioma. There remains some residual tumour which is inoperable. He complains of headaches, mood swings, visual loss and increased appetite. He also appears to have difficulties in orientation (both time and place), and he appears to confabulate at times. More recently, he has become irritable, forceful and aggressive with episodes of low mood and crying. His concentration and energy are poor, sleep and appetite excessive. He also appears to have some psychotic symptoms, which include delusional ideas about the intracranial shunt, as well as visual hallucinations. He appears to be on large amounts of medication . . .'.

Pause for thought

- How far does this preliminary information prepare you for seeing the patient?
- What could have been the causes of the problems described in the previous letter? Dementia, organic affective state secondary to local effect of tumour (e.g. pressure), functional depressive disorder, complication of polypharmacy are all things to consider.
- Can you find out how successful the management of his psychiatric illness was on this previous occasion?
- What further information/resources might you want before seeing the patient?
- How are you going to deal with the fact that he does not speak English?

Initial assessment

The initial assessment was arranged with his wife, who came to translate. She reported that there were episodes of violence, once or twice per week, during which he would try to attack the family, sometimes with kitchen utensils. These seemed to be precipitated by rows in the family, which occurred fairly frequently because of frustration with his behaviour. She said that some of the most difficult behaviour included getting up in the middle of the night, because of insomnia, during which he wandered round in purposeless activity, or cleaning the house. The primary-care physician had already given advice regarding sleep hygiene, which hadn't been helpful.

The patient was only able to give minimal details. He said that he had 'nose problems and brain problems', and said that he 'would be dead soon'. This belief appeared to be linked to pessimism about diagnosis, rather than to any clear-cut depressive cognitions. He was on multiple centrally acting drugs, including thyroxine, steroids, desmopressin and temazepam.

On mental state examination he was clearly well cared-for, but his attention during the interview was impaired. It wasn't clear whether he knew why he was seeing the psychiatrist. There were no symptoms of anxiety or depression, and there were no psychotic symptoms. However, he was clearly disorientated in place and time.

Pause for thought

- How useful is previous information now?
- What problems arise if essential medication is also contributing to an abnormal mental state?
- What are the real key issues being presented?
- What might be the hurdles in the management plan?
- Could you differentiate between acute and chronic confusional states in a non-English-speaking patient?

Further information

Appointment with family: The family were seen again on two more occasions to get further information. They disclosed that the situation had suddenly worsened about three weeks prior to the referral on this occasion, when his two brothers (from Hong Kong) returned home after a two-month visit. During those two months, he had in fact seemed quite well.

The Young Dementia Service: Said that they would be unable to offer a service to a patient who spoke no English at all.

A Cantonese voluntary agency: was identified, but they said that they were not able to offer a service to a patient with behavioural impairment, as their principal function was to offer a befriending service to socially isolated residents.

Pause for thought

- It's now the second appointment, and the family are expecting a management plan . . . .
- What is your understanding of the difficulties being presented, and what potential solutions might there be?

Management and progress

Further review of the old psychiatric notes revealed that the previous similar episode had been satisfactorily improved using an atypical antipsychotic, which had led to improvement in the aggression and in the lability of mood. Antidepressants had not been required. However the antipsychotic had been discontinued by the family during the past year. The medication was reinstated, which led to a marked improvement in behaviour, as on the previous occasion. Apart from the behavioural difficulties, sleep disturbance was also contributing to the patient's and the family's distress. In view of the potentially long-term need, antihistamines were successfully used in preference to benzodiazepines.

The detailed assessment had also revealed that excess face-to-face contact with the family, and social isolation from others, appeared to be contributing to the episodes of aggression. As a result the family were getting frustrated, leading to even more difficulties. This was discussed in detail with the family, who were encouraged to find alternative sources of social support for themselves and the patient.

Education of the family, together with the changes in medication led to a significant improvement in the quality of life of both the patient and his family. They were reviewed on two further occasions when there had not been any further difficulties. Furthermore, the family were making arrangements for one of the patient's brothers to visit again from Hong Kong.

Final thoughts

- This case illustrates the benefits of scrutinizing all sources of information, particularly old notes, where the current situation may have been encountered before.
- How can you manage the long-term psychological consequences of physical illness in the absence of appropriate resources?
- Carbamazepine can sometimes be used in the management of aggression. What are the precautions and difficulties in prescribing psychotropic medication in patients with complex medical and pharmacological regimens?
- The psychiatric consequences of pituitary tumours (such as a craniopharyngioma) are multitudinous. They range from the consequences of target gland dysfunction (e.g. hypothyroidism) together with more generalized features such as altered mood and confusion. In some cases, the primary presentation of altered pituitary function is psychiatric. In this patient's case, the tumour had been incompletely excised, with evidence of local pressure effects. Complete management of the re-presentation should, in collaboration with the physicians, have included investigation of target organ hormonal levels as well as a brain scan.

Case 7: 'I am just tired all the time'

Referral information

The rheumatologists referred a 25-year-old woman who had been attending the clinic for several months. She had presented with a four-year history of fatigue, as a consequence of which she was largely confined to a wheelchair. The problems started when she had considerable work and relationship stress. She had already discussed with the physicians that there might be some connection between her physical and psychiatric symptoms.

Pause for thought

- How helpful is it for referrers to explore psychological issues with patients? What are the advantages of the physician discussing the reasons for referral with the patient?
- In what setting will you want to see this woman? What are the advantages and disadvantages of holding liaison clinics in the medical outpatients?
- To whom might you also want to speak at the first appointment?

Pre-assessment

Primary-care physician: Said that the patient had been well until the current episode of illness. He said that her sister had agoraphobia, and that her father had been treated for recurrent depressive disorder. He was aware that she had joined the local myalgic-encephalomyelitis (ME) society, and that she had seen several alternative therapists (homeopathy and acupuncture) in addition to the practice counsellor.

Referring physician: Said that she was 'one of the most disabled patients in the rheumatology clinic'. She had already seen several of the consultants, at two hospitals, including a 'second opinion' at a third hospital. He confirmed that all investigations had been normal. His view was that she was persisting to look for a physical cause for her symptoms.

Pause for thought

- How far does this preliminary information prepare us for seeing this woman?
- What do you know about the illness attribution patterns of patients who somatize?
- She had already seen several specialists and alternative therapists, as well as at least one support group. How does this guide your thinking with regard to her eventual management?

Initial assessment

The patient was seen in the clinic, sat in a wheelchair. She said that the joint pains had started about four years previously whilst working on an assembly line. At first, the unions had attributed her pain to a repetitive strain injury. She then started to feel increasingly tired, to the point of no longer being able to go to work. Over the course of a few months the pain had spread to most muscle groups, but particularly to her thighs which, in combination with the fatigue, had caused her to become increasingly reliant on a wheelchair.

At the initial assessment she reported some disturbed sleep, but no other symptoms of depression or anxiety.

During the first assessment, she also spoke a little of the circumstances at work prior to becoming ill. She said that the company had failed to secure a large order, and that there was the possibility of redundancies. However she had been made redundant by the time of the first assessment by the psychiatrist.

Pause for thought

- She presents with symptoms of fibromyalgia and fatigue — how commonly do these symptoms coexist?
- She doesn't appear to be depressed — what is the evidence for the effectiveness of antidepressants in such situations?
- Issues of primary gain have already appeared in the first consultation. How would you use that information?

Further information (summary of further consultations)

A few months prior to the difficulties at work, she had started to have difficulties with her partner with whom she shared a flat. He had called her 'lazy and unattractive' and she suspected him of seeing someone else. She felt less and less able to cope with this, and her physical symptoms, for which he appeared to show no sympathy. Eventually she decided to move back to her parents' house, who themselves had intermittent marital difficulties, possibly linked to her father's long-term mental illness.

After moving back home, the patient's health continued to deteriorate. She encountered hostility from her parents who would shout at her whenever she attempted to exercise, warning her that she would cause permanent damage to her muscles. This was reinforced by friends at the local support group who told her that they had deteriorated following the recommended physiotherapy. She started to feel increasingly trapped and isolated, resulting in frequent outbursts at home. Her family refused to take her to see healthcare professionals, stating that it was 'too far' or 'a waste of time', or 'inconvenient'.

Pause for thought

- What might be the goals of the first few sessions?
- Can you start to make sense of the psychological issues?

Management and progress

At the third interview the psychiatrist established boundaries about how often he would see her, and for how many sessions. The family were invited to each appointment, but they were unable to attend. She was told that she would have to make her own way to appointments and that neither a wheelchair nor a hospital taxi would be provided.

During subsequent interviews the patient became increasingly angry with the psychiatrist. She accused him of not understanding the enormous disability she was experiencing. At first, she challenged all attempts to discuss an exercise programme by giving graphic descriptions of the 'devastating' effects that even walking round furniture could cause. Nevertheless, after several months, she started to talk about her anger towards work, her boyfriend and her parents. She started to recognize that her symptoms had forced her parents and her boyfriend to pay her more attention, and that she had missed most of the difficulties at work because of her illness. As she had already acknowledged some connection between symptoms and stress, she agreed to keep a diary, in which she was able to identify the links between events and symptoms of fatigue.

Over the following 12 months she stopped attending the physicians and the support group. She was able to identify some structured and graded activities (with the help of a physiotherapist) which increased her independence from home, leading to her renting her own flat again after about 12 months of treatment.

Final thoughts

- What do you think are the key psychological components of this case? How could the primary and secondary gain issues be discussed?
- Initially, family therapy was considered the best way forward. How would you engage a family like this?
- As is often the case in liaison services which receive tertiary referrals, this patient lived in another Health Authority. From an organizational point of view, what extra complexity does this add to her management?

Case 8: 'It's just too strange to be true'

Referral information

The Medical Emergency Ward referred a 30-year-old woman. She had presented to Accident & Emergency with a two-day history of chest pain and coughing blood, having just returned 12 hours previously from doing a medical locum position in New Zealand. The clinical history was strongly suggestive of a pulmonary embolus, so she was admitted for further management. However, over the next 48 hours, all investigations were normal. During this time, the Greek medical registrar had been surprised by her surname — he said that her Greek-sounding name was probably false. After two days on the ward she started to express symptoms of low mood with suicidal cognitions. Concerned by the overall clinical picture, the physicians contacted liaison psychiatry for further advice.

Pre-assesment

Medical notes: Simply contained details of the normal investigations. The psychiatrist noticed that the 'next of kin' was not documented. The physicians had attemped to obtain old medical notes from another hospital at which she said she had been previously treated, but her details were not registered on the hospital database.

Nursing staff: Reported that there had been no difficulties and that she had not had any visitors.

Primary-care physician: Not at address given.

Initial assessment

The patient said that symptoms started after a spontaneous miscarriage (her fourth) which had occurred after her boyfriend hit her. She had to run away from home, thus presenting at a distant hospital with the symptoms of chest pain. She described severe symptoms of low mood and hopelessness, with biological symptoms. During the course of the interview, although her history to the A&E staff and her history to the psychiatrist were incompatible, she could not account for the differences. Furthermore she was unable to explain how she could have graduated in medicine in a town without a medical school.

On mental state examination she was very distressed and agitated. Her self-care was poor. Her vocabulary was poor and it had a strong regional accent. She expressed symptoms of low mood and hopelessness with no psychotic symptoms. Surprisingly, she seemed much brighter, moments later, when discussing the local nightclubs.

Further information

As she had a strong regional accent, the liaison team launched an extensive investigation of all hospitals, mental health trusts and health authorities in that region. However, they failed to find any match for date of birth or approximation to name. Eventually one hospital identified a similar patient who was very well known to them — even though the only similarity was the year of birth. When the hospital records were retrieved, the patient's current name was identified as one of many aliases. The primary-care physician she claimed to be registered with was in fact her early childhood doctor.

In total, the patient had attended 139 hospitals in the past four years, using one of four clinical presentations, and seven aliases. Some components of her history remained constant and true at each presentation (e.g. sibship, location of birth, schooling), whereas most of the remaining history was variable and factitious. Throughout, there were several themes (which were probably true) such as abusive peer relationships and poor relationships with her parents.

Management and progress

The patient was confronted with this information, which she denied. She left the hospital a few moments later, and presented at another hospital five miles away later the same day.

Final thoughts

- How should factitious disorders be managed?
- This patient stayed in hospital for two days, and had many investigations. On this occasion none were invasive, but in the past they had been. How could this be managed?
- Her identity was only found by chance, and required several hours of investigation by a team of staff. Multiple aliases made this more difficult. What strategies could be developed nationally to address this?
- This case was interesting because of the mixture of fictitious and real facts (e.g. her year of birth), some of which changed at each presentation, while others were constant. Why would she do this? What would be the advantage of having a few real 'anchor points'?
- What do you know about the hypothesized psychodynamic mechanisms in this disorder?

Case 9: 'Born in the wrong body'

Referral information

The primary-care physician referred a 33-year-old man for a gender reassignment assessment.

Pre-assessment

None made.

Initial assessment

The patient reported gender dysphoria since puberty, knowing that something was 'not right'. In his teens he developed a fetish for wearing female underwear which was associated with marked guilt. His adolescence was painfully shy and inhibited, and he was bullied at school for being 'different'. Unfortunately, issues of sexuality could not be discussed at home. In his early twenties he moved out of the family home, and soon discovered that he formed physical relationships more easily with men than with women, having had a number of unsatisfactory heterosexual relationships. Soon after leaving home he discovered transvestite clubs and shops, and started to socialize with the local gay community. His new relationships, always homosexual and while cross-dressed, provided him with the emotional strength and support he had been seeking. He found also relationships, platonic and sexual, easier to form whilst cross-dressed.

He had continued to live in this way for several years, permanently dressed as a woman except when visiting his parents and his family, none of whom were aware of the tension in his life. Tragically, both parents were killed in a road traffic accident a few months before requesting gender reassignment, whereupon he realized that they had been a dominating force in limiting the expression of his sexuality. Consequently, he decided to consider gender reassignment.

Management plan

He was referred to the gender reassignment clinic where he confirmed that he had been living as the opposite sex for two years. Following a second psychiatric opinion and extensive counselling, he was commenced on hormonal treatment, and eventually listed for gender reassignment.

Final thoughts

- What are the differences between fetishistic transvestism and gender dysphoria?
- What are the key points of the assessment?
- What is generally required of the patient before gender reassignment can occur?
- What might be your role as a liaison psychiatrist, and how would you have helped him deal with his family?

Summary

These cases have provided a different perspective and way of thinking about liaison psychiatry which is more familiar to the clinician. It is important to remember that liaison psychiatrists cannot possibly be familiar with the latest developments across the whole of the field of medicine, but they may well be expected to provide advice about patients with a wide range of physical and psychological problems. The literature, databases and web-based resources are all useful ways of accessing information quickly. Many liaison psychiatry services are quite small and individual consultants may work in isolation. It is helpful to be able to discuss complex cases with other colleagues from different services who may bring a new perspective or particular experience of dealing with certain kinds of problems. In the UK, there is an email discussion group in which clinicians can present cases to other colleagues in confidence for advice and consideration.

Mentoring is also useful for newly appointed consultant liaison psychiatrists, where a more experienced liaison psychiatrist can provide support and guidance, without actually acting as a supervisor. This system can work very well, even if the newly appointed psychiatrist and mentor are based in separate hospitals or even localities.

Part V

Different treatment settings

36

Developing links with primary care

Richard Morriss, Linda Gask, Christopher Dowrick, Peter Salmon and Sarah Peters

Introduction

Most liaison psychiatry is practised in the general-hospital setting, but increasingly services for the physically ill are becoming community based. Family practitioners play a key role in identifying patients with comorbid physical and psychological distress. This chapter describes the developments over the last 10 years in the detection and treatment of patients with medically unexplained symptoms in a primary-care setting.

Medically unexplained symptoms in primary care

Medically unexplained symptoms (MUS) are defined as physical symptoms that doctors cannot explain by physical pathology, which distress or impair the functioning of the patient (Peveler *et al.* 1997). Patients with MUS seek help from the family doctor and are frequently unwilling to consult mental health professionals or non-medical personnel because many of these patients believe that they have a physical health problem (Kirmayer & Robbins 1996). Around 75% of patients with MUS persisting for more than six months (persistent medically unexplained symptoms or PMUS) are still distressed and/or function-ally impaired by them 12 months later (Kroenke & Spitzer 1998; Moore *et al.* 2000). Persistent MUS is the most common reason for frequent attendance to the family doctor (Jyvasjarvi *et al.* 1998), and a frequent source of family doctor frustration (Mathers & Gash 1995). Family doctors express lower satisfaction with care for patients with PMUS than patients with psychological problems (Hartz *et al.* 2000).

Persistent MUS is similar in definition to the DSM-IV diagnostic category of undifferentiated somatoform disorder, except that it includes patients with mood disorder, anxiety disorder and other somatoform disorders (American Psychiatric Association 1994). PMUS is a term that is popular with family doctors because it is utilizable without requiring lifetime symptom counts, which are impractical in busy surgeries. The term PMUS does not require the family doctor to reveal prematurely a diagnosis of mood or anxiety disorders, which many patients, who present with physical symptoms and physical health attributions for their symptoms, do not readily accept. Family doctors recognize PMUS patients primarily on the basis of two criteria: (a) they have medically unexplained symptoms; and (b) they regularly attend over a period of months (Schilte *et al.* 2000). There was poor agreement (kappa = 0.27) between family doctors' definition of patients with somatization (Schilte *et al.* 2000) and a commonly applied psychiatric definition (Lipowski 1988).

There is now a lot of empirical evidence suggesting that PMUS or somatoform disorders frequently coexist with mood or anxiety disorder cross-sectionally and longitudinally (Allen *et al.* 2001; Fink *et al.* 1999; Kroenke *et al.* 1997; Simon *et al.* 2001). For example, individuals with depression at baseline and a poor view of their overall health were likely to develop somatoform disorders within the next 12 months (Gureje & Simon 1999). Overlapping psychopathology may exist along a spectrum of anxiety, depression and somatization in primary care (Piccinelli *et al.* 1999). Often persistent and disabling psychopathology does not fit with the high symptom thresholds required for the current diagnostic system for mental disorders (Piccinelli *et al.* 1999). For instance, compared to other primary-care patients, undifferentiated somatoform disorder patients had impaired role function and poorer general health perception and were also four times more likely to be rated as difficult to manage by their family doctors (Kroenke *et al.* 1997). Therefore, the use of the term PMUS appears to be justified empirically as well as on the grounds of clinical utilizability by family doctors.

A large part of the family doctor's workload consists of patients with PMUS who are too numerous to refer to other health professionals or services. A survey of the French general population estimated that PMUS had a point prevalence of 19% (Hardy 1995). Estimates of PMUS/somatoform disorders in the community with a duration of six months or more suggest a point prevalence of 19.6% in Nigeria (Gureje & Obikoya 1992) and one-year prevalence of 21.7% in Italy (Faravelli *et al.* 1997). Patients with high levels of somatization or health anxiety accounted for 33–50% more visits to primary care doctors, 20–50% greater outpatient costs, and one-third more hospitalizations than other US primary-care patients over two years (Barsky *et al.* 2001). Not surprisingly in the UK, the management of PMUS is the second most popular topic for primary-care education in relation to mental health (Kerwick *et al.* 1997).

Given constraints on their time, it is important that family doctors have simple effective interventions for PMUS at their disposal. These simple interventions should be compatible with the working models and normal working practices of family doctors if they are to be widely used by family doctors.

Working models of practice held by family doctors

Family doctors are faced with the whole range of physical and psychosocial health problems. Modern practice is to teach family doctors to carry out 'patient-led' communication that reacts to and explores the patient's needs rather than 'doctor-led' communication based on the doctor's first conceptualization of the patient's problems (Levenstein et al. 1986; Morriss 1992). In 'patient-led' interviews, doctors are taught to ask open questions, followed by directive questions, according to verbal and non-verbal cues from their patients. History taking for physical problems is usually followed by a focused physical examination of the affected area of the body or system. Any approach to the management of MUS must be compatible with starting a consultation with a patient in this way.

Patient-centred management has become established as an ideal in primary care and typically displays five characteristics:

1. It explores the patient's main reason for the visit, concerns and need for information
2. It seeks an integrated understanding of the patient's world, i.e. their whole person, emotional needs and life issues
3. It finds common ground on what the problem is and mutually agrees on management
4. It enhances prevention and health promotion
5. It enhances the continuing relationship between the patient and doctor (Little et al. 2001; Stewart et al. 1995).

Again any approach to managing MUS should be compatible with such patient-centred management in primary care.

However, there are some significant barriers to achieving fully patient-centred care in any patient. First of all, patients' agendas are complex and it is probably impossible to establish all of the patient's agenda in one primary-care consultation (Barry et al. 2000). Second, neither patients nor doctors are passive communicators so that doctor–patient communication is inevitably a product of the agendas of both patient and doctor, and an ongoing dynamic process (Hunt et al. 1989). Third, doctors require sufficient time without interruption to systematically assess and attempt to meet patients' needs. Fourth, the doctor needs to have a positive attitude, the requisite communication skills, and sufficient general and local knowledge to address both medical and psychosocial needs.

There are specific barriers to addressing the needs of patients with PMUS. First, the patient and doctor may not share the same conceptualization of the patient's problems. The patient believes their symptoms to be partly or totally physically caused while the doctor is aware that an organic physical problem is unlikely to be the main explanation for their symptoms. The doctor may feel powerless to meet the patient's needs (Mathers & Gask 1995) so patient-centred care is not attempted (Salmon *et al.* 1999). Accurately addressing the health needs of patients presenting with physical symptoms is associated with improved patient satisfaction at two weeks, and improved symptoms and function at three months (Jackson *et al.* 2001). Thus, doctors and patients need to communicate so that there is common agreement about the conceptualization of the patient's problems and the patient's needs can be addressed through joint decision-making by the doctor and patient.

Second, the patient's past experience of illness will shape the patient's current agenda (Epstein *et al.* 1999; Hunt *et al.* 1989); patients with PMUS may have had an extensive, complex and sometimes negative experience of both illness and health service responses to illness (Salmon *et al.* 1999). Such experience has shaped the patient's beliefs about the cause and severity of their symptoms, and their ability to trust the assessments, explanations or treatments offered by health professionals (Walker *et al.* 1998).

Third, age, gender and culture may play a role in detection of PMUS in primary care. Younger people presenting with five or more MUS may be more likely to have greater psychiatric morbidity and harmful use of alcohol across cultures (Kisely *et al.* 1997). Males may offer fewer psychological interpretations of their symptoms and more concern about the serious physical health implications of their bodily symptoms (Jyvasjarvi *et al.* 1999). On the other hand, women present with more MUS even after adjusting for coexisting depressive and anxiety disorder (Kroenke & Spitzer 1998). However, the effects of gender and culture on the presentation of MUS may not be as great as the presence or absence of coexisting depressive or anxiety disorder (Piccinelli & Simon 1997).

Fourth, primary care is often organized so that patients do not see the same doctor on a regular basis, with the result that more somatic presentations of mental disorder and less consistent management are found in such primary-care services (Simon *et al.* 1999). Family doctors who were most satisfied with the care of patients with PMUS were more likely to work alone and have stayed in the same place of work for five years or more (Hartz *et al.* 2000), suggesting that consistency of care is important. Patients with MUS will try out a doctor's explanation for their illness and test it against past and ongoing experience over a period of days or weeks before rejecting or incorporating it into their own health-related beliefs (Hunt *et al.* 1989). Thus, a series of consultations between the patient and the same doctor may be required to establish a dialogue that may modify the patient's beliefs. Furthermore, psychological explanations for mental disorder are acquired over time as mental disorders become more chronic and severe in patients with mental disorder that initially presents somatically (Patel *et al.* 1998).

Routine care for patients with PMUS

Family doctors usually talk to PMUS patients about their symptoms in an unstructured way, investigate, provide reassurance, sanction time off from work, prescribe symptomatic relief, prescribe hypnotics, sedatives and antidepressants, and refer to hospital medical and surgery care, physiotherapy, dietitian, community nursing and counselling services (Morriss *et al.* 1998; Salmon *et al.* 1999). There is little short-term evidence of improved symptoms or function with the intervention of the family doctor delivering treatment as usual (Morriss *et al.* 1999).

The most common intervention for patients with MUS is reassurance. Reassurance may provide patients with a temporary reduction in anxiety about their health, lasting less than 24 hours, with a return to previous levels of health anxiety that persists for many months (Lucock *et al.* 1997; McDonald *et al.* 1996). Doctors who adopt a warm, friendly and reassuring manner are more effective than formal consultations providing little reassurance (Di Blasi *et al.* 2001). However, patients interpret reassurance in the light of their own views and perceptions, and successful reassurance is only achieved when the doctor accurately acknowledges the patient's perspectives of their difficulties (Donovan & Blake 2000). Lack of reassurance by a doctor's explanation for their symptoms contributes to the persistence of the MUS over 12 months, no matter how many visits are made to the doctor (Speckens *et al.* 2000). Poor communication by the doctor in a consultation may contribute to the persistence of MUS in a number of ways: (a) patients are not told the results of physical examinations or investigations (Bruster *et al.* 1994); (b) the reality of the patients' concerns are denied (Salmon *et al.* 1999); (c) the patient's own explanations for their symptoms are passively accepted (Salmon *et al.* 1999); (d) the doctor gives a double message that there is no reason for concern while giving the patient symptomatic medication or precautionary advice (McDonald *et al.* 1996); (e) explanations given by the doctor are poorly defined and vague (Cope *et al.* 1994).

Often routine care for patients with PMUS appears to be unstructured, inconsistently applied, and ineffective, or possibly even iatrogenic as a result of unnecessary investigations, treatments or referrals. Communication from the doctor to the patient with PMUS is often intangible, does not meet the patient's needs or expectations, and is not empowering (Salmon *et al.* 1999).

Naturalistic studies of outcome

There are only a small number of observational studies of determinants of outcome in patients with all types of MUS. In 215 patients with somatized presentations of mental disorder, negative changes in outcome of physical symptoms at one and three months were associated with the severity of baseline physical and psychiatric symptoms, prescription of hypnotics and benzodiaze- pines, the presence of DSM-IV anxiety disorders, and the presence of comorbid physical pathology (Downes-Grainger *et al.* 1998). The determinants of change in outcome of psychiatric symptoms at one and three months were similar, except that the patient's perception that the GP understood how they felt emotionally was associated with improved outcome at one month, and the patient's perception of the quality of the GP's explanation was associated with improved outcome at three months. Changes in functional outcome were associated with the same factors as for physical symptoms at one and three months with additional worse outcome effects of inpatient or outpatient care, invalidity benefit and absence of a job at both time points. Up to 35% of the variance in outcome could be explained by the factors that were measured.

In a Danish study of 905 patients with musculoskeletal symptoms in primary care who were referred to physiotherapy, psychological distress and somatization adversely predicted physical health change, patient self-rated improvement, sick leave and change in use of medication (Jorgensen *et al.* 2000).

Psychosocial predictors of outcome at one and two years in terms of subjective health, sick leave, number of healthcare visits and number of medicines were explored in a Dutch study of 376 frequent attenders with somatization (Schilte *et al.* 2001a). Absence of social support predicted subjective health, sick leave and number of healthcare visits at both time points while baseline subjective health and number of medicines prescribed were the best overall predictors of outcome (Schilte *et al.* 2001a).

In conclusion, naturalistic studies suggest that short- to medium-term outcome might be associated with interventions that improve empathy and explanations for symptoms by doctors to patients, reduce psychological distress, improve social support, and reduce unnecessary medication, investigations or referrals.

Symptom beliefs and outcome in observational studies

Patients with PMUS in primary care often have beliefs about symptoms that are discrepant with medical knowledge, but carefully reasoned and firmly held, after prolonged reflection and information gathering from many sources such as the media and family (Hunt *et al.* 1989; Peters *et al.* 1998; Salmon *et al.* 1999).

Doctors' views may not contribute much to the formation of these symptom beliefs by the patient if the doctor is not seen as knowledgeable or interested in the PMUS (Clements *et al.* 1997; Salmon *et al.* 1999). The patient's symptom beliefs reflect both individual experiences and cultural themes such as invasion of the body, wearing out of body parts or imbalance of bodily processes (Peters *et al.* 1998). Nevertheless, patients with PMUS (Peters *et al.* 1998), like patients with medically explained symptoms (Salmon *et al.* 1996), accept or suspect that psychological or behavioural factors, particularly stress or lifestyle may be contributing at least in part to their symptoms. Associated with these beliefs is the widespread expectation that discussion and advice from the family doctor will be helpful (Salmon *et al.* 1996; Woloshynowych *et al.* 1998). In practice, however, medical explanations for PMUS are commonly rejected by patients, especially explanations that attribute symptoms to psychological factors (Peters *et al.* 1998). There may be two reasons for this. First, patients' direct sensory knowledge of their symptoms provides a sense of authority over doctors who are seen as relying on inaccurate or mistaken evidence. Second, symptoms are experienced as evidence of an alien disease entity so patients value doctors who acknowledge the reality of this threat and form an alliance against it.

In primary-care patients with somatized mental disorder or medically unexplained fatigue, patient-held beliefs that their symptoms have a physical health cause were likely to persist over 12 months (Garcia-Campayo *et al.* 1997; Ridsdale *et al.* 1994). Beliefs that there may be an underlying serious physical health problem predicted frequent attendance in primary care with MUS (Jyvasjarvi *et al.* 2001). Sometimes patient-held beliefs about the cause of their symptoms are not strong determinants of outcome (Cathebras *et al.* 1995). Instead other aspects of patient-held beliefs concerning symptoms (Weinman *et al.* 1996) have been shown to predict clinical outcome and health utilization in patients with physical illness. Hence patient-held beliefs about the severity, future duration, consequences and controllability of their symptoms or illness predicted symptomatic, functional and health-service resource use in patients at three and six months who suffered a myocardial infarction (Petrie *et al.* 1996), and over one year in patients with psoriasis (Scharloo *et al.* 2000). Catastrophizing beliefs about the seriousness of bodily symptom change, together with negative affect (depression, anxiety, 'stress', and irritability) and high absorption (attention and preoccupation with the body), predicted patients who tended to present with PMUS according to the family doctor (McGrady *et al.* 1999).

In conclusion, some aspects of a patient's beliefs about their symptoms (the nature, consequences, time course and controllability of symptoms) may be modifiable by the family doctor through empathic and carefully reasoned explanation.

The effectiveness of simple interventions for PMUS

Four approaches to the management of PMUS that might be employed by family doctors have been explored in randomized controlled trials (RCTs): antidepressants, exercise, psychiatric consultation and emotional disclosure.

A meta-analysis of 94 RCTs of tricyclic, selective serotonin reuptake inhibitor and other antidepressants, in patients with six PMUS or syndromes involving MUS (chronic headache, fibromyalgia, functional gastrointestinal disorders, idiopathic pain, tinnitus and chronic fatigue), found that the pooled odds ratio was 3.4 (95% confidence intervals, 2.6–4.3; number needed to treat = 4) for a benefit of antidepressants (O'Malley *et al.* 1999). Benefits of antidepressants were shown in chronic headache, fibromyalgia, functional gastrointestinal disorders and idiopathic pain but not in tinnitus or chronic fatigue. The presence of depression was not necessary for improvement in MUS. However, the vast majority of these RCTs were conducted with chronic patients in secondary care rather than primary care. Moreover, the median duration of follow-up was only nine weeks.

Exercise therapies may be prescribed by the family doctor at a local gymnasium or sports centre. A meta-analysis of 39 RCTs of exercise therapies (Van Tulder *et al.* 2001), e.g. low-impact aerobics (Mannion *et al.* 2001), found that for chronic non-specific low back pain, exercise therapy was more effective than usual care by the family doctor and equally effective as conventional physiotherapy or inactive treatments for back pain, e.g. massage (Cherkin *et al.* 2001) on pain and disability. While some studies have demonstrated advantages of exercise therapies over conventional physiotherapy and other inactive treatments, the effects are inconsistent and may be non-specific (Van Tulder *et al.* 2001). A meta-analysis of graded exercise programmes for fibromyalgia (Rossy *et al.* 1999) and chronic fatigue syndrome (Fulcher *et al.* 1997; Wearden *et al.* 1998) have demonstrated improved symptomatic, and sometimes improved functional outcomes, but probably require the direct supervision of a trained therapist. A meta-analysis of 25 RCTs for chronic pain suggested that interventions that tackled illness beliefs were more effective than behavioural interventions, such as graded exercise, for pain, positive coping measures and behaviour related to pain, such as distance walked, but there were no significant differences in mood, negative coping or social function (Morley *et al.* 1999). The same conclusion was reached in a meta-analysis of 49 RCTs for fibromyalgia (Rossy *et al.* 1999).

In three RCTs, psychiatric consultation advice was sent in letters to family doctors suggesting that they provide regular brief appointments (initially weekly, later monthly) with the same doctor to patients with chronic somatoform disorders. In addition the family doctors should listen supportively, carry out a brief physical examination for any change in symptoms, and avoid unnecessary investigations and referrals (Rost *et al.* 1994; Smith *et al.* 1986, 1995). In each RCT, there were important savings in healthcare costs, and also benefits to physical health in two out of three trials. However, there were no effects on impaired general health perception, mental health or social functioning, which are important aspects of quality of life. Furthermore, these RCTs were prone to selection bias because the family doctor selected the patients for the trial and then carried out the intervention. A fourth randomized controlled trial of a joint diagnostic consultation between a psychiatrist and family doctor followed by care from the family doctor for distressed high utilizers of care (not confined to patients presenting with MUS) found no improvements in emotional distress, self-reported health status or number of healthcare visits (Katon *et al.* 1992). There was a significant increase in the use of antidepressants, but the clinical benefits of such prescribing were not evident in the trial.

The only randomized controlled trial of interviews by family doctors to disclose emotionally important events in a patient's life revealed no significant changes in symptoms, emotional distress, function, sickness or health visits among somatizing patients in primary care (Schilte *et al.* 2001b).

In conclusion, antidepressants have short-term symptomatic benefits to patients with painful or gastrointestinal PMUS, but not necessarily other types of PMUS. There is an absence of evidence for the long-term benefit of antidepressants and for benefits in terms of function, quality of life or healthcare costs. Graded exercise may be effective for certain PMUS complaints such as back pain, widespread body pain and fatigue, but tackling illness beliefs may make these interventions more effective. More severe, persistent and disabling PMUS complaints of widespread body pain and fatigue may require supervision by a therapist. A partly effective method of managing a patient with more numerous and chronic PMUS is for a single family doctor to see the patient on a regular and consistent basis, avoiding unnecessary investigations or referrals. This approach reduces physical disability (improved activities of daily life and mobility) and health costs but not other important aspects of patients' health or function. Disclosure of emotionally meaningful life events does not appear efficacious for patients with PMUS.

Cognitive-behaviour therapy and other similar therapist interventions for PMUS

A systematic review of 31 controlled trials (29 randomized) of cognitive-behaviour therapy (CBT) for somatization symptoms and syndromes, e.g. chronic fatigue syndrome, demonstrated that, compared to control or treatment-as-usual conditions, CBT improved physical symptoms in 71%, functional status in 47% and emotional distress in 38% of patients for up to 12 months (Kroenke & Swindle 2000). Five sessions of CBT and group interventions were efficacious. However, there are only a small number of randomized controlled trials of CBT as an intervention for somatoform disorders or PMUS in primary care (Lidbeck 1997; Moore *et al.* 2000; Sumithipala *et al.* 2000). Cognitive-behavioural therapy, requiring five or more 30–60 minute sessions and a high level of training, specialist therapeutic skill and supervision, is impractical for use by most family doctors in routine practice. However, CBT intervention studies inform us about the therapeutic ingredients of effective interventions that family doctors might use in consultations with PMUS patients. These approaches are also suitable for use by other health professionals working sessionally in primary care in a group setting (Kroenke & Swindle 2000; Lidbeck 1997) or individually with the aid of patient self-help manuals (Powell *et al.* 2001). However, there is still a need for interventions that can be used directly by family doctors because many primary-care patients with PMUS will not consult mental health professionals (Kirmayer & Robbins 1996) or enter psychotherapy groups (Hellman *et al.* 1990).

Studies of CBT and similar interventions have demonstrated the efficacy of the following explanations and techniques that might be used by family doctors to reduce PMUS such as pain, fatigue and symptoms related to overbreathing:

- live demonstration of hyperventilation and reattribution to psychological or physiological causes (Han *et al.* 1996)
- exercises to reduce time pressures on patients and relieve muscle tension (Clark *et al.* 1978a)
- evidence gathering followed by explanations relating symptoms physiologically or temporally to psychosocial factors (Bouman & Visser 1998; Clark *et al.* 1998; Fava *et al.* 2000)
- problem solving of interpersonal issues (Wilkinson *et al.* 1994)
- setting consistent sleep and rest patterns (Powell *et al.* 2001) to relieve fatigue and muscle aches.

Treatment approaches, which initially incorporate explanations that are compatible with the patient's symptom beliefs, then modify them as a result of the patient's experience of symptom relief, rather than directly challenge the symptom beliefs at the beginning of treatment, may require less time from the therapist (Powell *et al.* 2001).

Reattribution for managing PMUS

Reattribution was first described in 1989 by Goldberg and Gask (Goldberg *et al.* 1989) and was based on observation of over 1000 family doctor–patient interviews, and feedback from family doctors in Britain and Australia about explanations that worked for patients who somatize. It is a treatment designed to be used by family doctors with patients who have somatized mental disorder (SMD). Patients with SMD have depressive or anxiety disorders, present to the family doctor with somatic symptoms, and believe the symptoms to be wholly or partly due to physical health problems (Morriss *et al.* 1998, 1999). Such patients constitute about 4% of consultations with family doctors (Downes-Grainger *et al.* 1998; Weich *et al.* 1995). However, reattribution may have wider application to patients with MUS, especially PMUS. In its original format, reattribution had three stages, described in Table 36.1.

Table 36.1. Stages of the original reattribution model.

---

1. Feeling understood

The family doctor elicits a history of:
- the presenting physical symptom(s) – onset, duration, nature, severity, aggravating and relieving factors
- associated physical symptoms
- associated emotional symptoms
- associated psychosocial factors (antecedents and consequences): social, occupational, family, legal, financial, housing/neighbourhood
- patient's beliefs about the cause of their symptoms
- past episodes of similar symptoms and management
- brief physical examination of part of body or system relevant to presenting symptom.

2. Broadening the agenda

The family doctor:
- feeds back the results of the physical examination (including no/minor abnormalities)
- feeds back the results of any investigations (including no/minor abnormalities)
- explains the implications of the findings, i.e. lack of serious underlying pathology
- acknowledges the reality of the patient's presenting symptoms despite the absence of a clear physical cause
- explores with the patient the possibility that physical symptoms might be linked to psychosocial factors.

3. Making the link

The family doctor links the physical symptom to an underlying psychosocial explanation using one of the following physiological, temporal or social links:
- Autonomic symptoms in the 'stress' response
- Muscular tension can cause pain
- Depression lowers the pain threshold/causes fatigue
- Symptoms repeatedly occur after life 'stressors'
- Symptoms develop 'here and now' as patient talks about psychosocial situation
- Symptoms can be brought on by doctor, e.g. book on outstretched hands causes muscle tension
- Symptoms are present in family member/friend at times of 'stress'

Reattribution may be a useful therapeutic intervention for family doctors with patients with PMUS because it is compatible with the working practice of many family doctors. An interview by a family doctor using reattribution starts by taking a history of presenting symptoms, their symptom beliefs and related psychosocial factors from the PMUS patient (allowing family doctors to address organic physical, emotional or PMUS health presentations equally easily). It uses patient-centred management (Blankenstein *et al.* 2001a; Little *et al.* 2001; Stewart *et al.* 1995), and is completed within single (Morriss *et al.* 1998) or multiple (Blankenstein *et al.* 2001a) 10–20-minute consultations (Blankenstein *et al.* 2001a; Gask *et al.* 1989; Kaaya *et al.* 1992; Morriss *et al.* 1999). Reattribution does not require previous experience of mental health or specialist communication skills beyond those required for 'patient-led' communication (Blankenstein *et al.* 2001a; Gask *et al.* 1989; Kaaya *et al.* 1992; Morriss *et al.* 1999).

The effectiveness of reattribution for managing PMUS

Three before-and-after studies have demonstrated that around 90% of trainee and established family doctors can learn the skills required for reattribution and deliver them in role-played 10- or 15-minute videotaped interviews with actors playing somatizing patients, according to blinded, independent assessors (Gask *et al.* 1989; Kaaya *et al.* 1992; Morriss *et al.* 1998). These studies show improvements in the following aspects of family doctor-to-patient communication: exploration of social and family factors, exploration of health beliefs, acknowledgement of the reality of symptoms, summary of mood symptoms, summary of life stressors, and improvement in both the number and quality of statements making links between physical symptoms and psychosocial problems or mental disorder.

A Dutch study reported that reattribution and techniques to reduce illness worry were used in 70% of all consultations between family doctors, trained in reattribution and illness worry, and frequently attending patients with somatization (Blankenstein *et al.* 2001b).

There have been three studies reporting outcome. In a case series of 11 somatizing patients, there were significant improvements in self-rated somatization, psychiatric symptoms and psychosocial problems immediately after reattribution and problem-solving treatment with reduced numbers of contacts with primary care in the following three months (Wilkinson *et al.* 1994). Symptoms only improved if problems were successfully addressed; sometimes problems were addressed but symptoms showed limited improvement.

In a before-and-after training study (Morris *et al.* 1998, 1999, 2002) with eight family doctors and 215 patients with SMD, reattribution was associated with: at one month, greater patient satisfaction with the care that they received from the family doctor, and less psychiatric disorder in patients who did not attribute their symptoms to only physical causes; at three months in all patients, less self-rated psychiatric disorder, changes in symptom attributions from physical to non-physical causes, and reduced contacts and costs of healthcare outside the primary-care team; at three months, improved function (physical, social and occupational) in patients without entirely physical health beliefs; at three months, reduced major depression in patients with entirely physical health beliefs. There was no effect of reattribution on family doctor-initiated primary-healthcare contacts, investigations, prescribing (analgesics, sedatives, antidepressants or drugs in total), nor referrals. The reduction in secondary-healthcare contacts after reattribution might have been due to fewer continuing care arrangements with secondary care and fewer patient-initiated contacts with secondary care as patient needs are more frequently met in primary care.

A Dutch randomized controlled trial (Blankenstein *et al.* 2001b) of 17 family doctors and 162 frequently attending patients with somatization (including somatization disorder) showed improvements with reattribution and illness worry training compared to treatment as usual in subjective health, somatization, sick leave and visits to all healthcare providers over 24 months. There was no evidence of misdiagnosis of organic physical illness in these patient outcome studies (Blankenstein *et al.* 2001b; Morriss *et al.* 1999).

However, there remain a number of unanswered questions that call into question the evidence for the effectiveness of reattribution. First, there are major shortcomings in all the studies of reattribution in primary care such as lack of randomization (Morriss *et al.* 1998, 1999, 2002) or adequate allowance for cluster effects in the analysis of the results (Blankenstein *et al.* 2001a). Second, no RCT of reattribution or any other intervention for PMUS or somatization in primary care has used inclusion/exclusion criteria that are compatible with the family doctor's working definition of PMUS (Schilte *et al.* 2000). Unless they do, the external validity and generalizability of the findings are in doubt. Third, only one study has explored the long-term effects of reattribution over 12 and 24 months (Blankenstein *et al.* 2001a). Fourth, no study of reattribution has examined its effects on the patient's quality of life, nor on cost effectiveness from the perspective of society (costs to patients and family as carers or dependents, costs of lost work, provision of benefits and social care as well as direct health costs). Fifth, even after reattribution training, family doctors themselves report that they require help in negotiating further treatment for some patients with PMUS.

Modifications to reattribution to improve its efficacy and feasibility

Modifications have been proposed to reattribution such as asking family doctors to tackle illness worry and use diary records, but family doctors report that these techniques are alien to their usual practice and were used sparingly (Blankenstein *et al.* 2001a). Such modifications might discourage the routine use of reattribution by family doctors, but they may be useful occasionally for family doctors wanting to employ more advanced skills.

In response to recent empirical evidence, and feedback from family doctors who have learnt how to use reattribution, six modifications are proposed:

1. Feeling understood. The patient's beliefs about the nature, time course, severity, consequences and controllability of their symptoms are explored (Clements *et al.* 1997; Peters *et al.* 1998; Salmon *et al.* 1996, 1999; Weinman *et al.* 1996; Woloshynowych *et al.* 1998).
2. The pace of reattribution process is slower in patients with fixed and entrenched symptom beliefs (Blankenstein *et al.* 2001a). The end of the first consultation may end in two ways: (a) it ends with further investigation (feeling understood); (b) the patient is asked to monitor or discuss with family or friend their symptoms in relation to the timing of psychosocial stressors or lifestyle habit (broadening the agenda). The making-the-link explanation is made at a later stage and may also involve further monitoring, discussion with others, or information gathering, before acceptance by the patient is possible.
3. Using symptom beliefs in making the link. Explanations are compatible with existing symptom beliefs held by patients. Agreement is made where possible. For instance, the family doctor and PMUS patient may agree that 'stress' or depression impairs the PMUS patient's ability to control their symptoms. However, the family doctor and PMUS patient might not agree if discussion centred on the original cause of the patient's back pain.
4. Greater range of explanations in making the link. A greater range of lifestyle and physiological explanations are available such as adverse effects of prolonged bed rest or daytime sleep on fatigue and generalized muscle pain (Fulcher *et al.* 1997; Powell *et al.* 2001; Wearden *et al.* 1998).
5. The addition of a fourth stage to the reattribution model, termed 'negotiating further treatment'. The family doctor negotiates further management options with the patient including:
    i. exploring the patient's views about treatment;
    ii. acknowledging patient's worries and concerns;
    iii. promoting problem-solving and coping strategies;

    iv. appropriate use of muscular relaxation and slow breathing exercises for tension pains and other symptomatic relief, including painkillers such as paracetamol and antidepressants (O'Malley *et al.* 1999);

    v. appropriate treatment of depressive, anxiety or substance misuse disorders;

    vi. agreeing specific plans for follow-up.

Further management would normally fall into three types:

    i. no further follow-up or treatment if the patient accepts the family doctor's explanation concerning the absence of pathology, and reconstrues the physical symptoms as a warning sign of problems in their life that they should monitor or manage on their own. The family doctor should only accept this if there are no comorbid depressive, anxiety or substance misuse disorders requiring treatment;

    ii. further follow-up with the same family doctor so that the family doctor and patient can review progress of symptoms and psychosocial problems, and the patient leaves to consider or test the explanation given by the family doctor;

    iii. further active treatment by the family doctor (including strategies to address psychosocial problems and/or treatments for mental disorders such as antidepressant medication for depressive disorder) or other health professionals.

6. The family doctor may need to repeat reattribution on a number of occasions as the PMUS patient presents with different bodily symptoms. Gradually the PMUS patient may reattribute their symptoms to psychosocial or lifestyle factors by themselves (Patel *et al.* 1998).

Practical approaches to dissemination

Effective methods of disseminating reattribution to family doctors need to be devised and tested in RCTs. Reattribution requires the development of new skills and a positive attitude to helping patients with PMUS. These will require dissemination through skills-based training rather than lectures, seminars, workshops or clinical guidelines, which are relatively ineffective for teaching skills and attitude (Davis & Taylor-Vaisey 1997; Davis *et al.* 1995, 1997; Gask & Morriss 1999; Thomson *et al.* 2000). All previous studies of reattribution have involved the training of family doctor volunteers by experts from academic psychiatry or primary care. Such experts will not deliver reattribution training on a large scale or an ongoing basis. Reattribution will have a limited effect on public health unless it involves family doctors who do not normally volunteer for such training.

Many family doctors believe that they should play a major role in managing PMUS patients but are negative about their chances of therapeutic success with these patients (Garcia-Campayo *et al.* 1998; Hartmann 1989; Hartz *et al.* 2000; Mathers & Gask 1995). Such attitudinal shifts can be produced by:

- making the family doctor aware of the problem
- providing evidence that successful and rewarding management is feasible and does not cause harm, e.g. the doctor will miss organic physical health problems
- explaining that most PMUS patients are not expecting to be cured but hope for a sympathetic discussion of their problems with the doctor (Salmon *et al.* 1999)
- exploring practical issues preventing attendance for training or the use of reattribution in the surgery, e.g. patient acceptance or time
- encouraging reflection on these matters (Hartmann 1989).

Attitudinal shifts persuading most family doctors to embark on reattribution training may require academic detailing or educational outreach visits. These are brief face-to-face encounters between an educational outreach worker and the family doctor at their place of work. The success of academic detailing as part of a multifaceted educational programme to promote changes in behaviour of doctors, such as communication with patients and prescribing, has been demonstrated in a number of systematic reviews (Davis & Taylor-Vaisey 1997; Davis *et al.* 1995, 1997; Thomson *et al.* 2000).

Skills-based training involves the modelling of communication behaviours (a specially prepared videotape of reattribution demonstrating the skills of the family doctor is available), rehearsal of the component microskills under supervision during the training session, and employment of reattribution in videotaped or audiotaped consultations with PMUS patients with feedback in the training sessions. The feedback is often best delivered in a group of family doctors with a supervisor, who keeps the group focused on the tasks. Such groups help to build confidence, more positive attitudes towards helping these patients, and provide the opportunity for reflection on their own use of these skills with a peer group of family doctors. A written manual provides background knowledge about PMUS and reminders of how to use reattribution.

In addition to reattribution training family doctors do need simple advice on how to manage and organize care for people with more chronic symptoms. Our advice, summarized from relevant reviews and based around the concept of 'setting limits' (Bass & Benjamin 1993; Goldberg *et al.* 1992; O'Dowd 1988) can be found in Box 36.1.

Studies of medium-term or long-term patient outcome have yet to be performed with multifaceted education interventions involving academic detailing. Nevertheless, the teaching of reattribution using the model seems the most

Box 36.1 Advice for family doctors on the management of patients with chronic MUS.

- *Reassurance that nothing is wrong does not help*. Clear information should be provided about clinical findings, which can then provide a basis for the provision of appropriate reassurance.
- Contrary to what initially may appear to be the case, *the patient does not want simple straightforward symptom relief, but understanding*. Many patients can communicate distress only in the form of somatic symptoms and there may be a history of abuse or maltreatment in childhood. It can take a long time to change the agenda, but this may ultimately be achieved by empathizing with the patient's past experiences of distress and gradually helping them to feel understood.
- What the patient wants is for the doctor to agree that he or she is sick. *Avoid challenging the patient but instead agree that there is a problem*, and show a willingness to help to identify it.
- *Little is gained by a premature explanation that the symptoms are emotional*. Such an explanation must be presented in such a way that the patient does not experience it as a rejection.
- *A positive organic diagnosis will not cure the patient*. The emphasis should be on function not symptoms, with an assessment of how the patient copes and responds.
- *Try and be direct and honest with the patient about areas that you agree on and those that you disagree on*. Be explicit about what you think he or she is capable of doing despite the symptoms and negotiate mutually agreed goals (e.g. how far to walk, carrying out chores, helping family and so on). Spurious organic diagnoses only lead to a subsequent breakdown in trust and less likelihood that the patient will accept an appropriate referral. Never give treatment for disorders that the patient has not got; this only confirms the patient's view that something is wrong.
- *Regular scheduled appointments are required* so that the patient does not have to manifest symptoms in order to seek help. This can, paradoxically, be less time consuming than frequent short visits that are taken up with fruitless reassurance.
- *Clear agenda setting can be helpful in each consultation*. It can be very useful to work out a list of problems with the patient and agree to tackle one or two on each visit.
- *Diagnostic tests should be limited:* some focused examination can be helpful, with reliance more on signs than symptoms.
- *Provide a clear model for the patient:* which demonstrates that it is possible to have both organic pathology, which needs treatment, and emotional problems. It is important to challenge the dualistic model which assumes that illness is either physical or mental but never both, which many patients (and doctors) believe.
- *Involve the patient's family* so that spouse or children are aware of your treatment plan and can be involved in it if they wish to be.
- *Involve colleagues in the primary-care team* in discussion of the management plan so that the practice can present a consistent and agreed approach to management. Such practice meetings can provide essential support in the face of managing a difficult patient.
- *Don't expect a cure*. Damage limitation is a more realistic ultimate goal but it may be a difficult one for the doctor to accept. Peer-group discussion and support can help a doctor to understand their own reactions to such patients and learn how to deal with them.

> **Box 36.2 Plan of service linking to primary care.**
> 1. Family doctor: reattribution, antidepressants, exercise, limit setting.
> 2. Attached professionals in primary care: group cognitive-behaviour therapy (CBT) extended individual reattribution.
> 3. Referral to hospital: specialist liaison psychiatry and/or psychotherapy individual CBT, psychodynamic interpersonal psychotherapy.

likely to produce large-scale public health improvements over a relatively short time scale.

A further challenge is to integrate primary care and secondary mental health care so that supervision, support and advice or sometimes specialist care can be provided to more difficult PMUS patients. A possible model for this is summarized in Box 36.2.

Conclusion

There is a need for simple, effective, evidence-based interventions that family doctors can provide for patients with PMUS who are common, seek out family doctors, and do not return quickly to normal function. Such interventions must be compatible with the normal process, length and philosophy of primary-care consultation, and utilizable by family doctors without too much extra training. Reattribution, modified in the light of feedback from family doctors and empirical findings, is currently a viable candidate for such an intervention. It structures a consultation with a PMUS patient so that all the key features of a recently recommended approach to clinical care to patients with MUS can be achieved (Epstein *et al.* 1999): exploring the patient's life context, finding mutually meaningful language, normalizing the patient's bodily experience of distress, using a chronic disease model attending to functioning and the doctor's need for certainty and efficacy, and appropriate control of access to medical services to prevent iatrogenic harm. However, more evidence is required of its feasibility, generalizability, and clinical and cost effectiveness, before reattribution can be recommended for wide-scale use.

REFERENCES

Allen, L. A., Gara, M. A., Escobar, J. I., *et al.* (2001). Somatization: a debilitating syndrome in primary care. *Psychosomatics*, **42**, 63–7.

American Psychiatric Association. (1994). *Diagnostic and Statistical Manual of Mental Disorders*, 4th edn. Washington DC: American Psychiatric Association.

Barry, C. A., Bradley, C. P., Britten, N., *et al.* (2000). Patients' unvoiced agendas in general practice consultations: qualitative study. *British Medical Journal*, **320**, 1246–50.

Barsky, A. J., Ettner, S. L., Horsky, J., *et al.* (2001). Resource utilization of patients with hypochondriacal health anxiety and somatization. *Medical Care*, **39**, 705–15.

Bass, C. and Benjamin, S. (1993). The management of chronic somatization. *British Journal of Psychiatry*, **162**, 472–80.

Blankenstein, A. H., van der Horst, H. E., Schilte, A. F., *et al.* (2001a). Development and feasibility of a modified reattribution model for somatising patients applied by their own general practitioners. In *Somatising Patients in General Practice: Reattribution, a Promising Approach*, ed. A. H. Blankenstein. Ph.D. Thesis. Amsterdam: Vrije University, pp. 33–48.

Blankenstein, A. H., van der Horst, H. E., Schilte, A. F., *et al.* (2001b). Effectiveness of reattribution for somatisation in general practice, a randomized controlled trial. In *Somatising Patients in General Practice: Reattribution, a Promising Approach*, ed. A. H. Blankenstein. Ph.D. Thesis. Amsterdam: Vrije University, pp. 49–65.

Bouman, T. K. and Visser, S. (1998). Cognitive and behavioural treatment of hypochondriasis. *Psychotherapy and Psychosomatics*, **67**, 214–21.

Bruster, S., Jarman, B., Bosanquet, N., *et al.* (1994). National survey of hospital patients. *British Medical Journal*, **309**, 1542–9.

Cathebras, P., Jacquin, L., le Gal, M., *et al.* (1995). Correlates of somatic causal attributions in primary care patients with fatigue. *Psychotherapy and Psychosomatics*, **63**, 174–80.

Cherkin, D. C., Eisenberg, D., Sherman, K. J., *et al.* (2001). Randomized trial comparing traditional Chinese medical acupuncture, therapeutic massage, and self-care education for chronic low back pain. *Archives of Internal Medicine*, **161**, 1081–8.

Clark, D. M., Salkovskis, P. M., Hackmann, A., *et al.* (1998). Two psychological treatments for hypochondriasis. A randomized controlled trial. *British Journal of Psychiatry*, **173**, 218–25.

Clements, A., Sharpe, M., Simkin, S., *et al.* (1997). Chronic fatigue syndrome: a qualitative investigation of patients' beliefs about the illness. *Journal of Psychosmatic Research*, **42**, 615–24.

Cope, H., David, A., Pelosi, A., *et al.* (1994). Predictors of chronic 'post-viral' fatigue. *Lancet*, **344**, 864–8.

Davis, D. A. and Taylor-Vaisey, A. (1997). Translating guidelines into practice. A systematic review of theoretic concepts, practical experience and research evidence in the adoption of clinical practice guidelines. *Canadian Medical Association Journal*, **157**, 408–16.

Davis, D. A., Thomson, M. A., Oxman, A. D., *et al.* (1995). Changing physician performance. A systematic review of the effect of continuing medical education strategies. *Journal of the American Medical Association*, **274**, 700–5.

Di Blasi, Z., Harkness, E., Ernst, E., *et al.* (2001). Influence of context effects on health outcomes: a systematic review. *Lancet*, **357**, 757–62.

Donovan, J. L. and Blake, D. R. (2000). Qualitative study of interpretation of reassurance among patients attending rheumatology clinics: 'just a touch of arthritis, doctor?' *British Medical Journal*, **320**, 541–4.

Downes-Grainger, E., Morriss, R., Gask, L., *et al.* (1998). Clinical factors associated with short-term changes in outcome of patients with somatized mental disorder in primary care. *Psychological Medicine*, **28**, 703–11.

Epstein, R. M., Quill, T. E. and McWhinney, I. R. (1999). Somatization reconsidered: incorporating the patient's experience of illness. *Archives of Internal Medicine*, **159**, 215–22.

Faravelli, C., Salvatori, S., Galassi, F., *et al.* (1997). Epidemiology of somatoform disorder: a community survey in Florence. *Social Psychiatry and Psychatric Epidemiology*, **32**, 24–9.

Fava, G. A., Grandi, S., Rafanelli, C., *et al.* (2000). Explanatory therapy in hypochondriasis. *Journal of Clinical Psychiatry*, **61**, 317–22.

Fink, P., Sorensen, L., Engberg, M., *et al.* (1999). Somatization in primary care. Prevalence, health care utilization, and general practitioner recognition. *Psychosomatics*, **40**, 330–8.

Fulcher, K. Y. and White, P. D. (1997). Randomised controlled trial of graded exercise in patients with the chronic fatigue syndrome. *British Medical Journal*, **314**, 1647–52.

Garcia-Campayo, J., Larrubia, J., Lobo, A., *et al.* (1997). Attribution in somatizers: stability and relationship to outcome at 1-year follow-up. Grupo Morbilidad Psiquica y Psicosomatica de Zaragoza (GMPPZ). *Acta Psychiatrica Scandinavica*, **95**, 433–8.

Garcia-Campayo, J., Sanz-Carrillo, C., Yoldi-Elcid, A., *et al.* (1998). Management of somatisers in primary care: are family doctors motivated? *Australia and New Zealand Journal of Psychiatry*, **32**, 528–33.

Gask, L. and Morriss, R. (1999). Training general practitioners in mental health skills. *Epidemiologia e Psichiatria Sociale*, **8**, 79–84.

Gask, L., Goldberg, D., Porter, R., *et al.* (1989). The treatment of somatization: evaluation of a teaching package with general practice trainees. *Journal of Psychosomatic Research*, **33**, 697–703.

Goldberg, D., Gask, L. and O'Dowd, T. (1989). The treatment of somatisation; teaching techniques of reattribution. *Journal of Psychosomatic Research*, **33**, 689–95.

Goldberg, R. J., Novack, D. H. and Gask, L. (1992). The recognition and management of somatisation: what is needed in primary care training. *Psychosomatics*, **33**, 55–61.

Gureje, O. and Obikoya, B. (1992). Somatization in primary care: pattern and correlates in a clinic in Nigeria. *Acta Psychiatrica Scandinavica*, **86**, 223–7.

Gureje, O. and Simon, G. E. (1999). The natural history of somatization in primary care. *Psychological Medicine*, **29**, 669–76.

Han, J. N., Stegen, K., De Valck, C., *et al.* (1996). Influence of breathing therapy on complaints, anxiety and breathing pattern in patients with hyperventilation syndrome and anxiety disorders. *Journal of Psychosomatic Research*, **41**, 481–93.

Hardy, P. (1995). Epidemiology of somatoform disorders in the general French population. *Encephale*, **21**, 191–9.

Hartmann, P. M. (1989). A pilot study of a modified Balint group using cognitive approaches to physician attitudes about somatoform disorder patients. *International Journal of Psychosomatics*, **36**, 86–9.

Hartz, A. J., Noyes, R., Bentler, S. E., *et al.* (2000). Unexplained symptoms in primary care: perspectives of doctors and patients. *General Hospital Psychiatry*, **22**, 144–52.

Hellman, C. J. C., Budd, M., Borysenko, J., *et al.* (1990). A study of effectiveness of two group behavioral medicine interventions for patients with psychosomatic complaints. *Behavioral Medicine*, **16**, 165–73.

Hunt, L. M., Jordan, B. and Irwin, S. (1989). Views of what's wrong: diagnosis and patients' concepts of illness. *Social Science and Medicine*, **28**, 945–56.

Jackson, J. L., Chamberlin, J. and Kroenke, K. (2001). Predictors of patient satisfaction. *Social Science and Medicine*, **52**, 609–20.

Jorgensen, C. K., Fink, P. and Olesen, F. (2000). Psychological distress and somatisation as prognostic factors in patients with musculoskeletal illness in general practice. *British Journal of General Practice*, **50**, 537–41.

Jyvasjarvi, S., Keinanen-Kiukaanniemi, S., Vaisanen, E., *et al.* (1998). Frequent attenders in a Finnish health centre: morbidity and reasons for encounter. *Scandinavian Journal of Primary Health Care*, **16**, 141–8.

Jyvasjarvi, S., Joukamaa, M., Vaisanen, E., *et al.* (1999). Alexithymia, hypochondriacal beliefs, and psychological distress among frequent attenders in primary health care. *Comprehensive Psychiatry*, **40**, 292–8.

Jyvasjarvi, S., Joukamaa, M., Vaisanen, E., *et al.* (2001). Somatizing frequent attenders in primary health care. *Journal of Psychosomatic Research*, **50**, 185–92.

Kaaya, S., Goldberg, D. and Gask, L. (1992). Management of somatic presentations of psychiatric illness in general medical settings: evaluation of a new training course for general practitioners. *Medical Education*, **26**, 138–44.

Katon, W., Von Korff, M., Lin, E., *et al.* (1992). A randomized trial of psychiatric consultation with distressed high utilisers. *General Hospital Psychiatry*, **14**, 86–98.

Kerwick, S., Jones, R., Mann, A., *et al.* (1997). Mental health care training priorities in general practice. *British Journal of General Practice*, **47**, 225–7.

Kirmayer, L. J. and Robbins, J. M. (1996). Patients who somatize in primary care: a longitudinal study of cognitive and social characteristics. *Psychological Medicine*, **26**, 937–51.

Kisely, S., Goldberg, D. and Simon, G. (1997). A comparison between somatic symptoms with and without clear organic cause: results of an international study. *Psychological Medicine*, **27**, 1011–19.

Kroenke, K. and Spitzer, R. L. (1998). Gender differences in the reporting of physical and somatoform symptoms. *Psychosomatic Medicine*, **60**, 150–5.

Kroenke, K. and Swindle, R. (2000). Cognitive-behavioral therapy for somatization and symptom syndromes: a critical review of controlled clinical trials. *Psychotherapy and Psychosomatics*, **69**, 205–15.

Kroenke, K., Spitzer, R. L., deGruy, F. V., 3rd, *et al.* (1997). Multisomatoform disorder; an alternative to undifferentiated somatoform disorder for the somatizing patient in primary care. *Archives of General Psychiatry*, **54**, 352–8.

Levenstein, J. H., McCracken, E. C., McWhinney, I. R., *et al.* (1986). The patient-centered clinical method. 1. A model for the doctor-patient interaction in family medicine. *Family Practice*, **3**, 24–30.

Lidbeck, J. (1997). Group therapy for somatization disorders in general practice: effectiveness of a short cognitive-behavioural treatment model. *Acta Psychiatrica Scandinavica*, **96**, 14–24.

Lipowski, Z. J. (1988). Somatization: the concept and its clinical application. *American Journal of Psychiatry*, **145**, 1358–68.

Little, P., Everitt, H., Williamson, I., *et al.* (2001). Preferences of patients for patient-centred approach to consultation in primary care: observational study. *British Medical Journal*, **322**, 468–72.

Lucock, M. P., Morley, C., White, C., *et al.* (1997). Responses of consecutive patients to reassurance after gastroscopy: results of self-administered questionnaire study. *British Medical Journal*, **315**, 572–5.

Mannion, A. F., Muntener, M., Taimela, S., *et al.* (2001). Comparison of three active therapies for chronic low back pain: results of a randomised clinical trial with one year follow-up. *Rheumatology*, **40**, 772–8.

Mathers, N. and Gask, L. (1995). Surviving the 'heartsink' experience. *Family Practice*, **12**, 176–83.

McDonald, I. G., Daly, J., Jelinek, V. M., *et al.* (1996). Opening Pandora's box; the unpredictability of reassurance by a normal test result. *British Medical Journal*, **313**, 329–32.

McGrady, A., Lynch, D., Nagel, R., *et al.* (1999). Application of the high risk model of threat perception to a primary care population. *Journal of Nervous and Mental Disease*, **187**, 369–75.

Moore, J. E., von Korff, M., Cherkin, D., *et al.* (2000). A randomized controlled trial of a cognitive-behavioral program for enhancing back pain self care in a primary care setting. *Pain*, **88**, 145–53.

Morley, S., Eccleston, C. and Williams, A. (1999). Systematic review and meta-analysis of randomized controlled trials of cognitive behavior therapy for chronic pain in adults, excluding headache. *Pain*, **80**, 1–13.

Morriss, R. K. (1992). Interviewing skills and the detection of psychiatric problems. *International Review of Psychiatry*, **4**, 287–92.

Morriss, R. and Gask, L. (2002). The effects of reattribution training for patients with somatized mental disorder on outcomes under the direct control of the family doctor. *Psychosomatics*, **43**, 394–9.

Morriss, R., Gask, L., Ronalds, C., *et al.* (1998). Cost-effectiveness of a new treatment for somatized mental disorder taught to GPs. *Family Practice*, **15**, 119–25.

Morriss, R. K., Gask, L., Ronalds, C., *et al.* (1999). Clinical and patient satisfaction outcomes of a new treatment for somatized mental disorder taught to general practitioners. *British Journal of General Practice*, **49**, 263–7.

O'Dowd, T. (1988). Five years of heartsink patients in general practice. *British Medical Journal*, **297**, 528–30.

O'Malley, P. G., Jackson, J. L., Santoro, J., *et al.* (1999). Antidepressant therapy for unexplained symptoms and symptom syndromes. *Journal of Family Practice*, **48**, 980–90.

Patel, V., Pereira, J. and Mann, A. H. (1998). Somatic and psychological models of common mental disorder in primary care in India. *Psychological Medicine*, **28**, 135–43.

Peters, S., Stanley, I., Rose, M., *et al.* (1998). Patients with medically unexplained symptoms: sources of patients' authority and implications for demands on medical care. *Social Science and Medicine*, **46**, 559–65.

Petrie, K., Weinman, J., Sharpe, N., *et al.* (1996). Role of patients' views of their illness in predicting return to work and functioning after myocardial infarction: longitudinal study. *British Medical Journal*, **30**, 747–57.

Peveler, R., Kilkenny, L. and Kinmonth, A. L. (1997). Medically unexplained symptoms in primary care: a comparison of self-report screening questionnaires and clinical opinion. *Journal of Psychosomatic Research*, **42**, 245–52.

Piccinelli, M. and Simon, G. (1997). Gender and cross-cultural differences in somatic symptoms associated with emotional distress. An international study in primary care. *Psychological Medicine*, **27**, 433–44.

Piccinelli, M., Rucci, P., Ustun, B., *et al.* (1999). Typologies of anxiety, depression and somatization symptoms among primary care attenders with no formal mental disorder. *Psychological Medicine*, **29**, 677–88.

Powell, P., Bentall, R. P., Nye, F. J., *et al.* (2001). Randomized controlled trial of patient education to encourage graded exercise in chronic fatigue syndrome. *British Medical Journal*, **322**, 387–90.

Ridsdale, L., Evans, A., Jerrett, W., *et al.* (1994). Patients who consult with tiredness: frequency of consultation, perceived causes of tiredness and its association with psychological distress. *British Journal of General Practice*, **44**, 413–16.

Rossy, L. A., Buckelew, S. P., Dorr, N., *et al.* (1999). A meta-analysis of fibromyalgia treatment interventions. *Annals of Behavioural Medicine*, **21**, 180–91.

Rost, K., Kashner, T. M. and Smith, G. R. (1994). Effectiveness of psychiatric intervention with somatization disorder patients: improved outcomes at reduced costs. *General Hospital Psychiatry*, **16**, 381–7.

Salmon, P., Wolonyshynowych, M. and Valori, R. (1996). The measurement of beliefs about physical symptoms in English general practice patients. *Social Science and Medicine*, **42**, 1561–7.

Salmon, P., Peters, S. and Stanley, I. (1999). Patients' perceptions of medical explanations for somatisation disorders: qualitative analysis. *British Medical Journal*, **318**, 372–6.

Scharloo, M., Kaptein, A. A., Weinman, J., *et al.* (2000). Patients' illness perceptions and coping as predictors of functional status in psoriasis: a 1-year follow-up. *British Journal of Dermatology*, **142**, 899–907.

Schilte, A. F., Portegijs, P. J. M., Blankenstein, A. H., *et al.* (2000). Somatisation in primary care: clinical judgement and standardised measurement compared. *Social Psychiatry and Psychiatric Epidemiology*, **35**, 276–82.

Schilte, A. F., Blankenstein, A. H., Portegijs, P. J. M., *et al.* (2001a). Predictors of prognosis in long-term somatisation in primary care, the role of stress. In *Somatising Patients in General Practice: Reattribution, a Promising, Approach*, ed. A. H. Blankenstein. Ph.D. Thesis. Amsterdam: Vrije University, pp. 67–78.

Schilte, A. F., Portegijs, P. J. M., Blankenstein, A. H., *et al.* (2001b). Is disclosure of emotionally important events effective in somatisation in primary care? A randomized controlled trial. *British Medical Journal*, **323**, 86−9.

Simon, G., von Korff, M., Piccinelli, M., *et al.* (1999). An international study of the relation between somatic symptoms and depression. *New England Journal of Medicine*, **341**, 1329−35.

Simon, G. E., Gureje, O. and Fullerton, C. (2001). Course of hypochondriasis in an international primary care study. *General Hospital Psychiatry*, **23**, 51−5.

Smith, G. R., Monson, R. A. and Ray, D. C. (1986). Psychiatric consultation in somatization disorder: a randomized controlled study. *New England Journal of Medicine*, **314**, 1407−13.

Smith, G. R., Rost, K. and Kashner, T. M. (1995). A trial of the effect of a standardized psychiatric consultation on health outcomes and costs in somatizing patients. *Archives of General Psychiatry*, **52**, 238−43.

Speckens, A. E. M., Spinhoven, P., van Hemert, A. M., *et al.* (2000). The Reassurance Questionnaire (RQ): psychometric properties of a self-report questionnaire to assess reassurability. *Psychological Medicine*, **30**, 841−7.

Stewart, M., Brown, J. B., Weston, W. W., *et al.* (1995). *Patient-centered Medicine Transforming the Clinical Method*. Thousand Oaks: Sage Publications.

Sumithipala, A., Hewege, S., Hanwella, R., *et al.* (2000). Randomized controlled trial of cognitive behavior therapy for repeated medically unexplained complaints: a feasibility study in Sri Lanka. *Psychological Medicine*, **20**, 747−57.

Thomson O'Brien, M. A., Oxman, A. D., Davis, D. A., *et al.* (2000). Educational outreach visits: effects on professional practice and health care outcomes. *Cochrane Database Systematic Review*, **2**, CD000409.

Van Tulder, M. W., Malmivaara, A., Esmail, R., *et al.* (2001). Exercise therapy for low back pain. *Cochrane Database Systematic Review*, 4.

Walker, E. A., Unutzer, J. and Katon, W. J. (1998). Understanding and caring for the distressed patient with multiple medically unexplained symptoms. *Journal of the American Board of Family Practice*, **11**, 347−56.

Wearden, A. J., Morriss, R. K., Mullis, R., *et al.* (1998). Randomised, double-blind, placebo-controlled treatment trial of fluoxetine and graded exercise for chronic fatigue syndrome. *British Journal of Psychiatry*, **172**, 485−90.

Weich, S., Lewis, G., Donmall, R., *et al.* (1995). Somatic presentation of psychiatric morbidity in general practice. *British Journal of General Practice*, **45**, 143−7.

Weinman, J., Petrie, K. J., Moss-Morris, R., *et al.* (1996). The Illness Perception Questionnaire: a new method for assessing the cognitive representation of illness. *Psychological Health*, **11**, 457−63.

Wilkinson, P. and Mynors-Wallis, L. (1994). Problem-solving therapy in the treatment of unexplained physical symptoms in primary care; a preliminary study. *Journal of Psychosomatic Research*, **38**, 591−8.

Woloshynowych, M., Valori, R. and Salmon, P. (1998). General practice patients' beliefs about their symptoms. *British Journal of General Practice*, **48**, 885−9.

37

Frequent attenders in primary care

Navneet Kapur

Introduction

Why do people consult their doctors? Some individuals never consult medical practitioners while others consult unusually frequently. A number of factors contribute to patients' help-seeking behaviour (Campbell & Roland 1996; Gill & Sharpe 1999). Organizational factors such as distance from the surgery, the appointment system and access to other healthcare facilities may influence the decision to seek care. Doctor-related factors are also likely to be important. For instance, there is evidence that some doctors appear to attract a disproportionate number of frequently attending patients, and it is possible that some doctors actively encourage frequent attendance (Neal *et al.* 2000a). This chapter reviews the patient factors associated with frequent attendance in primary care and suggests strategies for managing patients who attend unusually frequently.

Concepts and definitions

There are two conceptual issues which have important implications for the interpretation of research findings.

The first concerns the concept of 'a consultation'. There is no standard definition. Different approaches include defining consultations as entries in primary care notes or computerized records, contact with any member of the primary-care team, or face-to-face consultation with a general practitioner. Some studies have included only patient-initiated consultations. Others have excluded attendance for 'routine' reasons such as contraception and pregnancy. Home visits have been counted as consultations in some studies but not in others.

The second issue is more complex and concerns the definition of 'frequent consultation'. Three main approaches have been adopted in the literature.

Handbook of Liaison Psychiatry, ed. Geoffrey Lloyd and Elspeth Guthrie. Published by Cambridge University Press. © Cambridge University Press 2007.

The first involves selecting an arbitrary cutoff point for number of consultations (usually 8–12 consultations per year). Patients consulting more frequently than this are automatically defined as frequent consulters. The second approach is a distributional one, with the top quartile, decile, or 3% of patients in terms of consultation frequency defined as frequent consulters. The third and perhaps most sophisticated definition takes into account the higher base rates for consultation among women and in certain age groups. Frequent consulters are defined on the basis of age and sex norms for consultation rates in the study practice. For example one study defined 'high users' as those visiting the health centre more than the mean plus one standard deviation for that age and sex group (Bellon *et al.* 1999).

Prevalence of frequent attendance and association with sociodemographic factors

What is the prevalence of frequent attendance in primary care and what sociodemographic factors are associated with it? Table 37.1 presents findings from selected studies carried out in a variety of settings. The prevalence of frequent attendance varies across settings and with the different definitions of frequent attendance that are used. However, one remarkably consistent finding is that a relatively small proportion of patients account for a relatively large proportion of workload. This is expressed graphically in Figure 37.1. For example, 3% of patients account for 15% of the workload, 5% of patients account for 20% of the workload, and 15% of patients account for as much as half the workload. This suggests that a definition of frequent attendance based on a distributional cutoff (for example, patients who are in the top decile of consultation frequency) might have most validity across settings.

There are also fairly consistent findings when we compare data from studies which have examined the sociodemographic characteristics of frequent attenders. Frequent attenders are more likely to be female, older, less likely to be married, and less likely to be in paid employment. Frequent attendance is also associated with relative socioeconomic deprivation.

Frequent attendance and psychiatric morbidity

A number of studies have examined the association between frequent attendance and psychiatric morbidity. Table 37.2 presents findings from selected studies. Some used case notes to assess psychiatric disorder, others used self-report questionnaires, and a small number used standardized psychiatric interviews.

Table 37.1. Prevalence and demographic characteristics of frequent attenders in studies using different definitions of frequent attendance.

Study and setting	Subjects	Consultation	Frequent consultation	No. of frequent attenders	Prevalence (%)	% of workload	Demographic characteristics	Cases	Controls
Browne et al. (1982), Ontario, Canada	All patients enrolled in a prepaid practice	Contacts with primary-care physicians, nurse practitioners and a family therapist	≥9 visits in one year	200	4.5	21	*Mean age*	—	—
							% female	22	15
							% single	22	15
							% working	46	58.5
Ward et al. (1994). Three practices (urban, rural, mixed) in Western Australia	All patients	Surgery and home visits only	≥7 visits during the first six months of the study	562	7.8	—	*Mean age*	—	—
							% age > 45	60	25
							% female	66	58
Andersson et al. (1995), Umea, Sweden	All patients	All contacts excluding child healthcare and antenatal consultations and out-of-hours visits	≥5 times during 1991	179	1.7	15	*Mean age*	—	—
							% age 22–64	64	—
							% female	62	—
							% females divorced	25	9
							% moved house	16	3
Heywood et al. (1998), Leeds, England	Adults aged 20–64	Face-to-face contacts including home visits and out-of-hours contact	≥12 visits in previous year	214	3.1	15.4	*Mean age*	44.5	40.9
							% female	85.6	51.7
							% married	59.8	77.5
							% social class 1/2	62	78

Table 37.1. (*cont.*) Prevalence and demographic characteristics of frequent attenders in studies using different definitions of frequent attendance.

Study and setting	Subjects	Consultation	Frequent consultation	No. of frequent attenders	Prevalence (%)	% of workload	Demographic characteristics	Cases	Controls
Neal *et al.* (1998). Four practices in Leeds, England	All patients registered 1991–95	Face-to-face contacts including home visits and out-of-hours contact	Top 3% consulters (1991–95)	1369	3	15.0	*% living alone*	25	14.7
							Median age	56.6	40.8
							% female	72.5	52
Baez *et al.* (1998). Nine practices in the Basque Country, Spain	Adults (18–80)	Patient-initiated only, i.e. consultations in which the doctor considered that at least one of the reasons for encounter was not generated by the physician.	Upper decile of consultation frequency for each physician	102	9.5	27.5	*Mean age*	–	–
							% age >45 years	70.6	30
							% female	64.7	52
							% widow/divorced	15.7	3
							% unemployed	21.6	42
McFarland *et al.* (1985). West USA	All enrollees of a prepaid practice 1967–1973	Doctor office visits (pregnancy-related contacts excluded)	Upper quartile of consultation frequency for age- and sex-matched group, over five or more years during study period	185	13	31	*Mean age*	50.0	50.0
							% female	44	57
							Utilization 'unrelated to marital, status, occupation and social class'		

Study	Population	Definition			
Bellon et al. (1999). Granada, Spain	Adults (>14) who had consulted at least once between 1985 and 1991	—	>mean +one standard deviation for age- and sex-matched group	285	14	—
			Mean age	—	—
			% female	—	—
			% widow/sep.	26.7	15.2
			% social class 1/2/3	22	19
			% unemployed	78.4	61.4
Dowrick et al. (2000). Practices in Liverpool, England and Granada, Spain	Adults (>16)	Patient- and doctor-initiated contacts, including telephone contacts and home visits (antenatal contacts excluded)	Annual rate of consultation twice as high as the age- and sex-related mean	127	—	—
			Mean age	46.1	45.1
			% female	73	50
			% widow/divorced	18	10
			% social class V	22	9

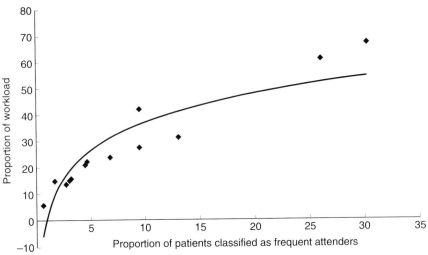

Figure 37.1. Comparing the proportion of frequent attenders with the proportion of the workload they generate across studies. Each data point represents one study ($n = 21$).

There seems to be a strong association between frequent attendance and psychiatric disorder, although studies have been largely cross-sectional in design. Using routinely collected case-note data has generally led to lower estimates for the prevalence of psychiatric disorder than using self-report or interview measures. The latter indicate clinically significant psychological distress in approximately half of frequent attenders and a quarter of normally attending controls. The most common psychiatric disorders in frequent attenders are episodes of minor depression or anxiety. When such disorders are recognized by the doctor, this may lead to an increase in subsequent consultation but it is possible that this association is due to general practitioners being more likely to identify disorders of the greatest severity (Ronalds et al. 2002). It may be that the psychiatric disorder in frequent attenders is relatively difficult to treat, with one study suggesting that a quarter of frequent attenders had been tried on three or more antidepressants without success (Mehl-Madrona 1998). The mean number of depressed days was 119 for frequent attenders in one study (Robinson & Granfield 1986). Those patients with longer-lasting psychiatric disorder may attend the doctor more frequently because they continue to be troubled by their symptoms.

Studies in this area have a number of methodological shortcomings including non-response bias and selection bias (for example, in some studies subjects were only eligible for inclusion if they had consulted once, thus under-representing very infrequent attenders). By contrast, other studies selected very infrequently consulting controls, which may lead to an overestimate of the difference

Table 37.2. Studies examining the association between frequent attendance and psychiatric disorder using case notes, self-report measures and standardized psychiatric interviews.

Study and setting	Subjects	n	Frequent consultation	Source of data	Outcome measures	Psychiatric disorder		
							Cases	Controls
Svab et al. (1993). Rural Slovenia	All registered patients	508	Upper quartile of consultation frequency for age group	Case notes	% Psychiatric complaints		5.3	1.5
					% Psychiatric diagnoses (ICD-9 criteria)		5.3	1.6
Mehl-Madrona (1998). Rural New England, USA	All registered patients	461	211 most frequent users	Case records	% Adjustment reaction		55	7
					% Anxiety state		35	10
					% Depressive disorder		35	4
					Half of frequent users were taking psychotropics, a quarter were worse despite medication, a quarter had tried three or more antidepressants			
Robinson & Granfield (1986). Single practice in South Wales	Adults aged 18–59	72	≥20 consultations in the previous year	Monthly interviews	Self-report of psychiatric symptoms			
					% Psychotropic medication		80	0
					Mean n days low mood		119	44

Table 37.2. (*cont.*) Studies examining the association between frequent attendance and psychiatric disorder using case notes, self-report measures and standardized psychiatric interviews.

Study and setting	Subjects	n	Frequent consultation	Source of data	Outcome measures	Psychiatric disorder	
						Cases	Controls
Heywood *et al.* (1998). Leeds, England	adults 20–64	202	≥12 visits in previous year	Case notes, self report questionnaire	Psychiatric disorder (notes)	*% Psychiatric disorder*	9	2
					Psychotropic medication	*% Psychotropic medication*	48	6
					GHQ 28	*% General Health Questionnaire (GHQ) cases*	52	29
					Nottingham Health Profile (NHP)	*% NHP cases*	35	10
Bellon *et al.* (1999). Granada, Spain	Adults (>14 years) who had consulted at least once between 1985 and 1991	656	>mean +one standard deviation for age- and sex-matched group	Patient report self-report questionnaire	Psychiatric problems	*% Psychiatric disorder (patient)*	57	29
					GHQ 28	*% GHQ cases*	85	30
						Mean GHQ score	11.9	5.4
Karlsson *et al.* (1994). Two practices in Turku, Finland	Adults (18–64)	562	≥11 consultations in previous year	Patient report, GP report, self-report questionnaire, psychiatric interview	Psychiatric symptom	*% Psychiatric symptoms*	25	14
					Psychiatric disorder (GP)	*% Psychiatric problems (GP)*	26	15
					Symptom Checklist (SCL) 25	*SCL 25 cases*	44	21.5

Reference	Sample	N	Definition of frequent attendance	Assessment	Instrument	Findings
Baez et al. (1998). Nine practices in the Basque Country, Spain	Adults (18–80)	202	Upper decile of consultation frequency for each physician	Psychiatric interview	PSE 9; Schedule for Clinical Assessment in Psychiatry-Present State Examination (SCAN–PSE) 10	% PSE 9 cases 54 20 Most common diagnoses among frequent attenders: anxiety state, neurotic depression; % SCAN cases 51 28 Most common diagnoses among frequent attenders: mood disorders (ICD-10 F3), and neurotic disorders (ICD-10 F4)
Ronalds et al. (2002). Practice in Manchester, UK	Adults (>16) with DSM-III psychiatric disorder	148	≥7 consultations in the following six months	Psychiatric interview, self-report measures	Psychiatric Assessment Schedule (PAS) Hamilton Depression Scale (HDS) Clinical Anxiety Scale	One-third of the sample were frequent attenders. Positive correlation between consultation rate and: HDS ($r = 0.16$), and Clinical Anxiety Scale ($r = 0.3$) Recognition of disorder by the general practitioner was associated with higher subsequent consultation rate (six-month consultation rate: 6 vs. 4)

between cases and controls. Very few studies have used standardized psychiatric interviews.

Most studies indicate that at least half of frequent attenders do not have psychiatric disorder. Equally, some studies show that not all subjects who have psychiatric disorder are frequent attenders. Although psychiatric disorder is undoubtedly associated with attendance in general practice it is likely that other factors are important in determining consultation behaviour, for example physical disorder and other psychosocial variables.

The association between frequent attendance and physical disorder

Studies that have examined the association between frequent attendance and physical disorder have used case-note data, self-report measures or physiological measures. Two studies in particular warrant further discussion.

In Robinson and Granfield's study (1986) of 35 frequent attenders and 37 controls in Wales, the subjects were interviewed monthly. Frequent attenders reported that over a 12-month period they were symptom-free just 7% of the time and had four or more symptoms for over 30% of the time. The corresponding figures for infrequent attenders were 35% and 0%. Frequent attenders were particularly likely to report symptoms of catarrh, headache, nausea and heartburn. Frequent attenders were taking over-the-counter medication for 92% of the time, and 40% of the time they were taking three or more drugs. The infrequent attenders were taking medication 20% of the time and no patients took three or more over-the-counter medications over the study period. For frequent consulters 381/643 (59%) of illness episodes led to drug treatment compared with just 75/411 (18%) of illness episodes for infrequent attenders. Although this study provides a uniquely detailed insight into the symptoms and treatment habits of frequent attenders over a 12-month period the results should be interpreted cautiously. The number of subjects was comparatively small and the authors did not state their response rate. The selection of infrequent consulters as controls will have exaggerated any between-group differences.

In Morris and colleagues' three-year follow-up study of middle-aged men in the UK (Morris *et al.* 1992), symptoms of angina, bronchitis, breathlessness and wheeze were assessed using standardized questions. The presence of ischaemic heart disease was determined on the basis of an electrocardiogram, lung function was assessed by measuring the forced expiratory volume, and blood pressure and cholesterol levels were also measured. The subjects were also asked about their smoking and drinking habits and the diagnosis their doctor had given them. The body mass index of all subjects was also calculated. Of the 306 frequent consulters 50% had at least one of the listed symptoms compared with

27% of average consulters and 23% of non-consulters. Of frequent consulters 14% had evidence of ischaemic heart disease compared with 6% of men in the other groups. Of frequent users 12% had poor lung function (compared with 9–10% of others) and 45% had high blood pressure (compared to 23–24% of men in the other groups). The prevalence of high cholesterol levels ranged from 13% in frequent consulters to 9% in average consulters to 6% in non-consulters. Of the frequent attenders 47% were current smokers, 15% were heavy drinkers; 29% of frequent consulters recalled a diagnosis of high blood pressure and 11% a diagnosis of angina, a much higher proportion than in the other groups. Of frequent attenders 12% were obese compared to 8–9% of average or non-consulters. This study confirms the importance of physical factors in determining consultation patterns, and is the only study to date to have used physiological measures.

Research suggests that frequent attenders report a greater number of physical symptoms than controls. Cardiovascular, musculoskeletal and digestive complaints may be particularly common (Heywood *et al.* 1998; Ward *et al.* 1994). Frequent attenders are significantly affected by their symptoms with up to one-fifth reporting chronic disability. Frequent attenders receive greater amounts of medication than controls. Studies suggest that anything up to 70% of frequent attenders have evidence of chronic physical disorder (Heywood *et al.* 1998) and physiological measures confirm poor cardiovascular and respiratory function. Frequent attenders may have a higher prevalence of harmful health behaviours and higher mortality rate than normal attenders (Nighswander 1984).

Studies examining the association between frequent attendance and physical disorder have a number of methodological difficulties. The distinction between self-reported and observed physical problems is often unclear. There are very few data regarding the proportion of symptoms that are due to organic disease and the proportion that are medically unexplained. Studies are subject to non-response bias and the selection of cases and controls from the extremes of consultation frequency may exaggerate between-group differences.

The association between frequent attendance and psychosocial factors

A number of studies have examined the association between frequent attendance and psychosocial factors other than psychiatric morbidity.

Studies suggest that frequent attenders have poorer perceived health and greater concerns about their health. For example, in McFarland's large US study (McFarland *et al.* 1985) a Household Interview Survey was used and included measures of health concerns and an item regarding the patient's perceived health.

The mean health concern scores were 4.1 for consistently high users, 3.8 for medium users and 3.2 for consistently low users ($p = 0.003$, one-way analysis of variance), suggesting that the frequent users were more concerned about their health. Similarly the proportion of patients perceiving their health as fair or poor ranged from 32.9% for frequent users to 9.1% for low users. Dowrick and colleagues (Dowrick *et al.* 2000) asked patients to rate their own health on a five-point scale. Only 40/127 frequent attenders (31%) reported their health as good or excellent compared with 136/175 controls (78%). In a study carried out at two practices in Dublin, Ireland (Conroy *et al.* 1999) there was a strong association between health anxiety (concerns and anxieties centred around the possibility of illness) and consultation rate.

Frequent attenders may be more likely to interpret common bodily sensations as abnormal. Sensky and colleagues (Sensky *et al.* 1996) studied the causal attributions of 14 frequent attenders and 14 controls at a large general practice in West London. Participants were presented with six statements from the Symptom Interpretation Questionnaire and asked to rate on 7-point Likert scales how worried they were about a symptom, how often they had experienced it in the past, and how likely they were to experience it in the future. They were then given a minute to generate as many reasons as they could why each symptom might happen to them. These attributions were classified by the investigators as normalizing (due to external or environmental factors), somatic (due to physical factors), or psychological. In the second part of the study the patients were presented with six different symptoms from the Symptom Interpretation Questionnaire together with a somatic explanation (e.g. 'if I had a hard time catching my breath I would probably think that this is because my lungs were congested because of irritation, infection or heart trouble'). They were then given one minute to think of as many reasons as they could why the given explanation might be true ('true reasons') or not true ('not true reasons') for them.

Frequent attenders were more worried about their health than infrequent attenders (mean scores 3.3 compared with 2.1, $p < 0.001$), and were more likely to have past experience of individual symptoms, and to believe they would experience them in the future. The frequent attenders gave fewer normalizing attributions than controls (mean number of attributions (SD):1.3(0.7) compared with 2.3(1.1), $p < 0.05$) and were less likely to give a normalizing reason as their first response. The frequent attenders provided significantly fewer 'not true' reasons than controls in the second part of the study. The findings of this study need to be interpreted cautiously because of the small sample size. However it is one of the few studies to examine cognitive factors in frequent attenders in primary care. The results suggest that frequent attenders might be less likely to think of external or environmental reasons for their symptoms, and may be less able to refute somatic explanations for bodily sensations.

Several studies have reported an association between alexithymia (having no words for feelings), the tendency to express distress by means of somatic symptoms and consultation rate (Jyvasjarvi *et al.* 1999, 2001). However, these associations may disappear when psychiatric and physical disorder are taken into account (Joukamaa *et al.* 1996).

There is some evidence linking frequent attendance and social stress (Baez *et al.* 1998; Robinson & Granfield 1986). It may be that chronic stressors are more important than acute ones (Ronalds *et al.* 2002). It has also been suggested that it is the way the subject copes with stressors rather than the stressors themselves which influences consultation. Frequent attendance may run in families and US studies suggest there may be an association between family dysfunction and consultation behaviour (Fiscella *et al.* 1997).

The evidence linking frequent attendance and psychosocial factors comes from a few heterogeneous studies in different settings. Some studies have had very low response rates and so these findings should be interpreted cautiously.

Frequent attendance and resource use

Research evidence consistently suggests that frequent attenders account for a disproportionate amount of the general practitioner's workload. Some studies have focused on non-primary care resource use of frequent attenders.

Frequent attenders use more medical and social care resources both in and out of their primary-care practices. In one study (Corney 1990) respondents were asked about contact with agencies during the previous year. Frequent attenders had double the rate of contact with other medical agencies and social agencies. Heywood and colleagues (Heywood *et al.* 1998) determined the use of hospital services by examining the primary care case notes. The use of 25 therapy and support services was ascertained by interviewing the patients. They found that 84/132 frequent attenders (64%) had been referred to a hospital consultant over a 12-month period compared with 13/102 controls (12.7%). Nineteen percent of frequent attenders but just 2% of controls had been referred to two or more specialists. The mean referral rate for frequent attenders was over five times that for controls.

Frequent attenders are referred for more investigations and have a greater incidence of hospitalization. McFarland and colleagues (McFarland *et al.* 1985) used computerized records to ascertain resource use over a seven-year period. They found that 13% of the sample (consistently frequent users) accounted for

27% of resource use with respect to laboratory tests, 26% of X-ray costs, and 30% of surgery costs. Use of mental health services was also determined from the database. The low-user group had 0 mental health contacts per person, the medium-user group had a mean of 0.43 contacts per person, and the high-user group had a mean of 0.82 contacts per person during the study period.

Frequent attenders use more out-of-hours as well as daytime services (Vedsted & Olesen 1999a) and tend to see certain doctors more than others. Neal and colleagues (Neal et al. 2000a) used their consultation dataset obtained from four practices in Leeds over a 41-month period to investigate frequent attenders consulting patterns with general practitioners. The authors found that some doctors at each practice saw a greater proportion of frequent attenders than expected. This difference was highly statistically significant. They also found that frequent attenders consulted with a greater number of doctors at each practice than normal attenders. Frequent attenders had a significantly greater proportion of same-doctor consultations than normal attenders. The results suggest that frequent attenders are more likely to consult with some doctors than others, and receive greater continuity of care than normal attenders. Frequent attenders see more doctors overall, perhaps because of a higher overall number of consultations or a tendency to 'doctor shop'. This study highlights the potential importance of both doctor and patient-related factors in perpetuating frequent attendance.

The outcome of frequent attendance

There is a relative lack of evidence concerning the course of frequent attendance. Between 30% and 50% of individuals who are frequent attenders in any one year will remain frequent attenders during the next year (Heywood et al. 1998; McFarland et al. 1985). Perhaps because of restricted definitions, patients tend not to remain frequent attenders for extended periods of time, but research that suggests frequent attendance is a short-lived and transitory phenomenon has significant methodological problems (Kapur et al. 2001). The best available evidence is that patients who are frequent attenders do have an increased propensity to consult frequently during future years. For example, a study from Oxford suggested over three-quarters of those who were frequent attenders in the index year consulted frequently during at least one of the subsequent four years (Gill et al. 1998). This suggests that frequent attendance may be a 'trait' to which patients are predisposed, rather than merely a 'state' that they slip in to. Long-term frequent attendance is associated with chronic disease, such as psychiatric and circulatory disorders, and older age (Ward et al. 1994). Each consecutive year of frequent attendance increases the chances of a subject remaining a high user in the subsequent year. McFarland and colleagues (McFarland *et al.* 1985) examined consultation rates in 1400 subjects over a seven-year period. They found the incidence of high utilization in the following year was 65% for those with two consecutive years of high utilization, 70% for those with three consecutive years of high utilization, 76% for those with four consecutive years of high utilization, and 80% of those with five consecutive years of high utilization.

Frequent attendance and childhood factors

Few studies have examined the association between frequent attendance in primary care in adulthood and childhood experience. By contrast, there is convincing evidence that adverse childhood exposures are associated with psychiatric disorder in adulthood (Kessler *et al.* 1997). A few studies have examined the association between childhood exposures and illness behaviour in adulthood. Two types of childhood exposure appear to be particularly important – childhood adversities such as abuse and neglect, and illness experiences in childhood such as significant illness in the subject themselves or household members.

Frequent attendance and childhood adversity

Newman and co-investigators (Newman *et al.* 2000) investigated the relationship between a specific childhood adversity (sexual abuse) and health utilization in a sample of women from a single health-maintenance organization attending internal medicine clinics in California. A quarter (26%) of the whole sample reported some type of sexual abuse although this included 'non-contact' abuse. Women who indicated a history of sexual abuse reported a greater number of symptoms than other women (mean (SD): 10.6 (4.7) compared with 8.1 (4.4)) and had a greater number of doctor visits over two years (mean (SD): 17.3 (14.0) compared with 11.7 (8.3)). There was no difference in the number of psychiatric consultations between groups. Walker *et al.* (1999a,b) sent self-report questionnaires to 1963 women in a large health-maintenance organization in Washington State. Measures included the Childhood Trauma Questionnaire, a self-administered instrument that enquires about childhood maltreatment in five areas: emotional abuse, physical abuse, sexual abuse, emotional neglect and physical neglect. Women who reported any form of maltreatment had median healthcare costs that were higher than those who did not report maltreatment. Women who reported sexual maltreatment had median healthcare costs that were higher than those without sexual maltreatment. When mental health costs were removed the differences between groups were no longer statistically significant. Women with maltreatment were twice as likely to make mental health visits in the five years before the study (OR 2.29 (95% CI 1.7–3.1)). Women with a history of maltreatment were more likely to report poor health, had greater physical and mental functional disability, reported more physical symptoms, had a greater number of high-risk behaviours and more physician diagnosis (Dickinson *et al.* 1999). There was a stepwise relationship between the degree of adversity experienced in childhood and adult health outcomes including utilization.

Both these US studies involved women only and used self-report measure of childhood adversities. They used what was essentially a cross-sectional design and so could not investigate issues of causation. Also, they did not measure other childhood variables that might have effected adult healthcare use such as childhood illness or parental psychiatric or physical illness. The Washington study did not measure adult psychiatric disorder which might act as a further confounder. Despite this, these studies provide some evidence that childhood adversity is associated to high adult healthcare use.

Frequent attendance and childhood illness experience

A number of studies have investigated the relationship between childhood illness exposures and adult outcome but perhaps the best evidence in this area comes from a series of studies carried out using a national birth cohort involving large numbers of subjects and a prospective design. Hotopf and colleagues explored a number of hypotheses related to childhood risk factors and adult outcomes (Fearon & Hotopf 2001; Hotopf *et al.* 1998, 1999a,b, 2000). The authors controlled for a number of potential confounding variables including gender, father's socioeconomic class, highest educational level attained and marital status aged 36. There was a clear association between parental ill health and unexplained symptoms in adulthood, which remained after controlling for sociodemographic variables and psychiatric disorder. 'Nervous problems' in fathers (but not mothers) were associated with unexplained symptoms in adulthood. Childhood physical illness, defined as a physical disorder that led to a hospital admission of a least three weeks' duration, was not associated with adult medically unexplained symptoms, but reports of persistent abdominal pain in childhood were.

Although some of the outcome measures were based on arbitrary classifications or *post hoc* judgements about the aetiology of symptoms, these studies provide some of the best available data regarding the link between childhood experience of illness and adult outcome. The authors suggest that defined physical illness in childhood is not associated with unexplained symptoms in adulthood, and previous studies suggesting such adults recall more childhood illness may reflect the presence of unexplained symptoms in childhood rather than defined physical disease. Parental illness does appear to be an important factor with regards to adult outcome. However this work was not able to explore the role of other adverse childhood exposures (such as abuse or parental care) in the aetiology of adult disorders, as this data was not collected as part of the survey.

It seems likely that both types of childhood exposure (adversity and illness experience) are important in determining adult outcomes. However very few studies have measured both types of exposures, making it difficult to elucidate differential effects and suggest possible mechanisms. A small retrospective study carried out in London suggested it was the interaction between childhood adversity and childhood experience of illness which was of aetiological importance in adults who presented with somatic symptoms of psychological distress (Craig *et al.* 1993). A more recent UK study suggested that both adveristy and experience of illness in childhood were related to adult consultation behaviour (Kapur *et al.* 2004a).

Models of attendance

Why do patients consult their doctors? This section briefly reviews quantitative, qualitative and theoretical models of frequent attendance.

Quantitative models of frequent attendance

Only a minority of studies have attempted to measure a large number of variables simultaneously in order to construct multivariate models of frequent attendance. Such models suggest that poor physical and mental health, poor perceived health, health anxiety, negative illness attitudes, medically unexplained symptoms, older age, female sex, family membership and social stress may be important determinants of consultation rate (Baez *et al.* 1998; Bellon *et al.* 1999; Kapur *et al.* 2004b; Little *et al.* 2001). Negative attitudes to doctors make repeated attendance less likely. Past consultation behaviour has also consistently been shown to be significant (Vedsted & Olesen 1999a). There may be different models of frequent attendance for men and women, with psychiatric symptoms being more important in women (Corney 1990).

Studies have identified different subgroups of frequent attenders based on reasons for consulting or pattern of consulting. However, these classifications have not been verified in independent samples.

Karlsson and colleagues (1997) attempted to establish a classification of frequent attenders and divided them into five groups that seemed to have face validity: those with physical (i.e. related to organic disease) reasons for consulting, those with psychiatric reasons for consulting, crisis patients, somatizing patients, and patients with multiple problems. The authors found differences between the groups. Crisis patients were younger. Crisis patients and somatizing patients were more likely to be female. Crisis patients and those with physical reasons for consulting reported higher levels of general life satisfaction.

Neal and colleagues (2000b) produced consultation timelines for the 100 most frequently attending patients at one practice in Leeds over a 44-month period. A panel of 12 experts was recruited and asked to sort the patients into groups. The data were analysed by collating them in a matrix and then carrying out a cluster analysis. Six clusters were identified: regular frequent attenders without bursts, supernovas (prolonged bursts of consultations with low numbers of consultations outside the bursts), a mixed diverse group, a gap-and-prolonged group, a burst-and-sporadic group, and a regular-as-clockwork group. The authors argue that their study shows that the natural history of frequent attending is unpredictable, and that cross-sectional snapshots of attendance are likely to be unreliable. The existence of a large mixed and diverse group (45 subjects) is consistent with the view that the decision to consult with the general practitioner is a multifactorial and complex one.

Qualitative and theoretical models of frequent attendance

Neal *et al.* (2000c) carried out a qualitative study of frequent attenders from three practices in Leeds. They included both regular frequent attenders and frequent attenders who attended in bursts. Non-random, purposive sampling was used to ensure that the final sample contained sufficient numbers of both types of frequent attender and a diverse age and sex mix. Semi-structured interviews were conducted by a single investigator, and covered areas such as experience of recent consultations, attitudes to consulting in general and their own consulting in particular, and perceptions of the general practitioner and the practice, health beliefs. The sampling was informed by themes that emerged from the analysis and data collection continued until no new themes arose from the data. A standard approach to analysis of qualitative data was used. Twenty-eight patients took part in the study (43% response rate). Non-responders were more likely to be women, were younger and had a higher consultation rate. Several key issues emerged from the interviews (Box 37.1).

The main themes that emerged from the data were incorporated into a two-part model. The first part of the model dealt with individual consultations and was very similar to the revised version of the Health Belief Model discussed by Campbell and Roland (1996). This model identified four key psychological characteristics as determinants of behaviour: perceived susceptibility, perceived severity, perceived costs and perceived benefits of action. The second part of the model looked at a wider outcome, that is the pattern of consulting over time and influences on it. This part of the model had similarities to the Network Episode Model (Pescosolido & Boyer 1996), a non-linear model which emphasizes the importance

> **Box 37.1   Findings from a qualitative study by Neal *et al.* (2000c).**
> - The processes by which frequent attenders make a decision to consult are complex and are informed by their experience of symptoms and of consulting in the past.
> - Chronic physical and psychiatric illnesses have a major influence over consultation.
> - The general practitioner has a great deal of perceived power in the control of medication and when and if the patient needs to return.
> - Consultation patterns over time are the result of more than just the result of individual decisions to consult. Consultations are not finite and discrete independent events.
> - Some frequent attenders discussed themes of passivity and external control in relation to consulting behaviour.
> - Familiarity with the whole process of consultation made it easier for frequent attenders to consult in the future.

of chronic illness and ongoing care, individual and social models of decision making, and formal and informal systems of care. One of its key assertions is that illness careers do not occur in a vacuum.

Other theoretical models of attendance include the folk belief model (Helman 1981) and the sociobehavioural utilization model (Anderson 1995).

Interventions for frequent attendance

The evidence from research studies

A number of studies have investigated interventions for frequent attendance. None have shown a clear benefit in terms of reducing consultation rate.

O'Dowd (1992) identified 28 'heartsink patients' (referring to the emotions triggered in doctors by certain frequently attending patients) at his practice with the help of his partner and the receptionist. Their case notes were reviewed in detail, the reasons for consulting summarized, and the current management recorded. A patient was then selected from the list (starting with the most 'heartsink') and the partners, a health visitor, a trainee, and occasionally a psychologist discussed them in depth at a lunchtime meeting. In addition follow-up information was presented on cases discussed at previous meetings. The main purpose of this intervention was to formulate a management plan to provide support for the professional dealing with the patient. This was recorded in the case notes. The meetings ended after six months due to time constraints, which meant that 9 patients had been discussed in detail and 19 patients had not. Consultation rates fell for both groups but those who had had a management plan showed a greater reduction (from 19 to 7 consultations per year compared with from 16 to 11 consultations per year). The author suggests that patients in the intervention group were more severely impaired at the outset of the study. This is a very small, non-randomized, open trial so the results should be treated with caution.

Katon *et al.* (1992) carried out a randomized trial in two clinics recruiting patients from 18 physicians. Two hundred and fifty-one frequently attending patients with defined psychological distress were randomized to receive a consultation-liaison psychiatry assessment or usual treatment. There were no significant differences between groups at 6- and 12-month follow-up with respect to psychiatric distress, functional disability or use of primary- or secondary-care services. However patients in the intervention group were more likely to be prescribed antidepressants and to continue antidepressants once they had been prescribed.

Jiwa (2000) undertook a prospective controlled study of 104 frequent attenders at one UK practice. Frequent attenders were defined as those who had attended 11 or more times in a year and were identified by examining practice lists of attenders and by asking the general practitioners to identify patients by memory. All patients had their clinical notes summarized, particularly with respect to current physical, social and psychological problems. In the intervention group summaries were displayed prominently in the notes and notes had a distinctive label. The general practitioners were asked to read and initial the summaries. In the control group the notes were not highlighted in any way and the summaries were not included in the notes. The main outcome measure was consultation rate at five months follow-up. The intervention failed to reduce the consultation rate of the frequent attenders. In the intervention group there was little difference between patients for whom there was evidence the general practitioner had looked at the summaries (that is, the summaries were signed) and patients whose notes were not endorsed in this way.

Simon and co-workers (2001) recruited adult patients from primary-care clinics in three health-maintenance organizations in the United States. Patients were eligible if they had been continuously registered for two years, were not receiving treatment for depression, and had made more than seven outpatient medical visits per year (that is, they were among the most frequently consulting 15% of patients). Participants were randomized to either usual care, or a depression-management programme. For patients in the usual-care group, their practices were informed that screening suggested they might be suffering from major depression. The depression management programme consisted of educational components for the patients and their physicians, pharmacotherapy where this was indicated, and psychiatric referral for those who did not respond to initial management. The main outcome measures were 'depression-free days' over the following 12 months and utilization and cost data obtained from health plan databases.

The intervention programme increased the number of depression-free days over 12 months by almost 50 days. Patients in the intervention group made more outpatient visits during the following 12 months and had a greater number of hospital admissions, and their health service costs were considerably higher.

Vedstead and Oleson (1999b) carried out an ecological time-trend study of the effects of a reorganization of out-of-hours family practice services in Denmark. Consultation data were obtained from the Public Health Insurance Database for Aarhus county. Contacts were taken to include telephone advice, home visits and office consultations. The main change introduced during the study period was the introduction of a mandatory county-wide telephone triage system staffed by general practitioners. The general practitioners would decide whether the patient required a home visit, a consultation at an out-of-hours medical centre, or simple telephone advice. The reorganization led to a 12% decrease in the number of attenders, a 16% decrease in the number of contacts, and a 29% decrease in costs. Much of this was attributable to a change in frequent attenders' behaviour. For the frequent attenders the reduction of face-to-face contacts did not lead to a compensatory increase in telephone contacts.

A pragmatic approach to intervention

Many primary-care doctors adopt a biopsychosocial approach to practice and this may also be the appropriate strategy for working with frequently attending patients. General practitioners need to be alert to the possibility of such diverse risk factors as psychiatric disorder, chronic physical disease, negative illness attitudes and childhood adversity. Should such risk factors be detected, appropriate treatment could then be instituted. What might such treatment look like? Promising interventions might include rigorous treatment for mood disorder and physical illness. Cognitive behavioural therapy for negative illness attitudes (Clarke *et al.* 1998) and symptom re-attribution for medically unexplained symptoms (Morriss *et al.* 1998), could also reduce healthcare use (see Chapter 36). Some studies suggest that written disclosure of emotionally important events, including events in childhood, reduces consultation rates (Pennebaker 1997; Smyth 1998). However a recent randomized controlled trial of face-to-face disclosure therapy in frequent attenders failed to show any benefit (Schilte *et al.* 2001). A promising alternative might be Psychodynamic Interpersonal Therapy (Hobson 1985). This treatment involves exploring interpersonal problems which cause or exacerbate psychological distress. The patient—therapist relationship is considered a valuable tool for identifying and helping to resolve interpersonal difficulties. In randomized controlled trials of patients with the irritable bowel syndrome and high utilizers of psychiatric services, it has been shown to significantly reduce the consultation rate (Guthrie *et al.* 1991, 1999). An important limiting factor, of course, is that many of these more specialized treatment options may not be easily available in primary-care settings.

Conclusion

Frequent attendance in primary care has been observed in a variety of settings across the world but one remarkably consistent finding across studies is that a small number of patients account for a disproportionate amount of the general practitioner's workload. Consistent associations have been reported between frequent attendance and female sex, older age, unemployment, socioeconomic deprivation, marital status, psychiatric disorder, physical illness, and health concerns. There are relatively few studies which investigate the outcome of frequent attendance or response to interventions, but the most useful treatment strategies are likely to be those which involve a biopsychosocial approach to management.

REFERENCES

Anderson, R. (1995). Revisiting the behavioural model and access to care: does it matter? *Journal of Health and Social Behaviour*, **36**, 1–10.

Anderson, S.O., Mattson, B. and Lynoe, N. (1995). Patients frequently consulting general practitioners at a general practice in Sweden – a comparative study. *Scandinavian Journal of Social Medicine*, **23**, 251–7.

Baez, K., Aiarzaguena, J. M., Grandes, G., *et al.* (1998). Understanding patient-initiated frequent attendance in primary care: a case-control study. *British Journal of General Practice*, **48**, 1824–7.

Bellon, J.A., Delgado, A., Luna, J.D., *et al.* (1999). Psychosocial and health belief variables associated with frequent attendance in primary care. *Psychological Medicine*, **29**, 1347–57.

Browne, G.B., Humphrey, B., Pallister, R., *et al.* (1982). Prevalence and characteristics of frequent attenders in a prepaid Canadian family practice. *Journal of Family Practice*, **14**, 63–71.

Campbell, S. and Roland, M. (1996). Why do people consult the doctor? *Family Practice*, **13**, 75–83.

Clarke, D. M., Salkovskis, P. M., Hackmann, A., *et al.* (1998). Two psychological treatments for hypochondriasis. A randomized controlled trial. *British Journal of Psychiatry*, **173**, 218–25.

Conroy, R. M., Smyth, O., Siriwardena, R., *et al.* (1999). Health anxiety and characteristics of self-initiated general practitioner consultations. *Journal of Psychosomatic Research*, **46**, 45–50.

Corney, R. H. (1990). Sex differences in general practice attendance and help seeking for minor illness. *Journal of Psychosomatic Research*, **34**, 525–34.

Craig, T. K., Boardman, A. P., Mills, K., *et al.* (1993). The South London Somatisation Study. I: Longitudinal course and the influence of early life experiences. *British Journal of Psychiatry*, **163**, 579–88.

Dickinson, L. M., deGruy, F. V. III, Dickinson, W. P., *et al.* (1999). Health-related quality of life and symptom profiles of female survivors of sexual abuse. *Archives of Family Medicine*, **8**, 35–43.

Dowrick, C. F., Bellon, J. A. and Gomez, M. J. (2000). GP frequent attendance in Liverpool and Granada: the impact of depressive symptoms. (See comments.) *British Journal of General Practice*, **50**, 361–5.

Fearon, P. and Hotopf, M. (2001). Relation between headache in childhood and physical and psychiatric symptoms in adulthood: national birth cohort study. *British Medical Journal*, **322**, 1145.

Fiscella, K., Franks, P. and Shields, C. G. (1997). Perceived family criticism and primary care utilization: psychosocial and biomedical pathways. *Family Process*, **36**, 25–41.

Gill, D. and Sharpe, M. (1999). Frequent consulters in general practice: a systematic review of studies of prevalence, associations and outcome. *Journal of Psychosomatic Research*, **47**, 115–30.

Gill, D., Dawes, M., Sharpe, M., *et al.* (1998). GP frequent consulters: their prevalence, natural history, and contribution to rising workload. *British Journal of General Practice*, **48**, 1856–7.

Guthrie, E. A., Creed, F., Dawson, D., *et al.* (1991). A controlled trial of psychological treatment for the irritable bowel syndrome. *Gastroenterology*, **100**, 450–7.

Guthrie, E. A., Moorey, J., Margison, F., *et al.* (1999). Cost effectiveness of brief Psychodynamic Interpersonal Therapy in high utilizers of psychiatric services. *Archives of General Psychiatry*, **56**, 519–26.

Helman, C. G. (1981). Disease versus illness in general practice. *Journal of the Royal College of General Practitioners*, **31**, 548–52.

Heywood, P. L., Blackie, G. C., Cameron, I. H., *et al.* (1998). An assessment of the attributes of frequent attenders to general practice. *Family Practice*, **15**, 198–204.

Hobson, R. F. (1985). *Forms of Feeling*. London: Tavistock Publications.

Hotopf, M., Carr, S., Mayou, R., *et al.* (1998). Why do children have chronic abdominal pain, and what happens to them when they grow up? Population based cohort study. (See comments.) *British Medical Journal*, **316**, 1196–200.

Hotopf, M., Mayou, R., Wadsworth, M., *et al.* (1999a). Childhood risk factors for adults with medically unexplained symptoms: results from a national birth cohort study. *American Journal of Psychiatry*, **156**, 1796–800.

Hotopf, M., Mayou, R., Wadsworth, M., *et al.* (1999b). Psychosocial and developmental antecedents of chest pain in young adults. *Psychosomatic Medicine*, **61**, 861–7.

Hotopf, M., Wilson-Jones, C., Mayou, R., *et al.* (2000). Childhood predictors of adult medically unexplained hospitalisations. Results from a national birth cohort study. *British Journal of Psychiatry*, **176**, 273–80.

Jiwa, M. (2000). Frequent attenders in general practice: an attempt to reduce attendance. *Family Practice*, **17**, 248–51.

Joukamaa, M., Karlsson, H., Sohlman, B., *et al.* (1996). Alexithymia and psychological distress among frequent attendance patients in health care. *Psychotherapy & Psychosomatics*, **65**, 199–202.

Jyvasjarvi, S., Joukamaa, M., Vaisanen, E., et al. (1999). Alexithymia, hypochondriacal beliefs and psychological distress among frequent attenders in primary health care. Comprehensive Psychiatry, 40, 292–8.

Jyvasjarvi, S., Joukamaa, M., Vaeisaenen, E., et al. (2001). Somatizing frequent attenders in primary health care. Journal of Psychosomatic Research, 50, 185–92.

Kapur, N., Macfarlane, G. J. and Creed, F. (2001). Frequent attenders in general practice. British Journal of General Practice, 51, 756–7.

Kapur, N., Hunt, I. and Macfarlane, G., et al. (2004a). Childhood experience and healthcare use in adulthood. Nested case-control study. British Journal of Psychiatry, 185, 134–9.

Kapur, N., Hunt, I., Lunt, M., et al. (2004b). Psychosocial and illness-related predictors of consultation rates in primary care – a cohort study. Psychological Medicine, 34, 719–28.

Karlsson, H., Lehtinen, V. and Joukamaa, M. (1994). Frequent attenders of Finnish public primary care: socio-demographic characteristics and physical morbidity. Family Practice, 11, 424–30.

Karlsson, H., Joukamaa, M., Lahti, I., et al. (1997). Frequent attender profiles: different clinical subgroups among frequent attender patients in primary care. Journal of Psychosomatic Research, 42, 57–66.

Katon, W., Von Korff, M., Lin, E., et al. (1992). A randomized trial of psychiatric consultation with distressed high utilizers. (See comments.) General Hospital Psychiatry, 14, 86–98.

Kessler, R. C., Davis, C. G. and Kendler, K. S. (1997). Childhood adversity and adult psychiatric disorder in the US National Comorbidity Survey. Psychological Medicine, 27, 1101–19.

Little, P., Somerville, J., Williamson, I., et al. (2001). Psychosocial, lifestyle and health status variables in predicting high attendance among adults. British Journal of General Practice, 51, 987–94.

McFarland, B. H., Freeborn, D. K., Mullooly, J. P., et al. (1985). Utilization patterns among long term enrollees in a pre-paid group practice health maintenance organization. Medical Care, 1221–33.

Mehl-Madrona, L. E. (1998). Frequent users of rural primary care: comparisons with randomly selected users. Journal of the American Board of Family Practice, 11, 105–15.

Morris, J. K., Cook, D. G., Walker, M., et al. (1992). Non-consulters and high consulters in general practice: cardio-respiratory health and risk factors. Journal of Public Health Medicine, 14, 131–7.

Morriss, R., Gask, L., Ronalds, C., et al. (1998). Cost-effectiveness of a new treatment for somatized mental disorder taught to GPs. Family Practice, 15, 119–25.

Neal, R. D., Heywood, P. L., Morley, S., et al. (1998). Frequency of patients' consulting in general practice and workload generated by frequent attenders: comparisons between practices. British Journal of General Practice, 48, 895–8.

Neal, R. D., Heywood, P. L. and Morley, S. (2000a). Frequent attenders' consulting patterns with general practitioners. British Journal of General Practice, 50, 972–6.

Neal, R. D., Heywood, P. L. and Morley, S. (2000b). Freight trains and supernovas: the use of a sorting task to determine patterns within long-term frequent attendance to general practitioners. Primary Health Care Research and Development, 1, 39–50.

Neal, R. D., Heywood, P. L. and Morley, S. (2000c). 'I always seem to be there' — a qualitative study of frequent attenders. *British Journal of General Practice*, **50**, 716–23.

Newman, M. G., Clayton, L., Zuellig, A., *et al.* (2000). The relationship of childhood sexual abuse and depression with somatic symptoms and medical utilization. *Psychological Medicine*, **30**, 1063–77.

Nighswander, T. S. (1984). High utilizers of ambulatory care services: 6 year follow up at Alaska Native Medical centre. *Public Health Reports*, **99**, 400–4.

O'Dowd, T. C. (1992). Five years of heartsink patients in general practice. *British Medical Journal*, **297**, 528–32.

Pennebaker, J. (1997). Writing about emotional experiences as a therapeutic process. *Psychological Science*, **8**, 162–6.

Pescosolido, B. and Boyer, C. (1996). From the community into the treatment system — how people use health services. In *The Sociology of Mental Illness*, ed. A. Horwitz and T. Scheid. New York: Oxford University Press.

Robinson, J. O. and Granfield, A. J. (1986). The frequent consulter in primary medical care. *Journal of Psychosomatic Research*, **30**, 589–600.

Ronalds, C., Kapur, N., Stone, K., *et al.* (2002). Determinants of consultation rate in patients with anxiety and depressive disorders in primary care. *Family Practice*, **19**, 23–8.

Schilte, A. F., Portegijs, P. J., Blankenstein, A. H., *et al.* (2001). Randomised controlled trial of disclosure of emotionally important events in somatisation in primary care. *British Medical Journal*, **323**, 86.

Sensky, T., MacLeod, A. K. and Rigby, M. F. (1996). Causal attributions about common somatic sensations among frequent general practice attenders. *Psychological Medicine*, **26**, 641–6.

Simon, G. E., Manning, W. G., Katzelnick, D. J., *et al.* (2001). Cost-effectiveness of systematic depression treatment for high utilizers of general medical care. *Archives of General Psychiatry*, **58**, 181–7.

Smyth, J. M. (1998). Written emotional expression: effect sizes, outcome types and moderating variables. *Journal of Consulting and Clinical Psychology*, **66**, 174–84.

Svab, I. and Zaletel-Kragelj, L. (1993). Frequent attenders in general practice: a study from Slovenia. *Scandinavian Journal of Primary Health Care*, **11**, 38–43.

Vedsted, P. and Olesen, F. (1999a). Frequent attenders in out-of-hours general practice care: attendance prognosis. *Family Practice*, **16**, 283–8.

Vedsted, P. and Olesen, F. (1999b). Effect of a reorganized after-hours family practice service on frequent attenders. *Family Medicine*, **31**, 270–5.

Walker, E. A., Unutzer, J., Rutter, C., *et al.* (1999a). Costs of health care use by women HMO members with a history of childhood abuse and neglect. *Archives of General Psychiatry*, **56**, 609–13.

Walker, E. A., Gelfand, A., Katon, W. J., *et al.* (1999b). Adult health status of women with histories of childhood abuse and neglect. *American Journal of Medicine*, **107**, 332–9.

Ward, A. M., Underwood, P., Fatovich, B., *et al.* (1994). Stability of attendance in general practice. *Family Practice*, **11**, 431–7.

38

Major disaster planning

Jonathan I. Bisson, Jim Bolton, Kevin Mackway-Jones and
Elspeth Guthrie

Introduction

In the last few decades there have been a number of high-profile disasters, memories of which can be evoked by the mention of a place name. For example, Zeebrugge, Lockerbie, Bradford, Bali, New York and Madrid. Disasters affect many people. Victims and their families, survivors, witnesses and the personnel of agencies involved in the emergency response are perhaps the most obvious groups, but disasters often affect whole communities, countries and, as we have seen following the terrorist attacks on 11 September 2001, the whole world.

Emergency plans

There have been criticisms regarding the unplanned and uncoordinated nature of psychosocial input following several disasters, leading to calls for the creation of multiagency planning groups that include mental health professionals to plan appropriate responses before disasters occur (Bisson 2003). Every local authority in England and Wales has an emergency planning officer whose key role is to develop an emergency plan. The emergency planning officer co-ordinates the *Disaster Management System*, a multiagency, multiprofessional partnership with the emergency services (ambulance, fire and police) being central to it. Other agencies including the local authority, social services, health services and voluntary agencies support the emergency services. In order for their input to be effective this support should be delivered in a preplanned co-ordinated manner integrated into the central plan.

Disaster plans often include a well-developed 'non-psychological' emergency response but little, if any, detail about the psychological response, perhaps reflecting the Home Office's (1998) *Dealing with Disasters* document that merely

Handbook of Liaison Psychiatry, ed. Geoffrey Lloyd and Elspeth Guthrie. Published by Cambridge University Press. © Cambridge University Press 2007.

states 'victims of disasters should be offered psychological support'. Health and social services have specific responsibility for making arrangements for the appropriate social and psychological support of survivors, relatives, casualties and other affected individuals. Other key roles of health and social services include the co-ordination of the activities of agencies and organizations involved, and the appropriate training and supervision of them. Liaison psychiatry services that cover Accident and Emergency departments are ideally placed to provide input to emergency planning along with traumatic stress services and child and adolescent mental health services.

Social and psychological care incorporates the emotional and practical help that individuals caught up in a disaster may require. This support ranges from providing immediate comfort and practical help through to longer term psychological support. Many individuals will receive excellent support from their family and friends. Any formal response should complement this. For most people involved in a disaster help may only be needed during the rescue phase and the immediate aftermath. Nevertheless, in planning the provision of care the need to make support services available in the medium and long term must be recognized. There may be the need to establish a dedicated support team, or referral services, after an incident. These services may need to be provided for 18 to 24 months, or even longer, and it is therefore essential that funding is identified, and protected, from the outset.

Every district should have a disaster plan in place. The exact nature of a response will vary in terms of size, management and the extent to which it will be proactive or reactive, depending on the specific circumstances of the disaster. An early meeting of those responsible for co-ordinating the psychosocial response should be held following a disaster to determine the level of input. The response should then be closely monitored to ensure that the planned service is being delivered and to make changes as necessary.

Prevalence of psychiatric disorder

Unfortunately there have been few high-quality studies of the prevalence of psychiatric disorder following disaster. Those that have been done show that the majority of individuals involved will not go on to develop psychiatric disorder. Post-traumatic stress disorder (PTSD) is the most discussed psychiatric disorder following disaster but it is important to remember that it is not the only psychiatric disorder or emotional response experienced following a disaster (see Box 38.1). In over 50% of cases of PTSD another comorbid psychiatric diagnosis will be present. The commonest codiagnoses are depressive disorders, anxiety disorders and substance-use disorders.

Box 38.1 Mental health presentations post-disaster.

Normal reaction	Grief reactions
Acute stress disorder	Pre-existing difficulties
Post-traumatic stress disorder	Generalized anxiety disorder
Specific phobias	Depression
Adjustment disorders	Substance misuse
Psychosis	Medically unexplained symptoms

Following the Oklahoma City bombing, North *et al.* (1999) interviewed 182 survivors six months after the event. Of these, 45% were suffering from a diagnosable psychiatric disorder, 34% were suffering from PTSD. Yule *et al.* (2000) reported the results of a follow-up study of the sinking of the *Jupiter*, a ship touring the Mediterranean whose passengers were mainly teenage school-children. They interviewed 217 survivors and 87 controls five to eight years later, when they were in their early twenties. Fifty-two per cent of the survivors had suffered from PTSD following the sinking compared to 3.4% of the controls. Of those with PTSD 30% recovered within a year and 34% had ongoing PTSD at follow-up.

There has been some high-quality research published following the 9/11 terrorist attacks in the USA. Galea *et al.* (2002) studied 1008 adults who lived south of 110 Street in Manhattan. They performed a survey using a random-digit telephone dialing methodology five-to-eight weeks after the attacks. They found that 7.5% reported symptoms consistent with current PTSD and 9.7% with current depression. Those individuals who lived closer to the site of the attack (south of Canal Street) had a 20% rate of PTSD. In a subsequent study Galea *et al.* (2003) considered a different sample of 2752 adults and at six months found a current prevalence of PTSD of 0.6%. The symptoms were again found to be higher in those more directly involved but, importantly, several individuals who were not directly affected reported significant PTSD symptoms. Unfortunately there have been no studies to date of those who actually escaped from the World Trade Centre.

Course of traumatic stress symptoms

The studies of Yule *et al.* (2000) and Galea *et al.* (2003) suggest that the natural course of traumatic stress symptoms following disaster is to reduce over time. This is supported by epidemiological research within the general population on the natural course of PTSD. For example, Kessler *et al.* (1995) studied 5877 15–54-year-olds in the United States' national comorbidity survey and found that individuals who satisfied the criteria for PTSD reported the sharpest decrease in symptoms during the first 12 months with a more gradual decrease to six years and then little change thereafter. There appeared to be a 50% chance of remission at two years. At six years after diagnosis over a third of those who suffered from PTSD continued to satisfy the diagnostic criteria.

It is widely agreed that a strong emotional response following a disaster can be a normal response that resolves naturally over time. However there is very limited evidence to suggest that to experience no emotional response, or a limited emotional response, is pathological. Indeed it appears that lack of a marked reaction predicts a better rather than a worse outcome. Recently, there has been increasing interest in the concept of resilience. Bonanno (2004) considered the differing trajectories of recovery in individuals who developed a marked initial emotional response following a traumatic event, but then recovered without any intervention and those who did not develop a marked response. The latter group had a much flatter recovery curve leading to discussion of the concept of resilience. He argued that we should not be thinking of response in dichotomous terms (classically recovery and non-recovery) but add a third resiliency group who do not develop marked psychological distress at all.

Given the rapid recovery of many individuals who do develop a psychological reaction following a traumatic event can we predict those who are going to develop PTSD? The answer appears to be yes, to a degree, but not very well. In large epidemiological trials there are fairly consistent and strongly statistically significant associations between various factors including pretrauma variables (e.g. past psychiatric history and childhood trauma), peritraumatic variables (e.g. life threat and early psychological distress) and post-traumatic factors (e.g. social support). The two largest and best designed systematic reviews in this area (Brewin *et al.* 2000; Ozer *et al.* 2002) found that lack of perceived social support following a trauma was the best predictor but only accounted for some 20% of the overall variance and therefore is unlikely to be of great predictive value for specific individuals or as a mass-screening method.

Intervention

Despite the high profile of disasters there has been no good systematic research on exactly what to do in the aftermath, and in reality, it is very difficult to organize and implement high-quality research in such sudden and often chaotic circumstances. Research of early interventions following traumatic events has focused on smaller-scale major traumas such as road traffic accidents and assaults. Caution must clearly be exercised when extrapolating the results of these studies to the disaster situation, but in the absence of disaster research they should be used to inform a general approach.

Three main models of early intervention have been researched to date. Single-session early interventions such as critical incident stress debriefing (Mitchell 1983) have been the most widely discussed interventions following major traumatic events, although their popularity has reduced over the last decade. Multiple-session early interventions have been increasingly researched in the last few years. These usually employ cognitive-behavioural techniques with imaginal exposure to the traumatic experience as a key component. Education and some form of cognitive restructuring are also frequently included. Psychodynamic interpersonal therapy has also been used for patients whose traumatic experiences have a clear link to underlying interpersonal dilemmas (Guthrie *et al.* 1999). Finally, three randomized controlled trials of medication following traumatic events have recently been published.

Single-session early interventions

There have now been 12 randomized controlled trials of single session early interventions including a total of 1836 individuals. All of these have been of interventions following smaller-scale traumatic events and therefore the results are difficult to generalize. Eleven of them have been scrutinized as part of a systematic review of single session early interventions following a traumatic event (Rose *et al.* 2003).

Bordow and Porritt (1979) studied 70 male inpatients within one week of a motor vehicle accident. Individuals either received no intervention, 'immediate assessment' which reviewed the experience of injury and hospitalization and the subject's emotional reactions to these, or a social worker intervention which lasted between two and 10 hours over three months. At three-to-four month follow-up the social worker group fared best followed by the immediate-review group and then the no-intervention group. Bunn and Clarke (1979) found that relatives of seriously ill or injured individuals admitted less than 12 hours previously benefited from a 30-minute semi-structured counselling session where subjects were encouraged to express their feelings, compared to no intervention, although unfortunately follow-up was only five minutes after the intervention was completed.

Hobbs *et al.* (1997) (three year follow-up reported by Mayou *et al.* 2001) found that individuals who received individual debriefing 24–48 hours after a motor vehicle accident fared worse than those who received no intervention at three years. Lee *et al.* (1996) found that a one-hour individual debriefing approximately two weeks after miscarriage had no advantage over no intervention at four months.

Stevens and Adshead (1996) found that a standardized interview that reviewed the emotions associated with sustaining a physical injury within 24 hours of attendance at an Emergency Room was no better than no intervention at three-month follow-up. Bisson *et al.* (1997) found individual psychological debriefing 2–19 days after acute burn trauma was associated with worse outcome at 13 months than no intervention. Conlon *et al.* (1999) found no difference between a 30-minute manualized counselling session immediately after a brief assessment and no further intervention in 40 ambulant trauma clinic attenders following a motor vehicle accident. Lavender and Walkinshaw (1998) found that a midwife-facilitated intervention within 48 hours of a normal delivery of a healthy baby that comprised discussion of labour, questions and exploration of feelings was beneficial to women at three-week follow-up.

Dolan *et al.* (unpublished data) found no differences between individual psychological debriefing less than 14 days post-trauma and no intervention in 100 patients who had presented to an Accident and Emergency Department following a motor vehicle accident, assault or other traumatic injury. Rose *et al.* (1999) found no difference between individual debriefing within one month of trauma and standard care in victims of violence at 11-month follow-up. Small *et al.* (2001) conducted by far the largest study with 1041 women who had given birth by caesarean section, forceps or vacuum extraction randomized to a midwife-facilitated psychological debriefing held less than 48 hours following the birth, or usual post-partum care. There were no significant differences between the two groups but like the other post-partum study (Lavender & Walkinshaw 1998) depression was used as the primary outcome measure and the generalizability is debatable. Campfield and Hills (2001) have published the only true randomized controlled trial of group debriefing in individuals who had recently been exposed to a robbery at work. Individuals assigned to an immediate debriefing group within 10 hours of the robbery (mean = 5 hours) fared better than those assigned to a delayed debriefing group at least 48 hours post-trauma (mean = 62 hours).

The studies of single-session early psychological interventions vary greatly in their quality, but overall the quality of the studies is only moderate. Common methodological shortcomings are small sample sizes, lack of concealment of randomization, failure to account for dropouts, and lack of use of standardized measures or manualized interventions. Eleven studies were of individual or couple interventions, one included group interventions. The consideration of individual or couple psychological debriefing has been criticized as the technique was primarily designed as a group intervention.

The randomized controlled trials available provide little evidence that early single-session interventions prevent psychopathology following trauma. Some negative outcomes were found but intervention appeared to make no difference to later psychological outcome when the studies were considered collectively.

In addition to the methodological issues already discussed other factors can be postulated to explain the apparent lack of effectiveness of single session interventions. For some individuals early re-exposure may disrupt normal processing, challenge individuals' usual coping mechanisms and result in re-traumatization. A further concern is that the introduction of a belief that a structured intervention is required for everyone following a traumatic event may interfere with natural social support systems and create an expectation that formal counselling is necessary for recovery.

Multiple-session early psychosocial interventions

There are eight completed randomized controlled trials of multiple-session early psychosocial interventions including a total of 625 individuals. As discussed earlier Bordow and Porritt (1979) found practical social work input more beneficial than immediate review or standard care. Brom *et al.* (1994) found that three to six sessions of cognitive-behavioural therapy and education starting one month post-trauma was no better than no intervention in 151 motor vehicle accident victims at six-month follow-up. Andre *et al.* (1997) found that assaulted bus drivers benefited from one to six sessions of cognitive-behavioural therapy from two weeks post-trauma, compared to a no-intervention group at six-month follow-up. Bryant *et al.* (1998, 1999) conducted two similar studies with a total of 69 motor vehicle accident, industrial accident and assault victims. Five 90-minute sessions of prolonged exposure or anxiety management commencing two weeks post-trauma were found to be superior to supportive counselling. Bisson *et al.* (2004) found that individuals who received four 60 minute sessions of cognitive-behavioural therapy, including prolonged exposure between 2 and 10 weeks post-trauma, fared better than individuals who received no intervention following physical injury at 13-month follow-up. Zatzick *et al.* (2001) found that four months of collaborative care to support individuals following physical injury requiring inpatient care did not reduce PTSD rates compared to standard care at four-month follow-up. Gidron *et al.* (2001) found that two sessions of a telephone-delivered 'memory-structuring intervention' (this involved listening and clarifying an individual's narrative and then structuring it for them to practice) 24—48 hours post-trauma fared better than two sessions of supporting listening in a small study of motor vehicle accident victims.

Four of the studies (Andre *et al.* 1997; Bordow & Porritt 1979; Brom *et al.* 1994; Zatzick *et al.* 2001) included all individuals irrespective of psychological distress reported. Two studies (Bryant *et al.* 1998, 1999) included only individuals who satisfied the criteria for acute stress disorder (ASD); one study (Bisson *et al.* 2004) included only individuals displaying evidence of acute psychological distress, and one study included only individuals with elevated heart rates (Gidron *et al.* 2001).

The overall methodological quality of these studies is better than that of the single-session interventions. However there remain problems in terms of sample size, lack of replication, absence of control condition, nature of control condition if present, and lack of inclusion of drop-outs in the final analysis.

The randomized-controlled trials to date suggest that multiple-session early psychosocial interventions, particularly those targeted at symptomatic individuals and usually commencing later than the single-session studies, are more effective than single-session early interventions. It is however clear that there is no panacea and it is well recognized in clinical practice that not everyone can tolerate direct psychological re-exposure to the traumatic event they have been involved in (Pitman *et al.* 1991).

Medication

Three randomized controlled trials of medication in adults shortly after a traumatic event have been published. The sample sizes have been very small but other aspects of methodological quality have been quite good. Schelling *et al.* (2001) randomized 20 victims of septic shock on an intensive treatment unit to intravenous hydrocortisone or placebo. One of the nine individuals who received hydrocortisone developed PTSD within the 31-month follow-up period compared to 7 of the 11 in the placebo group. It is obviously very difficult to generalize this result to individuals without severe physical disorder.

Pitman *et al.* (2002) hypothesized that early administration of propranolol following trauma may address the postulated role of excess epinephrine release in the development of PTSD. Thirty-one trauma victims were randomized to receive propranolol 40 mg four times per day for 10 days starting within six hours of the trauma, or to a placebo condition. Despite some evidence that physiological arousal was reduced in the propranolol group, the overall results were neutral. Mellman *et al.* (2002) considered 22 individuals with PTSD symptoms and sleep initiation difficulties 14 days after various traumas. They were randomized to receive temazepam 30 mg at night for five days and then 15 mg at night for two days, or to placebo. This did not appear to have an impact on the development of PTSD, but those on temazepam slept better after one night. There was no difference in sleep duration after one week.

Perhaps one of the most important findings from the above studies is that the medications researched to date have not been shown to impede the normal recovery process shortly after a traumatic event. There have been no randomized controlled trials of antidepressants to date but given the fact they have been shown to have some effectiveness in treating established PTSD they would seem worthy of research in the future.

A general-hospital psychosocial disaster plan

We shall now consider specific issues concerning the planning and delivery of the psychosocial component of a general hospital disaster plan. However, it must be remembered that disasters affect whole communities and not just the hospitals that serve them. Staff involved in planning and delivering psychosocial care within the general hospital are likely to have a wider remit to contribute to district planning and to liaise closely with those responsible for the district plan.

A review of general hospital major incident plans in the UK found that a psychosocial response was often not explicitly included (Adshead *et al.* 1994). Instead there was an assumption that psychosocial support would be provided by hospital chaplains and social workers. The separate provision of acute and mental health services may contribute to psychosocial care being inadequately addressed. Liaison psychiatry services are well placed to remedy this problem, but where these are not available a named local mental health professional should be involved.

Disasters are unpredictable and the number and type of casualties will depend on the nature, scale and complexity of the event. Hence a major incident plan must be both flexible and comprehensive. Other factors which contribute to a high quality psychosocial response are shown in Box 38.2.

Planning

Planning for a psychosocial response to a major incident should be multi-disciplinary. The core team should include representatives from the emergency unit, local mental health services (ideally liaison psychiatry and child and adolescent services), social services, pastoral services, voluntary organizations and the occupational health department. Additional team members will depend on local circumstances and may include hospital psychologists, counsellors and nursing staff. Advance planning should identify who these individuals will be and provide them with training on how to provide support to individuals involved in a disaster. The team should decide on a chairman who will co-ordinate the planning process, and will probably take the lead role during a major incident. The proposed psychosocial plan must be incorporated into the overall hospital

---

Box 38.2 Factors that contribute to a high-quality psychosocial disaster response.

- Comprehensive planning to include psychological, social and spiritual care
- Multiagency liaison to ensure integrated care
- A flexible response to a range of situations
- An immediate response to a diasaster
- A proactive approach to identifying and managing problems

major incident plan and the psychosocial planning group should be represented on the hospital's major incident committee. The plan should ensure that everyone involved in dealing with those involved in major incidents are aware of psychosocial issues and how to provide basic emotional support.

The planning group co-ordinates the response immediately following a major incident and in the aftermath. Practical considerations are listed in Box 38.3. The immediate psychosocial response will be part of the overall hospital major incident plan. The roles of key personnel, called into the hospital once a major incident has been declared, are detailed in 'action cards'. The aims of the longer-term response can be discussed in advance, but the details will be established by the core team following the incident.

The planning group should consider where the psychosocial response will be based in the event of an incident. The 'psychosocial control centre' will be the site where staff meet after a major incident is declared. An appropriate site is an outpatient clinic, where seating is available for casualties and their friends and relatives, and where there are rooms for private meetings. The overall hospital plan should include a system where news is brought directly from the area where the injured are being treated, so that members of the psychosocial response team can update those waiting. This area will require administrative staff to manage paperwork, and the clinic receptionists are ideal for this role. The importance of a supply of refreshments should not be underestimated, and should be included in planning.

Provision of a telephone helpline as part of the acute response should be discussed as part of the overall hospital plan. Generally, the hospital will have

---

Box 38.3 Practical considerations in planning for a psychosocial disaster response.

- Identification of a core multidisciplinary team
- Identification of a team leader
- Identification of secretarial and IT support
- Definition of roles and responsibilities of the response team in the event of an incident
- Preparation of telephone cascades to contact additional staff
- Compilation of action cards for the acute response
- Planning of support for telephonists, or the establishment of a separate emotional support telephone helpline
- Compilation of written information on the psychological response to a trauma
- Preliminary planning for a longer-term response
- Rehearsal of the psychosocial response
- Staff training where necessary

designated telephone lines to receive enquiries about the incident. One option is for a member of the psychosocial response team to be based with the telephonists, in order to provide support for distressed callers. Staff with this role should be aware of confidentiality issues which will limit what information can be given out. Some areas will have a plan to develop a separate telephone helpline for emotional support. In one area a partnership with the local Samaritans has been formed to provide this (Bisson *et al.* 2003).

During an incident, additional staff may be required. Telephone numbers should be collected in advance and kept at the psychosocial control centre. Similarly, predetermined telephone cascade systems can be used to call in pastoral workers of different faiths and denominations. Once the core team have identified the roles of key personnel, and have compiled action cards, the psychosocial response should be rehearsed. In the first instance this can be done as a table-top exercise. A mock incident with role players is helpful in identifying potential problems. This may be part of a full-scale hospital exercise, with casualties played by professional role players.

Following an incident, the core team should meet to co-ordinate, monitor and support the immediate response and to plan the longer-term response. The provision of written information on the psychological response to trauma can be prepared in advance. The Red Cross leaflet *Coping with Crisis* has been widely used following disasters and can be adapted for local use. Contact details for local help organizations and the telephone helpline should be included in the leaflet. Leaflets can be kept in the psychosocial control centre, and given out to casualties following a major incident.

The plan should be reviewed annually to take account of changes in organization and personnel that could affect the response to a major incident.

Immediate psychosocial response

Once a major incident has been declared, key staff on a predetermined list will be called in by the hospital switchboard. Staff arriving at the hospital will register at a central point and be given preliminary information about the incident. The psychosocial response team will gather at the psychosocial control centre. If necessary, additional staff can be called in using the telephone cascade list. The team leader, or a deputy, will take charge of staff response. The key roles of the response staff are listed in Box 38.4 and should be detailed on action cards.

In the hours following a disaster psychosocial care should predominantly comprise basic emotional and practical support and information giving rather than any form of structured intervention. Individuals should be offered the opportunity to discuss their experiences and feelings if they want to, but should not be forced to talk about their experiences. This input is most appropriately

> **Box 38.4 Key psychosocial roles immediately following a disaster.**
> · Respond to needs of distressed survivors: walking wounded and more severely injured
> · Respond to needs of distressed friends and relatives
> · Identify groups with special needs, e.g. children
> · Target trained staff at those with more complex needs
> · Record information on team activities

provided by non-mental-health professionals. Mental-health professionals should be available to deal with individuals who may require specialist mental-health assistance, for example for severe acute anxiety states or psychotic reactions, but their main role at this stage is to co-ordinate the response and support and supervise the management and other staff who are providing it.

Information should be conveyed regularly by a 'runner' from the areas where the physically injured are being treated to the psychosocial control centre and the waiting area. Those attending the waiting area, both families and casualties, should be booked in and basic information taken on individual record sheets. This enables staff to keep families informed about injured relatives and also provides opportunities to proactively offer further support in the future. Walking wounded can also attend this area to be reunited with family and to receive psychosocial support if required. It is important that the details of any discussions, or assistance given to family or casualties, are recorded.

Individuals involved in the disaster should be given verbal and written information about the normal emotional responses to such events. Individuals should be reassured that difficult feelings, and physical and emotional symptoms, are often part of a normal response to an abnormal situation. These subside over days or weeks after the traumatic event. Individuals should be encouraged to continue with normal activities within reason, and to discuss their feelings with those around them. They should be warned to avoid the excessive use of drugs or alcohol to deal with difficult feelings. If symptoms persist beyond a few weeks, or cause marked distress, patients should consult their GP, the telephone helpline, or other locally identified resources. Staff should be advised about the option of contacting the occupational health department.

Psychosocial response in the aftermath of an incident

In the aftermath of a disaster the psychosocial planning team should meet to co-ordinate the longer-term psychosocial response (Burns & Hollins 1991). This meeting should take place 24–48 hours after stand-down of the acute response. The response required will depend on the nature of the disaster, but key roles are listed in Box 38.5, and can be described in an additional action card within the major incident plan.

Box 38.5 Key roles of the psychosocial response team in the aftermath of an incident.

- Review the provision of services after the stand-down of the acute response
- Liaise with hospital staff in A&E and on the hospital wards
- Provide psychosocial support for hospital inpatients
- Support or establish a telephone helpline
- Liaise with traumatic stress services, and local bereavement services
- Liaise with community services and organizations
- Send written information to casualties and staff, describing the normal response to a trauma, and the availability of counselling services
- Liaise with services for out-of-area patients
- Consider the organization of a screening system for survivors and staff (may be via the occupational health department)
- Facilitate research

The psychosocial team should have proactive involvement with hospital wards caring for patients involved in the incident, to establish the availability of psychosocial and pastoral care in the minds of staff (Burns & Hollins 1991). This is the period following a disaster when the liaison psychiatry team are likely to be most involved. Hospital staff can be helped to recognize the potential impact of psychological symptoms on patients' functioning and recovery. Accident and Emergency (A&E) staff should also be made aware of services available. Patients with longer-term psychological reactions to a trauma may present to the A&E department several months later. Following certain incidents, such as those involving a real or perceived chemical, radiological and biological threat, there may be an increase in A&E attenders who fear contamination, or present with medically unexplained symptoms.

As discussed above, universal counselling for victims of trauma is not appropriate. The availability of psychosocial support should be communicated to those involved and co-ordinated by the psychosocial response team. Early intervention research suggests that offering symptomatic individuals a brief cognitive behavioural intervention at a month after the disaster is probably the most appropriate intervention with the current evidence base.

REFERENCES

Adshead, G., Canterbury, R. and Rose, S. (1994). Current provision and recommendations for the management of psychosocial morbidity following a disaster in England. *Criminal Behaviour and Mental Health*, **4**, 181–208.

Andre, C., Lelord, F., Legeron, P., *et al.* (1997). Controlled study of outcomes after 6 months to early intervention of bus drivers of aggression. *Encephale*, **23**, 65−71.

Bisson, J. I., Jenkins, P. L., Alexandra, J., *et al.* (1997). Randomised controlled trial of psychological debriefing for victims of acute burn trauma. *British Journal of Psychiatry*, **171**, 78−81.

Bisson, J. I., Roberts, N. and Macho, G. (2003). The Cardiff traumatic stress initiative: an evidence-based approach to early psychological intervention following traumatic events. *Psychiatric Bulletin*, **27**, 145−7.

Bisson, J. I., Shepherd, J. P., Joy, D., *et al.* (2004). Early cognitive-behavioural therapy for post-traumatic stress disorder symptoms after physical injury. Randomised controlled trial. *British Journal of Psychiatry*, **184**, 63−9.

Bonanno, G. A. (2004). Loss, trauma, and human resilience. Have we underestimated the human capacity to thrive after extremely aversive events? *American Psychologist*, **59**, 20−8.

Bordow, S. and Porritt, D. (1979). An experimental evaluation of crisis intervention. *Social Science and Medicine*, **13**, 251−6.

Brewin, C. R., Andrews, B. and Valentine, J. D. (2000). Meta-analysis of risk factors for posttraumatic stress disorder in trauma-exposed adults. *Journal of Consulting and Clinical Psychology*, **68**, 748−66.

Brom, D., Kleber, R. J. and Hofman, M. C. (1994). Victims of traffic accidents: incidence and prevention of post-traumatic stress disorder. *Journal of Clinical Psychology*, **49**, 131−40.

Bryant, R. A., Harvey, A. G., Dang, S. T., *et al.* (1998). Treatment of acute stress disorder: a comparison of cognitive-behavioral therapy and supportive counselling. *Journal of Consulting and Clinical Psychology*, **66**, 862−6.

Bryant, R. A., Sackville, T., Dang, S. T., *et al.* (1999). Treating acute stress disorder: an evaluation of cognitive behavior therapy and supportive counselling techniques. *American Journal of Psychiatry*, **156**, 1780−6.

Bunn, T. and Clarke, A. (1979). Crisis intervention: an experimental study of the effects of a brief period of counselling on the anxiety of relatives of seriously injured or ill hospital patients. *British Journal of Medical Psychology*, **52**, 191−5.

Burns, T. and Hollins, S. C. (1991). Psychiatric response to the Clapham rail crash. *Journal of the Royal Society of Medicine*, **84**, 15−19.

Campfield, K. M. and Hills, A. M. (2001). Effect of timing of critical incident stress debriefing (CISD) on posttraumatic symptoms. *Journal of Traumatic Stress*, **14**, 327−40.

Conlon, L., Fahy, T. J. and Conroy, R. (1999). PTSD in Ambulant RTA Victims: A Randomized Controlled Trial of Debriefing. *Journal of Psychosomatic Research*, **46**, 37−44.

Galea, S., Ahern, J., Resnick, H., *et al.* (2002). Psychological sequelae of the September 11 terrorist attacks in New York City. *New England Journal of Medicine*, **346**, 982−7.

Galea, S., Vlahov, D., Resnick, H., *et al.* (2003). Trends of probable post-traumatic stress disorder in New York after the September 11 terrorist attacks. *American Journal of Epidemiology*, **158**, 514−24.

Gidron, Y., Gal, R., Freedman, S., *et al.* (2001). Translating research findings to PTSD prevention: results of a randomised controlled pilot study. *Journal of Traumatic Stress*, **14**, 773−80.

Guthrie, E., Wells, A. and Pilgrim, H. (1999). The Manchester bombing: providing a rational response. *Journal of Mental Health*, **8**, 149–57.

Hobbs, M., Mayou, R., Harrison, B., *et al.* (1997). A randomised trial of psychological debriefing for victims of road traffic accidents. *British Medical Journal*, **313**, 1438–9.

Home Office (1998). *Dealing with Disasters*. Livepool: Brodie Publishing.

Kessler, R. C., Sonnega, A., Bromet, E., *et al.* (1995). Post-traumatic stress disorder in the national comorbidity survey. *Archives of General Psychiatry*, **52**, 1048–60.

Lavender, T. and Walkinshaw, S. A. (1998). Can midwives reduce postpartum psychological morbidity? A randomized trial. *Birth*, **25**, 215–19.

Lee, C., Slade, P. and Lygo, V. (1996). The influence of psychological debriefing on emotional adaptation in women following early miscarriage: a preliminary study. *British Journal of Medical Psychology*, **69**, 47–58.

Mayou, R. A., Ehlers, A. and Hobbs, M. (2000). Psychological debriefing for road traffic accidents: three-year follow-up of a randomised controlled trial. *British Journal of Psychiatry*, **176**, 589–93.

Mellman, T. A., Bustamante, V., David, D., *et al.* (2002). Hypnotic medication in the aftermath of trauma. *Journal of Clinical Psychiatry*, **63**, 1183–4.

Mitchell, J. T. (1983). When disaster strikes . . . the critical incident debriefing process. *Journal of Emergency Medical Services*, **8**, 36–9.

North, C. S., Nixon, S. J., Shariat, S., *et al.* (1999). Psychiatric disorders among survivors of the Oklahoma City bombing. *Journal of the American Medical Association*, **282**, 755–62.

Ozer, E. J., Best, S. R., Lipsey, T. L., *et al.* (2002). Predictors of posttraumatic stress disorder and symptoms in adults: a meta-analysis. *Psychological Bulletin*, **129**, 52–73.

Pitman, R. K., Altman, B., Greenwald, E., *et al.* (1991). Psychiatric complications during flooding therapy for post-traumatic stress disorder. *Jounal of Clinical Psychiatry*, **52**, 17–20.

Pitman, R. K., Sanders, K. M., Zusman, R. M., *et al.* (2002). Pilot study of secondary prevention of posttraumatic stress disorder with propranolol. *Biological Psychiatry*, **51**, 189–92.

Rose, S., Brewin, C. R., Andrews, B., *et al.* (1999). A randomised controlled trial of individual psychological debriefing for victims of violent crime. *Psychological Medicine*, **29**, 793–9.

Rose, S., Bisson, J. and Wessely, S. (2003) A systematic review of single-session psychological interventions ('debriefing') following trauma. *Psychotherapy and Psychosomatics*, **72**, 176–84.

Schelling, G., Briegel, J., Roozendaal, B., *et al.* (2001). The effect of stress doses of hydrocortisone during septic shock on posttraumatic stress disorder in survivors. *Biological Psychiatry*, **50**, 978–85.

Small, R., Lumley, J., Donohue, L., *et al.* (2000). Midwife-led debriefing to reduce maternal depression following operative birth: a randomised controlled trial. *British Medical Journal*, **321**, 1043–47.

Stevens Hobbs, M. and Adshead, G. (1996). Preventive psychological intervention for road crash survivors. In *The Aftermath of Road Accidents: Psychological, Social and Legal Perspectives*, ed. M. Mitchell. London: Routledge, pp. 159–71.

Yule, W., Bolton, B., Udwin, O., *et al.* (2000). The long-term psychological effects of a disaster experienced in adolescence: I: the incidence and cause of PTSD. *Journal of Child Psychiatry and Psychiatry and Allied Disciplines*, **41**, 503–11.

Zatzick, D. F., Roy-Byrne, P., Russo, J. E., *et al.* (2001). Collaborative interventions for physically injured trauma survivors: a pilot randomized effectiveness trial. *General Hospital Psychiatry*, **23**, 114–23.

Other sources of information

More information on stress following a trauma is available on the following websites:

- UK Trauma Group: www.uktrauma.org.uk.
- European Society for Traumatic Stress Studies: www.estss.org.

More information on anxiety and depression and their treatment is available on the Royal College of Psychiatrists website: www.rcpsych.ac.uk.

Useful publications include:

- *Understanding Your Reactions to Trauma* by Claudia Herbert, which can be obtained from the Psychology Department, Warneford Hospital, Headington, Oxford OX3 7JX.
- *Overcoming Traumatic Stress* by Claudia Herbert and Ann Wetmore, published in 1999 by Robinson Publishing Limited.

Index

ABI *see* acquired brain injury
abnormal illness behaviour, psychological
    reactions to illness 79–80
abortion 650–1
academic issues 19–20
acne vulgaris 725
acquired brain injury (ABI) 332–7
  cognitive deficits 335
  emotional disorders 335
  executive dysfunction 336
  incidence 332
  outcomes 333, 334
  prognosis 336–7
  PTA 333–5
  severity measures 333
acute organic brain syndrome, legal issues 59
Addenbrooke's Cognitive Examination 314
adjustment difficulties
  diabetes 462–3
  physical illness 114, 115
  renal disease 514–15
adjustment disorder
  ICU 679–81, 685
  psychological reactions to illness 72
adolescents
  renal disease 521–2
  self-harm 251
  suicide 256
AED *see* antiepileptic drugs
affective dysprosodia, stroke 338
ageing effects
  delirium 271
  psychological reactions to illness 66–7
agnosia 313
AID *see* amputee identity disorder
AIDS *see* HIV infection
alcohol 149–64
  acamprosate 166–7
  alcohol-related diseases 149–52
  anxiety 156–7, 168–9
  benzodiazepines 159–60
  blood test markers 154–6

brief intervention (BI) 163–8, 171–2
CAGE screening questionnaire 153–4
cardiovascular service 169–70
children 294–5
chlordiazepoxide 159
clomethiazole 159
delirium tremens 282
dementia 329
dependence detection 152
dependence symptoms 153
depression 156–7
detection 152–7
diabetes 459
diagnosis 152–4
diazepam 159
disulfiram 167–8
emergency department (ED) 170–2
Fast Alcohol Screening Test (FAST) 155
first seizure in adulthood 172–3
FRAMES 164
haloperidol 159
hazardous drinking 151–4
head injury 169
head/neck cancer 566
HIV infection 485–6
injury 169
interventions 161–8
liver disease 421–3
medication 159–60
motivational interviewing 164–6
obstetric service 170
older people 173
opiate antagonists 167
organizational issues 173
physical signs 154
presentations 150–1
requests for 'drying out' 171
screening 153–4
sexual problems 237
treatment 162–3
vitamins 160–1, 282, 331
Wernicke's syndrome 160–1

alcohol (cont.)
  withdrawal 157–60, 200–1
  WKS 331
alopecia areata 726
amineptine
amnesia
  amnestic syndromes 331–2
  PTA 333–5
  TGA 332
amoxapine 774
amputee identity disorder (AID) 628
ancillary support, drug misuse 208
anorexia nervosa
  diabetes 458–9
  follow-up study 292–3
  legal issues 61
  psychological reactions to illness 78–9
anosagnosia, stroke 338
antidepressant drugs 768–76
  depression 197–8
  drug misuse 197–8
  fibromyalgia 537
  indications 776–7
  liver disorders 428
  pregnancy 775–6
  puerperium 775–6
  risks 774–5
  side-effects 774–5
  and women 660
antiepileptic drugs (AED) 352–3
  mood stabilizers 788–90
anxiety
  alcohol 156–7, 168–9
  cancer 556–7
  causes 93
  CHD 367–8
  children 293
  detection 91–4
  diabetes 459–60
  eliciting mood symptoms 92
  genitourinary disorders 740–1
  head/neck cancer 568, 575
  history 93–4
  HIV infection 484–5
  management 603–4
  palliative care 602–4
  Parkinson's disease 344
  physical illness 113
  pregnancy 648–9
  problem case 827–30
  psychological reactions to illness 65–6, 72–4
  renal disease 516
  stroke 340
  symptoms 93
  treatment 648–9
apathy, stroke 338
aphasia
  delirium 276
  stroke 338
apraxia 313
arithmetic, neurological disorders 312–13
assessment/intervention liaison service 36

asthma
  COPD 375–6
  panic disorder 379–80
  psychological illness 379–80
asylum psychiatrists (alienists), specialization
    beginnings 5
atopic dermatitis 727–8
attention, neurological disorders 309–10

back pain *see* chronic low back pain
BDD *see* body dysmorphic disorder
Beck Depression Inventory (BDI) 97
Beck Suicidal Intent Scale 255
behaviour, abnormal illness behaviour 79–80
behaviour changes, physical illness 114
benzodiazepines 791
  alcohol 159–60
  delirium 281–2
  drug misuse 198
  mood stabilizers 789–90
  symptoms 199
  withdrawal 199
bereavement, children 297–8
best interests
  see also capacity
  legal issues 55, 59, 61–2
bipolar disorder
  perinatal management 644–5
  pregnancy 642–5
  treatment 642–5
body dysmorphic disorder (BDD)
  CBT 627–8
  cosmetic procedures 620–8
  in cosmetic surgery clinics 623–6
  in psychiatric clinics 622–3
  psychocutaneous disorders 722–4
  screening 621
Bolam test, Common Law 56
Borderline Personality Disorder (BPD), childhood
    experiences 291
BR *see* breathing retraining
breathing disorders 380–3
breathing retraining (BR) 381–3
Brief Symptom Inventory (BSI) 97–8
Broca's dysphasia 311–12
BSI *see* Brief Symptom Inventory
bulimia
  diabetes 458–9
  psychological reactions to illness 78–9
bupropion 771
burn trauma 697–711
  delirium 707
  early intervention 707–8
  later intervention 708–9
  liaison service 709–11
  management 707–9
  predictors, psychological reactions 704–5
  prevalence, psychological symptoms
    699–701
  psychiatric sequelae 697–704
  relatives 706–7
  self-inflicted 705–6

burning mouth syndrome
  see also functional somatic syndromes
    treatment 140–1
business case, liaison service 42–4
buspirone, COPD 383

CAM *see* complementary and alternative medicine
cancer 547–61
  see also head/neckcancer
  anxiety 556–7
  CAM 561
  communication 553–4
  counselling 558–9
  delirium 556
  depression 560–1
  effects of treatment 549–50
  emotional support 557–8
  factors predisposing to psychiatric disorders
      548–55
  fertility 551
  gastrointestinal 408–10
  information provision 559
  management 556–61
  nature of the illness 548–9
  organic factors 551–2
  problem cases 827–30, 833–6
  prognosis influencing 555–6
  psychiatric disorders 556–61
  psychological therapies 559–60
  screening 554–5
  sexual problems 231–2, 551, 557
  stress 552–3
  suicide 557
  treatment effects 549–50
cannabis
  differential diagnosis 203
  pharmacotherapy 196–7
  symptoms 199
  treatment 203
  withdrawal 199
capacity
  see also best interests
  assessment 54, 606–7
  assumption 53
  Mental Capacity Act (2005) 56–8
  mental capacity assessment 606–7, 611
carbamazepine 788
cardiac rehabilitation (CR) 372–3
cardiorespiratory disorders 365–83
cardiovascular disorders 365–9
  see also coronary heart disease
  drug treatment 374–5
  sexual problems 230
care aspects, nursing 115
care planning, nursing 112–13
catastrophic reactions, stroke 341
causes
  anxiety 93
  depression 76
CBD *see* corticobasal degeneration
CBT *see* cognitive behaviour therapy
cerebellar dysfunction 317

cervical smear 658–9
CHD *see* coronary heart disease
child abuse 291–2
childhood experiences 290–9
  BPD 291
  FSS 133
childhood factors, frequent attendance 885–7
childhood influences 291–5
children
  adjustment 293–4
  alcohol 294–5
  anxiety disorders 293
  bereavement 297–8
  Common Law 54–5
  comorbidity 290–1
  current practice variation 18
  depression 290–1, 293
  depression, maternal 296–7
  drug misuse 209–10, 294–5
  eating disorders 292–3
  eating disorders, maternal 297
  HIV infection 295, 479
  implications for the adult liaison psychiatrist
      298–9
  mental health difficulties, parental 296–7
  parental influences 295–8
  physical illness 293–4
  physical illness, parental 295–6
  psychiatric disorders 292–5
  PTSD 293
  sexual abuse 291–2
  somatization 293–4
chorea 315
  Huntington's disease 323–4
chronic fatigue syndrome
  see functional somatic syndromes;
      persistent medically unexplained
      symptoms
  interventions 854–6
  treatment 139
chronic inflammatory skin disease 726–8
chronic low back pain (CLBP) 539
  depression 539–40
  psychological distress 539–40
  treatment 540–1
chronic obstructive airways disease, problem case
    819–22
chronic obstructive pulmonary disease (COPD)
    375–8
  asthma 375–6
  depression 378
  drug treatment 383
  psychological illness 376–7
chronic pancreatitis (CP) 405–7
CJD *see* Creutzfeldt−Jakob disease
CL *see* consultation-liaison psychiatry
CLBP *see* chronic low back pain
cognition-improving drugs 790–2
cognitive approaches, sexual problems 240
cognitive behaviour therapy (CBT)
  BDD 627–8
  HIV infection 494

cognitive behaviour therapy (CBT) (cont.)
  physical illness 810–12
  PMUS 855–6
  problem case 821–2
cognitive behavioural approach, drug misuse 207
common disorders, detection, psychiatric
    disorders 86–96
Common Law 52–6
  best interests 55
  Bolam test 56
  capacity assessment 54
  capacity assumption 53
  children 54–5
  duty of care 55
  necessity 51
  principles 53
communication
  cancer 553–4
  decision making 71
  dissatisfaction 70
  good 70
  liaison psychiatry 842–3
  physical illness 114, 116
  psychological reactions to illness 70–1
comorbidity
  children 290–1
  physical illness 113
  psychiatric disorder, FSS 131
comparisons, international 12–13
competencies, nursing 105–6
complementary and alternative medicine (CAM)
  cancer 561
  fibromyalgia 537
comprehensive liaison service 37–8
consent, guidance 56
consultation-liaison psychiatry (CL), development
  8–13
consultation models 15
consultee-oriented consultation 15
conversational model therapy 804
conversion/somatoform disorders 357–9
COPD see chronic obstructive pulmonary disease
coping strategies, psychological reactions to illness
  64–5
coronary heart disease (CHD) 365–6
  anxiety 367–8
  depression 366–8
  hostility 367
  psychosocial interventions 370–1
  psychosocial risk factors 366
  psychosocial work characteristics 368
  social support 368–9
  Type A behaviour (TAB) 367
corticobasal degeneration (CBD) 326
corticosteroid induced psychiatric syndromes, RA
  530
cosmetic procedures 617–26
  AID 628
  assessment 618–19, 626
  availability 617–19
  BDD 620–8
  body sculpting 628–9

  contraindications 619–21
  decision criteria 618–19
  DIY 625–7
  eating disorders 620
  psychosocial effects 619–22
cost effectiveness, liaison service 27
costs
  drug misuse 194–5
  self-harm 261–2
counselling
  cancer 558–9
  drug misuse 205–7
  HIV infection 494
  physical illness 799–800
CP see chronic pancreatitis
CR see cardiac rehabilitation
Creutzfeldt–Jakob disease (CJD) 326–7
crisis-oriented, therapeutic consultation 15
Crohn's disease 393–7
current practice variation 13–19
  children 18
  clinical methods 14–15
  clinical problem types 13, 14
  emergency department (ED) 17
  inpatients 16, 17
  other disciplines 18–19
  outpatients 16–17
  primary care 17–18
  service models 16
  settings 16–18
  sub-specialization 18
  trends 14

DALT see Drug and Alcohol Liaison Team
decision making, communication 71
delirium 270–8
  acute psychotic states 276
  aetiology 272
  ageing effects 271
  aphasia 276
  benzodiazepines 281–2
  burn trauma 707
  cancer 556
  causes 272
  causes, finding 279–80
  classification 277–9
  clinical features 272–7
  clinical management 279–84
  clonidine 282
  concept 270
  death risk 277
  defining 277
  delirium tremens 282
  delusions 274
  dementia 275–6, 318
  diagnosis 275–7
  diagnostic criteria 278
  differential diagnosis 275–7
  donepezil 282
  ECT 282
  EEG abnormalities 275
  endogenous causes 273

environmental interventions 282–3
epidemiology 270–2
exogenous causes 273
hallucinations 274
haloperidol 280–1
HIV infection 272
ICU 676–9
immunology 282
liaison issues 283–4
management 605
medications 273, 280
mood disturbances 274–5
morbidity 277
neurological symptoms 275
neurovegetative symptoms 275
non-pharmacological interventions 282–3
older people 271
outcomes 276–7
palliative care 604–5
phenothiazines 281
physostigmine 282
pre-existing brain condition 271
prevention 279
prognosis 272–7
psychomotor disturbances 274
psychopharmacological intervention
    280–2
risk factors 270–2
sleep–wake cycle 274
stroke 337
surgery 271
therapeutic issues 279–84
demand estimation, liaison service 27–34
dementia 318–30
alcohol 329
atypical 322
causes 320–1
causes, reversible 322
CBD 326
CJD 326–7
cortical vs. subcortical 319
delirium 275–6, 318
diagnosis 318–19, 325
DLB 343
FTDs 325–6
HIV infection 482
Huntington's disease 323–4
infective 326–7
inflammatory 327–8
inherited 323–5
investigations 319–23
leucodystrophies 325
miscellaneous causes 329
neoplastic 328
OSA 329
palliative care 605–6
Pick's disease 325–6
primary degenerative 325–6
pseudodementia 329–30
PSP 326
reversible causes 322
structural 328

subcortical vs. cortical 319
traumatic 328
vitamins 329
Wilson's disease (hepatolenticular
    degeneration) 324
dementia with Lewy bodies (DLB) 343
depression
    see also antidepressant drugs
    alcohol 156–7
    cancer 560–1
    causes 75
    CHD 366–8
    children 290–1, 293
    CLBP 539–40
    COPD 378
    detection, psychiatric disorders 86–91
    diabetes 456–8
    diagnosis 598–9
    diagnostic criteria 90
    differential diagnosis 599
    drug misuse 197–8
    ECT 777
    eliciting mood symptoms 87
    epilepsy 352–3
    HADS 94, 97, 568
    head/neck cancer 568, 575, 581
    HIV infection 484
    ICU 674–5, 685–6
    impact 600
    liver disorders 418–19
    medications 89
    MI 369–70
    myths 87–8
    palliative care 597–602
    Parkinson's disease 343–4
    perinatal management 640–1
    physical illness 74–7, 88–91, 113–14
    pregnancy 638–42
    prevalence, advanced disease 599–600
    problem case 827–30
    prognosis 600
    psychological reactions to illness 74–7
    psychotherapy 602
    psychotropic drugs 601–2
    RA 528–32
    recognition 599
    renal disease 512–14
    screening 599
    stress 89
    stroke 338–9
    symptoms 76, 90–1
    treatment 600–2
dermatitis artefacta 718–19
dermatological disorders see psychocutaneous
    disorders
detection, psychiatric disorders 83–98
    anxiety 91–4
    clinical skills 83–6
    common disorders 86–96
    depression 86–91
    psychosis 95–6
    questionnaires 94, 96–8

diabetes 454–67
    adjustment difficulties 462–3
    alcohol 459
    anxiety 459–60
    clinical features 454–5
    depression 456–8
    drug misuse 459
    eating disorders 458–9
    family factors 463
    health beliefs 463
    hypoglycaemia fear 462
    interventions 464–6
    personality disorders 461
    pharmacological interventions 464
    psychiatric disorders 456–61
    psychological problems 462–3
    psychotherapy 464–6
    psychotic disorders 460–1
    self-harm 463
    sexual problems 230–1
diagnosis consequences, physical illness 113–14
diagnostic criteria, depression 90
disability, defining 306
disaster planning 896–911
    aftermath 907–8
    emergency plans 896–7
    general hospital plan 904
    immediate psychosocial response 906–7
    information sources 911
    interventions 899–903
    medications 903
    planning services 904–8
    prevalence, psychiatric disorders 897–8
    PTSD 897–903
DLB see dementia with Lewy bodies
doctor−patient relationship, FSS 131–2
Drug and Alcohol Liaison Team (DALT) 214
drug misuse 180–215
    abstinence syndromes 198–205
    accident and emergency units 185
    acute general medical settings 185–6
    acutely disturbed patients 201–3
    addiction, pharmacotherapy for 196–7
    Addicts Index 187
    alcohol withdrawal syndromes 200–1
    ancillary support 208
    antidepressant drugs 197–8
    antipsychotics 197
    assessment 188–93
    benzodiazepines 198
    cannabis differential diagnosis 203
    cannabis pharmacotherapy 196–7
    cannabis treatment 203
    children 209–10, 294–5
    classes, Misuse of Drugs Act (1971) 212
    classification 181
    cognitive behavioural approach 207
    compulsory treatment 211
    convulsions 201
    costs 194–5
    counselling 205–7
    criteria 182–3
DALT 214
dependence syndrome 183
depression 197–8
diabetes 459
diagnosis 181, 203–5
differential diagnosis 203–5
emergency department (ED) 752–3
epidemiology 182–4
evidence base 194–6
family therapy 207
group therapies 207–8
hallucinogens differential diagnosis 203
hallucinogens treatment 203
health care professionals 209
HIV infection 485–6
liaison team 214
Misuse of Drugs Regulations (2001) 213
morbidity 182–4
mortality 182
motivational interviewing 206–7
obstetric units 187–8
older people 210–11
opiate abstinence syndrome 198–200
opiates pharmacotherapy 196
outcome research 194–6
paediatric units 187–8
pain management 205
pharmacotherapy for addiction 196–7
phencyclidine differential diagnosis 204
phencyclidine treatment 204
planning services 214
police liaison 211
policy initiatives 180
pregnant users 208–9
prevalence 185–8
psychiatric disorders and drug treatment 197–8
psychiatric patients 186–7
psychological interventions 205–7
questions 189–92
residential treatments 207–8
sedative abstinence syndrome 200
sedatives differential diagnosis 204–5
sedatives treatment 204–5
self-harm 184
service delivery framework 188
severe mental illness 194
social network behaviour therapy 207
solvents differential diagnosis 205
solvents treatment 205
special groups 208
stimulants differential diagnosis 203–4
stimulants pharmacotherapy 196–7
stimulants treatment 203–4
suicide prevention 184
symptoms 181, 199
treatment 203–5
twelve-step programmes 207–8
withdrawal 198–205
drugs
    and women 660
    overdoses 681–2
    pharmacodynamics 763–764

pharmacogenetics 767
pharmacokinetics 765–7
psychotropic drugs 764, 767–76
selection principles 764
drugs, recreational, sexual problems 237
dying/death
    see also palliative care
    HIV infection 479
dyskinesias, neurological examination 315
dyspepsia, functional 397–405
    diagnosis 399
dysphasias 311–12
    classification 312
dyspraxia 313
dystonias 315, 354–5

eating disorders
    see also anorexia nervosa; bulimia
    BDD 620
    children 292–3
    cosmetic procedures 620
    diabetes 458–9
ECT see electroconvulsive treatment
Ekbom's disease 715–17
elderly see older people
electroconvulsive treatment (ECT), depression
    777
elements, liaison service 33–4
eliciting mood symptoms
    anxiety 92
    depression 87
    panic disorder 92
emergency department (ED) 764–5
    alcohol 170–2
    clinical skills 753–5
    current practice variation 17
    drug misuse 752–3
    epidemiology 763–7
    management 755–8
    outcomes 758–60
    presentations 752–3
    resourcing 755–8
emotionalism, stroke 340
endocrine disorders 432–49
    acromegaly 449
    Addison's disease 435, 437, 439, 447–8
    clinical aspects 433–9
    clinical relevance, psychiatric syndromes 434–5
    correlation, biochemical variables 436–7
    Cushing's syndrome 435, 437, 439, 445–7
    diabetes 434
    epidemiology 432–3
    hyperparathyroidism 434, 439, 442–4
    hyperprolactinaemia 435, 437, 439, 445
    hyperthyroidism 436, 439, 441–2
    hypoparathyroidism 435, 439, 444–5
    hypothyroidism 434, 439–41
    phaeochromocytoma 448–9
    prevalence, psychiatric disorders 436–7
    prevalence, psychiatric syndromes 434–5
    problem case 833–6
    somatic symptoms 439

epilepsy 346–53
    absence seizures 348–9
    antiepileptic drugs (AED) 352–3, 788–90
    complex partial seizures 348
    depression 352–3
    EEG 351
    etiology 346–7
    incidence 346
    NEAD 349–51
    partial seizures 347
    prevalence 346
    pseudo seizures 349–51
    psychiatric aspects 351–3
    psychogenic 349–51
    tonic-clonic seizures 347
euthanasia
    legal issues 58, 609
    palliative care 609–11
executive function
    neurological disorders 311
    stroke 341
expanded psychiatric consultation 15
'expert patients' 66
extrapyramidal signs 317
eye movement abnormalities 315–16

factitious disorders, problem case 839–41
family therapy, drug misuse 207
Fast Alcohol Screening Test (FAST) 155
fatigue
    see also functional somatic syndromes;
        persistent medically unexplained
        symptoms
    chronic fatigue syndrome 139
    interventions 854–6
    liver disorders 418
    multiple sclerosis 345–6
    problem case 836–9
fertility
    cancer 551
    treatment 636–7
fibromyalgia 533–8
    see also functional somatic syndromes
    aetiology 534–5
    antidepressant drugs 537
    CAM 537
    clinical features 533
    clinical management 536–8
    course 534
    diagnosis 533
    prevalence 533–4
    problem case 822–4
    psychiatric disorders 535–6
    treatment 139–40
finance see funding issues
focus of care 15
foetal anomaly 651
frequent attendance 871–92
    childhood adversity 885–6
    childhood factors 885–7
    childhood illness experience 886–7
    concepts 871–2

frequent attendance (cont.)
  definitions 871–2
  interventions 889–92
  models of attendance 887–9
  outcomes 884–5
  physical illness 880–1
  prevalence 872–5
  psychiatric disorders 877–9
  psychiatric morbidity 872–80
  psychosocial factors 881–3
  qualitative models 888–9
  quantitative models 887–8
  resource use 883–4
  sociodemographic factors 872–5
  theoretical models 888–9
frontal lobe disorders 311
frontal release signs 316
frontotemporal dementias (FTDs) 325–6
FSS *see* functional somatic syndromes
FTDs *see* frontotemporal dementias
functional gastrointestinal disorders 397–405
functional somatic syndromes (FSS) 125–41
  aetiology 132–8
  central dysfunction 136–7
  childhood experiences 133
  comorbid psychiatric disorder 131
  conceptual issues 125–32
  deconditioning 135
  defining 125
  doctor–patient relationship 131–2
  epidemiology 129–30
  five-factor model 127–8
  gender 130–1
  genetics 132–3
  heterogeneity 128
  illness beliefs 137–8
  infection 134
  injury 134
  maintaining factors 134–8
  neuroendocrine changes 135
  precipitating factors 134
  predisposing factors 132–3
  social factors 138
  by specialities 126
  stress 134
  symptom amplification 137–8
  symptomatic overlap 127–9
  symptoms 126–7
  terminology 125
  treatment 139
funding issues
  cost effectiveness 27
  liaison service 40–2

gabapentin 789
gait
  abnormalities 315
  neurological examination 314
gastrointestinal disorders 390–2
  abuse 403
  cancer 408–10
  CP 405–7

functional 397–405
GORD 397
IBS 140, 397–405
inflammatory bowel disease 393–7
palliative care 409–10
pathophysiological mechanisms 401
peptic ulcer disease 390–2
prevalence 399–400
psychological factors 401–4
reviews 405
Rome criteria 397–9
stomas 407–8
stress 401
treatment 404–5
gastro-oesophageal reflux disease (GORD) 397
GCS *see* Glasgow Coma Scale
gender reassignment, problem case 841–2
genetics, FSS 132–3
genitourinary disorders 733–6
  affective illnesses 739–40
  anxiety 740–1
  assault 742–3
  clinical recommendations 748–9
  epidemiology 744–5
  explanations/aetiology of psychological distress
    743–7
  herpes genitalis 746–7
  historical perspective 733–5
  hypochondriacal disorders 740–1
  illness behaviour 744
  personality disorders 742
  prevalence of psychiatric morbidity in GUM
    clinics 735–7
  prevalence, psychiatric problems 763–92
  psychotic illnesses 737–9
  qualitative studies 745
  recognition, psychological distress 747–8
  referrals 747–8
  sexual dysfunction 742–3
  sexual risk taking behaviour 745–6
  somatoform/conversion disorders 740–1
  syphilophobia 733–5
Gilles de la Tourette's syndrome (GTS) 353–4
Glasgow Coma Scale (GCS) 309, 310
  ABI 333
GORD *see* gastro-oesophageal reflux disease
group therapies, drug misuse 207–8
GTS *see* Gilles de la Tourette's syndrome
gynaecological disorders 632–45

HADS *see* Hospital Anxiety and Depression Scale
hallucinogens
  differential diagnosis 203
  treatment 203
haloperidol
  alcohol 159
  delirium 280–1
handicap, defining 306
head injury
  see also acquired brain injury
  alcohol 169
  outcomes 334

head/neck cancer 564–76
  alcohol 566
  anxiety 568, 575
  appearance 578–9
  chemoprevention 566
  depression 568, 575, 581
  diagnosis, psychological morbidity 567–9
  diet 566
  HADS 568
  high-risk behaviour 576–7
  information provision 572–3
  investigations 565
  moderators, psychological distress 569
  oral hygiene 567
  prevention 566
  psychological interventions 580–2
  psychological morbidity 567–9
  public health issues 565–7
  quality of life studies 569–72
  recurrence fears 573–5
  recurrence reactions 577–8
  risk factors 566–7
  screening for depression 581
  self-care behaviour 575–6
  sexual practices 567
  smoking 576–7
  social support 579–80
  statistics 564
  tobacco 566
  treatment 565
  treatment, psychological morbidity 567–9
headache 355–7
  cervicogenic 356
  chronic 355–6
  cluster 356–7
  migraine 355
  SAH 355
heart disease *see* coronary heart disease
heart transplantation, psychiatric aspects 375
hepatic encephalopathy 417–8
hepatitis 419–20
hepatolenticular degeneration 324
herpes genitalis 746–7
HIV infection 474–95
  adverse effects, medication 491
  affective disorders 484
  alcohol 485–6
  alternative medications 490
  anticonvulsants 491
  antipsychotics 490–1
  anxiety 484–5
  anxiolytics 491
  assessment 486–7
  biological aspects 475
  CBT 494
  children 295, 479
  clinical presentations, psychiatric illnesses 476
  cognitive impairment 483
  counselling 494
  delirium 272
  dementia 482
  depression 484

  drug misuse 485–6
  dying/death 479
  epidemiology, psychiatric morbidity 474–6
  general management 487
  interactions, drug 491–3
  landmark events 476
  lifestyle issues 485
  mania 484
  models of care 495
  monoamine oxidase inhibitors 488
  mood stabilizers 491
  neuropsychiatric disorders 480–3
  older people 480
  opportunistic infections 477–8
  organic disorders 480–3
  outcomes 495
  personality issues 485
  pharmacotherapy 487–91
  physical treatments 487
  problem case 830–3
  professionals involved 487
  prognosis 495
  psychiatric disorders 481
  psychological aspects 475
  psychological treatments 492–4
  psychosis 483–4
  psychotherapy 494
  sexual problems 235
  side-effects, medication 489
  social aspects 475
  social interventions 494–5
  SSRIs 488–90
  suicide 486
  test notification 476–7
  treatment 486–95
  tricyclic antidepressants 488
hormone replacement therapy (HRT) 657–8
Hospital Anxiety and Depression Scale (HADS)
  94
  head/neck cancer 568
HPV *see* human papilloma virus
HRT *see* hormone replacement therapy
human papilloma virus (HPV) 658–9
Huntington's disease 323–4
Hypericum perforatum (St John's wort) 774
hypertension 373–4
hyposexuality, stroke 341

IBS *see* irritable bowel syndrome
ICU *see* intensive care unit
impairment, defining 306
inflammatory bowel disease 393–7
information gathering skills 83–4
information provision
  cancer 559
  head/neck cancer 572–3
information sources
  disaster planning 911
  PTSD 911
inpatients
  current practice variation 16
  liaison service 37

intensive care unit (ICU) 673–92
  adjustment disorder 679–81, 685
  approaches, psychiatric liaison 691–2
  delirium 676–9
  depression 674–5, 685–6
  discharge 684–9
  epidemiology 674–6
  ICU psychosis 682–3
  ICU syndrome 682–3
  mechanical ventilation 683–4
  neurocognitive deficits 688–9
  overdoses 681–2
  psychiatric reactions 676–82
  PTSD 675–6, 686–8
  quality of life studies 676
  relatives' distress 690–1
  sedatives 680
  staff psychiatric problems 689–90
  stress 679–81
  suicide 681–2
interactions, drug 91, 491–3
  neuroleptics 781
international comparisons 12–13
interpersonal therapy (IPT) 803
intervention
  liaison service 36
  nursing 114–15
  physical illness 118
interviewing patients
  see also motivational interviewing
  single item screening interview 98
  skills 84–5
IPT *see* interpersonal therapy
irritable bowel syndrome (IBS) 397–405
  see also functional somatic syndromes
  diagnosis 399
  treatment 140

job descriptions, liaison service 39–40
job plans, liaison service 39–40

lamotrigine 789
language, neurological disorders 311–12
legal issues 47–58
  acute organic brain syndrome 59
  anorexia nervosa 61
  best interests 55, 59, 61–2
  clinical situations 58–62
  Common Law 52–6
  euthanasia 58, 609
  Mental Capacity Act (2005) 56–8
  MHA 47–52
  schizophrenia 61
  self-harm 59–61
  Statute Law 47–8
  treatment refusal 47–58
leucodystrophies 325
liaison psychiatry
  defining 3
  role 3

liaison service
  assessment/intervention 36
  business case 42–4
  comprehensive 37–8
  cost effectiveness 27
  demand estimation 27–34
  discussions 26–7
  elements 33–4
  establishing 24–33
  funding issues 40–2
  initial negotiations 25–7
  job descriptions 39–40
  job plans 39–40
  limited 38
  location 34
  management issues 40–2
  models 16, 34–7
  multidisciplinary team 38–9
  personnel 25–6
  preparatory work 25–7
  referrals 27–34
  restricted/unrestricted 35
  size/workload 11
  types 16, 34–7
liaison team, drug misuse 214
limbs, neurological examination 314–15
limited liaison service 38
lithium 787–8
liver disorders 416–29
  alcoholic liver disease 421–3
  antidepressant drugs 428
  antipsychotics 428–9
  anxiolytics 429
  chronic hepatocerebral degeneration 419
  cirrhosis 420–1
  depression 418–19
  fatigue 418
  hepatic encephalopathy 417–18
  hepatitis 419–20
  hepatolenticular degeneration 324
  hypnotics 429
  liver transplantation 424–7
  primary biliary cirrhosis 420–1
  psychiatric symptoms 416–19
  psychotropic drugs 427–9
  Wilson's disease (hepatolenticular
    degeneration) 324, 423–4
location, liaison service 34
lower motor neurone signs 317

malformed infants 652
management issues, liaison service 40–2
MAOI *see* monoamine oxidase inhibitors
MDP *see* monosymptomatic delusion of
    parasitosis
medically unexplained symptoms (MUS) 847–64
  see also persistent medically unexplained
    symptoms
memory, neurological disorders 310–1
menopause 653–5

menstrual disturbances 655
menstruation 633–6
Mental Capacity Act (2005) 56–8
Mental Health Act (1983) (MHA) 47–52
    holding orders 49–50
    managerial arrangements 52
    place of safety orders 51–2
    police 51–2
    role 48–9
    section 63; 25–6
mental health liaison nurse (MHLN) 102–19
    see also nursing
mental state examination
    sexual problems 226
    skills 86
mentoring 842–3
MHA see Mental Health Act (1983)
MHLN see mental health liaison nurse
MI see myocardial infarction
migraine see headache
Mini-Mental State Examination (MMSE) 275,
    309–10, 313–14
minors see children
mirtazapine (Remergil®) 772–3
miscarriage 650–1
Misuse of Drugs Act (1971), classes
Misuse of Drugs Regulations (2001), schedules
    213
MMSE see Mini-Mental State Examination
    models
    consultation 15
    liaison service 16
monoamine oxidase inhibitors 773–4
monosymptomatic delusion of parasitosis (MDP)
    715–17
mood disorders
    postnatal 652–3
    pregnancy 638–42
mood disturbances
    delirium 274–5
    multiple sclerosis 345
    Parkinson's disease 344
mood stabilizers 787–8
    HIV infection 491
motivational interviewing
    alcohol 164–6
    drug misuse 206–7
multidisciplinary team, liaison service 38–9
multiple sclerosis 344–6
    cognitive impairment 345
    fatigue 345–6
    mood disturbances 345
    pain 346
    problem case 824–7
MUS see medically unexplained symptoms
musculo-skeletal disorders 527–41
    CLBP 539
    fibromyalgia 533–8
    OA 538–9
    RA 527–33

myocardial infarction (MI)
    advice 371–2
    depression 369–70
    health beliefs 371
myoclonus 315
myths, depression 87–8

NARIs see selective noradrenaline reuptake
    inhibitors
narratives, patient 799
NEAD see non-epileptic attack disorder
nervous disorder, specialization beginnings 5–6
neuroleptic malignant syndrome (NMS) 784–5
neuroleptics 777–87
    choosing 778–80
    DA-antagonistic effects 779
    dose 780–1
    indications 778
    interactions, drug 781
    liaison settings 786–7
    longer term effects
    NMS 784–5
    pregnancy 785
    puerperium 785
    side-effects 781–5
neurological disorders 305–59
    ABI 332–7
    amnestic syndromes 331–2
    clinical assessment 306–18
    conversion/somatoform disorders 357–9
    dementias 318–30
    dystonias 354–5
    epilepsy 346–53
    headache 355–7
    multiple sclerosis 344–6
    Parkinson's disease 342–4
    sexual problems 231
    somatoform/conversion disorders 357–9
    stroke 337–42
    tic disorders 353–4
neurological examination 314–15
neuropsychiatric history 307–9
NMS see neuroleptic malignant syndrome
non-epileptic attack disorder (NEAD) 349–51
NRIs see selective noradrenaline reuptake
    inhibitors
nursing 102–19
    activities 106
    aims 104–5
    assessment 115
    care aspects 115
    care planning 112–13
    competencies 105–6
    development 103–4
    focus of clinical practice 107–13
    holistic approach 103–4
    intervention point 114–15
    physical illness 113–15
    practice 104–15
    practice domains 106–7

nursing (cont.)
  rehabilitation 114–15
  risk assessment 110–13
  role 102–19
  self-harm 107–10
  skills 105–6
  suicide prevention 107–10
  suicide risk assessment 114

OA *see* osteoarthritis
obsessive-compulsive disorder (OCD), stroke 341
obstructive sleep apnoea (OSA) 329
OCD *see* obsessive-compulsive disorder
olanzapine 783
older people
  alcohol 173
  delirium 271
  drug misuse 210–11
  HIV infection 480
  self-harm 257
  suicide 257
oncology *see* cancer
opiates
  abstinence syndrome 198–200
  antagonists, alcohol 167
  pharmacotherapy 196
  symptoms 199
  withdrawal 199
orientation, neurological disorders 309
OSA *see* obstructive sleep apnoea
osteoarthritis (OA) 538–9
outpatients, current practice variation 16–17

Paediatric Autoimmune
    Neuropsychiatric Disorders associated
    with Streptococcal Infection (PANDAS)
    353–4
palliative care 592–608
  anxiety 602–4
  assessment 596–7
  context 592–3
  delirium 604–5
  dementia 605–6
  depression 597–602
  disturbed behaviour 604–6
  Endicott substitution criteria 598
  euthanasia 609–11
  gastrointestinal disorders 409–10
  history 596–7
  Kübler–Ross model 594
  mental capacity assessment 606–7, 611
  models of coping 593–6
  presentations 597
  psychotic illness 606
  referrals 596
  self-harm 607–9
  spirituality 610
  stages of dying 594
  suicide 607–9
  task-based models 594–6
  will-to-live changes 609–10

pancreatitis, chronic 405–7
PANDAS *see* Paediatric Autoimmune
    Neuropsychiatric Disorders associated with
    Streptococcal Infection
panic disorder
  asthma 379–80
  eliciting mood symptoms 92
  psychological reactions to illness 73
paranoid traits, psychological reactions to illness
    66
Parkinson's disease 342–4
  anxiety 344
  depression 343–4
  features 342
  incidence 342
  mood disturbances 344
patient-centred care, PMUS 849–51
patient narratives, physical illness 799
patient-oriented consultation 15
PCOS *see* polycystic ovary syndrome
pelvic pain 656–7
peptic ulcer disease 390–2
perception, neurological disorders 313
perinatal disorders 632–45
persistent medically unexplained
    symptoms (PMUS) 847–64
  see also somatoform/conversion disorders
  CBT 855–6
  criteria 848
  exercise 854–5
  interventions 854–6
  links 857
  observational studies 852–3
  outcomes 852
  patient-centred care 849–51
  primary care 849–51, 854–6, 863–4
  reattribution 856–64
  routine care 851
  symptom beliefs 852–3
  working models 849–51
personality disorders
  diabetes 461
  genitourinary disorders 742
phencyclidine
  differential diagnosis 204
  treatment 204
phenothiazines, delirium 281
phobic anxiety disorder, psychological reactions
    to illness 73
physical illness
  adjustment difficulties 114, 115
  anxiety 113
  assessment 116
  behaviour changes 114
  CBT 804–9
  comorbidity 113
  cognitive factors 807
  communication 114, 116
  depression 74–7, 88–91, 113–14
  diagnosis consequences 113–14
  frequent attendance 880–1
  intervention 118

nursing 113–15
  preventive psychological care 116–17
  psychiatric disorders following 72–80
  psychological interventions 795–812
  SCTF 796
  stress 114
  suicide risk assessment 91, 114
  supportive techniques 798–801
  therapeutic alliance 796
physician-assisted suicide 609–11
Pick's disease 325–6
planning services, drug misuse 214
PMDD see premenstrual dysphoric disorder
PMUS see persistent medically unexplained
    symptoms
police liaison, drug misuse 211
polycystic ovary syndrome (PCOS) 655–6
post-traumatic amnesia (PTA) 333–5
post-traumatic stress disorder (PTSD)
  children 293
  disaster planning 897–903
  ICU 675–6, 686–8
  information sources 911
  psychological reactions to illness 73–4
postnatal mood disorders 652–3
practice domains, nursing 106–7
practice variation see current practice variation
praxis 313
pregnancy 637–8
  antidepressant drugs 775–6
  anxiety 648–9
  bipolar disorder 642–5
  depression 638–42
  mood disorders 638–42
  neuroleptics 785
  schizophrenia 646–8
  teenage 649–50
  violence 650
pregnant users, drug misuse 208–9
premenstrual dysphoric disorder (PMDD) 634–6
  criteria 634
  symptoms 634
  treatment 635–6
preventive psychological care
  physical illness 116–17
  suicide prevention 107–10
previous psychiatric illness, psychological
    reactions to illness 71–2
primary care
  current practice variation 17–18
  PMUS 849–51, 854–6, 863, 864
problem cases 818–43
  anxiety 827–30
  cancer 827–30, 833–6
  chronic obstructive airways disease 819–22
  depression 827–30
  endocrine disorders 833–6
  factitious disorders 839–41
  fatigue 836–9
  fibromyalgia 822–4
  gender reassignment 841–2
  HIV infection 830–3

multiple sclerosis 824–7
  self-harm 822–4
  somatoform/conversion disorders 824–7, 836–9
problem-solving therapy (PST), physical illness
    800–1
progressive supranuclear palsy (PSP) 326
pruritus 720–2, 724–5
pseudodementia 329–30
psoriasis 726–7
PSP see progressive supranuclear palsy
PST see problem-solving therapy
psychiatric patients, drug misuse 186–7
psychocutaneous disorders 714–29
  acne vulgaris 725
  alopecia areata 726
  BDD 722–4
  chronic inflammatory skin disease 726–8
  dermatitis artefacta 718–19
  dermatological disorders affected by
      psychological factors 724–8
  Ekbom's disease 715–17
  MDP 715–17
  pruritus 720–2, 724–5
  psoriasis 726–7
  psychogenic parasitosis 714–5
  psychogenic purpura syndromes 725–6
  psychological reactions 728–9
  self-inflicted skin disorders 717–22
  trichotillomania 722
  urticarias 724–5
psychodynamic interpersonal therapy 804
psychodynamic therapy 802–3
psychogenic parasitosis 714–15
psychogenic purpura syndromes 725–6
psychological interventions
  drug misuse 205–7
  head/neck cancer 580–2
  physical illness 795–812
  principles 795–8
  relational therapies 801–4
  supportive techniques 798–801
psychological reactions to illness 64–81
  abnormal illness behaviour 79–80
  adjustment disorder 72
  ageing effects 66–7
  anxiety 65–6, 72–4
  communication 70–1
  depression 74–7
  drug treatment 68–9
  eating disorders 78–9
  'expert patients' 66
  factors influencing 65–72
  minimizing the significance 66
  nature of the illness 67
  paranoid traits 66
  personal factors 65–7
  physical factors 69
  previous psychiatric illness 71–2
  psychotic reactions 77
  sexual dysfunction 77–8
  special procedures 68
  stress 71–2

psychological reactions to illness (cont.)
    terminal illness 67
    treatment environment 68
psychopharmacological treatment
psychosis
    detection 95–6
    HIV infection 483–4
    stroke 341
psychosomatic medicine, development 7
psychotic disorders, diabetes 460–1
psychotic reactions, psychological reactions to
    illness 77
psychotropic drugs 764, 767–76
PTA *see* post-traumatic amnesia
PTSD *see* post-traumatic stress disorder
puerperium
    antidepressant drugs 775–6
    neuroleptics 785
pyramidal signs 316

questionnaires
    see also information gathering skills
    BDI 97
    BSI 97–8
    detection, psychiatric disorders 96–8
    HADS 94, 97, 568
    SCL-90 97–8
    SF36 and SF12 98
    single item screening interview 98

RA *see* rheumatoid arthritis
reactions to illness, psychological *see* psychological
    reactions to illness
reattribution
    PMUS 856–64
    techniques 801
referrals
    criteria 37–8
    genitourinary disorders 747–8
    liaison service 27–34
    palliative care 596
    rates 28–33
refusal, treatment *see* treatment refusal
rehabilitation, nursing 114–15
relational therapies, physical illness 801–4
renal disease 506–22
    adjustment difficulties 514–15
    adolescents 521–2
    advice sources 517
    anxiety 516
    depression 512–14
    dialysis 507–9
    family factors 511–12
    healthcare limitations awareness 511
    loss
    mortality awareness 510–11
    non-adherence 520–1
    organic disorders 515–16
    overview, renal medicine 506–7
    pharmacotherapy 517–19
    prescribing rules 518
    psychiatric disorders 512–16

psychological issues 509–12
    psychological themes 509
    psychosocial interventions 519–20
    psychotropic drugs 517
    transplantation 507–9
    treatment 516–20
    triggers 509
    uncertainty 510
repetitive strain injury
    see also functional somatic syndromes
    treatment 140
research 19
residential treatments, drug misuse 207–8
respiratory disorders 375–83
    asthma 375–6, 379–80
    breathing disorders 380–3
    COPD 375–8
    OSA 329, 380
restricted/unrestricted liaison service 35
reversible and selective inhibition of monoamine
    oxidase type A (RIMA) 773
rheumatoid arthritis (RA) 527–33
    aetiological factors, psychiatric disorders
        528–30
    assessment, psychiatric disorders 531–2
    corticosteroid-induced psychiatric syndromes
        530
    depression 528–9
    impact, psychiatric illness 530–2
    neuroticism 529–30
    pain 528
    prevalence, psychiatric disorders 528
    social stress 529
    social support 529
    treatment, psychiatric disorders 531–3
    treatments problems 530
RIMA *see* reversible and selective inhibition of
    monoamine oxidase type A
risk assessment
    see also suicide risk assessment
    attitudes 111
    nursing 110–13
    principles 110–11
roles
    liaison psychiatry 3
    MHA 48–9
    nursing 102–19

SAH *see* subarachnoid haemorrhage
schizophrenia
    legal issues 61
    pregnancy 646–8
    suicide 250
    treatment 647–8
SCL-90 37–8 *see* Symptom Checklist 90
SCTF *see* specific Common Therapeutic
    Factors
sedatives
    abstinence syndrome 200
    differential diagnosis 204–5
    ICU 680
    treatment 204–5

selective noradrenaline reuptake
  inhibitors (NARIs or NRIs) 770
selective serotonin reuptake inhibitors (SSRIs)
  770
self-harm 245–62
  see also suicide
  adolescents 251, 256
  aetiological models 251–3
  aetiology 248–53
  assessment 254–7
  assessment topics 254
  burn trauma 705–6
  costs 261–2
  defining 245
  diabetes 463
  drug misuse 184
  epidemiology 246–7
  frequent repeaters 257
  general population 250–1
  guidelines 257–8
  hospital management 258–9
  legal issues 59–61
  long-term outcome 261
  mentally ill 256–7
  motives 255
  nursing 107–10
  older people 257
  palliative care 607–9
  problem case 822–4
  psychological models 253
  reasons 255
  repetition risk factors 256
  risk factors 250–1
  services 257–8
  suicide links 247–8, 255
  treatment interventions 259–60
self-inflicted skin disorders 717–22
sensory signs 317–18
serotonergic syndrome 765
serotonin and noradrenaline reuptake inhibitors
  (SNARIs) 770–1
service, liaison *see* liaison service
sexual abuse, children 291–2
sexual desire disorders 659–60
sexual dysfunction 659
  genitourinary disorders 742–3
  psychological reactions to illness 77–8
sexual problems 221–40
  aetiology, medical vs. psychological 229–30
  alcohol 237
  anatomy 221–2
  apomorphine 239
  arousal 223
  assessment 223–6, 228
  cancer 231–2, 551, 557
  cardiovascular disorders 230
  classification 222–3
  cognitive approaches 240
  contraceptive history 225
  current sexual preferences/practices 225
  current sexual relationship 224
  desire 223, 659–60

diabetes 230–1
drugs, prescribed 233–5
drugs, recreational 237
family environment 225
gender reassignment 841–2
genital and reproductive organs 232–3
HIV infection 235
hormone levels 237–8
hyposexuality 341
medical conditions, other 235
medical disorders 228
medical history 225–6
medical patients 228–9
mental state examination 226
neurological disorders 231
non-medical difficulties 223
obstetric history 225
orgasm 223
pain 223
past sexual relationships 225
physical examination 226
physical treatments 238–9
physiology 221–2
prescribed drugs 233–5
presenting problems 224
prevalence 227
prostaglandin-E 239
psychological treatments 239–40
screening investigations 237–8
sexual development 224
sexual education/knowledge 225
sildenafil 238
spinal injuries 231
tadalafil 238
testosterone therapy
transexualism 235–6
treatments 238–40
SF36 and SF12 *see* Social Function Scales
'shell shock' 6
side effects, medication 69
  antidepressant drugs 774–5
  HIV infection 489
  neuroleptics 781–5
single item screening interview 98
situation-oriented consultation 15
skills
  detection, psychiatric disorders 83–6
  information gathering 83–4
  interviewing patients 84–5
  mental state examination 86
  mix 38–9
  nursing 105–6
skin disorders *see* psychocutaneous disorders
SNARIs *see* serotonin and noradrenaline reuptake
  inhibitors
Social Function Scales (SF36 and SF12) 98
social network behaviour therapy, drug misuse
  207
'soldier's heart' 6
solvents
  differential diagnosis 205
  treatment 205

somatoform/conversion disorders 357–9
  see also persistent medically unexplained
     symptoms
  aetiology 358
  diagnosis 358
  genitourinary disorders 740–1
  history 357–8
  management 358–9
  problem cases 824–7
specialization beginnings
  asylum psychiatrists (alienists) 5
  history 5–6
  nervous disorder 5–6
specific common therapeutic factors (SCTF),
    physical illness 796
spinal injuries, sexual problems 231
SSRIs *see* selective serotonin reuptake inhibitors
standard instruments, neurological disorders
    313–4
Statute Law 47–8
stillbirth 652
stimulants
  differential diagnosis 203–4
  pharmacotherapy 196–7
  symptoms 199
  treatment 203–4
  withdrawal 199
stomas 407–8
stress
  see also post-traumatic stress disorder
  cancer 552–3
  depression 89
  FSS 134
  gastrointestinal disorders 401
  ICU 679–81
  physical illness 114
  psychological reactions to illness 71–2
stroke 337–42
  anxiety 340
  behavioural changes 338–9
  catastrophic reactions 341
  defining 337
  delirium 337
  dementia 338
  depression 338–9
  emotionalism 340
  empathy loss 342
  executive function 341
  hyposexuality 341
  inhibition control deficit 342
  OCD 341
  psychosis 341
subarachnoid haemorrhage (SAH), headache 355
subspecialization, current practice variation 18
substance misuse *see* drug misuse
suicide 245–62
  see also self-harm
  adolescents 256
  aetiology 248–53
  Beck Suicidal Intent Scale 255
  behaviour 252–3
  biological aspects 252

cancer 557
defining 245
epidemiology 246
frequent repeaters 257
general population 249
HIV infection 486
ICU 681–2
older people 257
palliative care 607–9
physician assisted suicide 609–11
psychiatric disorders 249–50
risk factors 249–50
schizophrenia 250
self-harm links 247–8, 255
social characteristics 252–3
suicide prevention
  drug misuse 184
  nursing 107–10
  strategies 248
suicide risk assessment 91, 254–7
  nursing 114
  physical illness 91, 114
Symptom Checklist 90 (SCL-90) 97–8
symptoms, MUS 847–64
syphilophobia 733–5

teaching 19–20
terminal illness
  psychological reactions to illness 67
  single item screening interview 98
TGA *see* transient global amnesia
tianeptine 774
tic disorders 315
  GTS 353–4
  PANDAS 353–4
  treatment 354
topiramate 789
transient global amnesia (TGA) 332
trazodone 773
treatment refusal, legal issues 47–58
tremor 315
trends, current practice variation 14
trichotillomania 722
tricyclic antidepressants 772
twelve-step programmes, drug misuse
  207–8

UK, liaison psychiatry development 10–12
ulcerative colitis 393–7
United States CL 9–10
urticarias 724–5

valproate 788
variation, current practice *see* current practice
  variation
visual field abnormalities 315–16
vitamins
  alcohol 160–1, 282, 331
  dementia 329
  WKS 331
vulvodynia 657
vulvovaginitis 657

wakefulness, neurological disorders 309
war
    First World War 6
    Second World War 7–8
ways of working 17
websites
Wernicke–Korsakoff syndrome (WKS) 331–2
Wernicke's dysphasia 311–12

Wernicke's syndrome, alcohol 160–1
Wilson's disease (hepatolenticular degeneration)
    324, 423–4
withdrawal
    alcohol 157–60, 200–1
    drug misuse 198–205
WKS *see* Wernicke–Korsakoff syndrome